Swartz
Textbook of
Physical Diagnosis

History and Examination

NINTH EDITION

Swartz Textbook of Physical Diagnosis

History and Examination

MARK H. SWARTZ, MD, FACP

Professor of Medicine
State University of New York Downstate Medical Center
Brooklyn, New York

Adjunct Professor of Clinical Medicine
Albert Einstein College of Medicine
Bronx, New York

Professor of Medicine
New York College of Podiatric Medicine
New York, New York

President/CEO
C3NY—Clinical Competence Center of New York
New York, New York

Visiting Professor of Medicine
Taipei Medical University
Taipei, Taiwan

Lecture Professor of Medicine
Xiangya Hospital of Central South University
Changsha, China

ELSEVIER

Elsevier
1600 John F. Kennedy Blvd.
Ste 1800
Philadelphia, PA 19103-2899

SWARTZ TEXTBOOK OF PHYSICAL DIAGNOSIS, NINTH EDITION ISBN: 978-0-443-23506-1

Notice

Practitioners and researchers must always rely on their own experience and knowledge in evaluating and using any information, methods, compounds, or experiments described herein. Because of rapid advances in the medical sciences in particular, independent verification of diagnoses and drug dosages should be made. To the fullest extent of the law, no responsibility is assumed by Elsevier, authors, editors, or contributors for any injury and/or damage to persons or property as a matter of products liability, negligence, or otherwise or from any use or operation of any methods, products, instructions, or ideas contained in the material herein.

Previous editions copyrighted 2021, 2014, 2010, 2006, 2002, 1998, 1994, 1989.

Senior Content Strategist: Marybeth Thiel
Publishing Services Manager: Catherine Albright Jackson
Project Manager: Doug Turner
Design Direction: Margaret Reid

Printed in India

Last digit is the print number: 9 8 7 6 5 4 3 2 1

One of the essential qualities of the clinician is interest in humanity,
for the secret in the care ***of*** *the patient is in caring* ***for*** *the patient.*

Francis Weld Peabody (1881–1927)

To ***Vivian Hirshaut, MD****, my wife, for her unwavering love,*
endless patience, support, and profound understanding;

To ***Talia H. Swartz, MD, PhD****, my loving and brilliant daughter,*
for her encouragement and sustained devotion;

To ***Ofer Nagar****, my wonderful son-in-law, who helped produce two of the*
most delightful granddaughters anyone could wish for;

and

To ***Yael Nagar*** *and* ***Karen Nagar****, my granddaughters,*
who have brought so much joy into my life.

To the memory of my parents,
Hilda *and* ***Philip Swartz****;*

and

To my ***students and patients****,*
from whom I am always learning.

PREFACE

Welcome to the Ninth Edition of the ***Swartz Textbook of Physical Diagnosis: History and Examination***. It is hard to believe that 36 years have passed since the first edition of this textbook graced the shelves of medical libraries and the eager hands of aspiring healthcare professionals. Over the past several decades, this venerable textbook has served as an indispensable resource for all healthcare professionals providing a comprehensive guide to the art and science of physical diagnosis.

The field of medicine is constantly evolving, marked by innovative technologies, emerging clinical guidelines, and a deeper understanding of the intricacies of the human body. Yet, amid this ever-changing landscape, one constant remains—the fundamental importance of clinical skills: the history, the physical examination, and good communication in the practice of medicine. The ability to elicit and interpret clinical signs and symptoms through the artful touch of a skilled healthcare professional remains a cornerstone of accurate diagnosis and patient-centered care.

In this Ninth Edition, we continue to honor the legacy of our earlier editions while embracing the dynamic nature of modern healthcare. Our humanistic goal remains unwavering: to equip healthcare professionals with the knowledge and skills necessary to perform thorough and accurate clinical skills, fostering a deep connection between patient and practitioner.

Like its predecessors, this edition is meticulously crafted to provide a comprehensive, evidence-based, and up-to-date exploration of clinical skills. We incorporate the latest advances in medical education to ensure that the information within these pages reflects the field's current state. However, we are mindful of the enduring value of the fundamentals and the timeless wisdom passed down through generations of healthcare professionals.

The ***Swartz Textbook of Physical Diagnosis: History and Examination*** is organized with the needs of both novice and experienced healthcare professionals in mind. It serves as an invaluable resource for all seeking to develop their foundational skills and understanding of the clinical encounter and for seasoned healthcare professionals looking to refine their diagnostic abilities and keep pace with evolving best practices.

In this edition, we continue to emphasize the importance of the patient–healthcare professional (i.e., patient-first) relationship, clinical reasoning, and empathy in the practice of medicine. We delve into the art of communication, teaching the subtle nuances of patient interaction that can make all the difference in providing comprehensive, compassionate care. Additionally, we explore integrating technology into the physical examination, acknowledging its potential to enhance our diagnostic capabilities while maintaining the primacy of the human touch.

But this edition is not just an update; it is a transformation. We have reviewed and revised all the chapters to reflect the latest advances in medical education. Moreover, we are excited to introduce three new chapters that address critical topics at the forefront of modern healthcare:

The Transgender Patient: In recognition of the evolving understanding of gender identity and the unique healthcare needs of transgender individuals, this chapter provides guidance on the sensitive and inclusive care of transgender patients.

Artificial Intelligence in Clinical Encounters: Opportunities & Challenges: As artificial intelligence continues to shape the landscape of medicine, this chapter examines both the potential transformative benefits and pitfalls of AI in healthcare.

Telehealth: Adapting Clinical Assessment: The advent of telehealth has reshaped how healthcare is delivered. This chapter delves into the intricacies of conducting patient assessments remotely.

Videos are crucial in this textbook as invaluable visual tools, enriching the educational journey. Many original videos have been remade to ensure their current relevance. Most videos are short and linked to specific paragraphs, demonstrating specific examinations.

Besides the improvements made to the videos, most chapters now incorporate multiple-choice questions. These questions are strategically crafted to reinforce crucial information and concepts covered in the text. They direct your understanding and self-assessment, offer a valuable resource for healthcare professional students, and evaluate their grasp and recall of essential knowledge.

As we look ahead to the future of medicine, we remain committed to the enduring principles of clinical excellence, ethical practice, and lifelong learning. We hope this Ninth Edition of our textbook will inspire a new generation of healthcare professionals to embrace the art and science of physical diagnosis, recognizing that the patient's history and examination remain the bedrock of exceptional medical care.

We invite you to embark on this journey through the pages of our Ninth Edition as we explore the rich tapestry of physical diagnosis, embracing the traditions of the past while forging ahead into the exciting possibilities of the future. Together, we will continue to advance the noble mission of healing and the pursuit of knowledge in the service of humanity.

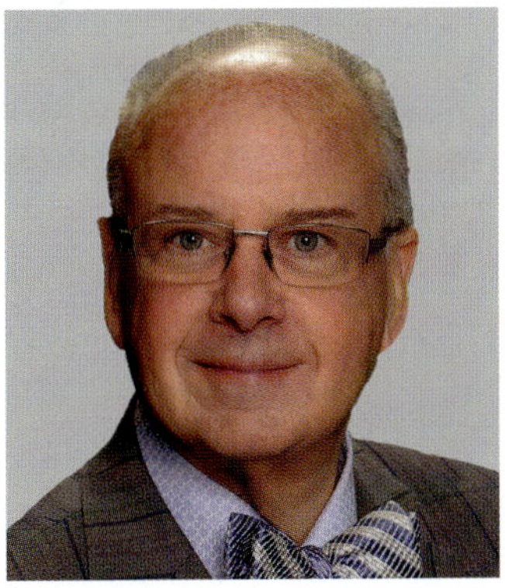

Mark H. Swartz, MD, FACP

CONTRIBUTORS

I want to express my profound gratitude to my colleagues for their invaluable support and expertise, which played a pivotal role in making the Ninth Edition of the ***Swartz Textbook of Physical Diagnosis: History and Examination*** so exceptional. Equally significant, I extend my heartfelt appreciation to my teachers, students, and patients. Their contributions have enriched my comprehension of medicine, and I am profoundly thankful for their influence.

I wish to convey my utmost gratitude to the following individuals whose indispensable contributions have been instrumental in crafting this edition. Their unwavering commitment to excellence and their painstaking focus on detail have proven vital in guaranteeing that this publication adheres to the most exacting standards of quality and precision.

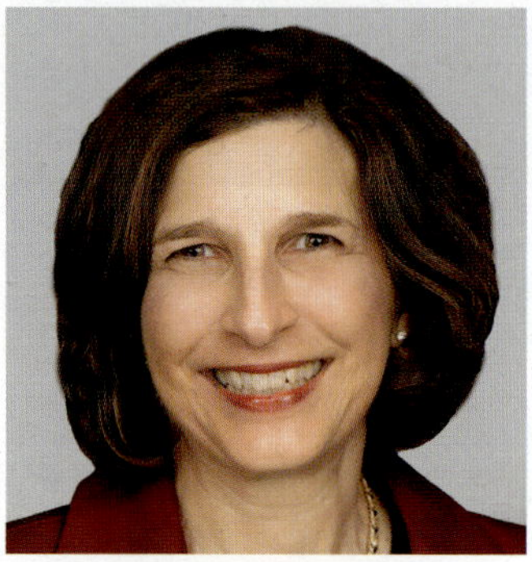

Marcy B. Bolster, MD
Professor of Medicine
Harvard Medical School
Director, Rheumatology Fellowship Training Program
Massachusetts General Hospital
Boston, Massachusetts

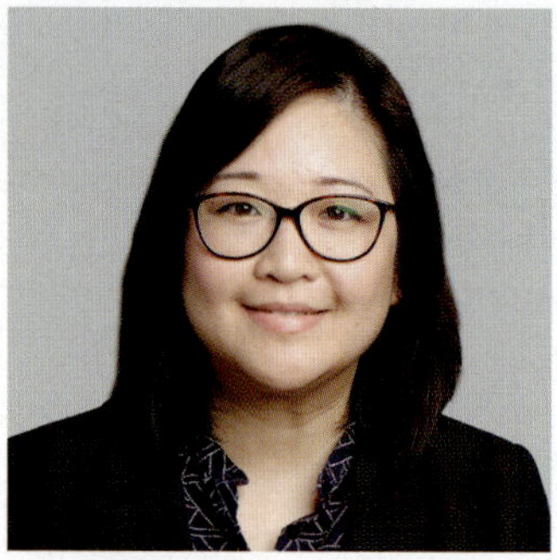

Lili Chan, MD, MSCR
Associate Professor of Medicine (Nephrology)
Icahn School of Medicine at Mount Sinai
New York, New York

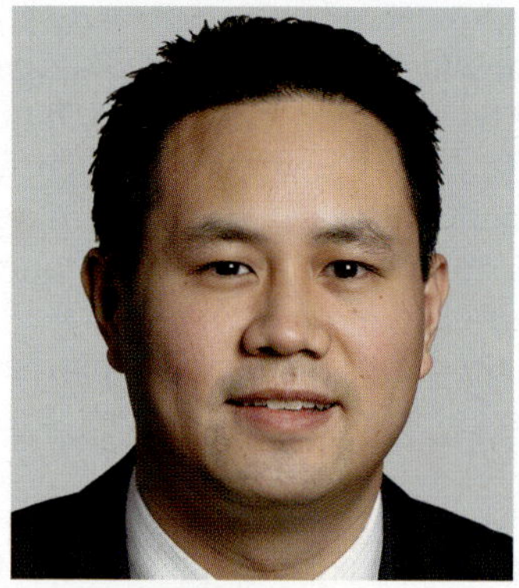

Darwin Chen, MD
Associate Professor of Orthopedic Surgery
Icahn School of Medicine at Mount Sinai
New York, New York

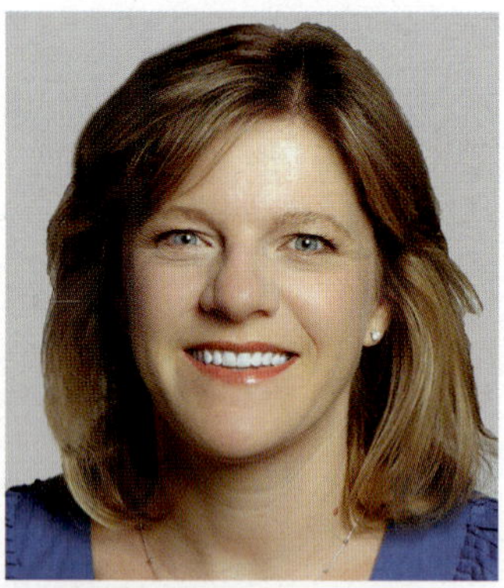

Barbara Deli, MD
Assistant Professor of Obstetrics, Gynecology, and Reproductive Science
Icahn School of Medicine at Mount Sinai
New York, New York

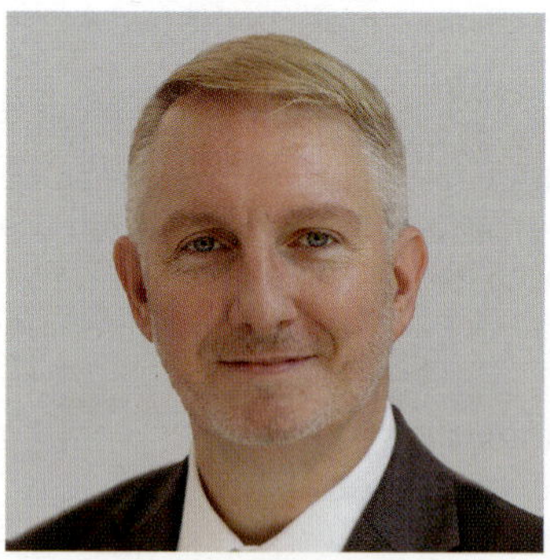

Patrick D. Herron, DBe, HEC-C
Montefiore Einstein Center for Bioethics
Associate Professor of Family & Social Medicine
Associate Professor of Epidemiology & Population Health
Albert Einstein College of Medicine
Bronx, New York

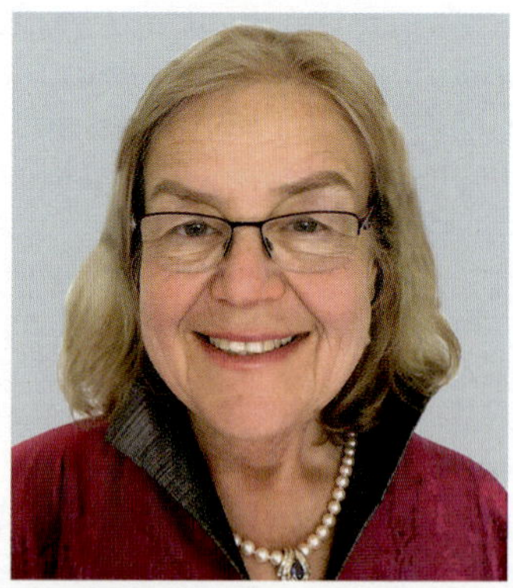

Vivian Hirshaut, MD
Assistant Professor of Ophthalmology
Mount Sinai Medical Center
New York, New York
Courtesy Staff, Department of Ophthalmology and Visual Sciences
Montefiore Medical Center
Bronx, New York

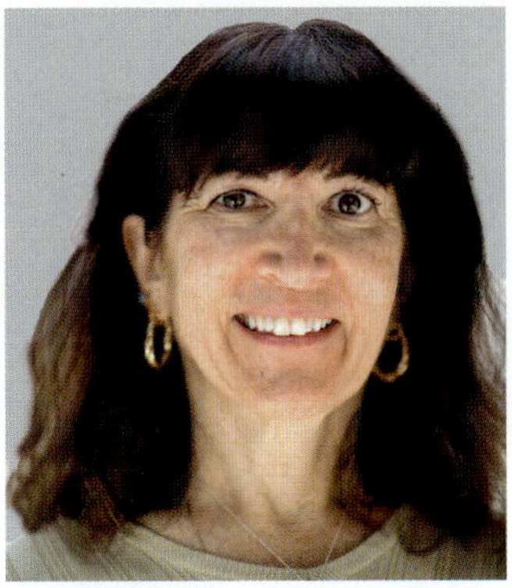

Joanne R. Hojsak, MD
Professor of Pediatrics & Medical Education
Icahn School of Medicine at Mount Sinai
Pediatric Intensivist
Mount Sinai Kravis Children's Hospital
New York, New York

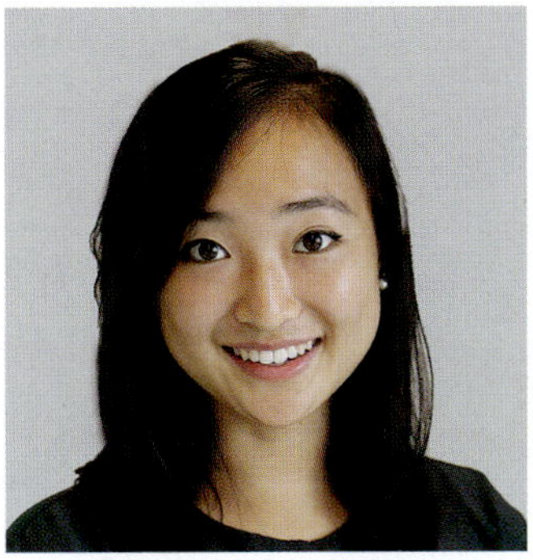

Joy J. Jiang, MD-PhD Student
Medical Scientist Training Program
Charles Bronfman Institute for Personalized Medicine
Icahn School of Medicine at Mount Sinai
New York, New York

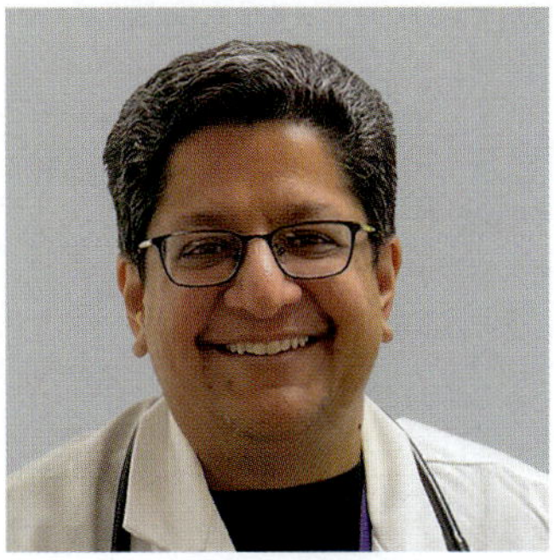

Reena Karani, MD, MHPE
Professor of Medicine, Medical Education and Geriatrics and Palliative Medicine
Director, Institute for Medical Education
Icahn School of Medicine at Mount Sinai
New York, New York

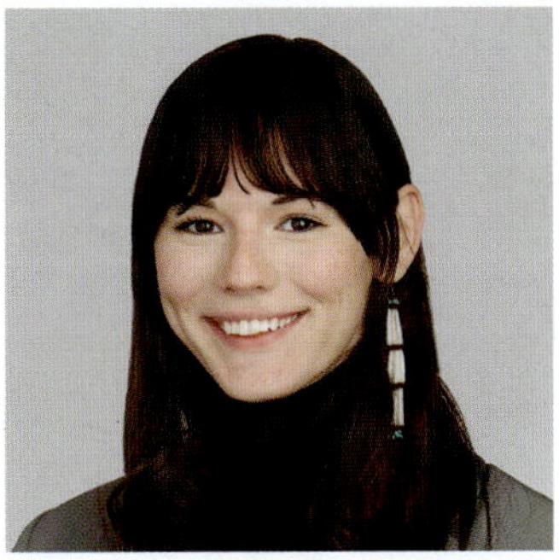

Sky Kihuwa-Mani, MD-PhD Student
Medical Scientist Training Program
Icahn School of Medicine at Mount Sinai
New York, New York

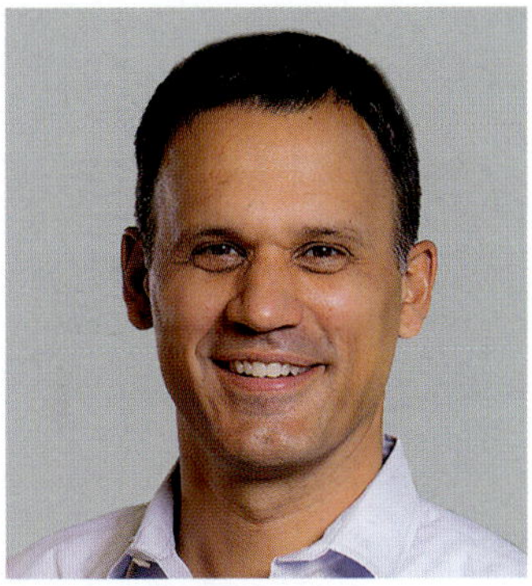

Jason R. Kolfenbach, MD
Associate Professor of Medicine (Rheumatology)
University of Colorado
Denver, Colorado

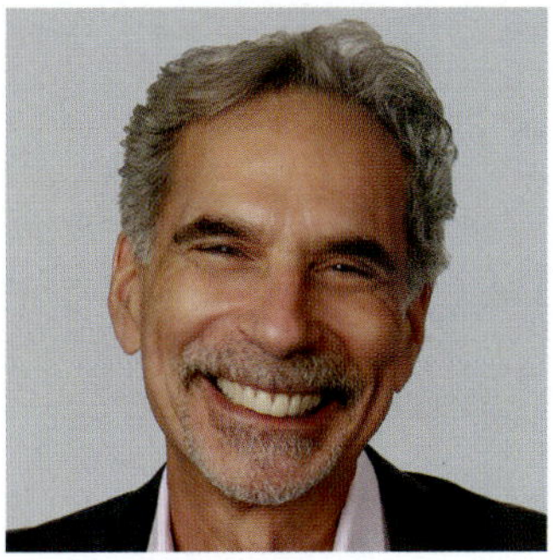

Robert F. Kushner, MD
Professor of Medicine
Northwestern University Feinberg School of Medicine
Director, Center for Lifestyle Medicine
Northwestern Medicine
Chicago, Illinois

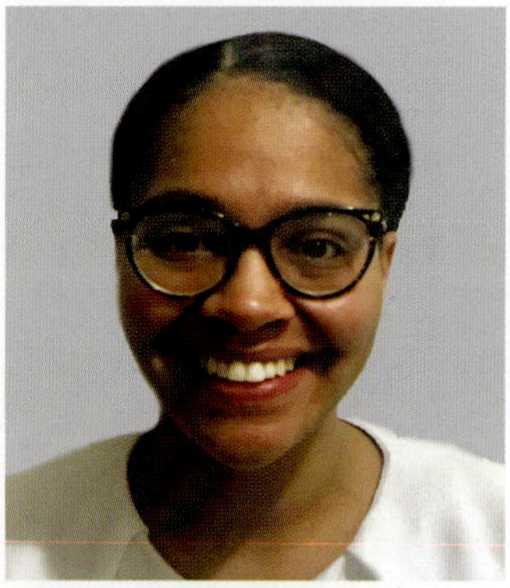

Giselle N. Lynch, MD
Glaucoma Fellow
Department of Ophthalmology
Columbia University
New York, New York

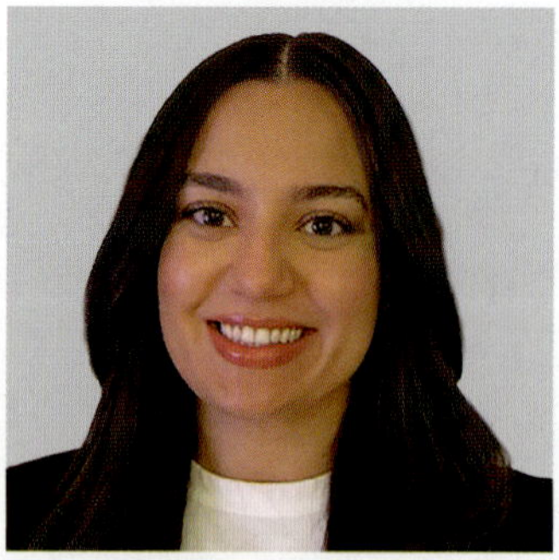

Maxiell Medina, MS
Assistant to the Dean for Clinical Clerkships and Affiliations
New York College of Podiatric Medicine
New York, New York

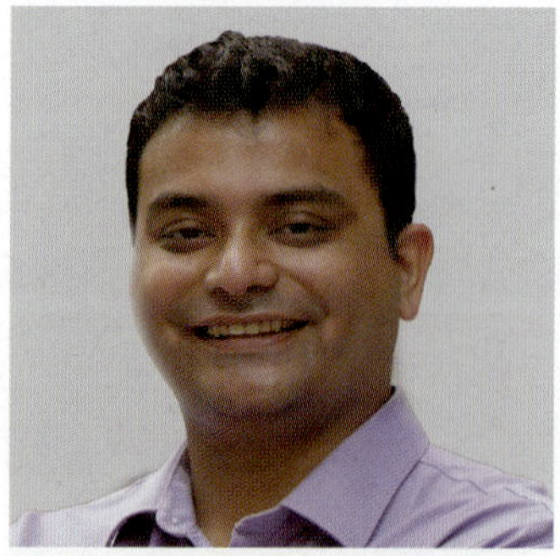

Girish N. Nadkarni, MD, MPH
Irene & Dr. Arthur M. Fishberg Professor of Medicine (Nephrology)
System Chief, Division of Data Driven and Digital Medicine
Co-Director, Mount Sinai Clinical Intelligence Center
Director, Charles Bronfman Institute for Personalized Medicine
Icahn School of Medicine at Mount Sinai
New York, New York

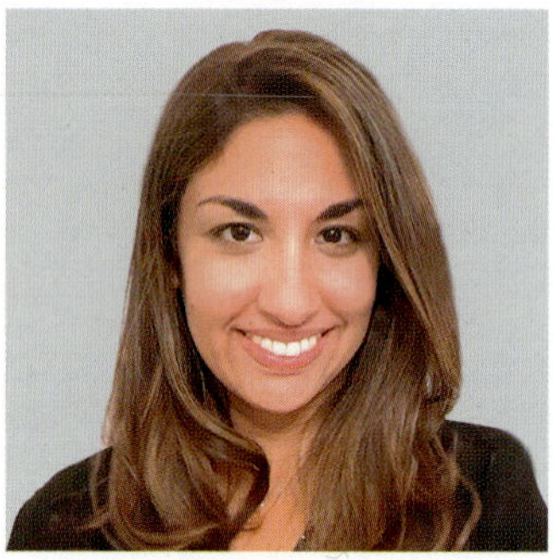

Farida G. Nentin, MD
Associate Professor of Obstetrics, Gynecology and Reproductive Sciences
Icahn School of Medicine at Mount Sinai, Mount Sinai Hospital
New York, New York

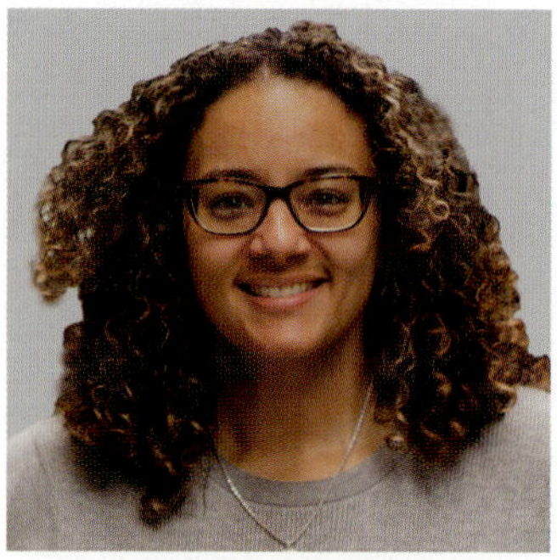

Ann-Gel S. Palermo, DrPH, MPH
Associate Professor of Medical Education
Senior Associate Dean for Diversity, Equity, and Inclusion
Patricia Levinson Center for Multicultural and Community Affairs
Icahn School of Medicine at Mount Sinai
New York, New York
Chief Diversity, Equity, and Inclusion Officer in Education and Research
Office for Diversity & Inclusion
Mount Sinai Health System
New York, New York

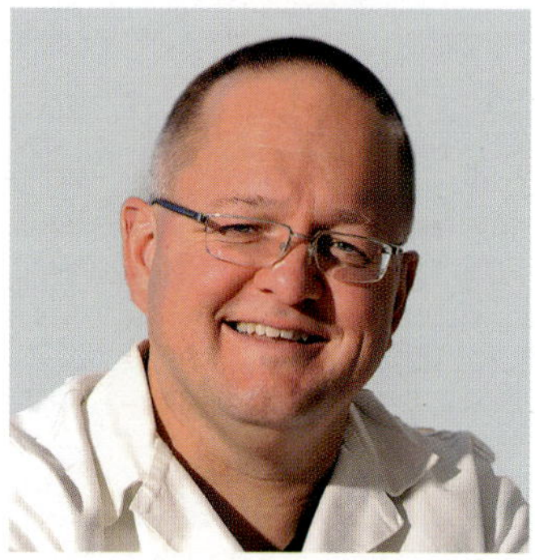

Paul E. Phrampus, MD, MBA, FACEP, FSSH
Professor of Emergency Medicine
Director, Winter Institute for Simulation, Education and Research (WISER)
University of Pittsburgh
Medical Director, Patient Safety
UPMC Health System
Pittsburgh, Pennsylvania

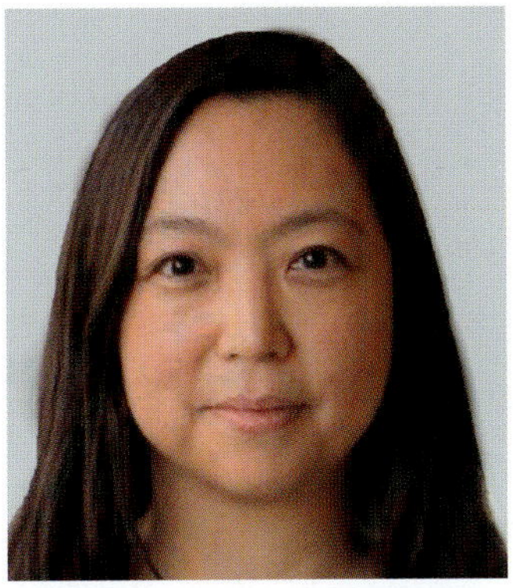

Hai Jung Helen Rhim, MD, MPH, MHPE
Associate Professor (Clinical) of Pediatrics
NYU Grossman School of Medicine,
New York, NY

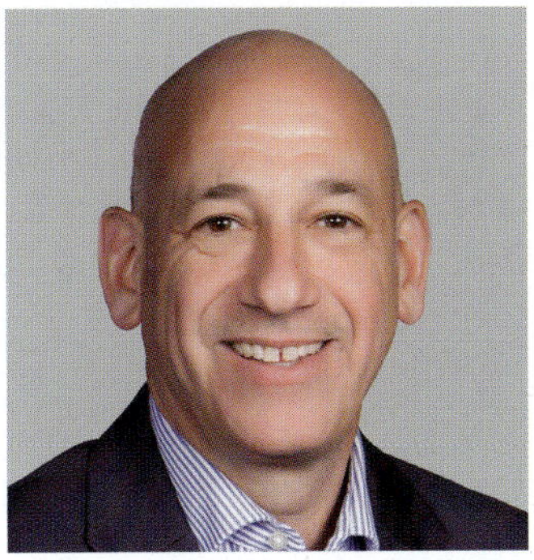

Joshua D. Safer, MD, FACP, FACE
Professor of Medicine, Endocrinology, Diabetes, and Bone Disease
Executive Director, Center for Transgender Medicine and Surgery
Mount Sinai Health System System
Icahn School of Medicine at Mount Sinai
New York, New York

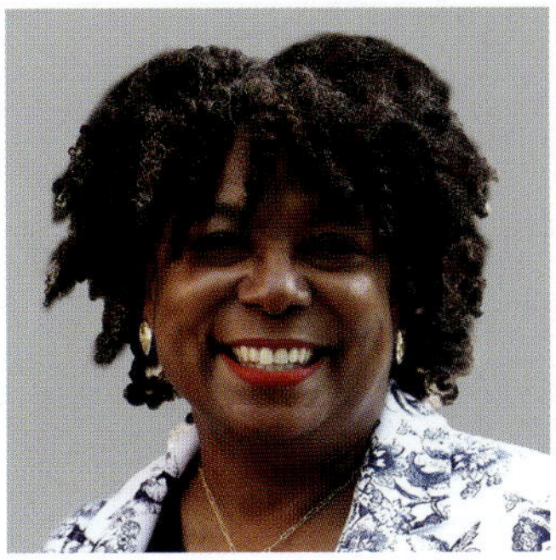

Michelle Sainté-Willis, BS
Senior Associate Dean for Medical Education Administration
Department of Medical Education
Icahn School of Medicine at Mount Sinai
New York, New York

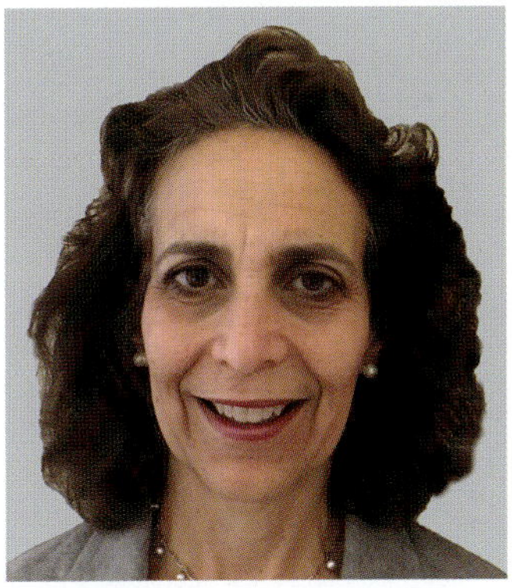

Miriam Schechter, MD
Associate Professor of Pediatrics
Albert Einstein College of Medicine
Bronx, New York

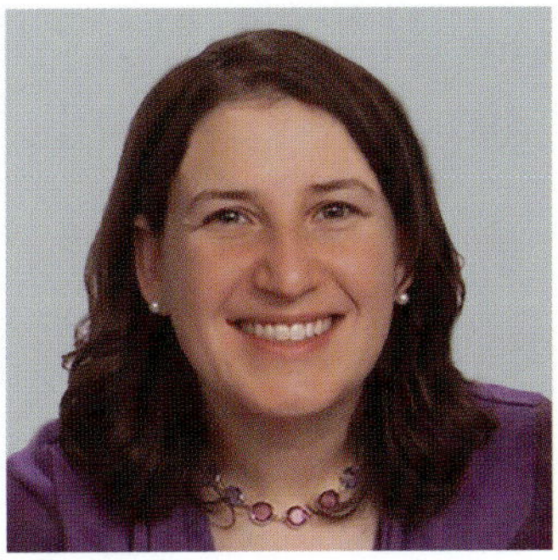

Talia H. Swartz, MD, PhD
Associate Professor of Medicine (Infectious Diseases)
Senior Associate Dean for MD-PhD Education
Director, Medical Scientist Training Program
Icahn School of Medicine at Mount Sinai
New York, New York

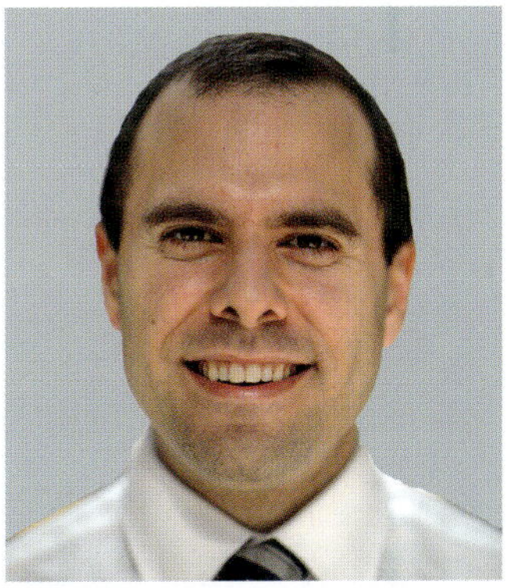

Joseph Truglio, MD, MPH
Associate Professor of Internal Medicine, Pediatrics and Medical Education
Icahn School of Medicine at Mount Sinai
New York, New York

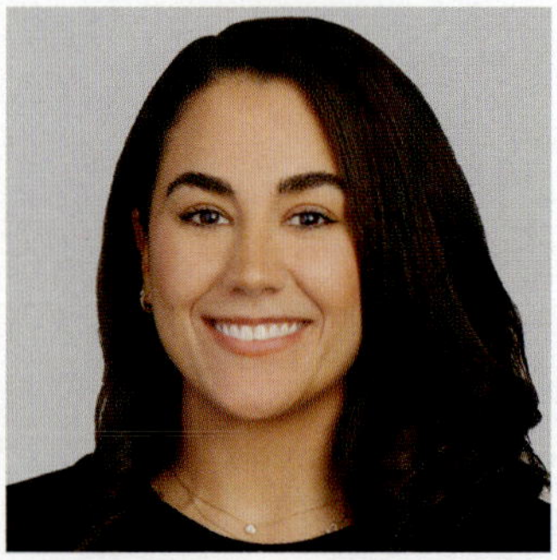

Christine S. Williams, MD
Orthopedic Surgery, PGY-5
Icahn School of Medicine at Mount Sinai
New York, New York

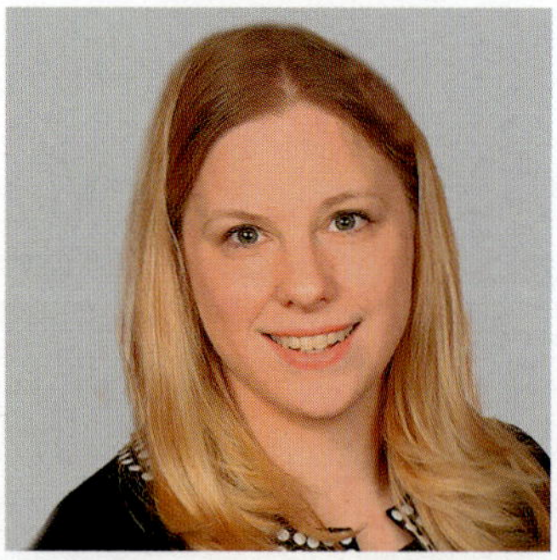

Lisa Zickuhr, MD, MHPE
Assistant Professor of Medicine
Washington University in St. Louis School of Medicine
St. Louis, Missouri

And to the following people who helped in previous editions:

James R. Bonner, MD
Dennis W. Boulware, MD
Jerry A. Colliver, PhD
Tracie L. DeMack
Siobhan M. Dolan, MD, MPH
Ethan D. Fried, MD
Margaret Clark Golden, MD
Jessica L. Israel, MD
Mark A. Kosinski, DPM
Ellen Landsberger, MD
Peter B. Liebert, MD
Robert W. Marion, MD
Mimi McEvoy, RN, CPNP

ACKNOWLEDGMENTS

Special thanks are due:

To Wendy Beth Jackelow, whose artistic illustrations have graced all nine editions of this textbook.

To Tamara Thomas, Mary Lang, and Karen Kim, whose outstanding performances brought life to the patients and doctor in our video presentations.

To the many Elsevier employees for their expert assistance and collaboration. A special acknowledgment goes to Marybeth Thiel, Senior Content Strategist for Education Content, whose invaluable contributions shaped this edition. I also want to thank Douglas Turner and Abdul Gaffar, our dedicated Project Managers, and Margaret Reid for her exceptional Design Direction.

Lastly, I am deeply grateful to my wife, Dr. Vivian Hirshaut, whose unwavering love and support have been instrumental in bringing these nine editions to fruition.

CONTENTS

SECTION 4 Evaluating Specific Patients

VIDEO CONTENTS

SECTION 1

Mastering the Art of Interviewing

1

The Interviewer's Questions

Mark H. Swartz and Sky Kihuwa-Mani

What is spoken of as a "clinical picture" is not just a photograph of a man sick in bed; it is an impressionistic painting of the patient surrounded by his home, his work, his relations, his friends, his joys, sorrows, hopes and fears.

Francis Weld Peabody (1881–1927)

BASIC PRINCIPLES

Effective communication is crucial in providing quality medical care. Despite the advancements in technology since 2000, the way healthcare professionals communicate with their patients remains a critical factor. Research has demonstrated that good communication can enhance health outcomes by alleviating symptoms, psychological distress, and anxiety in patients. Shockingly, 85% of all medical malpractice lawsuits in the United States stem from inadequate communication skills. It is not a matter of insufficient medical knowledge but rather the inability of healthcare professionals to communicate effectively with their patients.

While technologic medicine is important, it cannot replace the importance of effective communication and behavior when caring for the sick. Patient care greatly relies on the healthcare professional's ability to communicate and conduct a proper interview. This is because the relationship between a patient and a healthcare professional is unique and intimate, as personal details about the illness are discussed within a short amount of time. A strong therapeutic alliance must be established through trust for the patient to feel comfortable sharing their personal information.

During an interview, the goal is to gather important information about the patient's illness and how they are coping with it. This helps in assessing the patient's condition. A skilled interviewer considers all aspects of the patient's situation and focuses on the areas that need the most attention. The interviewer should also be aware of the influence of social, economic, and cultural factors in shaping the nature of the patient's problems. Other important aspects of the interview are educating the patient about the diagnosis, negotiating a management plan, and counseling about behavioral changes.

When a patient seeks consultation from a healthcare professional(s), it is important for the professional to evaluate the patient thoroughly. The provider should be aware of all clues, whether they are obvious or subtle. While body language is important, the spoken word remains the primary diagnostic tool in medicine. Therefore, speaking and active listening skills are crucial for the healthcare professional–patient interaction. Active listening requires practice and involves paying attention to both verbal and nonverbal cues. For inexperienced interviewers, it can be easy to focus solely on their next question instead of observing the entire patient picture, as Peabody eloquently explained in the quote that introduces this chapter. After gathering all the necessary clues from the patient's history, assimilating them into a final diagnosis is relatively straightforward.

To conduct a successful interview, clear communication is crucial. The interviewer should be able to ask questions freely and ensure that they are easily understood by each patient. In some cases, using slang words to describe certain conditions can help facilitate communication and prevent any misunderstandings.

The success of any interview depends on it being patient-centered and *not* healthcare professional-centered. Encourage the patient to tell their story and follow the patient's leads to better comprehend the problems, concerns, and requests. Do not have your own list of "standard questions" as would occur in a symptom-focused, healthcare professional–centered interview. **Patients are not standard; don't treat them as such.** Allow the patient to tell their story in their own words. In the words of Sir William Osler (1893), "Listen to your patient. He is telling you the diagnosis… The good physician treats the disease; the great physician treats the patient who has the disease." No truer words have been spoken.

After the patient has shared their story about their illness, it is common practice to transition from open-ended questions to more direct and specific ones. Begin with broader questions and gradually narrow them down to create a differential diagnosis. Start with general inquiries and then ask more specific questions to gain a better understanding of the patient's symptoms and history.

USING AN INTERPRETER

Healthcare professionals are now frequently providing medical care to patients who speak different languages. The term "native language" refers to the language that a person learned from birth, also known as their mother tongue. **Mother tongue** is not only about the language that a person learns from birth. It is also the person's dominant language and their "home language." This means that the person learns not only to speak the language but also gain the ability to know the communicative and linguistic aspects of it. Since it is the only language the person knows since birth, it is of high importance in the person's life.

As of 2022, there are 7106 languages that are still actively in use (i.e., living languages) and spoken by people. Among these, there are 23 languages that serve as the mother tongue for at least 60 million first-language speakers. The **mother tongue** languages that dominate are Chinese, Spanish, and English. Chinese might be spoken in 37 countries and has 1.284 billion speakers compared to English spoken in 106 countries with 327 million speakers. Spanish might be spoken in 31 countries and has 437 million speakers. Arabic and Hindi are the next most commonly spoken mother tongues.

In 2020, the United States Census Bureau reported that the number of people in the United States who speak a language other than English at home tripled between 1980 and 2019. About one in five people in the United States speak a second language at home, which is about 68 million people! While most of these individuals also spoke English with native fluency or very well, about 41% (25.1 million) were considered Limited English Proficient (LEP). LEP refers to anyone over the age of 5 who reported speaking English less than "very well" as classified by the U.S. Census Bureau. Though most LEP individuals are immigrants, nearly 19% (4.7 million) were born in the United States, most to immigrant parents. Overall, the LEP population represented 8% of the total U.S. population ages 5 and older.

Not being proficient in English can have harmful consequences. If a patient speaks a language other than the healthcare professional, it is crucial to have a trained medical interpreter present. Even if the healthcare professional knows the patient's language and culture, an interpreter should still be used. The interpreter acts as a bridge, connecting the provider and patient's ideas, values, biases, emotions, and difficulties. Effective communication between the patient, interpreter, and provider depends on their shared understanding and beliefs about the patient's issue. Interpreters who are familiar with the patient's culture are most effective. Discussing sensitive topics like sexual history or substance abuse can be difficult. That's why it can be helpful to have a neutral third party act as an interpreter. Sometimes, the patient may prefer to have a family member act as the interpreter. In this situation, the healthcare professional should honor the patient's request. It is not recommended to depend on friends of the patient for translation during emergencies as their translation skills are unknown and confidentiality may be compromised. Healthcare professionals should learn some important words and phrases in different languages to establish trust and respect with their patients. When using an interpreter, healthcare professionals should remember the following guidelines:

1. Choose an individual trained in medical terminology.
2. Choose a person of the same gender as the patient and of comparable age.
3. Talk with the interpreter beforehand to establish an approach.
4. When speaking to the patient, watch the patient, not the interpreter.
5. Do not expect a word-for-word translation.
6. Ask the interpreter about the patient's fears and expectations.
7. Use clear, short, and simple questions.
8. Use simple language.
9. Keep your explanations brief.
10. Avoid hypothetical questions using *if, would,* and *could* because these require nuances of language.
11. Avoid idiomatic expressions.

The U.S. Department of Health and Human Services has put together a useful mnemonic ***(INTERPRET)*** for working with interpreters in a cultural setting (Table 1.1).

Even with a trained translator, healthcare professionals are ultimately responsible for ensuring safe and effective communication with their patients. An article from 2008 describes a conceptual framework of when to call for an interpreter and what to do when one is not available.[1]

TABLE 1.1 Interpreters Mnemonic: INTERPRET

I – Introduction	Make sure to introduce all the individuals in the room. During introductions, include information as to the role individuals will play.
N – Note Goals	Note the goals of the interview: What is the diagnosis? What will the treatment entail? Will there be any follow-up?
T – Transparency	Let the patient know that everything said will be interpreted throughout the session.
E—Ethics	Use qualified interpreters (not family members or children) when conducting an interview. Qualified interpreters allow the patient to maintain autonomy and make informed decisions about their care.
R—Respect Beliefs	LEP patients may have cultural beliefs that need to be incorporated as well. The interpreter may be able to serve as a cultural broker and help explain any cultural beliefs that may exist.
P—Patient Focus	The patient should remain the focus of the encounter. Providers should interact with the patient and not the interpreter. Make sure to ask and address any questions the patient may have before ending the encounter. If you don't have trained interpreters on staff, the patient may not be able to call in with questions.
R—Retain Control	It is important as the provider that you remain in control of the interaction and not allow the patient or interpreter to take over the conversation.
E—Explain	Use simple language and short sentences when working with an interpreter. This will ensure that comparable words can be found in the second language and that all the information can be conveyed clearly.
T—Thanks	Thank the interpreter and the patient for their time. On the chart, note that the patient needs an interpreter and who served as an interpreter this time.

During the interview with the patient, it's important to not only identify their primary medical issues but also understand their reaction to the illness. It's crucial to determine how the illness has impacted the patient, how they have responded to it, and the effect it has had on their family, work, and social life.

A successful interview involves an interviewer who is cheerful, friendly, and genuinely concerned about the patient's well-being. This approach is much more effective than an interrogator who shoots questions from a standard list at the patient, making them feel vulnerable. Patients should not be bombarded with rapid-fire questions.

IMPORTANT INTERVIEWING CONCEPTS

At the start of a session, patients typically bring up topics that are less difficult to talk about. However, tactful questioning can help bring up more painful experiences. New interviewers will need to gain experience to feel at ease asking about delicate or unpleasant subjects. Timing is crucial when asking such questions.

When conducting an interview with a patient, it's important to let them share their story using their own words. This can reveal a lot about the nature of their illness. Additionally, paying close attention to their facial expressions and body language can provide valuable nonverbal clues. As the interviewer, using body language such as smiling, nodding, remaining silent, making hand gestures, or giving a questioning look can encourage the patient to keep sharing their story.

Listening without interruption is important and requires skill. If given the chance, patients often disclose their problems spontaneously. Interviewers need to *hear* what is being said. They must allow the patient to finish their answer even if there are pauses while the patient processes their feelings. All too often, an interview may fail to reveal all the clues because the interviewer did not listen adequately to the patient. Several studies have shown that healthcare professionals commonly do not listen adequately to their patients. One study showed that healthcare professionals interrupt the patient within the first 15 seconds of the interview. The interviewers are abrupt, appear uninterested in the patient's distress, and are prone to control the interview.

As mentioned earlier, the best clinical interview focuses on the patient, not on the healthcare professional's agenda.

An important rule for improved interviewing is *to listen more, talk less,* and *interrupt infrequently*. It's best not to interrupt the patient during the interview as it can cause them to lose their train of thought. It's important to allow the patient to have some control over the conversation.

During the interview, it's important for the healthcare professional to pay close attention to the way the patient chooses their words to express their thoughts and history. Interviewers should be cautious of overly positive statements like "Everything's fine," "I'm very happy," or "No problems," as they may be used to hide underlying issues. If the interviewer suspects that a patient may not be completely truthful, they can ask follow-up questions like "Is everything really as fine as it could be?" to encourage more open communication.

If the history given is vague, the interviewer may use direct questioning. Asking "how," "where," or "when" is generally more effective than asking "why," which tends to put patients on the defensive. Often replacing the word "Why" with "What's the reason" will allow for better, less confrontational dialogue. During an interview, it is important for the interviewer to avoid disapproving of any parts of the patient's story. It's crucial to recognize that different cultures have different norms, and the interviewer should listen without displaying any hint of bias.

Always treat the patient with respect. Do not contradict or impose your own moral standards on the patient. Knowledge of the patient's social and economic background will make the interview progress more smoothly. Treat all patients with respect, regardless of their age, gender, beliefs, intelligence, educational background, legal status, practices, culture, illness, body type, emotional state, or financial situation.

Effective interviewing in healthcare requires professionals to be compassionate and interested in the patient's story. They should create an open and comfortable atmosphere where patients feel encouraged to describe their problem. These guidelines serve as the foundation for successful interactions between healthcare professionals and patients.

The interviewer's appearance can influence the success of the interview. Patients have an image of healthcare professionals. Neatness counts; a slovenly interviewer might be considered immature or careless, and their competence may be questioned from the start. Surveys of patients indicate that patients prefer medical personnel to dress in white coats and wear shoes instead of sneakers or sandals.

Patients often tend to answer questions in a manner that they believe will please their healthcare professional and gain their approval, which may stem from fear. It is important for professionals to be aware of this phenomenon.

The interviewer must be able to question patients about subjects that may be distressing or embarrassing to the interviewer, the patient, or both. Answers to many routine questions may cause embarrassment to interviewers and leave them speechless. Therefore, there is a tendency to avoid such questions. The interviewer's ability to be open and frank about such topics promotes the likelihood of discussion in those areas.

During interviews, patients may feel at ease discussing behaviors that could be perceived as antisocial, such as drug addiction, unlawful actions, or sexual behavior. It's important for interviewers to avoid passing judgment on these behaviors. If an interviewer is judgmental, the patient might not feel comfortable opening up to them. On the other hand, if the interviewer is accepting, the patient will perceive them as being empathetic. However, it's crucial not to give the impression that one approves of destructive behavior, as this could encourage the patient to continue engaging in it.

When conducting an interview, it's helpful to follow the "***rule of five vowels***." This rule suggests that a thorough interview should include elements of *a*udition, *e*valuation, *i*nquiry, *o*bservation, and *u*nderstanding. During an interview, it's important to pay close attention to the patient's story *(Audition)*. Evaluating the information given is crucial to distinguish between relevant and irrelevant data *(Evaluation)*.

Asking further questions to clarify important areas *(Inquiry)* can provide a deeper understanding of the patient's situation. Nonverbal communication *(Observation)* is also important to consider, as it can convey emotions and feelings that may not be expressed verbally. By *(understanding)* the patient's concerns and apprehensions, the interviewer can show empathy and provide better support.

Speech Patterns

During an interview, the way someone speaks can be just as important as what they say. This is because the tone, speed, emphasis, and volume of their voice can communicate a lot about their emotions. Both the interviewer and patient can use these **paralanguage components** to convey important information. The way a person speaks, including their tone and intonation, can greatly affect the meaning of their words. These aspects of speech may also reveal important information about the individual's personality, even if they are not aware of it. The use of audible parameters can help detect a patient's anxiety, depression, and other emotional states. When the interviewer uses a warm and soft tone, it can be soothing for the patient and improve communication.

Body Language

The study of body language, also known as *kinesics*, has become increasingly popular due to its importance in modern communication and relationships. This type of nonverbal communication, when combined with spoken language, can offer a more complete understanding of a patient's behavior. Both your own body language and that of your patient can reveal emotions and intentions. The exchange of these signals occurs on both conscious and unconscious levels.

It is a commonly accepted fact that an interviewer can gather more information about a patient by observing the way they narrate their story rather than just the story itself. When a patient is fidgeting in their chair and appears embarrassed, it is a sign that they are uncomfortable. A frown often suggests annoyance or disapproval, while furrowed brows may indicate a lack of understanding. The body, excluding the face, can convey emotions through gestures. For example, a person who hits a table while speaking is emphasizing their point. A patient who slips a wedding band on and off may be ambivalent about their marriage. A palm placed over the heart asserts sincerity or credibility. When individuals are presented with something they don't want to accept, they often rub or cover their eyes. Sometimes patients may disapprove of something said by the interviewer but choose not to speak out. In these situations, they may instead begin to remove dust or lint from their clothing. See https://www.businessballs.com/self-awareness/body-language/, which is a wonderful reference about body language. Be aware that various body language behaviors may have different meanings with different cultures!

There are six facial expressions that are universally recognized as representing different emotions. These expressions are genetically inherited rather than learned through social conditioning. While slight variations exist among isolated populations, these basic human emotions are generally recognized as part of our genetic makeup. They are:

- Happiness
- Sadness
- Fear
- Disgust
- Surprise
- Anger

Fig. 1.1 shows some typical emotions. Of interest, Charles Darwin was first to make these claims in his book *The Expressions of the Emotions in Man and Animals,* published in 1872.

Body language includes the act of smiling, which is quite significant. A true smile is characterized by symmetry and the formation of wrinkles around the eyes and mouth, while a false smile usually involves only the mouth.

When your arms are crossed, it shows that you are being defensive. However, when your arms are in an open position with your palms facing up, it indicates that you are feeling open and secure. Arms can reveal a lot about your mood and emotions, especially when paired with other body language cues. For example:

- Crossed arms may indicate defensiveness.
- Crossed arms and crossed legs probably indicate defensiveness.
- Crossed arms, crossed legs, frowning, and clenched fists definitely indicate defensiveness and probably hostility.

The term "*proxemics*" refers to the personal space aspect of body language. This refers to the distance that individuals feel comfortable having between themselves and others. Personal space can be experienced through visual, auditory, or kinesthetic means, among others. The size of personal space can vary depending on an individual's cultural and personal background, as well as their relationships and the situation. People from different cultures have different personal space boundaries and often don't realize the extent of these differences.

To fully understand someone's body language, it's essential to consider their cultural and ethnic background as different cultures may have varying expectations for nonverbal communication. The interviewer shows interest in what the patient is saying by leaning forward and paying close attention to their description. This attentiveness is essential for effective communication.

Body language can have different meanings in different situations. Sometimes, what someone's body language appears to convey is not actually what they are feeling. For example:

- Someone rubbing their eye might have an irritation rather than being disbelieving or upset.
- Someone with crossed arms might be keeping warm rather than being defensive.
- Someone scratching their nose might actually have an itch rather than concealing a lie.

Interpreting a single body language signal is not as reliable as considering several signals. To accurately determine the meaning conveyed by body language, it is necessary to look for groups of signals that support an overall conclusion. Relying on only one or two signals in isolation can be misleading, especially when a signal can have different interpretations. However, it is important to remember that body language is not an exact science.

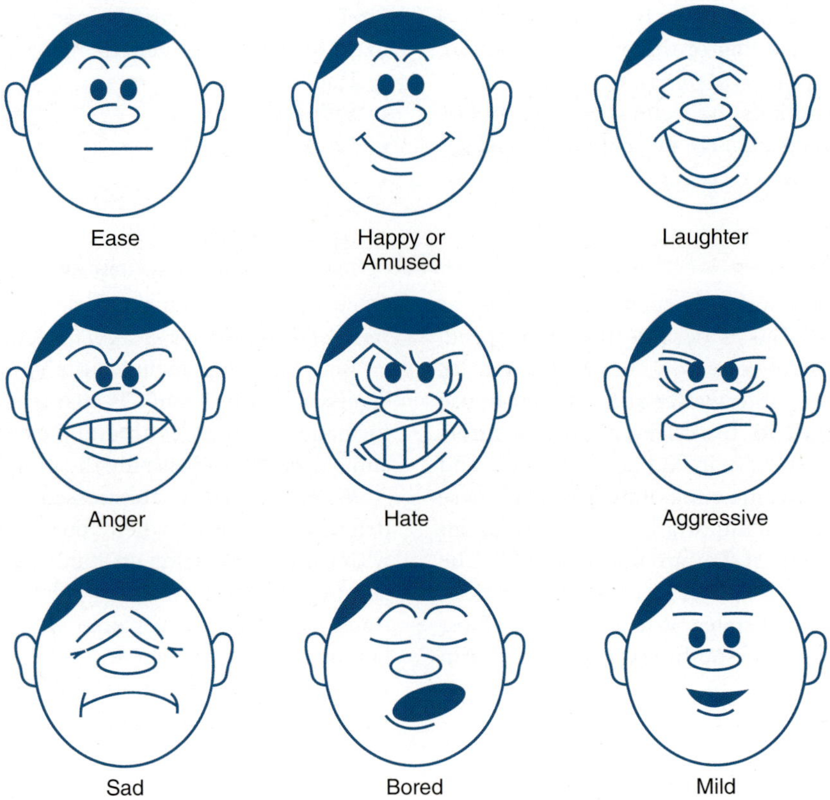

Fig. 1.1 Emotions. (From Babu S: Emotions and stress. In Babu S, Gayathri T, editors: *Psychology for Nurses*, ed 2, 2018, Elsevier.)

Touch

Physical touch can be a powerful tool for conveying warmth, affection, care, and understanding to patients. However, the use of touch can vary based on factors such as gender, culture, and the location of the touch. For example, in general, Latinos and people of Mediterranean descent tend to use more physical contact, while British, Asians, and people from India tend to use less. Scandinavians and Anglo-Saxon Americans fall in the middle of this spectrum.

It's important to be aware that certain religious groups prohibit physical contact with individuals of the opposite sex. In general, placing a hand on a patient's shoulder is the safest body part to touch to indicate support. It's important to **avoid placing a hand on a patient's leg or thigh,** which can be perceived as threatening.

Depersonalization of the Healthcare Professional–Patient Relationship

As biomedical technology advances, a new issue has emerged: a lack of personal connection between healthcare professionals and patients. Healthcare professionals often end up spending more time staring at a computer screen than interacting with their patients. Sometimes healthcare professionals may order computed tomography scans or sonograms without taking the necessary time to discuss the tests with the patient. Both professional and patient may feel increasingly neglected, rejected, or abused. Patients may feel dehumanized on admission to the hospital. Many find themselves in a strange environment, lying naked while clothed people march in and out of the room and touch them, tell them what to do, and so forth. They may be apprehensive because they have a problem that their healthcare professional considers too serious to be treated on an outpatient basis. Their future is filled with uncertainty. A patient admitted to the hospital is stripped of clothing and often dentures, glasses, hearing aids, and other personal belongings. A name tag is placed on the patient's wrist, and they become "the patient in 9W-310." This lowers the morale of the patient even more. At the same time, healthcare professionals may be pressed for time, overworked, and sometimes unable to cope with everyday pressures. They may be irritable and pay inadequate attention to the patient's story. They may eventually come to rely on the technical results and reports. This failure to communicate weakens the healthcare professional–patient relationship.

Inexperienced interviewers not only must learn about the patient's problems but also must gain insight into their *own* feelings, attitudes, and vulnerabilities. Such introspection enhances the self-image of the interviewer and results in them being perceived by the patient as a more careful and compassionate human being to whom the patient can turn in a time of crisis. This is discussed further in Chapter 5, Anti-Racist and Anti-Oppressive Clinical Skills.

During an interview session with patients, it's important to understand their perception of their own health problems. It's not enough to simply rely on the diagnosis given. It's crucial to ask specific questions about what the patient thinks is happening to them. Additionally, it's important to inquire about the impact the illness has on their work, family, and finances. Does the patient feel a loss of control? Do they feel guilty about their illness? Are they worried about dying? By asking these questions, you can gain valuable insight into the patient as a whole person, not just another statistic in the hospital.

Medical Malpractice and Communication Skills

According to studies, there has been a significant rise in malpractice lawsuits. Maintaining a positive relationship between healthcare professionals and patients is crucial in preventing such claims. It's worth noting that most lawsuits stem from issues with communication and patient dissatisfaction rather than actual medical negligence. Patients who are more likely to sue are those who have become dissatisfied with their provider and lost respect for them. Patients may feel disconnected from their healthcare professionals due to several factors. These barriers can include a shortage of time on the provider's end, a perceived lack of concern for the patient's issues, difficulty reaching the provider, an attitude of superiority or indifference, and insufficient information provided about the patient's condition. When healthcare professionals fail to communicate clearly about a patient's illness and treatment, it can make the patient feel rejected. Additionally, having friendly and competent office staff can help prevent malpractice lawsuits. Healthcare professionals who have not faced legal action tend to have longer visits with patients and use techniques such as orienting patients to the visit process, asking for their opinions, using humor and laughter, and making facilitative comments. It is widely recognized that a relationship built on honesty and understanding between provider and patient is crucial for good medical practice and the patient's well-being.

Novice interviewers may sometimes struggle to refrain from diagnosing every piece of information gathered during an interview. It is important to accept all the clues and analyze them later when attempting to establish a diagnosis.

If during the interview you cannot answer a question, do not. You can always act as the patient's advocate; listen to the question and then find someone who can provide an appropriate answer.

Healthcare Professional–Patient Engagement

A very important task of communication is to engage the patient. A helpful way of building rapport with a patient is to be curious about the person as a whole. Ask, "Before we begin, tell me something about yourself." When the patient returns, mention something personal that you learned from a previous visit—for instance, "How was your trip to Seattle to see your son?" Another part of engagement is to determine the patient's expectations from the visit; for instance, ask, "What are you hoping to accomplish today?" At the conclusion of the visit, ask "Is there anything else you are concerned about?" If the patient has several problems, it is acceptable to say, "We might need to discuss that problem at another visit. I want to be certain that we completely evaluate your main concern today."

Privacy Standards

In 2003, the U.S. Congress established federal privacy standards to safeguard the medical records and health information of patients. These standards were issued by the Department of Health and Human Services as part of the Health Insurance Portability and Accountability Act (HIPAA) of 1996. HIPAA regulations aim to promote electronic transactions and ensure the security and confidentiality of health information. The regulations apply to health plans, healthcare clearinghouses, and providers who conduct financial and administrative transactions electronically. To put it briefly, rules on patient confidentiality restrict how healthcare professional, plans, pharmacies, hospitals, clinics, and other organizations can utilize personal medical information. These regulations guarantee the safety of medical records and other identifiable health data, whether it's on paper, computers, or communicated orally. See Chapter 33, Clinical Ethics and Professionalism, and https://www.hhs.gov/hipaa/index.html for further information about privacy standards.

The medical interview requires a combination of cognitive and technical skills from the interviewer while also considering the personalities and emotions of both the patient and the interviewer. It is important for the interview to be flexible and not come across as an interrogation. When utilized properly, it is a highly effective diagnostic tool.

SYMPTOMS AND SIGNS

The healthcare professional must be able to elicit descriptions of, and recognize, a wide variety of symptoms and signs. *Symptom* refers to what the patient feels. Symptoms are described by the patient to clarify the nature of the illness. Shortness of breath, chest pain, nausea, diarrhea, and double vision are all symptoms. These labels help the patient describe the discomfort or distress that they are experiencing. Symptoms are not absolute; they are influenced by culture, intelligence, and socioeconomic background. As an example, consider the symptom of pain. Patients have different thresholds of pain.

Constitutional symptoms are symptoms that often accompany problems in any of the body systems. They may include fever, chills, weight loss, or excessive sweating.

A *sign* is what the examiner finds. Signs can be observed and quantified. Certain signs are also symptoms. For example, a patient may describe episodes of wheezing; this is a symptom. In addition, an examiner may hear wheezing during a patient's physical examination; this is a sign.

The major task of the interviewer is to sort out the symptoms and signs associated with a specific illness. A major advantage that the seasoned interviewer has over the novice is a better understanding of the pathophysiologic processes of disease states. The novice operates under the limitation of not knowing all the signs and symptoms of the associated diseases. With experience and education, the novice will recognize the combination of symptoms and signs as they relate to the underlying illness. For any given disease, certain symptoms and signs tend to occur together. When there is only an isolated symptom, the interviewer must be careful in making a definitive assessment.

CONDUCTING AN INTERVIEW

Getting Started and Introduction

The process of diagnosing a patient starts as soon as you meet them. It is important to dress professionally, wearing a white coat and a name badge that identifies you as a healthcare team member. Patients anticipate this level of professionalism, and dressing casually might come across as disrespectful.

At the beginning of a patient encounter, it is crucial to evaluate their sex, gender identity, preferred name, and pronouns. This helps avoid making assumptions about their gender identity, reduces the risk of potential biases, and creates a comfortable environment for the patient to discuss their gender identity. This also prevents using a salutation that does not correspond with the patient's gender identity, such as addressing a female-identifying patient as "Mr. Doe." For more information on this topic, refer to Chapter 5, Anti-Racist and Anti-Oppressive Clinical Skills.

It is crucial to understand the distinction between sex and gender. The term "sex" refers to the classification of male or female based on reproductive organs and chromosomal complement (XX for female and XY for male). On the other hand, "gender" pertains to a person's self-identification.

Introduce yourself, greet the patient by name, make eye contact, shake hands firmly (if appropriate), and smile. You may wish to say something like:

> *"I don't like to assume anything about my patients, so I always start my initial encounters by asking their name and how they would like to be addressed. My pronouns are she, her, and hers. If you are comfortable sharing, may I ask what pronouns you use? I am a medical (nursing, osteopathic, podiatric, dental, etc.) student at the XXX School of XXX. I've been asked to interview and examine you in the next hour."*

Use of Names and Pronouns

Pronouns and names are used all the time in everyday communication, both verbally and in writing. They are used often without thinking. Because names and pronouns are the two ways people call and refer to others, they are very personal and important; they are key facets of identity. Therefore, calling someone by the wrong name or "misgendering" them by using incorrect pronouns can make them feel disrespected.

Names are a crucial aspect of our identity as they are linked to our personal, cultural, familial, and historical roots. They provide us with a sense of belonging and a clear understanding of our position in society. A person's name may consist of several parts, such as name prefixes, given and middle names, surnames (family names), maiden or married names, and name suffixes. A name is a window into someone's world, opening a connection that reveals who they are and how they perceive others. By addressing someone by their name, we establish a bridge to make a positive impact on their life.

There are various reasons why people may choose to change their name, such as combining surnames, preferring an ethnic or non-ethnic name, changing names for transgender reasons, or due to religious beliefs.

There are people who may be uncomfortable with the name they were given at birth, or may want to change their name to match their gender identity. This can involve changing the name to a masculine or feminine form of their current name or choosing a completely new name. Sometimes, transgender individuals[a] may also choose to change their surname, especially if their parents do not react positively to their decision to "come out."[b]

Many cisgender (cis) people (people whose gender identity aligns with their sex assigned at birth) have never had to think about their **pronouns**… They take it for granted! Some people whose identities do not fit the binary or whose gender doesn't align with their sex assigned at birth, however, face being called by the incorrect pronoun(s) on a daily basis. It is one of many experiences that can make them feel rejected. Using the correct pronoun is an important way of showing that one recognizes, acknowledges, and accepts their gender. In addition, understanding that a pronoun does not tell you everything about a person's gender is an important way to show that you understand that gender identity is very complex, and a person's gender identity and expression may be different.

Years ago, children were taught that pronouns should follow specific rules along the gender binary: "*she, her, and hers*" for females and "*he, him, and his*" for males. However, since our society has progressed in understanding gender identity, our language must be updated. It should be accurate and convey understanding and respect for all people, especially for those who are transgender, gender non-conforming, and non-binary.

The following is a list of pronouns commonly used as of this writing. It is not a comprehensive list and other pronouns, or no pronouns at all, might be preferred by some transgender people. Be mindful that cisgender as well as transgender, gender non-conforming, and non-binary people may use any of these pronouns (see Fig. 1.2).

Feminine: She, her, hers
Masculine: He, him, his
Gender Neutral: They, them, theirs

At the start of the encounter, ask the patient to clarify their gender identity and establish the patient's preferred name and pronouns. See Chapter 26, The Transgender Patient, for more detail.

When addressing patients, it's important to use their preferred titles such as "Mr.," "Mrs.," "Miss," "Dr.," "Mx.," or "Ms." However, if they are adolescents or younger, it's best to avoid using any formal titles. Addressing a female as "Ms." is the default unless she explicitly requests to be called "Miss," "Mx.," or "Mrs." Avoid using name substitutes like "dear," "honey," or "grandpa." It's also best to avoid using "Sir" or "Ma'am" when addressing patients. Using a formal address helps to maintain a professional atmosphere during the interview. The term

[a]There are individuals who identify with a gender that does not align with the sex they were assigned at birth. This is commonly referred to as being transgender. It is important to note that the term "transsexual" is considered outdated and offensive by many.

[b]The phrase "coming out" is a way of describing when LGBTQ+ individuals discover and embrace their sexual orientation, romantic orientation, or gender identity.

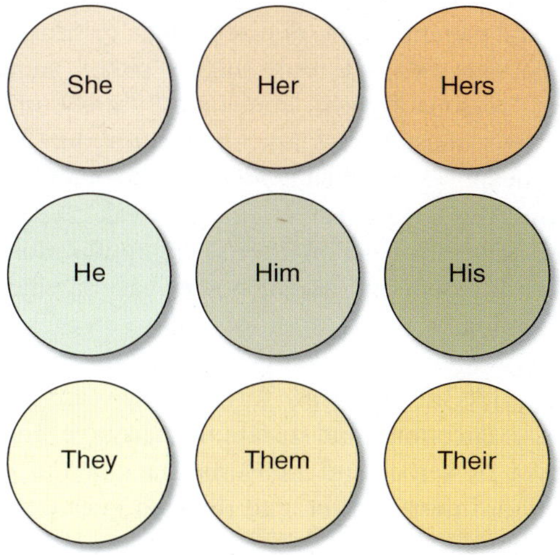

Fig. 1.2 Pronouns.

"Ma'am" is largely outdated, but there are a few specific situations where it may still be used. It is commonly used to address any female in the southern or southwestern areas of the United States. Use the patient's name. If you are uncertain about the pronunciation of a patient's name, kindly ask them to pronounce it correctly.

During their first meeting, the patient can choose to address the interviewer by their first name. However, it is generally not appropriate for the interviewer to use the patient's first name unless the patient specifically requests it, as this may affect the professional tone of the interaction.

Healthcare professionals should use inclusive language that avoids assumptions when determining a patient's sexual orientation and practices. It's best to use terms like "partner" instead of "husband" or "wife" until the patient's preferred terminology is known. Much more about this important subject is discussed in Chapter 5, Anti-Racist and Anti-Oppressive Clinical Skills.

The term *student doctor* or *student healthcare professional* should generally be avoided because patients may not actually understand this term; they may hear only the word *doctor* or *healthcare professional*. The introduction also includes a statement of the purpose of the visit. The welcoming handshake can serve to relax the patient. It establishes a contract between the patient and the healthcare professional. Of course, we need to remember cultural and religious reasons for not shaking hands.

If the patient is having a meal, ask whether you can return when they have finished eating. If the patient is using a urinal or bedpan, allow privacy. Do not begin an interview in this setting. If the patient has a visitor, you may inquire whether the *patient* wishes the visitor to stay. Do not assume that the visitor is a family member. Allow the patient to introduce the person to you.

The success of an interview can be influenced by the location in which it takes place. Ideally, a quiet and well-lit room is preferred. However, in most cases, hospital rooms do not meet these criteria, especially in teaching hospitals where patients are often housed in shared rooms. Despite this, it is important to make the most of the environment available. For the patient's privacy and to avoid any unnecessary distractions, it is recommended to close the curtains around the bed. You can also ask the nearby patients to lower their radios or televisions if needed. To reduce glare or shade, you can adjust the lights and window shades. Make sure to position the patient's bed light in a way that doesn't make them feel like they're being interrogated.

You should make the patient as comfortable as possible. If the patient's eyeglasses, hearing aids, or dentures were removed, ask whether the patient would like to use them. It may be useful to use your stethoscope as a hearing aid for hearing-impaired patients. The ear tips are placed in the ears of the patient, and the diaphragm serves as a microphone. The patient may be in a chair or lying in bed. Allow the patient the choice of position. This makes the patient feel that you are interested and concerned, and it allows the patient some control over the interview. If the patient is in bed, it is a nice gesture to ask whether the pillows should be arranged to make them more comfortable before the interview begins.

To Stand or to Sit?

Normally, the interviewer and patient should be seated comfortably at the same level. Often, it is useful to have the patient sitting even higher than the interviewer to give the patient the visual advantage. In this position, the patient may find it easier to open up to questions. If the patient is seated on the examination table, the interviewer should sit on the stool or in a chair, slightly off center, facing the patient to make good eye contact. Sitting down while speaking to the patient conveys the unspoken understanding that the interviewer is not in a rush and has time to spend with the patient. Sitting on the bed is too familiar and not appropriate. It is generally preferred that the interviewer sit at a distance of about 3 to 4 feet from the patient. Distances greater than 5 feet are impersonal, and distances closer than 3 feet interfere with the patient's "private space." The interviewer should sit in a relaxed position without crossing arms across the chest. The crossed-arms position is not appropriate because this body language projects an attitude of superiority and may interfere with the progress of the interview. If the patient is lying on the examination table, it is preferable for the interviewer to stand, as it may be uncomfortable for the patient to turn their head to speak to the interviewer.

When attending to a bedridden patient, it's important to position yourself properly. Either raise the head of the bed or have the patient sit up so that you are at eye level with them. Avoid standing directly over them. Also, remember to lower the bed rail to facilitate communication, but be sure to put it back up at the end of the session.

Regardless of whether the patient is sitting in a chair or lying in bed, make sure that they are appropriately draped with a sheet or robe.

The Opening Statement

Once the introduction has been made, the interview may begin with a general, open-ended question, such as "How may I help you?" or "What medical problem has brought you to the hospital?" or "I understand you are having… Tell me more about the problem." This type of opening remark allows the patient to speak first. The interviewer can then determine the patient's *chief concern:* the problem that is regarded as paramount. If the patient asks, "Haven't you read my records?" it is correct to say, "No, I've been asked to interview you without any prior information." Alternatively, the interviewer could say, "I would like to hear your story in your own words."

It's important to make patients feel comfortable and cared for during medical consultations. You can establish a good relationship with patients by asking them about themselves before getting into medical questions. Take a few minutes to chat and get to know them. If the patient is not in an urgent condition, try asking them to share a little about themselves before discussing their medical issue. This helps them relax and share positive experiences rather than just focusing on their medical problems. It also shows that you care about them as a person, not just as a patient.

The Narrative

Novice interviewers are often concerned about recalling the patient's history. Nevertheless, it is considered bad practice to take detailed notes while conducting the interview. It is important to concentrate on what the patient is saying and not on writing everything down. Moreover, if the interviewer takes notes, they may miss vital information conveyed through facial expressions and body language. It is acceptable to use a notepad to jot down significant dates, medications, or names that might easily be forgotten.

After the introductory question, the interviewer should proceed to questions related to the chief concern. These should naturally evolve into questions related to the other formal parts of the medical history, such as the present illness, past illnesses, social and family history, and review of body systems. Patients should largely be allowed to conduct the narrative in their own way. The interviewer must select certain aspects that require further details and guide the patient toward them. Overdirection is to be avoided because this stifles the interview and prevents important points from being clarified.

Engaging in small talk, also referred to as "*chit-chat*," can enhance the narrative of a conversation. Despite its name, small talk is not meaningless or haphazard, and research in conversation analysis has shown that it serves a beneficial purpose in communication. It has been shown that during conversations, the individual who tells a humorous anecdote is the one who is in control. For example, if an interviewer interjects a humorous remark during an interview and the patient laughs, the interviewer is in control of the conversation. If the patient does not laugh, the patient may take control.

It's important to stay attentive when a patient begins a conversation with phrases like "Let me ask you a hypothetical question" or "I have a friend with...; what do you think about...?" as these types of questions are likely related to the patient's own worries.

A patient often uses utterances such as "uh," "ah," and "well" to avoid unpleasant topics. It is natural for a patient to delay talking about an unpleasant situation or condition. Pauses between words, as well as the use of these words, provide a means for the patient to put off discussing a painful subject.

When patients use vague terms such as "often," "somewhat," "a little," "fair," "reasonably well," "sometimes," "rarely," or "average," the interviewer must always ask for clarification: "What does *sometimes* mean?" "How often is *often?*" Try to quantify a qualitative adverb. Even terms such as "dizzy," "weak," "diarrhea," and "tired" necessitate explanation. Precise communication is always desirable, and these terms, among others, have significant variations in meaning.

The interviewer should be alert for subtle clues from the patient to guide the interview further. There are a variety of techniques to encourage and sustain the narrative. These guidelines consist of verbal and nonverbal facilitation, reflection, confrontation, interpretation, and directed questioning. These techniques are discussed in this chapter.

The Closing

It is important that the interviewer pace the interview so that adequate time is left for the patient to ask questions and for the physical examination. About 5 minutes before the end of the interview, the interviewer should begin to summarize the important issues that were discussed.

By the conclusion of the interview, the interviewer should have a clear impression of the reason why the patient sought medical help, the history of the present illness, the patient's past medical history, and the patient's social and economic position. At this time, the interviewer may wish to say, "You've been very helpful. I am going to take a few notes." If any part of the history needs clarification, this is the time to obtain it. The interviewer may wish to summarize for the patient the most important parts of the history to help illuminate the important points made.

When a patient asks for your opinion, it's best to respond by saying, "I'm still a student. It would be better to ask your healthcare professional." This way, you don't give the patient the wrong information or a different opinion, and you don't harm the relationship between the healthcare professional and the patient.

At the conclusion, it is polite to encourage the patient to discuss any additional problems or to ask any questions: "Is there anything else you would like to tell me that I have not already asked?" "Are there any questions you might like to ask?" Usually, all possible avenues of discussion have been exhausted, but these remarks allow the patient the "final say."

Thus, a good closure should consist of the following four parts:

- Provide a summary.
- Provide an opportunity for questions. Does the patient have any questions, and have you answered them?
- Provide reassurance only as appropriate. You could say, "It's a good thing that you came in today; I will do everything possible to help you." Patients like to know that they did the right thing to seek medical attention. Do not give false reassurances.
- What happens next? Instruct the patient to get dressed and leave, wait for the nurse to draw blood, wait for the technician to do an electrocardiogram, or other activity.

BASIC INTERVIEWING TECHNIQUES

A successful interview should be natural and effortless. The interviewer needs to pay attention to subtle cues and respond accordingly. The interviewer should keep the conversation going smoothly. There are various techniques that can be employed to encourage the patient to keep talking, which we will discuss in this section. It's important to note that each technique has its own limitations and not all of them may apply to every interview.

Questioning

The secret of effective interviewing lies in the art of questioning. The wording of the question is often less important than the tone of voice used to ask it. In general, questions that stimulate the patient to talk freely are preferred.

Open-Ended Questions

When conducting the interview, open-ended questions are used to gather general information. These questions are best used at the beginning of the interview or when changing topics. Open-ended questions prompt the patient to tell their story without assuming a specific answer. It can be beneficial to allow the patient to speak freely. Open-ended questions cannot be answered with a simple "yes" or "no." Examples of open-ended questions are the following:

"How may I help you today?"
"What kind of medical problem are you having?"
"How has your health been?"
"Are you having stomach pain? Tell me about it."
"Tell me about your headache."
"How was your health before your heart attack?"
"Can you describe your feelings when you get the pain?"
"I'm curious about…"

Too much rambling, however, must be controlled by the interviewer in a sensitive but firm manner. This freedom of speech should obviously be avoided with overtalkative patients, whereas it should be used often with silent patients.

Direct Questions

After a period of open-ended questioning, the interviewer should direct the attention to specific facts learned during the open-ended questioning period. These *direct questions* serve to clarify and add detail to the story. This type of question gives the patient little room for explanation or qualification. A direct question can usually be answered in one word or a brief sentence; for example:

"Where does it hurt?"
"When do you get the burning sensation?"
"How do you compare this pain with your ulcer pain?"

Care must be taken to avoid asking direct questions in a manner that might bias the response.

Symptoms are classically characterized according to several dimensions or elements, including *bodily location, onset* (and *chronology*), *precipitating* (and *palliating*) *factors, quality, radiation, severity, temporal,* and *associated manifestations*. These elements may be used as a framework to clarify the illness. Examples of appropriate questions follow.

Bodily Location

"Where in your back do you feel pain?"
"Can you tell me where you feel the pain?"
"Do you feel it anywhere else?"

Onset (and Chronology)

"When did you first notice it?"
"How long did it last?"
"Have you had the pain since that time?"
"Then what happened?"
"Have you noticed that it is worse during your menstrual period?"

Precipitating Factors

"What makes it worse?"
"What seems to bring on the pain?"
"Have you noticed that it occurs at a certain time of day?"
"Is there anything else besides exercise that makes it worse?"
"Does exercise increase the shortness of breath?"
"Does stress precipitate the pain?"

Palliating Factors

"What do you do to get more comfortable?"
"Does lying quietly in bed help you?"
"Does rest help?"
"Does aspirin help the headache?"
"Does eating make it better?"

Quality (Looking for Descriptors of Pain)

"What does it feel like?"
"Can you describe the pain?"
"What do you mean by a 'sticking pain'?"
"Was it sharp (pause), dull (pause), or aching?"
"When you get the pain, is it steady or does it change?"

Radiation

"When you get the pain in your chest, do you feel it in any other part of your body at the same time?"
"When you experience your abdominal pain, do you have pain in any other area of your body?"

Severity (or Quantity)

"On a scale from 1 to 10, with 10 the worst pain you can imagine, how would you rate this pain?"
"How has the pain affected your lifestyle?"[c]
"What do you mean by 'a lot'?"
"How many sanitary napkins do you use?"
"How many times did you vomit?"
"What kind of effect does the pain have on your work?"
"How does the pain compare with the time you broke your leg?"
"Can you fall asleep with the pain?"

[c]This is probably a better question than the first question since it eliminates cultural differences in describing pain.

Temporal

"Does it ever occur at rest?"
"Do you ever get the pain when you are emotionally upset?"
"Where were you when it occurred?"
"Does the pain occur at any specific time of your menstrual cycle?"
"Does it awaken you from sleep?"
"Have you noticed any relationship of the pain to eating? Does it occur before meals, while eating, or after meals?"

Associated Manifestations

"Do you have any other symptoms?"
"Do you ever have nausea with the pain?"
"Have you noticed other changes that happen when you start to sweat?"
"Before you get the headache, do you ever experience a strange taste or smell?"

The mnemonic *O-P-Q-R-S-T*, which stands for *o*nset (chronology), *p*recipitating (or *p*alliative), *q*uality, *r*adiation, *s*everity, and *t*emporal, is useful in helping the interviewer remember these important dimensions of a symptom. The *setting* is also important to determine. Did the symptom occur when exposed to certain environmental conditions, during specific activities, during emotional periods, or under other circumstances?

Question Types to Avoid

There are several types of questions that should be avoided. One is the *suggestive* question, which provides the answer to the question. For example:

"Do you feel the pain in your left arm when you get it in your chest?"

A better way to ask the same question would be as follows:

"When you get the pain in your chest, do you notice it anywhere else?"

The *why* question carries tones of accusation. This type of question almost always asks a patient to account for their behavior and tends to put the patient on the defensive; for example:

"Why did you stop taking the medication?"
"Why did you wait so long to call me?"

The answers to such questions, however, are important. As mentioned previously, try rephrasing, such as *"What is the reason…?"* The "why" question is useful in daily life with friends and family, with whom you have a relationship different from that with your patients; do not use it with patients.

The *multiple* or *rapid-fire* question should also be avoided. In this type of question, there is more than one point of inquiry. Don't barrage the patient with a list of questions. The patient can easily get confused and respond incorrectly, answering no part of the question adequately. The patient may answer only the last inquiry heard; for example:

"Have you had night sweats, fever, or chills?"
"How many brothers and sisters do you have, and has any one of them ever had asthma, heart disease, pneumonia, or tuberculosis?"

Asking multiple questions can lead to confusion as patients may only answer part of the question. For instance, if you inquire about chills, as in the first question earlier, and the patient responds with a "No," it may not necessarily mean they do not have any symptoms (i.e., sweats or fever). By asking about each symptom separately, you can obtain more accurate information, such as discovering that the patient experiences night sweats.

Questions should be concise and easily understandable. The context should be free of *medical jargon*. Frequently, novice interviewers try to use their new medical vocabularies to impress their patients. They may sometimes respond to the patient with technical terms, leaving the patient feeling confused or put down. By using medical jargon, the interviewer distances himself or herself from the patient. This use of technical medical terms is sometimes called *doctorese* or *medicalese*. For example:

"You seem to have a homonymous hemianopsia."
"Have you ever had a myocardial infarction?"
"We perform Papanicolaou smears to check for cervical carcinoma in situ."
"I am going to order a CBC with differential."
"The MUGA scan shows that you have congestive heart failure."

Medical terminology, as a rule, should not be used in conversations with patients. Technical terms scare patients who are unfamiliar with them. Every healthcare professional student understands the term *heart failure,* but a patient might interpret it as failure of the heart to pump—that is, cardiac standstill or death. Although patients should be given only as much information as they can handle, adequate explanations must always be provided. A partial explanation can leave the patient confused and fearful. Conversely, patients may try to use medical terms themselves. Do not take these terms at face value; ask patients to describe what they mean. For example, some patients may use "heart attack" to describe angina, "stroke" to describe a transient ischemic attack, "spells" to describe dizziness, or "water pills" or "heart pills" when referring to their medication.

A *leading* or *biased* question carries a suggestion of the kind of response for which the interviewer is looking. For example, "You haven't used any recreational drugs, have you?" suggests that the interviewer disapproves of the patient's use of drugs. If the patient has used recreational drugs, they may not admit it under this line of questioning. Instead, ask, "Do you use recreational drugs?" Questions should be asked in the positive or affirmative mode, not the negative. Questions asked in the affirmative or positive mode convey a nonjudgmental approach and encourage the patient to answer more candidly without the fear of being blamed for an action.

It is also incorrect to ask, "*You don't have* diabetes, do you?" or "*You haven't been* wheezing, have you?" Instead, the interviewer should ask in the positive affirmative mode, "Do you have diabetes?" or "Have you been wheezing?" A leading question may also invite a particular answer. For example, "Did you notice that the pain came on after you vomited?"

In addition to avoiding certain types of questions, the interviewer should avoid certain situations. For example, patients may respond to a question in an unexpected manner, resulting in a period of unexpected silence on the part of the interviewer. This "stumped silence" can be interpreted by the patient in a variety of ways. The interviewer must be able to respond quickly in such instances, even if it means broaching another topic.

If a patient suggests that a test not be performed, perhaps because of an underlying fear of the test, the interviewer should never respond by stating, "I'm the healthcare professional. I'll make the decisions." The interviewer should recognize the anxiety and handle the response from that point of view. They should ask the patient, "What are your concerns about taking the test?"

If a patient appears overweight, ask first whether there has been any change in the patient's weight before asking whether they have tried to lose weight. The patient may have lost 30 pounds already but is still overweight. Never refer to an overweight person as obese.

The word "change" is your best friend in interviewing! Ask "Has there been a change in weight," "a change in appetite," "a change in your menstrual cycle," "a change in your mood," "a change in your diet," "a change in your skin," "a change in your bowel movements," etc.

Finally, assume nothing about patients' knowledge of their disease, their sexual orientation or experiences, their education, their family, or their knowledge of illness in general. People come from different backgrounds and have different beliefs based on culture, religion, and experience. It is incorrect to assume that if a medicine has been prescribed for an illness, the patient is taking it correctly or takes it at all. Do not even presume that a patient is happy or sad about an event in their life or in the lives of friends and family. It is much safer to ask questions in the following manner:

"How do you feel about it?"
"What do you know about...?"
"How often do you take this medication?"
"How do you remember to take this medication?"
"How does that make you feel?"

Silence

Silence is most useful with silent patients. Silence should never be used with overtalkative patients, because letting them talk continuously would not allow the interviewer to control the interview. This difficult type of communication, when used correctly, can indicate interest and support. Silence on the part of the patient can be related to hostility, shyness, or embarrassment. The interviewer should remain silent, maintaining direct eye contact and attentiveness. The interviewer may lean forward and even nod. After no more than 2 minutes of silence, the interviewer may say,

"What are you thinking about?"
"You were saying...?"
"These things are hard to talk about."
"You were about to say...?"

If the patient remains silent, another method of sustaining the interview must be chosen.

The interviewer must use silence when the patient becomes overwhelmed by emotion. This act allows the patient to release some of the tension evoked by the history and indicates to the patient that it is acceptable to cry. Handing the patient a box of tissues is a supportive gesture. It is inappropriate for the interviewer to say, "Don't cry" or "Pull yourself together" because these statements imply that the patient is wasting the interviewer's time or that it is shameful to show emotions.

Using silence correctly is crucial when conducting an interview. If the interviewer remains silent, fidgets, reviews notes, or evaluates the patient's facial expressions, it can make the patient feel uncomfortable. The frequent use of silence may also be perceived as aloofness or a lack of knowledge by the patient.

Facilitation

Facilitation is a communication technique that encourages a patient to keep talking without controlling the direction of the conversation. Verbal facilitations like "Uh huh," "Go on," "Tell me more about that," "And then?" and "Hmm" are commonly used.

Nonverbal cues, such as nodding the head or making a hand gesture, are important ways to show interest and encourage patients to continue speaking. However, it's important to be mindful of nodding too much, as it may give unintended approval in some situations. Moving closer to the patient can also signal interest, but should be done with care.

Often, a puzzled expression can be used as a nonverbal facilitation to indicate, "I don't understand."

Confrontation

Confrontation is a response based on an observation by the interviewer that points out something striking about the patient's behavior or previous statement. This interviewing technique directs the patient's attention to something of which they may or may not be aware. The confrontation may be either a statement or a question; for example:

"You look upset."
"Is there any reason why you always look away when you talk to me?"
"You're angry."
"You sound uncomfortable about it."
"What is the reason you are not answering my questions?"
"You look as though you are going to cry."

Confrontation is particularly useful in encouraging the patient to continue the narrative when there are subtle clues given. By confronting the patient, the interviewer may enable the patient to explain the problem further. Confrontation is also useful to clarify discrepancies in the history.

Confrontation must be used with care; excessive use is considered impolite and overbearing. If correctly used, however, confrontation can be a powerful technique. Suppose a patient is describing a symptom of chest pain. By observing the patient, you notice that there are now tears in the patient's eyes. By saying sympathetically, "You look very upset," you are encouraging the patient to express emotions.

Interpretation

Interpretation is a type of confrontation that is based on inference rather than on observation. The interviewer interprets the patient's behavior, encouraging the patient to observe their own role in the problem. The interviewer must fully understand the clues the patient has given before they can offer an interpretation.

The interviewer must look for signs of underlying fear or anxiety that may be indicated by other symptoms, such as recurrent pain, dizziness, headaches, or weakness. Once these underlying fears have been discovered, the patient may be led to recognize the inciting event during future interviews. Interpretation frequently opens previously unrecognized lines of communication. Examples are the following:

"You seem to be quite happy about that."
"Sounds as if you're scared."
"Are you afraid you've done something wrong?"
"I wonder whether there's a relation between your dizziness and arguments with your wife."

Interpretation can demonstrate support and understanding if used correctly.

Reflection

Reflection is a response that mirrors or echoes that which has just been expressed by the patient. It encourages the patient to expound further on details of the statement. The tone of voice is important in reflection. The intonation of the words may indicate entirely different meanings. For example:

Patient: *"I was so sick that I haven't worked since October 2023."*
Response: *"Haven't worked since 2023?"*

In this example, the emphasis should be on "2023." This asks the patient to describe the conditions that did not allow them to work. If the emphasis is incorrectly placed on "worked," the interviewer immediately puts the patient on the defensive, implying, "What did you do with your time?" Although often very useful, reflection can hamper the progress of an interview if used improperly.

Support

Support is a response that indicates an interest in or an understanding of the patient. Supportive remarks promote a feeling of security in the healthcare professional–patient relationship. A supportive response might be "I understand." An important time to use support is immediately after a patient has expressed strong feelings. The use of support when a patient suddenly begins to cry strengthens the provider–patient relationship. Two important subgroups of support are *reassurance* and *empathy.*

Reassurance

Reassurance is a response that conveys to the patient that the interviewer understands what has been expressed. It may also indicate that the interviewer approves of something the patient has done or thought. It can be a powerful tool, but false reassurance can be devastating. Good examples of reassurance are the following:

"That's wonderful! I'm delighted that you started in the rehabilitation program at the hospital."
"You're improving steadily."
"That's great that you were able to stop smoking."
"It's understandable why you are so upset after your accident."
"It's good you came in today. We will do everything to help you."

The use of reassurance is particularly helpful when the patient seems upset or frightened. Reassurance must always be based on fact. Reassurance is very important because it tells the patient that their fears are understandable and real.

It's natural for a patient to seek reassurance before undergoing a procedure. However, it's important to be honest about the risks involved, rather than making false promises of success. Simply reassuring the patient without acknowledging the potential complications can be misleading, illegal, and may not reflect the reality of the situation. As a helpful and fair assistant, I advise being transparent about the known morbidity and mortality rates, if known, associated with the procedure while still offering support and encouragement.

It's important to avoid telling a patient to relax or calm down. Patients have the right to feel nervous or worried, so it's inappropriate to dictate their emotions. Instead, focus on building their confidence and trust. Telling a patient to calm down might make them feel like you don't understand the severity of their problem or that you're uncomfortable dealing with it.

Empathy

Empathy is a response that recognizes the patient's feeling and does not criticize it. It is understanding, *not* an emotional state of sympathy. You try to put yourself in the shoes of the patient. The empathic response is saying, "I hear what you're saying." The use of empathy can strengthen the healthcare professional–patient relationship and allow the interview to flow smoothly. Studies have shown that high levels of empathy have been linked to better patient outcomes![2]

Examples of empathy are the following:

"I'm sure your daughter's problem has given you much anxiety."
"The death of someone so close to you is hard to take."
"I guess this has been kind of a silent fear all your life."
"You must have been very sad."
"I know it's not easy for you. I'm delighted to see that you're trying to eat everything on your tray."
"That's wonderful that you have stopped smoking."

The last two examples illustrate an important point: it is critical to give credit to patients to encourage *their* role in their own improvement.

It is impossible, however, to put yourself in the shoes of the patient because of a difference in age, gender, life experiences, education, culture, religion, and other factors. An extremely empathic statement, which sounds counterintuitive, is "It's impossible for me to fully understand how you are feeling, but how can I help you? How can we work together to get past this difficult problem?"

Empathy can be expressed without using words. A simple nod or a reassuring touch on the shoulder can communicate support and understanding to someone who is upset. In some situations, it's important for the interviewer to show empathy without displaying too much emotion themselves.

Transitions

Transitional statements are used as guides to allow the patient to understand better the logic of the interviewer's questioning and for the interview to flow more smoothly from one topic to another. An example of a transitional statement might be, after learning about the current medical problem, the interviewer's statement, "Now I am going to ask you some questions about your health history." Other examples while the history is documented might be, "I am now going to ask you some questions about your family," and "Now we are going to talk about your lifestyle and your activities in a typical day."

Usually, the line of questioning being pursued is obvious to the patient, so transitions are not always needed. Transitioning to the sexual history, however, often requires a transitional statement. As an example, a transitional statement such as "I am now going to ask you some routine questions about your sexual health" may bridge to this area comfortably for both the patient and interviewer. An alternative transitional statement might be, "To determine your risk for several diseases, I am now going to ask you some questions about your sexual health [or sexual activity, or sexual habits]." Avoid phrases such as "personal habits," "personal life," or "personal history," because these expressions send the message of what the interviewer considers these habits to be ("personal"); the patient may be more open to discuss this area and may not consider it "personal." It is better to ask about "sexual habits," "sexual activity," or "sexual health" rather than "sexual life." Other words to be avoided include "like to," "want to," "need to," or "have to" (e.g., "I would now like to ask you some questions about your sexual habits" or "I now have to ask you some questions about your sexual habits"). As will be discussed in subsequent chapters, always use specific language. Refer to the genitalia with explicit terms such as vagina, penis, uterus, and so on; do not use the term "private parts."

FORMAT OF THE HISTORY

The information obtained by the interviewer is organized into a comprehensive statement about the patient's health. Traditionally, the history has been obtained by using a *disease-oriented* approach emphasizing the disease process that prompted the patient to seek medical advice. For example, a patient may present with shortness of breath; the interview would be conducted to ascertain the pathologic causes of the shortness of breath.

An alternative approach to obtaining the history is a *patient-oriented* one. This entails evaluating the patient and their problems more holistically. By using this approach, the healthcare professional can elicit a more complete history, keeping in mind that other symptoms (e.g., pain from arthritis, weakness, depression, anxiety) may affect the patient's shortness of breath. For example, if a patient has arthritis and cannot walk, shortness of breath may manifest as less severe than if the patient were able to walk and experienced shortness of breath with minimal activity. In this way, the entire patient is considered.

The major traditional sections of the history, with some patient-oriented changes, are as follows:

- Source and reliability
- Chief concern
- History of the present illness and debilitating symptoms
- Past medical history
- Health maintenance
- Occupational and environmental history
- Biographic information
- Family history
- Psychosocial and spiritual history
- Sexual, reproductive, and gynecologic history
- Review of systems

Source and Reliability

The source and reliability section contains identifying data—source of the history and, if appropriate, the source of the referral. The identifying data consist of the age and gender of the patient. The source of information is usually the patient. If the patient requires a translator, the source is the patient and the translator. If family members help in the interview, their names should be included in a single-sentence statement. The source could also be a medical record.

The reliability of the interview should be assessed. Is the patient competent to provide a history? Often, determination of orientation to person, time, and place (discussed in Chapter 21, The Nervous System) is done early in the interview to assess the cognitive function of the person. If the patient is not oriented to person, time, and place, a statement such as, "The patient is a 76-year-old male with a moderate cognitive impairment as manifested by a lack of orientation to person, time, and place who presents with…." This indicates that the rest of the history needs to be taken with "a grain of salt" or that some or all the history that follows may be inaccurate. The date and time of the interaction is also vital for the record.

Chief Concern

The chief concern is the patient's brief statement explaining why they sought medical attention. **Try to fully quote the patient's own words.** It is the answer to the question, "What is the medical problem that brought you to the hospital?" or "How can I help you today?" The chief concern might then be:

"I've been having chest pain for the past 5 hours."
"I have had terrible nausea and vomiting for 2 days."
"I've got a splitting headache for the last few days."
"I'm here for my routine examination for school."
"I just don't feel well."

Patients sometimes use medical terms. The interviewer must ask the patient to define such terms to ascertain what the patient means by them.

History of Present Illness and Debilitating Symptoms

The *history of the present illness* refers to the recent changes in health that led the patient to seek medical attention at this time. It describes the information relevant to the chief concern. It should answer the questions of *what, when, how, where, which, who,* and *why.* It provides a clear, chronologic explanation of the patient's symptoms accounting for the reason the patient has sought medical attention.

Chronology is the most practical framework for organizing the history. It enables the interviewer to comprehend the sequential development of the underlying pathologic process. In this section, the interviewer gathers all the necessary information, starting with the first symptoms of the present illness and following its progression to the present day. To establish the beginning of the present illness, it is important to verify that the patient was entirely well before the earliest symptom. Patients often do not remember when a symptom developed. If the patient is uncertain about the presence of a symptom at a certain time, the interviewer may be able to relate it to an important or memorable event, for example, "Did you have the pain during your summer vacation?" In this part of the interview, mainly open-ended questions are asked because these afford the patient the greatest opportunity to describe the history.

In the patient-centered evaluation, the interviewer must determine whether any debilitating symptoms are also present and what effect they have on the patient. These symptoms include pain, constipation, weakness, nausea, shortness of breath, depression, and anxiety.

The effect of the symptom or condition on the patient's life must be assessed. One can simply ask, "How has your problem interfered with your daily life?"

Pain

Pain is one of the most debilitating symptoms and has traditionally been under-recognized. Unrelieved pain is very common and is one of the most feared symptoms of illness. Surveys indicate that 20% to 30% of the U.S. population experiences acute or chronic pain, and it is the most common symptom experienced by hospitalized adults. More than 80% of patients with cancer and more than two-thirds of patients dying of noncancer illnesses experience moderate to severe pain. There are approximately 75 million episodes of acute pain per year resulting from traumatic injuries and surgical procedures. Acute pain is caused by trauma or medical conditions, is usually brief, and abates with a resolution of the injury. Chronic pain persists beyond the period of healing or is present for longer than 3 months.

The effect of pain on the quality of life is important to understand. Untreated or undertreated pain impairs physical and psychological health, functional status, and quality of life. In particular, pain may produce unnecessary suffering; decrease physical activity, sleep, and appetite, which further weakens the patient; may increase fear and anxiety that the end is near; may cause the patient to reject further treatment; may diminish the ability to work productively; may diminish concentration; may decrease sexual function; may alter appearance; and may diminish the enjoyment of recreation and social relationships. In addition, pain has been associated with increased medical complications, increased use of healthcare resources, decreased patient satisfaction, and unnecessary suffering. In the United States, the economic costs of undertreated pain approach $80 billion per year in treatment, compensation, and lost wages.

Patients often experience inadequate pain control due to various factors such as healthcare professionals' limited knowledge about analgesics, negative attitudes toward pain management, lack of understanding about addiction, drug regulations, and the cost of effective pain treatment. A study of medical inpatients and the use of narcotic analgesics revealed that 32% of patients were continuing to experience "severe" distress despite the analgesic regimen, and 41% were in "moderate" distress. It was also revealed that pain was dramatically undertreated in ambulatory patients with acquired immune deficiency syndrome (AIDS).[3] Of patients experiencing severe pain, only 7.3% received opioid analgesics at the recommended doses. Approximately 75% with severe pain received no opioid analgesics at all. The Study to Understand Prognoses and Preferences for Outcomes and Risks of Treatment (1995) indicated that 50% of conscious patients who died in a hospital suffered "moderate-severe" pain during their last week of life.

Whatever the cause of pain, healthcare professionals must repeatedly ask about the presence of pain and the adequacy of its control:

"Are you having pain?"
"Have you had pain in the past week?"
"Tell me where your pain is located."
"How has the pain affected your life?"
"Are you satisfied with your pain control?"
"Tell me a little more about your pain."

When working with elderly patients, a helpful approach is to acknowledge that pain is a common experience, and ask if they have anything specific they would like to share about their own pain. For those with cognitive impairments, it's important to focus on their current pain levels rather than pain they may have experienced in the past few days.

Patients must be able to assess pain with easily administered rating scales and should document the efficacy of pain relief at regular intervals after the initiation or modification of treatment. In addition, it is vital to teach patients and their families how to promote effective pain management at home. The interviewer should ask patients to quantify their pain and should try using some form of pain rating scale. There are four commonly used scales:

- Simple Descriptive Pain Intensity Scale
- 0 to 10 Numeric Pain Intensity Scale
- Visual Analog Scale
- Face Scale

These scales are illustrated in Fig. 1.3. International pain scales are also very common, as shown in the simplified Chinese version in Fig. 1.4. On the back of the scale are grounding statements for each of the 10 points of pain. I saw this scale while lecturing at the Xiangya Hospital of Central South University in Changsha, China.

In addition to individual descriptions of the severity of pain, many studies have also indicated cultural differences in the description of pain. There is considerable evidence demonstrating substantial ethnic disparities in the prevalence, treatment, progression, and outcomes of pain-related conditions.[4] Campbell and Edwards describe "the experience of pain differentially activates stress-related physiological responses across various ethnic groups, members of different ethnic groups appear to use differing coping strategies in managing pain complaints, providers' treatment decisions vary as a function of patient ethnicity and pharmacies in predominantly minority neighborhoods are far less likely to stock potent analgesics." Culture shapes many aspects of the experience of pain, including pain expression, lay remedies, social roles, expectations, perceptions of the medical system, when/how/where to

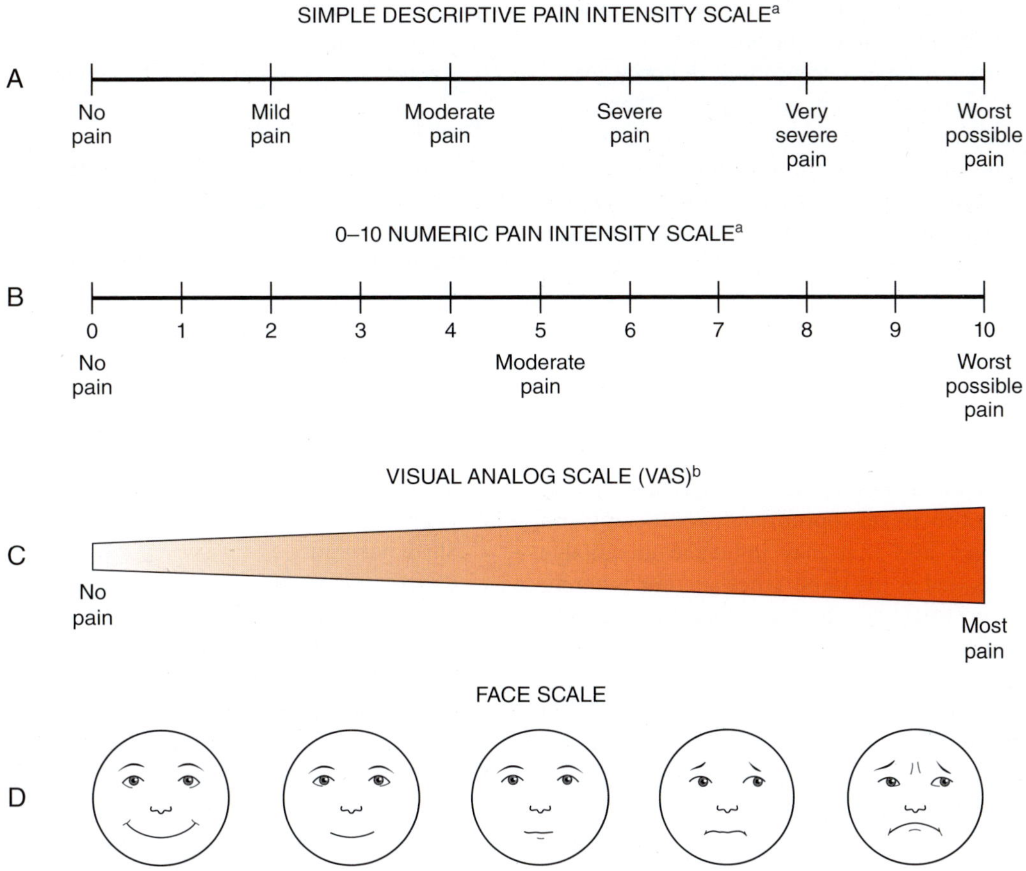

[a]If used as a graphic rating scale, a 10-cm baseline is recommended.
[b]A 10-cm baseline is recommended for VAS scales.

Fig. 1.3 Examples of Pain Scales. (A) Simple descriptive pain intensity scale. (B) 0 to 10 numeric pain intensity scale. (C) Visual analog scale. (D) Face scale.

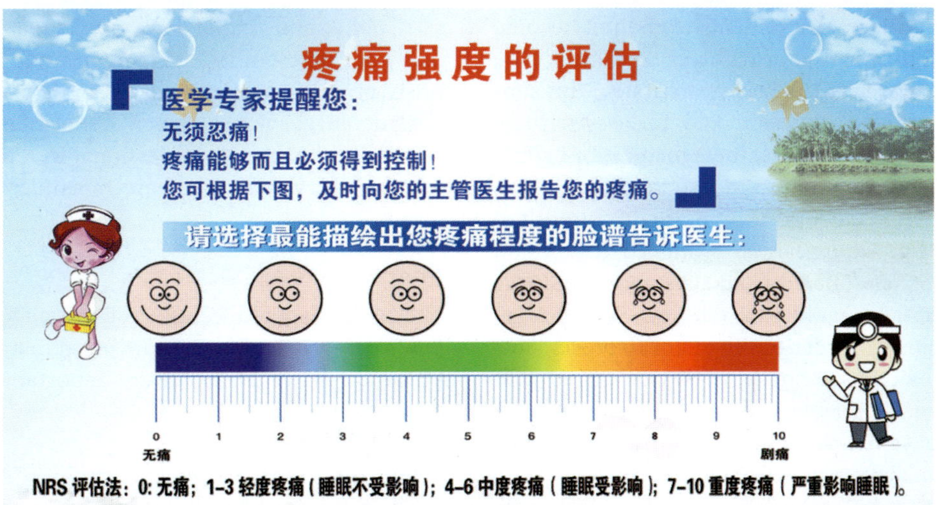

Fig. 1.4 International Pain Scales in Simplified Chinese. (Courtesy of Xiangya Hospital of Central South University, Changsha, China.)

seek care, healthcare practices, illness beliefs and behaviors, and receptivity to medical care interventions.[5]

A 1997 study reported that members of ethnic minority groups are likely to receive inadequate treatment for pain.[6] Their study showed that minority patients were three times more likely to be undertreated for pain. Sixty-five percent of minority patients did not receive guideline-recommended analgesic prescriptions. Latino patients reported less pain relief than did African American patients. A 2000 study investigated the availability of commonly prescribed opioid analgesics in pharmacies in New York City.[7] They found that 50% of a random sample of pharmacies surveyed did not stock sufficient medications to treat patients with severe pain adequately. Pharmacies in predominantly non-White areas were less likely to stock opioid analgesics than were pharmacies in predominantly White neighborhoods.

Regardless of a patient's demographic characteristics, healthcare professionals must focus on appropriate pain therapy and one's potential personal bias that may influence inequitable treatment decisions as well as the importance and our inherent obligation to take appropriate action when faced with an individual suffering in pain.

It's important to provide pain relief to patients, but it's crucial to keep in mind that pain medications can be addictive. Opioid pain relievers are safe when taken as prescribed by a healthcare professional for a short duration. However, their euphoric effects can lead to misuse. Dependence is possible even with regular use as prescribed by a physician. Misuse of opioid pain relievers can result in addiction, overdose, and even death.

There are different types of opioid medications, including misused substances like heroin and synthetic opioids such as fentanyl. Some pain relievers that fall under this category are oxycodone (OxyContin®), hydrocodone (Vicodin®), codeine, morphine, and many more, which are only available with a prescription. See Appendix B, Commonly Misused Substances.

Since the 1990s, opioids have been increasingly used to treat chronic pain. In the late 1990s, pharmaceutical companies reassured the medical community that patients would not become addicted to prescription opioid pain relievers, and healthcare professionals began to prescribe them at greater rates. This subsequently led to widespread diversion and misuse of these medications before it became clear that these medications could indeed be highly addictive. Opioid overdose rates began to increase. In 2021, more than 80,000 Americans died as a result of an opioid overdose. That same year, an estimated 2.2 million people in the United States suffered from substance use disorders related to prescription opioid pain relievers, and 652,000 suffered from a heroin use disorder. Seven out of 10 preventable opioid overdose death victims are male, 53,992 compared with 21,793 female deaths in 2021. However, since 1999, female opioid overdose deaths have increased at a faster pace than male deaths—1608% for females versus 1076% for males.

Every day, more than 130 people in the United States die after overdosing on opioids. The misuse of, and addiction to, opioids is a serious national crisis that affects public health as well as social and economic welfare. The Centers for Disease Control and Prevention estimates that the total "economic burden" of prescription opioid misuse alone in the United States was $1.04 trillion in 2018 and nearly $1.5 trillion in 2020, including the costs of healthcare, lost productivity, addiction treatment, and criminal justice involvement.

Past Medical History

The past medical history consists of the overall assessment of the patient's health before the present illness. It includes all the following:

- General state of health
- Past illnesses
- Prior injuries and accidents
- Hospitalizations
- Surgery
- Allergies
- Immunizations
- Substance abuse
- Diet
- Sleep patterns
- Current medications
- Complementary and alternative therapies

General State of Health

To begin discussing the patient's past medical history, the interviewer may ask, "How has your health been in the past?" If the patient gives a vague answer such as "Excellent" or "Fair," the interviewer can ask for more details by saying, "What does 'excellent' mean to you?" It's important for the interviewer to ask specific questions to gain a better understanding of the patient's medical history.

Past Illnesses

The record of *past illnesses* should include a statement of childhood and adult problems. Recording childhood illnesses is obviously more important for pediatric and young adult interviewees. All patients should nevertheless be asked about measles, mumps, whooping cough, rheumatic fever, chickenpox, polio, and scarlet fever. Older patients may respond, "I really don't remember." It is important to remember that a diagnosis given to the interviewer by a patient should never be considered absolute. Even if the patient was evaluated by a competent healthcare professional in a reputable medical center, the interviewer may have misunderstood the information given.

Prior Injuries and Accidents

The patient should be asked about any *prior injuries* or accidents: "Have you ever been involved in a serious accident?" The type of injury and the date are important to record.

Hospitalizations

When discussing *hospitalizations*, it's important to cover all types: medical, surgical, and psychiatric. It's crucial not to avoid asking about psychiatric illnesses out of embarrassment, as it only reinforces the stigma surrounding mental health. Interviewers should learn to ask direct questions sensitively, such as "Have you ever had therapy or counseling?" or "What nervous or emotional problems have you experienced?" Another option is to inquire if the individual has ever been hospitalized for a nonmedical or nonsurgical reason.

Surgery

All *surgical procedures* should be specified. The indication, type of procedure, date, hospital, and surgeon's name should be documented, if possible.

Allergies

All *allergies* should be described. These include environmental (including insects), ingestible, and drug-related reactions. The interviewer should seek specificity and verification of the patient's allergic response. "How do you know you're allergic?" "What kind of problem did you have when you took...?" The specific symptoms of an allergy (e.g., rashes, nausea, itching, anaphylaxis) should be clearly indicated.

Immunizations

Knowing the *immunization history* of every patient is crucial. Fewer than 25% of adults have immunity against tetanus and diphtheria, and even fewer targeted groups receive annual influenza vaccines. Fortunately, these diseases are preventable, and it's recommended to use combined toxoid when considering either immunization. Patients who have never received this toxoid will receive an initial injection, followed by doses at 1 month and 6 to 12 months. A booster dose is necessary every 10 years.

COVID-19. Regarding vaccination against COVID-19, everyone 5 months of age and older should be vaccinated. Since this is a rapidly changing field, please refer to the CDC website for the most up-to-date information: https://www.cdc.gov/coronavirus/2019-ncov/vaccines/stay-up-to-date.html. Last updated April 25, 2024.

Influenza. During the 2022–2023 influenza season, there were approximately 50,000 deaths from flu-related illnesses in the United States. According to the CDC, 50 million individuals suffered from flu illnesses with more than 500,000 hospitalizations related to the flu. Everyone 6 months and older is recommended for annual influenza vaccination with rare exceptions. Different influenza vaccines are approved for people of different ages. Some vaccines are only approved for adults. For example, the recombinant influenza vaccine is for people aged 18 years and older, and the adjuvanted[d] and high-dose inactivated vaccines are for people aged 65 years and older. Fluzone High-Dose vaccine contains four times the amount of antigen contained in regular flu shots. The additional antigen is intended to create a stronger immune response. Influenza shots are also recommended for pregnant women. All patients with chronic cardiovascular, pulmonary, metabolic, renal, or hematologic disorders and patients with immunosuppression should be vaccinated yearly against influenza.

[d]An adjuvant, like MF59, is an ingredient added to a vaccine that helps create a stronger immune response to vaccination.

Pneumococcal. In the United States, numerous infections like meningitis, bloodstream infections, pneumonia, and ear infections are caused by pneumococcal disease every year. The CDC recommends pneumococcal vaccination for all children younger than 2 years old and all adults 65 years or older.[8] Pneumococcal vaccines are very good at preventing severe disease and death. However, vaccination is not guaranteed to prevent infection and symptoms in all people. There are two kinds of pneumococcal vaccines available: *pneumococcal conjugate vaccine* and *pneumococcal polysaccharide vaccine.* The *pneumococcal conjugate vaccine* (PCV13 or Prevnar 13) protects against 13 types of pneumococcal bacteria. The CDC recommends PCV13 for use in infants, young children, and adults 65 years or older. Older children and adults younger than 65 years old who are at increased risk for getting pneumococcal disease may also need a dose of PCV13. The *pneumococcal polysaccharide vaccine* (PPSV23 or Pneumovax) protects against 23 types of pneumococcal bacteria. The CDC recommends pneumococcal polysaccharide vaccine for all adults 65 years or older, people 2 through 64 years old with certain medical conditions, and adults 19 through 64 years old who smoke cigarettes. In addition, patients with multiple myeloma, lymphoma, alcoholism, cirrhosis, and functional or anatomic asplenia should receive the vaccine. This vaccine usually provides lifelong immunity. Revaccination every 6 years is necessary only in asplenic patients because they are at high risk for pneumococcal infection.

Hepatitis. Hepatitis A is a liver disease caused by the hepatitis A virus that can be easily prevented with a vaccine. It is commonly acquired during travel and can affect anyone. The virus is transmitted through the fecal-oral route. Hepatitis A can occur in various situations in the United States, ranging from isolated cases to widespread epidemics. Practicing good personal hygiene and proper sanitation can help prevent hepatitis A. Additionally, vaccines are available for individuals 12 months and older to prevent long-term hepatitis A virus infection. The first dose of hepatitis A vaccine should be administered as soon as travel to countries with high or intermediate endemicity is considered. It has been noted that adults and children attain protective antibody levels ranging from 94% to 100% 1 month after receiving the initial dose of monovalent hepatitis A vaccine. To ensure long-term protection against hepatitis A, it is important to receive the second dose of the vaccine series. For short-term prevention of the virus, people of all ages can use immune globulin.

Hepatitis B vaccine should be given to all healthcare professionals, staff of institutions for developmentally disabled patients, intravenous drug abusers, patients with multiple sexual partners, hemodialysis patients, sexual partners of hepatitis B carriers, and patients with hemophilia. To achieve full immunization, three injections are required. These include an initial dose and two follow-up doses, one after a month and another after 6 to 12 months. There is no need for booster doses. It is recommended that individuals who are at high risk of exposure, such as medical, dental, podiatric, osteopathic, and nursing students, receive immunization before any possible exposure for optimal protection.

Haemophilus influenzae. *Haemophilus influenzae* type B (Hib) vaccine is now used routinely in children to prevent invasive *H. influenzae* diseases. The World Health Organization estimates that Hib causes three million episodes of serious disease, notably pneumonia and meningitis, and 400,000 deaths annually worldwide. Most cases are among non-immunized children and in economically developing countries. Meningitis and other serious infections caused by Hib disease can lead to brain damage or death. Hib disease is preventable by immunizing all children younger than 5 years with an approved Hib vaccine. Several Hib vaccines are available. The general recommendation is to immunize children with a first dose at 2 months of age and to follow with additional doses according to the schedule for the vaccine being used. Three to four doses are needed, depending on the brand of Hib vaccine used. Hib vaccine should never be given to a child younger than 6 weeks, because this might reduce their response to subsequent doses.

Shingles (herpes zoster). For the prevention of shingles,[9] it is recommended that two doses of recombinant zoster vaccine (RZV) (Shingrix) be given 2 to 6 months apart to adults aged 50 years or older regardless of past episodes of herpes zoster, receipt of the earlier live zoster vaccine (ZVL) (Zostavax), or receipt of the varicella (chickenpox) vaccine. Shingrix provides strong protection against shingles and post-herpetic neuralgia (PHN). In adults 50 years and older who have healthy immune systems, Shingrix is more than 90% effective at preventing shingles and PHN. As of November 18, 2020, the live shingles vaccine zoster (Zostavax) is no longer available for use in the United States.

Measles. Between 1991 and 1992, there was a 75% decrease in the number of cases of measles, mumps, and rubella (MMR), presumably because of the use of the MMR vaccine. This vaccine is now typically given in childhood, but it should also be given to adult healthcare professionals who have not had the diseases. Because the vaccine contains a live virus, it should not be given to pregnant patients, those with generalized malignancies, those receiving steroid therapy, those with active tuberculosis, or those receiving antimetabolites.

Since 2017, cases of measles have been increasing in several countries around the world, with a 300% rise in measles cases globally over the same period in 2018, according to the World Health Organization. The countries most affected are India, Yemen, Indonesia, and Ethiopia. As of March 2023, India's health officials recorded 68,473 measles cases, Yemen experienced 7554 cases, Indonesia 5754 cases, and Ethiopia 4505 cases.

The reasons for outbreaks differ in each country, from vaccine hesitancy[e] to problems with healthcare access or access to vaccines, to civil unrest and low awareness about the need to vaccinate. What is common in all these cases is the decreasing rate of vaccination.

Measles had been eliminated in the United States in 2000, but it is now back. According to the latest measles numbers from the Centers for Disease Control and Prevention, health officials recorded, as of April 28, 2023, 10 cases of measles that were confirmed in eight states.

[e]A reluctance or refusal to be vaccinated or to have one's children vaccinated.

The outbreaks in the United States have been concentrated in four states: New York, New Jersey, Washington, and California. The cases occurred mostly in Orthodox Jewish communities. There, a minority of people who are vaccine skeptics have been opting out of the vaccinations for their children, driving vaccine rates down and creating the space for the highly contagious virus to spread.

The Advisory Committee on Immunization Practices annually reviews the recommended adult immunization schedule to ensure that the schedule reflects the current recommendations for the licensed vaccines. It is advisable for the healthcare professional to review these guidelines regularly. The *Recommended Immunization Schedule for Adults Aged 19 Years or Older, United States* may be found on the Centers for Disease Control and Prevention website at https://www.cdc.gov/vaccines/schedules/hcp/adult.html.

Misused Substances

A careful review of any *misused substances* by the patient is included in the past medical history. Misused substances includes cigarette smoking and the use of alcohol and recreational drugs. In the United States in 2023, an estimated 42 million people (18.1% of the population) were smokers. Approximately 13 of every 100 adult males smoke (13.1%), and about 10 of every 100 adult females smoke (10.1%). As many as 30% of all deaths related to coronary heart disease in the United States each year are attributable to cigarette smoking; the risk is strongly dose related. Smoking also nearly doubles the risk of ischemic stroke. Smoking acts synergistically with other risk factors, substantially increasing the risk of coronary disease. Individuals who smoke are more likely to develop peripheral vascular disease, cancer, chronic lung disease, and other chronic illnesses. Cigarette smoking is the most controllable risk factor for premature morbidity and mortality in the United States, causing approximately 450,000 deaths each year.

During a patient interview, it is important for the interviewer to ask the patient about their smoking history. The interviewer should ask if the patient uses nicotine in any form, such as cigarettes, cigars, pipes, e-cigarettes, or chewing tobacco, and for how long they have used it. To determine the patient's smoking history, the interviewer can calculate the *pack-year*, which is the number of years the patient has smoked multiplied by the number of packs per day. For example, if a patient has smoked 2 packs of cigarettes a day for 25 years, their smoking history would be 50 pack-years. If the patient reports that they do not currently smoke, the interviewer should also inquire about whether they have ever smoked and if they have quit, for how long.

It has been estimated that the incidence of hazardous alcohol drinking in the United States ranges from 4% to 5% among females and 14% to 18% among males. In primary care settings, the prevalence rates range from 9% to 34% for hazardous drinking. Although studies have shown the beneficial effects of

E-cigarette, or vaping, products can be used to deliver nicotine, cannabis (THC, CBD), flavorings, chemicals, and other substances. Devices may be referred to as "e-cigs," "vapes," dab pens," "tanks," "mods," or "ENDS" (electronic nicotine delivery systems). Use of e-cigarette is often referred to as "juuling," named for the most popular brand of e-cigarettes.

moderate alcohol consumption (one to two drinks daily), these effects are lost at higher doses. Heavy alcohol consumption is associated with many medical problems (e.g., hypertension, decreased cardiac function, arrhythmias, hemorrhagic stroke, ischemic stroke, liver disease, increased risk of breast cancer), as well as behavioral and psychiatric problems. According to the American Psychiatric Association and the National Institute on Alcohol Abuse and Alcoholism, "moderate drinking" for males is defined as less than two drinks per day; for females and persons older than 65 years, it is defined as less than one drink per day.[10]

The history of alcohol consumption and dependency should be integrated into the general history immediately after the interviewer inquires about less threatening subjects such as smoking. It is easy to miss alcohol dependency unless specific direct questions are asked. It is acceptable to broach the topic of alcoholism by asking, "Please tell me about your drinking of alcohol." The interviewer should focus not on the quantity of alcohol consumed but rather on the adverse effects of drinking. By asking, "How much do you drink?" the interviewer may put the patient on the defensive. This type of question may also create an unnecessary power struggle between patient and interviewer. You might ask instead, "How much *can* you drink?" which puts the patient and interviewer in a position of alliance. Most individuals who drink heavily also underestimate the quantities they consume. The interviewer can often learn more about the quantity of alcohol consumed by asking about the patient's feelings and interpersonal relationships than by asking directly about the amount. The interviewer should determine whether the patient drives while intoxicated, has suffered amnesia of events that occurred during drinking, neglects or abuses their family, or has missed work as a result of alcohol consumption.

Ewing and Rouse (1970) developed the ***CAGE*** questionnaire as a formal screening instrument to help identify patients in primary care with alcohol problems. The acronym *CAGE* helps the interviewer remember the four clinical interview questions that focus on the social and behavioral aspects of alcohol problems: the effect alcohol has on one's lifestyle. Once it is established that a patient drinks alcohol, the following questions (CAGE) should be asked:

"Have you ever felt you should ***C****ut down on your drinking?"*
"Have people ***A****nnoyed you by criticizing your drinking?"*
"Have you ever felt bad or ***G****uilty about your drinking?"*
*"Have you ever taken a drink first thing in the morning (****E****ye-opener) to steady your nerves or get rid of a hangover?"*

The CAGE questionnaire is a highly effective screening tool for detecting alcoholism, proven since its introduction. In a primary care setting, CAGE scores of 2 (two positive responses) have a sensitivity of 77% to 94% and a specificity of 79% to 97% for a current diagnosis of alcohol abuse. One positive CAGE response has a sensitivity of 21% to 71% and a specificity of 84% to 95%. The history of alcohol consumption and dependency can be further assessed by using the sets of questions referred to by the acronyms *HALT, BUMP,* and *FATAL DT.*

The HALT questions are as follows:

"Do you usually drink to get ***H****igh?"*
"Do you drink ***A****lone?"*
"Do you ever find yourself ***L****ooking forward to drinking?"*
"Have you noticed whether you seem to be becoming ***T****olerant of alcohol?"*

The BUMP questions are as follows:

"Have you ever had ***B****lackouts?"*
"Have you ever used alcohol in an ***U****nplanned*[f] *way?"*
"Do you ever drink alcohol for ***M****edicinal*[g] *reasons?"*
"Do you find yourself ***P****rotecting*[h] *your supply of alcohol?"*

The final acronym reminds the interviewer about other major associations with alcoholism.

The FATAL DT questions are as follows:

"Is there a ***F****amily history of alcoholic problems?"*
"Have you ever been a member of ***A****lcoholics Anonymous?"*
"Do you ***T****hink you are an alcoholic?"*
"Have you ever ***A****ttempted or had thoughts of suicide?"*
"Have you ever had any ***L****egal problems related to alcohol consumption?"*
"Do you ever ***D****rive while intoxicated?"*
"Do you ever use ***T****ranquilizers to steady your nerves?"*

These questions provide the interviewer with a useful, thoughtful, and organized approach to the interview strategy designed to identify patients with a drinking problem.

When someone reaches the advanced stages of alcoholism, they may experience delirium tremens (DTs). It's important to note that DTs are not the same as the hallucinations that occur earlier on. DTs typically occur within 24 to 96 hours after withdrawal from alcohol and can include tremors, hallucinations, and seizures. However, trembling is a common symptom among all patients experiencing DTs. It's crucial to seek medical attention as DTs are the most severe form of alcohol withdrawal and can be fatal in 25% of cases.

The interviewer must ask all patients about the misuse of substances, other than smoking and alcohol, as well. People who use such substances often engender negative feelings or anger in the healthcare professional. These feelings are often unavoidable. The interviewer must not allow this bias to interfere with empathetic interviewing. Healthcare professionals should avoid stigmatizing terms (e.g., addict, addiction, user, junkie, habit, abuse) when discussing substance misuse. Even though some of these terms may be used in certain social communities of individuals with substance use disorder, healthcare professionals can set an example using language that reduces stigma and negative bias toward this disorder. When communicating with individuals who struggle with substance misuse, as well as their friends and family, and fellow professionals, it is important to use language that is free of stigma, reflects a scientific understanding of substance misuse, and aligns with our professional responsibilities.

In addition, always try to use person-first language (e.g., "a person with a substance use disorder"[11] or "a person with diabetes," not a "diabetic patient"). This statement maintains a neutral tone and emphasizes the individual rather than their

[f]Drink more than you intended or have an additional drink after you decided you had had enough.
[g]As a cure for anxiety, depression, or the "shakes."
[h]Buying enough alcohol just in case "company" arrives.

medical condition. Using person-first language means treating individuals as complete human beings by avoiding stigmatizing terminology that reduces them to their medical problem, thus ensuring their integrity and dignity. Using person-first language emphasizes that a person "has" a problem rather than "being" the problem![12]

A useful way of approaching this topic is to ask,

"Have you ever misused medications or other substances other than those required for medical reasons?"
"Do you use substances other than those prescribed by a physician?"
"Have you misused prescription drugs?"

If the answer to any of these questions is affirmative, the interviewer should determine the types of substances used, the routes of administration, and the frequency of use. In contrast to alcohol abusers, people who misuse nonalcoholic substances are more likely to magnify their use. The interviewer must ask all patients with a *history of substance misuse* the following questions:

"What type of substances do (or did) you use?"
"At what age did you start using them?"
"What was your period of heaviest use?"
"What is your recent pattern of use?"
"Are larger doses necessary to get the same effect now?"
"What do you feel when you take the substance?"
"Have you ever tried to quit? What happened?"
"Have you ever had any convulsions after taking the substance?"
"Do you use more than one substance at a time?"
"Do you use these substances on a continuous basis?"
"Have you been in trouble at work because of their use?"
"Have you ever had withdrawal symptoms due to using them?"

It is important to use simple words and expressions when inquiring about substance misuse. It may also be more appropriate to use slang (i.e., street names) than more formal terms. For example, "Do you ever shoot up or snort coke?" may be better understood than "Have you ever taken cocaine intravenously or by insufflation?" Knowing slang for misused substances can be as important as knowing the pharmacologic effects and may provide a means of better communication. Don't forget to ask empathically! It should be recognized that slang often differs from place to place and changes occasionally. Appendix B, Commonly Misused Substances, lists their slang and the major symptoms and signs associated with each of the misused substances.

It should also be recognized that *any* medication can be misused. Propranolol and metoprolol are β-blockers mainly prescribed for hypertension treatment and are not known as "recreational" substances. However, actors often misuse them to alleviate performance anxiety or stage fright.

Diet

In questioning a patient about *diet*, it is useful to ask the patient to describe what they ate the day before, including all three meals plus any snacks. How many fish meals do they have each week? What is the proportion of red meat in the diet in comparison with fish or poultry? How much saturated fat is in the diet? Does the patient add salt when they cook, and do they add salt at the table? Has their diet changed recently? What kinds of foods does the patient like or dislike, and why? Are there any food intolerances? Does the patient eat foods with a high fiber content, such as whole-grain breads and cereals, bran, fresh fruits, and vegetables? Does the patient eat high-fiber snack foods (which include sesame bread sticks, date-nut bread, oatmeal cookies, fig bars, granola bars, and corn chips)? What is the consumption of sodium? Pickled foods, cured meats, snack foods, and prepared soups have a high sodium content. The consumption of caffeine-containing products such as coffee, tea, sodas, and chocolate is important to determine. Caffeine ingestion may produce a variety of symptoms, including heart palpitations, fatigue, lightheadedness, headaches, irritability, and many gastrointestinal symptoms. The symptoms associated with caffeine ingestion are discussed at length in Chapter 7, Assessment of Nutritional Status. The interviewer should also ascertain the amount of exercise the patient gets.

Sleep Patterns

Understanding a patient's sleep patterns can reveal valuable information about their psychological well-being. Sleep issues, such as insomnia and daytime drowsiness, affect a significant portion of the American population, ranging from 20% to 50%. Additionally, obstructive sleep apnea is a prevalent and critical health concern. Sleep apnea is discussed in Chapter 12, The Oral Cavity and Pharynx.

Disturbed sleep patterns are a common concern among patients with psychiatric problems, affecting over 60% of them. In patients with depression, this number increases to 80%. Patients with posttraumatic stress disorder often experience disturbed sleep as their most common issue, while over 50% of those with chronic pain also report sleep problems.

An estimated 200,000 automobile accidents a year are caused by excessive sleepiness on the part of drivers; 20% of drivers report that they have fallen asleep behind the wheel. The following questions should be asked:

"When do you go to bed?"
"Do you have trouble falling asleep?"
"Do you stay asleep the whole night, or do you awaken in the middle of the night, unable to go back to sleep?"
"Do you go to bed only when sleepy?"
"Do you adhere to a regular waking time?"
"Do you snore?"
"Has anyone told you that you have episodes of stopping breathing during the night?"

Medications

All current medications should be noted. The following questions should be asked:

"Do you use any prescription medications?"
"Do you use any over-the-counter medications?"
"Do you use any herbal medications or vitamins?"
"Do you use any recreational drugs?"

To ensure accurate recording, it's important to note down the name (generic or trade), dose, route of administration, and frequency of use of all medications. If possible, the patient should demonstrate how the medications are taken using the bottles. The interviewer should also verify if the patient is taking the medications as directed. It's common for patients to overlook over-the-counter medications like vitamins, laxatives, antacids, or cold remedies, so the interviewer should ask specifically about these types of drugs. Additionally, the interviewer should inquire about the type of contraception used, if any, and whether the patient has used or is using birth control pills.

Alternative Therapies

To encourage open discussion about alternative therapies, it's important to avoid using labels like "unorthodox" or "unconventional." Instead, try starting the conversation by acknowledging that many patients use different types of therapies to manage their symptoms. You could ask if they've ever considered using massage, herbs, chiropractic, acupuncture, vitamins, or other alternative therapies to address their concerns. This approach creates a more comfortable and non-judgmental environment for discussing these types of treatments. The use of alternative therapies is discussed further in Chapter 3, Understanding Complementary and Alternative Medicine.

Health Maintenance

Healthcare professionals have an important role in identifying and managing medical, social, and psychiatric issues. They can use counseling skills to establish a supportive therapeutic relationship with patients and their families. A patient's family can help confirm the diagnosis and create a treatment plan. Health maintenance involves three main areas: detecting diseases, preventing diseases, and promoting overall health.

Asking patients about their regular healthcare professionals and medical checkups, as well as their recent dental and eye exams, can provide important information. It's also helpful to ask if they are aware of their cholesterol levels and if they engage in regular exercise. For female patients, it's important to inquire about their gynecologist visits, breast self-exams, and when they last had a mammogram or Papanicolaou smear. For male patients, it's recommended to ask if they perform routine testicular self-examinations.

Tobacco use is probably the main avoidable cause of morbidity and mortality in the world, with nearly 6 million deaths per year.[13] In the United States alone, tobacco use is responsible for more than 480,000 deaths each year from cancer, heart disease, stroke, and lung disease. This figure includes more than 41,000 deaths from secondhand smoke exposure.[14] This is approximately one in every five deaths annually, or 1300 deaths every day! Smokers die 10 years earlier than nonsmokers.[14] There are more than 16 million Americans living with diseases caused by smoking. If smoking continues at the current rate among youth in the United States, 5.6 million of today's Americans younger than 18 years of age are expected to die prematurely from a smoking-related illness. This represents about 1 in every 13 Americans aged 17 years or younger who are alive today.[15]

Despite these facts, however, tobacco use is still prevalent. The Centers for Disease Control and Prevention estimates that 25% of all Americans still smoke and that more than 3000 children and adolescents become regular users every day. It is estimated that the cost of medical care for tobacco-related illness in the United States is more than $300 billion annually,[16] and the cost of lost productivity and forfeited wages resulting from disability is an additional $156 billion per year. Despite these staggering statistics, healthcare professionals often fail to treat tobacco use effectively. Healthcare professionals have unique access to patients who use tobacco, and yet studies show that fewer than half of individuals who use tobacco reported being urged to quit by their physicians.

As part of their standard procedure, healthcare professionals need to determine and document whether their patients use tobacco. Patients who do use tobacco should be offered smoking cessation treatment during every office visit. Research has shown that even a brief 3-minute discussion per visit can be effective. However, for more long-term results, more intensive treatment that involves medical therapies, social support, and specific skills is recommended. In addition to nicotine replacement therapy options like patches, gum, lozenges, nasal spray, and inhalers, there is also a non-nicotine prescription medicine called varenicline (Chantix®) that can help adults quit smoking. Varenicline was approved by the U.S. Food and Drug Administration in 2006. Unlike nicotine, it does not contain nicotine, but it works by targeting the same receptors as nicotine. The drug is believed to prevent nicotine from binding to these receptors. Research has shown that after 12 weeks of taking varenicline, 44% of patients successfully stopped smoking. This medication also decreased the desire to smoke.

It also has been demonstrated, however, that there are times when patients are unreceptive or even resentful if the issue is broached. According to the "stages of change" model, success is most likely when the healthcare professional is sensitive to the patient's stage. Stage 1 is the precontemplation stage in which the smoker is in denial about the hazards of smoking and is not willing to stop. Stage 2 is the contemplation stage, when the patient acknowledges a willingness to quit but has not determined when that will occur. Stage 3 is the action stage, during which the patient has prepared for a change, is engaged in changing behavior, and has a plan for smoking cessation. Stage 4 is the maintenance stage, during which the healthcare professional needs to encourage the patient about the experience of quitting. Stage 5 is the relapse. Smokers generally make three or more attempts to quit smoking before permanent success is achieved.

It is important to communicate to patients the necessity of quitting smoking in a clear and assertive manner. You can say something like, "I strongly believe that quitting smoking is crucial for your well-being, and I am here to support you. Please understand that quitting smoking is the most effective way to safeguard your health both now and in the future."

Also remember to ask the questions about alcohol consumption discussed in the previous section.

Counseling is very important, but interviewers must remember that a patient must *want* to change their behavior. If they do not, interviewers should indicate to the patient that they will provide support when the patient is ready.

Finally, do not forget to ask all patients whether they wear seat belts in cars or use helmets if they ride bicycles or motorcycles. Helmets reduce the risk of serious injury or death!

A study published in 2018[17] found that bike helmets reduced head injuries by 48%, serious head injuries by 60%, traumatic brain injuries by 53%, and injuries to the face by 23%! The number of seriously injured or killed cyclists was reduced by 34%!

Occupational and Environmental History

When considering a person's health history, it's important to ask about any exposure they may have had to substances or environments that can cause disease. In the United States, it's estimated that between 50,000 to 70,000 deaths each year are due to occupational exposure, with over 350,000 new cases of occupational disease being recognized annually. These diseases can affect any part of the body and can often be mistaken for other illnesses. A key challenge in accurately diagnosing occupational and environmental diseases is the significant delay between exposure and the onset of symptoms.

Many occupational diseases have been well described over the years: malignant mesothelioma in workers exposed to asbestos; cancer of the bladder in workers exposed to aniline dye; malignant neoplasms of the nasal cavities in woodworkers; pneumoconiosis in coal miners; silicosis in sandblasters and quarry workers; leukemia in those exposed to benzene; hepatic angiosarcoma in workers exposed to vinyl chloride; byssinosis in cotton industry workers; skin cancer in those chronically exposed to the sun, such as sailors; ornithosis in bird breeders; toxic hepatitis in solvent users and workers in the plastics industry; and chronic bronchitis in individuals exposed to industrial dusts. Studies have revealed that exposure to specific pesticides is linked to sterility in both males and females, and exposure to certain solvents is associated with dementia.

The environment is also responsible for significant morbidity and mortality rates. Lead, radon, pesticides, and air pollution cause illness and death. Examples include Chernobyl, with its widespread high levels of radiation; Minamata Bay in Japan, with its mercury poisoning; Hopewell, Virginia, with its poisoning pesticide chlordecone; and Bhopal, India, where a leak at an industrial plant exposed hundreds of thousands of people to toxic methyl isocyanate gas. In India, thousands died shortly after exposure, and more than 200,000 people have suffered illness from the gas. The long-range effects of these agents have yet to be determined.

To diagnose occupational and environmental diseases accurately, it is crucial to take a detailed history of the patient's work and surroundings. This includes asking about all previous occupations and the length of time spent in each one. The history should not just be a list of jobs but should also include specific details about the activities performed and the use of protective gear. It is also important to determine the cleanup practices followed and any work done in nearby areas. The job title, such as electrician or machine operator, may not accurately reflect whether the worker has been exposed to hazardous materials. Workplaces in industrial areas can be complicated, so it's crucial to determine where hazardous materials are being used in relation to other work areas. Living near industrial toxins has been linked to the development of diseases in the future, so it's important to ask patients if they currently live or have ever lived near mines, farms, factories, or shipyards. The following questions regarding occupational and environmental exposure should be asked of all patients:

"What type of work do you do?"
"How long have you been doing this work?"
"Describe your work."
"Are you exposed to any hazardous materials? Do you ever use protective equipment?"
"What kind of work did you do before you had your current job?"
"What was your wartime employment, if any?"
"Where do you live? For how long?"
"Have you ever lived near any factories, shipyards, or other potentially hazardous facilities?"
"Has anyone in your household ever worked with hazardous materials that could have been brought home?"
"What types of hobbies do you have? What types of exposures are involved?"
"Do you now have, or have you previously had, environmental or occupational exposure to asbestos, lead, fumes, chemicals, dusts, loud noise, radiation, or other toxic factors?"

Attention must be paid to any temporal relationship between the onset of illness and toxic exposure in the workplace. Did the symptoms start after the patient began a new job? Did the symptoms abate during a vacation and then recur when the patient resumed work? Were the symptoms related to the implementation of any new chemical or process? Is there anyone else at work or are there any neighbors with a similar illness?

Biographic Information

When gathering biographic information, it's important to ask about the date and place of birth, sex assigned at birth, gender, gender identity, race, and ethnic background. It's crucial to **avoid making assumptions** about any of these factors. Gender identity should be assessed at the beginning of each patient encounter, as discussed previously. It's important to note that race is a social construct, shaped by historical, political, social, and economic factors of a particular time and place. To gain a better understanding of a patient's racial identity, you might ask, "How would you describe your race or racial identity?" See Chapter 5, Anti-Racist and Anti-Oppressive Clinical Skills.

Family History

You can start the family history by asking about the patient's ancestry. Possible questions about a patient's ancestry might be:

"Tell me about your family."
"You mentioned you identify as an African American. Tell me more about your family's history."

When reviewing the family history, it's important to consider the health of both living and deceased relatives. It's especially crucial to look for any potential genetic or environmental factors that could impact the patient's health. Does the patient have any knowledge of any genetically determined diseases within their family? Has there been any history of cancer, specifically colon, breast, ovarian, or prostate? Has there been any history of premature cardiovascular disease? Additionally, has there been any history of diabetes, thyroid, liver, lung, blood, or renal disease, or rheumatologic disorders within the family?

To assess the patient's health, it is necessary to gather information about their immediate family members. This includes their age and current health status, as well as any deceased relatives, along with the cause of death and age at the time of passing. You can create a pedigree or family chart to document this information, which should list all immediate relatives such as parents, grandparents, siblings, children, and grandchildren. Additionally, it's important to ask how a family member's illness may impact the patient's psychological well-being.

To better understand the patient's background, it's essential to ask about their parents' and grandparents' birthplaces, whether they grew up in an urban or rural environment, and from which country their family originates. If the patient was born in a different country, it's important to know at what age they came to the United States. Additionally, it's helpful to inquire about the patient's contact with other family members and whether their original family name was changed. If the patient is married, it's relevant to know if their spouse belongs to the same ethnic group. Lastly, it's important to ask about the patient's mother tongue, discussed earlier in this chapter.

The answers to these questions provide valuable information as a heritage assessment.

Psychosocial and Spiritual History

The psychosocial history contains details about the patient's personal relationships, life experiences, and education. This section should cover the patient's lifestyle, the people living with them, their schooling, military service, religious beliefs (in relation to health and treatment), and their marital or significant-other relationships. You can start by asking one of the following questions:

"Tell me a little about yourself: your background, education, work, and family."

"Who are the important people in your life?"

"What do you do for fun?"

"How do you feel about the way your life is going?"

A statement regarding the patient's knowledge of symptoms and illness is important. Has the illness caused the patient to lose time from work? What kind of insight does the patient have about the symptom? Do they think about the future? If so, how does it look? An excellent question that can elicit a vast amount of information is "What is your typical day like?"

A patient's spiritual history sheds light on what brings meaning to their life and helps them deal with serious illnesses, debilitation, and end-of-life situations. It offers valuable insights into their spiritual needs and beliefs, and is an important part of their medical history. Meditation and prayer can complement medical care. Spirituality can offer hope to those with chronic disease and may even provide new meaning to their suffering. Several studies have revealed the beneficial effect of spirituality in stress reduction, recovery from illness, mitigation of pain, and faster recovery from surgery. Puchalski[18] suggested that a spiritual history might begin with introductory questions such as:

"Do you consider yourself spiritual or religious?"

"How important are these beliefs to you, and do they influence how you care for yourself?"

More questions about the spiritual history are discussed in Chapter 5, Anti-Racist and Anti-Oppressive Clinical Skills.

Sexual, Reproductive, and Gynecologic History

The sexual history has traditionally been part of the psychosocial history or review of systems. However, because the sexual, reproductive, and gynecologic history is so vital for the complete evaluation of the patient, these histories are now considered a separate part of the interview.

Having a documented sexual history is important for various reasons. Sexual health can be an indicator of one's overall well-being, and sexual dysfunction can be linked to anxiety, depression, and anger, as well as physical symptoms. It's also crucial to identify any risky behaviors. Documenting a sexual history allows healthcare professionals to establish sexual norms for each patient and offer education on topics such as sexually transmitted diseases, HIV-related illnesses, and pregnancy prevention. This is a great opportunity for healthcare professionals to provide valuable information to patients.

When interviewing individuals, it is crucial to inquire about their sexual activity, regardless of their age. This is because child abuse is unfortunately prevalent, and early identification is crucial. Additionally, it is important not to make assumptions about the sexual activity of older individuals. It is normal for older adults to engage in sexual activity and enjoy it.

It's important to customize your questions and language for each interview. However, you may wonder if it's appropriate to use colloquial terms. Both patients and interviewers may feel uncomfortable with using these terms due to their emotional weight. In some cases, patients may use incorrect medical terminology out of embarrassment about using certain terms. On the other hand, using informal language may lead to more open and informative conversations, particularly when speaking with younger adults.

The interviewer must inquire about sexual relationships in a nonjudgmental manner. Direct questions regarding vaginal, oral, and anal sex; sexual contacts; and sexual problems are very important for specific patients. Novice interviewers often find it harder to discuss sexual behavior compared to patients who are often more open and less inhibited. It is more appropriate to use the term "partner" rather than gender-specific terms like "husband" or "wife" until the patient's preferred terminology is known. There is no easy way to ask about sexual preference, but it is vital to know. It is appropriate to inquire whether the patient has been in contact with individuals who have AIDS or AIDS-related illnesses. The term *homosexual* as an adjective for gender (e.g., "homosexual male") should be avoided; it is a term describing sexual activity between individuals of the same sex but can often be offensive to people who identify as LGBTQ+.[i] It is best to allow your patient to self-describe their sexual

[i]LGBTQ+ stands for Lesbian, Gay, Bisexual, Transgender, and Queer & Questioning. It is an umbrella term to refer to those with marginalized sexual orientations and gender identities. The + signals that the acronym is not an all-inclusive nor exhaustive list, and other identities may fall under the umbrella that are not represented in the acronym. See Chapter 5, Anti-Racist and Anti-Oppressive Clinical Skills and Chapter 26, The Transgender Patient.

orientation. You can do this by simply asking, "What is your sexual orientation?" or "How do you describe your sexual orientation?"

There are several general questions that can help broach the topic of sexual activity. In general, the best way to introduce the sexual history is to say, "Now I am going to ask you some questions about your sexual health and practices." Because the question, "Are you sexually active?" can be ambiguous, it is better to ask, "Have you ever had intimate physical contact with anyone?" If the answer is "Yes," the next question should be "Did that contact include sexual intercourse?" The interviewer should also then ask, "Are your partners male, female, or both?"

It is not acceptable to ask whether the person has "had sex" or is "sexually active," because there is great variability in the way individuals define these phrases. In one study,[19] 599 college students attending a major midwestern university were asked, "Would you say you 'had sex' with someone if the most intimate behavior you engaged in was... (mark 'yes' or 'no' for each behavior)." There were 11 behavioral items on the list, including "deep kissing," "oral contact on your breasts/nipples," "you touch other's genitals," "oral contact with other's genitals," and "penile–vaginal intercourse." Although 99.5% agreed that penile–vaginal intercourse qualified as "had sex," 19% did *not* believe that penile–anal intercourse meant "had sex"; that is one out of five polled. Only 40% felt that they "had sex" if oral–genital contact was their most intimate behavior (60% would not). The study suggests that Americans hold widely divergent opinions about what behaviors do and do not constitute as having "had sex." Therefore, a better question to ask is "What is the most intimate physical contact you have had with someone else?"

Some of the following questions about specific sexual behaviors and satisfaction may also be helpful in acquiring a sexual history:

"Are you having any sexual problems?"

"Are you satisfied with your sexual performance?" "Do you think your partner is?" If not, *"What is unsatisfactory to you (or your partner)?"*

"Have you had any difficulty achieving orgasm?"

"How frequently does it occur that your partner desires sexual intercourse and you do not?"

"Are there any questions pertaining to your sexual performance that you would like to discuss?"

"Most people experience some disappointment in their sexual function. Can you tell me what disappointments you might have?"

"Many people experience what others may consider unusual sexual thoughts or wish to perform sexual acts that others consider abnormal. We are often bothered by these thoughts. What has been your experience?"

"Do you have protected sex?"

"Have you ever had a sexually transmitted disease?"

"Have you been tested for HIV?" If yes, *"What was the result?"*

Asking a patient "How many sexual partners do you have or have you had?" is rather intrusive and does not help very much. It is much better to determine whether a person routinely uses protection with condoms, if appropriate. It is true, however, that studies have shown that the more sexual partners a female has had, the greater is the chance that she will develop cervical carcinoma.

It is less appropriate to ask "What activities and positions does your sexual contact include?" than to ask *specifically* about oral–genital, penile–vaginal, or penile–anal contact *tailored specifically* to the individual patient.

Although it may seem innocuous to ask a person in the United States about their marital status, it should not be done. Since June 26, 2015, by a Supreme Court ruling *(Obergefell v. Hodges)*, same-sex marriages have been allowed in 50 states. In a landmark 5–4 decision, marriage equality became the law of the land and granted same-sex couples in all 50 states the right to full, equal recognition under the law. This ruling was hailed as a milestone decision and a huge victory that would see discrimination crumble and provide equality for lesbian, gay, bisexual, and transgender couples and their children. Therefore, ***finding out that a person is married tells you nothing of the gender of the spouse.*** A male married to another male has a husband; a female married to another female has a wife.

Healthcare professionals, regardless of their sexual orientation, must provide the highest standard of care to all patients. They must reconcile their own fears and prejudices about homosexuality. In 1978, only one-third of Americans believed that they knew a gay male or lesbian; in 1996, approximately two-thirds of Americans reported that they knew someone who was gay or lesbian. Despite this fact, there is a significant degree of homophobia in society. By definition, *homophobia* is the "irrational fear of, aversion to, or discrimination against homosexuality or homosexuals." The medical and psychological effects of homophobia can pose a significant health hazard to gay and lesbian patients and can be detrimental to establishing a strong healthcare professional–patient relationship. If a gay or lesbian patient senses this discrimination, they may become alienated from the healthcare system and not use standard screening modalities, thus risking higher mortality and morbidity from disease. One study revealed that 98% of gay and lesbian patients believed that it was medically important to inform their healthcare professionals of their sexual orientation, but 64% believed that in doing so, they risked receiving substandard care. In the same study, 88% of the patients reported that their healthcare professionals made disparaging remarks about gay and lesbian patients. Because homophobia is widespread in society, a gay or lesbian patient should have the confidence to speak candidly with their healthcare professional. The term *gay* may be replaced with the expression "men having sex with men."

Much more information about the sexual history is presented in Chapter 5, Anti-Racist and Anti-Oppressive Clinical Skills.

Violence and Abuse

Domestic violence, rape, child abuse, sibling violence, and *elder abuse* are rampant and have reached staggering proportions. Of all domestic violence victims, 90% to 95% are women, and the perpetrators are mostly men. Every year, females experience 4.8 million intimate partner-related physical assaults and rapes. The violence is often a combination of physical, sexual, and psychological abuse, and the signs and symptoms may be subtle or obvious. It is therefore important to ask all patients whether they have ever been emotionally, physically, or sexually abused.

Much of the violence against females is perpetrated by their intimate partners or in relationships that are commonly protective, such as that of father and daughter. U.S. Department of Justice studies indicate that a female is more likely to be raped, assaulted, or murdered by a male partner or ex-partner than by a stranger. Up to 45% of abused females are beaten during pregnancy. Four percent of all male homicide victims are killed by spouses or female partners. As many as one in seven females seen in emergency departments has symptoms related to abuse. A national survey indicated that more than 2 million females are severely beaten by their male partners each year. It is recognized that such violence is vastly underreported; the actual number of cases is probably double the number reported. Healthcare professionals frequently treat the injuries only symptomatically and often fail to recognize the abuse. Forty-four percent of rape victims are under the age of 18 years; 80% are under the age of 30 years. It has been estimated that every 2 minutes, someone in the United States is sexually assaulted, and each year there are about 207,754 victims of sexual assault. Only 46% of sexually assaulted individuals report it to the police. Approximately two-thirds of assaults are committed by someone known to the victim.

Although many females who are victims of abuse do not volunteer any information, they often discuss the incidents if asked simple, direct questions in a nonjudgmental way and in a confidential setting. Be aware of the possibility of domestic violence in any female with multiple medical visits for sexual dysfunction; multiple, unexplained bruises; chronic pelvic pain; fatigue; chest pain; gastrointestinal disturbances; headaches; depression; anxiety; panic attacks; eating disorders; substance abuse; suicidal attempts; and abdominal pain.

Because the perpetrator often accompanies the victim to the interview, ask any other person present to leave while you speak to the patient. Begin with the following direct question: "Since domestic violence is so common, I've begun to ask about it routinely. At any time, has your partner hit, kicked, or otherwise hurt or frightened you?" If the patient answers in the affirmative, encourage her to talk about it. Alternatively, you may ask, "Do you feel safe in your relationship?" Always listen nonjudgmentally to encourage the patient to continue talking about the episode. Showing support is very important. A statement such as "You are not alone" or "Help is available for you" shows empathy. It is crucial to assess the danger to the patient as quickly as possible before she leaves the medical facility. If the patient is in imminent danger, determine whether she can stay with friends or family. A shelter for battered females may be an alternative. Finally, provide the patient with the telephone number of the local domestic violence hotline.

If the patient answers "no" to your introductory query and you suspect some form of domestic violence, be aware of the clinical findings that may indicate abuse:

- Injury to head, neck, breasts, abdomen, or genitals
- Multiple injuries that seem inconsistent with the patient's story
- Delay in seeking treatment
- Unusual explanation for the injury
- Injury during pregnancy
- Repeated vaginal infections
- Fear of pelvic examination
- Vaginal bruises or lacerations
- Chronic pain syndrome
- Psychological distress
- A partner who seems overly protective and doesn't want to leave the room

Any of these injuries must have a plausible explanation. If there is none, it is appropriate to ask further questions, but the partner must not be present. You might say, "It looks as if you've been hurt. Can you tell me how it happened?" Another approach could be "Sometimes when people feel the way you do, it's because they may have been abused. Is this happening to you?" Even if a patient is in an abusive setting and she fails to acknowledge it once you have provided an opportunity, allow her to return to discuss it later. Serious injury and homicide often result once a person attempts to leave an abusive partner. Allow her to make the decision to leave. You will have indicated your support.

The global prevalence of child sexual abuse has been estimated at 19.7% for females and 7.9% for males, according to a 2009 study published in *Clinical Psychology Review* that examined 65 studies from 22 countries. According to the National Child Abuse and Neglect Data System (2018),[20] the number and rate of victims have fluctuated during the past 5 years. Comparing the national rounded number of victims from 2012 (656,000) to the national estimate of victims in 2016 (676,000) shows an increase of 3.0%. For 2016, a nationally estimated 1750 children died of abuse and neglect at a rate of 2.36 per 100,000 children in the national population. Seventy percent of all child fatalities were younger than 3 years. Boys had a higher child fatality rate than girls; 2.87 per 100,000 boys in the population compared with 2.11 per 100,000 girls in the population. Eighty-seven percent (87.4%) of child fatalities were White (45.1%), African American (28.5%), and Hispanic (13.8%). The rate of African American child fatalities (4.65 per 100,000 African American children) is 2.2 times greater than the rate of White children (2.08 per 100,000 White children) and nearly 3 times greater than the rate of Hispanic children (1.58 per 100,000 Hispanic children). Most perpetrators were caregivers of their victims. More than three-quarters (78.0%) of child fatalities involved parents acting alone, together, or with other individuals. In 2019, state agencies identified an estimated 1840 children who died as a result of abuse and neglect—an average of five children a day. More than 70% of the children who died as a result of child abuse or neglect were 3 years of age or younger. Around 80% of child maltreatment fatalities involve at least one parent as the perpetrator.

A history of childhood sexual abuse is nearly always associated with enduring physical and psychological sequelae. There are many somatic disorders that may result after abuse. These include eczema, sleep disorders, sexual dysfunction, substance abuse, eating disorders, headaches, "mystery" pain, depression, asthma, and a wide variety of phobias. Healthcare professionals have an ethical and legal responsibility to report all cases of suspected child abuse and to protect the child from further abuse. Any injury that cannot be adequately explained should raise concern about either nonaccidental injury or neglect. Injuries to the skin are seen in 90% of abused children. Multiple injuries in various stages of healing almost always indicate repeated beatings.

Male rape is also on the rise. According to the National Sexual Violence Resource Center, 1 in 71 males will be raped at some point in their lives.[21] Fifty-two percent of male victims report being raped by an acquaintance and 15.1% by a stranger. Every year, males experience 2.9 million assaults. Most male rape victims are raped by other men, in the sense that they are forced to submit to anal intercourse, masturbation of the offender, oral sex, or other sex acts. Information about male rape is scarce because male victims, like their female counterparts, feel humiliation and shame and are reluctant to report it. Many males believe that if they have been raped by another male, it implies that the victim has homosexual tendencies.

RAINN (Rape, Abuse & Incest National Network) is the nation's largest anti-sexual violence organization. RAINN created and operates the National Sexual Assault Hotline (800) 656-HOPE (http://online.rainn.org/), in partnership with more than 1000 local sexual assault service providers across the United States. In 27 years, RAINN has helped 3.7 million survivors and their loved ones.

Reproductive and Gynecologic History

The *reproductive and gynecologic history* obtains information about a female's age at menarche, regularity of menstrual flow, and duration of periods. In addition, the number of pregnancies, number of deliveries, number of abortions (spontaneous or induced), and complications of pregnancies are included in this part of the history. It is also vital to determine whether the female was exposed to diethylstilbestrol through her mother's use during pregnancy. This is particularly important in any female born before 1975. Other important questions are discussed in Chapter 19, Female Genitalia.

In the reproductive history for a male, it is important to inquire about sexual interest, function, satisfaction, and any sexual problems. Has the male been unable to procreate? If so, is he aware of the reason? Other questions for males are discussed in Chapter 18, Male Genitalia and Hernias.

Review of Systems

The *review of systems* summarizes in terms of body systems all the symptoms that may have been overlooked in the history of the present illness or in the medical history. By reviewing the list of possible symptoms in an orderly manner, the interviewer can specifically check each system and uncover additional symptoms of "unrelated" illnesses not yet discussed. The review of systems is best organized from the head down to the extremities, and the questions can be asked during the physical examination of that body area. Patients are told that they are going to be asked whether they have ever had a particular symptom and should answer "yes" or "no." If they answer in the affirmative, further direct questioning is appropriate. The interviewer need not repeat questions that were previously answered, unless clarification of the data is necessary.

Table 1.2 is the review of systems and which questions should be asked of all patients. The questions should be understandable

TABLE 1.2 Review of Systems

General	Skin	Chest	Cardiac
• Usual state of health	• Rashes	• Cough	• Chest pain
• Fever	• Itching	• Pain	• High blood pressure
• Chills	• Hives	• Shortness of breath	• Palpitations
• Usual weight	• Easy bruising	• Sputum production (quantity, appearance)	• Shortness of breath with exertion
• Change in weight	• History of eczema	• Tuberculosis	• Shortness of breath when lying flat
• Weakness	• Dryness	• Asthma	• Sudden shortness of breath while sleeping
• Fatigue	• Changes in skin color	• Pleurisy	• History of heart attack
• Sweats	• Changes in hair texture	• Bronchitis	• Rheumatic fever
• Heat or cold intolerance	• Changes in nail texture	• Coughing up blood	• Heart murmur
• History of anemia	• Changes in nail appearance	• Wheezing	• Most recent electrocardiogram
• Bleeding tendencies	• History of previous skin disorders	• Most recent x-ray film	• Other tests for heart function
• Blood transfusions and possible reactions	• Lumps	• Most recent test for tuberculosis	
• Exposure to radiation	• Use of hair dyes	• History of bacille Calmette-Guérin (BCG) vaccination	
	• Head "dizziness"		
Mouth and Throat	**Neck**	**Nose**	**Breasts**
• Condition of teeth	• Lumps	• Nosebleeds	• Lumps
• Date of most recent dental appointment	• Goiter	• Infections	• Discharge
• Condition of gums	• Pain on movement	• Discharge	• Pain
• Bleeding gums	• Tenderness	• Frequency of colds	• Tenderness
• Frequent sore throats	• History of "swollen glands"	• Nasal obstruction	• Self-examination
• Burning sensation of tongue	• Thyroid trouble	• History of injury	
• Hoarseness		• Sinus infections	
• Voice changes		• Hay fever	
• Postnasal drip			

TABLE 1.2 Review of Systems—cont'd

Vascular	Neurologic	Musculoskeletal	Urinary
• Pain in legs, calves, thighs, or hips while walking	• Fainting	• Weakness	• Frequency
• Swelling of legs	• "Dizziness"	• Paralysis	• Urgency
• Varicose veins	• "Blackouts"	• Muscle stiffness	• Difficulty in starting the stream
• Thrombophlebitis	• Paralysis	• Limitation of movement	• Incontinence
• Coolness of extremity	• Strokes	• Joint pain	• Excessive urination
• Loss of hair on legs	• "Numbness"	• Joint stiffness	• Pain on urination
• Discoloration of extremity	• Tingling	• Arthritis	• Burning sensation
• Ulcers	• Burning sensation	• Gout	• Blood in urine
	• Tremors	• Back problems	• Infections
	• Loss of memory	• Muscle cramps	• Stones
	• Psychiatric disorders	• Deformities	• Bed-wetting
	• Mood changes		• Awakening at night to urinate
	• Nervousness		• History of retention
	• Speech disorders		• Urine color
	• Unsteadiness of gait		• Urine odor
	• General behavioral change		
	• Loss of consciousness		
	• Hallucinations		
	• Disorientation		

Male Genitalia	Female Genitalia	Gastrointestinal	Headaches
• Lesions on penis	• Lesions on external genitalia	• Appetite	• Pain
• Discharge	• Itching	• Excessive hunger	• Fainting
• Erectile dysfunction	• Discharge	• Excessive thirst	• History of head injury
• Pain	• Date of most recent Pap smear and result	• Nausea	• Stroke
• Scrotal masses	• Pain on intercourse	• Swallowing	**Eyes**
• Hernias	• Frequency of intercourse	• Constipation	• Use of eyeglasses
• Frequency of intercourse	• Birth control methods	• Diarrhea	• Current vision
• Ability to enjoy sexual relations	• Ability to enjoy sexual relations	• Heartburn	• Change in vision
• Fertility problems	• Fertility problems	• Vomiting	• Double vision
• Prostate problems	• Hernias	• Abdominal pain	• Excessive tearing
• History of venereal disease and treatment	• History of venereal disease and treatment	• Change in stool color	• Pain
	• History of diethylstilbestrol (DES) exposure	• Change in stool caliber	• Recent eye examinations
	• Age at menarche	• Change in stool consistency	• Pain when looking at light
	• Interval between periods	• Frequency of bowel movements	• Unusual sensations
	• Duration of periods	• Vomiting blood	• Redness
	• Amount of flow	• Rectal bleeding	• Discharge
	• Date of last period	• Black, tarry stools	• Infections
	• Bleeding in between periods	• Laxative or antacid use	• History of glaucoma
	• Number of pregnancies	• Excessive belching	• Cataracts
	• Abortions/miscarriages	• Food intolerance	• Injuries
	• Term deliveries	• Change in abdominal size	**Ears**
	• Complications of pregnancies	• Hemorrhoids	• Hearing impairment
	• Descriptions of labor	• Infections	• Use of hearing aid
	• Number of living children	• Jaundice	• Discharge
	• Menstrual pain	• Rectal pain	• "Dizziness"
	• Age at menopause	• Previous abdominal x-ray films	• Pain
	• Menopausal symptoms	• Hepatitis	• Ringing in ears
	• Postmenopausal bleeding	• Liver disease	• Infections
		• Gallbladder disease	

to the patient. For example, a question regarding paroxysmal nocturnal dyspnea should be asked in this manner:

"Do you ever awaken in the middle of the night with sudden shortness of breath or sudden difficulty in breathing?"

Each of the organ- and system-specific chapters that follow discusses the review of symptoms in more detail. Hints about specific questioning and pathophysiologic features of the symptoms are also provided.

Sometimes, a patient may answer all the questions in the affirmative. If the interviewer detects that this is occurring, it may be useful to ask a question about a physiologically impossible condition. For example, if a patient answers "yes" when asked,

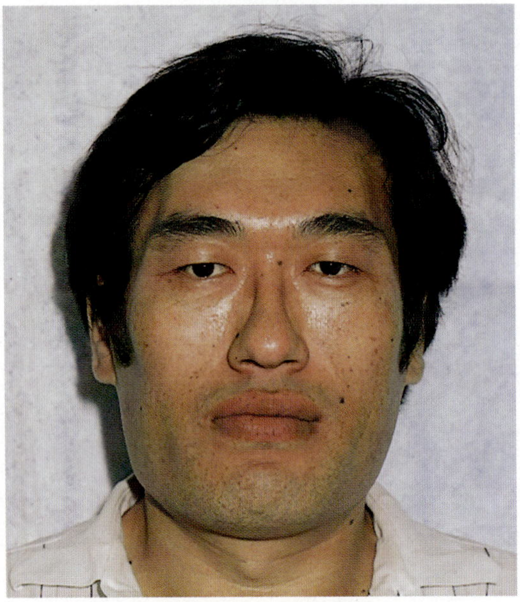

Fig. 1.5 Acromegaly: Facial Characteristics.

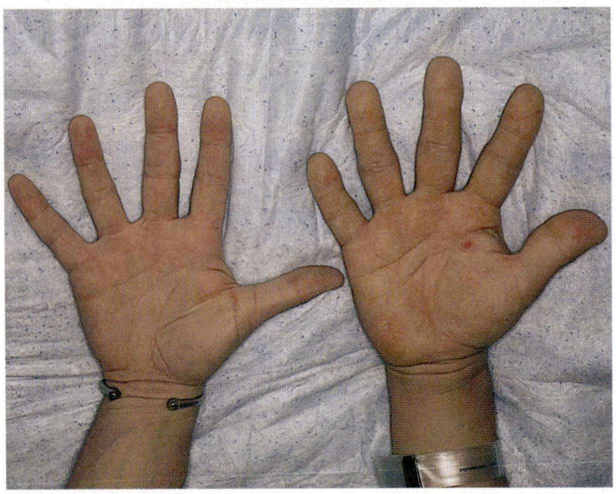

Fig. 1.6 Acromegaly: Characteristics of Hands. Note the stubby fingers of the patient on the right, compared to the fingers of a normal hand on the left.

"Do your stools glow in the dark?" the interviewer should not continue with the review of systems. The interviewer can state in the written history or in the verbal presentation that "the patient has a positive review of systems."

Because the goal of the medical history is to acquire as much information about each illness as possible, other specific questions related to a particular patient may be indicated. Look at the patient shown in Fig. 1.5. Note the large jaw and nose. If you saw such a patient, you might try to determine when the facial changes occurred. In such a case, you could ask the male whether he has noticed a change in his hat or baseball cap size and when he first noticed it.

Look at Fig. 1.6, in which the right hand of the same patient (on the right) is compared with the right hand of a normal individual. Asking about a change in glove size would be useful with this particular patient. It would be appropriate to inquire whether there has been a change in shoe size as well.

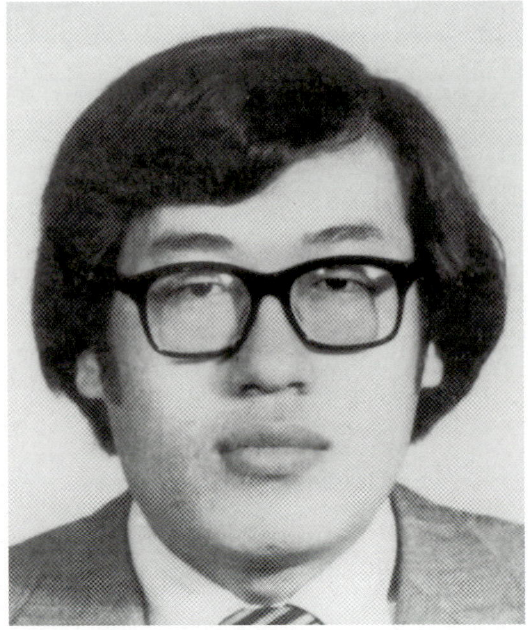

Fig. 1.7 Photograph of the patient shown in Fig. 1.5, taken 20 years earlier. Compare the facial features (i.e., nose and chin) in the two photographs.

A useful bit of information may be an old photograph of the patient to help determine when the suspected changes occurred. Compare Fig. 1.5 with the photograph in Fig. 1.7 (of the same patient taken 20 years earlier). Notice the bulging forehead and the prominent jaw in the later photograph. The patient has acromegaly, a condition of abnormal, excess growth hormone secreted by a pituitary tumor. The changes are insidious, occurring over many years. The photograph was helpful in determining the changes in bone and soft tissue structure.

TAKING NOTES

As mentioned earlier as a novice interviewer, you may feel like you need to write down every detail for fear of forgetting important information. However, it's far better to just jot down short phrases and dates and then write up the full history later. Don't focus too much on taking notes, and instead pay attention to what the patient is saying and their body language. If you are using electronic medical records, try to maintain eye contact by facing the patient as you take notes on the computer screen.

Summarizing the patient's story is important to maintain accuracy and show that you've been attentively listening. This allows the patient to correct any misunderstandings and helps you clarify details. You can summarize at various points during the interview, such as after the history or before/after the physical examination. Summarizing also helps in case of forgetting any important points during the interview.

CONCLUDING THOUGHTS

It's important to keep the medical history dynamic and tailored to the individual patient. While every patient is asked standard questions, they should also be evaluated on a case-by-case basis. There's no limit to the number of questions that can be asked to obtain a comprehensive medical history.

The patient's health history is documented in written form, which serves as a permanent and legal record. It is crucial that the information recorded is precise and unbiased. The interviewer summarizes all the data in a readable format based on the patient's history. It is important to note that anything written in the patient's record could be presented in a court of law, so only objective data should be included. Avoid any opinions or statements regarding previous care and therapy.

By convention, when the review of systems is stated or written, all symptoms that the patient has experienced are indicated first. Symptoms never experienced are indicated afterward. The *pertinent positive symptoms* are symptoms that have possible relevance to the present illness. *Pertinent negative symptoms* are symptoms that are not present but are often related to the present illness.

If information in the review of systems has been described previously—in the history of present illness, for example—it is correct to indicate under the systems review of that symptom, "see history of present illness."

As you proceed with the interview, you may sense that it is not going well. Is the patient comfortable? Is there a language barrier? Did you say or do something to interfere with the rapport? Is the patient intimidated? Is the patient concerned about confidentiality? Is the patient reluctant to talk in the presence of family members? Is the patient able to express their feelings? These issues reflect just a few of the common reasons for lack of progression of an interview. If you can alleviate the problems, do so. If you notice that the patient has suddenly become less communicative, you could say, "Is there anything that I have said or have asked that has made you upset?" Perhaps interviewing the patient on another day but using the same approach will be more successful.

Putting the Patient at Ease

Successfully conducting an interview requires the interviewer to make the patient feel comfortable. This can be achieved by the interviewer being relaxed. What methods can be utilized by both the interviewer and patient to promote relaxation? One useful approach is the visualization of color; for example, if the interviewer were to say, "Close your eyes and visualize the color blue," the patient would feel a definite response in body as well as in mind. If the patient were then to let that image dissolve, take a few breaths, close the eyes again, and visualize the color red, they would notice that the response to this color is quite different. Red creates a different state of mind than do blue, green, yellow, and so forth.

Whether this is entirely a result of psychological association is irrelevant to this discussion. The point is that because people respond strongly to color, interviewers can influence the state of mind of patients and themselves by suggesting an atmosphere of color that calms, warms, cheers, cools, and so forth, depending on what is called for in the situation. Because color can help a patient relax, it can have beneficial effects on blood pressure, heart rate, and other bodily functions.

To alleviate feelings of nervousness and tension, patients can visualize serene and tranquil surroundings. They can simply close their eyes and imagine being in a peaceful garden or a quiet pine forest for a few moments. It is increasingly recognized and acknowledged that relaxation is closely linked to good health. Research in the field of behavioral medicine has shown that meditation can be helpful in managing hypertension, certain heart conditions, depression, anxiety, and other health issues.

Visualization techniques have been around for a long time. The Tibetan approach to medicine, which was developed from the fourth to twelfth centuries, links a person's mental state to their physical health.

In the next chapter, the patient's responses to the questions are investigated, and the influence of background and age on those responses is observed.

REVIEW QUESTIONS

1. Which of the following statements is incorrect?
- **A.** Good communication skills are the foundation of excellent medical care.
- **B.** The success of any interview depends on its being healthcare professional-centered and not patient-centered.
- **C.** The main purpose of an interview is to gather all basic information pertinent to the patient's illness and the patient's adaptation to the illness.
- **D.** Any patient who seeks consultation from a healthcare professional needs to be evaluated in the broadest sense.
- **E.** Once the patient has told their story of the history of the present illness, it is customary to move from open-ended to direct, more focused questions.

2. Which statement is correct?
- **A.** Mother tongue is defined as the language spoken by a patient's mother.
- **B.** Limited language proficiency (LLP) refers to anyone at any age who reported speaking "poorly," as classified by the U.S. Census Bureau.
- **C.** It is always best to use a family member as an interpreter as they know the patient best.
- **D.** The healthcare professional should learn a few key words and phrases in several common languages to gain the respect and confidence of their patients.
- **E.** It is important to allow the patient or interpreter to take over the conversation.

3. Which of the following statements about interviewing skills is most correct?
- **A.** Use of speech patterns
- **B.** Use of body language
- **C.** Use of touch
- **D.** All of the above
- **E.** None of the above

4. Which of the following facial expressions is not one of the six universal emotional facial expressions?
A. Happiness
B. Fear
C. Disgust
D. Surprise
E. Boredom

5. Which of the following pairs is incorrect?
A. Crossed arms - defensiveness
B. Crossed arms and legs - defensiveness
C. Crossed arms, frowning, and clenched fists - defensiveness
D. Open palms - openness
E. Non-symmetric smile without creases around mouth - warmth

6. Which of the following is not a sign?
A. Jaundice
B. Rapid breathing
C. Shortness of breath
D. Hepatomegaly (liver enlargement)
E. Carotid bruit

7. Which of the following questions is not open-ended?
A. "How may I help you today?"
B. "Tell me about your headache."
C. "I'm curious about your..."
D. "What makes the pain better?"
E. "How has your health been?"

8. Which one of the following questions is the best?
A. "Do you feel the pain in your left arm when you get the pain in your chest?"
B. "Why did you stop taking the medications?"
C. "You don't have diabetes, do you?"
D. "Have you had night sweats, fever, or chills?"
E. "Do you have any siblings?"

9. Which of the following is an example of confrontation?
A. "How do you feel about it?'
B. "These things are hard to talk about."
C. "You look upset."
D. "Sounds like you're scared."
E. "You're improving nicely."

10. All of the following are part of the past medical history except:
A. General state of health
B. Hospitalizations
C. Surgeries
D. Abuse
E. Sleep patterns

REFERENCES

Available online.

BIBLIOGRAPHY

Available online.

2

The Patient's Responses

Mark H. Swartz

It is our duty to remember at all times and anew that medicine is not only a science, but also the art of letting our own individuality interact with the individuality of the patient.

Albert Schweitzer (1875–1965)

RESPONSES TO ILLNESS

Health is characterized by a state of well-being, enthusiasm, and energetic pursuit of life's goals. Illness is characterized by feelings of discomfort, helplessness, and a diminished interest in the future. Once patients recognize that they are ill and possibly face their own mortality, a series of emotional reactions occurs, including anxiety, fear, depression, denial, projection, regression, anger, frustration, withdrawal, and an exaggeration of symptoms. These psychological reactions are general and not specific to any particular physical illness. Patients must learn to cope not only with the symptoms of the illness but also with how life is altered by the illness.

Conflict

Conflict is an important medical and psychological concept to understand. Patients live with conflict. What is conflict? Conflict exists when a patient has a symptom and wants to have it evaluated by a member of the healthcare team, but the patient does not want to learn that it represents a "bad" disease process.

Conflict is widespread in medical practice. It is very common for patients to wait until the very end of the consultation to say something like, "Oh, there is one other thing I wanted to tell you!" That information is often the most important reason the patient sought consultation. The patient may have taken time off from work, paid the appropriate fees, and now does not want to return home without finding out the reason for the symptom. The patient may have hoped the healthcare professional would bring up the subject because it is often too painful for the patient to discuss it. One example of conflict occurs when patients with acute myocardial infarction suffer chest pain for several weeks before the actual event. They convince themselves that it is indigestion or musculoskeletal pain; they do not seek medical attention because they do not want to receive a diagnosis of coronary heart disease. Another example of conflict is a female with no family history of breast cancer who finds a breast mass during regular self-examination and does not seek medical attention for several months for fear that the diagnosis is cancer; she *wants* to find out what the mass is, but the conflict is that she does *not* want to find out that the mass is cancer. The patient may be unaware that statistics indicate that most breast masses in a female without a family history of breast cancer are usually benign (e.g., adenoma, fibroma, hematoma, etc.). The healthcare professional must be able to identify conflict, which is often a precursor of denial, to facilitate care of the patient.

Anxiety

Anxiety is a state of uneasiness in which the patient has a sense of impending danger. It is the fundamental response to stress of any kind, such as separation, injury, social disapproval, or decreased self-esteem. Anxiety and fear are common reactions to the stress of illness. The terms *anxiety* and *fear* are often used interchangeably. However, there are two important differences. First, fear tends to be specific and is triggered by a specific event or object; in contrast, anxiety tends to be more diffuse, often occurring without a specific trigger. Second, fear is more acute and tends to appear rapidly, whereas anxiety develops more slowly and takes longer to resolve. The feelings of loss of control, guilt, and frustration contribute to the patient's emotional reaction. Illness makes patients feel helpless. Recognizing the body's mortality leads patients to an intense feeling of anxiety. In addition to the emotional reaction, fear can be manifested physiologically by restlessness, gastrointestinal problems, or headaches. Other common symptoms of anxiety include difficulty falling asleep, nightmares, urinary frequency, palpitations, fatigue, vague aches and pains, paresthesias, sweating, trembling, nausea, a feeling of choking, chills, hot flashes, dizziness, and shortness of breath. It is not uncommon for patients to feel as if they are "falling apart."

Anxiety disorders can be manifested in many forms:

- *Generalized anxiety disorder*—lacks specific traumatic event or focus for concern
- *Panic disorder*—recurrent, unexpected attacks of fear or discomfort that develop abruptly and peak within 10 minutes
- *Agoraphobia*—anxiety about being in a place or situation from which escape may be difficult
- *Phobias*—uncontrollable fear about the presence or anticipation of something

- *Obsessive-compulsive disorder*—associated with obsessions and compulsions that cause marked distress or anxiety
- *Acute stress disorder*—symptoms occur within 4 weeks of the event and last from 2 weeks to a month
- *Posttraumatic stress disorder (PTSD)*—persistent reexperiencing of an event "outside the range of usual human experience" and lasts for months to years (discussed later in this chapter)

The young male who has been stricken with a heart attack feels helpless. As he lies in his intensive care unit bed, he begins to recognize that he really is mortal. The patient believes that he must depend on everyone and everything: the nurse, the health-care professional, the intravenous line, even the monitor. His anxiety, based on helplessness, is a normal response to his illness. His sudden illness and the threat of possible death oppose his belief that he is indestructible.

A 72-year-old male who has lived alone for years since his wife's death is admitted to a hospital for a transurethral prostatectomy. He is anxious that he may become dependent on his children. He may be more threatened by his fear of dependency than by the illness itself.

The hospitalized patient who is brought to the radiology department for a routine chest x-ray film and is forced to wait for 2 hours for a transporter to bring her back to her room suffers anxiety. She is angry that she has been left waiting and perhaps has missed some visitors, but she says nothing. Her anxiety is based on the fear of expressing anger to the nurses and staff members on the floor. She believes that if she were to express her anger, the hospital personnel might interfere with her medical care.

Some hospitalized patients cannot accept the love and care expressed by family or friends. This inability to accept tenderness is a common source of anxiety. Such patients feel threatened by these affectionate acts because they serve to reinforce their dependency.

All patients who are admitted to a hospital experience anxiety. The patients must put their most important commodity, their lives, into the hands of a group of strangers who may or may not be competent to assume responsibility for the patients' survival.

It is most important for the interviewer to identify the causes or roots of a patient's fear or anxiety, as well as to acknowledge the existence of the patient's feelings without expressing judgment. Whenever possible, the interviewer should provide some information to allay the patient's fear or anxiety.

Depression

Depression is a term used to describe a symptom of a chronic state of lowering of mood. Some patients have a predilection for depression, but depression is a common state, occurring in more than 20% of all patients with major illnesses, particularly cancer and cardiovascular disease.

In its chronic state, depression affects more than 8% of the United States population, or 15 million people, and is the leading cause of disability in the United States for people ages 15 to 45. Depression is twice as common in females as in males.

Depression is a common psychological response to a *loss of any kind*: death of a loved one, a relationship, health, autonomy, self-esteem, finances, a job, or even a hormone (such as thyroid). Certain degrees of depression probably accompany every chronic illness. There are many types of depression: reactive, neurotic, manic, melancholic, and agitated are only a few types. In general, patients with depression have pessimistic tones in speech and a downcast facial expression. They may express feelings of futility and self-accusation. They respond to questions with brief answers. Their speech is slow, their volume is low, and their pitch is monotonous. Depressed patients feel inadequate, worthless, and defeated. They also suffer profound feelings of guilt. A remark such as "You look sad" invites these patients to talk about their depression. Although many patients who are depressed cannot cry, crying can relieve some severe depressive feelings, even if only momentarily, and thus enables patients to continue their story. Although crying may be brought on by patients' concern for their own illness, crying usually occurs when patients think of an illness or death of a loved one or of a potential loss. They often have much hostility and resentment and suffer from rejection and loneliness. Self-accusative and self-deprecating delusions can occur in severely depressed patients. When these delusions are present, the feelings of worthlessness are so overwhelming that patients may believe that suicide is the only way out.

Depression may be the most common reaction to illness, as well as the most frequently overlooked. The most important diagnostic symptoms of depression are the following:

- Markedly diminished interest or pleasure in almost all activities *(anhedonia)*
- Insomnia
- Change in appetite or weight
- Fatigue or loss of energy
- Low self-esteem
- Agitation
- Feelings of guilt or worthlessness
- Decreased ability to think or concentrate
- Thoughts of death or suicide

As an example of severe depression, consider the following case of a 23-year-old law student. He is engulfed by anxiety when he is diagnosed with acquired immune deficiency syndrome (AIDS). When his friends and family learn of the illness, he is immediately excluded from all relationships. He has extreme feelings of guilt and low self-esteem. He is found later hanged in his parents' attic. His only way of coping with his illness has been through suicide.

Suicide is a major public health concern. More people die by suicide annually than by homicide. In 2020, there were 45,979 recorded suicides, according to the American Foundation for Suicide Prevention.[1] The age-adjusted suicide rate in 2020 was 13.48 per 100,000 individuals. The rate of suicide was highest in middle-aged males. In 2020, males died by suicide 3.88 times more than females. There were an estimated 1.20 million suicide attempts!

Suicide is often committed out of despair, the cause of which can be attributed to a mental disorder such as depression, bipolar disorder, schizophrenia, alcoholism, or drug abuse. Suicide ranks as the 12th leading cause of death in the United States. It is the second leading cause among 20- to 34-year-olds and the third leading cause among 10- to 19-year-olds.

The risk of suicide is greater if a behavior is new or has increased and if it seems related to a painful event, loss, or change. The following signs may mean someone is at risk for suicide:

- Talking about wanting to die or to kill themselves
- Looking for a way to kill themselves, such as searching online or buying a gun
- Talking about feeling hopeless or having no reason to live
- Talking about feeling trapped or in unbearable pain
- Talking about being a burden to others
- Increasing the use of alcohol or drugs
- Acting anxious or agitated; behaving recklessly
- Change in sleeping pattern
- Withdrawing or isolating themselves
- Showing rage or talking about seeking revenge
- Displaying extreme mood swings

For every person who dies by suicide annually, 316 people seriously consider suicide but do not kill themselves.

Suicide is tragic, but it is often preventable. Knowing the risk factors for suicide and who is at risk can help reduce the suicide rate. **Interviewers must not ignore any talk of suicide.** If patients bring up suicidal thoughts, interviewers must get the assistance of someone experienced in the field *immediately*. The 988 Suicide & Crisis Lifeline is a national network of local crisis centers that provides free and confidential emotional support to people in suicidal crisis or emotional distress 24 hours a day, 7 days a week in the United States. Since its founding in 2005, the Lifeline has received 23,044,100 calls through 2021![2]

Denial

Denial is a coping mechanism that consists of acting and thinking as if a part of reality is not true. It gives one time to adjust to distressing situations, but staying in denial can interfere with treatment and the patient's ability to tackle challenges. Denial is one of the most common psychological mechanisms of defense and can occur in both patients and healthcare professionals. Denial is often an emotional response to inner tension and prevents a painful conflict from producing overt anxiety. It is actually a form of self-deception. Denial is often observed in patients with terminal illnesses or with chronic, incurable diseases. In general, the more acute the illness, the greater is the patient's acceptance; the more insidious, the greater the denial.

If a patient is in denial, they are not being realistic about something that's happening in their life, although it might be obvious to those around the patient. A patient dying slowly from cancer can observe their weight decreasing and the side effects of medications. Frequent visits to the hospital for chemotherapy or radiation therapy confirm the severity of the illness; yet in spite of all this, the patient may continue to deny the illness. They make plans for the future and talk about the time when they will be cured. Denial is the psychological mechanism that keeps this patient going. The interviewer should not confront the patient's denial, despite its apparent absurdity. Telling such a patient to "face the facts" is cruel. Breaking down denial in such a patient serves only to add to the dying patient's misery. However, the patient's family must understand and accept the poor prognosis.

When a patient is in denial, they will:

- Refuse to acknowledge a stressful problem or situation.
- Avoid facing the facts of the situation.
- Minimize the consequences of the situation.

In its strictest sense, denial is an unconscious process. Denial can sometimes obstruct proper medical care. A female presents to a breast clinic with an orange-sized mass in one breast. The mass has already started to ulcerate, with a resultant foul-smelling infection. When asked how long she has had the mass, she responds that she noticed it "just yesterday." When a patient is in denial, it is often best to interview a reliable informant in addition to the patient.

Patients can be in denial about anything that makes them feel vulnerable or threatens their sense of control, such as:

- A chronic or terminal illness
- Depression or other mental health conditions
- Addiction
- Financial problems
- Job difficulties
- Relationship conflicts
- Traumatic events

Patients can be in denial about something that is happening to them or to someone else.

Fig. 2.1 illustrates another example of the tragic sequelae of denial. This male has a basal cell carcinoma of the face. As is discussed in Chapter 8, The Skin, basal cell carcinomas are very slow growing and rarely metastasize; they are locally invasive. Had the patient sought medical attention when the lesion first appeared (and was very small), he would have been totally cured. A person's denial can be so deep that it prevents them

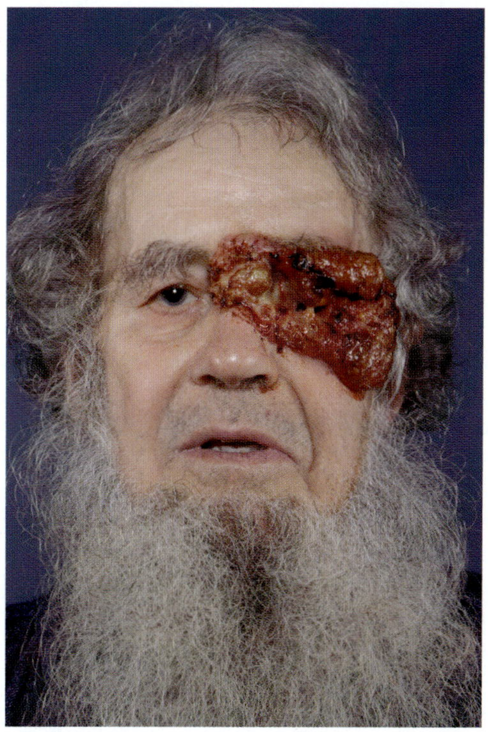

Fig. 2.1 A Portrait of Denial. This male has a locally invasive basal cell carcinoma.

from seeing reality and seeking medical attention. Therefore, it is important for the healthcare professional to be sensitive to this very powerful psychological mechanism. For another example of denial, see the unfortunate patient with inflammatory breast carcinoma shown in Fig. 16.8.

Projection

Projection is another common defense mechanism by which people unconsciously reject an unacceptable emotional feature in themselves and "project" it onto someone else. It is the major mechanism involved in the development of paranoid feelings. For example, hostile patients may say to interviewers, "Why are you being so hostile to me?" In reality, such patients are projecting *their* hostility onto the interviewers.

Projection is one of the defense mechanisms identified by Freud. According to Freud, projection is when someone is threatened by or afraid of their own impulses, so they attribute these impulses to someone else. Patients commonly project their anxieties onto healthcare professionals. For example, a person in psychoanalysis may insist to the therapist that he knows the therapist wants to rape some females, when in fact the client has these awful urges to rape. Patients who use projection are constantly watching the healthcare professional's face for subtle signs of their own fears.

As another example of projection, a 42-year-old female with a strong family history of early death from breast cancer has intense fears of developing the disease. During the inspection portion of the physical examination, the patient may be watching the healthcare professional's face for information. If the healthcare professional frowns or makes some type of negative gesture, the patient may interpret this as "They see something wrong!" The healthcare professional may have made this expression thinking about the amount of work still to be done that day or what type of medication to prescribe for another patient. The patient has projected her anxiety onto the healthcare professional. The healthcare professional must be aware of these silent "conversations."

In some instances, projection may have a constructive value, saving the patient from being overwhelmed by the illness.

Regression

Regression is a common defense mechanism by which the patient with extreme anxiety attempts unconsciously to return to earlier, more desirable stages of development. During these periods, the individual enjoyed full gratification and freedom from anxiety. Regressed patients become dependent on others and free themselves from the complex problems that have created their anxiety.

Behaviors associated with regression can vary greatly depending on which stage the person is fixated at:

- An individual fixated at the oral stage might begin eating or smoking excessively or might become very verbally aggressive.
- A fixation at the anal stage might result in excessive tidiness or messiness.

For example, consider a middle-aged married male who has recently been told that he has inoperable lung cancer that has already spread to his bones. He is stricken with grief and intense anxiety. There are so many unanswered questions. How long will he live? Will his last months be plagued with unremitting pain? How will his wife be able to raise their young child by herself? How will she manage financially without his income? Through regression, the patient can flee this anxiety by becoming childlike and dependent. The patient becomes withdrawn, shy, and often rebellious; he now requires more affection.

Another example is a teenager who learns that the cause of his 6-month history of weakness and bleeding gums is acute leukemia. He learns that he will spend what little time he has left in the hospital undergoing chemotherapy. His reaction to his anxiety may be regression. He now needs his parents at his bedside around the clock. He becomes more desirous of his parents' love and kisses. His redevelopment of enuresis (bedwetting) is part of his psychological reaction to his illness.

A final example is a 25-year-old female with inflammatory bowel disease who has had many admissions to hospitals for exacerbations of her disease. She fears the future and the possibility that a cancer may have already started to develop. She is engulfed by a feeling of terror and apprehension. She fears that someday she may require a colostomy and that she will be deprived of one of her most important functions: bowel control. She acts inappropriately, has temper tantrums, and is indecisive. Her dependency on her parents is a manifestation of regression.

RESPONSES TO THE INTERVIEWER

Much of the enjoyment of medical practice comes from talking with patients. Each patient brings a challenge to the interviewer. Just as there are no two identical interviews, there are no two people who would interview the same patient in the same manner. This section describes a few characteristically difficult patients and indicates some strategies for how the interview may be modified in each case.

Many of the patients to be described can arouse intensely negative feelings in the interviewer; as such, these patients have been collectively called "the patient who is hateful." The interviewer should recognize these feelings and deal with them directly so that they do not interfere with the interaction. The interviewer must recognize early in the interaction the general characteristics of these patient types so that they can facilitate the interview appropriately.

A variety of pejorative labels have unfortunately been given to many of these patient types. The labels serve only to reduce the interviewer's stress through the use of humor. This humor is demeaning to patients and can ultimately prevent them from receiving the proper medical care they deserve.

The Patient Who Is Silent

Some patients have a lifelong history of shyness. Some of these individuals lack self-confidence. They are very concerned about their self-image and do not want to say or do the wrong thing. These patients are easily embarrassed. Other individuals become hostile or silent as fear of illness develops. Many patients who are silent are seriously depressed, which may be a primary response as a result of the illness itself or a secondary response to it. These patients commonly have many of the other signs of depression, as seen in their attitude, facial expressions, and posture. The use of open-ended questions with these patients is usually of little value. Carefully directed questioning may yield some of the answers. You might ask, "Is there a reason for your not answering my questions?"

The young interviewer often has difficulty interviewing the silent patient; the interviewer may feel obligated to speak. Allow the patient periods of silence because the patient may need time to think and remember details. Always be attentive and respectful, and watch for nonverbal clues. As mentioned previously, patients who are depressed or worried about their health or lives are relatively silent. If you suspect depression, try refocusing the interview questions about depression and suicide.

The Patient Who Is Overtalkative

The patient who is overtalkative presents a challenge to the novice interviewer. These patients dominate the interview; the interviewer can hardly get a word in. Every question gets a long answer. Even the answers to "yes-no" questions seem endless. There is usually an aggressive quality to this patient's communications. Every answer is overdetailed. Do not show your impatience. A courteous interruption followed by another *direct* question helps focus on the subject of the interview. The use of open-ended questions, facilitations, or silence is to be avoided because these techniques encourage such a patient to continue speaking. You might say to the patient, "I am interested to learn more about…, but we have a limited time together, so I need to ask you some specific questions. Please answer them directly." If all else fails, the interviewer should try to relax and accept the problem.

The Patient Who Is Seductive

One of the most difficult types of patients for the novice to interview and examine is the seductive patient. In many ways, it is more difficult to deal with the patient who is seductive than with a patient who is hostile. Many of these patients have one of the personality disorders (e.g., histrionic, narcissistic) and harbor fantasies of developing an intimate relationship with their healthcare professional. These patients are often attractive and tend to be flashy in the way they dress, walk, and talk. They commonly offer inappropriate compliments to the interviewer to gain their attention. The patients are frequently emotionally labile. Not uncommonly, these patients expose themselves physically early in the interview. The interviewer may elect to cover the patient, but usually this is unsuccessful because the patient may expose themself again. It is difficult for the interviewer to cope with their own feelings when they are attracted to such a patient. The feeling of attraction is a natural one, and the interviewer must accept it. However, the interviewer must always maintain a strictly professional demeanor. Empathy and reassurance must be kept to a minimum because these supportive techniques stimulate further fantasies in the patient. The interviewer must always maintain professional distance. It may be necessary to say, "Thank you for your nice compliments, but for me to help you, we must keep our relationship strictly professional. I hope you understand." If necessary, the interviewer should get the advice of someone they trust.

The Patient Who Is Angry

Angry, obnoxious, or hostile patients are common. Some make demeaning comments or are sarcastic, whereas others are demanding, aggressive, and blatantly hostile. Some patients who are hostile may remain silent during most of the interview. At other times, they may make inappropriate remarks that are condescending to the novice or even to the experienced healthcare professional. The interviewer may feel resentment, anger, threatened authority, impatience, or frustration. **Reciprocal hostility must be avoided** because a power struggle can develop. Accept the patient's feelings and try to determine the cause of their behavior. Do not react to them.

The interviewer must realize that these reactions are the patient's responses to *illness* and not necessarily a response to the interviewer. These reactions may be deeply rooted in the patient's past. Every interviewer should be aware that the same emotions, such as rage, envy, or fear, are present in both the patient and the interviewer. A patient may express feelings toward the interviewer who must act in a detached, professional way and should not feel offended or become defensive.

Students of the healthcare professions may have been taught that they must like their patients to treat them appropriately. Ambivalence in the interviewer can be a problem. Healthcare professionals must treat patients medically correctly and with respect, but in fact, it is not necessary to like the patient to provide good care. Because of their illness, patients may have feelings of loss of control, threatened authority, and fear. Their anger is the mechanism by which they attempt to handle their fears. Once interviewers gain this insight and become aware of their own feelings, they can better treat such patients. Interviewers must accept and restrain their own negative feelings toward the patients so that their professional judgment is not distorted. Interviewers' awareness of their own anxieties and feelings aids in conducting a more productive interview. Conscious expression of the interviewer's own feelings in a frank and noninsulting manner facilitates the interviewing process. Regulation and control of the interviewer's feelings are the goals.

Confrontation may be a useful technique for interviewing such patients. By saying, "You sound very angry," the interviewer allows patients to vent some of their fears. Another confrontational approach is to say, "You're obviously angry about something. Tell me what you think is wrong." Maintain equanimity, and avoid becoming defensive. If at the beginning of the interview the patient is angry, try to calm the patient. Proceed slowly with questioning, avoid interpretations, and ask questions that are confined to the history of the present illness.

The Patient Who Is Paranoid

The patient who is paranoid constantly asks, "Why are you asking me that? Do I have…?" When the interviewer asks the many questions in the review of systems, the patient responds, "Who told you about that?" Paranoid patients think there is some devious plan and that people are constantly talking about them. The patient's suspiciousness can sometimes be handled by the interviewer's saying, "These are routine questions that I ask all my patients." Reassurance tends to be threatening to these patients and should not be used because it tends to produce more suspicion. The patient's delusion is beyond reason. The interviewer should therefore complete the questioning and not try to convince such patients about their false ideations. Avoidance of any anger by the interviewer is of paramount importance.

The Patient Who Is Insatiable

Patients who are insatiable are never satisfied. They have many questions, and despite adequate explanations, they feel that the interviewer has not answered all their questions. They tend to be very sensitive, anxious individuals. These patients are best handled with a firm, noncondescending approach. A definite closing statement is helpful, such as "We have reached the end of our time for today, but I will be back." Alternatively, the interviewer could say, "We have reached the end of our time for today. I will refer your concerns to Dr. ____."

The Patient Who Is Ingratiating

The patient who is ingratiating attempts to please the interviewer. Such patients believe that they must provide the "right" answers to satisfy the interviewer. They think that if they answer a question in a way that arouses the disapproval of the interviewer, the interviewer will abandon them. Intense feelings of possible rejection are present in this type of patient. The interviewer must recognize that anxiety is the cause of the patient's behavior and should try not to respond to that behavior. The interviewer should recognize the patient's tendency of trying to please and should stress to the patient how important it is to be accurate.

The Patient Who Is Aggressive

Many patients who are aggressive have a personality disorder. Such patients are easily irritated and often fly into a rage when dealing with the normal stresses of daily life. They are domineering and try to control the interview. However, if allowed to have their way, they may be quite pleasant. Frequently, patients with aggression have intense dependency needs that they cannot consciously handle. These patients mask the primary problem by becoming aggressive and hostile to disguise their anxiety and feelings of inadequacy and inferiority. Patients with aggression are difficult to interview. The interviewer must try to avoid areas provoking anxiety early in the interview. Once a rapport is established, the interviewer may attempt to delve into the deeper areas. In general, aggressive patients refuse any type of psychotherapy.

The Patient Who Is Help-Rejecting

Patients who are help-rejecting are usually not hostile. They describe having been seen by many "expert" healthcare professionals for help and often tell interviewers that no one can find out what is wrong with them. They return again and again to the healthcare professionals' offices, indicating that the healthcare professionals' suggestions "didn't work." Commonly, when a symptom appears relieved, another suddenly appears. These patients use their symptoms to enhance their relationship with their healthcare professionals. Such patients are often very depressed, although they may deny it. They believe that they have made many self-sacrifices and have had countless disappointments, which they attribute to their "illness." The best approach to these individuals is strong emotional support and gentle reasoning. Despite the need for psychiatric help, these patients usually refuse to accept it.

The Patient Who Is Demanding

The patient who is demanding makes demands of everyone: the healthcare professional, the student, the aide. These patients use intimidation and guilt to force others to take care of them. They view themselves as being neglected and abused. They may have outbursts of anger toward healthcare professionals, who may fear for their own reputations. A power struggle may result. Inform the patient that it is good that they came in and that you will do everything possible to help.

The Patient Who Is Compulsive

Patients who are compulsive are concerned about every detail of their lives. These patients pride themselves on their ability to solve all problems, but when their health deteriorates, they lose their composure because they cannot deal with ambiguity or uncertainty. They deny their feelings of anger and anxiety, and projection is a common reaction to their illness. In dealing with this type of patient, the interviewer must provide very detailed and specific information to the patient in a straightforward manner. The patient should be allowed as much control as possible, and all the possibilities discussed should be explained clearly.

The Patient Who Is Always Dependent

The patient who is always dependent finds life difficult without the help of others. Other persons provide the necessary support, both emotional and physical. If this support is removed, the patient feels hurt and deserted and demands even more help. When such persons become ill, they imagine that their illness will lead to loss of their support groups. Thus, these patients need to be cared for most closely. However, sometimes these patients can take advantage of a compassionate healthcare professional by demanding enormous amounts of time. Be as direct as possible when informing such patients of the appropriate limits without leaving them rejected. The interviewer might say, "You've given me a lot to think about. I do have to leave now. Please don't feel I'm rejecting you. I'll be back later to discuss some of your other problems."

The Patient Who Is Masochistic

The patient who is masochistic, or self-defeating, goes through life suffering. Although these patients need to continue to suffer mentally, they do not seek physical abuse or pain. This type of patient is dedicated to a life of self-sacrifice. In contrast to other types of patients, this type adapts well to illness and, in fact, may feel threatened by recovery. Thus, such patients often frustrate healthcare professionals. The goal for these patients is to be able to function despite their problems. Interviewers should not promise cures because this creates more problems for the patient and the healthcare professional.

The Patient Who Is Borderline

Patients who are borderline are individuals with a personality disorder who have an instability in their personal relationships, engage in impulsive behavior, and have unstable moods. Intense, fluctuating emotions of love and hate are typical of patients who are borderline. They need emotional support because they are constantly threatened by people and circumstances. It is often very difficult to develop a good healthcare professional–patient relationship with patients who are borderline because the swings of affect are rapid. These patients are always afraid, but this fear may be masked by outbreaks of anger. These patients are best handled with reassuring words.

The Transgender Patient

Transgender is an umbrella term that describes people whose gender expression or identity are different from their sex recorded at birth. Transmasculine, transfeminine, nonbinary, genderqueer, and other gender-diverse individuals occupy the same range of sexual orientations as cisgender individuals (people whose gender expression or identity are congruent with their sex assigned at birth). However, disparities in access to care and experiences of care in the **L**esbian, **G**ay, **B**isexual, and **T**ransgender (LGBT) community are often lumped together in homogenous issue briefs and research studies. Many people who are transgender have a unique need for specific medical treatments that will have meaningful short-term and long-term implications for their physical and/or mental health.

Due to rejection from family and friends related to transitioning, transgender individuals often have to create their own support systems *(families of choice)*. These close friends can serve the function of family. Consequently, when a transgender person comes to a clinic or hospital, they may not seek visitation from biological family members but rather from *family members of choice*.

Transgender people are often asked invasive questions about their bodies and transgender identity. Asking transgender patients what words they use to describe their body can help create a safe and affirming experience. Using transgender affirmative and inclusive language has a direct impact on healthcare and screenings. It can help transgender patients feel more comfortable talking about their bodies and overall health.

By educating oneself about transgender health, one can help remove barriers to care and create a safe, inclusive, and supportive healthcare environment for transgender patients.

See Chapter 26, The Transgender Patient, for more detailed information.

INFLUENCE OF BACKGROUND AND AGE ON PATIENT RESPONSE

Although disease is universal, patients respond to their illnesses differently. A particular question asked of different patients is answered in a style that is governed by the patient's ethnic background, emotions, customs, age, medical history, social history, and family history. These factors determine the way in which a patient perceives and responds to a question. As an example, consider a 42-year-old patient with increased thirst, increased urination, increased appetite, decreased weight, and blurry vision. The most likely diagnosis is diabetes mellitus. That same diagnosis will mean something very different if this patient has a parent or friend with diabetes who is doing well and is being managed with just a pill or diet versus a parent or friend with diabetes who is blind or has lost a limb as a result of the disease!

This section illustrates the importance of understanding a patient's background as an aid to better communication.

The Child Who Is Ill

Children tend always to be "on guard." Children who are ill are especially vulnerable and wary. First, they are taken from their "friendly" home environment. Second, healthcare professionals are constantly staring at them with a wide variety of facial expressions. Many older children believe that the healthcare professional has some sort of "magical eye" that can see through them and know everything about them. This all adds up to a frightening experience for youngsters. Frequently, tests that cause discomfort may have to be performed by those "people in white." The healthcare professional becomes a symbol of danger and pain.

When the healthcare professional takes a youngster for a test, the child experiences their greatest fear: separation from parents. This separation produces intense fear and anxiety, manifested by wailing, irritability, and aggressive behavior. The child's fear is that they will not see their parents again. This fear may actually be subconscious. Healthcare professionals should explain to the child, if old enough, that they know why the child is crying and should assure the child that they will see their parents soon. Parents should be urged to talk to their children, informing them that the healthcare professional is going to help them. The parents should be careful *not* to indicate that the professional will *not* hurt the child, because if the child has pain as a result of a test, the child–parent relationship may be jeopardized. The parent should be encouraged to stay with the child in the hospital as long as possible and even sleep in the child's room at night, if permitted. Studies have shown that when parents are permitted to stay with their children, the recovery is quicker, and there is less emotional trauma. An important part of caring for children is talking to the parents. If the parents understand the situation, they can do much to help the healthcare professional–child relationship.

Children who are disabled, like adults who are disabled, are extremely apprehensive of the atmosphere in the hospital. It reminds them of previous experiences. The interviewer must take time to play with the child while talking to the parent or the person accompanying the child. Complimenting the youngster with statements such as "How pretty you are" or "What a nice outfit you're wearing" seems to foster goodwill. These children crave love, affection, and attention. The parent has to be reassured that the staff members are reliable and caring. This will give the parent peace of mind. If a child wishes to keep a favorite toy or blanket, there should be no restrictions. Separation from home and family is a terrible experience for any child, but it is even more so for these children, who function better in familiar surroundings.

The Patient Who Is Aged

The patient who is aged requires a lot of attention. Depression is prevalent among older adults. These patients must frequently cope with the loss of loved ones and other important persons in their life. They are also stressed by changes in their own self-images and the way they are perceived by others. Deterioration in bodily function also contributes to depression in aged patients.

A patient's depression may be so severe that they may consider suicide a reasonable alternative to living with a severe chronic illness or living alone after the death of a spouse. Among this bereaved population, more deaths within the first 4 years after the spouse's death result from suicide than from all other causes.

The interviewer must never assume that older patients' complaints are natural for their age. **People do not die of old age; they die of illnesses.** Most of these patients are alert and capable of independent living. The ones who are unable to care for themselves are usually accompanied by a family member or an attendant. The interviewer must obtain as much information as possible from these sources. The interviewer should also refrain from using patronizing mannerisms that belittle the individual. A friendly, respectful approach reassures the patient. Older patients should be advised about everything that will be done to them. This makes patients confident that there will be no unpleasant surprises. Because of advanced age, such patients may be afraid of dying. Those who are afraid should be reassured that everything possible will be done to make them better. Many people survive an illness because of their desire to live and therefore fight to stay alive. Overzealous reassurance is not appropriate for all aged patients; many regard death as a reasonable outcome.

The Patient Who Is Widowed

Many patients who are widowed come to the hospital alone, with the thought that because their spouses are gone, nobody cares about them. They may be suffering from depression as a result of loneliness. The interviewer should inquire gently whether there are any children, relatives, or friends who can be contacted or will come to visit. Such a patient may be at odds with their children and may prefer that the children not know that the patient has entered a hospital. In other cases, the family may live far away. The patients do not want their family to worry, so they do not tell the family. In these cases, it is advisable for the healthcare professional to alert the social worker to the particular situation. Volunteers visiting the patient, as well as members of the clergy, can bring soothing counsel. A warm handshake and reassurance are effective ways of putting this patient in a relaxed state of mind. Many widowed patients are quite active. The clinician should not presume that all widowed individuals are isolated.

The Patient With Posttraumatic Stress Disorder

Although the effects of natural calamities and their aftermaths have been recognized since the time of ancient Greece, PTSD was not included in the American Psychiatric Association's handbook of psychiatric disorders, the *Diagnostic and Statistical Manual of Mental Disorders*, until 1980. One of the first descriptions of PTSD was made by the Greek historian Herodotus. In 490 BCE, he described an Athenian soldier who suffered no injury in the Battle of Marathon but became permanently blind after witnessing the death of a fellow soldier. Healthcare professionals are only beginning to recognize the enormous toll that trauma can take on personal suffering and functional impairment. PTSD may also have an effect on future generations through effects on parental or guardian behavior and competence. PTSD can be extremely debilitating, especially when complicated by comorbid depression and substance use.[3]

For many years, PTSD was considered only a wartime affliction. During World War I, PTSD was called "shell shock," and during World War II, it was referred to as "combat fatigue." After the Vietnam War, it was often mistakenly called the "post-Vietnam syndrome." The National Vietnam Veterans Readjustment Study reported that 15.2% of males and 8.5% of females who served in the war had current PTSD and that nearly 30% of the male and female veterans met lifetime criteria for PTSD.[4] These patients have a variety of symptoms, including nightmares, sleep disturbances, avoidance reactions, guilt, intrusive memories, and dissociative flashbacks.

In addition to the PTSD from the Vietnam War, as much as 9% to 10% of the U.S. population may have some form of PTSD. Almost 18% of 10 million females who were victims of physical assault have PTSD. Studies have shown that PTSD develops in 2% of people exposed to any type of accident, 30% of those exposed to a community disaster, 25% of those who have experienced traumatic bereavement, 65% of those experiencing nonsexual assault, 85% of battered females in shelters, and 50% to 90% of those who were raped. Of all psychiatric disorders, PTSD poses one of the greatest challenges to the healthcare professional because of its complexity and variability of signs and symptoms.

In 1987, the revised *DSM-III (DSM-III-R)* defined PTSD as caused by traumatic events that were "outside the range of usual human experience and that would be markedly distressing to almost anyone." PTSD is a normal reaction to an abnormal amount of stress. Although trauma is usually considered as an injury to a body part, it may be even more devastating to the psyche. Wounding of emotions, spirit, the will to live, dignity, and the sense of security can be traumatic. Some traumatic events may go on for months or years, whereas others may occur in a few seconds and have the same lasting effects as longer events. In minutes, a person's sense of self and sense of the world as a secure place can be shattered.

One problem with the *DSM-III-R* description is that it fails to recognize the importance of the subjective appraisal of the event; this includes the ethnocultural aspects of PTSD. The 1994 edition, *DSM-IV*, lists PTSD as the only diagnosis that identifies the origin of symptoms from external events rather than from within the individual. All the following *DSM-5* criteria must be met to make a diagnosis of PTSD:

- Experience of a traumatic event
- Experience of the trauma

- Evidence of numbing or other avoidance behavior
- Exhibition of signs of hyperarousal
- Evidence of symptoms for at least 1 month
- Experience of difficulties at home, work, or in other important areas of life as a result of the symptoms

Life is filled with many crises, such as losing a parent or being robbed. Although these events can be stressful, they are not considered "traumatic." A *traumatic event* is defined as an unusual occurrence that is not part of normal human experience and that evokes extreme helplessness, fear, and despair. Examples of traumatic events include a natural catastrophe, such as a tornado, hurricane, volcano, earthquake, fire, landslide, or flood; a human catastrophe, such as war, concentration camps, refugee camps, sexual assault, physical assault, or other forms of victimization; witnessing a death, rape, torture, or beating; a suicide of a family member or close friend; and any exposure to danger of one's own safety and life.

Experiencing the trauma can take many forms, including dreams, flashbacks, or situations that remind the person of the traumatic event. While dreaming, the person may shout, shake, or thrash about the bed. Although the person may awake suddenly, they may not remember the nightmare, but the intense emotion may persist for long periods.

Psychic or emotional numbing is a form of self-protection against unbearable emotional pain. After the event, the individual may experience periods of feeling emotionally dead or numb. That person may have great difficulty in expressing tenderness or loving feelings. *Avoidance behavior* is another important aspect of PTSD. People with PTSD often feel alienated and apart from others. They may lose interest in activities that once gave them pleasure. Others are unable to remember certain aspects of the traumatic event.

Hyperarousal symptoms include difficulty in falling or staying asleep, irritability, outbursts of anger, difficulty in concentration, overprotectiveness of oneself or others, and an exaggerated startle response. People who were abused in a bed commonly experience insomnia. People with an exaggerated startle response may jump at loud noises or if someone touches them on the back.

Duration of symptoms is variable, but according to the official diagnostic criteria for PTSD, the symptoms must endure at least 1 month.

The last criterion relates to the *influence of the psychic trauma on lifestyle.* Survivors of human-engendered catastrophes, in general, suffer longer than survivors of natural catastrophes. In addition, the devastating effects of emotional trauma may be influenced by exposure of the individual to one or more traumatic events. Rape is traumatic, but multiple rapes are even more traumatic. Do the person's symptoms interfere with their ability to work, study, socialize, or maintain healthy familial relationships?

Many trauma-related disorders have been recognized and include brief reactive psychosis, multiple personality disorder, dissociative fugue, dissociative amnesia, conversion disorder, depersonalization disorder, dream anxiety disorder, summarization disorder, borderline personality disorder, and antisocial personality disorder. Many other trauma-related disorders have been postulated. These disorders and the trauma that may precede them are indicated as follows:

- *Brief reactive psychosis:* Any one or more events that would be stressful to anyone
- *Multiple personality disorder:* Abuse or other childhood emotional trauma
- *Dissociative fugue:* Severe psychologically stressful event such as marital quarrels, military conflict, natural disaster, or personal rejection
- *Dissociative amnesia:* Severe psychologically stressful event such as the tragic death of a loved one, abandonment, or a threat of personal injury
- *Conversion disorder:* Extreme psychologically stressful event such as warfare or a recent tragic death of a loved one
- *Depersonalization disorder:* Severe stressful event such as military combat or an automobile accident
- *Dream anxiety disorder:* Any major life stress, depression, substance abuse, or substance withdrawal
- *Somatization disorder:* Early childhood abuse
- *Borderline personality disorder:* Early childhood trauma
- *Antisocial personality disorder:* Early childhood abuse

Learned helplessness syndrome is a condition frequently seen in trauma survivors, commonly females and children, prisoners of war, concentration camp survivors, refugee camp survivors, or other tortured survivors. The name developed from animal experiments by Seligman.[5,6] Animals subjected to electric shocks and unable to escape despite their attempts would sink into listlessness and despair. Later, they were reshocked, but although trained to press a lever to stop the shocks, the animals made no effort to do so. The animals had learned to be helpless. It has been postulated that there is an adrenal neurotransmitter problem in animals and humans exposed to severe, repeated traumatic events that may serve as the biologic basis for the hyperarousal and numbing phases of PTSD.

Although almost any symptom can result from PTSD, some of the more common ones are as follows:

- Eating disorders
- Anger or rage
- Self-condemnation
- Self-mutilation
- Depression
- Self-hatred
- Suicidal thoughts
- Homicidal thoughts
- Headaches
- Backaches
- Chronic gastrointestinal problems
- Worsening or activation of chronic medical problems (e.g., diabetes, hypertension)
- Drug abuse
- Overworking
- Self-isolation

The Holocaust is a classic example of a tragic, traumatic event that inflicted significant, permanent changes in the victims' physical and psychological responses to stress. Holocaust survivors who are still alive have complex problems that have affected them some for more than 85 years.[7] They are *survivors*;

therefore, they never stopped fighting for survival. They are especially frightened of becoming sick because, in the past, to survive meant to be in good health; the alternative was to face doom. These patients are afraid of losing control of their lives, as well as losing their dignity.

Barak and Szor described a high comorbidity of chronic PTSD (91.8%) with psychotic disorders many decades after the experience of the massive psychic trauma of the Holocaust. The occurrence of chronic PTSD of such magnitude for an extremely prolonged period is striking. It is significantly higher than the rate reported for war veterans, ranging from 12.4%[8] to 45%.[9] This difference, Barak states, may be related to the unique nature of the Holocaust trauma, combining dehumanization, confrontation with death, and massive loss for a prolonged period.

Patients who are Holocaust survivors may have many psychosomatic complaints commonly related to the gastrointestinal tract. Chest pain, often relieved by belching, may be related to frequent air swallowing. These patients experience vivid dreams and nightmares. They are suspicious and do not trust people readily because they suffered so much in the past. The interviewer must be especially kind and understanding. The majority of the survivors of the Nazi concentration camps are currently 95 years of age or older, and many still suffer from PTSD. Many suffer from severe depression, panic attacks, and anxiety. The interviewer must be careful when asking about family history and background. Most survivors lost entire families; many lost their first spouses and children. The psychological wounds are deep, and anything can trigger an outpouring of grief. It is frequently difficult to find out anything about the family medical history because the patients' parents and grandparents might have been killed at early ages. These patients should be reassured that they will be treated gently and competently. They, like all patients with PTSD, must be assured of security. Feeling safe is the highest priority in their lives.

On September 11, 2001, the United States was faced with one of its greatest tragedies. Many people were directly exposed to this massive traumatic event. Others were indirectly exposed through the extensive television coverage and/or stories from survivors of the attacks. It has become clear that individuals need not be present at a catastrophic event to experience stress symptoms. The events and their aftermath were shown in graphic detail repeatedly after the terrorist attacks. Many Americans identified with the victims directly or perceived the unprecedented attacks as directed at themselves as well. Thus, even people who were nowhere near the location of the attacks experienced substantial stress responses.[10]

In a study published in the *New England Journal of Medicine* shortly after the attacks,[11] 90% of the adults surveyed reported experiencing, to at least some degree, one or more symptoms of stress and 44% of the adults reported a substantial level of at least one symptom of stress. Although those closest to the sites of attack had the most substantial stress, respondents throughout the country, from large cities to small communities, reported stress symptoms: 36% of respondents more than 1000 miles from the World Trade Center reported substantial stress reactions, in comparison with 60% of those within 100 miles of the site. Among respondents who lived south of Canal Street in Manhattan (i.e., near the World Trade Center), the prevalence of PTSD was 20% after the attacks compared with 4% before the tragic event. The article notes that more than 130,000 Manhattan citizens suffered from PTSD, depression, or anxiety after the attacks. Other studies have shown that children who were exposed solely through television to horrifying events such as these attacks, the Challenger disaster, the Oklahoma City bombing, and the Gulf Wars experienced trauma-related stress reactions.

Approximately 5 to 8 weeks after the attack on the World Trade Center, a random telephone survey was conducted to estimate the prevalence of increased cigarette smoking, alcohol consumption, and marijuana use among residents of Manhattan.[12] Among 988 persons included, 28.8% reported an increase in use of any of these three substances; 9.7% reported an increase in smoking, 24.6% reported an increase in alcohol consumption, and 3.2% reported an increase in marijuana use. Persons who increased smoking of cigarettes and marijuana were more likely to experience PTSD than were those who did not (24.2% vs. 5.6% for cigarettes; 36.0% vs. 6.6% for marijuana). The study was repeated 6 months later, and the increases were sustained, suggestive of potential long-term health consequences as a result of such disasters.

The Healthcare Professional Who Is Ill

Perhaps the most difficult of all patients to care for is the healthcare professional who is ill. The expression "A little knowledge is a dangerous thing" applies to the healthcare professional who is ill. Every healthcare professional goes through the "student syndrome," which is the suspicion that they have been stricken with the disease about which they are learning. Imagine the anxiety that occurs when the healthcare professional actually is stricken. In addition to anxiety about health, there is the new role identification of being the patient. Healthcare professionals feel helpless and have great difficulty divorcing themselves from the role of healthcare professional. They constantly ask what the electrocardiogram shows and for the results of blood tests. They may suggest additional tests or even disagree with the tests that have been ordered. The novice interviewer should provide ample time for the sick healthcare professional to express fears and anxieties. With the interviewer's support, sick healthcare professionals eventually recognize and accept their new role as patient.

INFLUENCE OF DISEASE ON PATIENT RESPONSE

Just as background and age govern a patient's response, so do the patient's present illness and past medical illnesses. This section illustrates the influence of disease on the type of response.

The Patient Who Is Disabled

Patients who are disabled may come to the hospital with great apprehension and mistrust. They are usually familiar with the shortcomings of hospitals because they have probably been hospitalized for painful tests or surgery. They may be burdened with an inferiority complex and may feel unattractive. The interviewer must take all this into consideration and assure patients that everything will be done to make them comfortable. The interviewer must sort out the emotional problems of disabled persons from the physical ones that brought them to the hospital. A friendly smile or a few kind words can encourage these patients to cooperate, thereby securing a better healthcare professional–patient relationship.

Many people who are disabled have developed their own routines that work for them. They often do not want medical personnel to impose their way of doing something if the patient's way works.

Patients with a *hearing impairment* need to be treated differently from other patients who are disabled. Sit directly in front of these patients to allow them to benefit from lip reading. Make sure that the lighting in the room is correct so that your face is well illuminated. It is important to speak slowly with appropriate gestures and expressions to punctuate the question. Ask these patients whether it is necessary for you to speak louder. If a patient wears a hearing aid, speaking louder may not be necessary. It might be possible to use your stethoscope and place the earpieces in the patient's ears and speak into the diaphragm as a microphone. If all else fails, the use of written questions can be helpful.

Another special type of patient who is disabled is the *visually impaired* patient. Because the patient with limited or no vision has no reference for you in the room, it is useful for you to occasionally touch the patient on the arm or shoulder. This can be done instead of the more standard nonverbal facilitations, which are of no value in this patient. Always tell the patient who you are and why you are speaking to them.

The patient who is severely mentally challenged must be accompanied by a family member or guardian to provide a proper history.

The Patient With Cancer

The patient with cancer has five major concerns: loss of control, pain, alienation, mutilation, and mortality. Loss of control makes this patient feel helpless. The knowledge of something growing uncontrolled within a patient's body creates frustration, fear, and anger. Suffering with pain is one of the most feared aspects of cancer. The feeling of alienation stems from the reactions of people around the patient.

Fears of mutilation are common among patients with cancer. The fear of being perceived as lacking "wholeness" contributes to depression and anxiety. The young female with breast cancer who requires a mastectomy fears that she will be rejected as no longer being a complete female. Supportive family members are the key in reassuring this patient that they will love her just as they have before her surgery. A diagnosis of cancer makes a patient aware of mortality and leads to intense fear of unremitting pain.

Family members and friends often express grief before death occurs. Resentment and anger may be directed toward the patient with cancer. Healthcare professionals often harbor feelings of inadequacy about these patients and have difficulty speaking with them. The patients are thus rejected by their own healthcare professional. The healthcare professional is afraid that the patient may ask some questions, perhaps about death, that the healthcare professional cannot handle. The healthcare professionals must recognize their emotional and behavioral reaction and be realistic about the limitations of medical science.

The interviewer should allow the patient to vent anxieties and should promote dialogue. Listening to the patient enhances the healthcare professional–patient relationship.

The Patient With Acquired Immune Deficiency Syndrome

Patients with AIDS are fearful for their lives and of being stigmatized as a member of an undesirable group. The fear and misunderstanding common in high-risk groups result in delays in medical treatment. Denial is the important factor in most of these patients. The patient may have an intense fear of healthcare professionals, who may have strong emotions related to this disease and its risk groups. The patient's fear is paralleled by the anxiety of the hospital workers who have to treat an individual with this disease. Their fear of contracting the disease, even by casual contact, is formidable. These fears are also present among the patient's friends and family, who often banish the patient from all activities. The patient may have been fired from a job because the employer is afraid of catching the disease. There is an unsympathetic rejection of patients with AIDS. They suffer emotional turmoil, which contributes to intense anxiety, hostility, and depression.

The interviewer should be as supportive as possible without giving false reassurances. The patients should be given as many facts as appropriate, and the staff members tending to them must be educated about the disease.

The Patient Who Has Dysphasia

The patient with dysphasia has an impairment of speech and cannot arrange words correctly. Dysphasia is usually caused by a cerebral lesion, such as a stroke. The degree of dysphasia can vary enormously and can be as extensive as almost complete aphasia. Although patients may appear relatively unresponsive, they may be totally aware of all conversation. Therefore, all discussions conducted in the presence of such patients must be undertaken with the assumption that the patient can understand. Before the interview, the interviewer may give patients a pen and paper to determine whether they can respond by writing "Yes" and "No" answers.

The Patient Who Has Psychosis

Patients who have psychosis have an impairment of their reality-testing abilities. They have a gross inability to communicate effectively. They may also suffer from hallucinations, delusions, or feelings of persecution. These patients cannot deal with their fear. They are constantly struggling with the ever-changing demands of their environment. It is most important to recognize such patients early and remain as calm as possible. If the patient has had violent episodes, make sure assistance is standing by.

In general, interviewing patients with a psychosis presents a difficult task for the inexperienced interviewer. Some of these patients tend to be inarticulate and preoccupied with fantasies, whereas others are reasonably lucid. The symptoms and signs of their psychosis are not usually evident at first assessment. There are several clues to the existence of a psychosis. Interviewers should pay particular attention to the speech pattern and its organization. Is there a jumble of ideas? Psychotic patients are easily distracted, and the interviewer must constantly remind them of the subject. These patients fail to complete any chain of thought and cannot follow any idea to completion. They can have bizarre impressions about their bodies. They may complain that they have noticed that one arm has recently shortened or that their external genitalia have suddenly shrunk or enlarged. In addition, they may have evidence of an inappropriate affect; for example, a patient may laugh while telling about the death of a friend or relative.

A special type of psychotic personality disorder is found in patients with *Munchausen syndrome*. Such patients are the classic hospital malingerers. They are pathologic liars and travel from healthcare professional to healthcare professional and from hospital to hospital. They complain of a wide variety of symptoms and, in fact, *create* signs of illness to seek an advantage. Their histories are well rehearsed, and they have a masochistic perpetuation of self-injury. For example, the patient with Munchausen syndrome may actually prick the skin under a fingernail so that it will not be obvious, drop some blood into the urine, and call the healthcare professional, stating that there is blood in the urine. These patients frequently seek out painful diagnostic and therapeutic procedures. At times, they may even undergo unnecessary surgical procedures.

The Patient Who Has Dementia or Delirium

Patients who have dementia or delirium have lost previously acquired intellectual function, most typically memory. Patients who have dementia or delirium have a disorder of consciousness that does not allow them to interact correctly with their surroundings. Patients with dementia frequently become more confused when taken out of their normal environment, especially at night. The term *sundowning* is used in such circumstances. Fear is common in both types of patients. In interviewing these patients, healthcare professionals must try to be sensitive to their emotions as much as possible and, above all, try to allay their fears. Interviewers must be particularly aware of questions that may be possibly threatening to the patient.

Patients with an organic mental syndrome present a special problem. At times, these patients seem lucid; at other times, they are disoriented with regard to person, place, or time. If the patient is able to answer some of the questions, the interviewer should record the answers. The same questions should be asked again later to determine whether the patient will respond similarly. These patients have defects in attention span, memory, and abstract thought. Interviewers should be alert to inconsistent and slow, hesitant responses. On occasion, patients may interject some humor to try to cover up for their difficulty in memory. A careful mental status examination indicates the problem. It may be useful to remind the patient of your name and tell them that you will ask for the name in a few minutes. Frequently, such patients have forgotten it. **Never correct these patient errors,** and if they ask the same question again, never tell them that you already answered the question. This is a definite way to close down the interview because the patient will feel stupid and reluctant to answer other questions. Furthermore, because the histories these patients give may not be reliable, it is always useful to have another family member present when interviewing the patient with impaired cognitive abilities.

If the patient lacks the capacity for decision making, a determination of surrogacy will be necessary. In the best-case scenario, the patient may have previously appointed an agent; in the worst-case scenario, the court may need to become involved. Try to determine if the patient has a durable power of attorney for healthcare or a healthcare proxy (see Chapter 33 for a discussion of health proxies). If the patient does not have an advance directive or healthcare proxy, the surrogate will need to make decisions based on principles of "substituted judgment" (what the patient would have decided) or "best interest" (what the surrogate judges to be best for the patient).

The Acutely Ill Patient

The acutely ill patient merits prompt attention. In these situations, a concise history and physical examination are in order. A careful history of the present and past illnesses must be taken expeditiously so that the diagnosis may be made and treatment begun. It may be appropriate in this setting to interview the patient while performing the physical examination; time is of the essence. However, patients who are acutely ill may respond to questions more slowly than normal because of pain, nausea, or vomiting. Be considerate of their problems, and allow them time to answer questions. After a patient's condition has been stabilized, there will be time to go back and take a more complete history.

The Patient Awaiting Surgery

Patients faced with a surgical procedure may be frightened despite a calm appearance. They may feel helpless and out of control. The fear of anesthesia, disfigurement, disability, or death is always present. The fear of not awakening from the anesthesia can be devastating. When they awaken, will they find that their body is no longer "whole"? Did the surgeon find something that was not expected? These patients fear the unknown. A question about the surgeon's ability is an expression of the patient's anxiety. Often, patients have tests and are told the results are normal "except" for a small area: they will need surgery to "check it out." This lack of communication by the surgeon adds to the patient's anxiety. A surgeon's schedule is frequently erratic. Surgery may be delayed or postponed, which adds to the surgical patient's anxiety and anger. Many possible communication difficulties exist. The best way to avoid unnecessary anxiety-provoking situations is to maintain open communication among the patient, the healthcare professional, and the patient's family. In the postoperative period, the patient's relief over having lived through surgery may be displayed in a variety of ways. The patient may be apathetic and show a general lack of interest or may be moody, irritable, aggressive, angry, or tearful. Subconsciously, patients may wish to harm the surgeon for "cutting" into their bodies, whereas consciously they want to thank the surgeon. This dichotomy may be the root of the anger so commonly seen in postoperative patients. In other patients, depression may be seen as a result of the loss of part of the body. The best example of this is the "phantom limb." Patients who have undergone an amputation of a leg frequently claim sensation in their lost limb. Some of this may be physiologic, but certainly some of the phantom leg pain is related to depression. The caring interviewer should allow the patient time to release these tensions and feelings of loss.

The Patient Who Has Alcoholic Substance Misuse

Patients who have an alcoholic substance misuse are both physiologically and psychologically dependent on alcohol. Most of the time, interviewers conduct the sessions when the patient is not inebriated. Excessive drinking is often an attempt to deaden feelings of guilt and failure. The more patients drink, the more they are abandoned by their family and friends. They feel castigated and alone. They are left to their only "friend": alcohol. They are often ready to talk, and their account of their drinking habits may be interesting. Alcoholic patients generally have a low opinion of themselves. They may even be upset about their persistent drinking habits. Their hatred of themselves may be a manifestation of a self-destructive wish. Alcoholic patients may also have fears about sexual inadequacy or homosexuality. It is not easy to open up such topics because these patients are likely to respond explosively. The sensitive interviewer should approach these issues in a manner that is neither condescending nor moralistic.

The Patient With a Psychosomatic Illness

Just as physical illness can produce psychological problems, so can psychological problems create physical ailments. The intimate interaction of the mind and body is clearly demonstrated in the psychosomatic disorder.

Patients with a psychosomatic illness express emotional discomfort and distress in the form of bodily symptoms. They may be totally unaware of the psychological stress in their lives or the relationship of stress to the symptoms.

There are many ways of dealing with these patients. First, identify the disorder: Do not miss the possible diagnosis of an affective or anxiety disorder. Treatment of somatization is directed toward teaching the patient to cope with the psychological problems. Be aware that somatization operates unconsciously; the patient really is suffering. Above all, the patient should *never* be told that their problem is "in your head." Anxiety, fear, and depression are the main psychological problems associated with psychosomatic illness. The list of associated common symptoms and illnesses is long and includes chest pain, headaches, peptic ulcer disease, ulcerative colitis, irritable bowel syndrome, nausea, vomiting, anorexia nervosa, urticaria, tachycardia, hypertension, asthma, migraine, muscle tension syndromes, obesity, rashes, and dizziness. Answers to an open-ended question such as "What's been happening in your life?" often provide insight into the problems.

Finally, the interviewer should legitimize patients' suffering by acknowledging that their suffering is real. The interviewer must help patients recognize the way in which stress can create physical suffering. Giving patients the freedom to discuss hopes and fears is often more beneficial than a written prescription for medications.

The Patient Who Is Dying

Few patients are as conscious of taking up a healthcare professional's time as those who have less time remaining. Dying patients may initially have many questions, but as time goes by, they ask less and less of their healthcare professionals.

Many healthcare professionals have a dread of death that is so intense that they behave irrationally. They avoid patients who are dying or with incurable diseases. The emotional needs of the dying patients may be largely ignored. Many patients have a greater fear of the process of dying than of death itself. The fear of living as a chronically ill patient can be almost as intolerable as (and often more so than) the fear of death.

Patients who are dying may suffer from the pain, nausea, or vomiting caused by the disease or treatment. They may be rejected by their families, hospital staff members, or even their own healthcare professionals. Many patients have strong feelings of anger, guilt, resentment, and frustration: "Why me?" "It should have been diagnosed earlier." They may envy healthy individuals. They may deny their imminent death; this is the first stage of dying. Not uncommonly, a patient who is dying is interviewed and does not tell the interviewer about the illness. Even when asked specifically about the disease, the patient may deny any knowledge of having a fatal disease. This mechanism of denial allows the patient to cope with life as it is. Each person faces death differently. Some can deal with it head-on; others cannot. Some approach it with fear and tears, whereas others grow to accept it as an inevitable event. Given sufficient time and the necessary understanding, most patients who are dying can arrive at the final stage of dying: acceptance. This stage is characterized by apathy and social withdrawal. Counselors specifically trained in the grieving process are often helpful to the patient, family, and healthcare professionals.

Once a patient has come to grips with the fact that they have a terminal disease, the patient may ask, "Am I going to die?" The interviewer cannot answer this question as asked, and so they should then ask the patient, "What are you afraid of?" The patient may then indicate that they are afraid of dying in pain or dying alone. The interviewer can then answer these questions by saying that they will do everything possible to make sure that the patient will not have pain or that they or their associates will be with the patient throughout the duration of the illness.

The patient who is dying needs to speak with someone. The healthcare professional should be alert for subtle clues that the patient wishes to discuss the topic of death. For example, if a patient remarks that his "wife is well provided for," it is correct to pursue this point by making an interpretive statement such as, "I sense that you are very worried about your illness." Although the conversation that ensues might be emotionally draining for the interviewer, the interviewer must allow the patient to speak. Sometimes the most appropriate response to an expression of grief is a thoughtful period of silence.

REVIEW QUESTIONS

1. **Which of the following is *not* a response to illness?**
   A. Conflict
   B. Depression
   C. Anxiety
   D. Projection
   E. Aggressiveness
2. **Patients can be in denial by:**
   A. Loss of a job
   B. A chronic illness
   C. Relationship conflicts
   D. Traumatic events
   E. All of the above
3. **Which of the following behaviors is best for the angry patient?**
   A. Act in a detached, professional manner.
   B. Become offended and act accordingly.
   C. Do not accept the patient's feelings.
   D. Show your frustration.
   E. Show the patient that you like them despite any negative statement that patient may make.
4. **To make a diagnosis of posttraumatic stress disorder (PTSD), which of the following must be met?**
   A. Experience of a traumatic event
   B. Experience of the trauma
   C. Evidence of numbing or other avoidance behavior
   D. Exhibiting signs of hyperarousal
   E. All of the above
5. **Which of the following is *not* defined as a traumatic event?**
   A. Death of a parent due to a myocardial infarction
   B. Beating
   C. Suicide of a close friend
   D. Refugee camps
   E. Sexual assault
6. **Which of the following symptoms is *not* a symptom of posttraumatic stress disorder (PTSD)?**
   A. Eating disorder
   B. Depression
   C. Headache
   D. Urinary retention
   E. Drug misuse
7. **Which of the following statements is correct?**
   A. Demented patients have a disorder of consciousness that does not allow them to interact correctly with their surroundings.
   B. Delirious patients frequently become more confused when removed from their normal environment.
   C. At times, patients with organic mental syndrome seem lucid, and at other times they are disoriented.
   D. It is always best to correct patients with an organic mental syndrome.
   E. If a patient does not have an advance directive or a healthcare proxy, the healthcare professional may automatically assume that role.
8. **If a dying patient asks, "Am I going to die?", the best answer might be:**
   A. "*Yes, I think so. Everyone has to die sometime.*"
   B. "*No, I will keep you alive.*"
   C. "*What are you afraid of?*"
   D. "*Is your wife prepared for the future?*"
   E. "*Do you want your wife or children to be with you?*"

REFERENCES

Available online.

BIBLIOGRAPHY

Available online.

3

Understanding Complementary and Alternative Medicine

Mark H. Swartz

The natural healing force within each of us is the greatest force in getting well.

Hippocrates (460 BCE–377 BCE)

GENERAL CONSIDERATIONS

Complementary and alternative medicine (CAM) includes a group of diverse medical and healthcare systems, practices, and products taken from around the world that fall outside the realm of conventional medicine. Many aspects of CAM are rooted in ancient systems of healing from China, Tibet, India, Japan, Korea, Mongolia, Africa, and the Americas. Today, CAM alongside conventional medicine is widely used to treat and restore health to the sick and prevent disease in healthy individuals.

What is CAM? **Complementary medicine,** such as aromatherapy, is used *in conjunction with* conventional medicine, for example, to lessen a patient's postoperative discomfort. **Alternative medicine,** such as some herbal medicines, is used *instead of* conventional medicine to treat cancer, as an example. Alternative therapies include, but are not limited to, the following disciplines: folk medicine, herbal medicine, diet fads, homeopathy, faith healing, new age healing, chiropractic, acupuncture, naturopathy, reflexology, massage, and music therapy. **Integrative medicine** combines conventional medical and CAM therapies for which there is some scientific evidence of safety and effectiveness, regardless of their origin.

Studies have shown that the frequency of use of CAM therapy in the United States is far greater than previously reported. It has been estimated that 38.3% of the American population uses at least one of these healing methods to satisfy medical needs. The most common users of CAM therapy are more affluent people, females, those better educated, individuals born after 1950, and those who are concerned about emotional stress and the environment. According to the National Health Interview Survey (NHIS) of the Centers for Disease Control and Prevention,[1] the most common therapies are relaxation techniques (18%), massage (12%), herbal medicine (10%), and megavitamin therapy (9%). The perceived efficacy of these therapies ranged from 76% (hypnosis) to 98% (energy healing). The number of visits to providers of this healthcare is greater than the number of visits to all primary care healthcare professionals nationwide. More than 70% of these patients never mention using alternative therapy to their healthcare professionals. Out-of-pocket expenditures of more than $34 billion per year in the United States are a testament to a widely held belief that CAM therapies have benefits that outweigh their costs. This figure is in contrast to the $12.8 billion spent out of pocket annually for all hospitalizations in the United States.

One of the reasons patients seek CAM therapies may be a failure in the healthcare professional–patient relationship. Healthcare professionals often fail to discuss the use of these therapies because they lack adequate knowledge in this area and have poor insight into the cultures and beliefs of those who practice CAM. To many healthcare professionals, "alternative medicine" entails the threat of displacing conventional medicine for the sake of unproven therapies. It may lack organization and the rigorous, scientific standards of Western, evidence-based medicine. The response of the healthcare professionals ranges from outright dismissal of the practices to a gradual recognition that their extensive use can no longer be ignored. A lack of communication and knowledge in this area may also prove to be detrimental to the patient because the use of some forms of these therapies, if unsupervised, may be dangerous.

There has been an increasing interest throughout the world in the use of natural ingredients for health, especially tea. Tea is the world's second most popular beverage after water. Tea originated in the Southwest China provinces where it is used as a medicinal beverage. Green tea accounts for approximately 20% of all tea consumed. It has been claimed that overall health of the body, especially the oral cavity, can be maintained by the consumption of green tea. Green tea is rich in polyphenols, about 30% by weight, including large amounts of a catechin called epigallocatechin-3-gallate (EGCG).[2] EGCG is one of the most powerful compounds in green tea. It has been studied to treat various diseases and may be one of the main reasons green tea has such powerful medicinal properties. Catechins are natural antioxidants that help prevent cellular damage. They also reduce the formation of free radicals protecting cells from damage. These antioxidant properties have been touted to include lowering blood pressure, lowering cholesterol, stabilizing blood glucose, inhibiting bacterial growth, and blocking many carcinogenic agents. Green tea is not fermented; therefore, it contains *active* polyphenols that would be inactivated in the fermentation process of black tea production. Scientists have found that the catechins in green tea extract increase the body's ability to burn fat as fuel, which accounts for improved muscle endurance. These antioxidants might help protect against a large number of cancers, including breast,[3] colon, colorectal,[4] skin, lung, esophagus, stomach, small intestine, pancreas, liver, ovarian, prostate,[5] and oral cancer. Polyphenols have been shown to also inhibit the growth of *Streptococcus mutans*, the major etiologic bacterium associated with dental caries, and *Porphyromonas gingivalis*, the bacterium associated with periodontal disease.

In April 1995, the National Center for Complementary and Alternative Medicine (NCCAM)[a] of the National Institutes of Health (NIH) defined CAM as "a broad domain of healing resources that encompasses all health systems, modalities, and practices and their accompanying theories and beliefs, other than those intrinsic to the politically dominant health system of a particular society or culture in a given historical period." This group of therapeutics is not currently part of allopathic medicine, although some conventional healthcare professionals (those with an MD, DO, or other health-related degrees) are also practitioners of CAM. The CAM marketplace is currently valued at $24 billion or more, and the growth rate is close to 15% per year. Since 2010, Congress has provided more than $2.3 billion to promote CAM research. In fiscal year 2023, the funding for the National Center for Complementary and Integrative Health (NCCIH) was $170.3 million.[6]

The purpose of this chapter is to educate the reader about CAM. Medical schools in the United States are now including courses in which CAM treatments are taught, but 80% of medical students polled have indicated that they would like more information. Because several healthcare insurance companies in the United States now cover CAM therapies and 67% of health maintenance organizations now offer at least one form of CAM,[7-9] it is crucial for healthcare professionals to become more cognizant about these therapies. In the future, there will be more well-designed, randomized, controlled studies that will provide answers to many of today's questions regarding CAM.

CLASSIFICATIONS OF COMPLEMENTARY AND ALTERNATIVE MEDICINE

The NCCIH has classified CAM therapies into five major but overlapping categories:

1. Alternative medical systems
2. Mind–body interventions
3. Biologically based therapies
4. Manipulative and body-based methods
5. Energy therapies

Alternative Medical Systems

Alternative medical systems are complete, complex systems of healthcare practices that incorporate natural products, spiritual elements, diet, and other modalities. Some systems, such as homeopathic medicine and naturopathic medicine, have evolved in the Western world, whereas others, such as Chinese medicine and Ayurvedic medicine, have developed in non-Western cultures. *Ayurvedic medicine* was developed in India more than 5000 years ago and is the best known of the traditional approaches associated with Indian medicine. The system involves the use of diet and herbal remedies with emphasis on the mind, body, and spirit in disease prevention and treatment. *Homeopathic medicine* is based on the belief that "like cures like": minute doses of highly diluted animal, vegetable, and mineral substances can cure the symptoms that would be caused by higher concentrations of the same substance in a healthy person. It is believed that these minute doses stimulate the body's own defense mechanism to fight off illness. These natural substances are nontoxic and nonaddictive and have no known side effects. Homeopathic medications are regulated by federal law, and most are sold over the counter. *Naturopathic medicine* is based on the concept of natural healing and uses only natural, gentle, nontoxic treatments with the goal of having the body heal itself. Some of the naturopathic processes include dietary modifications, mineral and herbal supplements, exercise, massage, and acupuncture.

Mind–Body Interventions

Mind–body interventions entail a wide variety of techniques to improve the mind's capacity to affect bodily function and symptoms. Cognitive therapies, biofeedback, yoga, meditation, hypnosis, breathing techniques, prayer, Tai Chi, and creative outlets such as dance, music, and art are common examples of mind–body interventions. These all attempt to tap into the deep reservoir of the mind as a means to achieve therapeutic effects on the body. Mind–body interventions have been shown to influence favorably the practice of conventional medicine through placebo effects that are poorly understood.

Biologically Based Therapies

Biologically based therapies involve substances found in nature, such as herbs, vitamins, dietary supplements, and foods to treat illness and enhance health. Around the world, these products are extraordinarily popular, and billions of dollars are spent on them in the United States alone. The assumption is that natural products are healthier and better than synthetic chemicals for treating disease. Dietary supplements are considered foods and not drugs; therefore, they are not subjected to the same regulatory standards imposed by the U.S. Food and Drug Administration on pharmaceuticals. They can be marketed without any clinical evidence supporting their efficacy or safety. Without this regulatory oversight,

[a]In January 2015, NCCAM was renamed the National Center for Complementary and Integrative Health (NCCIH). It is the federal government's lead agency for scientific research on complementary and integrative health approaches. Its mission is to define, through rigorous scientific investigation, the usefulness and safety of complementary and integrative health interventions and their roles in improving health and healthcare.

these substances may contain impurities such as pesticides or other harmful products.

Manipulative and Body-Based Methods

Manipulative and body-based methods include modalities that move one or more parts of the body to produce a variety of health outcomes. These methods include massage therapy, chiropractic, osteopathy, reflexology, and movement therapies such as the Feldenkrais method[b] or Alexander technique.[c] *Chiropractic* is concerned with the relationship between structure and function. The primary structure is the spine, and the function is the nervous system; this relationship is thought to affect the restoration and preservation of health. The first chiropractic adjustment was given in 1895. The basic principle of chiropractic is that any interference with the transmission, reception, or application of impulses that travel over the nervous system causes functional abnormalities or disease. This interference may be the result of a vertebral subluxation. Over the years, numerous definitions have been formulated to describe the nature of subluxation. In all of these, there are at least four main criteria or characteristics:

1. Misalignment of the vertebra in relationship to the ones above and below it
2. Abnormal vertebral motion
3. Lack of joint play
4. Interference with the transmission of neural impulses

The vertebral subluxation may be the result of any of the following causes: trauma, toxins (infections, poisons), and autosuggestion (psychologic factors). Vertebral subluxation is treated with a chiropractic manipulation referred to as an *adjustment.* The chiropractic adjustment is a specific form of direct articular manipulation characterized by a dynamic, forceful, high-velocity thrust of controlled amplitude. These adjustments may be administered by hand or instruments directed at specific articulations. It is believed that chiropractic adjustments energize the life force that connects the spine to all parts of the body to promote healing and restore health.

Chiropractic has become one of the largest drug-free healing professions. It is estimated that chiropractors treat more than 35 million Americans (adults and children) annually.[10] Chiropractors are designated as healthcare professional–level providers in the vast majority of states and federal Medicare programs. Chiropractors are the highest-rated healthcare professionals for low-back pain treatments above physical therapists (PTs), specialist physician/MD (i.e., neurosurgeons, neurologists, orthopedic surgeons), and primary care physician/MD (i.e., family or internal medicine).[11] The market size, measured by revenue, of the chiropractor industry was $18.7 billion in 2022.

Osteopathy focuses on diseases arising in the musculoskeletal system. The belief is that all the body's systems work together, and disturbances in one system affect functions in another. The field involves understanding the entire patient, physically, psychologically, and emotionally, to uncover the underlying causes of symptoms. Osteopathic physicians use musculoskeletal manipulation, recommendations about diet and exercise, and general preventive medicine to alleviate pain, restore function, and promote health.

Reflexology[12] is a body-based therapy in which pressure is applied to the feet, hands, ears, and cranium to treat a variety of ailments and promote well-being and improved health. The therapist applies the tips of the fingers, the thumb, the elbow, and the hand firmly to areas of the recipient's body to assess the state of health and treat every part of the body. Dating back to as early as 2700 BCE, reflexology is believed to link every organ or gland in the body to a reflex point on the foot or hand; these areas are linked through a series of longitudinal and transverse zones that run from the feet or hands through the legs and arms, respectively, to the organ or gland. By manipulating the reflex area, most of which are found on the soles of the feet, as shown in Fig. 3.1, the therapist can treat that area of the body. It is believed that foot reflexology, which is not a simple foot massage, can relieve tension and blockages by stimulating sensory receptors in the nerves of the foot (see Fig. 3.2). As a result, energy is created that extends to the spinal cord and dispersed throughout the nervous system. Reflexology has been used for many conditions, including, among other things, improving the immune system, paralysis, arthritis, diabetes, and sleep disorders; lowering blood pressure; and stimulating circulation. A meta-analysis[13] in 2015 indicated a beneficial effect of massage for the relief of cancer pain. Foot reflexology appeared to be more effective than body massage or aromatherapy. The American Commission for Accreditation of Reflexology Education and Training (ACARET) sets the standards for education required for the reflexology profession. It also credentials those involved with educating students of reflexology. The American Reflexology Certification Board (ARCB) has a three-part examination process to ensure the practitioner has met the standards set by the board.

Energy Therapies

Energy therapies involve the detection and use of energy fields for therapeutic benefit. These therapies are categorized into three types: biofield therapies, bioelectromagnetic-based therapies, and acupuncture. The term *biofield* was coined in 1994 at a meeting at the NIH, and the biofield hypothesis purports that all objects radiate an electromagnetic field. If an object, such as part of a healer's body, a nutritional supplement, or an externally applied electromagnetic field, is brought near to or inside

[b]The Feldenkrais method of somatic education, which was developed in the 1950s, is a type of alternative exercise therapy that practitioners claim can repair impaired connections between the motor cortex and the body, thus benefiting the quality of body movement and improving well-being. The method directs attention to habitual movement patterns that are thought to be inefficient or strained and attempts to teach new patterns using gentle, slow, repeated movements. Today, there are more than 6000 Feldenkrais practitioners around the world.

[c]The Alexander technique, which was developed in the 1890s, is an educational process that was created to retrain habitual patterns of movement and posture. The technique is a method of re-education and self-awareness to change long-standing habits that cause unnecessary tension. One becomes aware of the habits of movement, tension, and reaction that interfere with natural and healthy coordination.

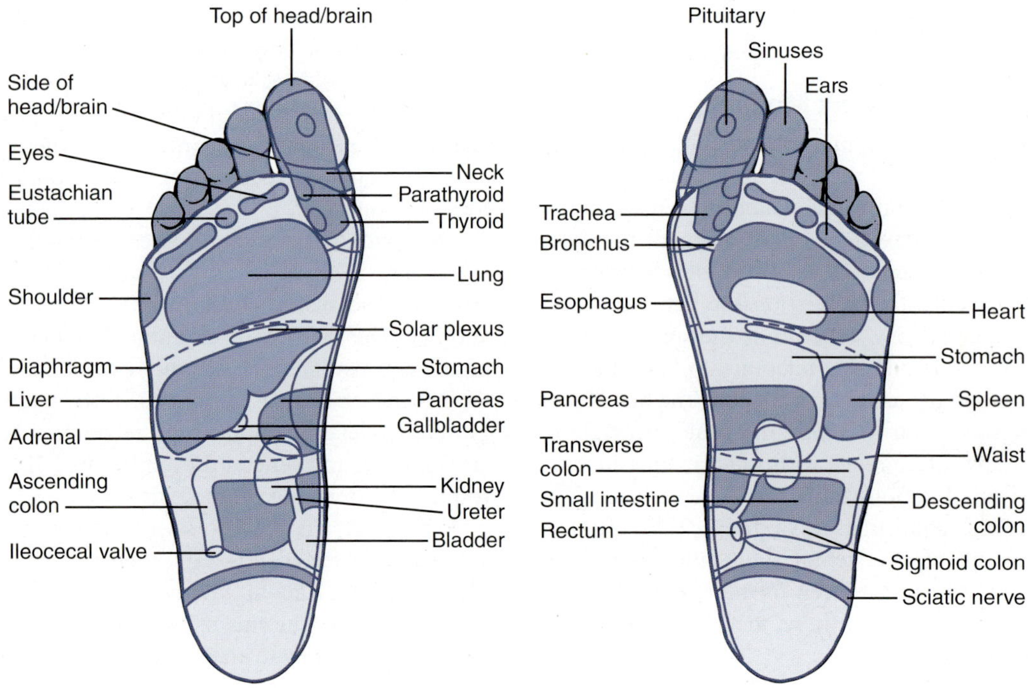

Fig. 3.1 Reflexology Foot Maps. The densest concentration of reflex areas is found on the soles of the feet.

the body of an individual, the frequencies radiated by the object or field interact with the individual's field. Biofields have been described traditionally by the ancient Indians as *prana,* by the Chinese as *qi* (or *chi*), by the Japanese as *ki*, by Jewish mysticism as "astral light," and by Christian painters as "halos." Current practices involving *biofield therapies* are intended to affect a patient's energy field for the purpose of healing by having a healer place their hands in or through them; the therapist's healing force restores the patient. Examples of this type of energy therapy include *Reiki*, *qi gong*, and therapeutic touch. *Reiki*, a Japanese word meaning "universal life energy," is an ancient form of healing by touch and is based on the belief that when spiritual energy is channeled through a Reiki practitioner, the patient's spirit is healed. It is a way of channeling this energy through one's hands, enabling the body to accelerate its own healing process. *Qi gong* is a Chinese technique that combines slow-moving meditative postures, meditation, stretching, and regulation of breathing to enhance the flow of *qi* in the body to enhance immune function, improve circulation, and achieve wellness.

Bioelectromagnetic-based therapies involve the unconventional use of electromagnetic fields. Positioning external magnetic fields near or around the person, usually by placing magnets on the body, into clothing, or in mattresses, is an example of this type of therapy.

Acupuncture is an age-old healing art of traditional Chinese medicine in which thin needles are placed into the body to allow *qi* (energy) to flow unimpeded. Advances in acupuncture allow for the attachment of electrodes to the needles through which small currents are passed. The dominant form of therapy in traditional Chinese medicine is acupuncture. To understand acupuncture, the reader must first understand the concept of meridians. Meridians are a unique part of Chinese medical theory; they are the channels through which *qi* flows among the organs, adjusting and harmonizing their activities. The meridians, which are not blood vessels, are 20 to 50 μm in diameter and link together all the fundamental substances and organs. They are bilateral and exist beneath the surface of the skin. The places at which the branches reach the skin surface are designated as acupuncture sites. Each meridian has an entry and exit point; energy enters through the entry point and flows through to the exit point. There are 12 primary meridians of the body, each running vertically, bringing *qi* and the other four essential substances to specific parts of the body. No part of the body is without *qi*; a blockage causes an imbalance in the flow of the life force. In Fig. 3.3, a male model demonstrates where the meridians and acupuncture sites are indicated. Fig. 3.4A depicts the clinician placing an acupuncture needle in the buttocks of a male with sciatica; Fig. 3.4B shows all the needles in position.

Shen is the energy unique to human life that is responsible for the spirit, consciousness, emotions, and thoughts. It is associated with the force of human personality. *Jing* is the fluid that is the basis of reproduction and development. *Xue* (pronounced "schwhey") moves in the same channels as *qi* and is similar to blood but is produced by food, refined in the spleen, and transported to the lungs, where nutritive *qi* turns it into *xue. Jin-ye* is all fluids other than *xue*. It includes sweat, urine, saliva, mucus, bile, and gastric juice. These five essential substances constitute the basis for the Chinese traditional medical system.

Acupuncture is used for prevention and treatment of disease and for maintenance of health by manipulating the flow of *qi* and *xue*, or body fluids, through the body channels. Although most Western clinicians have heard of acupuncture, few understand it. The Chinese have used acupuncture for more than 6000 years to stimulate or awaken the natural power within the body. It is estimated that there are more than 14 million individuals a year in the United States who try acupuncture. Acupuncture involves the use of nine types of fine needles, each with a specific purpose. There are as many as 2000 specific

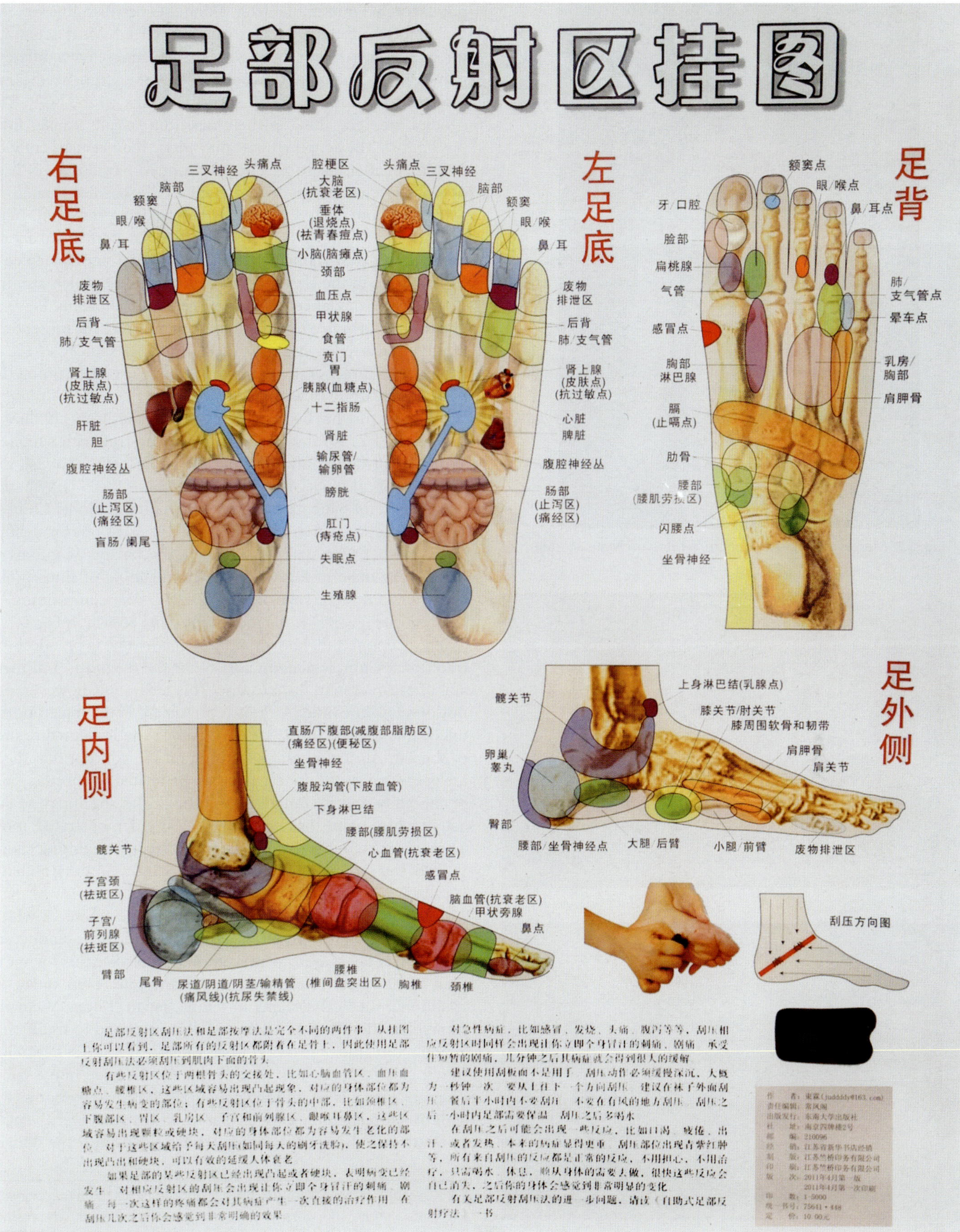

Fig. 3.2 As the title in Chinese reads, this is a poster of the reflex areas of the foot. (*Artist unknown.*)

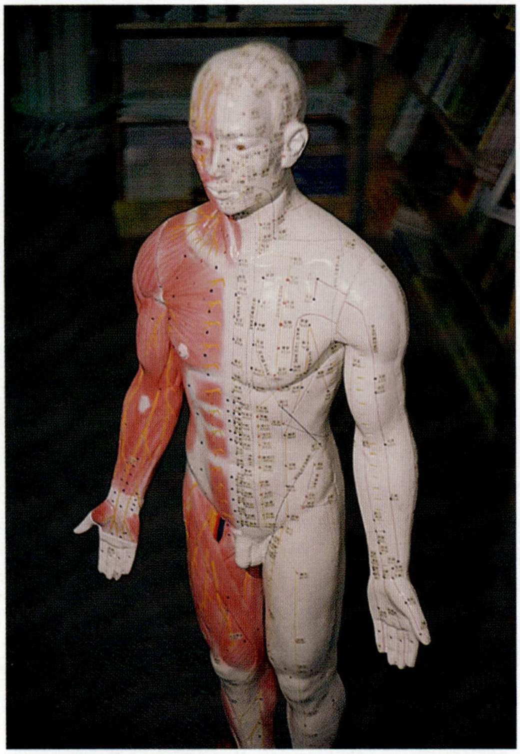

Fig. 3.3 Meridians and Acupuncture Sites on Male Model.

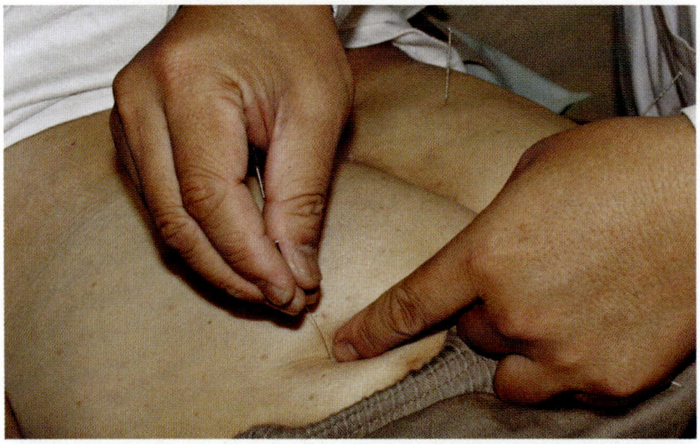

A

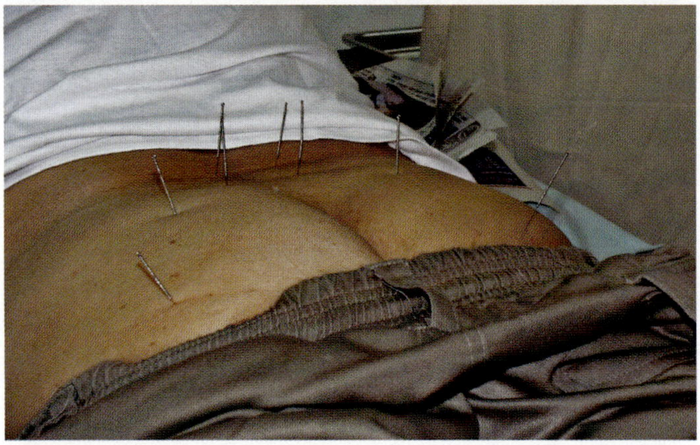

B

Fig. 3.4 Acupuncture. (A) Healthcare professional inserting needles into a patient with sciatica. (B) Needles in position.

points, each 3 mm in diameter, along the meridian lines on the skin into which these needles can be inserted. Most acupuncturists use only 150 of these points. The Chinese have different names for each acupuncture point. The acupuncture needles are inserted to various depths at strategic points on the body. The needles are very thin, so their insertion usually causes little discomfort. The acupuncturist may move the needles gently or twirl them after insertion. The practitioner may also apply heat or mild electric pulses to the needle. The needles remain in place for about 15 to 20 minutes before being removed. Acupuncture is generally considered safe when performed by an experienced, well-trained acupuncturist using sterile needles.

Examples of the classic acupuncture needles, which also include scalpel and lancet-like instruments, are shown in Fig. 3.5. The thin filiform needles marked "1" and "2" are the most commonly used needles in the United States. These needles act as antennae to direct *qi* to organs of the body. At other times, the needles may drain *qi* when it is excessive.

Acupuncture has been used to treat illnesses from childhood to old age. Fig. 3.6 depicts an acupuncture tray with supplies. While lecturing in Taiwan, I had the good fortune to visit the China Medical College in Taichung, where there is a special department for patients who wish to obtain traditional Chinese medical treatment. The child shown in Fig. 3.7A was brought in by his mother, who stated that her son was having symptoms of a cold. The male in Fig. 3.7B was complaining of sinus problems, and the older female in Fig. 3.7C was complaining of headaches. Fig. 3.7D is the foot of the child shown in Fig. 3.7A.

Ear acupuncture, known as *auriculotherapy*, is practiced by traditional Chinese acupuncturists for the diagnosis and therapy of organ system disharmony. This technique, however, did not develop in China. A French physician, Paul Nogier, introduced this concept in 1958. Fig. 3.8 shows the acupuncture sites of the ear. Auriculotherapy is based on the concept that there are specific parts of the ear that can be related to specific parts of the body and its functions. Although the specificity of ear acupuncture points has never been clearly demonstrated, most acupuncturists agree that ear acupuncture has a calming effect. Indeed, the most frequently cited ear point used in treatments is called *shenmen*, or spirit gate.

Moxibustion[14] is a specific form of acupuncture in which herbs, moxa,[d] are burned to stimulate specific acupuncture sites. It has been used to prevent and cure diseases for more than 2500 years. It plays an important role, even today, in traditional medical systems in China, Japan, Korea, Vietnam, Mongolia, and Tibet. If a disease fails to respond to traditional acupuncture, moxibustion is used. Moxa leaves are either rolled into a cigar-shaped stick or pulverized and made into a cone. The moxa stick is lit, and the glowing end is held over the vital spot to be treated; the cone is placed on the skin over the acupuncture site and ignited, letting it burn slowly near the skin, as

[d]A substance created from dried leaves of the herbs Chinese mugwort *(Artemisia argyi)* and wormwood *(Artemisia absinthium)*. Artemisia is a large genus of herbaceous plants of more than 300 species belonging to the daisy family. They are known for their powerful chemical constituents in their essential oils. Sagebrush is a member of this genus.

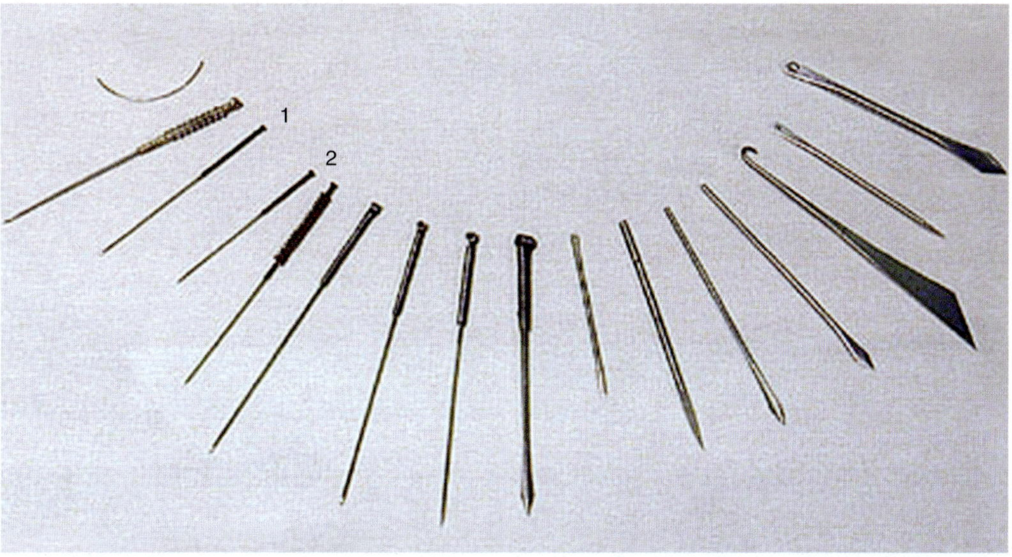

Fig. 3.5 Classic Acupuncture Needles. Thin filiform needles (#1 and #2) are most commonly used in the United States.

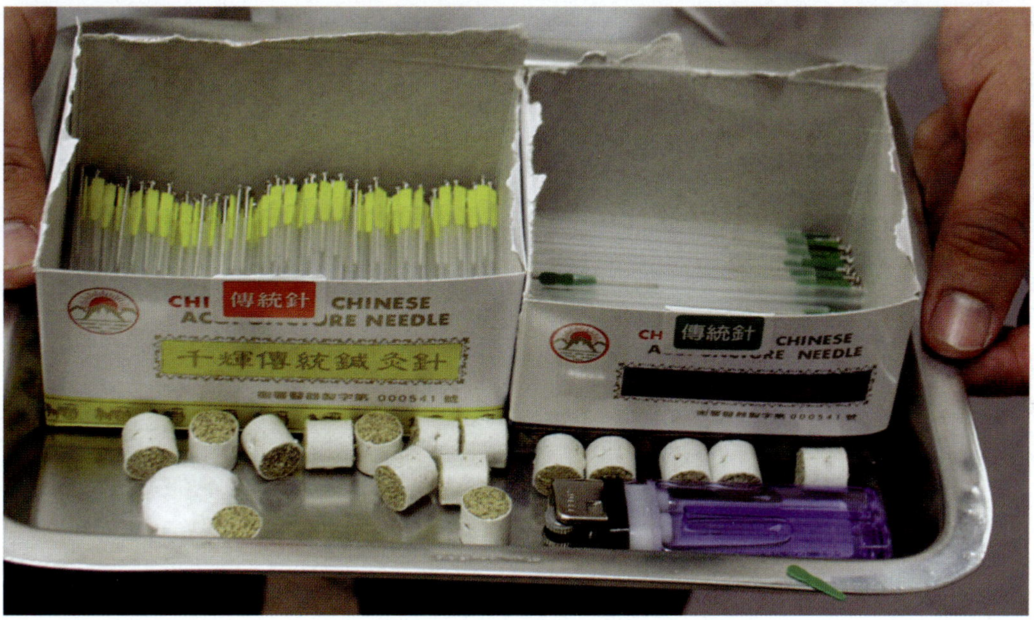

Fig. 3.6 Acupuncture Supplies.

shown in Fig. 3.9A. Often, the rolled moxa cone is placed on the end of an acupuncture needle and then lit to enhance the acupuncture therapy; this is shown in Fig. 3.9B in a patient complaining of lower back pain. According to alternative medicine providers, the heat generated during moxibustion helps increase the flow of *qi* throughout the body via the meridians. Stimulating *qi* is essential to achieving health and wellness. Moxibustion is used for treating a wide range of conditions in which there is an excess of *yin* (cold) and is contraindicated for heat and excess *yang* (warm) disharmonies. A bibliometric analysis[15] on the papers published from 1954 to 2007 in China showed that up to 364 kinds of diseases can be treated with moxibustion. The most common indications for moxibustion therapy are malposition, diarrhea, colitis, incontinence, and dysmenorrhea. It has also been used for knee osteoarthritis, temporomandibular joint disturbances, soft tissue injury, heel pain, asthma, urinary retention, and herpes zoster.[16]

In November 1997, the NIH[17] convened a panel of independent experts to review the clinical studies of all forms of acupuncture. The panel noted that the results of several studies, many sponsored by the NIH, were equivocal because of design, sample size, and other factors, complicated by inherent difficulties in the use of appropriate control subjects. The panel did agree that acupuncture has been shown to have promising results for relief of the following:

1. Adult postoperative nausea and vomiting
2. Nausea and vomiting secondary to chemotherapy
3. Postoperative dental pain

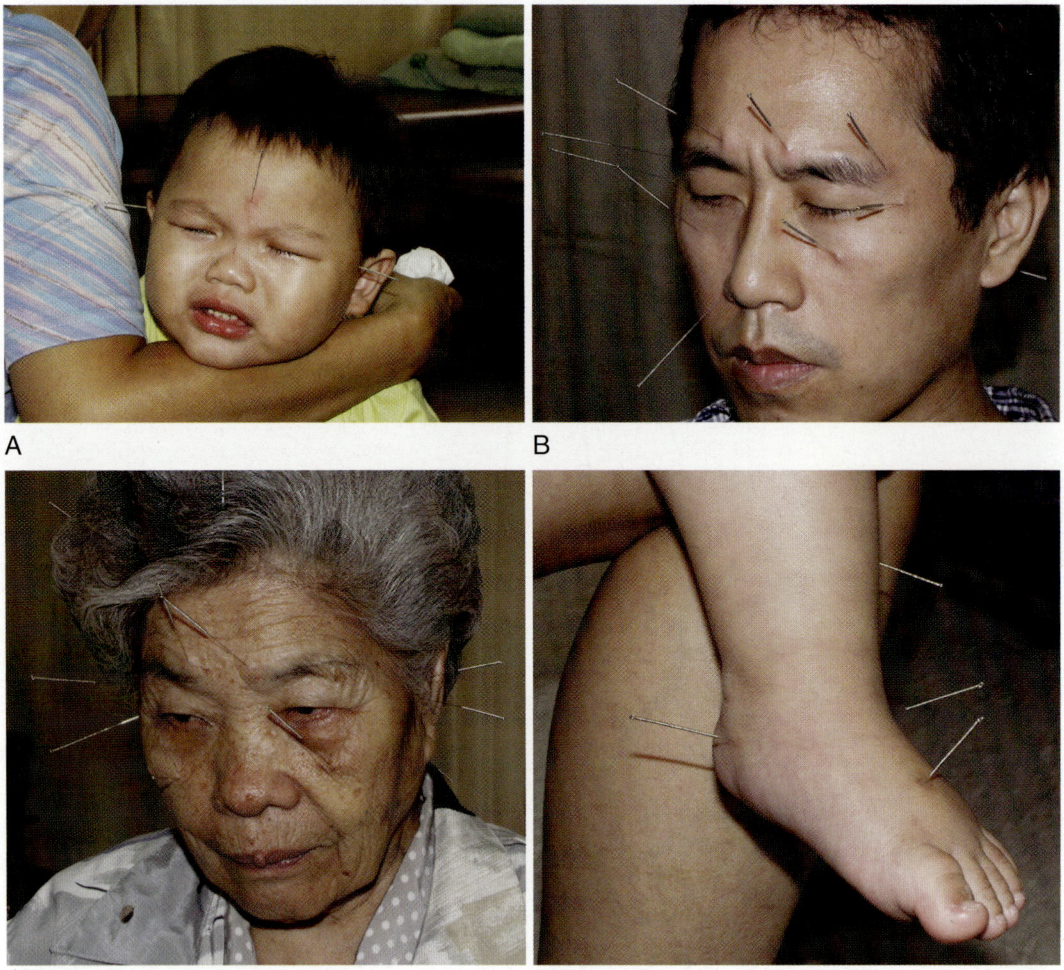

A B C D

Fig. 3.7 Acupuncture. (A) Child with upper respiratory infection, under treatment. (B) Male with sinus headache, under treatment. (C) Female with headache, under treatment. (D) Foot of the child with upper respiratory infection shown in (A).

The panel determined that acupuncture may be useful as an adjunct treatment, as an acceptable alternative, or as part of a comprehensive management program for addiction, stroke rehabilitation, headache, menstrual cramps, tennis elbow, fibromyalgia, myofascial pain, osteoarthritis, low back pain, carpal tunnel syndrome, and asthma. Further research is likely to uncover additional areas in which acupuncture interventions will be useful.

TRADITIONAL CHINESE MEDICINE

There are many traditional medical practices. Of particular note are the Chinese, Ayurvedic, and Greek systems of healing. Owing to the limitations of space in this chapter, one traditional system of healing, Chinese medicine, which has influenced so many other systems, is considered.

With more than 21.4 million people, the Asian and Pacific Islander group represents the third largest minority group in the United States in 2016.[18] The Chinese approach to healing is a rich and complex tradition. It emphasizes the importance of promoting balance and harmony in body, mind, and spirit, and has become the foundation for many other traditional medical systems. Chinese medicine had its origins more than 2500 years ago and is still in use to treat millions of people in China and throughout the world. As a result, to the traditional Chinese healers, allopathic medicine is new and experimental.

Chinese medicine is based on the idea that the human system is a microcosmic mirror of the macrocosmic universe. This means that no one thing can exist without the existence of the others. Each person is subject to the same laws that govern the stars, the planets, the trees, and the land. *Tao,* sometimes translated as "the infinite origin," is the single unified source from which all life and the entire universe originated; it is the way to ultimate reality. To follow the laws of nature is to be blessed with good health, long life, and good fortune. Because nature is the most enduring manifestation of *tao*, much of the traditional terminology of Chinese medicine is derived from natural phenomena, such as fire and water, wind and heat, and dryness and dampness. When the elements in the human body remain in balance, "fair weather" is said to prevail in the body, and the human is well both physically and mentally.

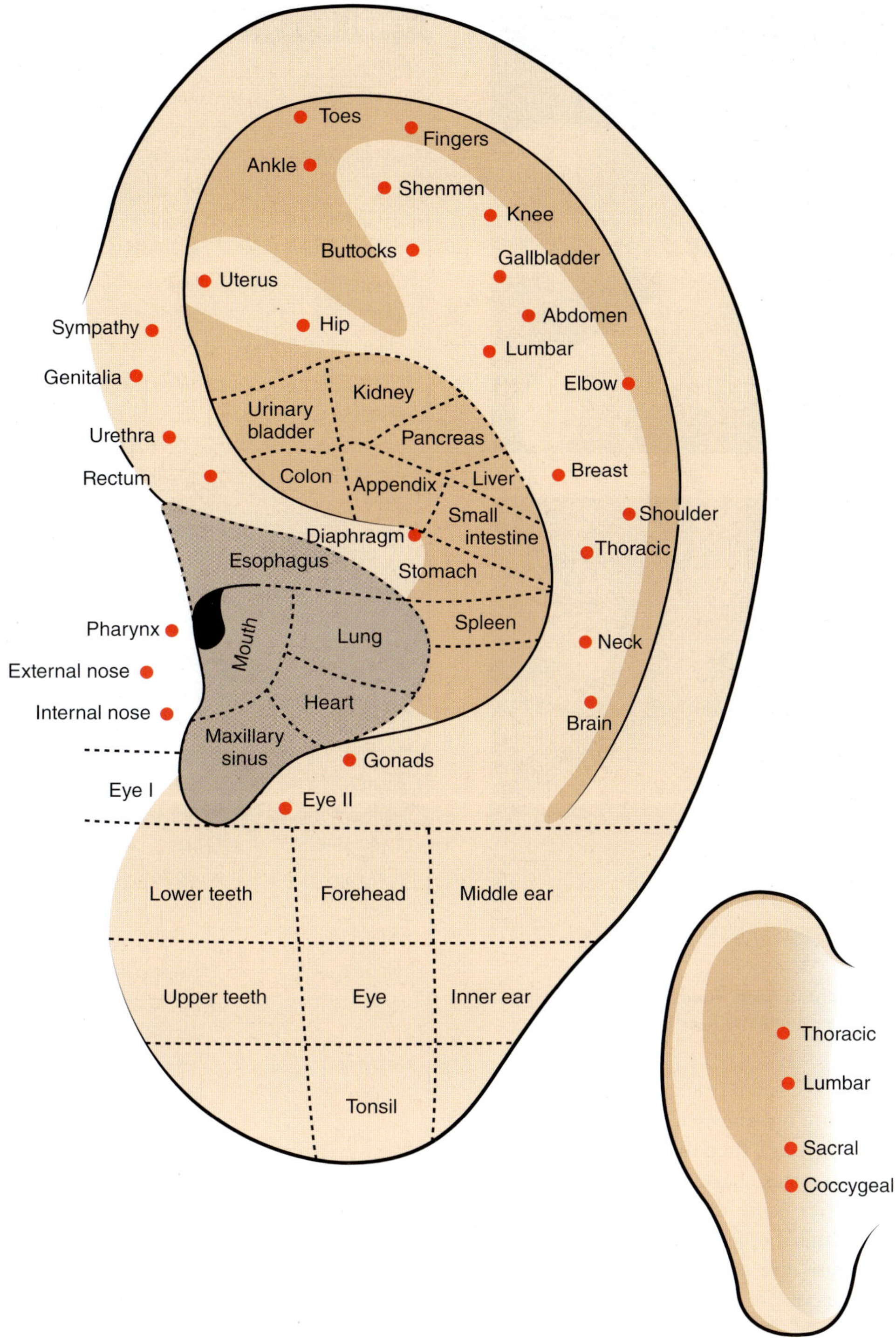

Fig. 3.8 Acupuncture Sites of the Ear. (Redrawn from Wensel LO, editor: *Acu-puncture in medical practice*, Reston, VA, 1980, Reston Publishing Co., Appleton & Lange.)

Yin and Yang

Tao created two opposing forces, *yin* and *yang*, which are opposites that combine to create everything in the world. The concept of *yin* and *yang* pervades all Chinese thinking and is fundamental to understanding Chinese medicine. They are two opposing forces. All phenomena in the world derive from the confrontation and interactions of these forces. *Yin* is a force of darkness and is associated with such qualities as earth, moon, night, water, interior body, femininity, cold, rest, passivity, emptiness, introverted, and negative energy. *Yang* is a force of brightness and is associated with heaven, sun, daylight, fire, exterior body, masculinity, heat, stimulation, activity, excitement, vigor, fullness, extroverted, and positive energy. *Yin* and *yang* must be properly balanced and harmonious to be healthy.

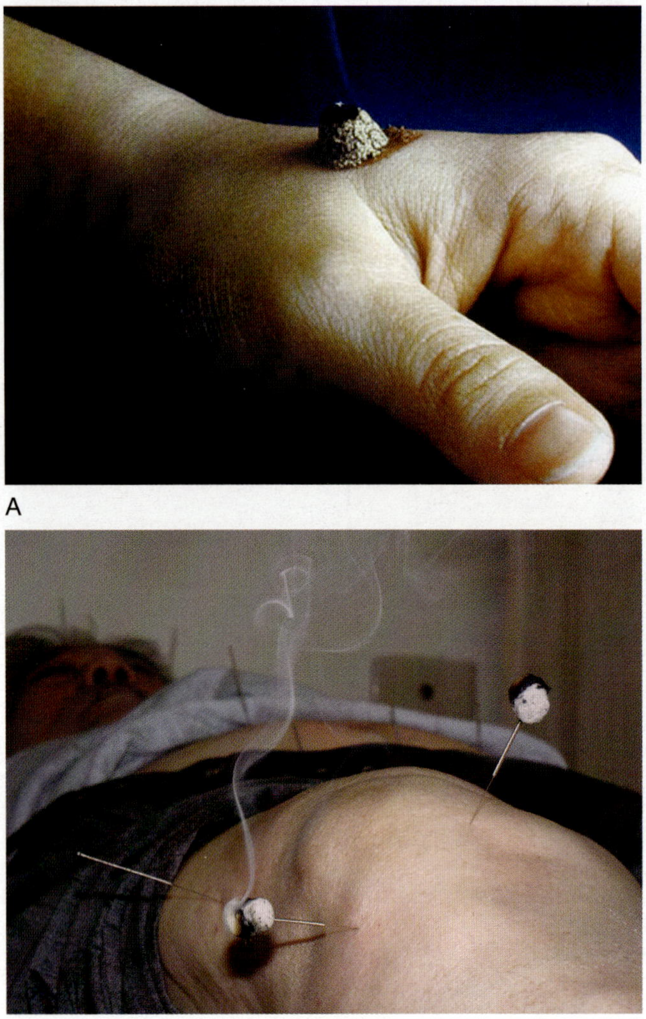

A

B

Fig. 3.9 Moxibustion. (A) Moxibustion cone. (B) Moxibustion and acupuncture therapy in a patient with low back pain.

TABLE 3.1 Aspects of *Yin* and *Yang* Polarity		
Aspect	***Yin***	***Yang***
Cosmic bodies	Moon	Sun
	Earth	Heaven
Energy condition	Passive	Aggressive
	Mentally active	Physically active
	Asleep	Awake
	Weak	Strong
	Empty	Full
	Deficient	Excessive
	Cold	Hot
Time of day	Night	Day
Season	Fall	Spring
	Winter	Summer
Magnetic pole	Negative	Positive
Speed	Slow	Fast
Body location	Interior	Exterior
	Lower torso	Upper torso
	Lower extremities	Upper extremities
	Feet	Head
	Right side	Left side
	Back	Front
Gender	Female	Male
Numbers	Even	Odd
Distance	Near	Far
Relative moisture	Very moist, saturated	Dry
Quality of light	Dark	Light
Acid/base	Alkaline	Acid
Speed	Slow	Fast
Metabolism	Anabolism	Catabolism
Psychic type	Contemplative	Active
	Introverted	Extroverted
	Gentle	Robust
Movement	Contraction	Expansion
Position	Descending	Ascending
	Below	Above
	Rest	Activity

Disease results when they are unbalanced. As an example, if a disease is recognized as hot *(yang)*, then medications and treatments must be cold *(yin)* to restore harmony and health.

General words to describe *yang* diseases include "warm," "hot," "inflamed," "spasm," "full," or "acute." Solid cancers, kidney stones, arthritis, and bursitis are examples of *yang* diseases. Words to describe *yin* diseases are "coolness," "laxity," "depletion," "emptiness," "deficiency," "weakness," "low energy," and "stasis." Osteoporosis, hypothyroidism, adrenal insufficiency, iron deficiency anemia, and depression are examples of *yin* diseases. An excess of *yin* (cold) can cause illnesses such as insomnia and dry mouth. Conversely, a *yang* (hot) deficiency can cause cold limbs and a sickly complexion. Table 3.1 lists the aspects of *yin* and *yang* polarity. Table 3.2 lists some important *yin* and *yang* signs in the body.

TABLE 3.2 *Yin* and *Yang* Signs in the Body		
Body Signs	**Yin Signs**	**Yang Signs**
Face	Pale face, low spirit, feels cold, cold limbs, tired and weak	Red face, fever, hot sensation, agitated
Voice	Low, soft voice	Strong voice
Appetite	Reduced	Increased
Urine	Copious, clear urine	Dark yellow urine
Bowels	Constipation	Diarrhea
Tongue	Pale, swollen tongue	Bright red tongue
Pulse	Slow, weak, frail pulse	Rapid, strong

Important Chinese Concepts of Medicine

There are two other important concepts in traditional Chinese medicine. The first is that the occurrence of disease represents a failure in preventive healthcare. The second is that health is a responsibility shared equally by the patient and healthcare professional. According to a Chinese proverb, "The superior physician teaches his patients how to stay healthy." In traditional Chinese medicine, the healthcare professional treats the patient as a whole system rather than dealing with separate parts, as is common in Western medicine. An important belief is that the mind is engaged to control and guide energy to heal and repair the body. Chinese medicine is a system of preserving health and curing disease that treats the mind, body, and spirit as a whole.

Whereas the Western healthcare professional starts with a symptom and tries to search for the cause of a specific disease, the traditional Chinese healthcare professional directs their attention to the whole patient and forms a "pattern of disharmony." This pattern describes the situation of "imbalance" in the patient's body. The traditional Chinese healthcare professional asks not "Which *A* is causing *B*?" but "What is the relationship between *A* and *B*?" The patterns of disharmony provide the framework for therapy. In Chinese medicine, a person does not catch the flu; a person develops a disharmony. If a patient requires an antibiotic, herbs or acupuncture may be used to dispel the disharmony. Regardless of the ailment, the mind, body, and spirit must be treated as a whole. Healing is achieved by rebalancing *yin* and *yang* and restoring harmony in the whole person.

The traditional Chinese healthcare professional inspects a patient in four stages: looking, listening or smelling, asking, and touching. Inspection of the tongue *(tongue diagnosis)* and palpation of the pulse *(pulse diagnosis)* are the two most important examinations. The tongue is believed to be the clearest indicator of the nature of the disharmony. The Chinese recognize more than 100 different conditions of internal energy imbalance, based on features of the tongue: the color, shape, moisture, coating, thickness, cracks, and texture of the tongue "fur." The condition of the five major organ-energy systems is evaluated according to their corresponding areas on the tongue. These systems are the kidneys, liver, spleen, lungs, and heart.

Pulse Diagnosis

In traditional Chinese medicine, *pulse diagnosis* is one of the major clinical diagnostic methods. It is predicated on the belief that disharmonies of the body leave a specific impression on the pulse. Fig. 3.10 depicts an ancient description, from a scroll, of pulse diagnosis. In traditional Chinese medicine, the radial pulse is divided into three positions on each wrist. The first pulse closest to the wrist is the *cun* position, the second is the *guan* position, and the third pulse position furthest away from the wrist is the *chi*. The strengths and weaknesses of these positions are assessed at three different depths. The traditional Chinese healthcare professional can evaluate the lungs, spleen, and kidney *yang* on the right wrist, and the heart, liver, and kidney *yin* on the left wrist.

The Chinese have used iron balls for health since the Ming Dynasty (1368–1644). The balls, originally solid, today are hollow with a sounding plate inside them. Each pair consists of one that produces a high tone and the other a low tone. The iron

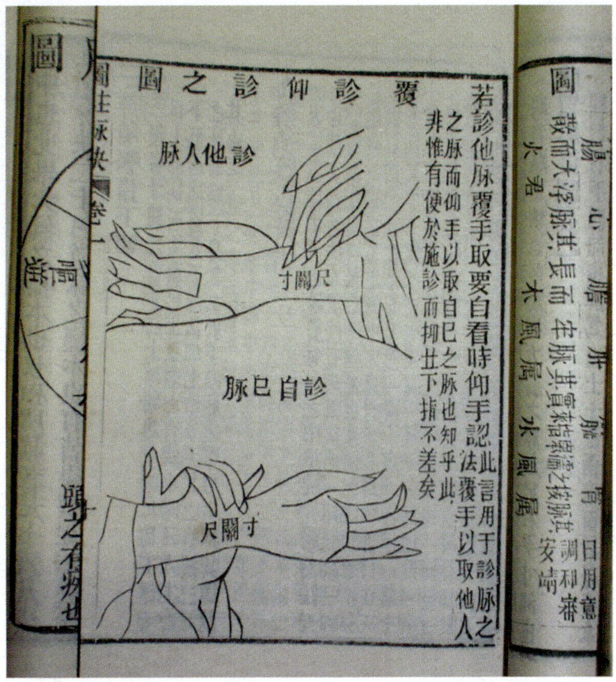

Fig. 3.10 Ancient Chinese Description of Pulse Diagnosis.

balls are believed to enhance the user's health and well-being. By moving the iron balls with the fingers, various acupuncture points on the hand are stimulated, resulting in increased circulation of vital energy and blood to the internal organs. Those who use these balls believe that, with daily use, the brain can be kept in good health with improved memory, fatigue will be relieved, and life will be prolonged.

Five Element Theory

Another major concept in traditional Chinese medicine is the *five element theory,* also known as the *five phases (wu xing)*. This theory is an attempt to classify phenomena in terms of five quintessential processes represented by wood, fire, earth, metal, and water. Each phase has qualities and functions that describe the various processes in the body and their interactions with the environment. The phases are as follows:

- *Wood:* proper and straight; characterizes the liver, gallbladder, anger, sour taste, and windy weather
- *Fire:* ascending and blooming; characterizes the heart, small intestine, joy, bitter taste, and hot weather
- *Earth:* solid and quiet; characterizes the spleen, stomach, melancholy, sweet taste, and damp weather
- *Metal:* firm and strong; characterizes the lung, colon, grief, pungent taste, and dry weather
- *Water:* inward and clear; characterizes the kidney, urinary bladder, fear, salty taste, and cold weather

Traditional Chinese healers use this theory to diagnose and treat illness. Often plotted on a circle, the five phases show a unity in the world and in the body. Many conditions correspond to the five phases. Table 3.3 lists some of the medically relevant somatic associations of the five phases.

TABLE 3.3 Somatic Associations of the Five Phases

	Wood	Fire	Earth	Metal	Water
Taste	Sour	Bitter	Sweet	Pungent	Salty
Yin organ	Liver	Heart	Spleen	Lungs	Kidney
Yang organ	Gallbladder	Small intestine	Stomach	Colon	Urinary bladder
Orifice	Eyes	Tongue	Mouth	Nose	Ears
Tissue	Tendons	Blood vessels	Flesh	Skin	Bones

Acupressure and Massage

In addition to acupuncture, acupressure and massage are also important aspects of the traditional Chinese healing arts. Acupressure, or *dian hsueh,* is the forerunner of the Japanese technique called *shiatsu.* Acupressure is the technique of transferring energy from the therapist's body directly into the patient's system by pressing thumb and hands into the patient's vital areas. Acupressure involves the application of deep pressure to the same points along the channels used in acupuncture. Once a point is located, rotating pressure is applied for 10 to 15 seconds, released, and then repeated as often as the therapist believes necessary. Massage *(tui na)*, in contrast, focuses primarily on the muscle masses, ear, abdomen, foot, and spine. Massage offers the energy of acupuncture, the serenity of meditation, and spiritual refreshment. *Tui na* stimulates circulation and energy within the body, activates and drains the lymph, tones the muscles, and enhances nerve function.

Tui Na Therapy

Tui na therapy is accompanied by cupping, a technique called *ba guan,* in which glass or bamboo cups containing small amounts of alcohol are applied to the areas of disease and the alcohol is ignited, creating a vacuum inside. The underlying tissue swells up, and the vacuum pressure draws out heat, damp, or wind energies. This technique has been adapted by many other ethnic groups. Fig. 3.11 shows the glass cups and a modern suction device for their application.

Chinese Herbal Therapy

Chinese herbal therapy encompasses eight methods: sweating, vomiting, purging, harmonizing, warming, removing, supplementing, and reducing. There are more than 5500 herbal remedies known in traditional Chinese medicine, fewer than 10% of which are commonly used. Different parts of plants, such as the leaves, roots, stems, flowers, and seeds are used as well as some animal products and minerals. Through clinical experience, Chinese medicine recognizes that each herbal remedy has an affinity for a particular meridian or organ. If an illness is caused by heat, cooling with herbal therapy is used; if caused by a deficiency, drugs that restore are used. In a manual of traditional Chinese herbal remedies, each herb is listed as to the part of the plant (P) used, the taste and nature (T&N), the meridian (M) or organ affected, the actions (Act), the amount and form (A&F) of use, and the cautions and contraindications (C&C). For example,[19]

- *Acorus gramineus* (Japanese sweet flag)
- Shichangpu
- P: Root stalk
- T&N: Acrid; slightly warm
- M: Heart, liver, spleen
- Act: To open ostia and conduits, to eliminate sputum, to regulate *qi,* to mobilize blood, to disperse wind, to excrete dampness
- A&F: 3 to 6 g (fresh 9 to 24 g) as decoction, pill, or powder
- C&C: Waning *yin* with waxing *yang,* restlessness with diaphoresis, cough, vomiting of blood, spontaneous semen emission

The photograph in Fig. 3.12 was taken in a traditional Chinese herbal pharmacy in San Francisco's Chinatown. Note the prescription written in Chinese, which is necessary to purchase these herbal medications. Fig. 3.13 shows the modern herbal pharmacy at the China Medical College in Taichung, Taiwan. Fig. 3.14 shows a computer-generated prescription for herbal medications.

The use of medicinal herbs is prevalent and growing. The healthcare professionals must be cognizant of the commonly used herbs and their benefits and limitations. Some herbs can interfere with prescribed medications and with surgery. Bleeding

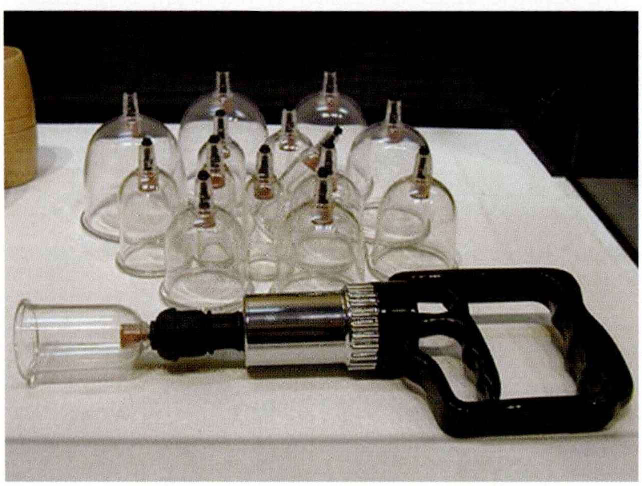

Fig. 3.11 *Ba guan* (Cupping) Devices.

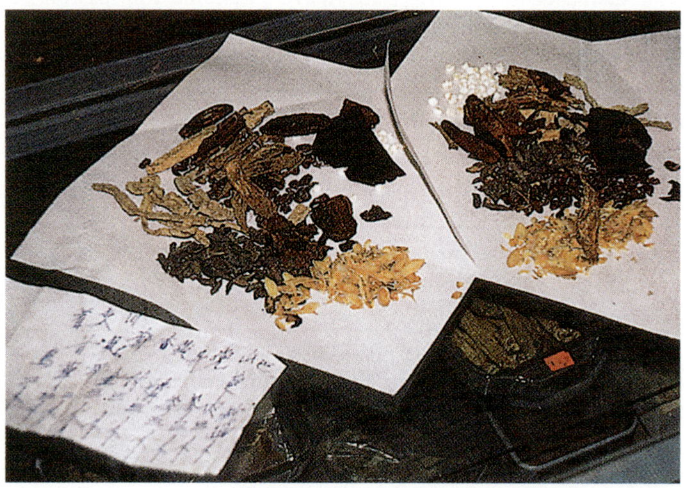

Fig. 3.12 Herbal Chinese Medications, With Prescription in Lower Left.

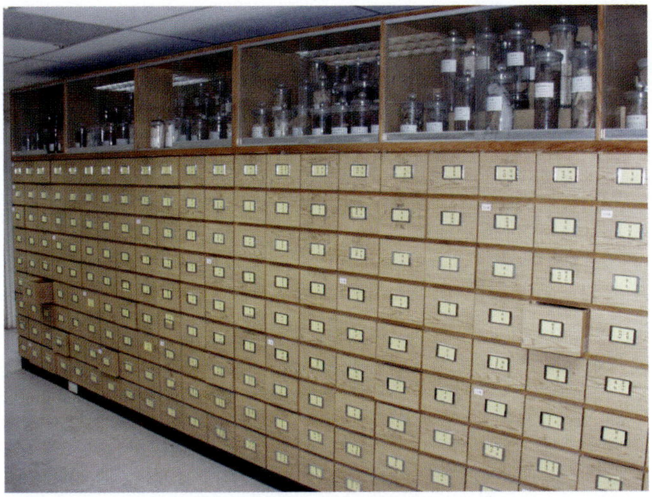

A

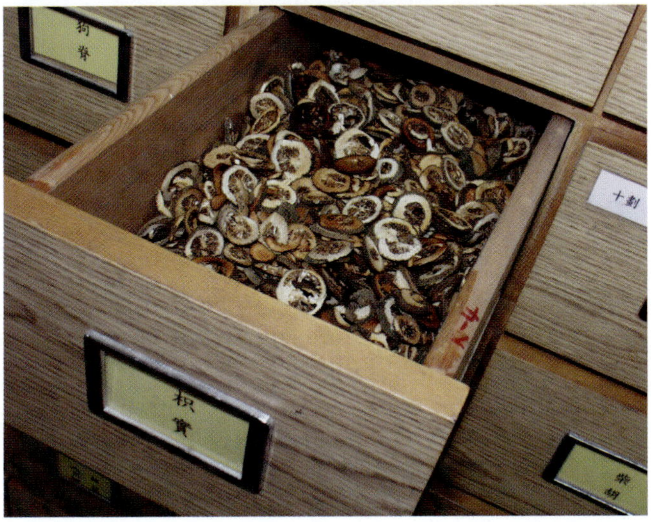

B

Fig. 3.13 (A) and (B) Modern herbal pharmacy at China Medical College in Taichung, Taiwan.

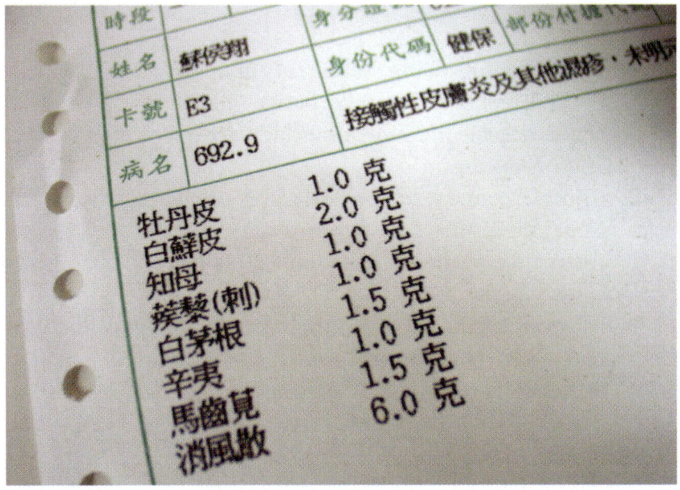

Fig. 3.14 Computer-Generated Prescription for Herbal Medications.

is a common problem. Certain antioxidants may interfere with chemotherapy. The use of medicinal herbs in the West goes back to the days of Paracelsus (1493–1541), who said, "The dose determines the poison." More clinical trials of safety and efficacy of medicinal herbs are needed to help understand the active ingredients and herb actions.

CONCLUDING THOUGHTS

CAM therapies have long played a key role in healthcare. Most healthcare professionals have failed to recognize the magnitude of these forms of healing. Many of the therapies, however, are not based on any sound medical knowledge. Some have been derived from ethnic and folk traditions, semireligious cults, metaphysical movements, and healthcare groups who rebel against technology and the perceived impersonality of 21st-century medical care. Unfortunately, marketing terms such as "miracle cure," "new discovery," and "satisfaction guaranteed" attract patients looking for cures for diseases for which there are no cures. "Purify," "detoxify," and "energize" sound impressive, but they are often used to cover up the lack of scientific proof of efficacy. Finally, healthcare professionals must advise patients that the word *natural* does not always mean that the therapy is safe, and these products may have drug-like effects that may be deleterious to their health and have dangerous interactions with prescribed medications. Therefore, healthcare professionals should look for solid scientific studies. A lack of solid evidence does not always mean these treatments do not work, but it does mean they have not been proven effective.

This chapter has introduced the healthcare professional to the richness of several of these CAM therapies. Ideally, the healthcare professional is better prepared now to deal with patients of diverse backgrounds who use CAM and with the challenges of caring for those patients in the United States. The healthcare professional must be open-minded with regard to these therapies and able to incorporate alternative and complementary therapies into Western medicine. All healthcare professionals must become familiar with CAM practices, the efficacies of the various practices, and the potential risks and benefits from their use.

REVIEW QUESTIONS

1. **Which of the following statements is *incorrect*?**
   - **A.** Complementary and alternative medicine (CAM) includes diverse medical and healthcare systems, practices, and products.
   - **B.** Complementary medicine is used in place of conventional medicine.
   - **C.** Alternative medicine is used instead of conventional medicine.
   - **D.** Integrative medicine combines conventional medical and CAM therapies for which there is some scientific evidence of safety and effectiveness.
   - **E.** About 40% of the American population uses at least one of the CAM therapies.
2. **Which of the following statements about tea is *incorrect*?**
   - **A.** Tea is the world's second most popular beverage.
   - **B.** Green tea accounts for about 20% of all tea consumed.
   - **C.** Green tea can improve the health of the entire body.
   - **D.** The heart and lungs benefit the most from green tea consumption.
   - **E.** Green tea is rich in active polyphenols.
3. **Antioxidants may help the body protect against many cancers. These include:**
   - **A.** Breast cancer
   - **B.** Colon cancer
   - **C.** Skin cancer
   - **D.** Prostate cancer
   - **E.** All of the above
4. **The National Center for Complementary and Alternative Medicine (NCCAM) has classified complementary and alternative medicine into several major categories. These include all the following *except:***
   - **A.** Biologically based therapies
   - **B.** Energy therapies
   - **C.** Acupuncture therapies
   - **D.** Mind–body therapies
   - **E.** Manipulative therapies
5. **All the following are body-based methods *except:***
   - **A.** Massage therapy
   - **B.** Chiropractic
   - **C.** Osteopathic
   - **D.** Reflexology
   - **E.** Moxibustion
6. **Reflexology is used to treat a variety of conditions. It includes pressure applied to:**
   - **A.** Hands
   - **B.** Feet
   - **C.** Ears
   - **D.** Cranium
   - **E.** All the above
7. **The greatest concentration of reflex areas is found on the:**
   - **A.** Soles of the feet
   - **B.** Occipital region of the cranium
   - **C.** Solar plexus
   - **D.** Axillae
   - **E.** Eyes
8. **Which of the following statements about acupuncture is *false*?**
   - **A.** Acupuncture is a traditional Chinese medicine in which thin needles are placed into the body to block energy flow.
   - **B.** Meridians are channels in which qi flows throughout the body's organs.
   - **C.** The meridians are not blood vessels and are 20–50 μm in diameter.
   - **D.** The meridians exist beneath the skin's surface.
   - **E.** There are 12 primary meridians of the body running vertically.
9. **The National Institutes of Health Consensus Statement of 1997 agreed that acupuncture has promising results for all of the following *except:***
   - **A.** Adult postoperative nausea and vomiting
   - **B.** Vomiting secondary to chemotherapy
   - **C.** Postoperative dental pain
   - **D.** Multiple sclerosis
   - **E.** Stroke rehabilitation
10. **Which of the following is *true*?**
    - **A.** Traditional Chinese medicine is based on the idea that the human system is a microcosmic mirror of the macrocosmic universe.
    - **B.** *Yang* is associated with the lower extremities, while *yin* is with the upper extremities.
    - **C.** *Yin* is a force of brightness.
    - **D.** *Yang* is a force of passivity.
    - **E.** If a disease is recognized as a *yang* disorder, then medications must be *yang* to restore harmony and health.

REFERENCES

Available online.

BIBLIOGRAPHY

Available online.

4

Putting the History Together

Mark H. Swartz

The doctor may also learn more about the illness from the way the patient tells the story than from the story itself.

James B. Herrick (1861–1954)

In the first two chapters, the interviewer's questions and the patient's responses were discussed. In this chapter, these materials are put together to create a mock interview. In the following interview, note the way in which the interviewer allows the patient to speak and the way various techniques are incorporated. The footnotes refer to the type of technique used and other important aspects of the interview.

In writing up the history, be precise and well-organized. The patient relates the history in their order; you need to reorganize the facts into the standard form discussed in Chapter 1 (i.e., chief concern, history of present illness, etc.). Your skill in writing up the history will evolve with time as you gather more experience. Make sure that you organize the history in chronological order. **Always record *all* the relevant data obtained.** If data aren't recorded, that data will be lost permanently. Be careful about using abbreviations; they may mean something different to others. As an example, PND often stands for paroxysmal nocturnal dyspnea; however, it is also used to mean postnasal drip (or discharge). Finally, **be objective;** the patient record is no place for editorial or judgmental comments. Your opinion should not be in evidence; **just state the facts.** For example, state "alcohol on breath," not "patient drunk."

INTERVIEW OF MR. JOHN DOE

Mr. John Doe, the patient, is lying comfortably in a two-bed room in St. Mary's Hospital. He is slightly overweight. Mr. Doe is watching television. The interviewer, wearing a white coat, enters the room.

(Interviewer smiles and extends hand for a firm handshake.)

Interviewer: Good morning, I'm Susan Smith, a second-year medical student. My pronouns are "she," "her," and "hers." Are you John Doe? For proper identification, may I ask your date of birth? What are your pronouns? How would you like me to address you?

(Pause; interviewer watches for response.)

Patient: Yes, I am. John is fine. I was born on June 15, 1979, and my pronouns are "he," "him," and "his."

(Extends hand to shake hand of John.)

Interviewer: Nice to meet you, John. I've been asked to interview and examine you today.

(Patient smiles, appearing friendly.)

Patient: Dr. James, the resident, told me you'd be coming to see me.

(Interviewer draws curtain around bed; pulls up a chair at the patient's bedside and sits down; arms in lap.)

Interviewer: Would you mind if we turn off the TV?

(Patient turns off television.)

Patient: Not at all.

Interviewer: How are you feeling today?

Patient: OK. No pain for the past 2 days.

Interviewer: Tell me about the problem that brought you to the hospital, John?[a]

Patient: I've been having terrible chest pain for the past 6 months…

(pause)

I guess I should start at the beginning. About 4 years ago, I started having this strange sensation in my chest. It wasn't pain, exactly. It was a dull, aching discomfort. I didn't pay any attention to it. I guess I should have… Well, anyway, I was able to go to work, play tennis, and have fun. Occasionally when I had an argument at work, I would get this sensation.

(looking sad)

My wife never knew anything about it. I never told her. No one knew. I didn't want to upset them. Then, all of a sudden on July 15, 2022, it happened.

(silence)

Interviewer: It happened?[b]

Patient: Yeah. I had my first heart attack.[c]

I was playing tennis when I got this awful pain. I never had anything like that before. I was just getting ready to serve when this pain hit me. All I could do was lie down on the court. My partner ran over to me, and all I remember was that pain. I woke up in Kings Hospital.

(pause)

They told me I lost consciousness and was taken to the hospital by ambulance. I remember when I came to in the hospital, I still had the pain. I was there for about 6 days.

[a]Inquiring about the chief concern by using an open-ended question.
[b]This is an example of reflection.
[c]The patient is now telling the history of the current illness.

Interviewer: How did you feel when you left the hospital?
Patient: I really felt fine. No more chest pain. My doctor there had given me some pills and said I would be fine.[d]
Interviewer: Then what happened?[e]
Patient: I went back to work after about 3 weeks. I really felt great!
(smiles)
Interviewer: What type of work do you do?
Patient: I'm a lawyer.
Interviewer: You mentioned that this was your first heart attack. Have you had others?
Patient: Unfortunately…
(looking down)
Yes.
Interviewer: Tell me about it.[f]
(leaning forward[g])
Patient: Six months later, I had my second attack.
(pause)
Interviewer: What were you doing?
Patient: Playing tennis.
(silence)
This time I don't remember anything…not even the pain. I remember being on the court and waking up in the intensive care unit of Kings Hospital. They said I had a massive heart attack and had some irregularity of my pulse that made me faint. But I left the hospital in about 6 days feeling much better. I went back to work after 4 weeks at home.
Interviewer: Did you have any tests while you were in the hospital?
Patient: No…
(pause, hand over mouth)
The doctor just gave me some pills to strengthen my heart and for the irregularity.
(silence for 10 seconds)
Interviewer: Your silence makes me think that you want to tell me something.[h]
Patient: I should have listened to him.
(pause, shaking head)
Interviewer: To whom?
Patient: My doctor suggested after my first heart attack that I should have cardiac catheterization. I told him that I was fine, I didn't need it. Even after my second attack, I didn't listen to him.
(pause)
I hope it's not too late.
Interviewer: Too late?
Patient: Yeah. That's why I'm here. I'm going to have the cardiac catheterization tomorrow. Emily finally convinced me to have it.
(pause)
I've really not been able to do anything for the past 6 months.
(pause, looking down)
I had to give up my work at the office. Sure, they still call me for advice, but it's not the same.
(pause, almost tearful)
The commuting by car just got to me.
(pause)
My son and his friends yelling around the house.
(longer pause)
I just can't take it anymore.
Interviewer: What did your doctor tell you about the test?[i]
Patient: The doctor told me if I have some blockage, he'll operate or fix it with a balloon or a type of Roto-Rooter. Will I be normal again?
(pause)
Interviewer: After the study, your doctor will be in the best position to answer that question.[j]
(pause)
Tell me about the pain you've been having.
Patient: It seems I have the pain all the time. I can hardly walk up the stairs at home without getting the pain.
Interviewer: What's the pain like now?
Patient: It's an awful tightness, like a vise…
(closes fist over chest[k])
Right here.
Interviewer: When you get the pain, do you feel it anywhere else?
Patient: Yeah. It goes straight to my back and my left arm. The arm feels so heavy.
Interviewer: Are there any other times when you get the pain?
Patient: It seems I get it with the slightest effort or emotion.
Interviewer: Do you get the pain during sexual intercourse?
Patient: I had to stop even that 6 months ago. I'd get the pain just when I'm about to come…and…and…I'd have to stop.
Interviewer: Have you had any difficulty breathing?
Patient: When I get the pain, I get short of breath.
Interviewer: Do you ever get short of breath without the pain?
Patient: I find I just can't walk far any more without getting winded.
Interviewer: How many level blocks can you walk now without getting short of breath?
Patient: About one block.
Interviewer: How much could you walk 6 months ago?
Patient: I guess about two to three blocks.
Interviewer: Since your heart attack, have you had any skipped beats or fluttering of your heart?

[d]Possibly false reassurance by the physician, or the patient heard what he wanted to hear.
[e]Interviewer continues obtaining information with another open-ended question about the current illness.
[f]An example of verbal facilitation.
[g]An example of nonverbal facilitation.
[h]An example of confrontation.
[i]Inquiring about the patient's understanding of the test.
[j]The interviewer does not want to give false reassurances. Therefore, she chooses not to answer the question directly. Notice how the interviewer gets the narrative back on course.
[k]This example of body language has been termed Levine's sign. It is discussed in Chapter 14, The Heart.

Patient: No, never.
Interviewer: Has anyone ever told you that your cholesterol or fats in your blood were high?[l]
Patient: No.
Interviewer: Have you ever smoked?
Patient: I stopped after my first heart attack.
Interviewer: That's great that you stopped smoking. Congratulations! How much did you smoke?
Patient: About two packs a day.
Interviewer: For how long?
Patient: Oh…since I was about 18.
Interviewer: Have you ever had high blood pressure?
Patient: Yep. My doctor gave me some medications for it, but…but…I never refilled the pills after they ran out. I felt fine.
Interviewer: Do you know how high your pressure was?[m]
Patient: Not really.
Interviewer: Do you have diabetes?
Patient: Thank goodness, I don't. My father does, though. He's been pretty sick lately. He's got some sort of a problem with his eyes. The doctor said that it's from his diabetes. He's going to see a specialist in a couple of weeks. He's had a lot of problems. He broke his hip a few years ago when he was walking our dog. Some big guy came pulling a cart out of the supermarket and knocked my father over. He was hospitalized for several weeks because he really couldn't take care of himself. His hip is fine now. He would…
Interviewer: *(interrupting)* I'm glad his hip is well healed. Is there anyone else in your family who has diabetes?[n]
Patient: No.
Interviewer: Anyone else in your family who's had a heart attack?
Patient: I think my mother's father died of a heart attack.
Interviewer: How old was he?
Patient: About 75.
Interviewer: What about your mother?[o]
Patient: She died when she was age 64…right after my first heart attack. She had stomach cancer. She really suffered…I guess it's a blessing.
Interviewer: Do you have any brothers or sisters?
Patient: My sister is 37 and she's fine.
Interviewer: Any other siblings?
Patient: My brother is 47. He had a heart attack when he was 40.
Interviewer: Do you have any children?
Patient: One boy who's 15.
Interviewer: How's your son's health?
Patient: No problem, except he's a little overweight.
Interviewer: Earlier you mentioned your wife. How are things going?[p]
Patient: Married to a great gal. Emily's the one who convinced me to have the test.[q]
Interviewer: Does anyone in your family have high blood pressure?
Patient: No.
Interviewer: Asthma?
Patient: No.
Interviewer: Tuberculosis?
Patient: No.
Interviewer: Birth defects or congenital diseases?
Patient: Not that I know of.
Interviewer: Have you ever been hospitalized here at St. Mary's Hospital?
Patient: No.[r]
Interviewer: Have you ever been hospitalized at any time other than for your heart attacks?
Patient: I had my appendix taken out when I was 15.
Interviewer: Do you remember the surgeon's name and the hospital?
Patient: I think it was a Dr. Ralph Meyers at Booth Memorial Hospital. We were living in Rochester.
Interviewer: Any other operations?
Patient: No.
Interviewer: Have you ever been hospitalized for any other nonmedical or nonsurgical problem?[s]
Patient: No, what do you mean?
Interviewer: Just a routine question. Do you have any allergies?
Patient: No.
Interviewer: How was your health as a child?
Patient: I guess OK. I had the usual sore throats and earaches that most kids get.
Interviewer: Did anyone ever tell you that you had rheumatic fever?[t]
Patient: No.

[l]The interviewer is now starting to ascertain whether the patient has any risk factors for coronary artery disease.

[m]Notice that the interviewer ignores the statement that the patient didn't take his medications. Questioning the patient "Why not?" would only put the patient on the defensive.

[n]Notice that the patient was beginning to ramble. The interviewer politely interrupted and redirected the interview. She is now inquiring about the family history.

[o]Notice that the interviewer does not assume anything about the mother's well-being or health. Because the patient approached the family's health history, the interviewer is now directing her questions to that history.

[p]Notice that the interviewer does not assume that John is married now, even though he referred to his wife at the beginning of the interview and has acknowledged "Emily." "Emily" may not be his wife.

[q]In this case, "Emily" is John's wife. It is extremely important for the patient to identify family members. The interviewer must never make an assumption that another person with the patient or described in the history is even related to the patient.

[r]Had the patient answered in the affirmative, the interviewer would have asked when, and the patient's record would have been reviewed later.

[s]The interviewer is specifically asking about nonmedical hospitalizations (e.g., for psychiatric reasons). This type of question is not offensive. If the patient has had such admissions to hospitals, he can usually describe them at this time. If not, as in this case, watch how the interview progresses. Notice how the interviewer continues directly with the next question.

[t]This question can follow nicely after the history of sore throats.

Interviewer: Did you have any of these illnesses?[u] Chickenpox? Measles? Diphtheria? Polio? Mumps? Whooping cough?
(Patient shakes head "no.")
Do you take any medications?
Patient: Just metoprolol and amlodipine.
Interviewer: Do you know the dosages?
Patient: I take 50 mg of metoprolol and 2.5 mg of amlodipine, each once a day.
Interviewer: Do you think the medications help you?
Patient: I guess so. I think I feel better with them.
Interviewer: Any other medications?
(pause)
Patient: Nitroglycerin…when I get the pain.
Interviewer: How long does the nitroglycerin take to work?
Patient: Real quickly.
Interviewer: How long is that?
Patient: About 4 to 5 minutes.
Interviewer: Do you take any other medications?
(pause)
Over-the-counter medicine? Herbal medicines? Anything else?
Patient: (thinks for a moment) I take Chlor-Trimeton when I get a cold…but that's about it.
Interviewer: Have you ever had any other health problems?
Patient: No.
Interviewer: Any problems with your liver? Kidneys? Stomach? Lungs?[v]
(Patient shakes head "no.")
How's your appetite?
Patient: Pretty good. I haven't been real hungry lately.
Interviewer: Starting with breakfast yesterday, what did you eat?
Patient: Toast, coffee, and juice for breakfast…
(pause)
A ham sandwich with a Diet Coke for lunch…
(pause)
Oh, yeah, blueberry pie for dessert…
(pause)
And…uh…steak with a baked potato and salad for dinner.
Interviewer: Any snacks between meals?
Patient: I had a cupcake with milk before I went to bed.
Interviewer: Do you eat fish?
Patient: Sometimes.
Interviewer: How often?[w]
Patient: Maybe…
(pause)
Once every 2 weeks.
Interviewer: Have you had any weight change recently?
Patient: I lost about 10 pounds in the past 3 months…
(pause)
But I wanted to…
Interviewer: Were you on a diet?
Patient: No, not exactly…I just haven't been too hungry lately.
Interviewer: How well do you sleep?[x]
Patient: Like a baby…
(pause)
Although I've been getting up pretty early recently.
Interviewer: Mmmm?
Patient: Yeah, recently I go right to sleep, but seem to get up about 3 in the morning and can't go back to sleep…
(pause)
I guess I've got a lot on my mind…
(pause, looking down, hand to mouth)
Interviewer: You seem depressed.[y]
(Patient pauses)
Patient: I guess I am… What's going to happen to me? I really want to live…
(beginning to cry)
I've been so stupid…
(pause)
My kid's only 15. He's a great kid… He needs me… What's the test gonna show? I hope I can have the surgery or the balloon to get relief from this pain.[z]
(Interviewer is silent, handing a box of tissues to the patient.)[aa]
(Patient is sobbing, trying to control his emotions.)
I'm sorry…I can't help it…
(wiping his tears)
I guess we'll have to wait till tomorrow.
Interviewer: I just have a few more questions for you. Do you drink alcohol?
(Patient shakes his head "no.")
Patient: Just socially…one drink…maybe after work, sometimes.
Interviewer: Do you ever feel that you have need of a drink as the day goes on?
Patient: Yeah, I sure do!
Interviewer: Have you ever felt the need to cut down on your drinking?
Patient: No.
Interviewer: Have people annoyed you by criticizing your drinking?
Patient: Never…but my wife doesn't like me drinking.
Interviewer: Have you ever felt bad or guilty about your drinking?

[u]The interviewer slowly asks about each illness, after which she pauses for the patient to respond.

[v]Because this patient has demonstrated so much denial, the interviewer wishes to ask specifically about diseases of the major organs. Each question is asked slowly, and the interviewer pauses after each question, waiting for a response.

[w]The interviewer is not satisfied with qualitative statements. She pursues each question to quantify as best as possible.

[x]The interviewer has now picked up some other somatic element of depression and will now pursue it.

[y]An example of interpretation.

[z]The interviewer could have elected to ask the patient his reactions if surgery cannot be performed. How will he face life? Is there a possibility of suicide? The interviewer chose not to create further anxiety at this time.

[aa]An example of empathetic support. The interviewer cannot answer the patient's questions, but she allows the patient to express his emotions. She is, in essence, saying, "I'm with you."

Patient: Yeah...Once about 10 years ago my friend's father made some wine. We got really drunk...it was terrible...but never again!
Interviewer: Do you drink in the morning?
Patient: Never.
Interviewer: Do you ever drive while intoxicated?
Patient: No! That's suicide.
Interviewer: Do you drink coffee or tea?
Patient: About three cups of coffee a day at work. I have tea only when I'm sick with a cold.
Interviewer: Have you ever used recreational drugs?
Patient: I've tried pot a couple of times...never did anything to me... Nothing else.
Interviewer: What's your usual day like?[bb]
Patient: Before I stopped working at the office, I got up about 5:30, dressed, and was at my desk in the office by 7:30. I usually left the office about 7 and got home by 8:15. We'd have dinner, and I'd be in bed by 11:30, after the news.
Interviewer: Sounds like you have a pretty busy day.
Patient: Yeah. I enjoy my work...or at least I used to.
Interviewer: How long have you been working with your present office?
Patient: I started right after law school. I guess I've been there... about...17 years. I'm one of the senior partners.
(pause)
I was just promoted... A lot of good that will do now.
Interviewer: Congratulations on your promotion! I now have several questions to ask you. You can answer just "yes" or "no" to each.[cc]
(pause)
Have you had any recent fevers?
Patient: No.
Interviewer: Chills?
Patient: No.
Interviewer: Sweats?
Patient: No.
Interviewer: Rashes?
Patient: No.
Interviewer: Changes in your hair or nails?
Patient: No.
Interviewer: Headaches?
Patient: Rarely, about once every 2 to 3 months.
Interviewer: For how long have you been having headaches?
Patient: Years...I guess about 20 to 25 years.
Interviewer: Can you describe them to me?
Patient: That's hard. They're right here.
(pointing to the center of his forehead)
They last about 1 to 2 hours.
Interviewer: What relieves them?
Patient: Usually aspirin.

[bb]Interviewer is inquiring about the patient's lifestyle and psychosocial history.

[cc]The interviewer now begins asking the review of systems. She asks about each symptom. If the patient answers in the affirmative, further questioning is appropriate.

Interviewer: Have you noticed a change in the pattern or severity of your headaches?
Patient: No.
Interviewer: Have you had any head injuries?
Patient: Never.
Interviewer: Have you ever fainted?
Patient: No.
Interviewer: Do you have any problems with...[dd]
(The interviewer completes the review of systems.)
Is there anything else you would like to tell me that I haven't asked about?
Patient: No...you've certainly been very thorough.
Interviewer: Let me summarize your history briefly to make sure I have the details correct before I proceed with your physical examination. This is your first time here at St. Mary's Hospital. You had your first heart attack on July 15, 2022, while playing tennis. You were hospitalized in Kings Hospital for about 6 days. Your second heart attack was 6 months later. You were again hospitalized in Kings Hospital again for about 6 days. Your medications since then have been metoprolol 50 mg once daily and amlodipine 2.5 mg once daily. Because of a worsening of your chest pain and an increase in your shortness of breath in the past 6 months, you're now being admitted for cardiac catheterization. Is that correct, John?
Patient: Exactly!
Interviewer: Do you have any questions for me before I begin your physical examination?
Patient: No...I can't think of any.
(The interviewer stands up, sets up the equipment on the night table, and goes to the sink to wash her hands. The physical examination then commences.)
(Interviewer concludes the physical examination.)
Interviewer: It's good you came in today; we are going to do everything possible to help you feel better.
Patient: Well...what do you think? Will I make it?
(Interviewer opens curtain around patient's bed)
Interviewer: Let me first speak to my preceptor whom I am going to meet now. Afterwards, we'll be back to discuss your medical condition.[ee]

WRITTEN HISTORY OF Mr. JOHN DOE

The preceding interview has revealed much about this 45-year-old lawyer. Superficially, he is a patient with coronary artery disease (CAD). Just as important as his physical illness is his emotional reaction to it. As the interview progressed, the interviewer recognized that the patient is frightened and anxious. What will

[dd]The interviewer continues through the entire review of systems, asking further questions when necessary.

[ee]By indicating to the patient that the interviewer and her preceptor will be back, the patient is less likely to press the interviewer for her opinion at this time. The interviewer should never provide an answer at this point without first speaking to their preceptor. False reassurances can be dangerous.

happen "after tomorrow"? Will he be a candidate for balloon angioplasty? Can it be performed? Is he a good candidate for bypass surgery? Will he live? The anxiety from these questions has resulted in his depression, which must be dealt with as well.

The written history is a summary of the information obtained during the interview. It is usually written after the interview and the physical examination have been completed. The following is an example of the written history of Mr. John Doe, based on the preceding interview.

Chief Concern: "Chest pain for the past 6 months."

History of Current Illness: This is the first St. Mary's Hospital admission for Mr. John Doe, a 45-year-old lawyer with CAD. His history dates back to approximately 3 years before admission, when he started to experience a vague discomfort in his chest. He describes it as "a dull ache" provoked by emotional upsets at work. He suffered his first heart attack on July 15, 2022, while playing tennis. He was hospitalized for about 6 days in Kings Hospital. After 4 weeks at home, he returned to work. Six months later, he suffered his second heart attack, again while playing tennis. He was again hospitalized at Kings Hospital and was told that he had "irregularity" of his heart. He was started on some medications for this irregularity. The patient denies any palpitations since then.

Over the past 6 months, the patient has had increasing chest pain with radiation down his left arm despite metoprolol 50 mg daily and amlodipine 2.5 mg daily.

The patient's chest pain is produced by exercise, emotion, and sexual intercourse. The patient takes nitroglycerin as needed, with relief within 5 minutes. One-block dyspnea on exertion is also present. This has worsened in the past 6 months, before which he could walk 2 to 3 blocks. The patient's risk factors for CAD include a history of untreated hypertension, a 40-pack-year history of smoking (2 packs per day for 20 years), and a brother with a myocardial infarction at the age of 40 years. The patient's brother is now 47 years of age. The patient denies any history of diabetes or hyperlipidemia. At his physician's and wife's request, he has entered the hospital for elective cardiac catheterization. The patient has a significant denial of his illness and a secondary depression.[ff]

Although cardiac catheterization was suggested after the patient's heart attacks, he refused to accept it until this admission.

Past Medical History: The patient was hospitalized at age 15 years for an appendectomy in Booth Memorial Hospital in Rochester, New York. The surgery was performed by a Dr. Ralph Meyers. The only other hospitalizations were for the patient's two heart attacks, as indicated previously. The patient is predominantly a red meat eater with little fish in his diet. Recently, presumably owing to depression, there has been a loss of appetite with a 10-pound weight loss. The patient admits to a sleeping problem. He falls asleep normally but awakens early and cannot go back to sleep. His only medications are indicated in the history of current illness. There is no history of renal, hepatic, pulmonary, or gastrointestinal disease. There is no history of allergy.

Family History: The patient's father is 75 years of age and has a history of diabetes. He apparently has some ocular problem related to diabetes. The patient's mother died at age 64 years from stomach cancer. The patient's older brother, as mentioned previously, is 47 years of age and has CAD (MI at age 40 years). The patient has a younger sister who is 37 years of age and is well. There is no history of congenital disease. The patient is married and has a 15-year-old son, who is well.

Psychosocial History: The patient is a "type A" personality. He admits to having a need to drink alcohol occasionally after work. He drinks coffee about three times a day. He has used only marijuana on rare occasions, and he denies the use of other recreational drugs.

Review of Systems: There is a 20- to 25-year history of headaches without any recent change in their pattern or severity. The patient denies any head injury. There is...[gg]

There is no history of claudication.[hh]

The remainder of the review of systems is noncontributory.[ii]

SUMMARY

The patient is a 45-year-old male attorney with CAD, status post myocardial infarction (MI) 3 years ago and a second MI 6 months later who presents now with recurrent angina for the past 6 months. His risk factors for CAD include untreated hypertension for years, 40-pack-year history of smoking, and a family history for CAD (brother with MI at age 40 years). The patient does not follow a regular low-fat diet. He is currently being medicated with atenolol 50 mg daily and amlodipine 2.5 mg daily. Following his two MIs, cardiac catheterization was recommended, but the patient refused. The patient is being admitted for elective cardiac catheterization. He has significant denial of his illness and a mild secondary reactive depression.

[ff]Notice that the history of the current illness summarizes all the information related to the current illness chronologically, regardless of when the information was obtained during the interview.

[gg]The review of systems would then indicate any of the other symptoms that may be present.

[hh]Notice that the positive symptoms are indicated first. The important, or pertinent, negative symptoms are then listed. A pertinent negative symptom in this patient is the lack of claudication. Coronary artery disease is often associated with peripheral vascular disease. The absence of a major symptom of peripheral vascular disease, claudication, makes claudication in this patient a pertinent negative symptom. Chapter 15, The Peripheral Vascular System, provides a further discussion of pertinent positives and negatives.

[ii]This statement indicates that none of the other symptoms is either present or contributes to the patient's current illness.

SECTION 2

Valuing Diversity: Race, Gender, and Ethnicity

5

Anti-Racist and Anti-Oppressive Clinical Skills

Joseph Truglio, Giselle N. Lynch, Ann-Gel S. Palermo, Joanne R. Hojsak, Michelle Sainté-Willis, and Reena Karani

The paradox of education is precisely this—that as one begins to become conscious, one begins to examine the society in which he is being educated.

James Baldwin (1924–1987)

INTRODUCTION

Like all American institutions, medicine is shaped by a legacy of racial injustice. Racism permeates clinical practice and medical education and results in dramatic health inequities. Healthcare professionals and the systems in which we practice are not passive observers of these processes but rather active participants. Healthcare professionals both practice in a system that creates and perpetuates oppression and also experience racism and oppression within clinical and educational environments. The result is poor health outcomes for patients and moral injury and fatigue for healthcare professionals. In recent years, the landscape of anti-racist and anti-oppressive pedagogy in medical education has mirrored prior periods of progression toward liberation with a subsequent backlash of oppression and resistance. The current post-pandemic and sociopolitical climates amplified the fissures in our system and revealed the longstanding impact on historically marginalized communities. In response to this climate, many health profession programs introduced or expanded upon their anti-racist and anti-oppressive curricula and pedagogy. However, this awareness was met with a systematic effort to roll back policies related to diversity, equity, inclusion, and justice. Further, broad legislative efforts across the country now work to eliminate resources dedicated to broadening diversity and removing all language related to racism from our educational environments. These measures cast into doubt the ability of many schools to teach anti-racism and anti-oppression. These attacks on this body of work are not newfound nor are they novel. This reaction is cyclical in nature and tracks back to post–Civil War, post-Reconstruction, and post–Civil Rights movements. Within this context, we hope this chapter provides educators and students with tools and resources to work toward dismantling racism and oppression in clinical practice. The weight of our effort is vast, and the lives of our patients and communities will depend on it.

Background and Frameworks

Racism and oppression do not exist in isolation within the clinical encounter. They operate within global and historical systems of colonialism, capitalism, and white supremacy.[1] Such systems are contemporary, ubiquitous forces. This chapter introduces concrete clinical skills designed to dismantle these systems as they manifest in individual patient encounters.

Such skills represent the work of many educators, healthcare professionals, students, community activists, and patients. Within this chapter, we organize these clinical skills into four groups. The first three follow the traditional arc of "before," "during," and "after" a face-to-face patient encounter. The last section presents those skills commonly used to navigate patients or caregivers demonstrating discriminatory behavior. The first step in learning each of these anti-racist and anti-oppressive clinical skills is recognition. This includes a recognition of the relationship between medicine and racism and a recognition of our positionality within this relationship.

In this updated version of the chapter, we have made an intentional effort to pivot away from centering the role of bias and toward exploring tangible and intangible ways that racism is enacted in interpersonal and institutional medical environments. This shift in pedagogy has the effect of (1) emphasizing the real and continued legacy of race and racism in medicine and (2) positioning individuals to be active participants in leveraging their own privilege to uplift oppressed communities and undo the harms of medicine's legacy.

Historically, healthcare professionals participated in the creation of race and racial hierarchies to sustain and justify colonial expansion, the genocide of indigenous communities, and the enslavement of Black people in the Americas. Racial hierarchies and ever-changing racial categories perpetuate inequities of racialized Americans through contemporary times (Fig. 5.1). Despite recent shifts away from race-based medicine, this scientific racism remains a dominant framework within medical literature, education, and clinical practice. Within this paradigm, healthcare professionals are taught to pay attention to race, along with the outcomes of health inequities, without any acknowledgment of the historical and sociopolitical forces that yield such inequitable outcomes. This is done explicitly—through guidelines and clinical prediction rules that employ

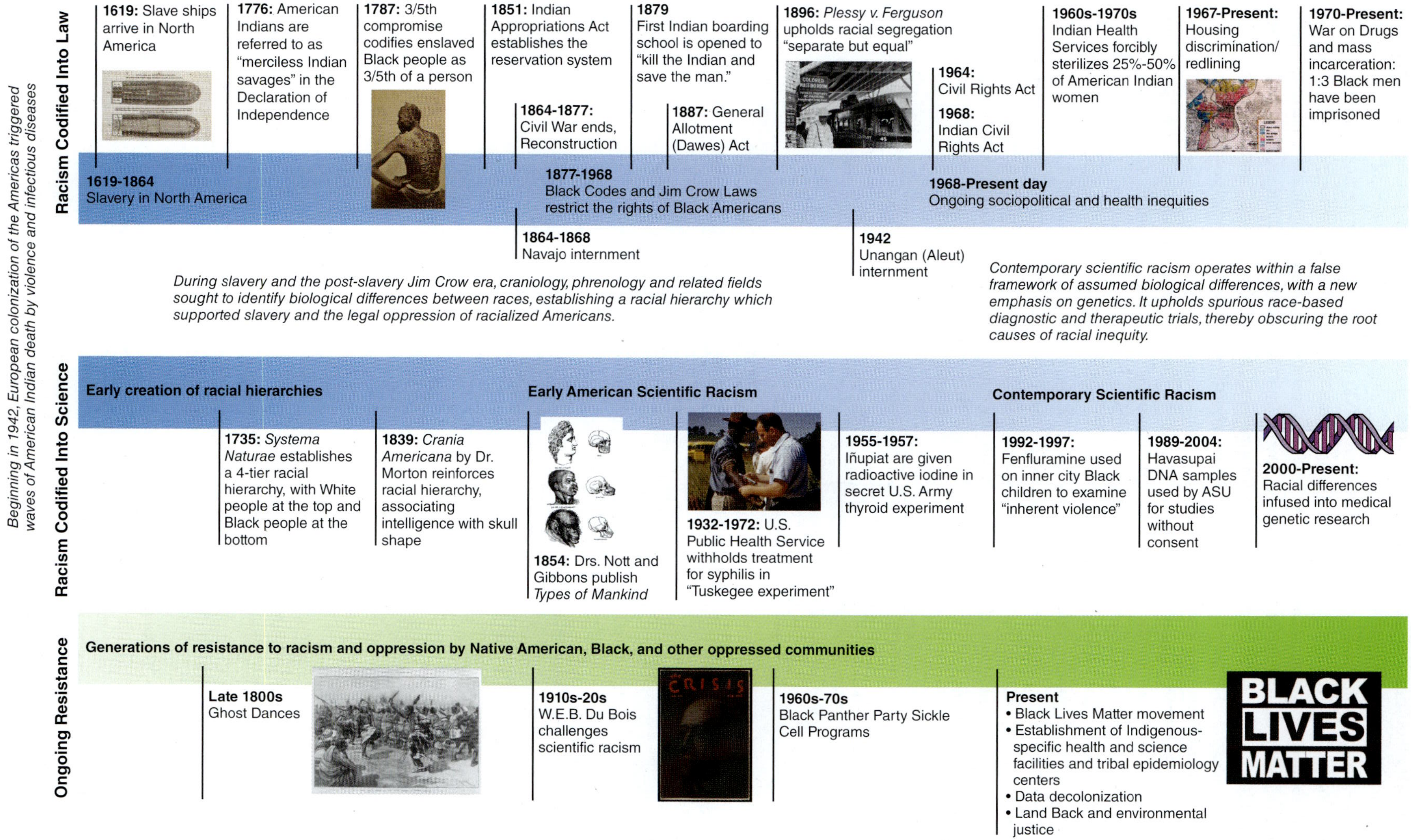

Fig. 5.1 The Relationship Between Scientific Racism and American Sociopolitical Culture. The roots of white supremacy and the development of medicine in America are both grounded in colonial exploitation. Scientists and physicians classified human anatomical variation and developed a specious, hierarchical concept of "race" to justify slavery and genocide. Since the end of slavery in the United States, laws and structures have been established to continue this legacy of racism. As Jim Crow receded, it was replaced by systemic and institutionalized social policies that produced conditions such as mass incarceration and housing discrimination. Similarly, explicit hierarchical concepts of race are replaced by contemporary scientific racism. The juxtaposition of these timelines underscores the co-development and interdependence of scientific racism and sociopolitical racism. Throughout this time, Native American, Black, and other marginalized and racialized groups maintained a resistance to systemic and scientific racism—preserving their health and spiritual practices and explicitly countering concepts of racial hierarchies. This provides the social and medical contexts within which we develop and employ anti-racist clinical skills—within a system interdependent with colonialism and white supremacy, yet grounded firmly in generations of Black and indigenous resistance to colonialism and oppression. (Sources of images 1619 Slave ship from https://loc.gov/pictures/resource/cph.3a34658/; 3/5th Compromise reused from Library of Congress, Prints & Photographs Division, LC-DIG-ppmsca-54375, https://loc.gov/pictures/resource/ppmsca.54375/; *Plessy v. Ferguson* reused from Library of Congress, Prints & Photographs Division, Farm Security Administration/Office of War Information Black-and-White Negatives LC-DIG-ppmsc-00199; Housing redlining reused from National Archives and Records Administration, Mapping Inequality; Dr. Notts and Gibbons from Nott, Josiah C, and George R Gliddon. Types of mankind: or, Ethnological researches based upon the ancient monuments, paintings, sculptures, and crania of races, and upon their natural, geographical, philological and biblical history: illustrated by selections from the unedited papers of Samuel George Morton and by additional contributions from L. Agassiz, W. Usher, and H.S. Patterson. Philadelphia: J.B. Lippincott, Grambo & Co, 1854. Pdf. https://www.loc.gov/item/49043133/; Public Health Service from the Centers for Disease Control and Prevention/Released; Ghost dances from Library of Congress, Washington, D.C. (Digital file no. cph 3a51166) https://www.britannica.com/topic/Ghost-Dance:/media/1/232793/150029; WEB DuBois from Walts, Frank, Artist, and Donor National Association for the Advancement of Colored People. Portrait of W.E.B. Du Bois., 1918. Feb. Photograph. https://www.loc.gov/item/2010718752/).

race as a biological construct—and implicitly—through observational studies that report on racial health inequities without providing a sociopolitical context for these outcomes. Healthcare professionals thus rely on their own assumptions and explanations, which include genetic and biological differences, as well as behavioral choices and innate abilities. Together, this manifests clinically as false beliefs about biological differences between races,[2] cycles of implicit bias (Fig. 5.2), and inequities in care management based on a patient's race.[3,4]

Racism can be defined as "a system of structuring opportunity and assigning values based on the social interpretation of how one looks (race), which unfairly disadvantages some individuals and communities, unfairly advantages other individuals and communities, and saps the strength of the whole society through the waste of human resources."[5] Racist policies and practices provide this structure and include any policy or practice that, regardless of intent, results in a shift in power, privilege, or opportunity away from racialized individuals or communities and toward those assigned as "White." Racist policies and practices in healthcare can exist on multiple overlapping levels (Table 5.1). Such policies and practices are supported by the hierarchy, values, beliefs, and norms of a predominantly White culture, also known as "white supremacy culture."

White supremacy culture is the organizing principle of American society. The features of white supremacy culture are well described and intimately linked to those forces that drive other forms of oppression. As such, anti-racist and anti-oppressive clinical skills are linked. Both require a recognition of white supremacy norms at play within the clinical environment. Select examples of these norms appear in Table 5.2, White Supremacy Culture and Anti-Racist Clinical Approaches. While race has no biological basis, white supremacy culture has biological effects and real consequences for people's health, wealth, social status, reputation, and opportunities in life.

White supremacy culture is thus embedded within medicine: influencing medical practice and perpetuated by scientific racism. White supremacy culture is also interdependent with medical culture through dominant narratives. A dominant

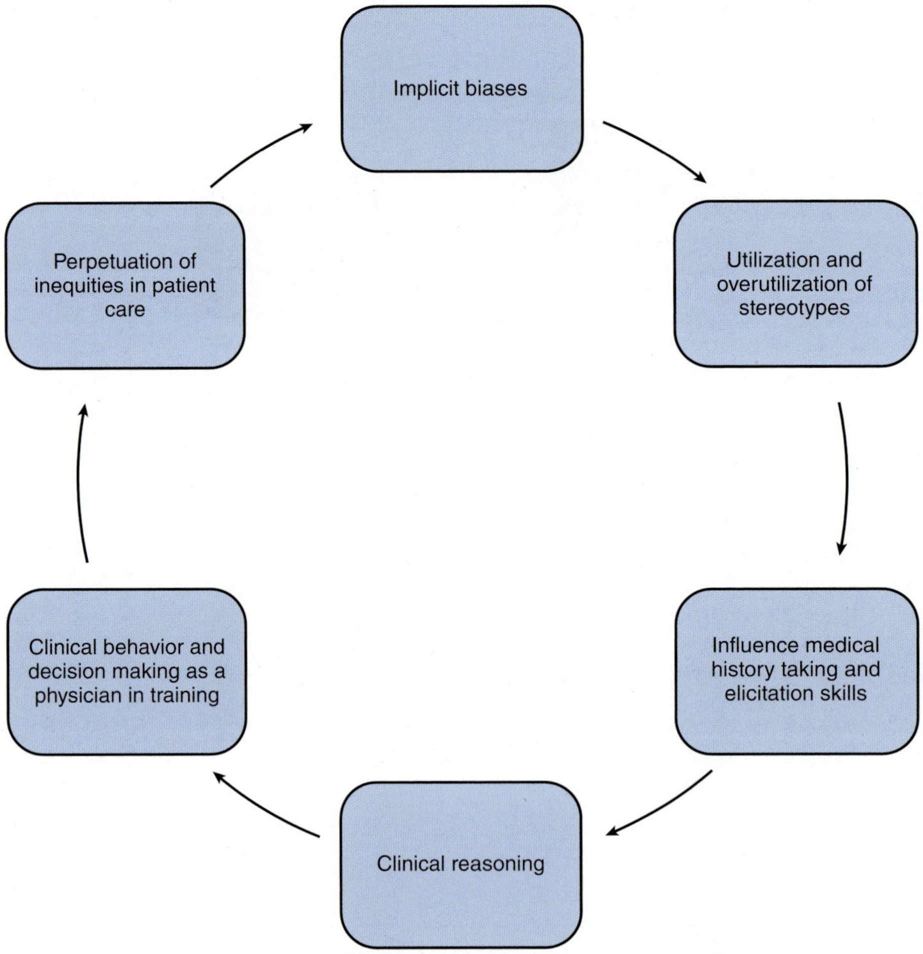

Fig. 5.2 The Cycle of Implicit Bias. Implicit biases underlie all aspects of clinical medicine. Trainees enter medical education primed with their own biases. These biases are reinforced, and new ones are created, through training within a structurally biased system. Healthcare professionals are thus primed to utilize and overutilize stereotypes and automatic associations, which directly influence the type of questions asked of patients. Consequently, clinical reasoning becomes embedded with shortcuts, pattern recognition, and biased clinical tools. This practice directly leads to the perpetuation of health inequities. Healthcare professionals have a responsibility to become aware of their own biases in an effort to break this cycle.

TABLE 5.1 Individual and Institutional Racism

Institutional Explicit	Individual Explicit
Policies that explicitly discriminate against a group	***Prejudice in action—discrimination***
Example: Segregated care via faculty practice vs. clinic-based healthcare system	**Example:** Healthcare professional states "these Mexicans are a waste of resources" while rounding on a patient in alcohol withdrawal
Policies that negatively impact one group unintentionally	***Unconscious attitudes and beliefs***
Example: Use of race embedded in clinical prediction rules and guidelines	**Example:** Healthcare professional spends less time with patients of color compared with White patients

Data from https://www.racialequityalliance.org/about/our-approach/.

TABLE 5.2 White Supremacy Culture and Anti-Racist Clinical Approaches

White Supremacy Culture	Anti-Racist Clinical Approach
Either/or Thinking	***Systems and Complexity Thinking***
Things are viewed as "either/or"—people are either "good or bad," patients are "adherent or nonadherent." Inequities are viewed as isolated incidents, and complex systems are simplified (i.e., poverty is due to lack of education, a flare of a chronic illness is due to nonadherence to medication).	Healthcare professionals strive for understanding context and intersectionality. Patients can be both nonadherent to a treatment recommendation (for reasons that are myriad) and deeply committed to their own health. Instances of inequities are viewed as manifestations of broader systems of oppression, and healthcare professionals search for the underlying causes for these observations within their patients and communities.
Power Hoarding and Paternalism	***Power Sharing***
Power is viewed as limited. Ideas from patients and communities are treated as not worthy of inclusion or seen as a threat (see "Defensiveness"). Healthcare professionals assume they have the best interests of patients in mind, and clinical information (lab results, chart notes, etc.) and clinical decision making processes (alternate approaches, levels of ambiguity, etc.) are not openly shared with patients. Patients recognize they do not have power and do not understand how clinical decisions are made.	Patient and family ideas are valued for the positional experience and expertise they represent. Healthcare professionals actively seek out and make space for them to be heard. Healthcare professionals openly share their own thought process with patients and prioritize collaborative decision making. Healthcare professionals and patients share a common and expressed goal, and healthcare professionals acknowledge that without the patient's explicit investment in the treatment plan, the plan is useless.
Defensiveness	***Vulnerability***
There is an absence of space to air grievances or concerns. Healthcare professionals and health systems focus on protecting power instead of addressing harms. Healthcare professionals spend time naming intentions instead of acknowledging harms. Either/or thinking contributes to clinicians viewing critique as inappropriate.	Healthcare professionals actively create space for patients and families to address concerns. Healthcare professionals respond to the concerns and include them in the decision making process.
Focus on Individuality	***Community and Group Connection***
Patients act as individuals, devoid of connection to a group or community, unless a pathological association about their behavior or genetics can be made. An individual is responsible for controlling their environment. Healthcare professionals act individually, with responsibility functioning "up-down" hierarchies as opposed to sideways to peers.	Healthcare professionals view patients as both autonomous agents AND still acting within a community that may be under oppressive economic, social, and political structures. Therefore, patients' concerns, interactions within the clinical encounter, and health are also viewed within the lens of that community's positionality. Teamwork is prioritized, and healthcare professionals include patients, families, and communities within that team.
Right to Comfort/Fear of Open Conflict	***Direct and Constructive Feedback/Growth and Learning***
Healthcare professionals value politeness over honesty. Healthcare professionals blame patients and communities that voice concerns or cause discomfort, labelling them as responsible for the problem or as "difficult" patients.	Healthcare professionals actively create a space where patients can question and challenge the healthcare professional and medicine at large. Specifically, healthcare professionals do not require patients to raise concerns in "acceptable" ways. Healthcare professionals openly admit to gaps in knowledge and experience and welcome challenges/questions from patients as opportunities for learning, growth, and improvement in care.
Worship of the Written Word	***Centering the Experiences of Patients/Communities***
Healthcare professionals rely almost exclusively on published data and do not take into account or value other ways in which information and experiences are shared.	Healthcare professionals take the time to understand how patients and communities get and share information, especially information about health and illness. Healthcare professionals strive to understand the stories of their patients and communities that are not always written and not always heard.

Modified from dRworks at www.dismantlingracism.org, https://resourcegeneration.org/wp-content/uploads/2018/01/2016-dRworks-workbook.pdf, accessed on August 25, 2019.

BOX 5.1 Characteristics of Dominant Narratives in Clinical Medicine

- Shifts blame from healthcare systems and society to the patient/community
- Obscures the true social and historic determinants of health driving the observed outcome
- Results in cognitive errors and ineffective, at times dangerous, patient care
- Perpetuates individual and institutional racism and bias

narrative refers to "an explanation or story that is told in service of the dominant social group's interests and ideologies." The concept of a "dominant narrative" is a useful lens through which we can understand how stories are told and how medical knowledge is transmitted (see Box 5.1). These narratives serve to perpetuate power hoarding within the dominant social group and are most often incomplete or false representations of complex social histories. For that narrative to be perpetuated, it must be told without consideration for alternative explanations and in service of those in power. These stories shape our perception and, as a consequence, our understanding of what should be done. Moreover, the repetition of these stories becomes pervasive, unquestioned, and seemingly objective.

Anti-racism is an active process for identifying and eliminating racism and white supremacy. Anti-racism recognizes racism in oneself and seeks to change systems, organizational structures, policies, practices, and attitudes so that power and privilege are redistributed and shared equitably.[a] In the context of clinical practice, anti-racism examines the power imbalances between racialized people and nonracialized/White people whether they are patients, learners, medical educators, or healthcare professionals. This approach decenters whiteness and requires healthcare professionals to shift from the role of "ally" to a more active identity as "accomplice" in dismantling systems of harm.

HOW TO USE THIS CHAPTER

The foundational clinical skills presented in this chapter are part of a larger practice of abolition medicine—a practice that seeks to abolish the systems of racism and oppression that prevent our communities from experiencing the health and wellness they deserve in all aspects of their lives. The development of these skills is an iterative process and can only be done in partnership with others, including patients and communities. While using this chapter, we recommend the following tips to promote your growth in anti-racist and anti-oppressive clinical skills:

- ***Do the exercises.*** Be mindful of the ways in which your discomfort could influence you to rush through the exercises or prevent you from engaging deeply. The exercises pose challenging questions to help you investigate what you know and the process of transformation.
- ***Take time.*** Choose a pace that works for you. Going too quickly through the content and exercises often results in missing some of the most useful and transformative experiences. It's fine if you need to revisit a concept, exercise, or case example. You will not find a linear path to an anti-racist future in a few days, weeks, or months. Give yourself the gift of time to allow for reflection and the opportunity for self-interrogation about the concepts and frameworks presented in this chapter. We invite you to disrupt the sense of urgency. Don't forget, there is so much to unlearn about how racism and white supremacy ideology work.
- ***Realize that people are at different stages of readiness.*** The goal isn't to get everyone to be at the same stage and marching in lockstep. Use the chapter as a roadmap and an opportunity to align people to the process, with permission to course correct when needed.
- ***Develop a community of practice.*** Disrupting racism and oppression in the clinical environment is a lifelong process and one that requires ongoing critical self-reflection and growth. A community of practice—a group of individuals from varied backgrounds and in varied roles, striving together toward this common goal—is a source of support, feedback, and strength to help you in this journey.
- ***Take ownership of your learning and growth with humility.*** This chapter is only an overview of centuries of colonialism, white supremacy, and the forces that resist such oppression. It should serve as a "jumping off point," providing structure and organization to your learning and growth. Explore the Key Terms (Table 5.3). Read the references. Apply the skills in real life. Revisit the exercises from time to time. Search for newly published work and humbly seek out unwritten knowledge from within the community you practice.

BEFORE THE CLINICAL ENCOUNTER (PRE-VISIT PREPARATION)

Deconstructing racism and oppression in a clinical encounter starts before you even meet the patient. It involves cultivating an awareness of one's own interconnected identities, positionality, power, biases, and likely triggers to those biases, as well as an awareness of potential structural forces at play in the clinical environment. By increasing awareness, the healthcare professional can develop clinical skills to actively dismantle them in advance of the patient encounter. Although described here as events that take place prior to a clinical encounter, this is a continuous process, wherein reflection and skill development are ongoing through personal reflection and feedback from colleagues, patients, and communities.

The following exercises will assist you in this process. By its nature, however, this process is ongoing and should be employed by you throughout your career. Furthermore, the most effective techniques involve a combination of self-reflection and discussion with others.

Practice Exercises

Exercise 1: Introduction to the Person-Role-System Framework

We all have personal and social identities that shape our worldview, and we take these views into every role we hold, personally

[a]While distinct from "insurgent multiculturalism," anti-racism shares many characteristics with this new clinical and educational paradigm, described here: Wear D. Insurgent multiculturalism: rethinking how and why we teach culture in medical education. *Acad Med* 78(6):549, 2003.

TABLE 5.3 Key Terms and Definitions

Term	Definition
Abolition	The action of abolishing a system, practice, or institution. Abolition centers on getting rid of prison, jails, police, courts, and surveillance. Abolitionist practice is also about establishing a system that is rooted in dignity and care for all people. A system that does not rely on punishment as accountability.[6]
Ancestry	A process-based concept, a statement about an individual's relationship to other individuals in their genealogic history; thus, it is a very personal understanding of one's genomic heritage.[7]
Bias	Judgment without question.
Biomedical model	A framework for healthcare that focuses on purely biological factors and excludes psychological, environmental, and social influences. It is considered to be the historically dominant model of medicine for healthcare professionals to diagnose and treat a condition in most Western countries.
Critical consciousness	The process of exploring unexamined assumptions that are held at individual, institutional, and cultural levels of healthcare and aim to raise awareness of the conditions of the people and communities served.[8]
Dominant narrative	An explanation or story that is told in service of the dominant social group's interests and ideologies.
Explicit bias	The attitudes and beliefs we have about a person or group on a conscious level.
Gender expression	The manner by which one chooses to express gender, through clothing, mannerisms, and other aspects of presentation, which may or may not align with societal expectations.
Gender identity	One's internal sense of gender at a given time.
Generational trauma	When trauma is passed down from generation to the next (also known as intergenerational trauma). Intergenerational trauma that is experienced by a systematically oppressed group is distinct and called historical trauma.[9]
Implicit bias	An automatic response or mental association that occurs without awareness, intention, or control.
Oppression	The systematic subjugation of one social group by a more powerful social group for the social, economic, and political benefit of the more powerful social group.[10]
Privilege	Unearned social power accorded by the formal and informal institutions of society to ALL members of a dominant group (e.g., White privilege, male privilege, etc.). Privilege is usually invisible to those who have it because we're taught not to see it, but nevertheless it puts them at an advantage over those who do not have it.[11]
Race	A social, cultural, and historical construct that artificially divides people into groups based on characteristics such as phenotype, ancestry, national origin, etc., to facilitate and justify exploitation.
	A specious classification of human beings created in the 1600s–1700s by Europeans, or people who we have come to call White, establishing White as the highest level of human worth and social status for the purpose of establishing and maintaining power and privilege.[12]
Racial bias	A person's identification with their racial in-group, which leads to preference for those of the in-group and negative preconceived notions about those of an out-group.
Racism	Economic, political, social, and cultural structures, actions, and beliefs that systematize and perpetuate an unequal distribution of privileges, resources, and power between White people and people of color.[12]
Religion	An organized system of beliefs, rituals, and practices with which an individual identifies and associates and includes a relationship with a divine being.[13]
Scientific racism	Scientific inquiry that stems from a belief in biological evidence of race and racial inferiority/superiority, and that Black people are biologically different and inferior to White people.
Sexual orientation	The presence and/or object of a person's romantic, sexual, physical, or spiritual attractions.
Spirituality	The aspect of humanity that refers to the way individuals seek and express meaning and purpose and the way they experience their connectedness to the moment, to self, to others, to nature, and to the significant and sacred.
Structural competency	The trained ability to discern how a host of issues defined clinically as symptoms, attitudes, or diseases represent the downstream implications of upstream decisions about such matters as healthcare and food delivery systems, zoning laws, urban and rural infrastructures, medicalization, or even about the very definitions of illness and health.
White supremacy	A global system that shifts power, privilege, and opportunity away from racialized groups and toward people called White. Its culture is the idea (ideology) that White people and the ideas, thoughts, beliefs, and actions of White people are superior to people of color and their ideas, thoughts, beliefs, and actions.[14]

and professionally. The person-role-system framework[15] recognizes the dynamic interplay between an individual, their role, and the system in which they function, in this case, the healthcare system.

See Box Practice Exercise 5.1.

Practice exercise 5.1 debrief. This exercise provides a way to reflect on how the multidimensionality of your own self-identity is associated with privilege and oppression and how to situate your personhood as a member of the healthcare profession. This multidimensionality can be appreciated through the concept of intersectionality.[17] *Intersectionality* is the interconnected nature of social categories such as race, class, and gender as they apply to a given individual or group, thus creating overlapping and interdependent systems of marginalization and oppression, power and privilege. While intersectionality has typically been used to understand the interconnected identities of marginalized groups, it is important to consider how this term clarifies how intersecting identities can work together to privilege or oppress groups of people, creating systems of power and advantage. After completing the exercise, you should consider how to reinforce the person-role-system framework as a longitudinal lens throughout your learning and leverage it as an opportunity to

PRACTICE EXERCISE 5.1 Introduction to the Person-Role-System Framework

Instructions

In this exercise, you will consider your personal and social identities, your evolving role as a healthcare professional, and the ways by which our healthcare system and broader systems of oppression influence you.

Part 1: Person

Exploring how your personal and social identities shape your sense of self as you become a healthcare professional.

A person represents an individual within a system. Every person has a mental model (way of thinking) encompassing unique beliefs and experiences that make them valuable contributors to the system. Thus, we must start here and assess how we show up, what we represent, and the ideas and cultures we perpetuate.

Consider the following questions. Write down your answers here or in a notebook or computer. Periodically return to these questions throughout your training and your career and reflect on the ways they might change or stay the same.

- *What are examples of your own personal and social identities? List at least five below.*
- *What ways are your identities linked to how you feel about practicing healthcare?*

You will now explore the relationship of intersecting social identities with regard to privilege, power, access, and resources. Social identities influence our beliefs, attitudes, and behaviors. Social identities impact how we perceive ourselves and others in day-to-day life and influence how we perceive social roles. You cannot enter a room as one identity—as one part of your full self. Your social identities work together simultaneously. Social identities overlap and create different degrees of advantages and disadvantages.

Your world experience is based on the interplay of your identities within multiple dimensions of societal privilege and societal oppressions (i.e., intersectionality).

Consider the interconnecting identities you described in the previous reflection questions. Use the following image to examine each identity and how it relates to power, privilege, and opportunity in your life. Write each identity in the circle: the closer to the center, the more privilege, access, power, and resources this identity tends to produce for you and other members of that social group, even if unearned. As we move out from the center, there is less proximity to privilege, access, power, and resources and increased marginalization and oppression.[16]

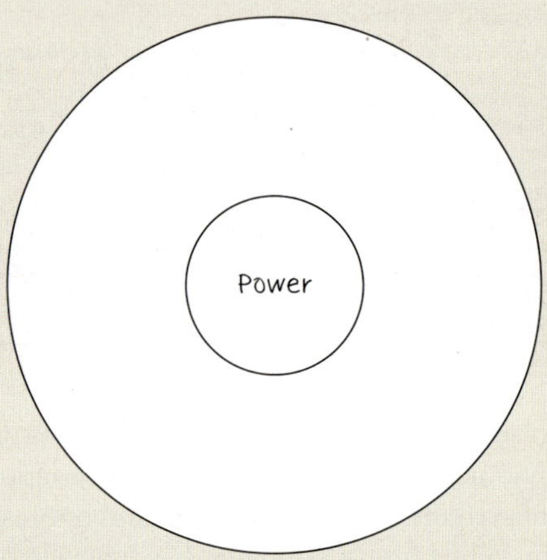

- *Where did you place your identities on this chart? Why?*
- *How does that affect how you identify most strongly?*
- *How might the might proximity or distance from the center of the wheel affect your experience as a healthcare professional?*
- *Where does your role as healthcare professional fall? Why?*
- *If you have moved countries or culture, have your identities shifted on this circle? In what ways?*

Although the identities explored are not intended to be exhaustive of all social identity categories, this exercise provides a powerful illustration of the complexity of intersectionality. It also must be interpreted through the lens of a particular culture at a particular time. For example, as shown in the following completed diagram, for chapter author Palermo, her reflection using the matrix of oppression illustrates the co-existence of privileged (English-speaking, able-bodied, Catholic) and oppressed social identities (Latina, lesbian, female, working class). For Palermo, who was raised in the northeast United States from 1982 to the present day, the combined systemic social disadvantages of being a lesbian, Latina female from a working-class background outweighed the benefit of being a U.S. citizen and English-speaking because of the various forms of systemic oppression including, but not limited to, racism, sexism, and homophobia.

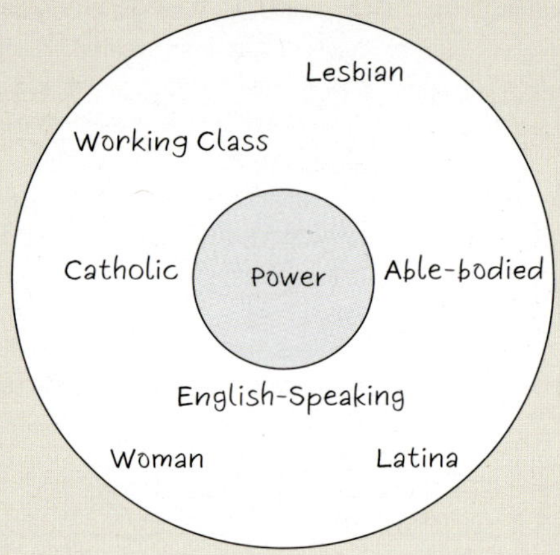

Part 2: Role

A role refers to the positions, functions, and responsibilities given or assigned to an individual within a system. We must consider our power, formal and informal, in the roles we occupy.

Consider the following questions. Write down your answers here or in a notebook or computer. Periodically return to these questions throughout your training and your career and reflect on the ways they might change or stay the same.

- *How might your personal and social identities shape your role as a healthcare professional?*
- *What do you expect of yourself as you work toward becoming a healthcare professional?*
- *At this moment in time, what will the profession expect of you?*

Part 3: System

A system is a larger environment in which the person and role exist. It provides context, constraints, and resources. We must consider how we use our positionality in the roles we possess within systems to produce outcomes. In the case of healthcare, how can we use our sphere of influence—considering our intersecting identities and personal/professional roles—to dismantle racism and oppression and improve health outcomes?

Consider the following questions. Write down your answers in a notebook or on a computer. Periodically return to these questions throughout your training and your career and reflect on the ways they might change or stay the same.

- *How have the healthcare systems and health education systems impacted your role as a health professions student so far?*
- *How might these systems shape your role as a healthcare professional?*
- *How might you use your sphere of influence as a healthcare professional to impact these systems?*

advance dialogue and reflection on specific social identities such as race.

Practice exercise 5.1 clinical correlation. Numerous studies demonstrate the impact of healthcare professional identities, and the systems in which they operate, on clinical outcomes.[18] By critically reflecting on one's own personal and social identities and how these identities shape one's role, learners can begin to see how power and privilege emerge formally and informally. Through critical and ongoing self-reflection, this inquiry about the meaning of your clinical role and professional expectations can reveal your relationship to power and privilege and your sphere of influence within healthcare. Developing a critical awareness about one's relationship to power and privilege is the first step in effectively using anti-racist clinical skills centered around your sphere of influence at any given time.

Exercise 2: How Did You Come to Know Your Race?

The following exercise adapts the person-role-system framework with an expanded reflection on how a specific social identity—racial identity—informs your role as a healthcare professional. You will explore how your role with this specific social identity may be perceived by patients, peers, and colleagues in the clinical environment. This exercise may be adapted by replacing the racial identity with other specific social identities such as gender, sexual orientation, spiritual/religious identity, and disability status to name a few.

See Box Practice Exercise 5.2.

Exercise 3: Self-Proclaimed vs. Perceived Identity

One cannot control the impact of a pre-existing perception, attitude, or judgment of another individual on themselves based on their visible social identities. We all carry deeply held beliefs and attitudes based on how we have been socialized to relate to individuals or groups with specific types of social identities. Thus, we all carry a self-proclaimed perception—a view of ourselves—that may or may not be aligned with how we are perceived by others. However, despite how we may view ourselves, our thinking and behaviors are often influenced by how we are perceived by others. The next exercise explores this dynamic that may play out to the benefit or detriment of our patients.

See Box Practice Exercise 5.3.

Practice exercises 5.2 and 5.3 clinical correlation and debrief. The clinical correlation from these exercises provides a learning path to deconstruct the impact of one or more social identities, how the formation of that identity is expressed in one's own life and with others, and the creation of new or reinforcement of existing biases in one's role as a healthcare professional. These exercises provide a way to link visible social identities with potential cognitive biases and behaviors in the clinical environment. While often ignored, the "multidimensionality" of both the healthcare professional and the patient creates nuanced interpersonal interactions that may play out in the clinical setting. The impact of these interactions on clinical reasoning, clinical decisions, and health outcomes will be further explored in subsequent exercises.

Exercise 4: The Priming Effect of Dominant Narratives

There are innumerable triggers for bias in a clinical encounter (Fig. 5.3). Here we explore biases based on a review of the patient's medical record that may activate specific dominant narratives and prime the thinking and behavior of the healthcare professional prior to even meeting the patient. The dominant narratives at play and suggested anti-racist clinical skills that can be used to disrupt these biases are described in the following table. The skills are described in more detail in the following section, During the Clinical Encounter.

PRACTICE EXERCISE 5.2 How Did You Come to Know Your Race?

Instructions

Reflect on the following questions regarding race and racial identity within the person-role-system framework:

Person

- *How did you first come to know your racial and/or ethnic identity?*
- *What was that exact moment like for you when you realized you were [Insert racial/ethnic identity]? Where were you? How old were you? What were the circumstances? How did it make you feel?*

Role

- *How might your racial identity shape your role as a healthcare professional?*
- *What concerns, if any, do you have about how your racial identity will be perceived by your patients?*
- *How might these biases inform your interaction with patients with shared or different racial and ethnic backgrounds from your own? What conscious and/or unconscious biases might be at play?*

System

- *How might the features of the clinical environment impact you as a healthcare professional?*
- *What do you think you might need personally and professionally to effectively navigate the healthcare environment given your racial identity?*

PRACTICE EXERCISE 5.3 Self-Proclaimed vs. Perceived Identity

Instructions

Imagine now that ***you are a patient***, in a hospital, lying in a hospital bed. A healthcare professional enters the room. How many assumptions might that healthcare professional make about your identity? What would be assumed of your racial identity? Gender identity? Ability or disability? Spirituality or religion? How would these assumptions align with your own priorities? In what ways might these assumptions impact your relationship with the healthcare professional and the care you receive?

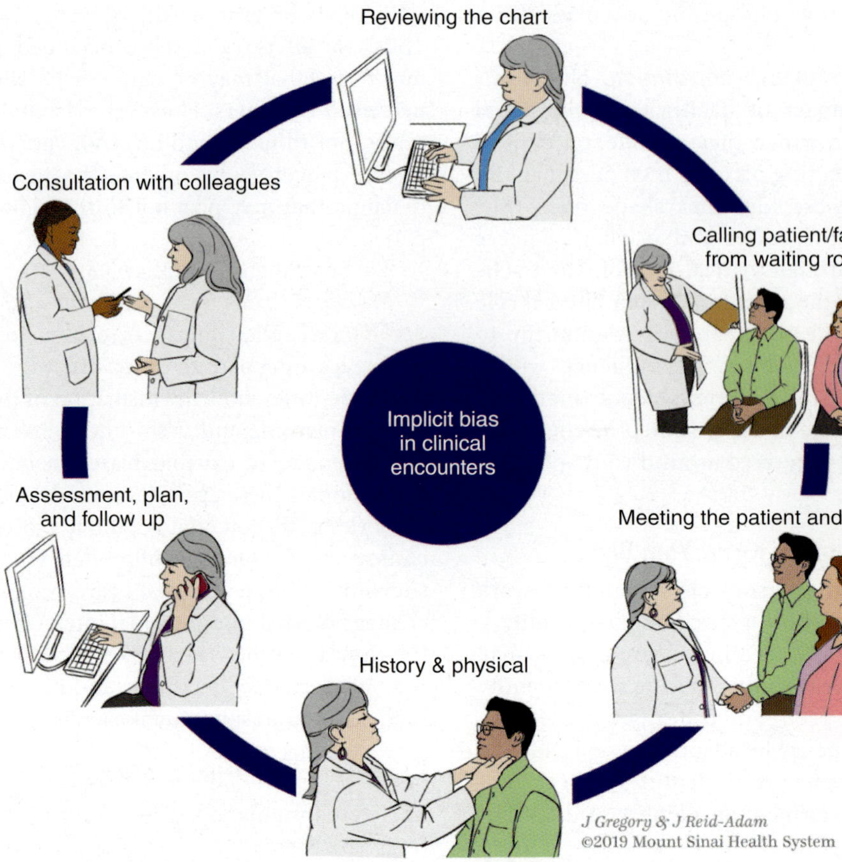

Fig. 5.3 Implicit Bias in the Clinical Encounter. Implicit bias can exist at every stage of a clinical encounter. When unchecked, these healthcare professional biases impact the patient encounter, the healthcare professional's cognitive reasoning, and post-visit communication with the patient and with colleagues. Healthcare professionals must develop anti-racist skills to deconstruct these biases and their impact on patient care. (Illustration by Jill Gregory. Used with permission from Mount Sinai Health System.)

See Box Practice Exercise 5.4.

Practice exercise 5.4 debrief and clinical correlation. Your individual reaction to each example will depend heavily on your own identity and lived experiences, and will be influenced by societal dominant narratives. Table 5.4 describes common dominant narratives that are connected to the clinical documentation examples. The anti-racist clinical skills suggested in the table are active processes you can use to disrupt the impact of such dominant narratives on your clinical reasoning, clinical decisions, and relationships with your patients.

As healthcare professionals, we will read and be influenced by the documentation of others in our profession. We also influence others via our own oral communication and written documentation. This will be further explored in the After the Clinical Encounter section.

PRACTICE EXERCISE 5.4 The Priming Effect of Dominant Narratives

Instructions

Imagine you are about to see a patient for the first time. You read the following clinical documentation in the chart before you enter the room. What societal dominant narratives are connected to each example? What feelings and emotions do each of these engender within you? How might this impact your relationship with the patient?

Chart Excerpt/Observation	Reflection
1. Multiple missed appointments seen on chart review.	
2. Previous doctor's history of present illness begins "45-year-old African American male with sickle cell disease and frequent emergency department visits for pain medication presents complaining of chest pain."	
3. Previous doctor's assessment and plan reads: "55-year-old male with poorly controlled type 2 diabetes. He refuses the addition of insulin despite extensive counseling on the necessity of this medication."	
4. Triage nurse note reads: "32-year-old HIV-negative gay male presents for routine physical."	
5. A body mass index (BMI) of 45 kg/m seen in last clinic note.	

TABLE 5.4 Common Dominant Narratives in Documentation

Chart Excerpt/Observation	Dominant Narrative(s)	Brief Discussion	Suggested Anti-Racist Clinical Skills and Approaches
1. Multiple missed appointments seen on chart review	Patients who miss appointments do not care about their health.	Missed visits often reflect structural barriers to care, including issues of access and issues of trust.	**Generate alternative hypotheses**—Develop a differential diagnosis as to why the patient may be missing appointments and prepare to explore these in the encounter.
2. Previous doctor's history of present illness begins "45-year-old African American male with sickle cell disease and frequent emergency department visits for pain medication presents complaining of chest pain."	Black males have higher pain thresholds than white males. Multiple visits for pain suggests the patient is a "drug abuser." Black males frequently abuse opioid pain medications.	This case demonstrates a common dominant narrative regarding Black males and pain, as well as a common example of scientific racism. There persists a false association between race (being Black) and hemoglobinopathies (including sickle cell). It is important to recognize hemoglobinopathies as a geographic and ancestral condition, to avoid premature closure in a differential diagnosis. The commentary on the patient's need for pain medication is pathologized in the chart, even though medicine recognizes that the pathophysiology of the disease will include pain due to vaso-occlusive crises.	**Question scientific racism**—Do not accept the association between a patient's assumed race and medical diagnosis. Consider more detailed family and ancestral history if diagnosis is in question. **Deconstruct the dominant narrative**—Recognize your own potential biases relating to how particular groups experience pain. Be aware of the impact of this bias throughout the encounter. **Generate alternative hypotheses**—Consider, "What else could be going on?" For this patient, frequent emergency department visits may represent poor access to care, inadequate pain control at baseline due to structural or individual racism of the healthcare professional, or inadequate patient education regarding management of his chronic illness. His chest pain may represent a flare of his chronic illness, a serious complication such as acute chest syndrome, or an unrelated diagnosis such as myocardial infarction.
3. Previous doctor's assessment and plan reads: "55-year-old male with poorly controlled type 2 diabetes. He refuses the addition of insulin despite extensive counseling on the necessity of this medication."	Patients who refuse medical care do not want to get well.	A patient deciding against a recommended treatment speaks to the need to better understand the patient's experiences. This case represents "either/or" thinking, with the healthcare professional "centered" with regard to power and value of opinion.	**Utilize complexity thinking**—Consider the innumerable reasons why a patient may not think insulin is the best option for them, even if they wish to get well. **Decenter the healthcare professional and center the patient**—Create a space for the patient to voice his concerns about insulin.
4. Triage nurse note reads: "32-year-old HIV-negative gay male presents for routine physical."	Gay men are at high risk for HIV or being gay is a risk factor for HIV.	This case represents two cognitive errors grounded in bias. The first is a conflation of identity with behavior (identifying as gay and having "risky sexual behavior"). The second is the placement of risk on the patient/community as opposed to identifying the structural causes for inequitable health.	**Deconstruct the dominant narrative**—Recognize your own potential biases, informed by this dominant narrative, prior to the encounter. Be aware of the impact of this bias throughout the encounter. **Personalize the patient**—Taking an effective history around the patient's identities and behaviors allows for a fuller understanding of the patient's true health needs. For example, despite current guidelines to offer HIV Pre-Exposure Prophylaxis (PreP) to "men who have sex with men," a male in a long-term monogamous relationship with another male has no indication for PreP.
5. A body mass index (BMI) of 45 kg/m seen in last clinic note	Obese patients are nonadherent to suggestions/therapies relating to lifestyle modification. Obese patients do not care about their health.	Patient may be unable to attain goals of BMI depending on other social determinants of health, like access to healthy food, exercise, and healthcare.	**Partner with the patient**—Consider a position that sees the patient as inherently invested in their health and well-being. Approach the encounter from a place of partnership and not antagonism: "I am glad that you're engaging in this discussion with me about your weight. How can I help support you in reaching your BMI goals?"

DURING THE CLINICAL ENCOUNTER

This section will discuss the ways racism and oppression impact the patient during a clinical encounter. Examples of biased behavior of a patient toward a healthcare professional will be discussed in the section Discriminatory Behavior from Patients or Caregivers. Healthcare professionals bring innumerable implicit biases into the clinical encounter. These biases can be triggered during the clinician's time with a patient and can influence the care delivered to the patient. In addition to these individual biases, there exist broad structural forces that impact the clinician-patient encounter. Next, we will address communication and interpersonal skills that can be used by a healthcare professional to disrupt the impact of some of the most common and pervasive individual and structural forms of racism and oppression that manifest during a clinical encounter.

Deconstructing Your Implicit Biases—Personalizing the Patient

We all have biases. It is a human function for survival. One goal of this chapter is to build skills and confidence to recognize, discuss, and disrupt bias in real time during clinical encounters. Research demonstrates healthcare professionals use implicit biases and unconscious associations, often without awareness, intention, or control, when first meeting a patient. A useful anti-racist skill to disrupt such implicit bias is to begin your encounter by "personalizing the patient."

A component of personalizing the patient is exploring the patient's identities and lived experiences. Recall your experiences with the exercises in the previous section (Before the Clinical Encounter [Pre-visit Preparation]). Despite the complexity of our many interconnected identities, healthcare professionals frequently and inaccurately experience our patients as a single or limited number of identities. Patients' identities are frequently simplified or assumed, as often occurs when patients with dark skin are described as "Black" or "African American" without any inquiry into their racial identity. At other times, misinformed associations can result in incorrect assumptions and the conflation of identity with behavior or risk. For example, patients from predominantly Muslim countries or regions are often assumed to be Muslim before obtaining a spiritual history, and patients who identify as gay are often assumed to be at risk for HIV before taking a sexual history.

Exploring a patient's identities through effective questioning techniques can prevent these assumptions from impacting patient care and can also begin to personalize the patient. This is an iterative process and unfolds over time as a healthcare professional develops a relationship with a patient. Much of this is done during the social and family histories, as described in Chapter 1, The Interviewer's Questions, or can be done through less "formal" but no less meaningful conversation with the patient. Approaching these portions of the history can and should be individualized based on style of the healthcare professional, patient preference, and the patient-healthcare professional relationship.

Racial Identity and Ancestry

Enumerable studies, guidelines, and prediction rules ask healthcare professionals to identify a patient's race. In general, healthcare professionals can categorize such recommendations as grounded in one or more of the following categories:

1. **Inaccurate or flawed data:** For example, physiologic corrections for "race" that are applied to estimated glomerular filtration rate and predicted pulmonary volumes are grounded purely in fictitious assumptions of biological differences between racial groups and flawed anthropomorphic data rooted in scientific racism.[19] National organizations now near-universally call for the removal of these "race corrections."
2. **A conflation of race and ancestry:** For example, the genetic variations resulting in sickle cell anemia include parts of Africa and the surrounding regions. Patients who may or may not identify as Black, or be perceived as Black, may have ancestry from these regions. Healthcare professionals often conflate geographic ancestry with sociopolitical categories of race and inappropriately overestimate the likelihood of this condition in patients labeled as "Black" and underestimate it in other populations.
3. **A manifestation of racism:** For example, "risk" calculators for conditions for atherosclerotic cardiovascular disease report a higher likelihood of heart attacks for patients who are labeled as Black compared with those labeled as White in the tool. The studies that support such tools generally observe real racial inequities in health outcomes. However, these inequities are due to racism and not inherent to race.

Navigating the contemporary landscape of race-based medicine therefore requires not only an understanding of the inherent flaws with the use of race as a biological construct (Table 5.5) but the ability to effectively discuss race, racism, and ancestry with patients. To do so, it is necessary to have a clear understanding of what we mean by "race" and what we mean by "ancestry." Race is a sociopolitical and economic construct, by

TABLE 5.5 Flaws With Use of Race as a Biological Construct

Genetic Flaws	Methodologic Flaws	Socio-Medical Implications
Genetic variation is usually distributed in a continuous, overlapping fashion among population, as opposed to being distributed into discrete, racially defined nonoverlapping categories[22]	Inconsistency in the definition and use of race	Promotes understanding of race as a biological concept and biological determinant of health, at the expense of identifying true and potentially modifiable structural and social drivers of inequities
Commonly defined racial groups are genetically heterogeneous and lack clear-cut genetic boundaries[20]	Failure of studies to distinguish between self-identified racial categories and assigned/assumed racial categories[23]	We can only point to a few diseases associated with White race (e.g., cystic fibrosis) and White heritage/Ashkenazi Jewish (e.g., lysosomal storage diseases) thus perpetuating an illness burden on Black bodies and erasing other non-White people from discussions of racially based diseases
Approximately 90% of genetic variation exists *within* Old World populations, as opposed to *between* populations, making the clinical utility of even geographic ancestry minimal[22,24]		Racial categories are historically created, originally suggested a scale of inferiority and superiority, and today continue to connote notions of human hierarchy[25]

which we mean race is a socially, politically, and economically defined category to which value and meaning are ascribed. Several definitions of race exist. A useful definition when considering how to explore a patient's racial identity is "a social, cultural, and historical construct that artificially divides people into groups based on factors such as phenotype, ancestry, national origin, etc., to facilitate and justify exploitation."[20] This definition is helpful when approaching a patient because it highlights the historic and contemporary significance of race and racial identity along with its very real social implications.[21] Ancestry, on the other hand, can be understood as "a process-based concept, a statement about an individual's relationship to other individuals in their genealogic history; thus it is a very personal understanding of one's genomic heritage."[20] We view ancestry as more than a family's genealogic or geographic history. It is a living history of a family's sociopolitical, medical, and environmental experiences and is related to, yet distinct from, the racial identities of the members of that family. Clinically, these experiences represent the cumulative structural drivers of health within a patient's family. They also inform the patient's understanding of health and wellness and the patient's relationship with the medical system. For example, consider two patients who both identify as Black. One patient's family was enslaved 200 years ago and participated in the Great Migration north to Central Harlem in New York City where the patient and her parents have lived for 60 years. The other patient also identifies as Black, yet her parents immigrated to Central Harlem from West Africa 40 years ago, before the patient was born. Each patient's individual and family medical and social histories have related yet distinct experiences of structural racism and other social and structural drivers of health, and each must be interpreted within these varying contexts. As such, while an individual patient may or may not distinguish race from ancestry in their minds, the healthcare professional should approach them separately during their history.

Generally, "self-identified race/ethnicity" is the gold standard used in medical research.[26] Most data collection tools that purport to collect "self-identified race" present patients with a list of options from which to choose. These options are finite, do not always align with an individual's understanding of racial identity, and often change over time as a society's or government's understanding of race changes. Further, two patients with the same self-identified race may appear and therefore be perceived, and often treated, differently within healthcare and society at large. When inequities are due to individual healthcare professional bias, perceived race is a more significant factor than self-identified race.

We recommend an open discussion that allows a deeper and richer understanding of the patient's own understanding of racial identity, ancestry, and personal and generational experiences of racism, oppression, and trauma. This approach allows for a useful understanding of the patient's self-identified and perceived race as this relates to their lived experience, as well as the patient's ancestry, as it relates to their genealogic history.

Potential questions to transition into a racial and ancestral history:

- *I'm going to ask you a few questions to better understand your background and that of your family. I ask these questions of all my patients.*
- *I don't want to assume anything about your identity, so I'm going to ask you a few questions so I can best take care of you.*

Potential questions to ask about a patient's racial identity include:

- *How would you best describe your race or racial identity?*
- *How about that of your family?*
    - This question can begin to transition into an ancestral history.
- *How do you feel others would describe your race or racial identity?*

Potential questions to explore a patient's lived experiences with respect to racial identity[27]:

- *Many of my patients experience racism in their healthcare. What has been your experience with racism when you seek out medical care?*
- *What have been your experiences within the healthcare system?*
- *Have you had any experiences that have caused you to lose trust in the healthcare system or your doctor?*

An ancestral history is often best asked coupled with either the social history or the family medical history. It is essentially a "family social and geographic history."

Potential questions to ask about a patient's ancestry:

- *Tell me about your family.*
- *Where is your family from?*
- *You mentioned you identify as an Irish-American. Tell me more about your family's history.*

We recommend discussing race and ancestry with all patients, regardless of their assumed or stated racial identities. This allows the healthcare professional to obtain invaluable historical information about a patient and the patient's family. Further, whiteness is often made "invisible" in medicine because it is assumed to be the normative identity without explicit reference; only people of color are identified and called by a racial/ethnic status. White patients are not perceived as racialized or as having any particular medical or social risk. Discussions of racial identity and ancestry with patients who identify as White serve to decenter whiteness in the healthcare professional's mind and promote a deeper, more authentic relationship with the patient.

Spiritual and Religious Identity

Discussing a patient's religion and spirituality improves patient satisfaction[28] and end-of-life decision making,[29,30] and it is generally preferred by patients.[31,32]

Spirituality can be defined as "the aspect of humanity that refers to the way individuals seek and express meaning and purpose and the way they experience their connectedness to the moment, to self, to others, to nature, and to the significant and sacred." *Religion*, on the other hand, can be defined as "an organized system of beliefs, rituals, and practices with which an individual identifies and associates and includes a relationship with a divine being."[33,34]

One well-validated tool to assess a patient's spiritual and religious identity is the *"FICA" tool* (Table 5.6). The FICA spiritual history tool provides a framework for healthcare professionals to explore a patient's spiritual identity, experiences, and beliefs with a particular focus on how these intersect with the patient's

TABLE 5.6 FICA Spiritual History Tool

The FICA Spiritual History Tool was developed by Dr. Puchalski and a group of primary care physicians to help physicians and other healthcare professionals address spiritual issues with patients. Spiritual histories are taken as part of the regular history during an annual exam or new patient visit but can also be taken as part of follow-up visits, as appropriate. The FICA tool serves as a guide for conversations in the clinical setting.

The acronym FICA can help structure questions in taking a spiritual history by healthcare professionals.

F–Faith and Belief

"Do you consider yourself spiritual or religious?" or "Is spirituality something important to you?" or "Do you have spiritual beliefs that help you cope with stress/difficult times?" (Contextualize to reason for visit if it is not the routine history.)

If the patient responds "No," the healthcare professional might ask, "What gives your life meaning?" Sometimes patients respond with answers such as family, career, or nature.

(The question of meaning should also be asked even if people answer yes to spirituality.)

I–Importance

"What importance does your spirituality have in your life? Has your spirituality influenced how you take care of yourself, your health? Does your spirituality influence you in your healthcare decision making (e.g., advance directives, treatment, etc.)?"

C–Community

"Are you part of a spiritual community?" Communities such as churches, temples, and mosques, a group of like-minded friends and family, or yoga can serve as strong support systems for some patients. Can explore further: "Is this of support to you and how? Is there a group of people you really love or who are important to you?"

A–Address in Care

"How would you like me, your healthcare professional, to address these issues in your healthcare?" (With the newer models including diagnosis of spiritual distress, A also refers to the "Assessment and Plan" of patient spiritual distress or issues within a treatment or care plan.)

medical care. When used routinely, the FICA tool also helps mitigate a healthcare professional's potential biases and assumptions regarding a patient's religious or spiritual beliefs and practices and helps identify structures and systems that may impact. It can also help healthcare professionals identify patients who may benefit from consultation or co-management with a chaplain.

Gender Identity and Sexual Orientation

Gender identity and sexual orientation are important aspects of a patient's personal identity. Sadly, healthcare professionals often fail to assess these identities appropriately. Various systemic factors contribute to the subpar healthcare provided to patients based on their gender identity and sexual orientation.

A sexual history is typically asked as a stand-alone part of the history or included within the social history. Prior to establishing the patient's sexual history, healthcare professionals should use inclusive terminology that avoids assumptions. For example, use terms such as "partner," as opposed to "husband or wife," until the patient's preferred terminology is established.

In Chapter 26 (The Transgender Patient), we delve into the intricacies of gender identity, sexual orientation, prejudice, and communication, all with the goal of creating an environment that fosters respect, dignity, and inclusivity.

Moving the Center to the Patient

Structural racism and oppression marginalize patients. Clinically, this process is deeply rooted in the history of racism in medicine (see Fig. 5.1) and the interdependence of white supremacy culture and medical culture and practice. Excellent communication and interpersonal skills can disrupt this by centering the voice and experience of the patient. There are additional skills, however, that move the center of the clinical encounter from the healthcare professional's perspective to that of the patient, thus balancing the dynamic within the relationship. These are active processes that have been described within the social context. Here we present them as applied to the clinical environment (see Table 5.2). Each of these approaches dovetails with the anti-racist clinical skills described in Table 5.7.

Disrupting Structural Racism and Oppression

Structural competency recognizes health outcomes as downstream effects of broad, structural forces. Several tools exist to help healthcare professionals identify proximal "social determinants of health" (SDH) including food insecurity, health literacy, and housing insecurity. When used within a structural competency framework, these tools help healthcare professionals partner with patients to explore areas of structural vulnerability,[35] identify individual and community-based strengths, and develop collaborative plans to improve health.[36] Comprehensive structural vulnerability assessments typically assess multiple domains including financial security, residence, environmental risks/safety, access to food, social networks, legal concerns, and education. Structural competency also assesses an individual's experience with racism, oppression, or discrimination, as well as clinician implicit bias.

Effective application of structural competency requires healthcare professionals to identify and disrupt white supremacy norms (Table 5.2) and challenge colonial systems. For example, structural competency requires healthcare professionals to identify and disrupt the biases they bring to a patient encounter; this runs counter to the "right to comfort," calling for vulnerability, growth, and learning within the healthcare

TABLE 5.7 Sample Anti-Racist Clinical Skills

Skill	Description	Example
Generate alternative hypotheses	Goal here is to identify and challenge the label that drives your bias, then identify the real structural forces at play.	Patient with multiple emergency department (ED) visits labeled as a "frequent flyer." View ED visits as a symptom and seek to identify broader structural barriers to care that force patient into using ED as an access point.
Personalize the patient	An active measure to reduce the impact of an identified implicit bias within the clinician triggered by patient name, socioeconomic status, and/or race (identified or presumed). This can also be used universally, with all patients, to reduce the impact of implicit biases of which the clinician may not be aware.	Healthcare professional recognizes an implicit bias regarding patients of color and pain medication seeking. The healthcare professional intentionally and purposefully engages in conversation and/or takes a more detailed social history to personalize the patient and reduce the impact of the bias on clinical decision making.
Deconstruct dominant narratives	A preparatory measure wherein the clinician seeks to learn about the historical and structural drivers of dominant narratives that support their implicit biases.	Healthcare professionals learn the historical relationship between their community and medicine to better interpret clinical observations. A patient complaining about long wait times for appointments and never seeing the same healthcare professional twice while receiving care in a resident clinic should be viewed in the context of the historic and contemporary segregation of care—once explicitly by race, now indirectly race via insurance status. Some patients' mistrust of the medical system should be viewed in the context of historic and contemporary experimentation upon individuals and communities of color.
Frame	Grounded in the well-documented cognitive theory of framing, in which the way a patient is presented can impact the clinical reasoning of the listener or reader. Healthcare professionals can use this as an anti-racist skill by reframing a patient to call attention to the structural drivers of an observed health outcome. This skill is also used to counter dominant narratives.	A Black mother who voices concerns about the care her child received in the hospital is labeled as disruptive or angry. The healthcare professional highlights mother's advocacy and uses language such as "invested in her child's health" and "advocate for her child" when describing the family to colleagues.

professional. *Structural humility* is only possible when healthcare professionals engage in authentic power sharing and center the experiences of patients and communities. Structural competency also calls for healthcare professionals to examine how they may leverage their professional status and positionality to intervene and disrupt structural violence and structural vulnerability for their patients and communities. The final goal of a structurally competent healthcare professional is developing a mindset of and practicing structural humility.

Structural humility is only possible when healthcare professionals engage in authentic power sharing and decenter themselves in their role as "omniscient" healthcare professionals. This involves not simply asking a checklist of questions but rather intentionally centering the lived experiences of patients. Together, the healthcare professional and patient recognize how structural forces embedded in systems and institutions engender structural violence, harm, trauma, and vulnerability. Neither can nor should one intervene in disrupting structural forms of oppression alone. Structural competency and structural humility can only be truly learned via relationships with patients. Consider using the following reflection exercise periodically throughout your training and career.

Practice Exercise

Exercise 5: Exploring Structural Humility

See Box Practice Exercise 5.5.

Practice exercise 5.5 debrief. Demonstrating structural humility is the personification of a mindset. This is an ongoing process and journey, not a destination or static state, because of the ubiquitous nature of structural oppression in all systems and institutions. Healthcare professionals may demonstrate structural competency through a motivational desire to distinguish the features of systems and structures, cautioning against the biomedical approach to patient care in their practice, and encouraging inquiry, reflection, partnership, and collaboration amongst traditional and nontraditional partners in patient care.[37]

Disrupting Trauma in the Clinical Encounter

Racism and oppression cause individual and generational trauma, which have profound effects on the health of individuals

PRACTICE EXERCISE 5.5 Exploring Structural Humility

Instructions

Reflect on the following question: What behaviors and/or ways of thinking have I experienced, as a healthcare professional or as a patient, that demonstrate structural humility? How do I know?

BOX 5.2 Elements of Structural Competency

1. Recognizing the structures that shape clinical interactions
2. Developing an extra-clinical language of structure
3. Rearticulating "cultural" presentations in structural terms
4. Observing and imagining structural interventions
5. Developing structural humility.

Based on data in Metzl JM, Hansen H: Structural competency: theorizing a new medical engagement with stigma and inequality, *Soc Sci Med* 103:126–133, 2014. https://doi.org/10.1016/j.socscimed.2013.06.032

and communities.[1,9] Structural competency and structural humility (Box 5.2) aid the healthcare professional and the patient in identifying sources of trauma, including those from within the healthcare system. In every clinical encounter, healthcare professionals have the opportunity to disrupt the impact of this trauma and partner with the patient to improve their overall health. *Trauma-informed care* (TIC) is an approach to care that includes organizational, structural, and interpersonal elements. TIC broadly refers to a set of principles that guide and direct how we view the impact of severe harm on an individual's mental, physical, and emotional health and encourages support and treatment to the whole person rather than focusing on only treating individual symptoms or specific behaviors. Fundamentally, TIC represents a holistic approach to shaping organizational culture, practices, and policies to be sensitive to the experiences and needs of traumatized individuals. It is oriented to an organizational change process centered on principles intended to promote healing and reduce the risk of retraumatization for individuals who experience structural vulnerability.[38]

The four aims of TIC include ***realizing*** the widespread impact of trauma, ***recognizing*** signs and symptoms of trauma, ***responding*** via policies and practices, and ***resisting re-traumatization***.[39] We recommend a trauma-informed approach for all patients. Formal TIC training is invaluable for healthcare professionals. Next, we outline general recommendations for before, during, and after clinical encounters.

Before:

- Reflect on the ways you as an individual, and within your role as a healthcare professional, experience and perpetuate trauma and violence.
- Recognize concrete implicit biases you carry and how these play out in individual patient encounters (i.e., word choice, assumptions about patient behavior or preferences, etc.).
- Recognize the way the system in which you practice perpetuates violence and trauma for patients (this can be as granular as a lack of appropriate gender options on a registration form to the propensity of a practice to call security or perform drug screening without consent on patients of color).
- Familiarize yourself with local and community resources commonly sought by your patients.

During:

- Take active steps to disrupt your own biases during the encounter (i.e., personalizing the patient).
- Use inclusive, patient-centered language throughout the encounter.
- Ask for permission and provide context for particularly sensitive aspects of the history and physical exam.
- Be mindful of body position (avoid approaching patients from behind) and draping (only expose the part of the body you need to examine and only while examining it).

After:

- Practice liberating documentation to prevent trauma/re-traumatization of patients through the care plan (see next section). Collaborate and share documentation with patients.
- Reflect on any trauma you may have experienced during the encounter (see the final section on Discriminatory Behavior from Patients and Caregivers).
- Advocate for system and institutional change based on individual experiences.

AFTER THE CLINICAL ENCOUNTER

Following the patient encounter, it is critically important for the healthcare professional to consider how racism and oppression impact oral communication about and written documentation of patients, as well as the clinical reasoning and clinical decisions made by the care team.

Oral Presentations and Written Documentation

Just as in the clinical encounter, one's unconscious associations must be consciously dismantled during the oral presentation and written documentation of patients. Healthcare professionals must consider the impact of how patients, their identities, their clinical problems, and the systems in which these exist are described.

Stigmatizing language in presentations and documentation results in ineffective management of chronic conditions, lowered patient trust in healthcare professionals, increased rates of depression and anxiety, and decreased follow-up and care-seeking.[40] Evidence-based recommendations for nonstigmatizing language include using person-first language, eliminating pejorative terms, making communication inclusive, avoiding labels, not using weaponizing quotes, and desisting from blaming patients.[41] Documenting all aspects of the clinical encounter in a way that is truthful and affirming to a patient is vitally important not only for clinical decision making but also to ensure that biased and subjective impressions are not perpetuated within a patient's medical record.

Anti-racist and anti-oppressive language is not simply a matter of word choice or omission of potentially biased language. Oral presentations and written documentation represent a distinct sphere of influence for healthcare professionals to disrupt the influence of racism and oppression in the clinical environment. Liberating language is an anti-racist practice wherein oral and written communications reflect a relationship with the patient grounded in authentic structural competency and structural humility.

Emerging literature provides in-depth discussions of anti-racist documentation practices.[42] Here we present concrete recommendations for common components of the oral presentation and written documentation (the opening statement, the family and social history, the physical exam, and the assessment and plan), followed by an exercise that illustrates moving from stigmatizing to liberating documentation.

Opening Statement

The opening statement frames the case for listeners and should include the patient's chief complaint framed by important clinical and social context. To minimize false stereotypes, biases, and assumptions made about the patient and to disconnect inaccurate associations of a patient's race with their clinical complaint or presenting illness, **the presenter should not include race in the opening line about a patient.** We are not advocating for being colorblind or ignoring a patient's race. Instead, the use of race should be used to frame the social context of a patient's lived experience. Traditionally race has been included in the opening statement of a presentation to call attention to presumed associations between race and prevalence of various conditions or differential responses to treatments based on race. Outside of these associations, race is also used to call attention to the assumed pathologic behavior of a patient (e.g., "Hispanic alcoholic," or "disruptive Black female"). It has become clear that race, however, is not a valid or useful proxy for genetics or family history. Instead of providing relevant and useful clinical context, the use of race in the opening statement risks engendering biases in the audience and obscuring the true drivers of health.

Additional patient characteristics often represented in the opening statement are sex and gender. Given the fluidity of gender identity, if the opening line about a patient includes sex, it should also specify the patient's current gender identity and note whether the patient identifies as cisgender, transgender, gender nonbinary, or other. This will avoid assumptions regarding the patient's current gender identity, normalize assessing and reporting the gender identity of all patients, and decenter the cisgender experience. **When deciding whether and how to include sex (and, therefore, current gender identity) in an opening statement, the healthcare professional should consider clinical relevance, patient preference, potential unintended consequences, and potential biases in the audience.**

Recommended opening statement:

RO is a 36-year-old cisgender female who presents with 3 days of a cough productive of yellow sputum.

Not recommended opening statement:

RO is a 36-year-old African American female who presents with 3 days of a cough productive of yellow sputum.

Family and Social Histories

When documenting the social and family histories of the patient in oral or written format, we recommend reporting a patient's chosen identity. A patient's description of their racial identity, that of their family, and their ancestral history as well as their answers to the FICA questions provide an opportunity for the written and oral record to more fully reflect the patient's voice.

Recommended social history:

RO identifies as a cisgender female, and her preferred pronouns are she/her/hers. Her self-identified racial identity is African American and that of her family is African American and Asian. Her father's family is from Atlanta, Georgia, and her mother's family is from Beijing, China. RO identifies as a cisgender female and describes her sexual orientation as bisexual. She is currently sexually active with two cisgender men; she always has her partners use condoms. Using the FICA Spiritual History Tool, RO indicates that she is spiritual but not religious and her family gives her a sense of meaning. Spirituality has not influenced her healthcare decision making, but it does influence how she approaches life and her family and friends. She is not part of a spiritual community at this time. She is not sure how her spirituality can be addressed by our team at this time.

Not recommended social history:

RO is African American, female, and bisexual. She is currently sexually active with two men; she always uses condoms. She says she does not practice any formal religion.

Physical Exam

The physical exam has the potential to trigger biases and assumptions as well. Ensuring accurate descriptions of findings in a descriptive manner is critical for the physical examination presentation and documentation, but it is imperative to avoid assumptions and inferences that may be stereotyping or biased. For example, the general appearance should not specify light- or dark-skinned (unless using standardized systems in descriptions of rashes), and *the description of a patient's hair should not specify how the hair is styled.* In addition, documentation of a patient's physical ability should be clinically relevant, specific, and empowering by including the patient's self-reported abilities.

Assessment and Plan

Medical decision making is a critical aspect of medical care and typically manifests in the assessment and plan portion of both the oral and written case presentation. Medical decision making represents the healthcare professional's analysis and interpretation of information gathered through the patient history and physical exam; from the family, team, and medical record; and any available test and study data. As described earlier in this chapter, harmful assumptions made about patients are pervasive in the medical record. Applying anti-racist techniques, such as developing alternative hypotheses to counter typical dominant narratives, is critically important. Addressing these in the assessment and plan as part of medical decision making is vital to an anti-racist approach to patient care. Documenting all aspects of the clinical encounter in a way that is truthful and affirming to a patient is vitally important not only for clinical decision making but also to ensure that biased and subjective impressions are not perpetuated within a patient's medical record.

When structural root causes of a clinical problem are identified, a prioritized structural problem list can be developed and documented.[43] Such documentation promotes consideration of health system and community resources that should be mobilized and documented in the assessment and plan for the patient. Lastly, many diagnostic algorithms, practice guidelines, and primary literature suggest that a patient's race be used to modify or adjust treatment plans. In the interpretation of such recommendations, healthcare professionals should remember that race is a sociopolitical and economic construct, but racism has very real health outcomes. Multiple tools and resources exist to guide the appraisal of such literature[44] and to discern if the application is likely to relieve or exacerbate inequities.[45] The ultimate assessment and plan should reflect these assessments.

Practice Exercise

Exercise 6: liberating documentation.

You are admitting a patient to the pediatric inpatient service after he presented to the emergency department (ED) due to a seizure. In reviewing the chart before seeing the patient, you read the following note from the neurology team:

"Patient is a 21-year-old Hispanic male with an epilepsy syndrome, generalized tonic-clonic seizures (GTC), who presented with multiple witnessed GTC seizures in the setting of marijuana and alcohol use. He has a history of noncompliance with his seizure medications and frequent visits to the emergency room for the same. In the ED, he was agitated and refused to answer questions. He was belligerent and urinated on the floor before having another seizure. He is now being admitted for further management."

See Box Practice Exercise 5.6.

Practice exercise 5.6 debrief and clinical correlation. Reflect back on Exercise 5.4 from Before the Clinical Encounter (Previsit Preparation). Recall the ways in which clinical documentation may engender bias in you as the reader. In this exercise, we explored the ways you can use clinical documentation as a

PRACTICE EXERCISE 5.6 Liberating Documentation

Part 1 Instructions

Identify examples of potentially stigmatizing language in this clinical documentation. In what ways might this language influence you, as the reader, and your approach to this patient? Consider alternative documentation.

You can use this table for your reflection or copy the table to a blank sheet of paper. Suggestions are provided on the following page.

Potential Stigmatizing Language	Impact on Reader	Alternative Documentation

Suggested responses for Part 1:

Potential Stigmatizing Language	Impact on Reader	Anti-Racist Approach
"Hispanic"	May trigger implicit bias in reader and perpetuate dominant narratives.	Do not include racial identity in this opening statement. The extent to which this patient's self-identified or perceived race impacts their experience of care (i.e., racism) can be elucidated from the patient and documented later in the history of present illness, the social history, and/or the assessment and plan.
"History of noncompliance with seizure medications." "Frequent visits to the emergency room for the same."	Can result in assumptions about patient's overall approach to care and/or premature closure (i.e., not considering other causes for current seizure).	Either omit until additional information available or include evidence of current seizure medication use and context/barriers to medication use (see Part 2) as elucidated from a discussion with the patient.
"...setting of alcohol and marijuana use..."	Can engender bias against the patient and result in assumptions regarding the association between alcohol or marijuana use and the patient's presenting symptoms. May cause reader to assume some behaviors are due to alcohol use rather than post-seizure changes.	May include recent or current use of alcohol or marijuana in the HPI if contextualized and done in a way to prevent premature closure of the differential diagnosis (see Part 2).
"He was agitated, refusing to answer questions... he was belligerent..."	This is stigmatizing language and also represents assumptions ("agitated," "belligerent") as opposed to observations. May trigger visceral bias in the reader.	Remove such stigmatizing language from clinical documentation. Include only clinically relevant observations without inferences or value-based statements.

Part 2 Instructions

Imagine you will be meeting the patient depicted in the consultant's note from Part 1. Consider the domains from a typical structural vulnerability assessment. What questions might you ask to better foster a relationship grounded in authentic structural humility? How might these questions impact his care?

Would you find these questions hard to ask? Why or why not?

PRACTICE EXERCISE 5.6 **Liberating Documentation—cont'd**

Domain	Questions	Reflection
Financial Security		
Residence		
Environmental risks/safety		
Access to food		
Social networks		
Legal concerns		
Education		
Bias		

liberating tool to frame your patients in a way that (1) disrupts dominant narratives, (2) is developed in collaboration with patients, (3) redirects attention away from race and toward racism/oppression as drivers of health inequities, and (4) assists in the effective, structurally competent care of patients.

Communication Within the Clinical Care Team

Healthcare professionals should continuously assess for the impact of racism and oppression on the clinical reasoning and decisions made by the care team, including themselves. Healthcare professionals at every stage in their career, from learners to supervisors, have a broad sphere of influence on the teams in which they practice. The following examples of effective anti-racist and anti-oppressive communication skills can help leverage this influence and disrupt racism and oppression in the clinical environment.

Probing questions for yourself:

- Would I be making this same decision if this patient was White?
- What factors about this patient could be influencing my clinical reasoning or the ways by which I interact with this patient?
- What assumptions am I making about this patient?

Probing questions for the care team:

- What assumptions are we making about this patient?
- What do you mean when you say…?
- Would we be calling child and family protective services if this were a White family?

Naming (simple statements that name observed oppression and promote ongoing discussion):

- I noticed our team tends to spend more time rounding on patients with private insurance than Medicaid/White patients compared with patients of color.
- I noticed we had not asked the patient for their goals/perspectives on this treatment.

"C.U.S." Language

Many team-based communication strategies also exist that can be applied within anti-racist and anti-oppressive frameworks when bias is identified on a team. "C.U.S." is part of "Team STEPPS"[46] training and includes a series of escalating statements that include "concerned," "uncomfortable," and "safety." For example:

- "I am ***concerned*** that our biases around this patient's race may be influencing our clinical decisions."
- "I am ***uncomfortable*** with how this patient is being described as 'aggressive.'"
- "Not offering this procedure because of her race is a ***safety issue***."

DISCRIMINATORY BEHAVIOR FROM PATIENTS OR CAREGIVERS

When faced with race-based mistreatment, learners and their teachers may be uncertain of an action plan. Their actions can be unclear and conflicted as there may be competing interests: duty to provide care versus duty to self and one's mental/physical safety versus duty to hospital policy. When not named and processed appropriately, such interactions with patients can undermine healthcare professional resilience and the very reasons for which a learner studies and works.

Learner mistreatment in the form of discrimination is a widespread, but not new, phenomenon. Throughout their training, healthcare professionals recall events with particular patients that were hurtful and undermined the good intentions to deliver compassionate patient care. Many of these events are internalized and preserved without full resolution of the interaction. At best, these events are debriefed with colleagues. Learners often receive no advice as to how to anticipate and address racism directed toward them. Without discussion with supervisors and faculty near the time of the event, the status quo remains.

A comment regarding a learner or healthcare professional's race or ethnic background or a patient's refusal of care based on the healthcare professional's race or ethnic background can be painfully personal, confusing, and scarring. As the United States healthcare professional population becomes more racially and ethnically diverse, it is speculated that race-based assignment demands may increase.[47] A study of nearly 400 first-year residents identified 93% as having experienced "disruptive behavior," which included racial and gender bias, berating, and exclusion from decision making.[48] Another study regarding the mistreatment of trainees found that 40% of this mistreatment was delivered by their patients.[49] In a study of over 300 internal medical residents from three academic medical centers, biased patient behavior is experienced frequently with a disproportionate burden of these incidents occurring among non-White and female residents. Incidents were frequent with nearly one-third of respondents experiencing biased patient behaviors at least once per month.[50] Residents rarely reported biased patient behavior to the institution or switched the patient to another healthcare professional, citing the need to prioritize clinical care and a sense of futility in reporting.

Students may be reluctant to bring forth their concerns regarding mistreatment and racism exhibited by patients. They may fear being labeled as "overly sensitive" and uncaring for certain patients. Additionally, students may be reticent to communicate the problematic nature of the interaction to their superior if the superior or team shares the same racial identity with the patient. When learners do express their concerns regarding discriminatory behavior from patients, they may not always receive adequate support and guidance. Faculty may not understand how to support learners and may advise them to "let it go" or accept that "you cannot change people." In the immediate period of time following a discriminatory event, learners have described that their learning stops.[51] In a survey performed at the Annual Medical Education Conference, residents who self-identified as Black, Hispanic, and/or Native American reported the need to downplay or hide their true identities to be accepted in the clinical arena. The challenges to their personal identities were heightened by limited social and professional support.[52]

The cumulative effect of these unacknowledged behaviors toward learners can be significant, with the occurrence of sustained residual effects such as increased vigilance, increased anxiety, avoidance of certain types of patients, and a change in career interest.[53]

Institutions are beginning to develop faculty education and programs in the realm of identifying, anticipating, and debriefing discriminatory patient encounters with medical trainees. Whitgob et al. have outlined strategies with which to address discrimination against students and residents.[54] Four themes emerge: (1) assess illness acuity, (2) cultivate a therapeutic relationship, (3) depersonalize the event, and (4) ensure a safe learning environment for trainees. Goldenberg et al. described a standardized approach to empower educators to recognize and respond to trainee mistreatment by patients.[51] The framework used is described by the acronym **ERASE**: ***E****xpect* that mistreatment will happen; ***R****ecognize* when mistreatment occurs; ***A****ddress* the situation in real time; ***S****upport* the trainee after the event; and ***E****stablish* a positive culture. Boutin-Foster has promoted the R.E.A.C.T. framework that provides educators with methods of how to role-model anti-racism to learners in the clinical environment. This acronym describes *Reflecting* on the educator's implicit biases; *Educating* oneself on historical and current forms of structural racism; *Assessing* the use of race in clinical practice and *Asking* how racism is impacting a clinical encounter; *Calling out* racism-perpetuating behaviors; and *Treating* everyone with dignity and respect.[55]

From the perspective of a healthcare professional, you should anticipate that discriminatory patient encounters will occur and be prepared with an algorithm on how to address the situation when they occur in real time.

Table 5.8 provides examples of discriminatory behavior from patients or caregivers. Problems listed include patients expressing that racial/ethnic minorities are inferior, are not worthy of respect, are assumed to be of inferior intelligence, and are not from the dominant culture. These encounters may be unrecognized by those in a supervisory position or are glossed over by faculty who are uncomfortable or uncertain of a trainee's reaction and do not want to "make a big deal about it" or distract from the clinical process. Utilizing the four themes set forth by Whitgob et al., Fig. 5.4 describes potential actions that students can take when confronted by discriminatory behavior from a patient or caregiver.

Assess the Illness Acuity of the Patient

The acuity of the patient's illness and the clinical role of the trainee can help determine the initial steps following a discriminatory encounter. Your primary role is that of a learner. You should consider if this encounter is of "high stakes" (i.e., Does this patient need their assistance or do you need to obtain particular components of the history and/or physical examination to provide treatment for the patient? Is there an assignment/grade required following this patient encounter? Are there other patients who can be interviewed instead?).

TABLE 5.8 Discriminatory Patient Encounters at the Bedside During Clinical Teaching

Problem	Example	Message
Inferiority of racial/ethnic minorities	"Can I speak to the doctor?" "Are you the nurse?"	Non-White people, particularly African Americans and Latinos, cannot be healthcare professionals.
Racial and gender stereotype	"Hi, Susan." (Dr. Smith)	Non-White healthcare professionals are not worthy of respect.
Assigning intelligence	"You're so articulate."	People of color assumed to be inferior in intelligence.
Othering	"Where are you from?" "Your English is good."	Inquiry into racial/ethnic background that implies that person is not part of the dominant culture; often a distracting line of questioning that does not relate to clinical encounter.
Racial unconscious bias and stereotyping	Patient only addressing or making eye contact with White healthcare professionals on the team	Non-White healthcare professionals are not worthy of respect or acknowledgment.

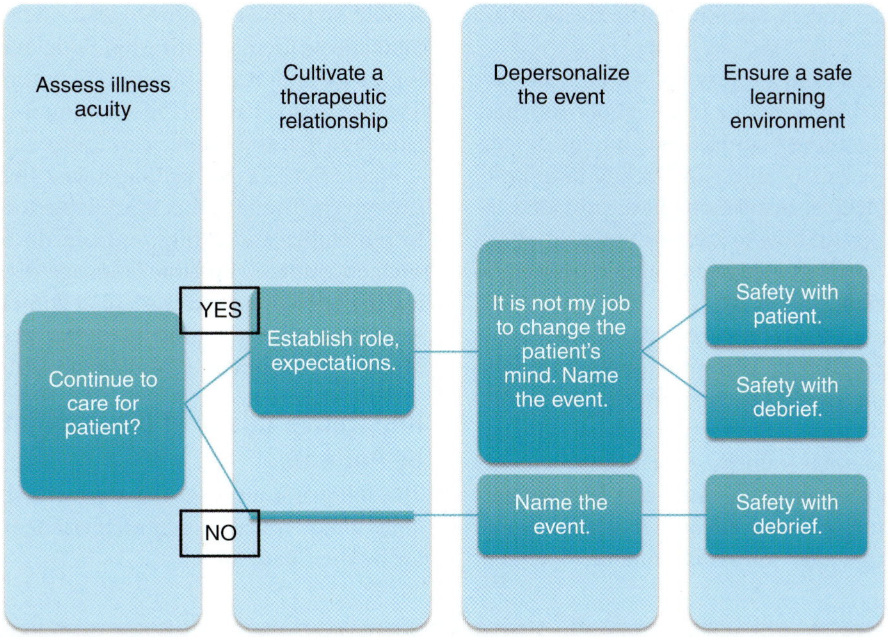

Fig. 5.4 A Learner Approach to Discriminatory Patient Behavior. It is vitally important to have a reliable approach when confronting discriminatory patient behavior. Above is a pathway you may use when weighing the sometimes competing interests of personal safety and duty to treat a patient. While this should be facilitated by the supervisor, here we empower you to take an active role in reflection and response.

Your options include continuing care for the patient, reaching out to another team member to assist with this patient, or removing yourself from the situation entirely. While this may not be the first response, you should be empowered to remove yourself from a hurtful situation and transfer patient care to another healthcare professional. When transferring patient care, you may say to your supervisor, "*During my encounter with Patient X, there were times during the conversation when I was made to feel uncomfortable by factors unrelated to the clinical situation; I would like to care for another patient at this time.*"

Cultivate a Therapeutic Alliance With the Patient

The key here is to recognize that it is not your role or other team members to change a patient's bias. If your intent is to continue to care for the patient, you can consider engaging the patient by asking about patient concerns. This might be best done with the assistance of a senior learner or supervisor/faculty. The medical team can define the roles and structures of the team for the patient. You, in the presence of your superior, are empowered to state "*I work as part of your medical team…*" as a way to start this conversation.

Identifying the Behavior

You can acknowledge that the discriminatory behavior may come from a patient's illness and the patient's/family's sense of lack of control. A patient's delirium or disorientation due to illness may play a role, but it does not make the behavior acceptable or any easier to handle or process. If the patient's family or caregiver exhibits the behavior, you should consider focusing on the patient and your role in caring for the patient. A senior learner or faculty/supervisor should name the behavior with the patient: "*Are you discriminating against this learner because of their skin color/gender/religion?*" If you choose to name the behavior with the patient/family, you should feel sufficiently comfortable or empowered to respond to the patient or family.

You may get into the habit of minimizing these events so as not to call further attention to them, create extra work for the medical team, or appear overly sensitive. In addition, if you are of a different race than the medical team, readdressing the event with a homogenous team can be doubly traumatic as senior members of the group represent another barrier and may respond without true empathy and understanding of the issues at play. You should be encouraged to reflect on these encounters and seek debriefing from faculty or supervisors who they identify as mentors in the time following the event.

Establishing a Supportive Learning Environment

The onus and responsibility of establishing a supportive learning environment should be on the faculty or supervisor. You, as a learner, need not be the person who owns this responsibility.

You should seek support and opportunities to debrief the event from their team or others with whom you feel comfortable. Longitudinal mentorship with a senior student or faculty member is particularly helpful for managing future encounters. So as not to feel helpless, you should also be educated as to how and to whom you can report these incidents. Following an event, you should consider what would be the ideal response or next steps. These may be different for various scenarios. You should be able to work with a mentor or faculty member and be empowered to come up with the next steps that may include commentary in post-rotation evaluations, communication with a dean or ombudsperson, and/or speaking with the rotation director.

Encounters with patients who express racism and bias are fraught with challenges. When being the recipient of bias, there is fear of retribution by grade or clinical assignment, uncertainty of what to say or do, lack of allies, and lack of familiarity with institution policy. Medical institutions have provided instruction and/or workshops on how to address these situations and determine what to say.[56-58] Active bystander training is provided at some institutions.[59,60]

Training or preparation on dealing with biased patients is helpful because it enables advanced planning for what to do in real time. As a learner, you should be empowered to name racism and set limits with the patient.[61] Opportunities to practice what to say are invaluable to all trainees so that those who are not members of minority groups can intervene and support their colleagues. Debriefing after an encounter with a biased patient best occurs shortly after an event, and medical staff should be trained on how to lead a debrief session. Finally, hospital and academic institution policies on biased patient behavior are an important source of institutional support for trainees. These policies can include communication scripts, providing language that the trainee can utilize in the moment.[62]

Table 5.9 is a Navigating Racist Behavior From Patients or Caregivers Toolkit. This modifiable toolkit provides key points to remember and things you can do before, during, and after such encounters. Possible language to use with the patient during the encounter and ways to acknowledge the event and offer support as an ally are included. We recommend modifying this toolkit with location, school, and institution-specific resources.

Illustrative Cases of Discriminatory Behavior by Patients

The following are two illustrative cases involving junior residents and medical students experiencing discriminatory behavior by their patients.

TABLE 5.9 Navigating Racist Behavior From Patients or Caregivers Toolkit

Before	During	After
Key Points to Remember		
These events are common in the clinical environment. Preparation helps you recognize and respond to these events. There is a system-level policy regarding discriminatory patient behavior.	It is not your job to "make the patient/family not racist." Priorities are your safety, your education and, if possible, a therapeutic alliance. As a student you get to decide what, if any, role you continue to play in the patient's care. Your response may vary based on the event and your emotional reserve in that moment—this is OK! You always have the option to leave the room.	While clinical status (fear, delirium, dementia, etc.) may influence a patient's behavior, this context is never an "excuse" and does NOT change the impact of such behaviors on you and your team. Multiple support structures are in place for students who experience and witness racist behavior—those in the room or on the team are the first-line of support. Student mistreatment pathways allow immediate review and intervention if desired.
Things You Can Do		
Discuss with your team that these events do occur. Familiarize yourself with the hospital/medical facility policies on discriminatory patient behavior. Discuss with colleagues how they would like to be supported in these situations. Identify reporting and escalation pathways. Identify your support structures: • Friends/Family • Clinical Team • Attending • Clerkship director • Faculty and/or Wellness Advisor • Student Affairs Leadership • Student/Trainee Mental Health or other local mental health resources • Student Mistreatment Panel • School Office for Diversity and Inclusion • Ombudspersons	**Assess illness acuity:** Rarely will students have to continue to provide care. **Provide opportunity to clarify the statement:** "What did you mean by that?" "Are you discriminating against my colleague because of her race?" **Cultivate a therapeutic alliance:** "As a student on your medical team, I am focused on your health and wellness. Can you tell me what concerns you?"[a] "We treat all of our patients, staff, and learners/trainees with respect, and we expect the same from our patients."[a] **Provide a statement of support for yourself or your teammate:** "Those comments have no place in this hospital. Our staff is well-trained and very capable of providing high-quality care, all are professionals and will be respected as such."[a] **Communicate the impact of the patient's behavior and leave the room:** "I'm not comfortable continuing this interview when you use that language toward me/my colleague. We're going to step out."[a]	**Acknowledge the event:** "I saw what happened in there. That was not OK, and I want to check in on you." "What the patient said/did in there was racist—I am sorry you experienced that." **Offer support:** "How can I support you?" "I can help you report if you like, or just be here to listen." **What not to say:** "They didn't mean it." "It was probably because he was sick/scared/has dementia." "I don't think it was because of your race/gender/religion—probably just because you're a student." **When it happens to you:** Discuss with your support system/those you trust. Debrief the incident with your team—discuss with your resident or attending to what extent and with what conditions you would (or would not) like to continue working with the patient/family. Identify the reporting mechanism for student mistreatment at the hospital/medical/school and report the incident.

[a]See *Mount Sinai Health System Policy and Procedure. Responding to Racist and Discriminatory Patient Behavior. February 2021.*

Case 1

Dr. Int is a 25-year-old intern training in pediatrics at an academic teaching hospital. During an evening shift in the emergency department (ED), a 10-month-old infant is brought in by her parents for evaluation following new-onset seizure activity. The infant's uncle is a prominent surgeon at this hospital, and the parents announce this to the ED staff and hospital administration.

As the child would require monitoring following the seizure, the ED staff arranges an admission with the intensive care unit (ICU) team. The attending physician in the ICU, Dr. Att, visits the patient in the ED and introduces herself to the patient's parents. Prior to transfer to the ICU, the patient requires a lumbar puncture (LP) to assess for potential cerebrospinal fluid (CSF) infection. Parents are informed of the need for this test; they confer with the infant's uncle, who confirms the need for an LP.

As Dr. Int obtains consent for the LP, the patient's father asks the ICU attending physician who will perform the LP. The father is tense, anxiously makes eye contact, and directs the question to Dr. Att. The attending attributes the father's unease to the fact that Dr. Int is a junior member of the team and still in training. Dr. Att remains firm as to her decision that Dr. Int performs the LP. The father is reluctant to consent until Dr. Att states that she will remain in the room with Dr. Int as the procedure is performed. Dr. Int performs the LP well, and there are no complications. The child is monitored in the ICU without further seizure activity.

The ICU attending compliments Dr. Int on her technical skills in performing the LP and her poise in dealing with a parent who makes demands from a position of presumed power. Dr. Att is sympathetic to Dr. Int's circumstance as a junior physician and interprets the father's behavior and reluctance to have Dr. Int treat his daughter as being due to her level of medical experience. What Dr. Att fails to acknowledge or address is that the patient's father is White, and Dr. Int is Black. As Dr. Att did not consider racism an issue in this encounter, she did not address this with Dr. Int. Conversely, although provided with the time and the space to debrief the encounter, Dr. Int did not bring up racial discrimination as a factor.

Discussion and questions. *How did Dr. Att handle the situation? How could the interaction have been improved upon?*

Outside of considerations about racial discrimination, are there other factors that could have contributed to why Dr. Att allowed the special requests of this family? Do all families have space to make similar requests?

By failing to acknowledge racism as a factor in the parent's behavior, Dr. Att unconsciously minimized the issue of racial discrimination. Ideally, rather than assume that the cause for concern was Dr. Int's young age and junior level of training, Dr. Att could challenge the parent and inquire as to his concerns about Dr. Int. Dr. Att can emphasize that Dr. Int is a vital member of the team and is fully trained and capable of performing the procedure. She could state that racial discrimination has no place in the care of his child and that the best care possible is being provided, regardless of his presumed elevated status in the hospital.

It is possible that Dr. Int might feel uncomfortable addressing this scenario with a team that is not Black and would feel further victimized and singled out if debriefing the encounter with a group who could not fully understand her feelings at the time. Dr. Int could work with a faculty mentor of her choice and consider her reactions and responses in future scenarios.

Acknowledging the event and debriefing potential responses would empower Dr. Int for future encounters.

In a busy emergency department, there are several physicians who could perform the LP. Should Dr. Int have handed the procedure off to another physician? Do patients or their guardians have a right to choose their physician, especially for an invasive procedure?

In this scenario, the parent of the patient used his assumed elevated status, as a surgeon's relative, to challenge the workflow in the ED and the physicians involved with his daughter's care. The parent did not have the right to select the physician of his choice based on unfounded reasoning. There may be circumstances in which acknowledging a patient's wishes regarding a physician may be appropriate. For example, certain cultures dictate a preference for a female physician for a gynecologic exam. This religious/cultural preference should be respected whenever possible, as a sign of respect for the patient and their spirituality or culture.

In this scenario, Dr. Int should consider the pros and cons of transferring care. The ED is staffed with many physicians who could perform the LP; therefore, the patient would have received the medical care that she required. However, Dr. Int would have missed the opportunity to hone her skills, which she requires to be a pediatrician. With the support of the medical team and Dr. Att, she chose to perform the procedure. The key is to have support from other members of the medical team before continuing the care of the patient.

Of note, the parent, who is White, assumes a degree of power and privilege because he is related to a prominent physician. The ED staff acknowledges this power and actively involves hospital administration for a straightforward procedure. Thus, this example brings to light the ways in which families with privilege may be given latitude to make requests that may not be in line with clinical care, while families with less privilege may be deemed demanding or excessive. Patients who have demands in their care and are labeled as being of a minoritized race may be considered as overstepping their race's boundaries and not worthy of the power portrayed by the White patient.

Case 2

Medical student A is rotating on a geriatrics rotation during his third-year clerkship. He is the only medical student on a team with a social worker, two residents, and an attending physician. The attending and medical student both identify as Black, while the rest of the team does not. They enter the room of their 67-year-old patient who is being evaluated for delirium in the setting of a complicated urinary tract infection. The attending greets the patient at the bedside, and immediately the patient demands to see the attending's hospital ID badge exclaiming, "You are not a real doctor! I need to see your badge or you cannot touch me!" The attending immediately complies and brings the badge closer to the patient's view. He remains professional and tells the patient that he will be providing her care and that he can come back later in the day to update the patient on the proposed plan for her urinary tract infection. The team exits the room. In the hallway, the attending asks, "Does anyone have any thoughts or concerns regarding that encounter?" While the medical student feels triggered and hurt, the residents and social worker make no comment. The attending begins to describe how both the patient's illness (delirium in the setting of acute illness) combined with racial bias may have provoked her outburst. He outlines a variety of ways that he could have responded and comments on why he chose to respond in the way that he did. The team remains silent, and they go to round on the next patient.

Discussion and questions. *What are other options for how the attending may have responded to the patient? What might the medical student be feeling throughout the encounter and during the attending's debrief with the team? Is there any responsibility on the rest of the team, and how could they have responded during the encounter or during the debriefing in the hallway?*

In this example, the patient's illness potentially uncovered a racial bias toward the attending. The attending decided to comply with the patient's request as an appropriate response to the clinical context of altered mental status and to de-escalate the situation. While the attending had the power to dictate the direction of the clinical encounter, the medical student was left to quietly internalize the situation. In this particular example, the student and the attending shared the same racial identity, which allowed the student to feel seen and understood during the attending's debriefing. There may have been a role for other members of the team to voice their support for the attending and to debrief with the medical student about the direct patient bias and emotional intensity of the encounter. Because that explicit support from the team was lacking, the student may be left to experience future encounters with that team without any evidence of past support and trust that a similar situation would be handled more appropriately.

CONCLUSION

Racism and oppression, historically rooted in medicine and ubiquitous in medical culture, have dramatic and harmful effects on patient outcomes. *Healthcare professionals also experience moral injury practicing within an unjust system and trauma via discriminatory behavior from patients.* It is incumbent on medical educators and healthcare professionals to transform medical culture into one that is rooted in anti-racism and anti-oppression to produce a future workforce of healthcare professionals that is equipped with strategies to promote liberation and justice within patient care. Seizing the opportunity to teach these skills, often in real time, requires a commitment to broadening the understanding of not only one's own biases and positional power but the historical impact that racism and oppression have had on one's self, trainees, and patients. Traditional medical education does not effectively address these topics or teach means to understand their historical roots and contemporary implications.

Healthcare professionals become embedded in this medical culture leading to the communication of unintended values and lessons about race and its clinical significance. Without clear tools to understand race and ancestry and the interconnected identities of religion, gender, sexuality, and much more, we will continue to perpetuate medical errors, scientific racism, and systems that obscure the true drivers of inequitable health outcomes. In this chapter, we offered tangible techniques and clinical skills to deconstruct and dismantle the impact of racism and oppression on the patient and on the healthcare professional. This work is challenging and requires ongoing self-reflection, dialogue, and an awareness of and engagement with the broader individual and structural forces that influence patient–healthcare professional encounters and relationships. Developing such skills as a healthcare professional requires professional and personal investment and growth. We hope that through each clinical encounter and step of self-reflection, you will become closer to actively and purposefully deconstructing racism individually, structurally, and together with the medical community. It is imperative that you take on this work to ensure and advance a liberating system of care for our patients and the communities in which we serve.

ACKNOWLEDGMENTS

The authors would like to acknowledge Dr. Barbara Warren, PsyD, for her assistance with the section on sexual orientation and gender identity; Rev. David Fleenor for his assistance with the section on spirituality and religion; Jill Gregory, CMI, and Dr. Gale Justin, PhD, for their illustration and content assistance; Gloria Willson, MLIS, MPH, for her reference and content assistance; DeAnalise Jones for her content assistance and assistance with Fig. 5.1; Adam Kraus, MD, and Luis Seija, MD, for their content assistance with liberating documentation; Beverly Forsyth, MD, for her content assistance with Table 5.8; Melody Walton, Patricia Burns, Anasthasia Thomas, and many other patients and community members for their inspiration and partnership in clinical skills and curricular development; and Yancy Aracena for his research assistance. We would also like to acknowledge Dr. Jessica Reid-Adam; Dr. Leona Hess, PhD, MSW; and Dr. Sharon Washington, EdD, MPH, for their guidance and inspiration. Lastly, we want to acknowledge the courageous and bold leadership of our medical students who catalyzed a movement to deconstruct and dismantle racism and bias in our medical education and clinical environments.

REVIEW QUESTIONS

1. **What is one key difference between race and ancestry when assessing a patient's background?**
   A. Race is a biological construct while ancestry is a social construct.
   B. Race is a sociopolitical and economic construct. Ancestry is a statement about an individual's relationship to other individuals in their genealogic history; thus, it is a very personal understanding of one's genomic heritage.
   C. Race is a fluid identity, while ancestry is a fixed identity.
   D. Race and ancestry are essentially synonyms in the medical context.
   E. Race is a useful proxy for genetics.

2. **Potential actions that trainees can utilize when confronted by a patient with discriminatory behavior include:**
   A. Assessing the acuity of the patient and removing yourself from care of that patient when there are others who can assist with the patient.
   B. Acquiring help from the medical team in defining your role as part of the care team.
   C. Naming the behavior with the patient or family.
   D. Seeking support and the time to debrief the encounter with a mentor.
   E. All of the above.
3. **Which of the following excerpts from clinical documentation best represents liberating documentation?**
   A. The patient complained of ongoing pain despite being in minimal visible discomfort.
   B. The patient describes multiple prior experiences of family members being asked to interpret rather than appropriate use of an interpreter phone. She reports this has reduced her trust in her healthcare team.
   C. The patient presented with his third asthma exacerbation this month in the setting of noncompliance to controller medications.
   D. The patient described difficulty making specialist appointments as he is the primary caregiver for his younger sibling, who has cerebral palsy. He reports prior specialists have not refilled his medications due to missed visits, resulting in frequent asthma flares. He states afternoon appointments are preferable due to transportation scheduling.
   E. B and D
4. **Which of the following questions should you routinely ask yourself and/or your team when making a decision that may be impacted by racism/racial bias?**
   A. Am I/are we racist?
   B. Am I/we sure this is the right decision?
   C. What would someone who shares a racial identity with this patient do?
   D. Would I/we be making this same decision if this patient were White?
   E. What decision makes me the most comfortable here?
5. **The FICA tool for spiritual assessment includes all of the following except:**
   A. Faith
   B. Importance
   C. Community
   D. Address in care
   E. Age began with current religion
6. **All of the following are elements of structural competency except:**
   A. Recognizing the structures that shape clinical interactions
   B. Developing an extra-clinical language of structure
   C. Rearticulating structural presentations in cultural terms
   D. Observing and imagining structural interventions
   E. Developing structural humility
7. **The inclusion of a patient's race in the opening statement of a presentation is most likely to result in which of the following?**
   A. A more accurate estimate of that patient's likelihood having certain medical conditions
   B. A more accurate estimate of how that patient may respond to certain medications
   C. An increase in cultural competency within the team
   D. An increase in likelihood for implicit bias and dominant narratives to impact that patient's care
   E. A decrease in likelihood for implicit bias and dominant narratives to impact that patient's care
8. **Which of the following is true regarding anti-racist clinical skills?**
   A. They should only be practiced once a healthcare professional senses that racism may be impacting a patient or the team.
   B. They were created by academics and contemporary healthcare professionals over the last decade in response to a growing recognition of racism in medicine.
   C. They build upon centuries of tradition, culture, and resistance of racialized and oppressed communities and should be infused into the daily practice of all healthcare professionals.
   D. Focused on the patient and health outcomes, they do not require any level of self-reflection.
   E. They are only valid if published in peer-reviewed journals.
9. **Which of the following statements is true about trauma-informed care?**
   A. It should be reserved for patients known to have experienced trauma.
   B. It is an approach to care that includes organizational, structural, and interpersonal elements.
   C. It is best performed only by individual healthcare professionals one-on-one with a patient.
   D. It is not effective in addressing racial trauma.
   E. It can only be practiced by social workers.
10. **Which of the following are true regarding gender identity?**
    A. Gender identity can be determined based on how someone looks.
    B. Gender identity is a fixed state and cannot change over time.
    C. The manner by which a patient's gender identity is documented in the medical record should be determined in partnership with the patient.
    D. A patient's gender identity should always be excluded from the medical record to avoid potential bias.
    E. A patient's gender identity should never be excluded from the medical record to avoid assumptions.

REFERENCES

Available online.

SECTION 3

Understanding the Science of the Physical Examination

6

The Physical Examination

Mark H. Swartz and Talia H. Swartz

Don't touch the patient—state first what you see; cultivate your powers of observation.

Sir William Osler (1849–1919)

VIDEOS

Video 6.1 Introduction to the Physical Examination

THE APPROACH

The previous chapters discuss the general rules for mastering the art of taking history. The specific skills necessary to perform a proper physical examination are discussed in this chapter (Video 6.1). The four principles of physical examination are as follows:

- Inspection
- Palpation
- Percussion
- Auscultation

To achieve competence in these procedures, the student must, in the words of Sir William Osler, "teach the eye to see, the finger to feel, and the ear to hear." The ability to coordinate all this sensory input is learned with time and practice.

Even though examiners only use some of these techniques for some organ systems, they should consider these four skills before moving on to the next area to be evaluated.

Inspection

Inspection can yield an enormous amount of information. Proper technique requires more than just a glance. Examiners must train themselves to look at the body by using a systematic approach. All too often, the novice examiner rushes to use the ophthalmoscope, stethoscope, or otoscope before the naked eyes have been used for inspection.

An example of what is meant by "teaching the eye to see" can be demonstrated in the following exercise. Read the sentence in the box. Then count the number of "f's" in the sentence.

> Finished files are the result of years of scientific study combined with the experience of years.

How many did you count? The answer is given at the end of this chapter. This example clearly shows that eyes must be trained to see.[a]

Upon entering a patient's room, whether in an ambulatory or in-patient setting, healthcare professionals should initiate a critical process of room assessment to ensure the patient's safety, well-being, and the delivery of appropriate medical care. First and foremost, safety precautions are imperative. Healthcare professionals should perform rigorous hand hygiene and don personal protective equipment, especially when infection control is paramount. Patient identification is another crucial step, where confirming identity with two unique identifiers[b] and cross-referencing with medical records is standard procedure. Additionally, adhering to infection control measures, such as isolating patients, is pivotal in minimizing cross-infection risks, so it is important to observe any precautionary signs before entering the room.

Another essential aspect is the positioning of the bed or examination table. Properly adjusting the bed or examination table is crucial to performing maneuvers or examinations safely and effectively. It ensures that the patient and healthcare professional have optimal access and visibility, reducing the risk of injury or discomfort during procedures. Returning the bed or table and side rails to their original positions after the procedure is equally important to ensure the patient's continued comfort and safety.

Moving on to the patient assessment, healthcare professionals must inspect medical devices like ventilators, IV infusion pumps, heart monitors, or dialysis machines; note this in the documentation; and be aware of misplacement or malfunction. Intravenous (IV) lines warrant scrutiny, focusing on fluid types, flow rates, IV site conditions, and complications. Drainage systems, including urinary catheters, surgical drains, and chest tubes, must be examined for functionality and the absence of leaks or infections. An assessment of the necessity of these devices and the possibility of removal should be discussed daily. Medication delivery, involving the administration route and pumps, requires a review of dosages, administration schedules, and allergy status. Furthermore, assessing nutritional support, wound care, and the condition of surgical dressings, incisions, sutures, and wounds is imperative for patient evaluation.

[a]This test has been circulated widely in the medical community. The original writer is unknown.

[b]To prevent errors, The Joint Commission requires two patient identifiers: name, date of birth, or medical record number (MRN).

The assessment extends to mobility and assistive devices. Healthcare professionals should observe whether patients require mobility aids such as wheelchairs, walkers, crutches, or orthopedic braces and ensure their accessibility and functionality. Assistive devices like hearing aids, eyeglasses, or prosthetic limbs should be present and operational as needed. Evaluating the presence of personal belongings and ensuring that patients have access to personal hygiene items, clothing, and footwear is also important.

The impact of family members or caregivers on the patient's well-being and comfort should be acknowledged. Lastly, psychosocial and cultural considerations are integral to holistic care. Observing the patient's emotional state and communication abilities helps gauge the need for psychosocial support. Additionally, vital steps include recognizing cultural or religious beliefs, identifying relevant artifacts or practices, and arranging interpreter services when language barriers exist.

Once the environment has been assessed, the examiner should observe the following aspects of the patient:

- General appearance
- State of nutrition
- Body habitus
- Symmetry
- Posture and gait
- Speech

The *general appearance* includes the state of consciousness and personal grooming. Does the patient look well or sick? Are they comfortable in bed, or do they appear in distress? Is the patient alert, or are they groggy? Do they look acutely or chronically ill? The answer to this last question is sometimes difficult to determine from inspection, but there are some helpful signs to aid the examiner. Chronic disease is associated with poor nutrition, sunken eyes, temporal wasting, and loose skin. Does the patient appear clean? Although the patient is ill, they do not have to appear unkempt. Is their hair combed? Do they bite their fingernails? The answers to these questions may provide useful information about the patient's self-esteem and mental status.

Inspection can evaluate the *state of nutrition*. Does the patient appear thin and frail? Is the patient obese? Most individuals with chronic disease are *not* overweight; they are cachectic. Long-standing ailments such as cancer, hyperthyroidism, or heart disease can result in a markedly wasted appearance. See Chapter 7, Assessment of Nutritional Status.

The *body habitus* is informative because certain disease states are more common in different body builds. The *asthenic*, or *ectomorphic*, patient is thin, has poor muscle development and small bone structure, and appears malnourished. The *sthenic*, or *mesomorphic*, patient is the athletic type with excellent muscular development and a large bone structure. The *hypersthenic*, or *endomorphic*, patient is a short, round individual with good muscular development but frequently has a weight problem.

Any asymmetry should be noted because the body's outward appearance is symmetric. Many systemic diseases provide clues that can be uncovered on inspection. For example, a noticeable unilateral supraclavicular swelling or a less obvious unilateral miotic pupil is a clue that can aid the examiner in reaching a final diagnosis. A left supraclavicular swelling in a 61-year-old male may represent an enlarged supraclavicular lymph node and could be the only sign of gastric carcinoma. A miotic pupil in a 43-year-old female may be a manifestation of interruption of the cervical sympathetic chain by a tumor of the apex of the lung. The recent onset of a left-sided varicocele in a 46-year-old male could be related to the development of a left hypernephroma.

The patient is usually in bed when introduced to the examiner. If the patient were walking about, the examiner could use this time to observe the patient's *posture* and *gait*. The ability to walk involves the coordination of the nervous and musculoskeletal systems. Does the patient drag their foot? Is there a shuffling gait? Does the patient limp? Are the steps asymmetrical?

The examiner can learn much about the patient from their *speech patterns*. Is the speech slurred? Does the patient use words appropriately? Is the patient hoarse? Is the voice unusually high or low in pitch? Is the patient moving their face symmetrically when speaking? If not, this could provide clues to some cranial nerve problems.

Is the patient oriented to person, place, and time? Tell the patient that you have some routine questions that you ask all your patients. Orientation can quickly be evaluated by asking the patient, "Who are you?" "Where are you?" and "What is the date, season, or month?" If the patient avoids answering the question, ask it again. For example, if the patient answers the question, "Where are you?" with an answer like "I'm in your office," ask, "But what is the address of my office?" Patients with cognitive impairment try to avoid the answer if they do not remember or know the answer. These questions certainly do not have to be asked at the beginning, but they should be asked sometime during the interview and examination. These questions provide an insight into the mental status of the patient. It would be best to preface these questions by stating, "I have some routine questions that I would like to ask you." The mental status examination is discussed further in Chapter 21, The Nervous System.

The examiner must recognize the cardinal signs of inflammation: swelling, heat, redness, pain, and disturbance of function. Swelling results from edema or congestion in local tissues. Heat is the sensation of increased blood supply to the involved area. Redness is also a manifestation of the increased blood supply. Pain often results from the swelling, which exerts increased pressure on the nerve fibers. Because of the pain and swelling, a disturbance of function may occur.

Palpation

Palpation is the use of touch to determine the characteristics of an area of the body, such as skin elevation or depression, warmth, tenderness, pulses, crepitus, and sizes of organs or masses. For example, an impulse may be palpated on the right side of the chest and could be related to an ascending aortic aneurysm. A pulsatile mass palpated in the abdomen might be an abdominal aneurysm. An acutely tender mass palpated in the right upper quadrant of the abdomen that descends with inspiration is probably an inflamed gallbladder.

Percussion

Percussion relates to the tactile sensation and sound produced when a sharp blow is struck to an area being examined. One finger delivers a sharp tap to another finger of the other hand. This provides valuable information about the structure of the underlying organ or tissue. A difference from the expected sensation may be related to fluid in an area that usually does not contain fluid. The collapse of a lung changes the percussion note, as does a solid mass in the abdomen. Percussion that produces a dull note in the midline of the lower abdomen in a male probably represents a distended urinary bladder.

Auscultation

Auscultation involves listening to sounds produced by internal organs. This technique furnishes information about an organ's disease process. The examiner is urged to learn as much as possible from the other methods before using the stethoscope. This instrument should corroborate the signs that were suggested by the other techniques. Auscultation should be used to examine the heart, chest, and abdomen, not alone but with inspection, percussion, and palpation. Listening for carotid, ophthalmic, thyroid, or renal bruits can provide lifesaving information. The absence of normal bowel sounds could indicate a surgical emergency.

PREPARATION FOR THE EXAMINATION

The physical examination usually begins after the history has been documented. You should have a portable case containing all the necessary equipment, including the items in Table 6.1.

Place the equipment on the patient's night table or bed stand. By laying out all the tools, you are less likely to forget to perform a specific examination. Adjust the lighting; good lighting is important for good inspection! If possible, daylight is preferable for illumination because skin color changes may be masked by artificial light. The patient's curtains should be closed for privacy at the start of the interview. Finally, adjust the bed to a convenient height. If you have elevated the bed, lower it after completing the examination.

Before examining the patient, wash your hands, preferably while the patient is watching. Washing with soap and water is the most effective way to reduce disease transmission. Be sure to lather for 15 to 20 seconds or more. Alternatively, a hand sanitizer may be used instead of soap and water. The Centers for Disease Control and Prevention (CDC) recommends using an alcohol-based hand sanitizer that contains at least 60% ethyl alcohol when soap and water are not available. Ethyl alcohol kills 99.99% of germs that may cause illness. Make sure that your hands are dry before touching the patient.

The patient should wear a gown that opens at the front or back. Pajamas are also acceptable for hospitalized patients. It is most important to consider the comfort of the patient. You should allow the patient the use of pillows if needed.

It is important that you become skilled in each organ system examination. Incorporate the individual evaluations into the complete examination with the least amount of movement of the patient. Avoid unnecessary changes, if possible. Regardless of age, patients tire quickly when asked to "sit up," "lie down," "turn on your left side," "sit up," "lie down," and so on. You should perform as much of the examination as possible with the patient in one position. It is also important that the patient is never asked to sit up in bed without support for any extended period. **Although you are learning physical examination by systems, the physical examination is conducted by body regions, not by systems.** When examining the head, for example, you will evaluate the skin, hair, eyes, nose, ears, throat, sinuses, and cranial nerves even though these involve many "systems."

By convention, the examiner stands to the *patient's right* as the patient lies in bed or on the examination table. The examiner uses their right hand for most maneuvers of the examination. It is common practice that even left-handed individuals learn to examine the right side using their right hand. Each of the subsequent chapters on organ systems discusses the placement of hands and is shown in the associated videos.

Although the patient must disrobe completely, the examination should be done by exposing only the areas being examined at that time without undue exposure to other areas. When a female's breast is examined, for example, it is necessary to check for any asymmetry by inspecting both breasts simultaneously. After inspection, you may use the patient's gown to cover the breast not being examined. The abdomen examination may be performed discreetly by placing a towel or a bed sheet over the genitalia. Examination of the heart with the patient in the supine position may be performed with the right breast covered. Respecting the patient's privacy goes a long way in establishing a good healthcare professional–patient relationship.

While performing the physical examination, you should continue speaking to the patient. You may wish to pursue various parts of the history and tell the patient what is being done. You should refrain from comments such as "That's good," "That's normal," or "That's fine" about any part of the examination. Although this is initially reassuring to the patient, if you

TABLE 6.1 Equipment for Complete Physical Examination

Required	Optional	Available in Most Patient Care Areas
Stethoscope	Nasal illuminator[a]	Sphygmomanometer
Otoscope and ophthalmoscope	Nasal speculum	Tongue blades
Penlight	Tape measure	Applicator sticks
Reflex hammer		Gauze pads
Tuning fork: 128 Hz		Gloves
Tuning fork: 512 Hz		Lubricant gel
		Guaiac card for occult blood
Pocket visual acuity card		Vaginal speculum
		Hand sanitizer

[a]Attachment for the otoscope handle.

fail to make such a statement during another part of the examination, the patient may automatically assume that there is something wrong or abnormal.

The following chapters discuss the individual organ system examinations. Chapter 22, Putting the Examination Together, then summarizes a method of combining all the individual evaluations into one smooth, continuous examination.

HEALTHCARE INFECTION PREVENTION PRACTICES

Any member of the healthcare delivery team who has exposure to patients has the potential for exposure to infections. The healthcare professional must be aware of the possible infections that may be transmitted and how certain organisms can be transmitted from patient to patient. Infection prevention practices aim to prompt the identification of individuals who harbor or are infected with transmissible agents; appropriate guidelines must be followed to protect both the patient and the healthcare professional.

Guidelines have been established by both the CDC and the Occupational Safety and Health Administration (OSHA). All healthcare professionals should follow these guidelines when exposure to potentially infectious materials such as blood or other body fluids is possible.

Universal precautions are infection prevention considerations that treat all human blood and other body fluids as if they are known to be infected with human immunodeficiency virus (HIV), hepatitis B virus (HBV), hepatitis C virus (HCV), and other blood-borne pathogens in the occupational setting. Blood is the most important source of HIV, HBV, and HCV infection; infection prevention methods should focus on limiting exposure and delivering HBV vaccination (CDC). Universal precautions dictate the use of protective barriers to reduce exposure to body fluids. Examples of barrier protection include gloves, gowns, masks, and eye protection. The use of protective equipment pertains to the specific nature of the patient contact and body fluid. Universal precautions serve to supplement recommendations for routine infection prevention, including handwashing and the use of gloves to prevent obvious contamination. Proper judgment and referral to appropriate guidelines are necessary. This applies to individuals in contact with body fluids, especially those performing procedures.

Standard precautions are recommended for all patients regardless of their disease status. These include handwashing and using the appropriate protective equipment for handling body fluids.

Transmission-based precautions are additional guidelines recommended to decrease the transmission of pathogens throughout the hospital. There are several categories:

- *Airborne precautions* are used for infectious agents that are spread through small particles in the air. This includes measles, varicella (chickenpox), influenza, severe acute respiratory syndrome (SARS), and tuberculosis. An N-95 or equivalent respiratory mask is necessary, and the patient must be isolated in a negative-pressure room.
- *Droplet precautions* are used to prevent the spread of agents that can be carried in large droplets, such as influenza, coxsackievirus, croup, severe acute respiratory syndrome coronavirus 2 (SARS-CoV-2), and respiratory syncytial virus (RSV). The bacteria or viruses travel on relatively large respiratory droplets that people sneeze, cough, talk, sing, or shout into the air. The droplets travel only short distances before settling, with most traveling only 3 to 6 feet. The infectious agents often land on hands, toys, mats, doorknobs, telephones, pens, or other surfaces where they can remain for hours or days. These surfaces become contagious to others. These inanimate objects are called **fomites**. A surgical mask and gloves are required in this situation.
- *Contact precautions* are used for infectious agents that can be spread by skin-to-skin contact and by contact with surfaces. Examples of these agents are multidrug-resistant organisms, chickenpox, conjunctivitis, hepatitis A and B, herpes simplex, influenza, measles, infectious mononucleosis, pertussis, adenoviruses, rhinoviruses, *Neisseria meningitidis*, mycoplasma pneumoniae, norovirus, *Clostridium difficile*, impetigo, pediculosis (head lice), polio, and roseola (German measles is also spread by direct contact). The use of gowns and gloves is required in this situation.

There are also circumstances where more than one type of precaution is recommended. The appropriate signage should be indicated on the door of the patient's room, and all proper guidelines should be followed.

Needlestick injuries[1] can occur in accidental situations. Healthcare personnel who use or may be exposed to needles are at increased risk of needlestick injury. Needlestick injuries can lead to severe or fatal infections with blood-borne pathogens such as hepatitis B virus, hepatitis C virus, or HIV. When a needlestick injury occurs, the individual should promptly flush the affected area with water vigorously and seek guidance from the hospital's needlestick coordinator. Every hospital and medical care facility has protocols; an individual should be available anytime to answer questions. If appropriate, postexposure prophylaxis for HIV is available and should be administered as soon as possible. Hepatitis B serologic testing should also be considered, as immunoglobulin can be considered in rare situations. Hepatitis C can likewise be spread via needlestick; serologic testing should be performed within 48 hours of exposure to determine the need for nucleic acid testing and possible treatment referral.[2]

Specific work practices may increase the risk of needlestick injury. Studies have shown that needlestick injuries are often associated with:

- Not using safety-engineered sharps or using them incorrectly
- Recapping needles
- Transferring a body fluid between containers
- Failing to dispose of used needles properly in puncture-resistant sharps containers

All healthcare professionals with direct contact with patients should complete appropriate vaccinations including hepatitis B and the annual influenza vaccine series. Typical pre-employment and student health service screening includes a purified protein derivative (PPD) test for tuberculosis and various serologic testing, including testing for hepatitis B.

It is also the responsibility of all healthcare professionals not to transmit disease to their patients. Professionals with a lesion on their hands should wear gloves; if sick, they should defer patient contact.

GOAL OF THE PHYSICAL EXAMINATION

The physical examination aims to obtain valid information concerning the patient's health. The examiner must be able to identify, analyze, and synthesize the accumulated information into a comprehensive assessment.

To enhance the clarity and precision of our descriptions, it is important to refrain from using the term "normal" when assessing physical findings. Instead, employing alternative expressions that convey specific characteristics is more informative. For instance, we can describe symmetry to indicate that a body part or feature appears balanced and proportionate. By focusing on what would be expected in a particular context, we can provide a more accurate representation of the findings. This approach enables us to convey information in a manner that is both descriptive and meaningful, facilitating a better understanding of the patient's condition.

The validity of a physical finding depends on many factors. Clinical experience and reliability of the examination techniques are most important. False-positive or false-negative results reduce the precision of the techniques. Variance can occur when different examiners with different equipment perform techniques on different patients. The concepts of validity and precision are discussed further in Chapter 28, Precision, Accuracy, and Critical Thinking in Clinical Assessment.

Unconscious bias is an important concept to understand. It has already been discussed in Chapter 5, Anti-Racist and Anti-Oppressive Clinical Skills. It is well known that unconscious bias in an examiner can influence the evaluation of a physical finding. For example, the ventricular rate is irregular in patients with rapid atrial fibrillation and varies from 120 to 150 beats per minute. The radial pulse rate is significantly lower, owing to a pulse deficit (explained in Chapter 14, The Heart). If examiners first record the apical heart rate, they find that it varies from 120 to 150 beats per minute. If they then check the radial pulse, they detect a faster pulse rate than if they had measured the radial pulse first. The first observation, therefore, biases the second observation. Alternatively, if examiners determine the radial pulse first and the heart rate second, the apical heart rate appears slower, but the chance of bias is lower because observer error is less at the apex.[3]

It is important to review the concepts of sensitivity and specificity. *Sensitivity* is the frequency of a positive result of a test or technique in individuals with a disease or condition. *Specificity* is the frequency of a negative result of a test or technique in individuals without a disease or condition. *Sensitivity* and *specificity* refer to the properties of the test or technique. In contrast, the healthcare professional is interested in the properties or characteristics of the patient, which are characterized by predictive values. The *positive predictive value* is the disease frequency in patients with positive test results. The *negative predictive value* is the frequency of lack of disease in patients with negative test results. The question "What is the possibility that a female with a stony-hard breast mass has cancer?" addresses the positive predictive value. Predictive value depends on the prevalence of disease in the respective population and the sensitivity and specificity of the test. In an individual from a population with a low prevalence of disease, a positive test result still yields a low positive predictive value.

For example, eliciting shifting dullness is a highly sensitive technique for detecting ascites. Thus, an examiner who does not detect shifting dullness in a patient's abdomen can be reasonably sure that this negative finding rules out ascites. In contrast, the finding of microaneurysms in the macular area of the retina is a highly specific finding for diabetes. Thus, an examiner who finds microaneurysms at the macula can be reasonably confident that this finding confirms diabetes because individuals without diabetes do not have macular microaneurysms; that is, the finding of microaneurysms at the macula has a high degree of specificity. Unfortunately, a technique is rarely both very sensitive and very specific. Several techniques must be applied together to make an appropriate assessment.

In summary:

1. A technique or test with high sensitivity can be used confidently to rule out disease for a patient with a negative finding.
2. A technique or test with high specificity can be used confidently to confirm disease for a patient with a positive finding.

Chapter 28, Precision, Accuracy, and Critical Thinking in Clinical Assessment, discusses these concepts in more detail.

SUMMARY

In conclusion, the physical examination is one of the cornerstones of clinical medicine, providing invaluable insights into a patient's health. It is a skill that requires knowledge, practice, and a compassionate approach. As we wrap up this chapter, remember that mastering this art is a continuous journey. The knowledge and techniques you have gained here will serve as the foundation for your clinical practice, enabling you to provide the best possible care to your patients. In the chapters that follow, we will delve into specific aspects of the physical examination in greater detail, equipping you with the tools needed to become a skilled and empathetic healthcare professional.

USEFUL VOCABULARY

The vocabulary of medicine is difficult and broad. Memorizing a term is less useful than determining the meaning by understanding its etymology, or roots. When etymology is understood, the spelling of terms will also be easier.

This box lists some general prefixes, roots, and suffixes that are important to understand. At the end of each chapter is a list of terminology for that area of the body. The following list should not be memorized at this time. It should be referred to in conjunction with the lists in subsequent chapters.

Prefix/Root/Suffix	Pertaining to	Example	Definition
ab-	away from	***ab***duction	Away from the body
ad-	toward	***ad***duction	Toward the body
aden-	gland	***aden***opathy	Glandular disease
an-	without	***an***osmia	Without the sense of smell
aniso-	unequal	***aniso***coria	Unequal pupils
asthen-	weak	***asthen***opia	Eye fatigue
contra-	against; opposite	***contra***lateral	Pertaining to the opposite side
diplo-	double	***diplo***pia	Double vision
duc-	lead	ab***duc***tion	Turning outward
dys-	bad; ill	***dys***uria	Painful urination
eso-	in	***eso***tropia	Eye deviated inward
eu-	good; advantageous	***eu***pnea	Easy breathing
exo-	out	***exo***tropia	Eye deviated outward
hemi-	half	***hemi***plegia	Paralysis of one side of the body
hydro-	water	***hydro***philic	Readily absorbing water
hyper-	beyond; excessive	***hyper***emia	Excess of blood
hypno-	sleep	***hypno***tic	Inducing sleep
hypo-	below	***hypo***dermic	Below the skin
idio-	separate; distinct	***idio***pathic	Of unknown cause
infra-	below	***infra***hyoid	Below the hyoid gland
intra-	within	***intra***cranial	Within the skull
ipsi-	self	***ipsi***lateral	Situated on the same side
iso-	equal	***iso***tonic	Equal tension
leuko-	white	***leuko***cyte	White blood cell
lith-	stone	***lith***otomy	Incision of an organ to remove a stone
macro-	larger than	***macro***cephaly	Head size larger than expected
micro-	smaller than	***micro***cephaly	Head size smaller than expected
neo-	new	***neo***plasm	New growth
pedia-	child	***pedia***trics	Branch of medicine treating diseases of children
peri-	around	***peri***cardium	Sac around heart
poly-	many	***poly***cystic	Many cysts
presby-	old	***presby***opia	Impairment of vision because of advancing age
retro-	situated behind	***retro***bulbar	Behind the eye
soma-	body	***soma***tic	Pertaining to the body
sten-	narrowed	***sten***osis	Narrowed
trans-	through	***trans***urethral	Through the urethra
-dynia	pain	cephalo***dynia***	Headache
-ectomy	removal of	append***ectomy***	Removal of the appendix
-gnosis	recognition	stereo***gnosis***	Recognizing an object by touch
-gram	something written	myelo***gram***	X-ray film of the spinal cord
-ism	state; condition	gigant***ism***	State of overgrowth
-itis	inflammation of	col***itis***	Inflammation of the colon
-kinesia	movement	brady***kinesia***	Slow movement
-lysis	dissolution	hemo***lysis***	Liberation of hemoglobin into solution
-malacia	softening	osteo***malacia***	Softening of bones
-megal-	enlargement	cardio***megaly***	Cardiac enlargement
-mycosis	fungus	blasto***mycosis***	A specific fungal infection
-oid	resembling	human***oid***	Resembling a human
-ologist	specialist in study of	cardi***ologist***	A specialist in heart disease
-oma	tumor; growth	fibr***oma***	A tumor of fibrous tissue
-osis	diseased state	endometri***osis***	Disease state of abnormally located uterine tissue
-otomy	cutting; incision	gastr***otomy***	Incision of the stomach

Continued

USEFUL VOCABULARY—cont'd

Prefix/Root/Suffix	Pertaining to	Example	Definition
-pathy	disease	uro***pathy***	Disease of the urinary tract
-phobia	fear; pain; intolerance	photo***phobia***	Intolerance of light
-plasty	repair	valvulo***plasty***	Surgical repair of a valve
-plegia	paralysis	hemi***plegia***	Paralysis of one half of the body
-ptosis	drooping	blepharo***ptosis***	Drooping eyelids
-rrhagia	hemorrhage	oto***rrhagia***	Hemorrhage from the ear
-rrhaphy	suture; repair	hernio***rrhaphy***	Repair of a hernia
-rrhexis	rupture	gastro***rrhexis***	Rupture of stomach
-scope	instrument for	ophthalmo***scope***	Instrument for examination of the eye
-spasmos	spasm	blepharo***spasm***	Twitching of the eyelids
-stom-	opening	ileo***stom***y	Surgical creation of an opening into the ileum
-tome	cut	micro***tome***	An instrument for cutting thin slices

There are *six* "f's" in the sentence in the box. Go back and count them. Many people may mistakenly perceive only three "f's." This illusion occurs due to two reasons. Firstly, our brain tends to overlook the "f" in the word "of" because its phonetic sound is closer to "ov." Generally, the letter "f" produces an "f" sound, as in the word "fill." However, in the word "of," it produces a "v" sound. Subconsciously, our mind registers it as "ov," while our conscious mind perceives it as "of," creating a conflict. The subconscious tends to prevail in such conflicts between the subconscious and conscious minds. Secondly, we tend to assign varying importance to words when processing language. We often skip over small words like "in," "on," "of," and "at," and instead focus more on nouns and verbs. This phenomenon is known as word skipping.

REVIEW QUESTIONS

1. **Which of the following is NOT one of the basic procedures of the physical examination?**
   A. Inspection
   B. Palpation
   C. Percussion
   D. Auscultation
   E. Olfaction
2. **According to Sir William Osler, what should be taught to achieve competence in physical examination procedures?**
   A. Teach the eye to see
   B. Teach the finger to feel
   C. Teach the ear to hear
   D. All of the above
   E. None of the above
3. **What is the first principle of physical examination?**
   A. Inspection
   B. Palpation
   C. Percussion
   D. Auscultation
   E. Olfaction
4. **Which of the following aspects should be observed during the inspection phase of the physical examination?**
   A. General appearance
   B. State of nutrition
   C. Body habitus
   D. Symmetry
   E. All of the above
5. **Which of the following is NOT part of the examiner's observation during the gait assessment?**
   A. Foot dragging
   B. Shuffling gait
   C. Limping
   D. Asymmetrical steps
   E. None of the above
6. **What can be determined from the patient's speech patterns during the inspection phase?**
   A. Slurred speech
   B. Word usage
   C. Hoarseness
   D. Facial symmetry when speaking
   E. All of the above
7. **Which of the following precautions is NOT part of the transmission-based precautions?**
   A. Airborne precautions
   B. Droplet precautions
   C. Contact precautions
   D. Universal precautions
   E. None of the above
8. **Which technique involves using touch to determine the characteristics of an area of the body?**
   A. Inspection
   B. Palpation
   C. Percussion
   D. Auscultation
   E. Olfaction
9. **What does percussion relate to?**
   A. Tactile sensation and sound produced by a sharp blow
   B. Feeling the organs through touch
   C. Listening to internal sounds of organs
   D. Evaluating the characteristics of the skin
   E. None of the above
10. **What does auscultation involve?**
    A. Observing the patient's general appearance
    B. Feeling the characteristics of the body
    C. Tapping on the body to elicit sounds
    D. Listening to sounds produced by internal organs
    E. None of the above

11. **What is the purpose of combining all the individual evaluations into one smooth, continuous examination?**
 A. To save time
 B. To avoid unnecessary changes in the patient's position
 C. To enhance patient comfort
 D. To establish a comprehensive assessment
 E. All of the above

12. **Which type of precautions should be used to prevent the spread of infectious agents carried in large droplets, such as influenza and respiratory syncytial virus (RSV)?**
 A. Airborne precautions
 B. Droplet precautions
 C. Contact precautions
 D. Universal precautions
 E. None of the above

13. **What should healthcare professionals do in the event of a needlestick injury?**
 A. Promptly flush the affected area with water
 B. Seek guidance from the hospital's needlestick coordinator
 C. Consider postexposure prophylaxis for HIV
 D. All of the above
 E. None of the above

14. **What are the cardinal signs of inflammation?**
 A. Swelling, heat, redness, pain
 B. Swelling, coldness, blanching, itching
 C. Numbness, tingling, redness, warmth
 D. Itching, burning, bruising, swelling
 E. None of the above

15. **What does sensitivity refer to in the context of diagnostic tests or techniques?**
 A. The ability of a test to accurately detect the presence of a particular condition or disease
 B. The ability of a test to accurately rule out the presence of a particular condition or disease
 C. The proportion of individuals with a positive test result who truly have the condition or disease
 D. The proportion of individuals with a negative test result who truly do not have the condition or disease
 E. None of the above

REFERENCES

Available online.

BIBLIOGRAPHY

Available online.

7

Assessment of Nutritional Status

Mark H. Swartz and Robert F. Kushner

One must eat to live, and not live to eat.

Jean Baptiste Molière (1622–1673)

VIDEO

Video 7.1 Counseling a Patient About Health Issues

Nutrition is one of the most important factors regarding development and treatment of disease in individuals because it affects almost every system. It has been shown that dietary habits contribute in important ways to the pathogenesis of many of the major noncommunicable causes of death in the United States. One of the most challenging nutritional problems in the world today is obesity. In 2020, an estimated 658 million adults, 18 years and older, had obesity.

In the United States, the prevalence of overweight and obesity was 30.3% and 42.8%, respectively, in 2017–2018.[1] Minority populations are particularly at risk, as Mexican Americans (50.4%) and non-Hispanic Blacks (49.6%) have the highest age-adjusted prevalence of obesity. Obesity is a risk factor for many diseases, including hypertension, coronary artery disease, diabetes, obstructive sleep apnea, osteoarthritis, cancers of the breast and endometrium, and hepatobiliary disease. There is an increased awareness of obesity, but it remains a major problem. The overall cost to society of obesity in the United States is estimated to be $172.74 billion per year.[2] In addition, obesity is associated with job absenteeism, costing approximately $4.3 billion annually.

Malnutrition is a significant issue in the United States. Studies have revealed that nearly 50% of patients admitted to hospitals for general medical and surgical interventions suffer from some form of malnutrition. Out of these, approximately 25% may have functional illnesses stemming from malnutrition, and 10% may have advanced malnutrition symptoms. Malnutrition affects various groups, including older individuals living alone, chronically ill patients, teenage individuals with erratic eating habits, and patients diagnosed with cancer who may experience nutritional problems due to chemotherapy and radiation treatments. Even patients with obesity may experience malnutrition, commonly caused by catabolic stress.

Healthcare professionals have a unique opportunity to educate patients and help modify their lifestyle and health behaviors. More than half of these health-promoting behaviors are diet and nutrition related. They include balancing caloric intake to match energy expenditure, limiting calories from added sugars and saturated fats, reducing sodium intake, and shifting to healthier foods and beverage choices. The healthcare professional must have a firm understanding of clinical nutrition and its influence on health and illness. A patient's ability to recover from an illness or surgery depends, in many cases, on their past and current nutritional status. Adequate protein-calorie nutrition is important for wound healing, recovery from infection, and responsiveness to treatment, and protein-calorie malnutrition may be a factor in the development of decubitus ulcers and wound disruption. Five of the leading causes of death in the U.S.—heart disease, cancer, stroke, diabetes mellitus, and atherosclerosis—are diet related. Therefore, knowing what patients eat, the nutritional adequacy of their diets, and their clinical nutritional status is a necessary component of physical diagnosis.

In this chapter, we will discuss the important aspects of history and physical examination that are essential for a nutritional assessment. Currently, there is no standardized set of questions for dietary history or a single method for assessing nutritional status. Nutritional assessment demands the integration of information gathered from the medical history and physical examination (Video 7.1). This chapter provides nutrition-focused questions and examples of diet-related ailments to help develop history-taking and physical examination skills. The chapter begins by reviewing the medical history and physical examination, highlighting the integration of nutritionally focused information. It then covers the nutritional evaluation of specific patient groups along with some pathophysiologic correlations.

MEDICAL HISTORY

Chief Concern

Often the chief concern is directly related to the patient's nutrition, which may affect treatment and prognosis. The most voiced nutritional concerns are "loss of appetite," "weight loss," "weight gain," "fatigue," and "weakness." Changes in dietary intake and weight are among the earliest signs of medical problems. These concerns should prompt a detailed inquiry about diet and related symptoms in the history of present illness.

History of Present Illness

After asking the patient to describe the symptoms or medical problem that caused them to seek medical attention, begin to explore any diet-disease relationship that may exist. The following self-directed questions should guide your inquiry:

- *Does nutrition contribute to the cause, severity, or treatment of the illness?*

  For example, type 2 diabetes is most often seen among patients with obesity and is diet responsive. Inquiry should be made into the patient's body weight history and diet, including calorie content, pattern of consumption, types of foods and beverages consumed, and relationship to blood glucose levels.
- *How has the illness affected the patient's diet and nutritional status?*

  For example, a patient with esophageal cancer typically experiences increasing difficulty swallowing solid foods (dysphagia), pain with swallowing (odynophagia), occasional vomiting, weight loss, and reduced muscle strength.
- *Does the patient see a relationship between diet and disease?*

  For example, is a patient with hypercholesterolemia aware that consumption of dietary saturated fats and cholesterol raises blood cholesterol, whereas intake of dietary soluble fiber lowers blood cholesterol?
- *Was the patient ever advised to follow a special diet or use other nutritional therapy, such as defined formula supplements, tube feedings, or intravenous (parenteral) nutrition? What were the aspects of this therapy? What was the patient's understanding of how the treatment works? What was the patient's understanding of its potential efficacy?*

  For example, a patient with celiac disease must learn to follow a strict gluten-free diet to control the immune response that attacks the small intestine. The patient must become knowledgeable concerning dietary grains that contain gluten (wheat, barley, or rye), how to read food labels (nutrition literacy), and how to make dietary substitutions. This commonly requires guidance from a registered dietitian nutritionist.

Body Weight History

Body weight is a global indicator for overall health. Any unexplained weight loss is a good general indication of the severity or systemic nature of the presenting symptoms, whether they are acute or chronic. Both low body weight and unintentional weight loss have been shown to be predictive of increased morbidity and mortality. Although the cause of weight loss is often linked to the presenting medical problem, often no identifiable physical cause is apparent. In all cases, the underlying reasons for the weight change should be explored and the amount of weight loss should be clearly defined. Information-yielding questions include the following:

"Has your weight changed, either up or down, over the past several weeks or months?" If so, *"In what way?"*
"Was the change in weight intentional?"
"How much weight did you lose or gain?"
"What was your weight before the symptoms started?"
"During what period did you experience the weight loss or gain?"
"How was your appetite over this time?"
"If not intentional, do you know what may have contributed to your change in weight?"

Rapid weight gain is often an indicator of fluid retention and may be accompanied by edema or ascites. Common diseases associated with rapid weight gain include congestive heart failure, liver disease, and renal disease. In contrast, rapid weight loss usually signifies loss of body tissue, unless the patient has been undergoing therapeutic diuresis (in which case the patient would report markedly increased urination) or is experiencing dehydration (in which case the patient would report decreased fluid ingestion, dry mouth, weakness, and dizziness). If the patient has experienced weight loss, it is useful to think in terms of the percentage of weight lost over a specific time frame. To convert absolute pounds into percentage lost, the following simple equation is used:

$$\%\ \text{weight change} = \left[\frac{\text{usual weight} - \text{current weight}}{\text{usual weight}}\right] \times 100$$

Significant involuntary weight loss is generally defined as more than 5% of usual weight during the preceding 6 months or 10% or more within the year. When a patient has experienced unintentional weight loss, it is useful to direct your questions toward the underlying causes. There are four physiologic categories (Table 7.1) for weight loss: (1) decreased caloric intake, (2) malabsorption or maldigestion, (3) impaired metabolism or increased requirements, and (4) increased losses or excretion.

Past Medical History

As patients list their past illnesses, the healthcare professional should consider the role of nutrition or diet in the cause or treatment. Common diet-related diseases include cardiovascular disease (e.g., coronary artery disease, peripheral vascular disease, cerebrovascular disease), hypertension, diabetes, obesity, hyperlipidemia, some forms of cancer, metabolic dysfunction–associated steatotic liver disease (MASLD),[a] and other gastrointestinal (GI) diseases. In addition to asking how the illness was diagnosed and what treatment was rendered, ask the patient whether they received dietary counseling or altered their diet in response to the diagnosis. Try to ascertain the patient's understanding of the role that diet plays in the condition.

Past Surgical History

It is important to document all surgical procedures in this section, including any significant complications like fistulas, abscesses, open wounds, and chronic blood loss. These complications can often lead to malnutrition, which requires specialized nutritional support such as enteral and parenteral feedings. If the patient is currently in the postoperative period, it is essential to consider the role of nutritional support in the recovery process and how the surgery has affected the patient's dietary needs. For instance, a patient who underwent total gastrectomy must adjust their diet to reduce simple sugars, eat several small meals throughout the day, and receive

[a]Formerly known as nonalcoholic fatty liver disease (NAFLD). It is the most common chronic liver disease worldwide, affecting 30% of the global population.

TABLE 7.1 Physiologic Categories Associated With Weight Loss

Category	Symptoms	Diseases
Decreased caloric intake	Loss of appetite (anorexia) or early fullness (satiety) Change in taste, dry mouth, or sore mouth and tongue Difficulty chewing or swallowing Nausea or vomiting Inability to feed self or obtain food Self-imposed diet	Social isolation, depression Dysmotility Gingivitis, poor dentition Gastroparesis Obstruction (esophageal, gastric, or intestinal) Anorexia nervosa Cancer
Maldigestion and malabsorption	Diarrhea Fatty, malodorous stools Change in bowel habits Food particles in stool	Pancreatic insufficiency Radiation enteritis Crohn's disease Short bowel syndrome Lactose intolerance Celiac disease
Impaired metabolism or increased requirements	Fever Increased or decreased appetite	AIDS Pneumonia, sepsis Major surgery or trauma Hyperthyroidism Chronic hepatic, renal, or pulmonary disease Pregnancy and growth
Increased losses or excretion	Draining fistulas or open wounds Diarrhea Increased urination Excessive vomiting	Burns Occult gastrointestinal bleeding (iron loss) Hemodialysis Diabetes (glucosuria)

AIDS, Acquired immune deficiency syndrome.

TABLE 7.2 Commonly Used Herbs and Their Side Effects

Herb	Common Use	Side Effect and Interaction
Echinacea	Treatment and prevention of upper respiratory infections, common cold	Rash, pruritus, dizziness
St. John's wort	Treatment of mild to moderate depression	Gastrointestinal upset, photosensitivity
Gingko biloba	Treatment of dementia	Mild gastrointestinal distress, headache; may have anticoagulant effects
Garlic	Treatment of hypertension, hypercholesterolemia, atherosclerosis	Gastrointestinal upset, gas, reflux, nausea, allergic reaction, antiplatelet effects
Saw palmetto	Treatment of benign prostatic hyperplasia	Uncommon
Ginseng	General health promotion, energy	High doses: diarrhea, hypertension, insomnia, nervousness
Goldenseal	Treatment of upper respiratory infections, common cold	Diarrhea, hypertension, vasoconstriction
Aloe	Topical application for dermatitis, herpes	Possible delay in wound healing after topical application; diarrhea and hypokalemia with oral use
Siberian ginseng	Similar to those of ginseng	May alter digoxin levels
Valerian	Treatment of insomnia, anxiety	Fatigue, tremor, headache, paradoxical insomnia

additional vitamin B_{12} and iron supplements to maintain optimal nutritional health.

Medications

The medication history should include both prescription and over-the-counter medications. Because complementary and alternative therapies have become popular, many patients take vitamins, minerals, herbs (Table 7.2), and other dietary supplements that they may not mention without prompting. A thorough review of alternative and integrative therapy use should be a standard part of the patient medication and lifestyle history. When eliciting this information, be careful not to be judgmental or accusatory. Many patients do not disclose this information because of fear of being censured. Suggested questions are as follows:

"Are you taking any vitamins, minerals, herbs, or other dietary supplements, either prescription or over-the-counter?" If so, *"What is the dosage?"*

"What is the reason you are taking the supplement?"

"Have you experienced any side effects or benefits from the supplements?"

"Is anybody monitoring you, such as your healthcare professional, nutritionist, or herbalist?"

"What is your consumption of grapefruit and grapefruit juice?"

Drugs and nutrients interact in many ways to affect both nutritional status and the effectiveness of drug therapy. Drugs may influence nutritional status by several physiologic mechanisms: altering food intake (through nausea, changes in appetite, altered taste sensations), producing malabsorption (through alterations in intestinal mucus, motility, or pH; competition with nutrients for absorption sites; binding of bile acids), or modifying excretion (through renal tubular reabsorption or secretion). Drug-induced nutrient deficiencies usually develop slowly and are more likely in patients who use drugs chronically, especially older adults. Other risk factors include high drug dosages, multiple drug dosages, multiple drug regimens, poor diets, and marginal nutrient stores. Table 7.3 lists examples of drug interactions and nutrient metabolism.

Studies by Bailey[3] and associates in 1998 revealed possible drug interactions involving grapefruit and grapefruit juice (fresh or frozen) with several common medications used to treat high blood pressure, anxiety, depression, cancer, gastroesophageal reflux disease, erectile dysfunction, angina, convulsions, and human immunodeficiency virus (HIV) infection and acquired immune deficiency syndrome (AIDS). In general, grapefruit juice tends to increase the drug's effect.

Grapefruit juice decreases the activity of the cytochrome CYP_3A_4 enzymes in the liver and intestines that are responsible for breaking down many drugs and toxins. Grapefruit juice contains compounds known as furanocoumarins that block the CYP_3A_4 enzymes. When grapefruit juice is consumed, the enzyme's ability to break down the drug for elimination is decreased, potentially leading to overdosage of the medication.[4] The advisory also cautioned that sour oranges and tangelos may also interfere with medication blood levels. Other citrus fruits were considered safe. Bailey's study indicated that as little as one 8-oz (0.26-mg) glass of grapefruit juice could increase the blood drug level, and the effects could last for 3 days or more. It is recognized today that grapefruit juice can interact with many medications including some statins,[b] antihistaminics,[c] calcium channel blockers,[d] psychiatric medications,[e] immunosuppressants,[f] pain medications,[g] medications for erectile dysfunction,[h] HIV medication,[i] antiarrythmics,[j] and corticosteroids.[k]

TABLE 7.3 Drug Interactions and Nutrient Metabolism

Drug Class and Examples	Nutrients Affected
Antacids	
Aluminum hydroxide	Phosphorus
Magnesium trisilicate	Iron
Antibiotics	
Tetracyclines	Calcium, magnesium, iron, vitamin B_{12}
Neomycin, kanamycin	Fat-soluble vitamins, vitamin B_{12}
Sulfasalazine	Folate
Anticonvulsants	
Phenobarbital, phenytoin	Calcium, vitamin D, folate
Hypolipidemics	
Cholestyramine, colestipol	Fat and fat-soluble vitamins
Cytotoxic Agents	
Methotrexate	Folate
Laxatives	
Mineral oil	Water, electrolytes, fat, and fat-soluble vitamins
Antituberculotics	
Isoniazid	Pyridoxine (vitamin B_6)
Anticoagulants	
Warfarin	Vitamin K
Analgesics	
Aspirin, nonsteroidal anti-inflammatory drugs	Iron
Diuretics	
Thiazides, furosemide	Potassium, magnesium, calcium, zinc
Antineoplastic Agents	
Cisplatin	Potassium, magnesium

Allergies and Food Intolerances

In addition to asking about allergies to medications and environmental allergens, the interviewer should inquire about allergies and intolerances to food. The most common allergenic foods among adults are peanuts, tree nuts, shellfish, fish, eggs, soy, wheat, and milk. The first four foods listed may cause life-threatening reactions. If the patient states that they have a food allergy, the interviewer should ask what happens when those foods are eaten. Allergic symptoms may affect the respiratory tract (rhinorrhea, sneezing, wheezing, chest tightness, laryngeal edema), skin (urticaria, angioedema, pruritus, erythematous macular rash), or GI tract (nausea, vomiting, diarrhea, abdominal cramping). It is also appropriate to ask if the patient carries an EpiPen® (Epinephrine Auto-Injector) in case of anaphylaxis.

A food allergy needs to be differentiated from *food intolerance*. Symptoms of food intolerance are usually confined to the GI tract and may be acute or chronic. Upper GI tract symptoms of belching and bloating may be due to aerophagia (swallowing air during the ingestion of food or drink), which is commonly associated with smoking, eating rapidly, or talking while eating, chewing gum and hard candy, or ingesting carbonated beverages.

[b]Lovastatin (Mevacor®), atorvastatin (Lipitor®), simvastatin (Zocor®) (Vytorin®).

[c]Fexofenadine (Allegra®)—Blood levels of the drug are lowered, and the effectiveness of this commonly used antihistamine may be reduced. This interaction occurs by a different mechanism than CYP_3A_4.

[d]Felodipine (Plendil®), nifedipine (Procarida®).

[e]Buspirone (BuSpar®), triazolam (Halcion®), carbamazepine (Tegretol®), diazepam (Valium®), midazolam (Versed®), sertraline (Zoloft®).

[f]Cyclosporine (Neoral®), tacrolimus (Prograf®).

[g]Methadone.

[h]Sildenafil (Viagra®) (Revatio®).

[i]Saquinavir (Invirase®).

[j]Amiodarone (Pacerone®).

[k]Budesonide (Entocort EC®) (Uceris®).

Chronic lower GI tract symptoms of bloating, cramping, flatulence, or diarrhea may result from the ingestion of sugar substitutes (e.g., sorbitol, xylitol) or fructose, high fiber intake, or lactase deficiency. The term *FODMAP*[5] is an acronym referring to "**F**ermentable **O**ligo-, **D**i-, **M**onosaccharides, **A**nd **P**olyols." These are complex names used to classify groups of fermentable carbohydrates that trigger potentially debilitating digestive symptoms like bloating, gas, and stomach pain in sensitive individuals. FODMAPs are short chain carbohydrates that are poorly absorbed in the small intestine. FODMAPs are found in a wide range of foods in varying amounts. Some foods contain just one type of FODMAP, while others contain several.[1] Of these potential causes of lower GI symptoms, lactose intolerance, however, is the most common, affecting 25% of the population in the United States and up to 80% of African Americans. In lactose-intolerant individuals, symptoms occur after the consumption of products containing lactose, including milk, cheese, ice cream, yogurt, and some processed foods.

Social History

Social determinants of health (SDOH) can affect the dietary and nutritional status of patients. For example, low socioeconomic status, low fixed income, homelessness, food insecurity (the uncertainty of having or being able to acquire enough food because of insufficient funds or other resources), or lack of access to a variety of food choices may contribute to nutritional deficiencies. Chronic alcohol and misused substances are two additional conditions that put people at high nutritional risk. The patient's attitudes about food and nutrition, religious observances, and cultural practices also determine eating patterns and the selection or avoidance of specific foods. This information is important to note and document.

Lifestyle Habits

The lifestyle habits section of the medical history includes the dietary history, physical activity history, alcohol use history, and smoking history. Questions related to alcohol use and smoking are discussed in Chapter 1, The Interviewer's Questions.

Dietary History

The dietary history provides information about the patient's food habits, diet, and any counseling they may have received. Depending on the patient's medical problems, the dietary history may be brief or comprehensive. It is often difficult to obtain accurate information about a patient's diet because of variability, general lack of focus on what is eaten, and forgetfulness. For this reason, the primary goal is to obtain a qualitative description of eating patterns and the foods and beverages that are habitually chosen, along with any dietary changes that occurred over the course of the illness. Three methods are commonly used: a 24-hour intake recall, a typical day, and food frequency.

A 24-hour intake recall is used extensively and may be broached as follows: *"Please tell me what you had to eat and drink for the entire day yesterday. Could you start with the first item you had to eat or drink, and bring me through the entire day? I would also like to know the times you ate and the amounts."* The advantage of this method is that patients can usually remember what they ate over the course of one recent day. The disadvantage is that one particular day may not adequately depict the patient's usual diet, especially if there has been a recent change.

The preferred method is to ask the patient to describe a typical day. A good opening is, *Please let me know about your usual or typical diet. Can you bring me through a typical day, starting with the first item you eat or drink? I would also like to know the times you eat and the amounts."* The advantage is that you are more likely to capture a picture of the patient's habitual diet. If the patient states that every day is different and there are no typical days, then ask them to describe 1 or 2 days as examples, such as one weekday and one weekend day. Note that in both of these methods, the diet history is taken using an open-ended question. Patients are *not* asked what they ate for breakfast, lunch, and dinner. Anchoring food intake to predefined meals may bias the patient to provide an inaccurate history.

The third method is *food frequency.* This refers to how often the patient consumes specific food groups or nutrients and other dietary practices. Examples of questions are *"How often do you eat fruits and vegetables: daily, every few days, weekly, or rarely?"* and *"When you do eat them, how many servings do you choose?"* The same qualitative questions can be extended to the consumption of dairy products, whole-grain breads and cereals, red meats, visible fats, and so forth. Examples of other informative questions for taking a dietary history are as follows:

"What are your favorite foods and snacks?"

"Are you following any special or prescribed diet (diabetic, low sodium, low fat, kosher, vegetarian, low protein, commercial)?" If so, *"What does this diet entail?"*

"How often are meals home-cooked? Who prepares the meals?"

"What sort of fats or oils (if any) do you use in cooking?"

"How often do you eat out or order food in?" (Meals prepared outside the home are generally higher in calories, fat, and sodium.)

"How is food usually prepared (baked, broiled, fried, boiled, steamed, poached)?"

"How often do you consume sugar-sweetened beverages?"

Targeted, disease-focused questions should be asked, depending on the patient's medical history. For example, if the patient has *osteoporosis,* you would probe for the consumption of calcium-containing foods such as milk, cheese, sardines, and greens. For a patient with *hypercholesterolemia* or *coronary artery disease,* you would ask about the intake of saturated fats, whole dairy products, egg yolks, fried foods, tropical oils, and fiber sources. For a patient with *diabetes mellitus,* you would ask whether meals and snacks are timed to correspond with insulin injections, whether the patient follows a carbohydrate-controlled diet and counts carbohydrate grams, and whether the patient knows the symptoms of hypoglycemia and how to treat it.

Patients should be asked whether they read nutrition labels and, if they do not, they should be instructed how to read them. **Nutrition literacy** is defined as the degree to which individuals have the capacity to obtain, process, and understand

[1]**Oligosaccharides:** Wheat, rye, legumes, and various fruits and vegetables, such as garlic and onions.

nutrition information and skills needed in order to make appropriate nutrition decisions. Since May 1994, nutritional labeling has been required for almost all foods. There are now uniform definitions for the terms "free," "low," "light," "reduced," "high," "lean," "extra lean," and so forth. The current food label, known as *Nutrition Facts* and updated in 2024[6], allows individuals to choose healthier foods more easily. Nutrition labeling provides the "% Daily Value," which shows how a food fits into the overall daily diet. This value is based on a 2000-calorie diet and informs the individual whether the food is high or low in the specific nutrient. These labels must include serving size, total calories, calories from fat, total fat, saturated fat, trans fat, cholesterol, sodium, total carbohydrate, dietary fiber, protein, and total and added sugars. The % Daily Value of four key vitamins and minerals (vitamin D, calcium, iron, and potassium) is also mandatory on these labels. Information about other vitamins and minerals is optional. The % Daily Value is only a guide; if a patient eats more than 2000 calories daily, the food would contribute a lower % Daily Value to the diet.

The Institute of Medicine of the National Academies[7] recommends that the following guidelines be used daily for achieving a healthful diet:

- **Carbohydrates:** 45% to 65% of calories
- **Fat:** 20% to 35% (<10% saturated fat)
- **Trans fat:** no more than 1% of total body calories
- **Protein:** 10% to 35% of calories
- **Sodium:** 2300 mg
- **Cholesterol:** no more than 300 mg each day
- **Fiber:** females need 21 to 25 g/d; males need 30 to 38 g/d

Most individuals on a balanced diet consume foods that contain all the vitamins and minerals they need. Some individuals, however, might benefit from vitamin supplementation. These individuals include those who habitually restrict their diet, ill patients (especially those with loss of appetite or impaired absorption), pregnant or lactating females, infants consuming formula, some vegetarians, older patients, and patients with anorexia nervosa.

Physical Activity

Both nutrition and regular physical activity play an important role in the overall health of the individual. It is recommended that all adults accumulate at least 150 minutes (2.5 hours) of moderate-intensity (or at least 75 minutes [1.25 hours] of vigorous-intensity) physical activity per week, preferably spread throughout the week. There are many benefits to regular physical activity: increasing physical fitness; building and maintaining healthy bones, muscles, and joints; improving endurance and muscle strength; lowering the risk of certain diseases (e.g., diabetes, cardiovascular disease, colon cancer); controlling blood pressure; promoting and improving a sense of well-being; reducing feelings of anxiety and depression; and managing excess weight.

Always ask patients about their current level of physical activity and functioning. Some helpful questions include the following:

"What is the most physically active thing you do in the course of the day?"

"How do you spend your working day and leisure time?"

"What types of physical activity do you enjoy? How often do you do them?"

"Do you exercise regularly?" If so, *"What exercises do you do regularly? How often?"*

"What gets in the way of you consistently doing physical activity?"

"How many hours of screen time do you have every day?"

"How many hours per day are you sitting?"

"Do you belong to (and attend) a health club or exercise classes?" If not, *"Do you have access to exercise equipment?"*

Review of Systems

When conducting a review of systems, the patient's medical history should be reexamined by organ system. It is important to include a general statement about the patient's body weight history and appetite in this section, especially if this information has not been previously mentioned in the history of the present illness or past medical history.

PHYSICAL EXAMINATION

Vital Signs

Besides the standard vital signs like heart rate, pulse, blood pressure, and temperature, it's important to also record the patient's height and weight. Even though height and weight aren't typically considered vital signs, they reveal significant information about the patient's overall health status and are often used for medication dosing. Measuring height and weight is the best option, but if not possible, estimated values are still better than no values at all. If you're estimating, note that these values are *reported* and *not measured.* Keep in mind that body weight can vary depending on the presence of clothing, wet dressings, and hydration status. Always measure the patient's height in stocking feet and note that conditions such as renal or liver failure or congestive heart failure can affect body weight.

The nutritional status of the patient based on height and weight is interpreted by the *body mass index (BMI).* BMI is an international designation of relative weight for stature and is a more reliable index of obesity than the older insurance-based height-weight tables. BMI is moderately correlated with the amount of fat mass in the general population but loses predictability when applied on the individual level. Although imperfect, it is used as a currently acceptable assessment of a person's risk for disease that can occur with more body fat. The higher the BMI, the greater the risk for certain diseases such as heart disease, high blood pressure, type 2 diabetes mellitus, gallstones, pulmonary problems, and certain cancers. It is calculated in one of the two following ways:

- **BMI** = weight (kg)/height (meters)^2
- **BMI** = weight (pounds)/height (inches)^2 × 703

The advantage of BMI is that it is relatively easy to calculate, is routinely included in the electronic medical record (EMR), and can be readily used for comparisons between females and males and persons of different heights. BMI can easily be determined from tables, as shown in Fig. 7.1.

A disadvantage of using BMI is that it does not directly measure body composition and therefore may yield a spurious

BMI	19	20	21	22	23	24	25	26	27	28	29	30	31	32	33	34	35
Height (inches)	Body Weight (pounds)																
58	91	96	100	105	110	115	119	124	129	134	138	143	148	153	158	162	167
59	94	99	104	109	114	119	124	128	133	138	143	148	153	158	163	168	173
60	97	102	107	112	118	123	128	133	138	143	148	153	156	163	168	174	179
61	100	106	111	116	122	127	132	137	143	148	153	158	164	169	174	180	185
62	104	109	115	120	126	131	136	142	147	153	158	164	169	175	180	186	191
63	107	113	118	124	130	135	141	146	152	158	163	169	175	180	186	191	197
64	110	116	122	128	134	140	145	151	157	163	169	174	180	186	192	197	204
65	114	120	126	132	138	144	150	156	162	168	174	180	186	192	198	204	210
66	118	124	130	136	142	148	155	161	167	173	179	186	192	198	204	210	216
67	121	127	134	140	146	153	159	166	172	178	185	191	198	204	211	217	223
68	125	131	138	144	151	158	164	171	177	184	190	197	203	210	216	223	230
69	128	135	142	149	155	162	169	176	182	189	196	203	209	216	223	230	236
70	132	139	146	153	160	167	174	181	188	195	202	209	216	222	229	236	243
71	136	143	150	157	165	172	179	186	193	200	208	215	222	229	236	243	250
72	140	147	154	162	169	177	184	191	199	206	213	221	228	235	242	250	258
73	144	151	159	166	174	182	189	197	204	212	219	227	235	242	250	257	265
74	148	155	163	171	179	186	194	202	210	218	225	233	241	249	256	264	272
75	152	160	168	176	184	192	200	208	216	224	232	240	248	256	264	272	279
76	156	164	172	180	189	197	205	213	221	230	238	246	254	263	271	279	287

BMI	36	37	38	39	40	41	42	43	44	45	46	47	48	49	50	51	52	53	54
58	172	177	181	186	191	196	201	205	210	215	220	224	229	234	239	244	248	253	258
59	178	183	188	193	198	203	208	212	217	222	227	232	237	242	247	252	257	262	267
60	184	189	194	199	204	209	215	220	225	230	235	240	245	250	255	261	266	271	276
61	190	195	201	206	211	217	222	227	232	238	243	248	254	259	264	269	275	280	285
62	196	202	207	213	218	224	229	235	240	246	251	256	262	267	273	278	284	289	295
63	203	208	214	220	225	231	237	242	248	254	259	265	270	278	282	287	293	299	304
64	209	215	221	227	232	238	244	250	256	262	267	273	279	285	291	296	302	308	314
65	216	222	228	234	240	246	252	258	264	270	278	282	288	294	300	306	312	318	324
66	223	229	235	241	247	253	260	266	272	278	284	291	297	303	309	315	322	328	334
67	230	236	242	249	255	261	268	274	280	287	293	299	306	312	319	325	331	338	344
68	236	243	249	256	262	269	276	282	289	295	302	306	315	322	328	335	341	348	354
69	243	250	257	263	270	277	284	291	297	304	311	318	324	331	338	345	351	358	365
70	250	257	264	271	278	285	292	298	306	313	320	327	334	341	348	355	362	369	376
71	257	265	272	279	286	293	301	308	315	322	329	338	343	351	358	365	372	379	386
72	265	272	279	287	294	302	309	316	324	331	338	346	353	361	368	375	383	390	397
73	272	280	288	295	302	310	318	325	333	340	348	355	363	371	378	386	393	401	408
74	280	287	295	303	311	319	328	334	342	350	358	365	373	381	389	396	404	412	420
75	287	295	303	311	319	327	335	343	351	359	367	375	383	391	399	407	415	423	431
76	295	304	312	320	328	336	344	353	361	369	377	385	394	402	410	416	426	435	443

Fig. 7.1 Body Mass Index (BMI). To find a specific BMI, (1) look down the left column to find the height (measured in inches); (2) look across that row and find the weight; and (3) look to the top of the column to find the number that is the BMI.

interpretation. For example, a malnourished patient with excessive fluid retention may be categorized incorrectly as having a healthy BMI, or a muscular body builder may be misclassified as obese (excess body fat). Additionally, BMI does not consider differences in body shape and heterogeneity across race and ethnic groups, sex, gender, and age span that are essential to consider when applying BMI as a measure of adiposity.

Nonetheless, by conventional practice, the standard weight categories associated with BMI ranges are shown in Table 7.4.[8]

For example, in Table 7.5 are the weight ranges, the corresponding BMI ranges, and the weight status categories for a person who is 5′9″.

Lower BMI thresholds for overweight and obesity have been proposed for Asians since this population appears to be at risk for glucose and lipid abnormalities at lower body weights.

If the person's BMI is equal to or less than 35, it is important to measure the waist circumference horizontally at the level of the anterior superior iliac crest of the pelvic bone using a flexible tape measure (Fig. 7.2). The measurement is made at normal minimal respiration making sure that the tape is horizontal

TABLE 7.4 Standard Weight Categories Associated With BMI Ranges

BMI	Weight Status
Below 18.5	Underweight
18.5–24.9	Normal or healthy weight
25.0–29.9	Overweight
30.0 and above	Obese

TABLE 7.5 Example of Weight Ranges for Person Who Is 5′9″

Height	Weight Range	BMI	Weight Status
5′9″	124 pounds or less	Below 18.5	Underweight
	125–168 pounds	18.5–24.9	Normal or healthy weight
	169–202 pounds	25.0–29.9	Overweight
	203 pounds or more	30 or higher	Obese

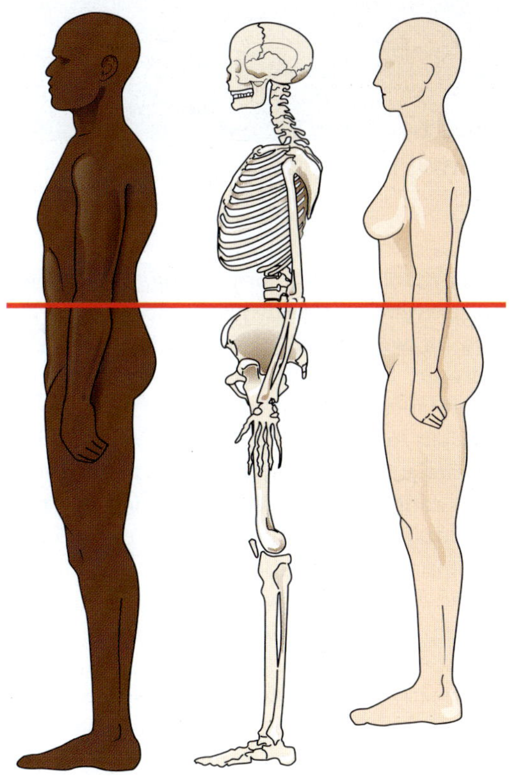

Fig. 7.2 Measuring Tape Position for Determining Abdominal Circumference.

around the waist. It should be snug around the waist and not compress the skin. If the waist circumference is 35 inches (88 cm) or more in nonpregnant females or 40 inches (102 cm) or more in males, the risk of developing hypertension, type 2 diabetes, coronary artery disease, and stroke increases significantly independent of BMI. Such individuals may have *metabolic syndrome. Metabolic syndrome* is a name for a group of risk factors that cluster together and increase the risk for the disease indicated. The metabolic syndrome is becoming more and more common in the United States. It is unknown whether the syndrome is due to one single cause, but **all of the risks for the syndrome are related to obesity.** The two most important risk factors for metabolic syndrome are:

- Extra weight around the middle and upper parts of the body (central obesity). The body may be described as "apple-shaped."
- Insulin resistance. The body uses insulin less effectively than normal. Insulin is needed to help control the amount of sugar in the body. As a result, blood sugar and fat levels rise. Other risk factors for insulin resistance include the following:
- Aging
- Genes that make you more likely to develop this condition
- Hormone changes
- Lack of exercise

People who have metabolic syndrome often have two other problems that can either cause the condition or make it worse:

- Excess blood clotting
- Increased levels of blood substances that are a sign of inflammation throughout the body

Appearance

A description of the patient's general appearance is always found at the beginning of the physical examination report; for example, "On examination, Ms. B. is a well-developed, thin, female." Other nutritionally descriptive terms are as follows:

- Emaciated
- Cachectic
- Malnourished
- Thin/slim
- Underweight
- Normal weight
- Fit
- Overweight
- Obese
- Edematous

Nutrition-oriented aspects of the physical examination focus on the skin, eyes, mouth, skeletal muscle, and fat stores. The skin provides an excellent barometer of clinical nutrition and is accessible to healthcare professionals in its entirety. Chronic wasting associated with loss of subcutaneous fat from calorie or protein deficiency results in a fine wrinkling of the skin. Easy bruising may result from vitamin deficiencies. In areas of the skin where sebaceous glands are dense, such as the nasolabial folds, neck, cheeks, and forehead, a deficiency of essential nutrients may result in disturbance of their secretory function and blockage of their ducts with plugs of dried sebum. Around hair follicles, there may be accumulations of keratin associated with vitamin and fatty acid deficiencies. Edema may result from protein deficiencies. This occurs as a consequence of low plasma albumin and reduced oncotic pressure. Excessive skin pigmentation may also be seen. In deficiencies of niacin or tryptophan, increased pigmentation occurs in areas of skin exposed to the sun. Changes in the hair and nails are also common in nutritional deficiencies. Blindness may result from vitamin A deficiency. Fissuring of the lips is indicative of riboflavin deficiency. The tongue may be large in iodine or niacin deficiency. Some of the more common physical signs of nutritional deficiency are listed in Table 7.6.

TABLE 7.6 Manifestations of Nutritional Deficiencies

Site	Sign	Deficiency
Skin	Dry and scaly, cellophane appearance	Protein (see Fig. 7.4)
	Flaking dermatitis	Zinc (see Fig. 7.10)
	Follicular hyperkeratosis	Vitamin A (see Fig. 7.5)
	Pigmentation changes	Niacin (see Fig. 7.9)
	Petechiae	Vitamin C (see Fig. 7.7)
	Purpura	Vitamin C (see Fig. 7.7), vitamin K
	Pallor	Iron, vitamin B_{12}, folate
	Nail changes	Iron (see Fig. 8.11)
Eyes	Night blindness	Conjunctiva pallor
	Vitamin A	Iron, vitamin B_{12}, folate
Mouth	Angular stomatitis	Riboflavin, pyridoxine, niacin
	Cheilosis (dry, cracking, ulcerated lips)	Riboflavin, pyridoxine, niacin
	Glossitis	Riboflavin, niacin, B vitamins, iron, folate (see Fig. 7.8)
	Bleeding gums	Vitamin C (see Fig. 7.6), riboflavin
Muscles	Interosseous muscle atrophy, squaring off of shoulders, poor hand grip and leg strength	Protein, calories (see Fig. 7.4)

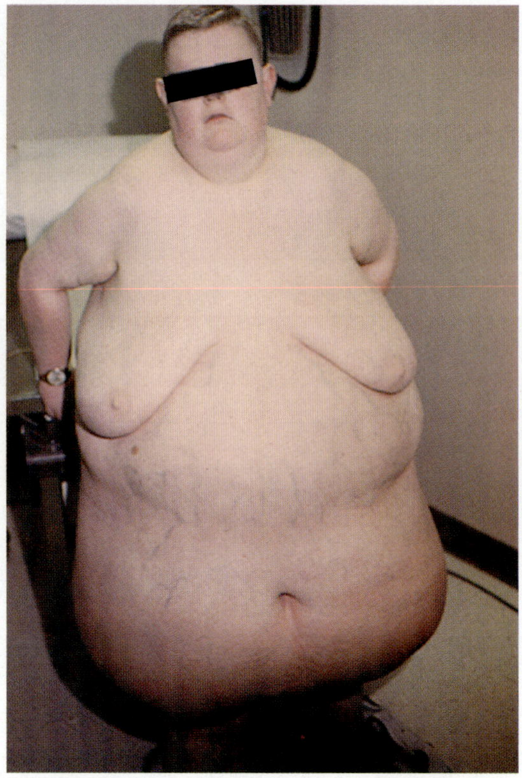

Fig. 7.3 Patient With Prader-Willi Syndrome. (From Morgan SL, Weinsier RL: *Fundamentals of Clinical Nutrition*, ed 2, St. Louis, 1998, Mosby.)

SPECIAL POPULATIONS

Patients With Obesity

Results from the 2017–2018 National Health and Nutrition Examination Survey (NHANES)[9] indicate that an estimated 42.4% of U.S. adults have obesity, including 9.2% with severe obesity (BMI $\geq$40 kg/m^2), and another 30.7% are overweight.[9,10] Thus, overweight and obesity represent the most significant diet-related health problems encountered by healthcare professionals.

Obesity results from the complex interplay of environmental, social, behavioral, genetic, and biological determinants that alter calorie balance. When calorie intake continuously exceeds requirements, obesity results. Although relatively uncommon, neuroendocrine abnormalities, such as hypopituitarism, adrenocortical excess, polycystic ovary syndrome, hypothalamic tumors, or other damage to this part of the brain, as well as some rare inherited conditions, result in obesity. *Prader-Willi syndrome* is a rare chromosomal microdeletion syndrome associated with childhood massive obesity, mental retardation, and failure of sexual development. A patient with Prader-Willi syndrome and severe obesity is pictured in Fig. 7.3.

Obesity-Focused History

An obesity-focused history provides a contextual understanding of how and when patients gained weight, what efforts were employed to take control, and the impact of body weight on their health and quality of life. For females, weight gain often occurs during adolescence, pregnancy, child-rearing years, and menopause. For many patients, weight gain is a consequence of smoking cessation or other changes in lifestyle, such as changes in marital status, occupation, or housing. The patient's history may be suggestive of, as already mentioned, several endocrinologic causes for weight gain. However, except for polycystic ovary syndrome, these conditions are uncommon causes of obesity. Several medications are known to cause weight gain as an iatrogenically unintended side effect. The most common drug groups are antidepressants (tricyclic agents and mirtazapine), lithium, antipsychotics (phenothiazines, butyrophenones, olanzapine, clozapine, risperidone, and brexpiprazole), anticonvulsants (valproic acid, carbamazepine), steroid hormones (corticosteroid derivatives, megestrol acetate), and antidiabetics (insulin, sulfonylureas, thiazolidinediones).

When a patient's weight history is documented, it is important to be sensitive. Many patients feel stigmatized by their obesity or feel ashamed and frustrated about not being able to control their weight. The mnemonic "OPQRST," commonly used for ascertaining the dimensions of a patient's symptoms, can be modified for taking an informative and comprehensive obesity-focused weight history by concentrating on the following six features: onset, precipitating events, quality of health, remedy, setting, and temporal pattern. Examples of questions that can be used to explore these features are provided in Table 7.7. The questions should be open-ended and nonjudgmental.

Obesity-Focused Physical Examination

According to the most recent American Association of Clinical Endocrinologists (AACE) guidelines, assessment of risk status according to overweight and obesity is based on the patient's

TABLE 7.7 Using the Mnemonic "OPQRST" to Take an Obesity-Focused Weight History

	Sample Questions
Onset	"When did you first begin to gain weight?" "Have your struggled with your weight since childhood?" "What did you weigh in high school, college, early 20s, 30s, 40s?" "Did the weight gain begin when you started taking a certain medication?"
Precipitating events	"What life events led to your weight gain, e.g., college, long commute, marriage, divorce, change in jobs, financial loss, depression, illness?" "How much weight did you gain with pregnancy?" "How much weight did you gain when you stopped smoking?" "How much additional weight did you gain when you started insulin?"
Quality of life	"At what weight did you feel your best?" "What is hard to do at your current weight?" "How does your weight affect how you feel and function?"
Remedy	"What have you done or tried in the past to control your weight?" "What is the most successful approach you tried to lose weight?" "What do you attribute the weight loss to?" "What caused you to regain your weight?"
Setting	"What was going on in your life when you last felt in control of your weight?" "What was going on when you gained your weight?" "What role has stress played in your weight gain?" "How important is social support or having a buddy to help you?"
Temporal pattern	"What is the pattern of your weight gain?" "Did you gradually gain your weight over time, or is it more cyclic (yo-yo)?" "Are there large swings in your weight, and if so, what is the weight change?" "What was your lightest weight and heaviest weight as an adult?"

BMI, waist circumference, and existence of complications/comorbid conditions.

Being overweight or having obesity substantially increases the risk of morbidity and mortality from hypertension, type 2 diabetes mellitus, dyslipidemia, coronary artery disease, stroke, gallstones, osteoarthritis, respiratory problems (including sleep apnea), several cancers, and metabolic syndrome, which is a clustering of risk factors for cardiovascular disease and diabetes. Factors characteristic of this syndrome are abdominal obesity, elevated triglyceride levels, low high-density lipoprotein cholesterol level, raised blood pressure, and impaired fasting blood glucose.

Excess abdominal fat, a hallmark of the metabolic syndrome, can be clinically defined as a waist circumference greater than 40 inches (102 cm) in males and greater than 35 inches (88 cm) in females. Lower waist circumference thresholds have been recommended for the Asian population. Proper measurement of waist circumference was described earlier in this chapter and is illustrated in Fig. 7.2. An increased waist circumference can indicate increased risk even at a healthy weight (BMI ≤25). In contrast, waist circumference is less useful as an independent marker of medical risk when the BMI is greater than 35. Table 7.8 lists the classification of weight status and risk of disease.

The physical examination process for patients with obesity is identical to that for other adult patients, except for specific measures to determine the obesity category (height, weight, and waist circumference) and the use of an appropriate blood pressure cuff. A bladder cuff that is not the appropriate width for the patient's arm circumference can cause a systematic error in blood pressure measurement; if the bladder is too narrow, the pressure will be overestimated and lead to a false diagnosis of hypertension. The most frequent error in measuring blood pressure is "miscuffing," with undercuffing large arms accounting for 84% of the "miscuffings." To avoid errors, the "ideal" cuff should have a bladder length that is 80% and a width that is at least 40% of arm circumference (a length-to-width ratio of 2:1). Therefore, a large adult cuff (16 × 36 cm) should be chosen for patients with mild to moderate obesity (or arm circumference of 14 to 17 inches [36 to 43 cm]), whereas an adult thigh cuff

TABLE 7.8 Classification of Weight Status and Risk of Disease

		RISK OF DISEASE[a,b]	
Classification	**Body Mass Index**	**Waist Circumference: Females: ≤35 inches (88 cm); Males: ≤40 inches (102 cm)**	**Waist Circumference: Females: >35 inches (88 cm); Males: >40 inches (102 cm)**
Underweight	<18.5	—	—
Healthy weight	18.5–24.9	—	—
Overweight	25–29.9	↑	↑↑
Obesity	30–34.9	↑↑	↑↑↑
Obesity	35–39.9	↑↑↑	↑↑↑
Extreme obesity	≥40	↑↑↑↑	↑↑↑↑

[a]Waist circumference is measured just above the iliac crest. An increased waist circumference may indicate increased disease risk even at a normal weight.

[b]Preventing and Managing the Global Epidemic of Obesity: *Report of the World Health Organization Consultation of Obesity*, Geneva, June 1997, WHO. Adapted from National Institutes of Health and National Heart, Lung, and Blood Institute: *Clinical guidelines on the identification, evaluation, and treatment of overweight and obesity in adults*, Rockville, MD, 1998, U.S. Department of Health and Human Services, Public Health Service.

(16 × 42 cm) must be used for patients whose arm circumferences are greater than 17 inches.

When the interviewer completes the review of systems section of the history and performs the physical examination, it is important to have a high index of suspicion for obesity-related diseases. Clinically, obesity affects at least nine organ systems. Obesity has been linked with an increased risk of breast and endometrial cancers in females. The mechanism is thought to be related to an increase in circulating estrogens as a consequence of increased conversion of androgens to estrogens in adipose tissue. Obesity increases the risk of gallstone formation by increasing gallbladder volume and bile stasis. Increased cholesterol production is also thought to play a role. Degenerative joint disease is seen in individuals with obesity more frequently than in persons of normal weight. Regardless of whether it is a causative factor, osteoarthritis aggravates joint symptoms. A positive association has been noted between serum triglyceride and low-density lipoprotein cholesterol levels and obesity. High-density lipoprotein cholesterol level tends to be lower in patients with obesity. The Pickwickian,[m] or obesity hypoventilation, syndrome is characterized by marked obesity, somnolence, periodic apnea (transient cessation of breathing), chronic hypoxemia (deficient oxygenation of the blood), hypercapnia (carbon dioxide retention), and polycythemia (increased number of red blood cells). Table 7.9 lists the symptoms and diseases that are directly or indirectly related to obesity. Although individuals vary, the number and severity of organ-specific comorbid conditions usually rise with increasing levels of obesity.

TABLE 7.9 Review of Obesity-Related Organ Systems

Cardiovascular	Hypertension Congestive heart failure Cor pulmonale Varicose veins Pulmonary embolism Coronary artery disease Atrial fibrillation
Endocrine	Metabolic syndrome Type 2 diabetes mellitus Dyslipidemia Polycystic ovary syndrome, androgenicity Amenorrhea, infertility, menstrual disorders
Musculoskeletal	Hyperuricemia and gout Immobility Osteoarthritis (knees and hips) Low back pain, carpal tunnel syndrome
Psychologic	Depression, low self-esteem Body image disturbance Social stigmatization
Integumentary	Striae distensae (stretch marks) Stasis pigmentation of legs Lymphedema Cellulitis Intertrigo, carbuncles Acanthosis nigricans, skin tags Hydradenitis suppurativa
Respiratory	Dyspnea Obstructive sleep apnea Hypoventilation syndrome Pickwickian syndrome Asthma
Gastrointestinal	Gastroesophageal reflux disease Metabolic dysfunction-associated steatotic liver disease (MASLD) Cholelithiasis Hernias Colon cancer
Genitourinary	Urinary stress incontinence Obesity-related glomerulopathy End-stage renal disease Hypogonadism (male) Breast and uterine cancer Pregnancy complications
Neurologic	Stroke Idiopathic intracranial hypertension Meralgia paresthetica

Malnourished Patients

Malnutrition (which is synonymous with undernutrition) is associated with slower wound healing, increased number of medical complications, longer length of hospital stays, higher healthcare costs, and increased mortality rate. By performing a nutritionally focused history and physical examination, you can identify individuals who are at high nutritional risk or are malnourished. Key elements from the history and physical examination were reviewed earlier in this chapter.

There is no single clinical or laboratory indicator of malnutrition. Rather, the comprehensive assessment includes the medical/surgical history and clinical diagnosis, dietary assessment, clinical signs and physical examination, functional outcomes, and anthropometric data. A Global Leadership Initiative on Malnutrition (2018)[11] sought to standardize the clinical practice of malnutrition diagnosis. Five assessment factors were identified: weight loss, reduced BMI, and reduced muscle mass were categorized as phenotypic criteria, and reduced food intake/assimilation and disease burden/inflammation as etiologic criteria. The diagnosis of malnutrition is made by the combination of at least one phenotypic criterion and one etiologic criterion.

Impairment of function secondary to loss of body protein and energy reserves along with identifying the presence or absence of systemic inflammation are important components of the assessment of nutritional risk. *Sarcopenia* is the gradual loss of muscle mass, strength, and function that more commonly affects the aging population. You can evaluate function while performing the physical examination and watching the patient's activity. You can assess grip strength by asking the patient to squeeze your index and middle fingers hard for at least 10 seconds. You can assess respiratory muscle function by asking the patient to exhale quickly or cough deeply. Shortness of breath may be noted at rest. You can assess leg muscle strength by asking the

[m]In the 1950s, scientists named the condition after a character, Pickwick, in a Charles Dickens novel that had symptoms of obesity hypoventilation. Obesity hypoventilation syndrome is a serious respiratory complication of obesity. It can cause life-threatening health issues.

patient to push their legs and feet against your hand and watching the patient ambulate. Indicators of inflammatory response include fever, elevated C-reactive protein, elevated white blood count, and negative nitrogen balance. Fig. 7.4 depicts three patients with protein-energy malnutrition or deficiency of macronutrients. Note the severe loss of subcutaneous fat reserves and muscle mass and the prominence of the bones.

Three of the previously discussed phenotypic criteria—percent weight loss, low BMI, and reduced muscle mass—can be used to categorize the severity grading of malnutrition into Stage 1 (Moderate) and Stage 1 (Severe) Malnutrition (Table 7.10).

Older Adult Patients

Older adults represent a diverse group who are at specific risk for a variety of nutritional problems. These problems are caused by a combination of environmental, social, and economic factors, and are compounded by numerous physiologic changes that occur at different rates as individuals age. The *Nutrition Screening Initiative,* a multidisciplinary effort to promote nutrition screening and better nutritional care in America's healthcare system, has identified the following risk factors associated with poor nutritional status in older Americans: inappropriate food intake, poverty, social isolation, dependency or disability, acute or chronic diseases or conditions, and chronic medication use.

These factors have been incorporated into a risk factor checklist with the acronym *DETERMINE,* which identifies several warning signs for individuals at risk for poor nutritional status:

- **D**isease: Any disease can cause the patient to change the way they eat or make it hard to eat, cook, or shop. Confusion or memory loss can make it hard for people to remember what or how to eat. Depression can lead to changes in appetite, energy level, and weight.

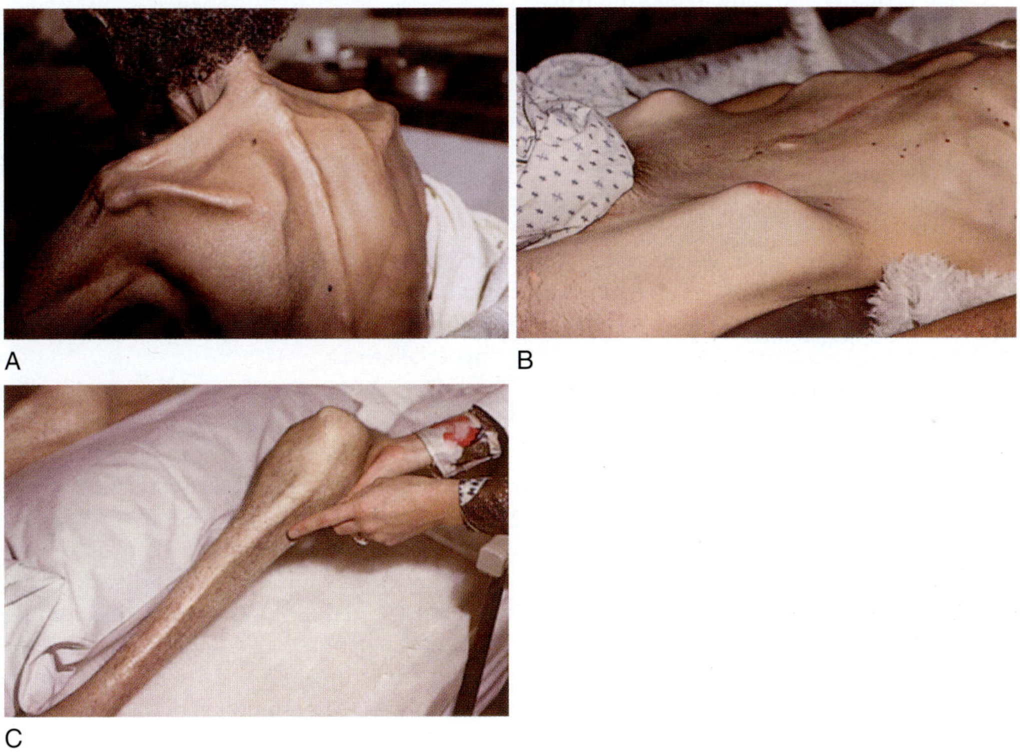

Fig. 7.4 (A to C) Loss of subcutaneous fat and muscle in three patients with protein-energy malnutrition. (From Morgan SL, Weinsier RL: *Fundamentals of Clinical Nutrition*, ed 2, St. Louis, 1998, Mosby.)

TABLE 7.10 Diagnosing Malnutrition Into Stage 1 (Moderate) and Stage 2 (Severe) Malnutrition

	PHENOTYPIC CRITERIA		
	Weight Loss (%)	**Low Body Mass Index (kg/m²)**	**Reduced Muscle Mass**
Stage 1/moderate malnutrition (requires 1 phenotypic criterion that meets this grade)	5%–10% within the past 6 months, or 10%–20% beyond 6 months	<20 if <70 years; <22 if ≥70 years	Mild-moderate deficit
Stage 2/severe malnutrition (requires 1 phenotypic criterion that meets this grade)	>10% within the past 6 months, or >20% beyond 6 months	<18.5 if <70 years; <20 if ≥70 years	Severe deficit

Adapted from Jensen GL, et al: GLIM criteria for the diagnosis of malnutrition: a consensus report from the Global Clinical Nutrition Community, *JPEN J Parenter Enteral Nutr* 43(1):32–40, 2019.

- Eating poorly: This may involve eating too little or too much, drinking too much alcohol, or not eating the foods needed for health every day. A diminished sense of taste and smell can decrease appetite and influence food choices. Many older people have a decreased ability to taste salt, which results in the liberal salting of foods. A reduced sense of smell may make it difficult for an older person to detect whether food has spoiled. Older patients should be advised to read all dates stamped on food products.
- Tooth loss or mouth pain: Some people do not eat well because they have lost teeth or have problems with their mouth, teeth, or gums.
- Economic hardship: When a patient has very little money to spend on food, they may not eat enough food or may eat foods that do not have enough vitamins, minerals, or calories to stay healthy. The individual may buy prepackaged or convenience foods that are typically high in sodium, potassium, and sugar.
- Reduced social contact: Cooking and eating alone are hard. Some people who live alone do not feel like shopping for or preparing the food they need. Loss of a spouse, retirement, or social isolation can lead to loneliness, depression, and lack of motivation to eat.
- Multiple medications or drugs: Drugs and other medications can depress the appetite and alter nutrient absorption and excretion. Drugs can further alter the sense of taste and smell, change the secretion of saliva, irritate the stomach, and cause nausea. Some drugs can contribute directly to dietary deficiencies; for example, antacids absorb folic acid and calcium, laxatives absorb fat-soluble vitamins, and aspirin increases the excretion of folic acid.
- Involuntary weight loss or gain: Assess changes in weight.
- Need for assistance with self-care: Assess self-care practices.
- Elderly years: Patients older than 80 years are considered "elderly."

Specific nutritional interventions are vital components of the healthcare delivery system for older patients. The older person may overeat as a way of coping with feelings of loneliness. Some of these individuals, however, can be overweight but malnourished; their diet consists of cake and candy, which are high in calories but low in nutrients. The National Institute on Aging suggests that the daily diet for the geriatric population include the following:

- Two servings of milk or dairy products low in lactose (3 cups per day)
- Two servings of high-protein foods (5 to 5½ ounces per day)
- Four servings of fruit and vegetables, including a citrus fruit and a dark green leafy vegetable (2 to 2½ cups per day)
- Four servings of bread or cereal products (3 ounces per day)

See Chapter 25, The Geriatric Patient, for additional information.

CLINICOPATHOLOGIC CORRELATIONS

There are myriad vitamin and trace element deficiencies, and it is beyond the scope of this book to describe them. There are, however, several worth considering.

Vitamin A, a fat-soluble vitamin, is an integral component of rhodopsin and iodopsin, the light-sensitive proteins in the rods and cones of the retina. A deficiency of vitamin A is associated with follicular hyperkeratosis and night blindness. Fig. 7.5 illustrates a patient with vitamin A deficiency and follicular hyperkeratosis.

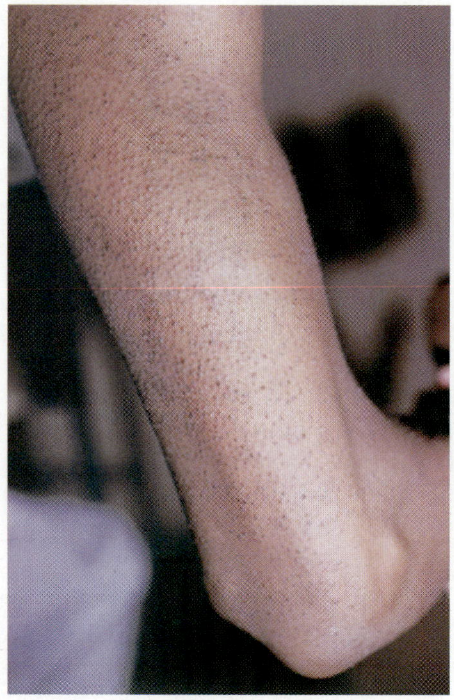

Fig. 7.5 **Effects of Vitamin A Deficiency.** (From Morgan SL, Weinsier RL: *Fundamentals of Clinical Nutrition*, ed 2, St. Louis, 1998, Mosby.)

Vitamin C, or ascorbic acid, is a biologic antioxidant and free radical scavenger. The biosynthesis of bile acids, collagen, and norepinephrine, as well as the normal functioning of the hepatic oxygenase system, depends on these antioxidant properties. Vitamin C deficiency is rarely found in the United States. The classic deficiency state is known as *scurvy.* It is characterized by depression, fatigue, and widespread abnormalities in connective tissue. Oral lesions (including inflamed gingiva), petechiae, hemorrhage, impaired wound healing, hyperkeratosis, and bleeding into body cavities are commonly seen. Fig. 7.6 depicts marked periodontal disease in two patients with scurvy. Fig. 7.7 illustrates perifollicular purpura and ecchymoses in a patient with vitamin C deficiency.

Folate is required for the synthesis of nucleotides and the metabolism of several amino acids. The inhibition of folate metabolism in bacteria and cancer cell growth is the mechanism of action of the sulfonamide antibiotics and chemotherapeutic agents such as methotrexate and 5-fluorouracil. Folate deficiency is seen in females of childbearing age and alcoholic patients. It manifests with a megaloblastic anemia reflecting ineffective DNA synthesis. Depapillation of the tongue and diarrhea are common findings. Fig. 7.8A depicts the classic glossitis of folate deficiency in an alcoholic patient; Fig. 7.8B illustrates the patient's tongue after folate replacement.

Niacin, a B-complex vitamin, is required as a coenzyme to form nicotinamide adenine dinucleotide or nicotinamide adenine dinucleotide phosphate. There are more than 200 enzymes that require the active coenzyme forms of niacin as electron

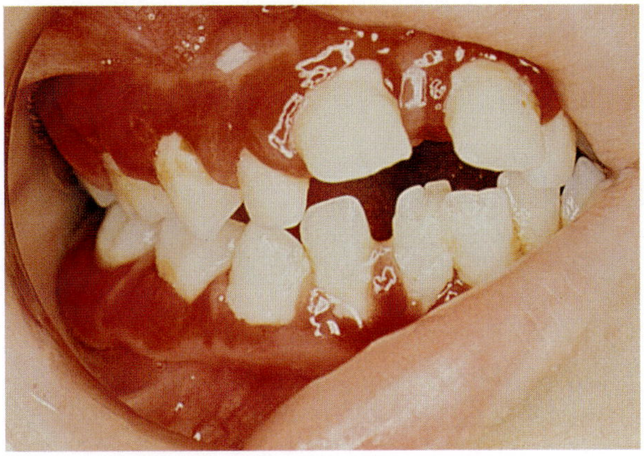

A

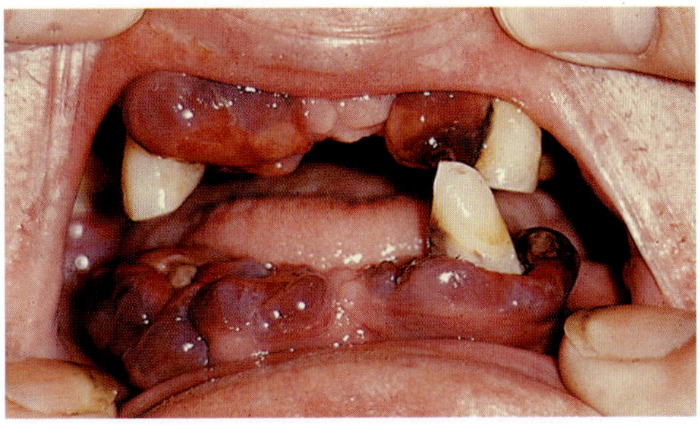

B

Fig. 7.6 (A and B) Marked periodontal disease in two patients with vitamin C deficiency. (A, From Morgan SL, Weinsier RL: *Fundamentals of Clinical Nutrition*, ed 2, St. Louis, 1998, Mosby. B, From Callen JP, Paller AS, Greer KE, et al: *Color Atlas of Dermatology*, ed 2, Philadelphia, PA, 2000, WB Saunders.)

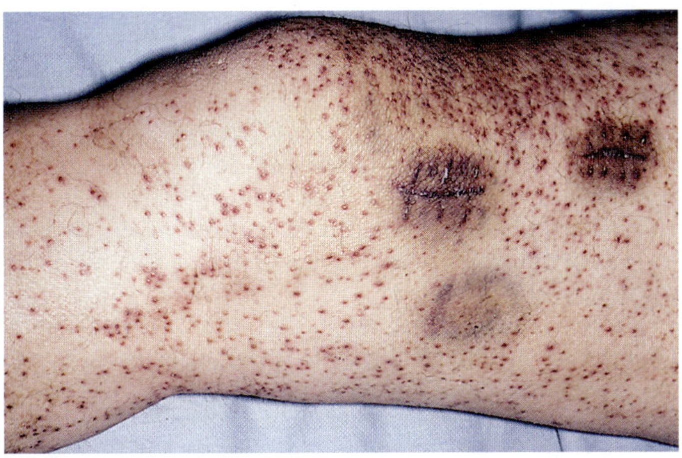

Fig. 7.7 Perifollicular Purpura and Ecchymoses Caused by Vitamin C Deficiency. (From Callen JP, Paller AS, Greer KE, et al: *Color Atlas of Dermatology*, ed 2, Philadelphia, PA, 2000, WB Saunders.)

acceptors or hydrogen donors. The classic deficiency of niacin is *pellagra.* It is seen in populations in China, Africa, and India, where rice is the major source of energy. The most common symptoms are diarrhea, dementia, and pigmented dermatitis in sun-exposed areas. Glossitis, stomatitis, vertigo, and burning paresthesias are also common. Fig. 7.9A illustrates marked pigmented dermatitis secondary to niacin deficiency in an alcoholic patient; Fig. 7.9B depicts the skin of the same patient after replacement therapy.

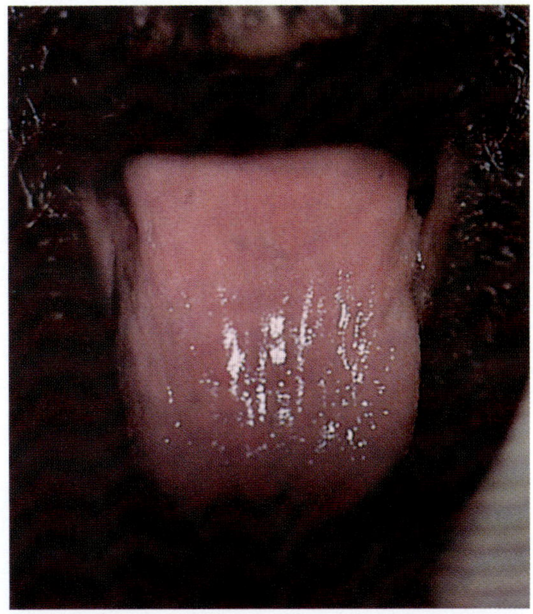

A

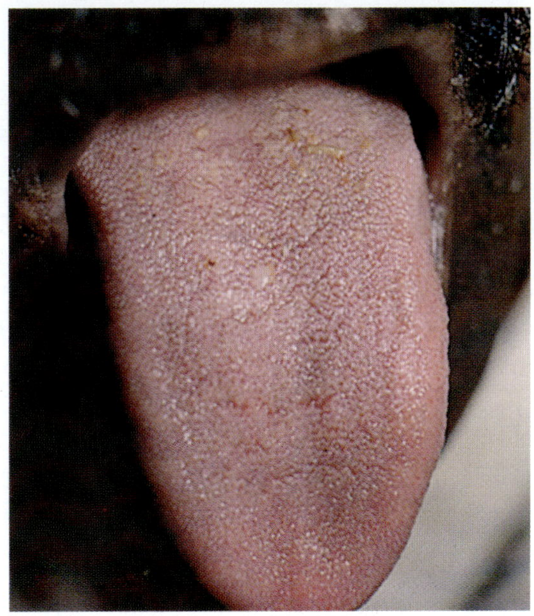

B

Fig. 7.8 Tongue of a Patient With Folate Deficiency. (A) Before folate therapy. (B) After folate therapy. (From Morgan SL, Weinsier RL: *Fundamentals of Clinical Nutrition*, ed 2, St. Louis, 1998, Mosby.)

Zinc is a trace element needed for a variety of metabolic processes. It is a component of more than 100 enzymes, including DNA polymerase, RNA polymerase, and transfer RNA synthetase. Zinc deficiency is associated with growth retardation and hypogonadism in children. In adults, infertility, poor wound healing, diarrhea, and dermatitis are frequent symptoms. Fig. 7.10A illustrates a widespread scaling dermatitis secondary to zinc deficiency in a patient with fat malabsorption; Fig. 7.10B illustrates the patient's skin after treatment with zinc. See Appendix C for the signs and symptoms of deficiency states.

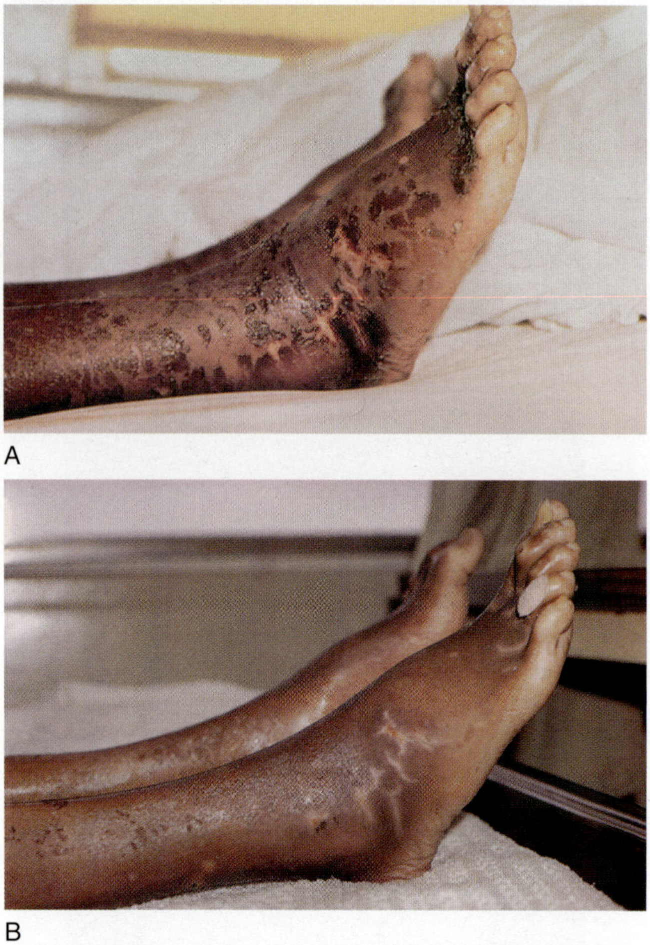

Fig. 7.9 **Legs and Feet of a Patient With Niacin Deficiency.** (A) Before niacin therapy. (B) After niacin therapy. (From Morgan SL, Weinsier RL: *Fundamentals of Clinical Nutrition*, ed 2, St. Louis, 1998, Mosby.)

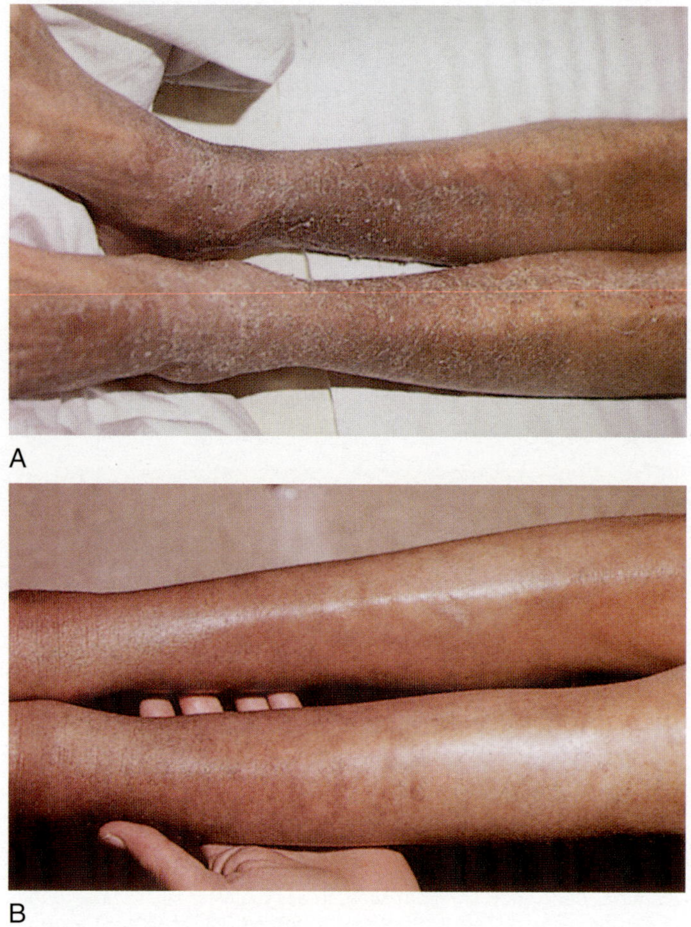

Fig. 7.10 **Legs of a Patient With Zinc Deficiency.** (A) Before zinc therapy. (B), After zinc therapy. (From Morgan SL, Weinsier RL: *Fundamentals of Clinical Nutrition*, ed 2, St. Louis, 1998, Mosby.)

Concluding Thoughts

Many people are interested in losing weight and are eager to purchase books on trendy diets, over-the-counter dietary supplements, and experimental treatments for illnesses. Unfortunately, most of these options are ineffective and only waste people's money. Instead, a competent healthcare professional should educate patients on how to adopt healthy eating habits. Any good diet should accomplish the following:

- Include a wide variety of foods to ensure adequate amounts of all essential nutrients
- Educate the person about proper nutrition
- Be based on sound biochemical facts
- Have no medical risks or metabolic side effects
- Be economical
- Be adaptable to a variety of lifestyles

For healthcare professionals, dealing with patients who are following diets of questionable nutritional value requires tact and skill. Your success often depends more on how you meet the patient's emotional needs than on your academic credentials. Always be informed about contemporary fad diets and cures. Discuss them openly with the patients; never condemn them out of your ignorance or unwillingness to learn about them.

Nutritional assessment cannot be conducted in isolation but must be incorporated into the overall patient history and physical examination. The extent and detail of the assessment should be tailored to the patient's specific medical conditions. This chapter has furnished a structure for integrating pertinent nutrition-related queries and concerns into patient evaluations.

REVIEW QUESTIONS

1. **A 42-year-old patient presents with fatigue, weakness, muscle pain, and difficulty walking. The patient has a history of consuming a predominantly polished rice-based diet for an extended period. Laboratory tests reveal an elevated heart rate, edema, and reduced deep tendon reflexes. Based on these findings, which of the following is the most likely diagnosis?**
   A. Scurvy
   B. Pellagra
   C. Rickets

D. Beriberi
E. Anemia

2. **A 30-year-old female presents with concerns of muscle weakness, fatigue, and bone pain for the past few months. She reports that she primarily works indoors, avoids sun exposure, and follows a vegan diet with limited fortified foods. On physical examination, you observe tenderness upon palpation of the sternum and ribs. Laboratory tests show a low serum calcium level and an elevated serum alkaline phosphatase level. What is the most likely diagnosis?**
   A. Iron-deficiency anemia
   B. Hypothyroidism
   C. Osteoporosis
   D. Vitamin D deficiency
   E. Hyperparathyroidism
3. **A 55-year-old male patient presents with concerns of fatigue, tingling sensations in his hands and feet, and difficulty walking. Upon examination, you observe pallor and a smooth, beefy-red tongue. The patient has been a vegetarian for several years. What is the most likely cause of the patient's symptoms?**
   A. Iron-deficiency anemia
   B. Folate deficiency
   C. Vitamin B_{12} deficiency
   D. Vitamin C deficiency
   E. Hypothyroidism
4. **What is a limitation of using BMI (body mass index) to diagnose obesity?**
   A. BMI cannot differentiate between muscle and fat mass.
   B. BMI is not readily available to the general population.
   C. BMI does not account for individuals who are above the 95th% for height.
   D. BMI does not account for individuals who are about the 95th% for weight.
   E. BMI is not correlated with population risk for morbidity and mortality.
5. **What is the major challenge in taking a dietary history?**
   A. Patients typically overestimate their portion sizes.
   B. Patients are reluctant to disclose their dietary habits.
   C. Dietary histories are time-consuming to obtain.
   D. Dietary histories do not account for genetic factors.
   E. Patients typically have difficulty recalling their dietary intake accurately.
6. **You are asked to take a patient's dietary history to provide personalized nutritional advice. What is the best method to take the dietary history from the patient?**
   A. Use a structured questionnaire with predefined food options and portion sizes.
   B. Probe the patient to recall what she ate last week and whether she prepares her own foods.
   C. Ask the patient to take you through an example of a typical day regarding what she eats.
   D. Administer a blood test to assess nutrient levels.
   E. Provide the patient with a list of recommended foods to assess her preferences.
7. **Using the Global Leadership Initiative on Malnutrition (GLIM) criteria, how would you define malnutrition in a patient?**
   A. A BMI below 18.5 kg/m^2
   B. Presence of at least one chronic disease
   C. Low dietary protein intake
   D. Inadequate energy intake
   E. Meeting at least one phenotypic criterion and at least one etiologic criterion
8. **What are the most important social determinants of health that lead to nutritional deficiency?**
   A. Genetic predisposition and family history
   B. Socioeconomic status, income, and education level
   C. Access to healthcare services and medical insurance
   D. Physical activity levels and fitness habits
   E. Geographic location and climate
9. **A 45-year-old patient presents with concerns of fatigue, muscle weakness, swollen gums, and small red spots on the skin. The patient's dietary history reveals a prolonged exclusion of fresh fruits and vegetables from their diet. Based on these findings, what is the most likely diagnosis for this patient's condition?**
   A. Iron-deficiency anemia
   B. Pellagra
   C. Rickets
   D. Scurvy
   E. Beriberi
10. **A 60-year-old patient presents with a history of unexplained weight loss over the past few months. The patient reports mild abdominal discomfort and steatorrhea (oily, foul-smelling stools). Physical examination reveals muscle wasting and pallor. Based on these findings, which of the following conditions is most likely responsible for the patient's weight loss?**
    A. Reduced caloric intake
    B. Increased urinary protein excretion
    C. Increased energy requirements
    D. Maldigestion or malabsorption
    E. Change in taste and food preference

REFERENCES

Available online.

BIBLIOGRAPHY

Available online.

8

The Skin

Mark H. Swartz

What is the hardest of all? That which you hold the most simple; seeing with your own eyes what is spread out before you.

Johann Wolfgang von Goethe (1749–1832)

GENERAL CONSIDERATIONS

The skin is the largest organ of the body and is one of the best indicators of general health. Even a person without medical training can detect changes in skin color and texture. The trained examiner can detect these changes and, at the same time, evaluate more subtle cutaneous signs of systemic disease.

Diseases of the skin are common. Approximately one-third of the United States population has a skin disorder that warrants medical attention. Nearly 8% of all adult outpatient visits are related to dermatologic problems. Basal cell carcinomas and squamous cell carcinomas (i.e., nonmelanotic skin cancers [NMSCs]) are by far the most common malignancies in the United States. One of every three new cancers is skin cancer; the vast majority are basal cell carcinomas. There are approximately 4.3 million cases of basal cell carcinoma diagnosed annually in the United States. The number of new basal cell carcinoma cases occurring every year (incidence) increased by nearly 50% in the 35-year period ending in 2010. Approximately 80% of the new skin cancer cases are basal cell carcinoma, 16% are squamous cell carcinoma, and 4% are melanoma. Most of these cases occur on the head and neck, which is evidence of the importance of sun exposure as a causative stimulus. Squamous cell carcinoma, the second-most common skin cancer after basal cell carcinoma, afflicts more than 200,000 Americans yearly. Approximately 1 million cases of squamous cell skin cancer are diagnosed annually in the United States. Although the cancer is treated and cured in most of these patients, skin cancer still causes more than 5000 deaths a year.

Even though invasive melanoma accounts for only about 1% of all skin cancers, it is responsible for the majority of deaths from skin cancer. In 2024, there were approximately 200,340 cases of melanoma diagnosed in the United States. Of those, 99,700 cases were in situ (noninvasive), confined to the top layer of skin (the epidermis), and 100,640 cases were invasive, penetrating the epidermis into the skin's second layer (the dermis). Of the invasive cases, 39,170 were in males, and 41,470 were in females. The number of new cases of melanoma has steadily increased for the last 30 years. In the past decade (2013–2023), the number of new invasive melanoma cases diagnosed annually increased by 27%. The reasons for this are unclear, but excessive sun exposure is a major factor. Melanoma is more than 20 times more common in Whites than in Blacks. Overall, the lifetime risk of getting melanoma is about 2.5% (1 in 40) for Whites, 0.1% (1 in 1000) for Blacks, and 0.5% (1 in 200) for Hispanics. The risk of melanoma increases as people age. The average age of people when melanoma is diagnosed is 65, but melanoma is not uncommon even among those younger than 30. In fact, it is one of the most common cancers in young adults, especially young females.

Early detection and treatment of malignant melanoma, as with most cancers, offers the best chance of a cure. Both basal cell carcinoma and squamous cell carcinoma have a better than 99% cure rate if detected and treated early. Among patients with a superficial melanoma (<0.76 mm in depth), the 5-year survival rate is more than 95%, whereas among those with a more significant lesion (>3.64 mm in depth), the 5-year survival rate is less than 40% because these cancers are more likely to spread to other parts of the body. The external nature of melanoma allows the examiner to detect these small, potentially more curable, lesions.

The skin's most important function is protecting the body from the environment. The skin has evolved in humans to be a relatively impermeable surface layer that prevents the loss of water, protects against external hazards, and insulates against thermal changes. It is also actively involved in the production of vitamin D. The skin appears to have the lowest water permeability of any naturally produced membrane. Its barrier to invasion retards potentially noxious agents from entering the body and causing internal damage. This barrier protects against many physical stresses and prohibits the invasion of microorganisms. By observing patients with extensive skin problems, such as burns, healthcare professionals can appreciate the importance of this organ.

STRUCTURE AND PHYSIOLOGIC CHARACTERISTICS

The three tissue layers of the skin, depicted in Fig. 8.1, are as follows:

- Epidermis
- Dermis
- Subcutaneous tissue

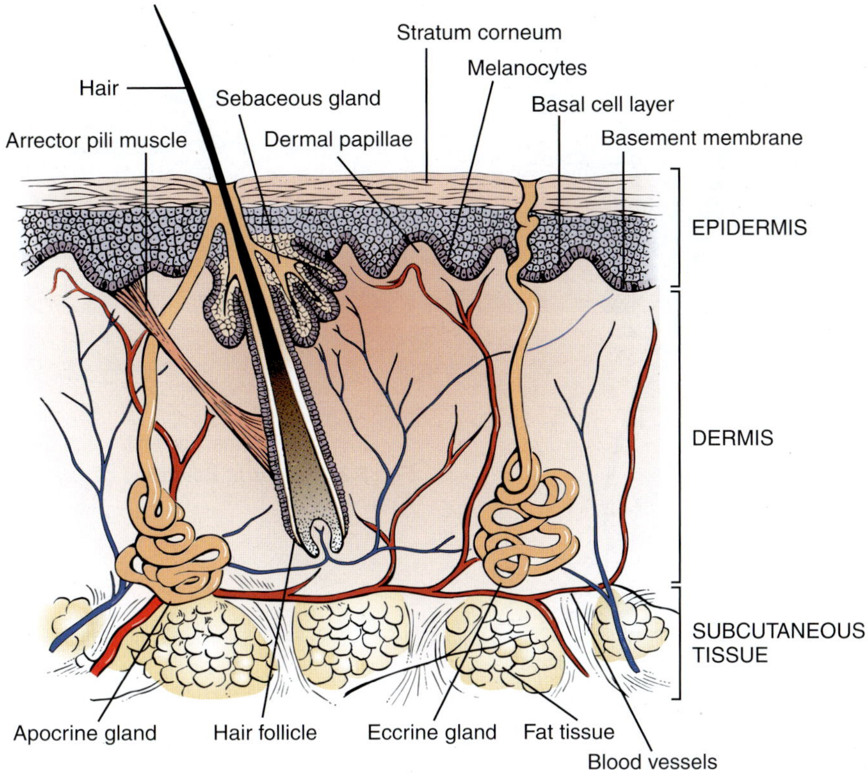

Fig. 8.1 Cross-Section Through the Skin, Illustrating the Structures in the Epidermis and Subcutaneous Tissues.

The *epidermis* is the thin, outermost layer of the skin. It is composed of several layers of keratocytes, or keratin-producing cells. Keratin is an insoluble protein that provides the skin with its protective properties. The *stratum corneum* is the outermost layer of the epidermis and serves as a significant physical barrier. The stratum corneum is composed of keratinized cells, which appear as dry, flattened, anuclear, and adherent flakes. The *basal cell layer* is the deepest layer of the epidermis. It is a single row of rapidly proliferating cells that slowly migrate upward, keratinize, and are ultimately shed from the stratum corneum. The process of maturation, keratinization, and shedding takes approximately 4 weeks.

The basal layer cells are intermingled with *melanocytes*, which produce *melanin*. The number of melanocytes is approximately equal in all people. Differences in skin color are related to the amount, size of particles, and type of melanin produced, as well as to its dispersion in the skin. Skin color is due primarily to the presence of a pigment called melanin, which is controlled by at least six genes. Both light- and dark-complexioned people have melanin. However, two forms of melanin are produced: pheomelanin, which is red to yellow in color, and eumelanin, which is dark brown to black. People with light-complexioned skin mainly produce pheomelanin, whereas those with dark-colored skin mostly produce eumelanin. Melanocytes have photosensitive receptors, similar to those in the eye, that detect ultraviolet radiation from the sun and other sources. In response, they produce melanin within a few hours of exposure.

Beneath the epidermis is the *dermis*, which is the dense connective tissue stroma forming the bulk of the skin. The dermis is bound to the overlying epidermis by fingerlike projections that project upward into the corresponding recesses of the epidermis. In the dermis, blood vessels branch and form a rich capillary bed in the dermal papillae. The deeper layers of the dermis also contain the hair follicles with their associated muscles and cutaneous glands. In addition, the dermis is supplied with sensory and autonomic nerve fibers. The sensory nerves end either as free endings or as special end organs that mediate pressure, touch, and temperature. The autonomic nerves supply the arrector pili muscles, blood vessels, and sweat glands.

The third layer of the skin is the *subcutaneous tissue*, which is mainly composed of fatty connective tissue. This highly variable adipose layer is a thermal regulator, as well as a protection for the more superficial skin layers from bone prominences.

The sweat glands, hair follicles, and nails are termed *skin appendages*. The sweat glands' evaporation of water from the skin provides a thermoregulatory mechanism for heat loss. Fig. 8.2 illustrates the types of sweat glands.

Within the skin, there are 2 to 3 million small, coiled *eccrine glands*. The eccrine glands are distributed over the body surface and are particularly profuse on the forehead, axillae, palms, and soles. They are absent in the nail beds and some mucosal surfaces. These glands can produce more than 6 L of watery sweat in 1 day. The eccrine glands are controlled by the sympathetic nervous system.

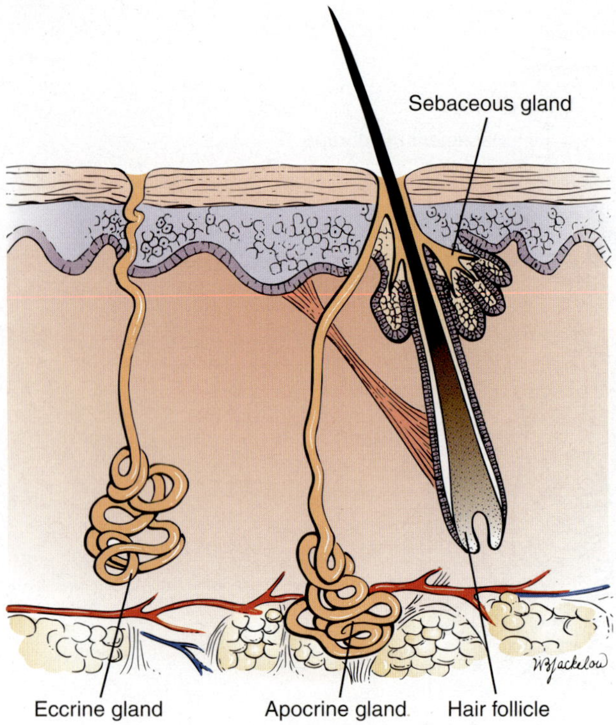

Fig. 8.2 Types of Sweat Glands.

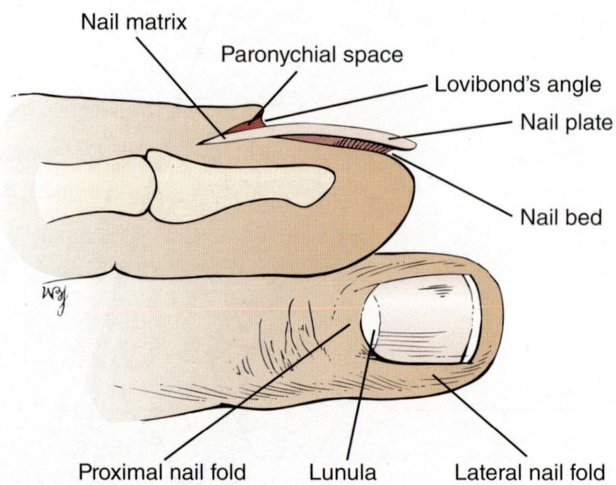

Fig. 8.3 Structural Relations of the Nail: Cross-Section and From Above.

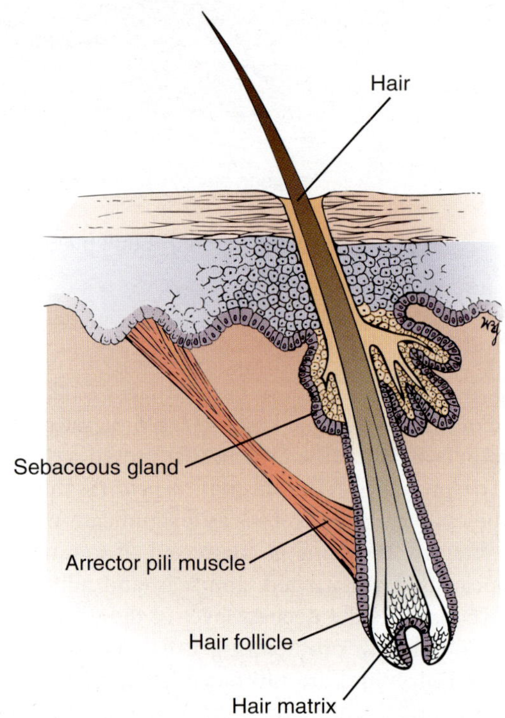

Fig. 8.4 The Hair Follicle and Its Surrounding Structures.

The *apocrine glands* are larger than the eccrine glands. The apocrine glands are closely associated with hair follicles but tend to be much more limited in distribution than the eccrine glands. The apocrine glands occur mostly in the axillae, the areolae, the pubis, and the perineum. They reach maturity only at puberty, secreting a milky, sticky substance. Apocrine glands are adrenergically mediated and appear to be stimulated by stress.

The *sebaceous glands* are also found surrounding hair follicles. The sebaceous glands are distributed over the entire body; the most prominent glands are found on the face and upper back. They are absent on the palms and soles. Their secretory product, sebum, is discharged directly into the lumen of the hair follicle, where it lubricates the hair shaft and spreads to the skin surface. Sebum consists of sebaceous cells and lipids. The production of sebum depends on gland size, which is directly influenced by androgen secretion.

Nails protect the tips of the fingers and toes against trauma. They are derived by keratinization of cells from the nail matrix located at the proximal end of the nail plate. The nail plate consists of the nail root embedded in the posterior nail fold, a fixed middle portion, and a distal free edge. The whitish nail matrix of proliferating epithelial cells grows in a semilunar pattern. It extends outward past the posterior nail fold and is called the *lunula*. The structural relationships of the nail are shown in Fig. 8.3.

A *hair shaft* is a keratinized structure that grows out of the hair follicle. Its lower end, called the *hair matrix,* consists of actively proliferating epithelial cells. The cells at this end of the follicle, along with those of the bone marrow and gut epithelium, are the most rapidly growing dividing cells in the human body. This is the reason that chemotherapy causes hair loss, along with anemia, nausea, and vomiting. Visible hair is present over the entire body surface except on the palms, soles, lips, eyelids, glans penis, and labia minora. In apparently hairless areas, the hair follicles are small, and the shafts produced are microscopic. Hair follicles show conspicuous morphologic and functional heterogeneity. Follicles and their developing shafts differ from location to location in shaft length, color, thickness, curl, and androgen sensitivity. Some follicles, those in the axilla and inguinal areas, are very sensitive to androgens, whereas those in the eyebrow are insensitive. The arrector pili muscles attach to the follicle below the opening of the sebaceous gland. Contraction of this muscle erects the hair and causes "goose bumps." The structure of a hair follicle is shown in Fig. 8.4.

REVIEW OF SPECIFIC SYMPTOMS

The main symptoms of disease of the skin, hair, and nails are the following:

- Rash or skin lesion
- Changes in skin color
- Itching (pruritus)
- Changes in hair
- Changes in nails

Rash or Skin Lesion

There are some important points to clarify when a patient is interviewed about a new rash or skin lesion. First, the specific time of onset and location of the rash or skin lesion is critical. A careful description of the first lesions and any changes is vital. The patient with a rash or skin lesion should be asked the following questions:

"Was the rash initially flat? Raised? Blistered?"
"Did the rash change in character with time?"
"Have there been new areas involved since the rash began?"
"Does the rash itch or burn?"
"Is the lesion tender or numb?"
"What makes the rash better? Worse?"
"Was the rash initiated by sunlight?"
"Is the rash aggravated by sunlight?"
"What kind of treatment have you tried?"
"Do you have any joint pains? Fever? Fatigue?"
"Does anyone near you have a similar rash?"
"Have you traveled recently?" If so, *"To where?"*
"Have you had any contact with anyone with a similar rash?"
"Is there a history of allergy?" If so, *"What are your symptoms?"*
"Do you have any chronic disease?"

Note whether the patient has used any medications that may have changed the nature of the skin disorder.

Inquire whether the patient uses any prescription medications or over-the-counter drugs. Ask specifically about aspirin and aspirin-containing products. The most common triggers for rashes include antibiotics, antiseizure medications, antigout medications (e.g., allopurinol), and even over-the-counter medications like nonsteroidal antiinflammatory drugs (NSAIDs). The most common type of drug reaction is hives, also known as urticaria. These are raised, swollen, red or flesh-colored bumps or welts that appear on the skin. They can take on many shapes and can be very itchy. They usually develop in groups and may cover large areas of skin. Patients can suddenly develop a reaction to medications that they have taken for many years. Do not ignore a long-standing prescription. Has the patient had any recent injections, vaccines, or taken any new medications? Does the patient use "recreational" drugs? Ask the patient about using soaps, deodorants, cosmetics, and colognes. Has the patient changed any of these items recently?

A family history of similar skin disorders should be noted. The effect of heat, cold, and sunlight on the skin problem is important. Could there be any contributing factors, such as occupation, specific food allergies, alcohol, or menses? Is there a history of gardening or household repair work? Has there been any contact with animals recently? The interviewer should also remember to inquire about psychogenic factors that may contribute to a skin disorder.

Determine the patient's occupation if it is not already known. Ascertain any avocational and recreational activities. This information is essential even if the patient has been exposed to chemicals or similar agents for years. Manufacturers frequently change the basic constituents without notifying the consumer. It may also take years for a patient to become sensitized to a substance. There are many occupational skin disorders. Healthcare workers, veterinary workers, hairdressers, agricultural workers, food handlers, construction workers, mechanics, automotive repair workers, and sanitation workers are potentially at risk of developing dermatologic conditions including contact and noncontact dermatitis, folliculitis,[a] hyperkeratosis,[b] burns, cuts, hyperpigmentation, xerosis,[c] miliaria,[d] frostbite, melasma,[e] allergic dermatitis, fungal infections, and skin cancer.

During the COVID-19 pandemic, healthcare workers needed to wear personal protective equipment (PPE). Most skin conditions seen throughout the pandemic were associated with using PPE like gloves, N95 masks, and goggles; frequent hand washing; and applying alcohol sanitizer.[1,2] Irritant contact dermatitis (ICD) was the most common dermatoses seen due to the frequent use of PPE during the COVID-19 pandemic.[3] Allergic contact dermatitis (ACD) to handwashing soaps, alcohol-based cleansers, moisturizers, masks, rubber gloves, gowns, etc., was also commonly reported. In addition, seborrheic dermatitis, acne, and rosacea occurred as a result of friction and sweating due to chronic mask wearing.

Changes in Skin Color

Patients may complain of a *generalized* change in skin color as the first manifestation of an illness. Cyanosis and jaundice are examples of this type of problem. Determine whether the patient is aware of any chronic disease responsible for these changes. *Localized* skin color changes may be related to aging or neoplastic changes. Certain medications can also be responsible for skin color changes. Inquire whether the patient is taking or has recently taken any medications. Antimalarials, chemotherapeutic agents, heavy metals, various medications (e.g., amiodarone, zidovudine, minocycline, clofazimine, psoralens), and psychotropic drugs are among the most commonly implicated medications in acquired **dyschromia**. Dyschromia refers to skin discoloration or patches of uneven color that can appear on the skin or nails. "Hyperchromia" refers to hyperpigmentation, and "hypochromia" refers to hypopigmentation.

Pruritus

Pruritus, or itching, may be a symptom of a generalized skin disorder or an internal illness. It can be associated with diabetes, dry skin, skin disorders, thyroid disease, parasites, arthropod

---

[a]Inflammation of the hair follicles.
[b]Abnormal thickening of the outer layer of the skin.
[c]Abnormally dry skin or membranes.
[d]Medical term for prickly heat.
[e]A skin condition that causes patches and spots, usually on the face, which are darker than your natural skin tone.

bites, pregnancy, inflammatory disorders, and cancer. Histamine is one of the most important itch mediators, although other chemical substances have also been implicated. Ask any patient with pruritus the following questions:

"When did you first notice the itching?"

"Did the itching begin suddenly?"

"Is the itching associated with any rash or lesion on your body?"

"Are you taking any medications?...such as antibiotics?...pain medications?"

"Has there been any change in the sweating or dryness of your skin?"

"Have you noticed any color changes to your skin?"

"Have you been told that you have a chronic illness like liver disease?...kidney disease?...diabetes?...HIV?"

"Have you traveled recently?" If so, *"To where?"*

If the patient is a female, *"Is it possible you might be pregnant?"*

Diffuse pruritus is observed in biliary cirrhosis and cancer, especially lymphoma. Many drugs have been associated with diffuse pruritus: antibiotics, allopurinol, amiodarone, angiotensin-converting enzyme inhibitors, estrogen, hydrochlorothiazide, opioids, and statins. Pruritus in association with a diffuse rash may be dermatitis herpetiformis.[f] Determine whether the pruritus has been associated with a change in perspiration or dryness of the skin because either of these conditions may be the cause of the pruritus.

Changes in Hair

Inquire whether there has been a loss or an increase in hair. Ascertain any changes in distribution or texture. If there have been changes, ask the following questions:

"When did you first notice the changes?"

"Did the change occur suddenly?"

"Is the hair loss symmetric?"

"Has the change been associated with itching? Fever? Recent stress?"

"Are you aware of any exposure to any toxins? Commercial hair compounds?"

"Have you changed your diet?"

"What medications are you taking?"

Changes in diet and medications are frequently responsible for changes in hair patterns. Hypothyroidism is frequently associated with the loss of the lateral third of the eyebrows. Vascular disease in the legs often causes hair loss on the legs. Alternatively, ovarian and adrenal tumors can cause an increase in body hair. Of course, aging causes a change in hair. As a person ages, the texture of their hair can change. Hair can also become thinner, and people may experience hair loss. Different people's hair changes in various ways as they age. Hair changes can also occur due to environmental exposure and physical stress.

[f]Dermatitis herpetiformis (DH) is a chronic, intensely pruritic, blistering skin manifestation of gluten-sensitive enteropathy, commonly known as celiac disease. Gluten is found in common foods such as wheat, rye, and barley. DH is a rash that affects about 10% of people with celiac disease. It can affect people of any age but typically first occurs in people in their 30s, is more common in males than females, and is rare in children.

Changes in Nails

Changes in nails may include splitting, discoloration, ridging, thickening, or separation from the nail bed. Ask the patient the following questions:

"When did you first notice the nail changes?"

"Have you had any acute illness recently?"

"Do you have any chronic illness?"

"Have you been taking any medications?"

"Have you been exposed to chemicals at work or home?"

Fungal disease causes thickening of the nail. Clues to systemic illness may be found by close examination of the proximal nail fold, the lunula, the nail bed, the nail plate, and the hyponychium. Acute illnesses are associated with lines and ridges in the nail bed and nail. Medications and chemicals are notorious for causing nail changes.

General Suggestions

All patients should be asked whether there have been any changes in moles, birthmarks, or spots on the body. Determine any color changes, irregular growth, pain, scaling, or bleeding. Any recent development of a flat, pigmented lesion is relevant information.

All patients should be asked whether any red, scaly, or crusted areas of skin do not heal. Has the patient ever had skin cancer? If the patient has had skin cancer, further questioning regarding the body location, treatment, and description is appropriate. Has anyone in the family had skin cancer? Melanoma can run in families. In fact, about 1 in every 10 patients diagnosed with melanoma has a family member with a history of the disease. Nonmelanoma skin cancers can run in families also. A primary risk factor for skin cancer is UV exposure. Exposure to UV light may be similar between members of the same family and may contribute to multiple family members being diagnosed with skin cancers.

EFFECT OF SKIN DISEASE ON THE PATIENT

Skin diseases play a profound role in how the affected patient interacts socially. If located on visible skin surfaces, long-standing skin diseases may actually interfere with the emotional and psychological development of the individual. The attitude of a person toward self and others may be markedly affected. Loss of self-esteem is common. An adult with a skin disorder often faces limitation of sexual activity. This disruption of intimacy can foster or increase hostility and anxiety in the patient. Skin is a sensitive marker of an individual's emotions. It is known that blushing can reflect embarrassment, sweating can indicate stress, and pallor or "goose bump" skin may be associated with fear.

Patients with rashes have always evoked feelings of revulsion. Rashes have been associated with impurity and evil. Even nowadays, friends and family may reject the individual with a skin disease. Patients with skin that is red, oozing, discolored, or peeling are rejected not only by family members but perhaps even by their healthcare professionals. At other times, skin lesions cause others to stare at the patient, which causes further discomfort. Some skin disorders may be associated with such extreme physical or emotional pain that marked depression may result and, on occasion, lead to suicide.

Skin diseases are often treated palliatively. Unfortunately, because numerous skin disorders have no cure, many patients go through life helpless and frustrated, as do their healthcare professionals.

The role of anxiety as a natural stressor in producing rashes is frequently observed. Stress tends to worsen certain skin disorders, such as eczema. This creates a vicious cycle because the rash then exacerbates the anxiety. Rashes are common symptoms and signs of psychosomatic disorders.

Healthcare professionals should discuss these anxieties with the patient in an attempt to break the cycle. The interviewer who tries to elicit the patient's feelings about the disease allows the patient to "open up." The fears and fantasies can then be discussed. The examiner should also be comfortable touching the patient for reassurance. This tends to improve the healthcare professional-patient relationship because the patient has a lesser sense of isolation.

PHYSICAL EXAMINATION

The only equipment necessary for the examination of the skin is a penlight. The examination of the skin consists of only two steps:

- Inspection
- Palpation

The skin examination depends on inspection, but palpation of a skin lesion must also be performed. Although most skin lesions are not contagious, it is prudent to wear gloves to evaluate any skin lesion. This is especially true because of the prevalence of skin disease associated with human immunodeficiency virus (HIV) infection. Palpation of a lesion helps define its characteristics: texture, consistency, fluid, edema in the adjacent area, tenderness, and blanching.

The patient and the examiner must be comfortable during the skin examination. The lighting should be adjusted to produce the optimal illumination. Natural light is preferable. Even in the absence of concerns related to the skin, a careful examination of the skin must be performed on all patients because the skin may provide subtle clues of an underlying systemic illness. Examining the skin may be performed as a separate system approach, or, preferably, the skin should be examined when other body areas are evaluated.

General Principles

The examiner should be suspicious of any lesion that the patient describes as having increased in size or changed in color. In addition, the development of any new growth warrants attention.

When examining the skin, the healthcare professional initially determines the general aspects of the skin: the *color, moisture, turgor,* and *texture.*

Any *color* changes, such as cyanosis, jaundice, or pigmentary abnormalities, should be noted.

Red vascular lesions may be either extravasated blood into the skin, known as *petechiae* or *purpura,* or malformed elements of the vascular tree, known as *angiomas.* When pressure is applied by a glass slide over an angioma, it blanches. This is a valuable test to differentiate an angioma from petechiae, which does not change when pressure from a glass slide is applied.

During the physical examination, inspect all pigmented lesions and be aware of the "**ABCDE**" warning signs associated with malignant melanoma:

- **A**symmetry of shape
- **B**order irregularity
- **C**olor variation
- **D**iameter larger than 6 mm
- **E**volving

Asymmetry means that half the lesion appears different from the other half. *Border irregularity* describes a scalloped or poorly circumscribed contour. The *color variation* refers to shades of tan and brown, black, and sometimes white, red, or blue. A *diameter* larger than 6 mm, the size of a pencil eraser, is considered a danger sign for melanoma. A lesion that is *evolving* always needs to be evaluated.

The healthcare professional should remember this axiom in dermatology: "*There are more errors made by not looking than by not knowing.*"

Excessive *moisture* may be seen in normal individuals, or it may be associated with fevers, emotions, neoplastic diseases, or hyperthyroidism. Dryness is a normal aging change but may also be seen in myxedema, nephritis, and certain drug-induced states. Look for excoriations, which might indicate the presence of pruritus as a clue to an underlying systemic illness.

When palpating the skin, evaluate its *turgor* and *texture.* Tissue turgor provides a mechanism for estimating the patient's general state of hydration. For example, if the skin over the forehead is pulled up and released, it should promptly reassume its normal contour. In a patient with decreased hydration, this response is delayed.

It is often difficult for the inexperienced examiner to evaluate the skin's texture because texture is a qualitative parameter. Has the patient noticed a change in his or her skin texture? Softness has occasionally been likened to skin texture over a baby's abdomen. "Soft"-textured skin is seen in secondary hypothyroidism, hypopituitarism, and eunuchoid states. "Hard"-textured skin is associated with scleroderma, myxedema, and amyloidosis. "Velvety" skin is associated with Ehlers-Danlos syndrome.

Examination With Patient Seated

When the patient is seated, examine the hair and the skin on the hands and upper extremities.

Inspect the Hair

The hair and scalp are evaluated for any lesions. Is alopecia or hirsutism present? Pay attention to the pattern of distribution and texture of hair over the body. The hair becomes sparse and coarse in certain diseases, such as hypothyroidism. In contrast, patients with hyperthyroidism have hair that is very fine in texture. Loss of hair occurs in many conditions: anemia, heavy metal poisoning, hypopituitarism, and some nutritional disease states, such as pellagra. Increased hair patterns are seen in Cushing disease, Stein-Leventhal syndrome, and several neoplastic conditions, such as tumors of the adrenal glands and gonads.

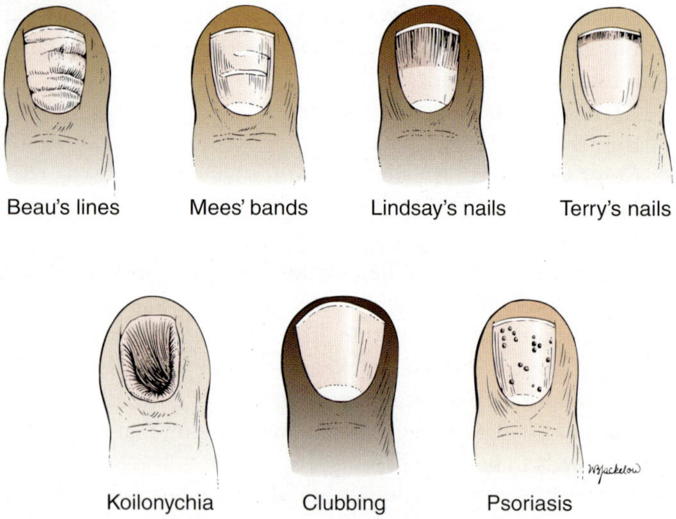

Fig. 8.5 Common Nail Findings Associated With Medical Diseases.

Inspect the Nail Beds

Evaluation of the nails can provide essential clues about diseases. The nails may be affected by many systemic and dermatologic conditions. Nail bed changes are usually not pathognomonic for a specific disease. Disorders stemming from renal, hematopoietic, or hepatic conditions may be evident from the nails. The nails should be inspected for shape, size, color, brittleness, hemorrhages underneath, transverse lines or grooves in the nail or nail bed, and an increased white area of the nail bed. Fig. 8.5 illustrates some typical nail changes associated with medical diseases.

Beau's lines are horizontal grooves or depressions parallel to the lunula. Any severe, systemic illness that disrupts nail growth can produce Beau's lines. They indicate that an illness, injury, or skin condition interrupted the nail growth. Treating the underlying cause will allow new, smooth nails to grow again. They are often associated with infections (typhus, acute rheumatic fever, malaria, acquired immune deficiency syndrome [AIDS]), nutritional disorders (protein deficiency, pellagra), circulatory problems (myocardial infarction, Raynaud disease), dysmetabolic states (diabetes, hypothyroidism, hypocalcemia), digestive diseases (diarrhea, enterocolitis, chronic pancreatitis, sprue), drugs (chemotherapy agents), operations, and alcoholism. Beau's lines are caused by conditions that cause the nail to grow slowly or even cease to grow for short intervals. These lines are most commonly seen in the thumbnails and toenails. Fig. 8.6A shows a patient's fingers with Beau's lines on the nails. Fig. 8.6B shows Beau's lines in the toenails of a patient who underwent major surgery 5 months earlier.

On occasion, a white transverse line or band results from poisoning or an acute systemic illness. These lines, called *Mees' bands,* are historically associated with chronic arsenic poisoning. Mees' lines or Aldrich–Mees' lines, also known as **leukonychia striata**, are white lines of discoloration across the nails of the fingers and toes. They are also seen in patients with Hodgkin disease, congestive heart failure, leprosy, malaria, chemotherapy, carbon monoxide poisoning, and other systemic insults. These lines or bands are also parallel to the lunula. By measuring the width of the line and approximating nail growth

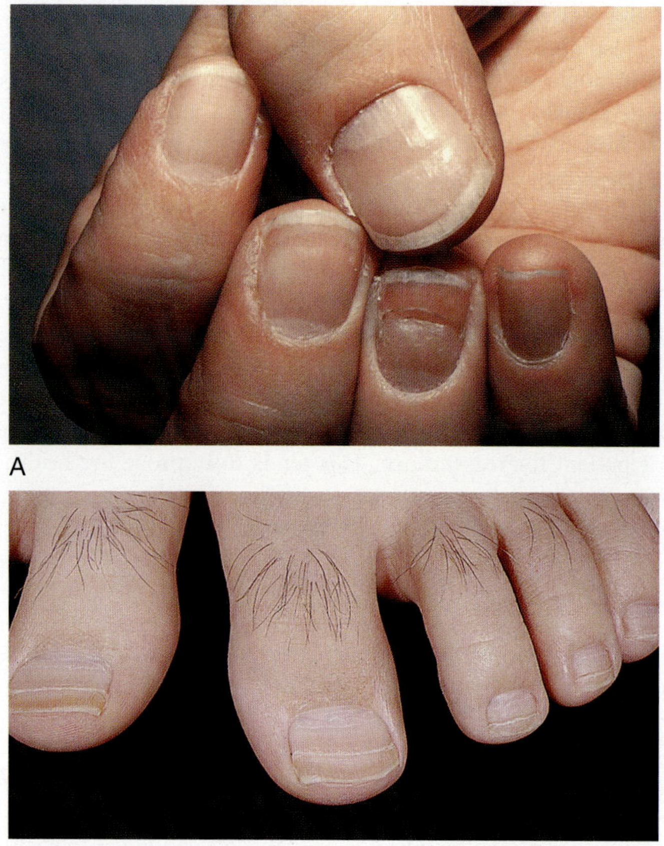

A

B

Fig. 8.6 Beau's Lines. (A) Fingernails. (B) Toenails. (A, From Callen JP, Greer KE, Hood AF, et al: *Color atlas of dermatology*, Philadelphia, 1993, WB Saunders. B, From Callen JP, Paller AS, Greer KE, et al: *Color atlas of dermatology*, ed 2, Philadelphia, 2000, WB Saunders.)

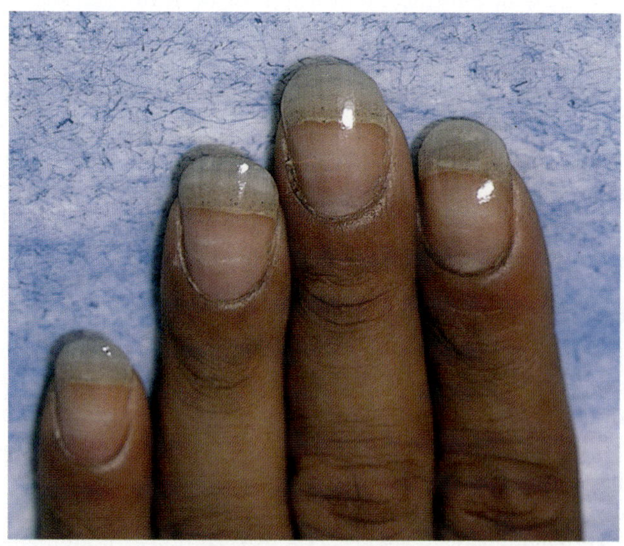

Fig. 8.7 Mees' Bands.

at 1 mm per week, the examiner may be able to determine the duration of the antecedent acute illness. Fig. 8.7 shows the fingernails of a patient who received chemotherapy several weeks earlier.

Lindsay's nails are also called "half-and-half nails." The proximal portion of the nail bed is whitish, whereas the distal part is

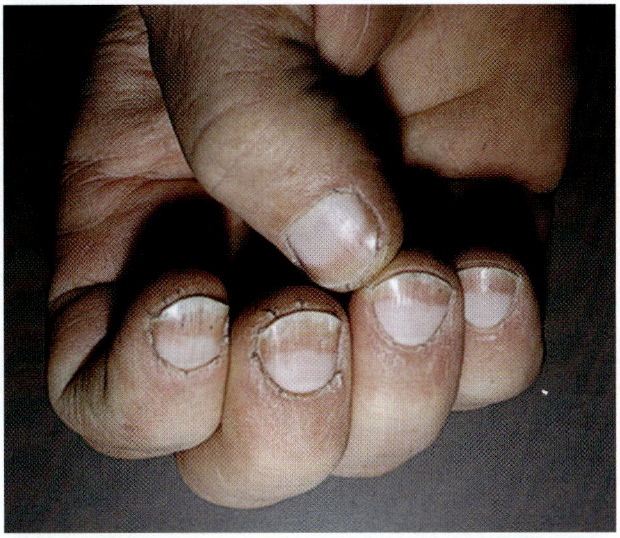

Fig. 8.8 Lindsay's Nails. (From Callen JP, Paller AS, Greer KE, et al: *Color atlas of dermatology*, ed 2, Philadelphia, 2000, WB Saunders.)

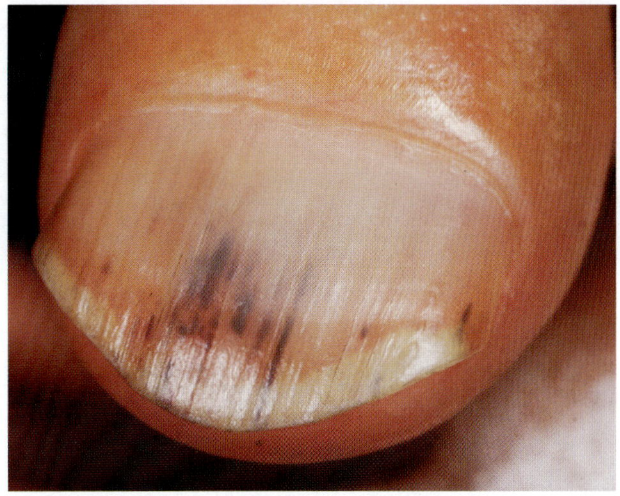

Fig. 8.10 Splinter Hemorrhages. (From Hordinsky MK, Sawaya ME, Scher RK: *Atlas of hair and nails*, Philadelphia, 2000, Churchill Livingstone.)

red or pink. Chronic renal disease and azotemia are the commonly associated conditions with this type of nail abnormality. This condition can be found in up to 40% of patients with chronic kidney disease. Fig. 8.8 shows Lindsay's nails secondary to chronic renal failure.

Terry's nails are white nail beds within 1 to 2 mm of the distal border of the nail. These nail findings are most commonly associated with hepatic failure, cirrhosis, hypoalbuminemia, chronic congestive heart failure, hyperthyroidism, malnutrition, and adult-onset diabetes mellitus. Fig. 8.9 shows classic Terry's nails.

Splinter hemorrhages are formed by the extravasation of blood from longitudinal nail bed blood vessels into adjacent troughs. Splinter hemorrhages are very common. It has been estimated that up to 20% of all hospitalized patients have splinter hemorrhages. Their presence is most often related to local, light trauma, but these hemorrhages are commonly associated with systemic disease. Classically associated with subacute bacterial endocarditis, splinter hemorrhages may also be seen in leukemia, vasculitis, infection, rheumatoid arthritis, systemic lupus erythematosus, renal disease, liver disease, and diabetes mellitus, among other conditions. Splinter hemorrhages are depicted in Fig. 8.10.

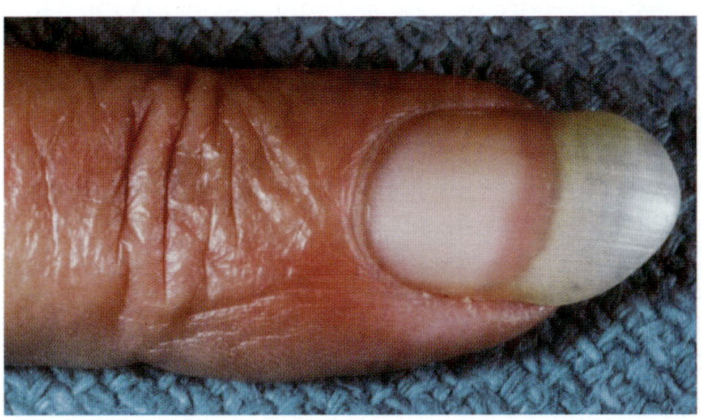

Fig. 8.9 Terry's Nails. (From Hordinsky MK, Sawaya ME, Scher RK: *Atlas of hair and nails*, Philadelphia, 2000, Churchill Livingstone.)

Is *koilonychia* present? Koilonychia, or "spoon nail," is a dystrophic state in which the nail plate thins and a cuplike depression develops. Spoon nails are most commonly associated with iron deficiency anemia but may be seen in association with thinning of the nail plate from any cause, including local irritants. Fig. 8.11 shows an average fingernail in comparison with koilonychia secondary to iron deficiency anemia.

Inspect the Nails for Clubbing

The angle between the normal nail base and the finger is approximately 160 degrees, and the nail bed is firm. The angle is referred to as the *Lovibond angle*. When clubbing develops,

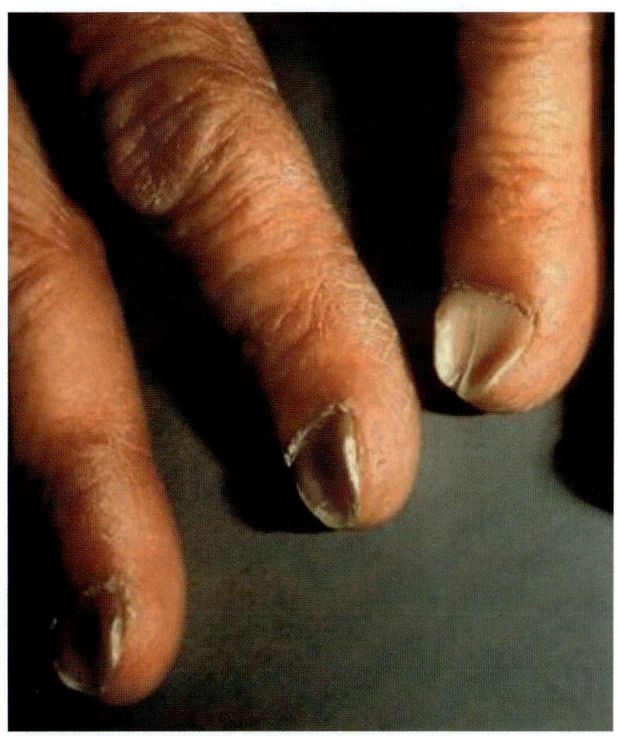

Fig. 8.11 Koilonychia. (Used with permission of Mayo Foundation for Medical Education and Research, all rights reserved.)

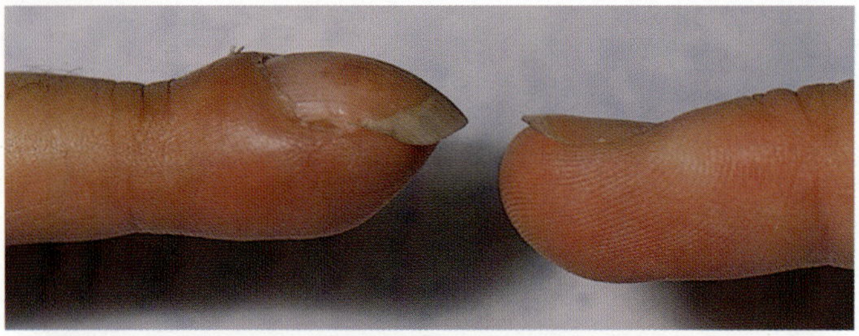

Fig. 8.12 Late-Stage Clubbing.

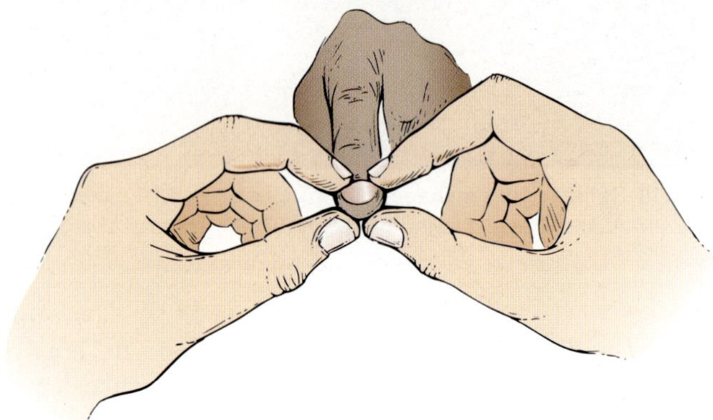

Fig. 8.13 Technique for Assessing Whether Clubbing Is Present.

this angle straightens out to greater than 180 degrees, and the nail bed, when palpated, becomes spongy or floating. As clubbing progresses, the base of the nail becomes swollen, and the Lovibond angle greatly exceeds 180 degrees. As a result, the nail has a bullous shape with exaggerated longitudinal and horizontal curvatures. A fusiform enlargement of the distal digit may also occur. In Fig. 8.12, an average finger is compared with a finger with nail clubbing.

To examine for clubbing, the patient's finger is placed on the pulp of the examiner's thumbs, and the examiner's index fingers palpate the base of the nail bed. If clubbing is present, the nail appears to float on the finger. The initial manifestation of clubbing is tissue softening over the proximal nail fold. Fig. 8.13 illustrates the technique for assessing whether early clubbing is present.

Since Hippocrates first described digital clubbing in patients with empyema,[g] digital clubbing has been associated with various underlying pulmonary, cardiovascular, neoplastic, infectious, hepatobiliary, mediastinal, endocrine, and gastrointestinal diseases. The pathogenesis of clubbing is unknown. Vascular endothelial growth factor (VEGF) from the continued impaction of shunted megakaryocytes and platelets in the digital vasculature, potentiated by hypoxia, is considered to drive the cellular and stromal changes in clubbing. Enhanced VEGF expression is common in various diseases associated with digital clubbing. Clubbing of the nails is most commonly acquired but may be inherited as an autosomal dominant trait. When not inherited as a familial trait, clubbing is most commonly seen associated with congenital cyanotic heart disease, cystic fibrosis, mesothelioma of the pleura, and pulmonary neoplasms. The most common acquired pulmonary cause is bronchogenic carcinoma; it is mainly seen in non–small cell cancer (54% of all cases) and not generally seen in small cell lung cancer (<5% of cases). Other causes, including bronchiectasis or bronchogenic carcinoma, should be sought in a patient with chronic obstructive pulmonary disease who manifests clubbing. Clubbing is also found in suppurative lung diseases, such as lung abscess, empyema, bronchiectasis, and cystic fibrosis.

[g]A collection of pus in the pleural cavity.

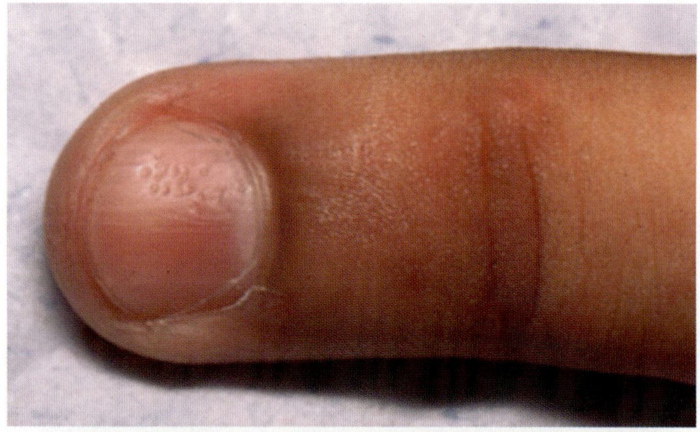

Fig. 8.14 Psoriasis: Nail Pitting.

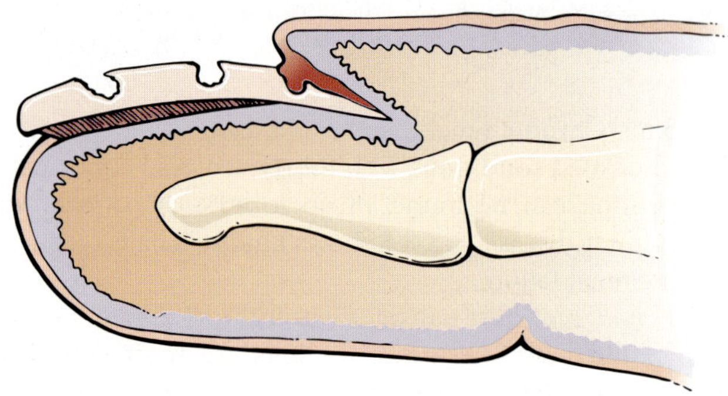

Fig. 8.15 Cross-Section of Nail Pitting.

Inspect the Nails for Pitting

Pitting of the nails is commonly associated with psoriasis and psoriatic arthropathy. Involvement of the nail bed and nail matrix by psoriasis causes the nail plate to be thickened and pitted. Nail involvement occurs in approximately 50% of all patients with psoriasis. Discrete psoriatic foci in the nail matrix produce multiple pits in the nail. Minor degrees of pitting is also seen in people with no other skin concerns. Pitting rarely occurs in toenails. Psoriatic nail pitting is shown in Fig. 8.14; Fig. 8.15 illustrates a cross-section of pitting. Fig. 8.16A shows psoriatic nail lesions in another patient. Notice the characteristically dystrophic nail changes caused by subungual hyperkeratosis. Fig. 8.16B is a close-up of a typical nail with psoriatic changes.

Inspect the Skin of the Face and Neck

Evaluate the eyelids, forehead, ears, nose, and lips carefully. Evaluate the mucous membranes of the mouth and nose for

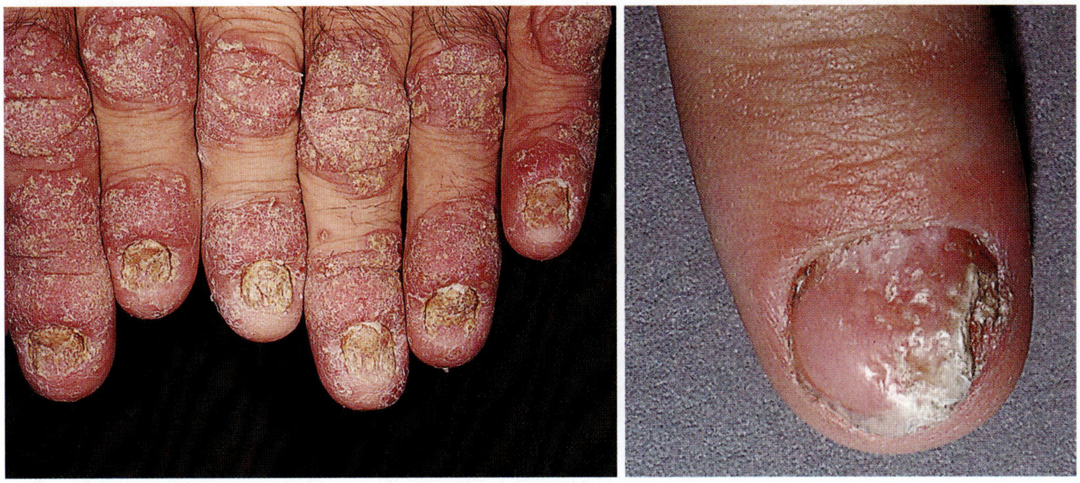

A B

Fig. 8.16 (A) and (B) Psoriatic nail lesions. (From Callen JP, Paller AS, Greer KE, et al: *Color atlas of dermatology*, ed 2, Philadelphia, 2000, WB Saunders.)

ulceration, bleeding, or telangiectasis. Is the skin at the nasolabial fold and mouth normal?

Inspect the Skin of the Back

Examine the skin of the patient's back. Are any lesions present?

Examination With Patient Lying Down

Inspect the Skin of the Chest, Abdomen, and Lower Extremities

Ask the patient to lie down so you can complete the skin assessment. Inspect the skin of the chest and abdomen. Pay particular attention to the skin of the inguinal and genital areas. Inspect the pubic hair. Elevate the scrotum. Inspect the perineal area. Evaluate the pretibial regions for the presence of ulcerations or waxy deposits.

Scrutinize the feet and soles for any skin changes. Spread the toes to evaluate the webs between them thoroughly.

Ask the patient to roll onto the left side so that you may examine the skin on the back, gluteal, and perianal areas.

DESCRIPTION OF LESIONS

If a skin lesion is found, it should be classified as a *primary* or *secondary* lesion, and its shape and distribution should be described. Primary lesions arise from normal skin. They result from anatomic changes in the epidermis, dermis, or subcutaneous tissue. The primary lesion is the most characteristic lesion of the skin disorder. Secondary lesions result from changes in the primary lesion. They develop during the course of cutaneous disease.

The first step in identifying a skin disorder is to characterize the appearance of the primary lesion. In describing the skin lesion, the healthcare professional should note whether the lesion is flat or raised and whether it is solid or contains fluid. A penlight is often helpful to determine whether the lesion is slightly elevated. If a penlight is directed to one side of a lesion, a shadow forms according to the height of the lesion.

The location of the lesion on the body is essential. Therefore, the distribution of the eruption is crucial in making a diagnosis. Inspecting a patient's clothing may be rewarding when contact dermatitis or pediculosis (infestation with lice) is suspected. Occasionally, occupational exposure may leave traces of contamination with oils or other materials that may be visible on the clothing and help in the assessment.

The three specific criteria for a dermatologic diagnosis are based on *morphologic characteristics, configuration,* and *distribution,* morphologic characteristics being the most important. The purpose of the following section is to acquaint the reader with the morphologic features of the primary and secondary lesions and the associated vocabulary.

Primary and Secondary Lesions

To facilitate reading, the primary lesions are listed here with regard to being flat or elevated and solid or fluid-filled (Figs. 8.17 to 8.20). A primary lesion has no "standard" size; the dimensions indicated are only approximate. The secondary lesions are grouped according to their occurrence below or above the plane of the skin (Figs. 8.21 and 8.22). Other significant skin lesions are shown and described in Fig. 8.23.

Configuration of Skin Lesions

The examiner doesn't have to diagnose all skin diseases definitively. A detailed description of the lesion, the pattern of distribution, and the arrangement of the lesion often point to a group of related disease states with similar manifesting dermatologic signs (e.g., confluent macular rashes, bullous diseases, grouped vesicles, papular rashes on an erythematous base). For example, grouped urticarial lesions with a central depression suggest insect bites. Fig. 8.24 lists the terms used to describe the configurations of lesions.

Primary Skin Lesions: Nonpalpable, flat

Lesion	Characteristics	Examples
Macule	Smaller than 1 cm	Freckles, moles
Patch	Greater than 1 cm	Vitiligo, café au lait spots

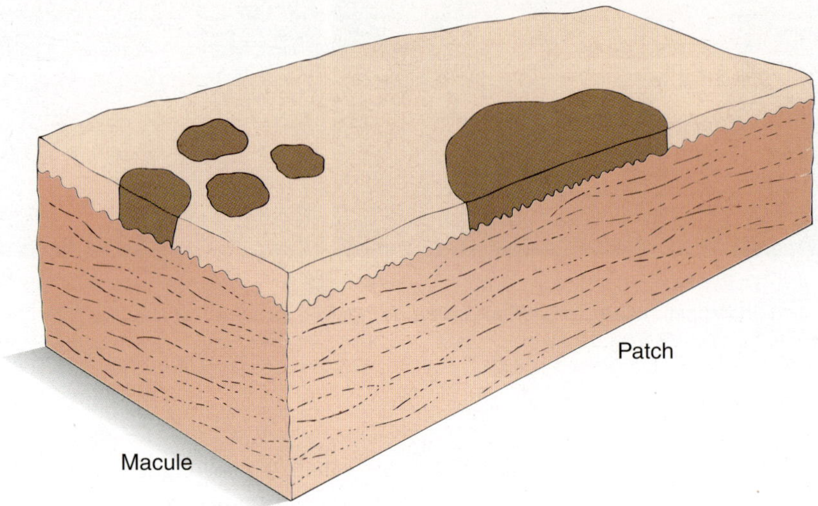

Fig. 8.17 Primary Skin Lesions: Nonpalpable, Flat.

Primary Skin Lesion: Palpable, Solid Mass

Lesion	Characteristics	Examples
Papule	Smaller than 1 cm	Nevus, wart
Nodule	1–2 cm	Erythema nodosum
Tumor	Greater than 2 cm	Neoplasms
Plaque	Flat, elevated, superficial papule with surface area greater than height	Psoriasis, seborrheic keratosis
Wheal	Superficial area of cutaneous edema	Hives, insect bite

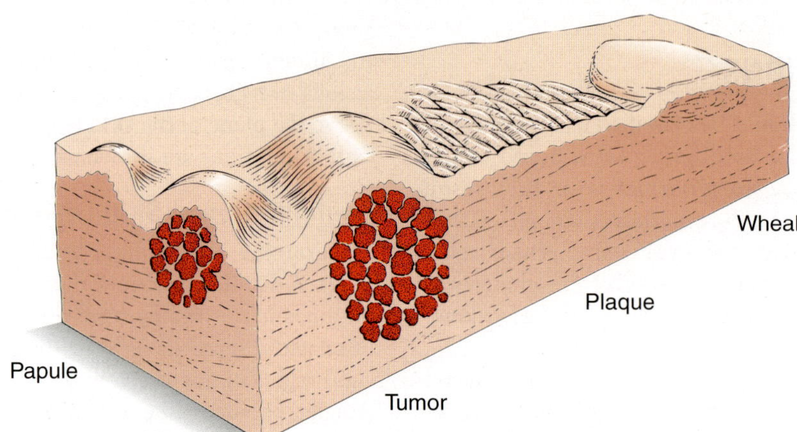

Fig. 8.18 Primary Skin Lesions: Palpable, Solid Mass.

Primary Skin Lesions: Palpable, Fluid-Filled

Lesion	Characteristics	Examples
Vesicle	Smaller than 1 cm; filled with serous fluid	Blister, herpes simplex
Bulla	Greater than 1 cm; filled with serous fluid	Blister, pemphigus vulgaris
Pustule	Similar to vesicle; filled with pus	Acne, impetigo

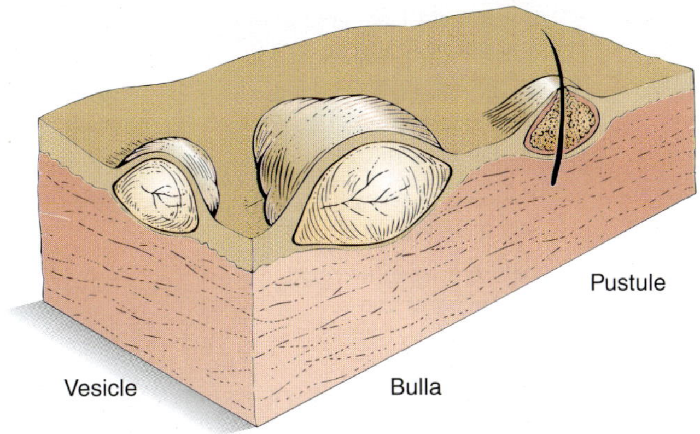

Fig. 8.19 Primary Skin Lesions: Palpable, Fluid-Filled.

Special Primary Skin Lesions

Lesion	Characteristics	Examples
Comedo	Plugged opening of sebaceous gland	Blackhead
Burrow	Smaller than 10 mm, raised tunnel	Scabies
Cyst	Palpable lesion filled with semiliquid material or fluid	Sebaceous cyst
Abscess	A specific type of primary lesion with localized accumulation of purulent material in the dermis or subcutis; in general, the accumulation is so deep that the pus is not visible from the skin's surface	
Furuncle	A specific type of primary lesion that is a necrotizing form of inflammation of a hair follicle	
Carbuncle	A coalescence of several furuncles	
Milia	Tiny, keratin-filled cysts representing an accumulation of keratin in the distal portion of the sweat gland	

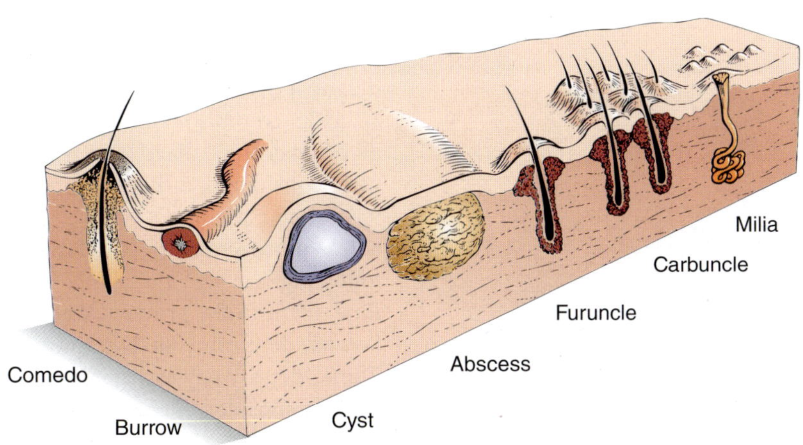

Fig. 8.20 Special Primary Skin Lesions.

Secondary Skin Lesions Below the Skin Plane

Lesion	Characteristics	Examples
Erosion	Loss of part or all of the epidermis; surface is moist	Rupture of a vesicle
Ulcer	Loss of epidermis and dermis; may bleed	Stasis ulcer, chancre
Fissure	Linear crack from epidermis into dermis	Cheilitis, athlete's foot
Excoriation	A superficial linear, or "dug out," traumatized area, usually self-induced	Abrasion, scratch mark
Atrophy	Thinning of skin with loss of skin markings	Striae
Sclerosis	Diffuse or circumscribed hardening of skin	

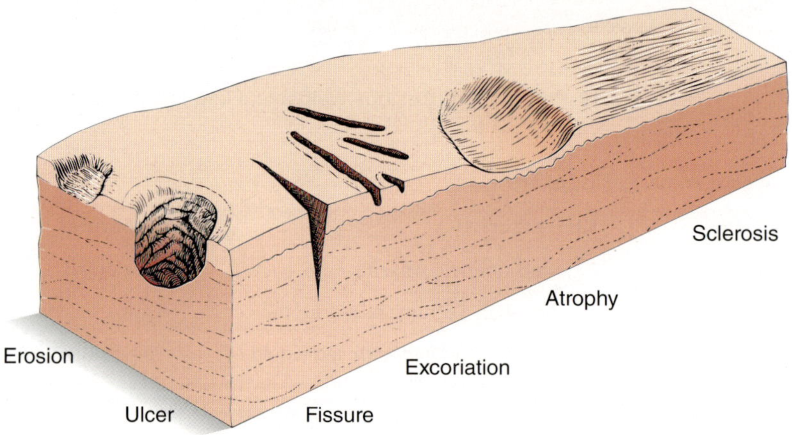

Fig. 8.21 Secondary Skin Lesions Below the Skin Plane.

Secondary Skin Lesions Above the Skin Plane

Lesion	Characteristics	Examples
Scaling	Heaped-up keratinized cells; exfoliated epidermis	Dandruff, psoriasis
Crusting	Dried residue of pus, serum, or blood	Scabs, impetigo

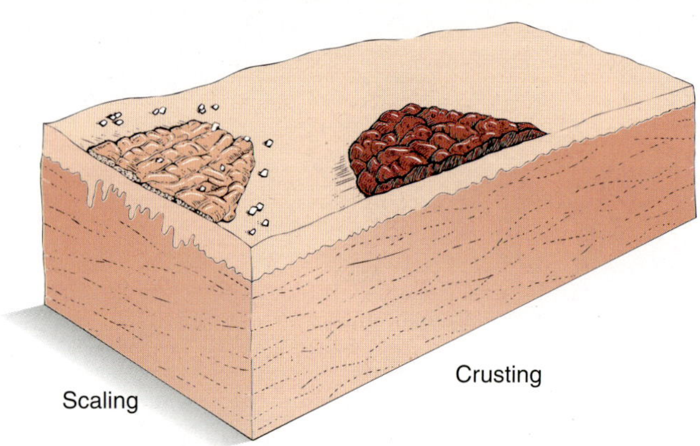

Fig. 8.22 Secondary Skin Lesions Above the Skin Plane.

CLINICOPATHOLOGIC CORRELATIONS

Skin disorders are frequently perplexing to the examiner. When an examiner sees a rash, the common thought is, "Where do I begin?" All too often, the examiner may become frustrated and not even attempt to make a diagnosis. Dermatologic terms are complicated, and the names of dermatologic disorders may be intimidating. Often the descriptions of skin disorders in textbooks are more confusing than helpful.

There are more than 2500 separately named dermatologic diagnoses. Most of these diseases occur in low frequencies; only 10 to 15 common conditions constitute approximately 50% of all dermatologic diagnoses. If the 50 most common conditions were considered, a diagnosis could be rendered for more than 95% of all patients.

In approaching a skin lesion, the examiner must do the following:

First, identify the primary lesion.
Second, determine its distribution.
Third, identify any associated findings.
Fourth, consider the age of the patient.

Vascular Skin Lesions		
Lesion	**Characteristics**	**Examples**
Erythema	Pink or red discoloration of the skin, secondary to dilatation of blood vessels, that blanches with pressure	
Petechiae	Reddish-purple; nonblanching; smaller than 0.5 cm	Intravascular defects
Purpura	Reddish-purple; nonblanching; greater than 0.5 cm	Intravascular defects
Ecchymosis	Reddish-purple; nonblanching; variable size	Trauma, vasculitis
Telangiectasia	Fine, irregular dilated blood vessels	Dilatation of capillaries
Spider angioma	Central red body with radiating spider-like arms that blanch with pressure to the central area	Liver disease, estrogens

Miscellaneous Skin Lesions		
Lesion	**Characteristics**	**Examples**
Scar	Replacement of destroyed dermis by fibrous tissue; may be atrophic or hyperplastic	Healed wound
Keloid	Elevated, enlarging scar growing beyond boundaries of wound	Burn scars
Lichenification	Roughening and thickening of epidermis; accentuated skin markings	Atopic dermatitis

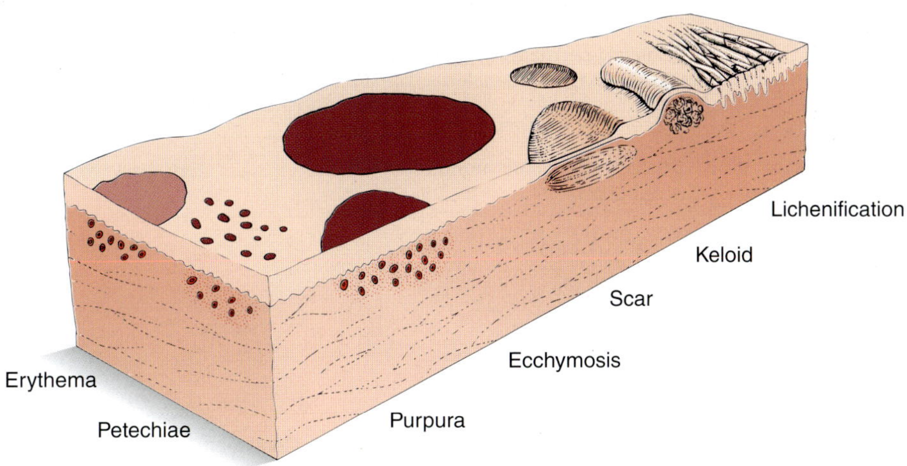

Fig. 8.23 Vascular and Other Miscellaneous Skin Lesions.

Skin diseases evolve, and their manifestations change. For example, a lesion may evolve from a blister to an erosion, from a vesicle to a pustule, or from a papule to a nodule or tumor.

The examiner should be familiar with many common skin disorders or lesions. Illustrated in the figures in this chapter are examples of some of these conditions; these cross-sectional diagrams illustrate the locations of these abnormalities in the skin and the involvement of the various skin layers in the pathogenesis of the diseases. In addition, the text describes the primary lesions.

Warts

A *common wart* is a common, benign growth usually caused by an infection of an epidermal cell by the human papillomavirus (HPV). There are more than 100 types of HPV, and different types of the virus cause different kinds of warts. Most types of HPV cause relatively harmless conditions such as common warts, whereas others may cause serious diseases such as cancer of the cervix. Wart viruses pass from person to person. Individuals can be infected by the virus indirectly by touching a towel or object used by someone who has the virus. Each person's immune system responds differently to HPV, so not everyone who comes in contact with HPV will develop warts. Warts are firm nodules with rough, keratinous surfaces ranging from a pinhead to pea size and can coalesce to form an extensive bed. There is vacuolation of the epidermis with scaling and upward growth of the dermal papilla. Fig. 8.25 illustrates a cross-section

Descriptive Dermatologic Terms

Lesion	Characteristics	Examples
Annular	Ring-shaped	Ringworm
Arcuate	Partial rings	Syphilis
Bizarre	Irregular or geographic pattern *not* related to any underlying anatomic structure	Factitial dermatitis
Circinate	Circular	
Confluent	Lesions that run together	Childhood exanthems
Discoid	Disc-shaped without central clearing	Lupus erythematosus
Discrete	Lesions that remain separate	
Eczematoid	An inflammation with a tendency to vesiculate and crust	Eczema
Generalized	Widespread	
Grouped	Lesions that are clustered together	Herpes simplex
Iris	Circle within a circle; a bull's-eye lesion	Erythema multiforme
Keratotic	Horny thickening	Psoriasis
Linear	In lines	Poison ivy dermatitis
Multiform	More than one type of shape of lesion	Erythema multiforme
Papulosquamous	Papules or plaques associated with scaling	Psoriasis
Reticulated	Lacelike network	Oral lichen planus
Serpiginous	Snakelike, creeping	Cutaneous larva migrans
Telangiectatic	Relatively permanent dilatation of the superficial blood vessels	Osler-Weber-Rendu disease
Universal	Entire body involved	Alopecia universalis
Zosteriform*	Linear arrangement along a nerve distribution	Herpes zoster

* Also known as *dermatomal.*

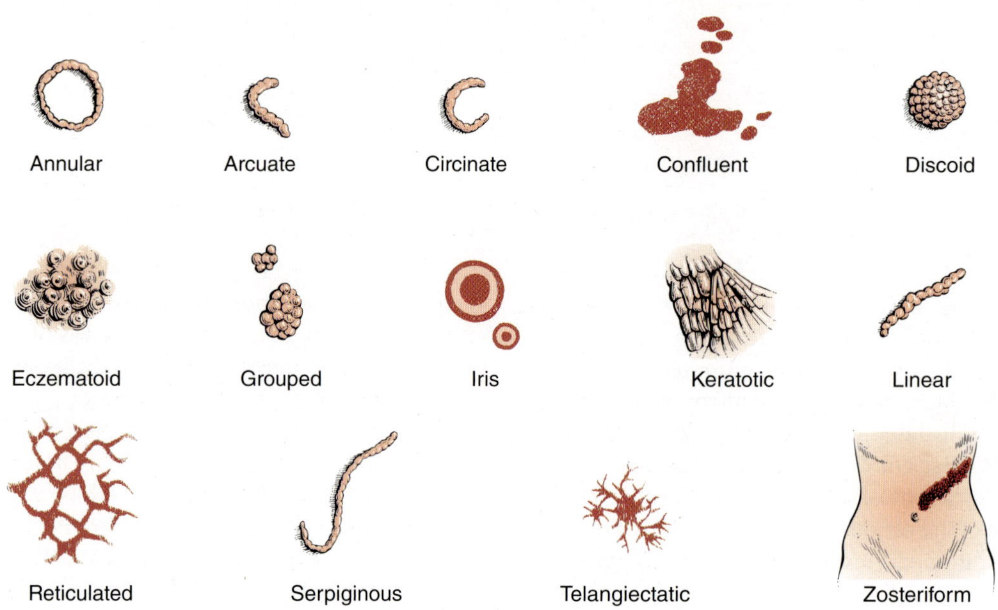

Fig. 8.24 Descriptive Dermatologic Terms.

through a wart. Two examples of finger warts are pictured in Fig. 8.26.

Warts can also occur on the soles of the feet (*plantar verruca*), which have a distinctive appearance because of constant pressure. In addition, they are very painful owing to the continuous pressure, which forces the keratinous material into the deeper tissue. An example of a plantar wart on the heel is shown in Fig. 8.27A. Notice the keratotic lesion with a yellow center, within which are visible areas of multiple red-to-black dots that represent hemorrhage from the tips of the dermal papillae. Classically, there is an interruption of the regular skin lines as well. Fig. 8.27B shows the excised lesion. Notice the depth of the lesion when viewed horizontally. Because warts are in the epidermis, excision to the dermis level is sufficient for complete removal with minimal scarring.

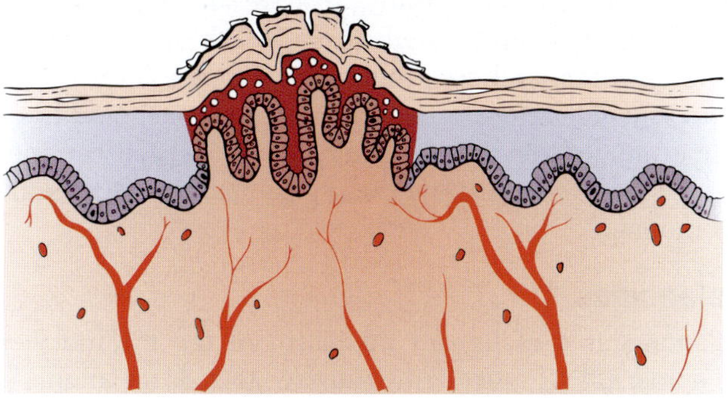

Fig. 8.25 Cross-Section Through a Wart. Note the thickened epidermis and hyperkeratosis.

Squamous Cell Carcinoma

A *squamous cell carcinoma* is a malignant neoplasm of keratocytes in the epidermis and is locally invasive into the dermis. The tumor results in a scaling, crusting nodule, or plaque that can ulcerate and bleed. Squamous cell carcinoma is a potentially dangerous lesion that can infiltrate the surrounding structures and metastasize to lymph nodes and other organs. The causes include ultraviolet radiation, x-radiation, polycyclic hydrocarbons (e.g., tar, mineral oils, pitch, and soot), mucosal diseases (e.g., lichen planus and Bowen disease), scars, chronic

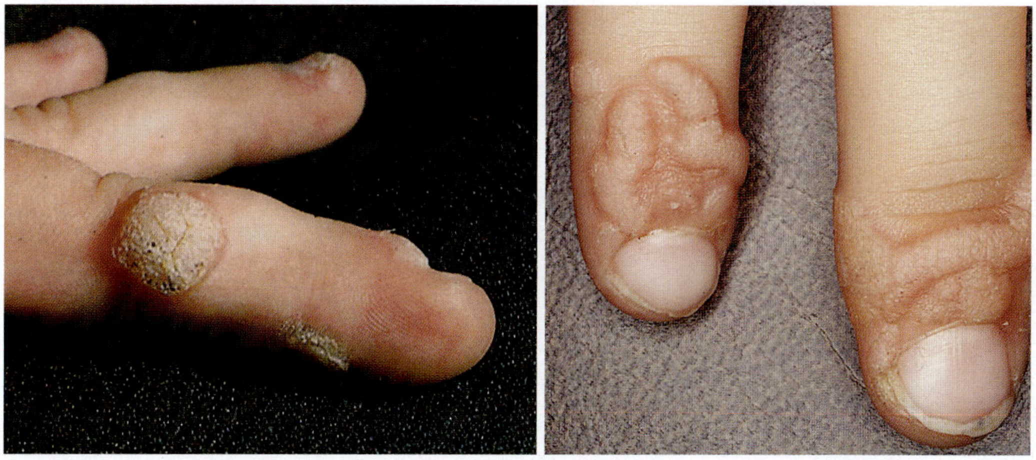

A B

Fig. 8.26 (A) and (B) Warts. (From Callen JP, Paller AS, Greer KE, et al: *Color atlas of dermatology*, ed 2, Philadelphia, 2000, WB Saunders.)

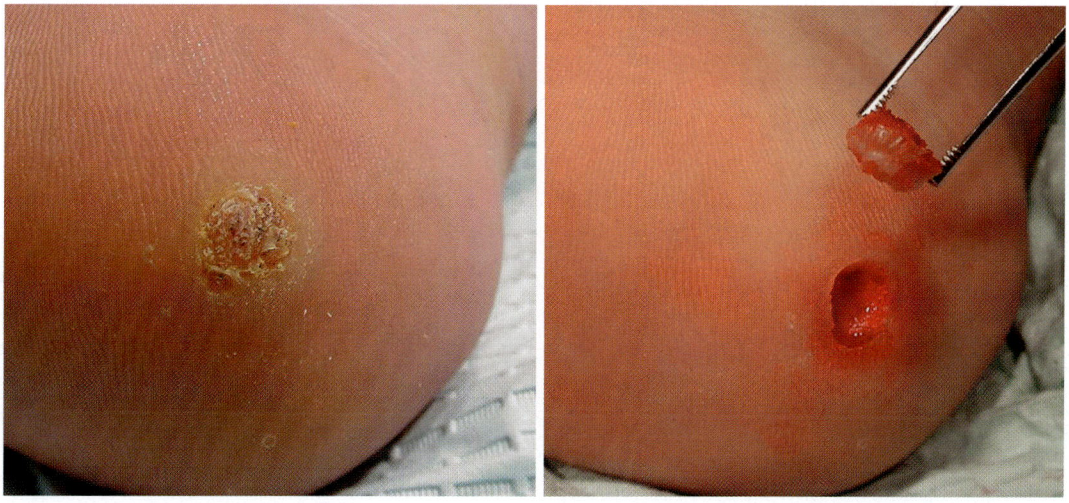

A B

Fig. 8.27 Plantar Wart. (A) Note the keratotic lesion with the yellow center and areas of hemorrhage within. (B) After excision.

skin disorders, genetic diseases (e.g., albinism and xeroderma pigmentosum), and HPV. The tumor develops predominantly on areas of skin exposed to sunlight. The latency from carcinogenic exposure to the development of the cancer may be as long as 25 to 30 years. Two examples of squamous cell carcinoma of the skin are pictured in Fig. 8.28. Notice that the lesions are ulcerated with firm, raised, indurated margins. Fig. 11.11 also shows a patient with squamous cell carcinoma and a malignant melanoma of the ear lobule. A squamous cell carcinoma on the lip of another patient is pictured in Fig. 8.29. Notice the round, centrally ulcerating tumor. Fig. 8.30 illustrates a cross-section through a squamous cell carcinoma. Although squamous cell carcinomas are usually found in sun-exposed areas, the lesion pictured in Fig. 8.31 is on the plantar aspect of the foot. A callus is also present under the head of the first metatarsal.

Basal Cell Carcinoma

A *basal cell carcinoma* is a malignant neoplasm of the basal cells of the epidermis and is the most common skin malignancy. The epidermis is thickened, and the malignant basal cells may invade the dermis. It may manifest as a lesion with a pearly, rolled, well-defined margin and a central ulcerated depression. Although sunlight is an important etiologic factor, basal cell carcinomas are almost always seen on the face and rarely in other sun-exposed areas. They are slow-growing tumors and rarely metastasize, unlike squamous cell carcinomas. They are locally invasive and may invade the cranial cavity when located near the eye or nose. If ulceration, bleeding, and crusting occur, a *rodent ulcer* is said to be present. Therefore, any nonhealing lesion should be carefully evaluated for the possibility of a basal cell carcinoma. Figs. 8.32 to 8.34 illustrate the typical features of a basal cell carcinoma.

Melanomas

Melanoma is a malignant neoplasm of the melanocytes of the epidermis. If untreated or unrecognized, melanoma progresses to fatal metastases. Most melanomas have a prolonged superficial or horizontal growth phase with progressive lateral

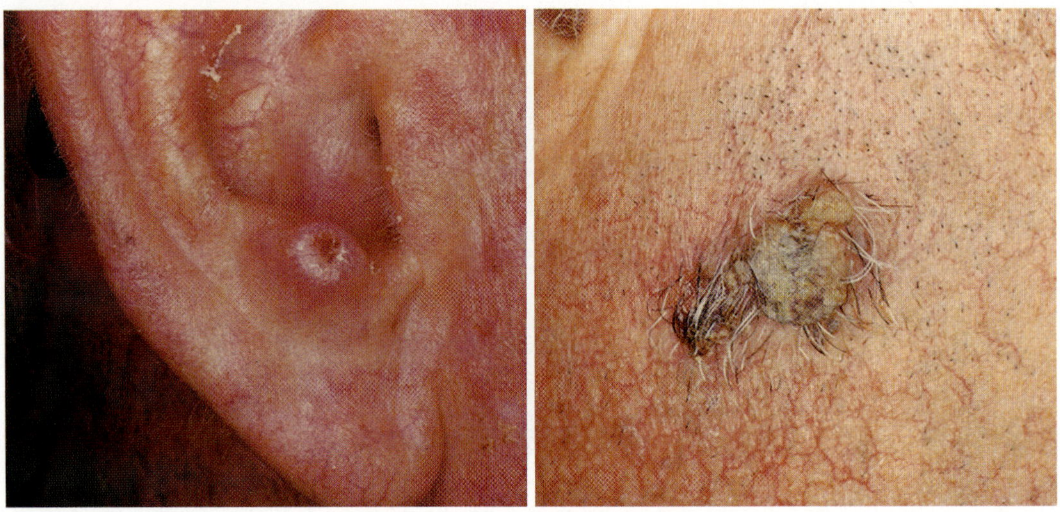

A B

Fig. 8.28 Squamous Cell Carcinoma of the Skin. (A) Ear. (B) Face. (From Callen JP, Greer KE, Hood AF, et al: *Color atlas of dermatology*, Philadelphia, 1993, WB Saunders.)

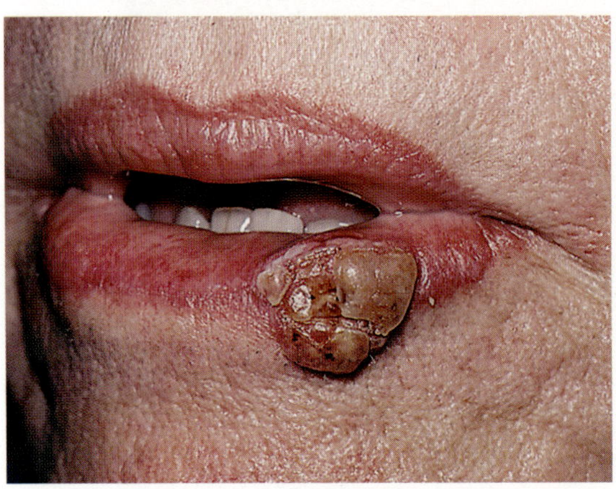

Fig. 8.29 Squamous Cell Carcinoma of Lip. (From Callen JP, Paller AS, Greer KE, et al: *Color atlas of dermatology*, ed 2, Philadelphia, 2000, WB Saunders.)

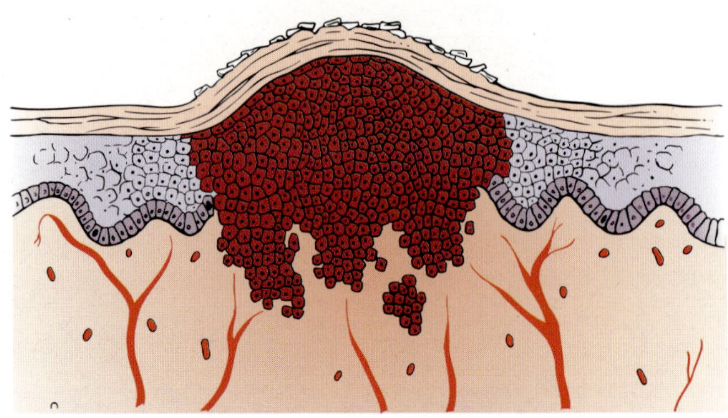

Fig. 8.30 Cross-Section Through a Squamous Cell Carcinoma. Note the invasion into the dermis.

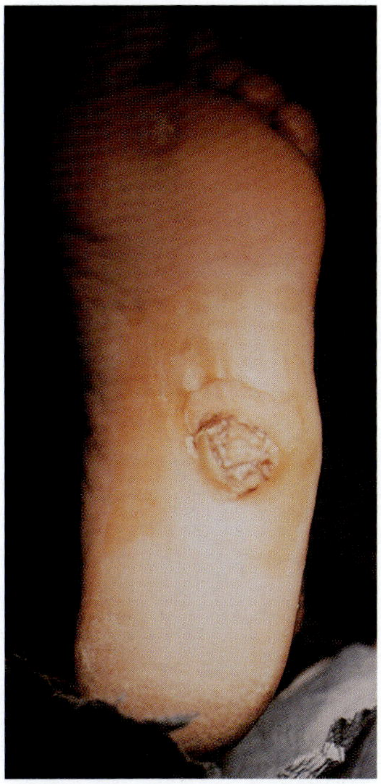

Fig. 8.31 Squamous Cell Carcinoma on the Plantar Surface of the Foot.

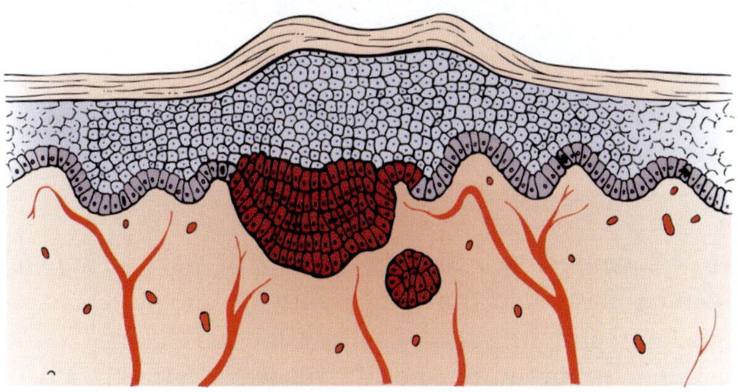

Fig. 8.32 Cross-Section Through a Basal Cell Carcinoma.

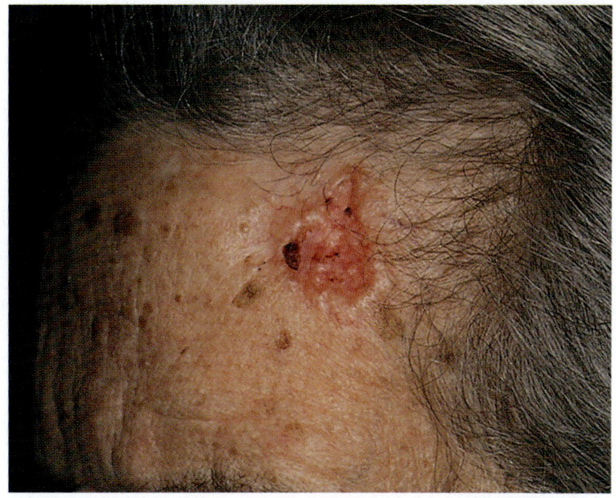

Fig. 8.34 Basal Cell Carcinoma. Notice the rolled, well-defined margin.

expansion. With time, the melanoma enters the vertical, or deep, phase by penetrating the dermis, and metastatic spread may occur.

Malignant melanomas are the most common malignancy seen by dermatologists. The incidence of malignant melanoma is increasing faster than any other malignancy. Most melanomas have atypical pigmentation in the epidermis, such as shades of red, white, gray, blue, brown, and black, all in a single lesion. There are four types of malignant melanoma: lentigo maligna melanoma, superficial spreading melanoma, nodular malignant melanoma, and acral-lentiginous malignant melanoma. Fig. 8.35 shows the typical features of a lentigo maligna melanoma on the face. Lentigo maligna melanoma is seen frequently in the geriatric population. This type of melanoma has a prolonged horizontal growth phase and appears in sun-exposed, sun-damaged skin areas. The superficial spreading variety (Fig. 8.36) is the most common type of melanoma (70% of all melanomas). Typically, an irregularly colored plaque has

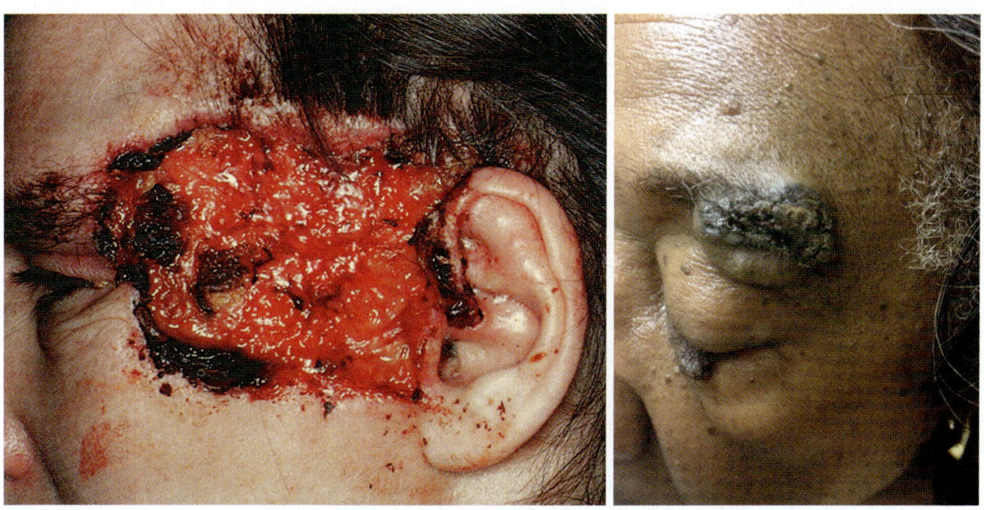

A B

Fig. 8.33 Basal Cell Carcinoma (Rodent Ulcer). (A, From Callen JP, Greer KE, Hood AF, et al: *Color atlas of dermatology*, Philadelphia, 1993, WB Saunders. B, From Abdulhak A, Moiin A: Cancers Arising in Black Skin. In: Moiin A (eds): *Atlas of black skin*, 2020, Springer, Cham. https://doi.org/10.1007/978-3-030-31485-9_10)

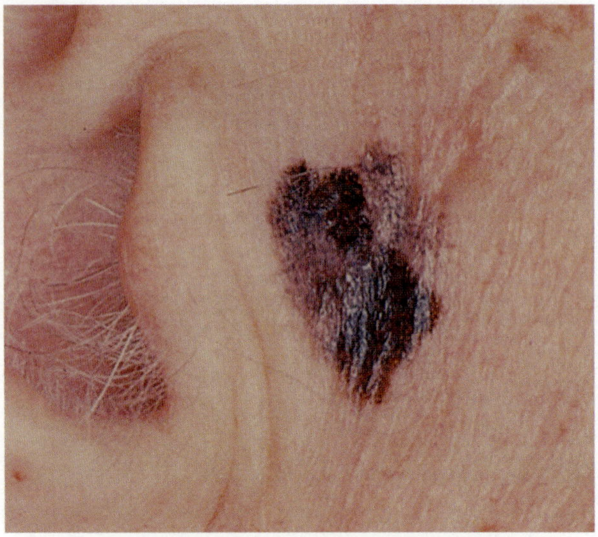

Fig. 8.35 Lentigo Maligna Melanoma.

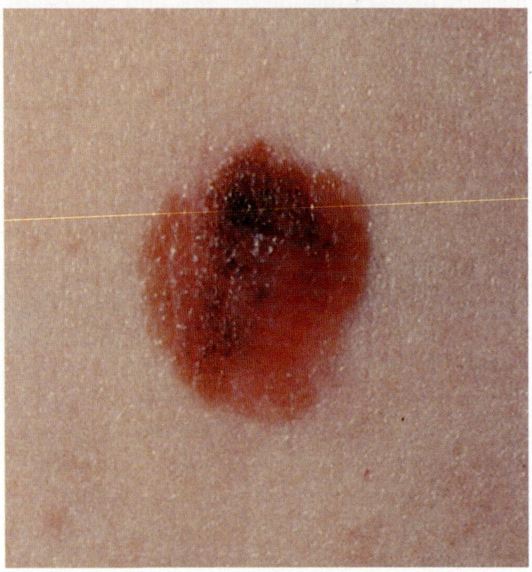

Fig. 8.36 Superficial Spreading Malignant Melanoma. (From Callen JP, Greer KE, Hood AF, et al: *Color atlas of dermatology*, Philadelphia, 1993, WB Saunders.)

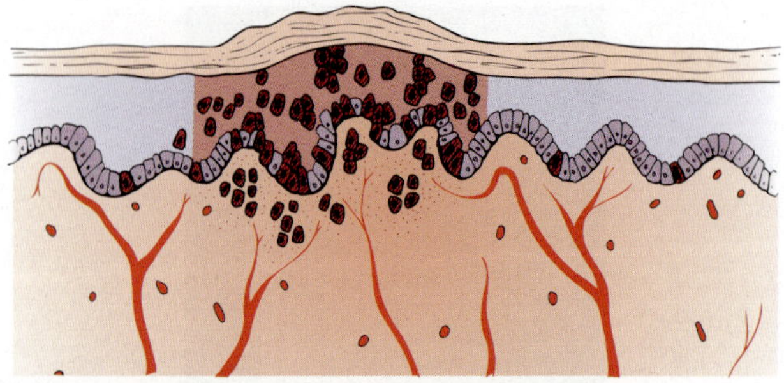

Fig. 8.37 Cross-Section Through a Melanoma. Note the nests of melanoma cells in the dermis.

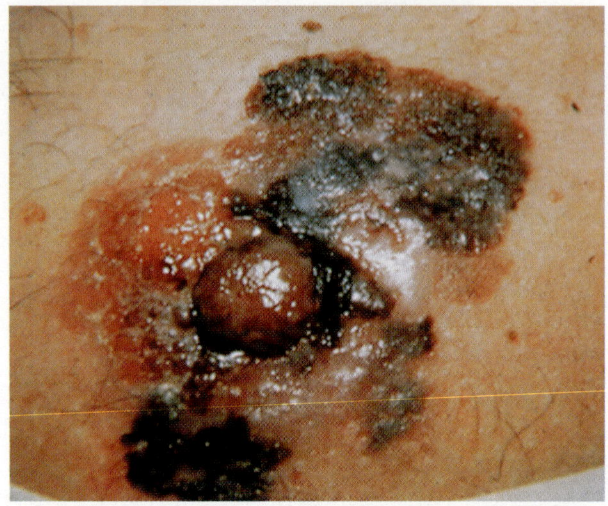

Fig. 8.38 Superficial Spreading Malignant Melanoma With Vertical Growth.

sharp notches and variegation of pigment. If diagnosed early, the prognosis is excellent, with a 5-year survival rate of 95%. Fig. 8.37 illustrates a cross-section through a melanoma. Vertical growth and deep invasion follow the spreading phase of superficial malignant melanomas. Fig. 8.38 shows another superficial spreading melanoma that has developed vertical growth. Nodular melanoma is the second-most common type, seen in approximately 15% of cases of melanoma. Unlike the superficial spreading type, these melanomas are usually black, brown, or dark blue and tend to grow rapidly for months.

Melanomas occur predominantly in White individuals and have a predilection for the back in males and females and for the anterior tibial areas in females. In general, lesions on the back, axillae, neck, and scalp (the so-called BANS area) tend to have a worse prognosis than melanomas on the extremities. A great contrast between the risk of acquiring melanoma and basal or squamous cell carcinoma is that basal and squamous cell carcinomas occur more frequently in individuals exposed to constant sunlight, such as sailors and agricultural workers. Melanomas occur more often in relatively fair-skinned individuals who experience brief, intense sun exposure, such as during vacations in the southern latitudes.

Fewer than 5% of all melanomas occur in the African American population. The acral-lentiginous melanoma is the most common form of melanoma in African Americans and Asians, occurring on non–hair-bearing parts of the body: palms, soles, beneath the nails, and in the oral mucosa. It is more common on toenails than on fingernails. Acral-lentiginous melanoma accounts for 29% to 72% of melanoma in dark-skinned individuals but less than 1% in fair-skinned people. Unlike other forms of melanoma, *acral-lentiginous melanomas do not appear to be linked to sun exposure.* The average age at diagnosis is between 60 and 70 years. However, melanoma can also occur in White populations and young people. These melanomas have a short, superficial growth phase and an early vertical growth phase and, as such, are associated with a poor prognosis. Typical signs of an acral-lentiginous melanoma include the following:

- Longitudinal tan, black, or brown streak on a fingernail or toenail
- Pigmentation of the proximal nail fold
- Areas of dark pigmentation on palms of hands or soles of feet

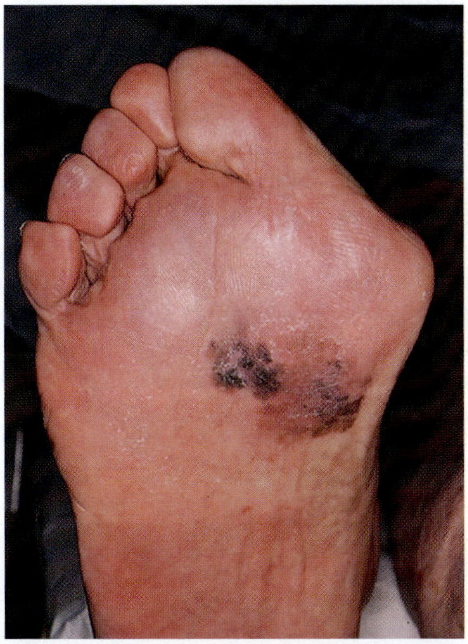

Fig. 8.39 Acral-Lentiginous Melanoma.

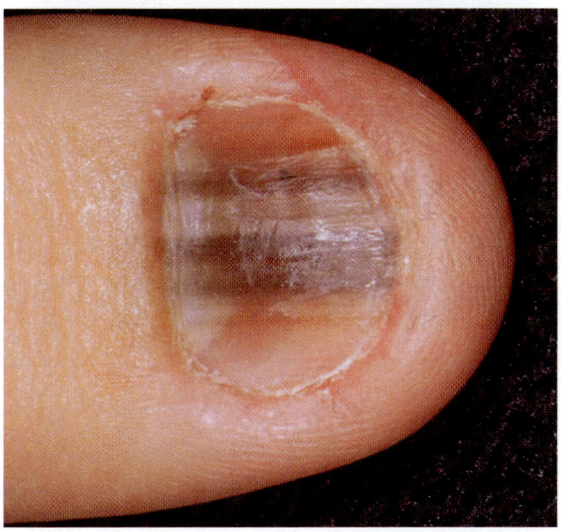

Fig. 8.40 Acral-Lentiginous Melanoma of the Nail Bed. (From Hordinsky MK, Sawaya ME, Scher RK: *Atlas of hair and nails*, Philadelphia, 2000, Churchill Livingstone.)

An acral-lentiginous melanoma on the sole of an African American patient is pictured in Fig. 8.39. The nail of the hallux (great toe) is a common site. The famous Jamaican (of African descent) singer-songwriter, musician, and revered performer of reggae music, Bob Marley, died at age 36 from metastatic acral-lentiginous melanoma that originated in one of his toenails. Fig. 8.40 shows an acral-lentiginous melanoma of the nail bed, with a broad longitudinal band and variegated colors. Fig. 8.41 shows another patient with an acral-lentiginous melanoma of the nail bed. Notice that the bandwidth is slightly wider at the base than at the tip, indicating a rapidly growing lesion. Even though acral-lentiginous melanoma is rare, given its atypical locations and poor survival rates, it is essential that healthcare professionals maintain a high index of suspicion in all ethnic groups and closely examine a patient's palms, soles, and nail beds.

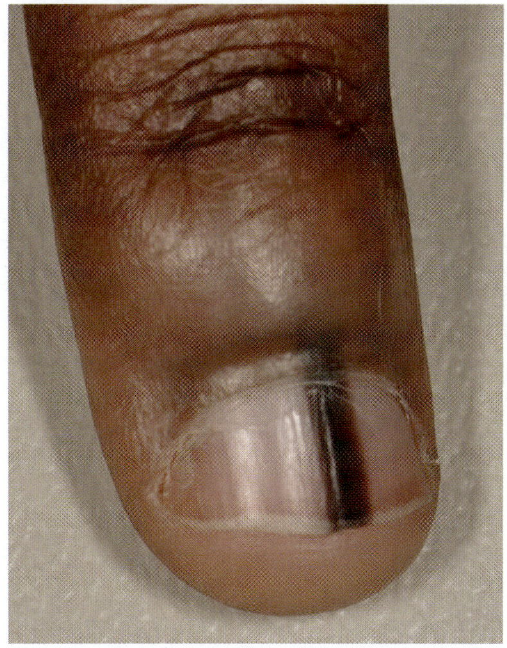

Fig. 8.41 Melanoma of the Nail Bed. (From Bellet JS: Nail discoloration in pediatric skin of color patients, *Pediatr Dermatol* 38:37–41, 2021. https://doi.org/10.1111/pde.14659)

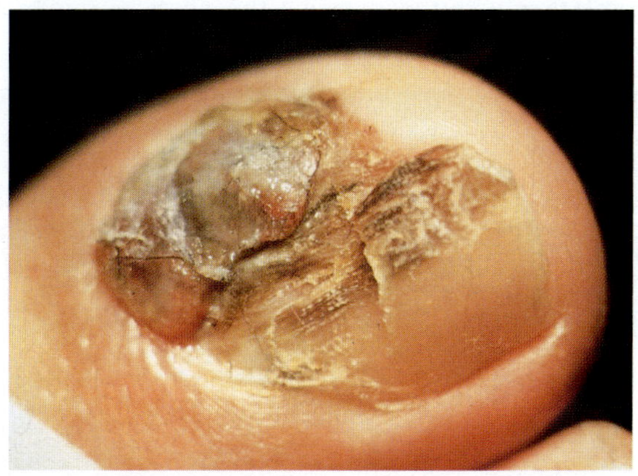

Fig. 8.42 Subungual Presentation of Malignant Melanoma of the Hallux.

Fig. 8.42 shows a subungual presentation of *malignant melanoma* of the hallux. Unusual pigmentation under the nail, especially if of long duration, should always be regarded with suspicion and biopsied. Subungual melanomas represent approximately 20% of melanomas in dark-skinned and Asian populations, compared with about 2% of cutaneous melanomas in White people. Ultraviolet radiation exposure seems to be an essential risk factor for cutaneous melanoma; however, because ultraviolet radiation is unlikely to penetrate the nail plate, it does not appear to be a risk factor for subungual melanomas. There is a considerable predominance of subungual melanoma localized on the thumb (58% of all affected fingers) and the hallux (86% of all affected toes).

Lipoma

A *lipoma* is a benign growth of subcutaneous fat and has a rubbery appearance. Lipomas are often found on the torso, neck, upper thighs, upper arms, and armpits, but they can occur almost anywhere in the body. One or more lipomas may be present at the same time. Lipomas are the most common noncancerous soft tissue growth. The epidermis is normal. Frequently, an encapsulated lipoma may grow considerably and elevate the overlying dermis and epidermis, as shown in Fig. 8.43; a cross-section through a lipoma is illustrated in Fig. 8.44. The examiner can easily push into the soft tissue tumor. Another example of a lipoma is shown on the arm of the patient in Fig. 8.45.

Café au Lait Spots

Café au lait spots are patch lesions that are well circumscribed and brownish. They may occur as a solitary birthmark in up to 10% of the average population. The café au lait macule or patch results from increased functionally hyperactive melanocytes. Many healthy people have one or two small café au lait spots. However, adults with six or more spots larger than 1.5 cm in diameter (0.5 cm in children) likely have neurofibromatosis. These spots may be the only symptom in most people with the condition. Fig. 8.46 shows a café au lait spot (patch) in a patient with neurofibromatosis.

Neurofibroma

A *neurofibroma* is a tumor produced by a focal proliferation of neural tissue in the dermis. The epidermis is normal. Neurofibromas may appear as papules or nodules. Cutaneous neurofibromas are soft in consistency. Neurofibromatosis is a disorder in which multiple neurofibromas are present, sometimes as many as several hundred. Although the tumors are benign, the occurrence of these space-occupying lesions may produce severe disfigurement or neurologic disease. Other dermatologic features of neurofibromatosis include multiple café au lait patches and axillary freckling. Fig. 8.47 shows several neurofibromas in a patient with neurofibromatosis; a cross-sectional view is illustrated in Fig. 8.48. Fig. 8.49 shows axillary freckling (Crowe sign) in a patient with neurofibromatosis. Fig. 8.50 shows multiple neurofibromas on the face of another patient with neurofibromatosis.

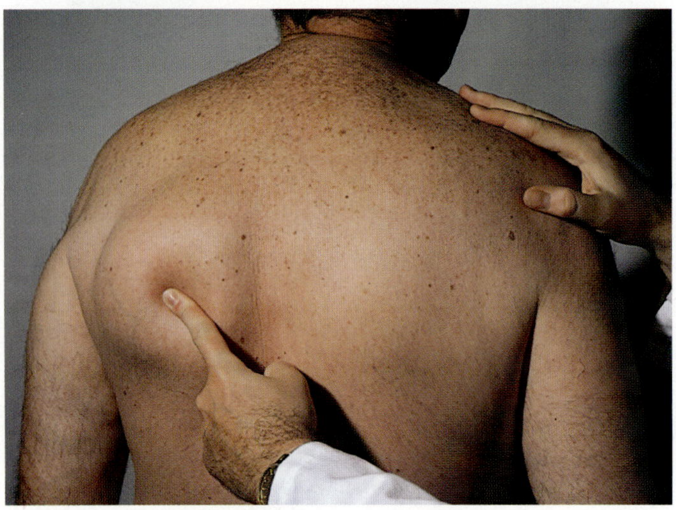

Fig. 8.43 Lipoma of the Back.

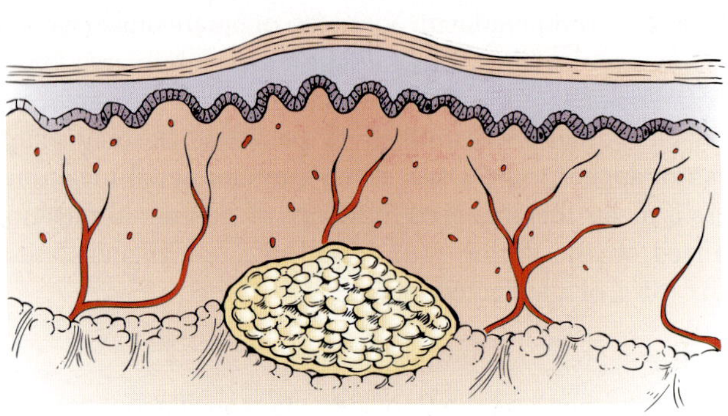

Fig. 8.44 Cross-Section Through a Lipoma.

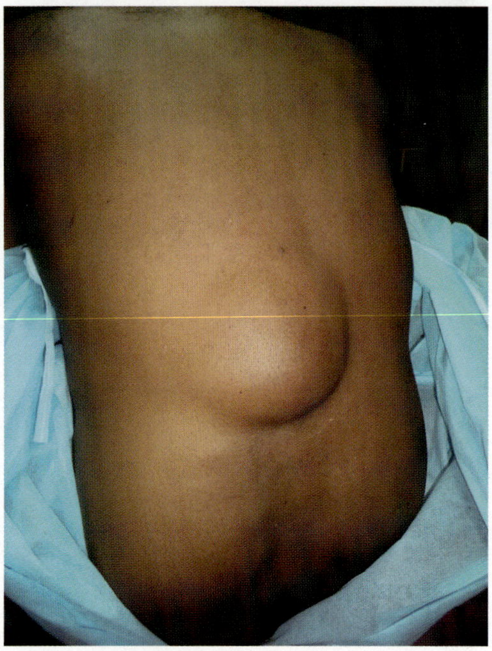

Fig. 8.45 Lipoma on Back. (From Rao S, Rao K: *Essentials of surgery for dental students,* ed 1, 2016, Elsevier.)

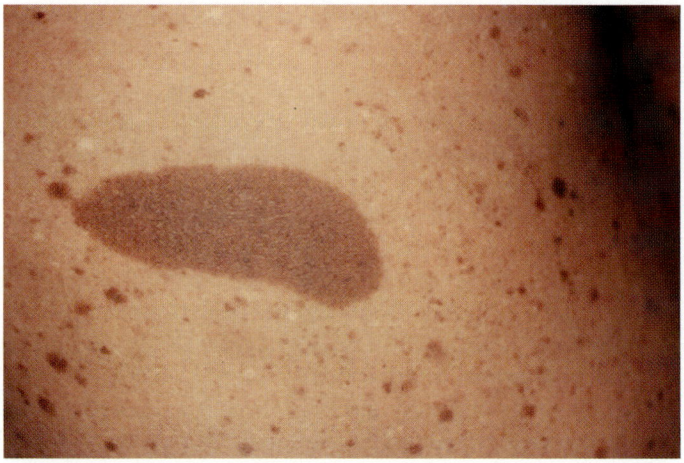

Fig. 8.46 Café au Lait Spot in a Patient With Neurofibromatosis. (From Callen JP, Greer KE, Hood AF, et al: *Color atlas of dermatology,* Philadelphia, 1993, WB Saunders.)

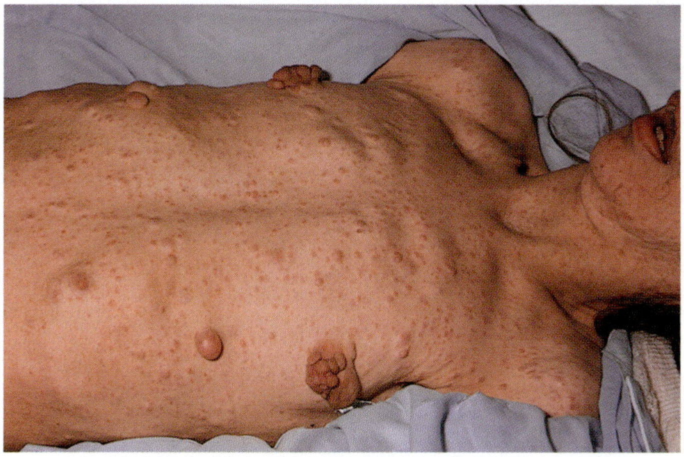

Fig. 8.47 Multiple Neurofibromas in a Patient With Neurofibromatosis.

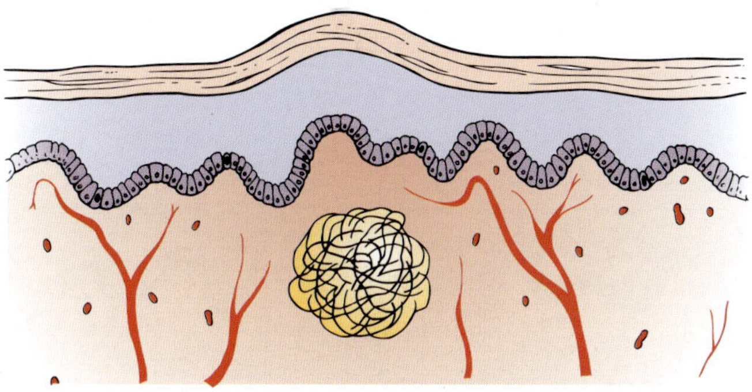

Fig. 8.48 Cross-Section Through a Neurofibroma. Note that the tumor is a well-delimited mass of loosely packed neural elements.

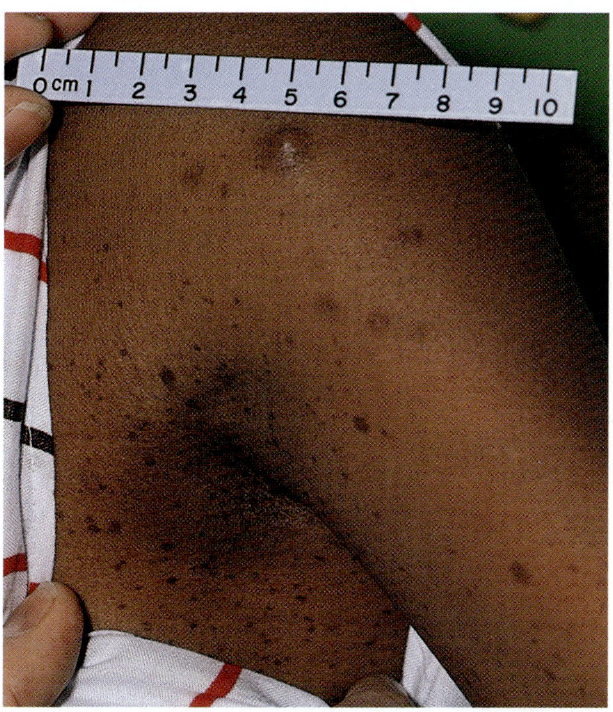

Fig. 8.49 Neurofibromatosis: Axillary Freckling (Crowe Sign).

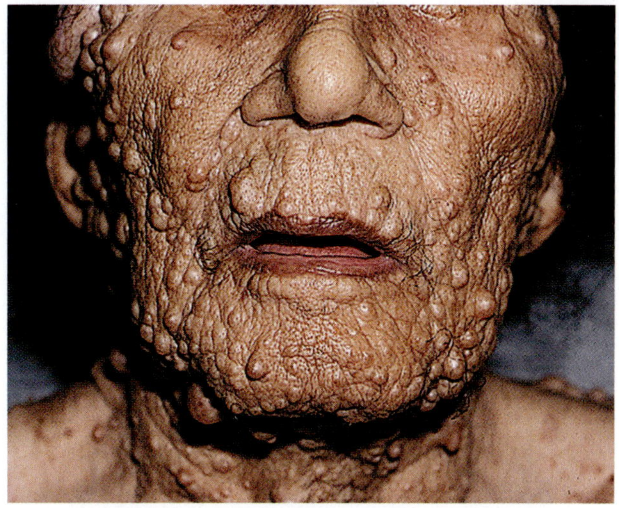

Fig. 8.50 Multiple Neurofibromas on the Face of a Patient With Neurofibromatosis. (From Callen JP, Paller AS, Greer KE, et al: *Color atlas of dermatology*, ed 2, Philadelphia, 2000, WB Saunders.)

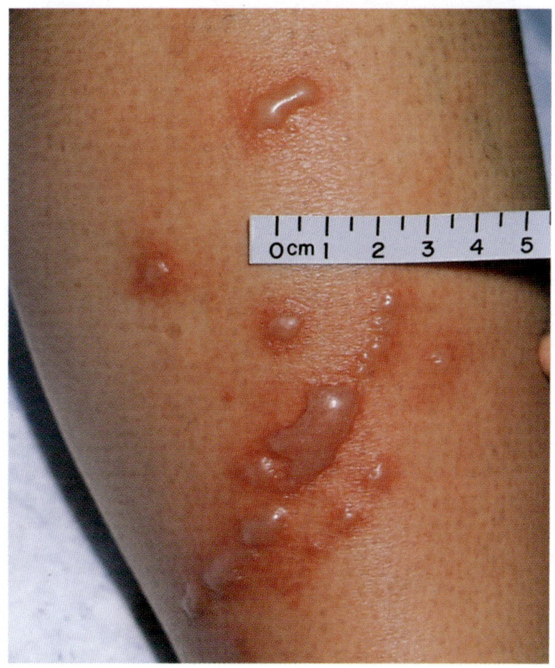

Fig. 8.51 Contact Dermatitis: Poison Ivy Reaction.

Contact Dermatitis

Contact dermatitis is an inflammatory skin reaction precipitated by contact with an irritant or allergen, such as detergents, acids, alkalis, plants, medicines, and solvents. Vesicles in the epidermis and perivascular inflammation result. Fig. 8.51 shows contact dermatitis in reaction to poison ivy; the area is illustrated in cross-section in Fig. 8.52. The characteristic linear distribution of vesicles and bullae is visible on this patient's calf, where the plant leaves rubbed against the leg. The distribution of the bullous lesions and their location strongly suggest the diagnosis.

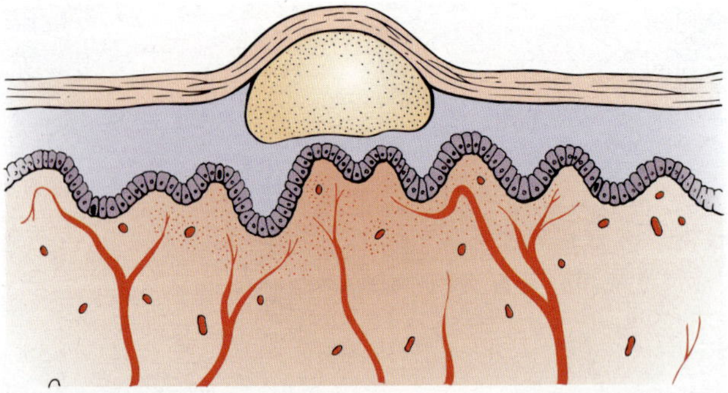

Fig. 8.52 Cross-Section Through an Area of Contact Dermatitis. Note the perivascular inflammation in the dermis and the vesicles and bullae in the epidermis.

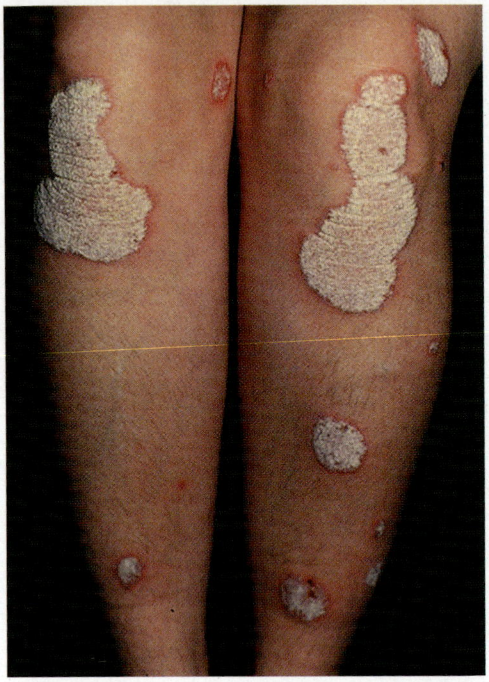

Fig. 8.53 Psoriatic Lesions on the Knees. (From Callen JP, Greer KE, Hood AF, et al: *Color atlas of dermatology*, Philadelphia, 1993, WB Saunders.)

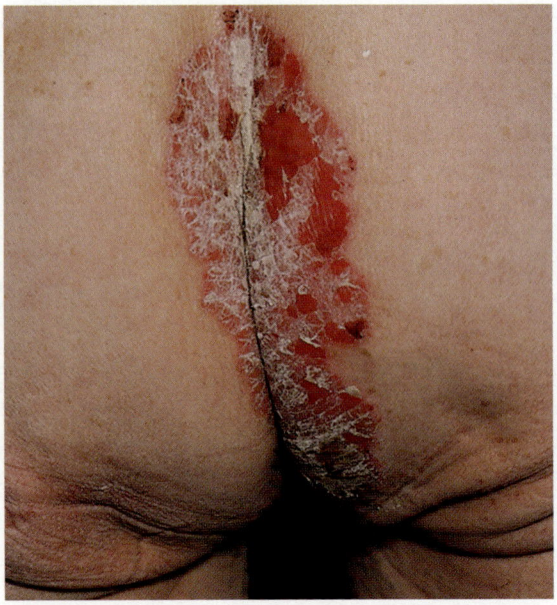

Fig. 8.54 Psoriatic Lesions on the Intergluteal Cleft.

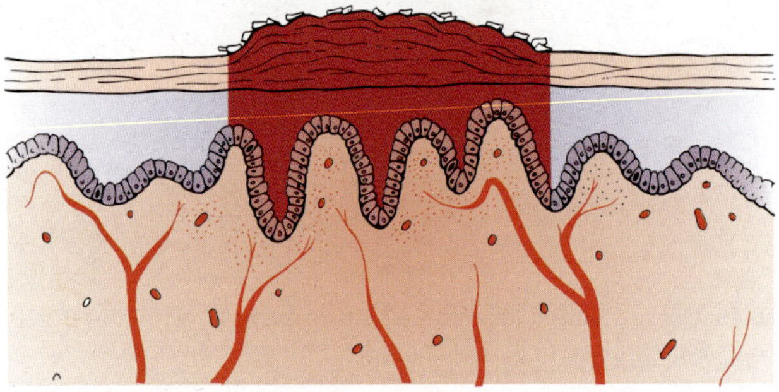

Fig. 8.55 Cross-Section Through an Area of Psoriasis. Note the area of hyperkeratosis.

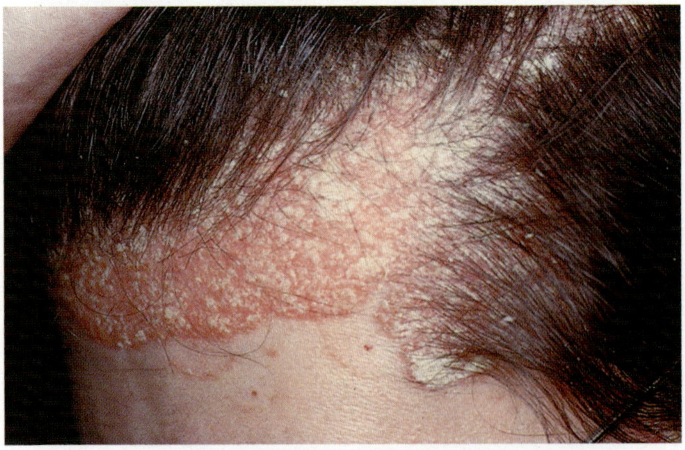

Fig. 8.56 Psoriasis of the Scalp.

Psoriasis

Psoriasis is one of the most common noninfectious skin disorders. It is frequently inherited, often chronic, and it, too, may affect the joints and nails. The rash is characterized by well-defined, slightly raised, hyperkeratotic (scaling) plaques. Small bleeding points appear if the lesion is scratched, a specific sign of the disease. The lesions are frequently symmetric and can be extremely itchy. The stratum corneum thickens, and erythematous plaques with silvery scales result. Within the dermis, there is capillary proliferation with perivascular inflammation. The lesions are characteristically located on the elbows, knees, scalp, and intergluteal cleft. Fig. 8.53 shows the typical, symmetric lesions on the knees of an affected patient. Fig. 8.54 shows the classic scaling lesions at the intergluteal cleft of another patient. Fig. 8.55 illustrates a cross-section through an area of psoriasis. Fig. 8.56 shows psoriasis of the scalp. The lesions commonly extend beyond the hair-bearing areas onto the adjacent skin. Surprisingly, this lesion rarely results in hair loss. Fig. 8.57 shows severe, diffuse psoriasis involving more than 85% of the body of a 56-year-old male. This patient suffered from persistent itching, burning, and bleeding with psoriasis for more than 35 years. Psoriasis may produce several nail changes. Pitting of

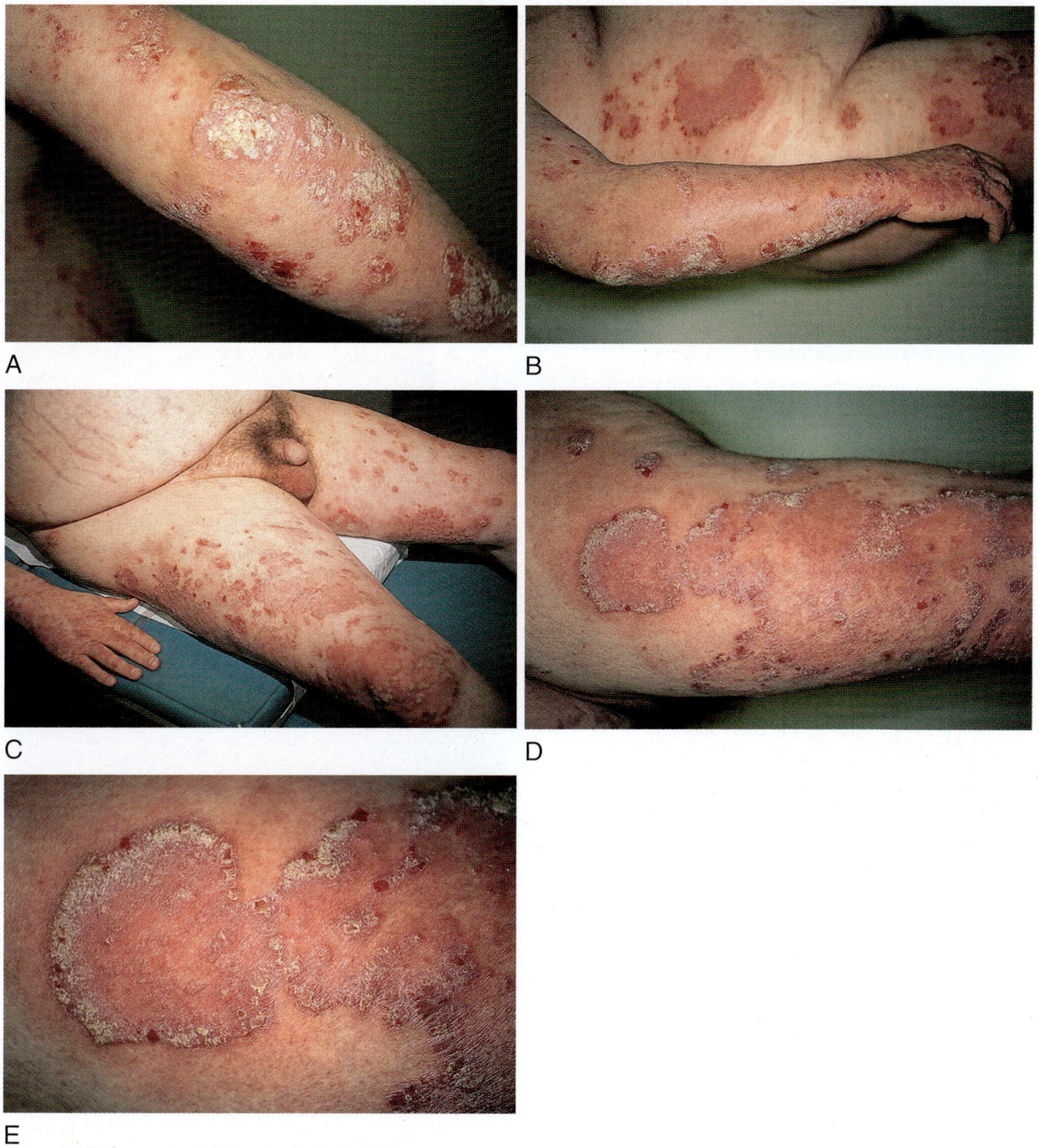

Fig. 8.57 Psoriasis. (A–E) Severe psoriasis in a 56-year-old patient.

the nail has already been discussed (see Figs. 8.14 and 8.15). There are several other nail changes: oily patches, onycholysis, subungual hyperkeratosis, and splinter hemorrhages.

Fungal Infections

Fungal infections of the skin, nails, and hair are prevalent. The primary fungi responsible for skin, hair, and nail diseases are dermatophytes of the genera *Trichophyton, Microsporum,* and *Epidermophyton.* Fungal infections of the skin produce a scaling, erythematous patch, often with a reddened, raised, serpiginous border. The term *tinea* indicates the fungal cause, and the second word denotes the area of the body involved: *tinea corporis* is an infection on the torso (also known as "ringworm"); *tinea pedis,* in the foot (also known as "athlete's foot"); *tinea faciale,* in the face; *tinea barbae,* in the beard and mustache area in men; *tinea cruris,* in the groin (also known as "jock itch"); and *tinea capitis,* in the head. The epidermis is thickened in all cases, and the stratum corneum is infiltrated with fungal hyphae. The underlying dermis displays mild inflammation. Figs. 8.58 and 8.59 illustrate the classic annular lesion of tinea corporis with its raised erythematous border and central clearing. Another example of tinea corporis is pictured in Fig. 8.60. Tinea faciale in a child is shown in Fig. 8.61. Tinea cruris is pictured in Fig. 8.62. This typical pruritic lesion is seen commonly in young men; it is unusual in females. It spreads outward from the groin down the thigh, leaving postinflammatory pigmentation. The advancing border is well-defined, red, scaly, and slightly raised. If untreated, the eruption can spread onto the lower abdomen, as shown, and the buttocks. The foot of a patient with tinea pedis is pictured in Fig. 8.63. Notice the maceration with erosions and scaling.

Bacterial and fungal infections are common in diabetic patients. Fig. 8.64 depicts bacterial cellulitis and tinea pedis in a diabetic patient. Tinea pedis produces macerated, scaling,

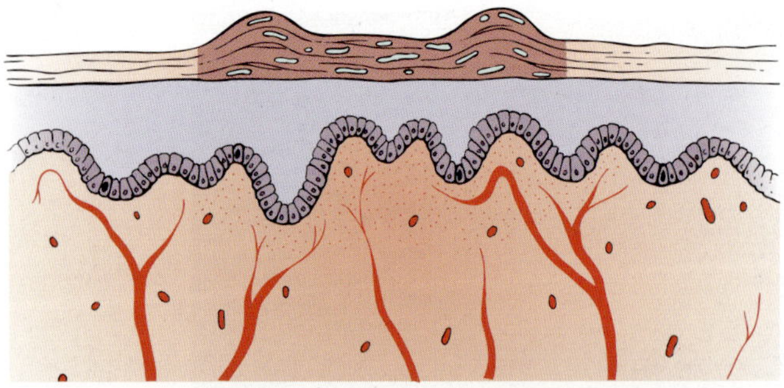

Fig. 8.58 **Cross-Section Through an Area of Tinea Corporis.** Note the thickened stratum corneum, which is infiltrated by the fungus.

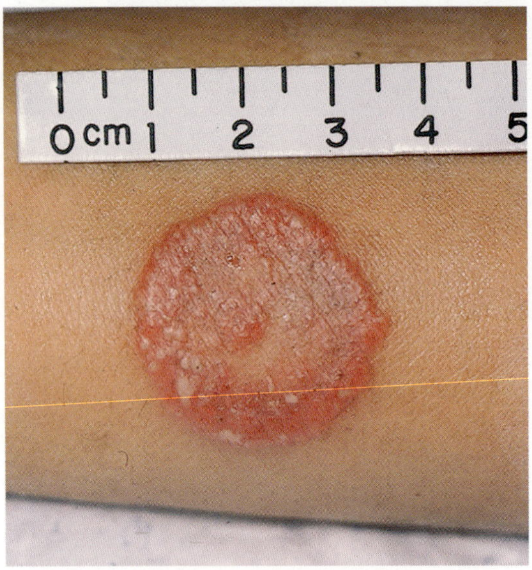

Fig. 8.59 **Tinea Corporis.**

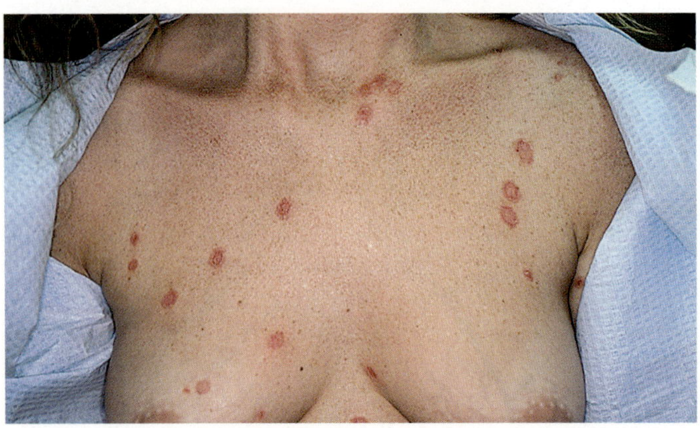

Fig. 8.60 **Tinea Corporis.** (From Callen JP, Paller AS, Greer KE, et al: *Color atlas of dermatology*, ed 2, Philadelphia, 2000, WB Saunders.)

fissured toe webs; inflammatory epidermis; and thick, hypertrophic, discolored nails.

Onychomycosis is an infection in which fungal organisms invade the nail bed and is the most common nail disorder. It accounts for nearly 50% of all nail problems. Its prevalence in the general population ranges from 2% to 14%. This infection causes progressive changes in the nail's color, structure, and

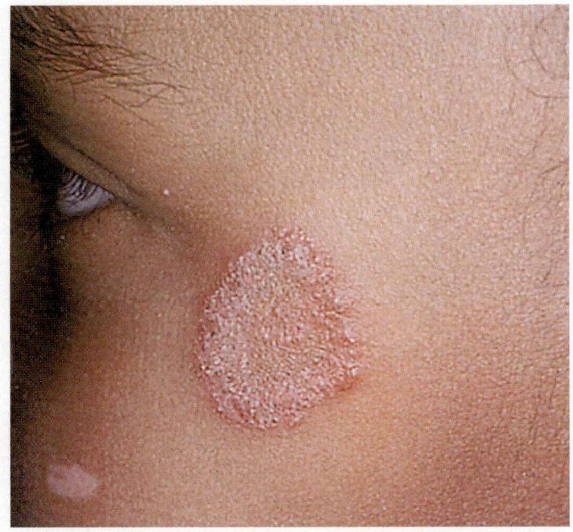

Fig. 8.61 **Tinea Faciale.** (From Callen JP, Paller AS, Greer KE, et al: *Color atlas of dermatology*, ed 2, Philadelphia, 2000, WB Saunders.)

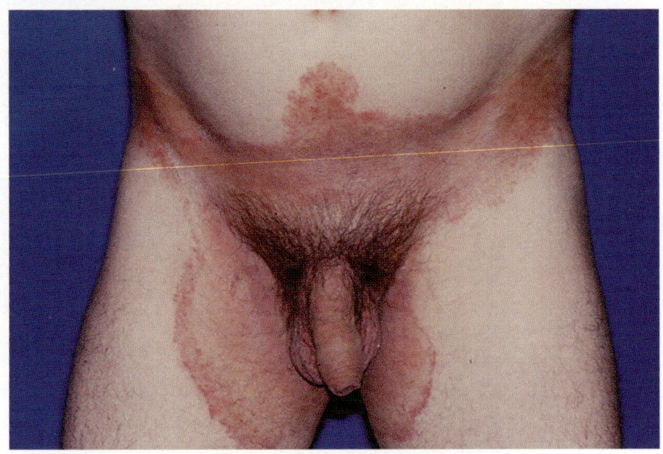

Fig. 8.62 **Tinea Cruris.** (From Callen JP, Greer KE, Hood AF, et al: *Color atlas of dermatology*, Philadelphia, 1993, WB Saunders.)

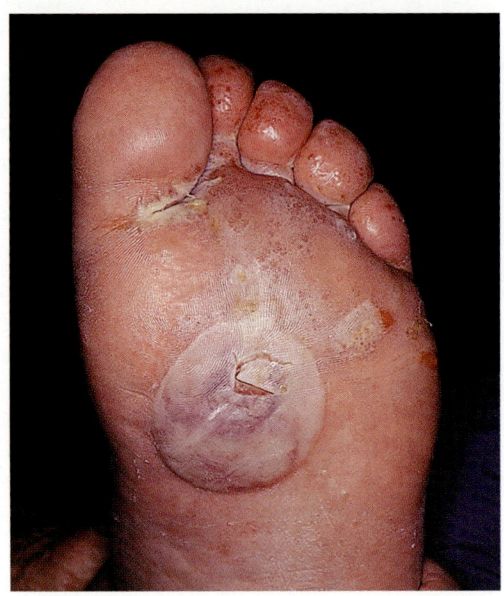

Fig. 8.63 **Tinea Pedis.** (From Callen JP, Paller AS, Greer KE, et al: *Color atlas of dermatology*, ed 2, Philadelphia, 2000, WB Saunders.)

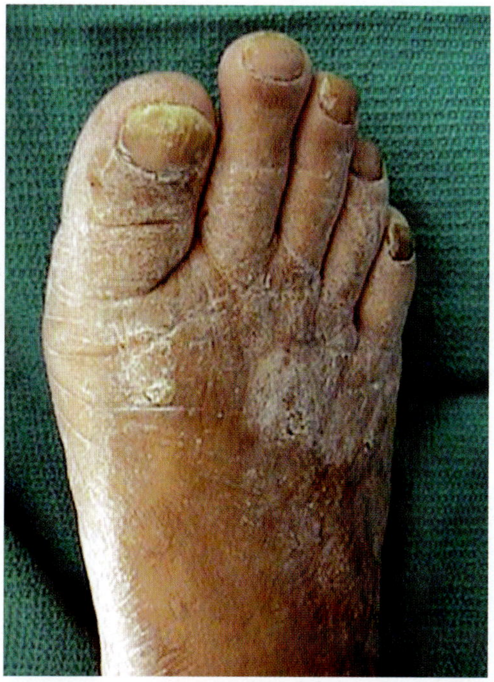

Fig. 8.64 Tinea Pedis and Bacterial Cellulitis in a Diabetic Patient.

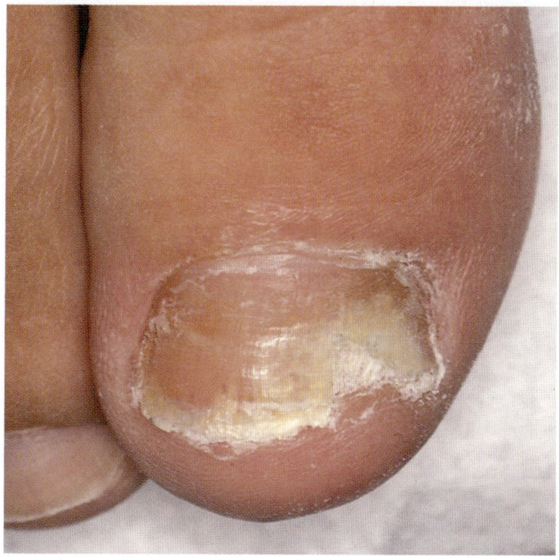

Fig. 8.65 Subungual Onychomycosis. (From Hordinsky MK, Sawaya ME, Scher RK: *Atlas of hair and nails*, Philadelphia, 2000, Churchill Livingstone.)

texture. It rarely resolves spontaneously; even with treatment, it may take months to years to clear. Figs. 8.65 and 8.66 show examples of distal and lateral subungual onychomycosis, the most common form of nail infection, caused by *Trichophyton rubrum*. Onychomycosis results in inflammation of the nail bed, which promotes hyperkeratosis of the nail bed epithelium and thickening. This may cause a lifting up of the nail plate, as shown in Fig. 8.67.

Pityriasis Rosea

Pityriasis rosea is a common, acute, self-limiting inflammatory disease of unknown cause that usually occurs during the spring. The generalized eruption is preceded by a "herald patch," a

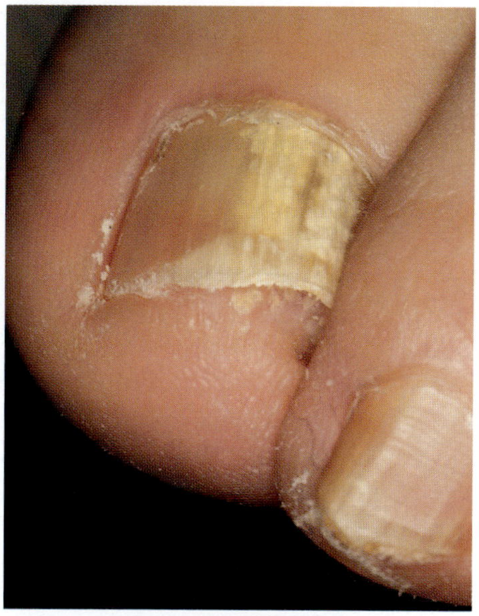

Fig. 8.66 Subungual Onychomycosis. (From Hordinsky MK, Sawaya ME, Scher RK: *Atlas of hair and nails*, Philadelphia, 2000, Churchill Livingstone.)

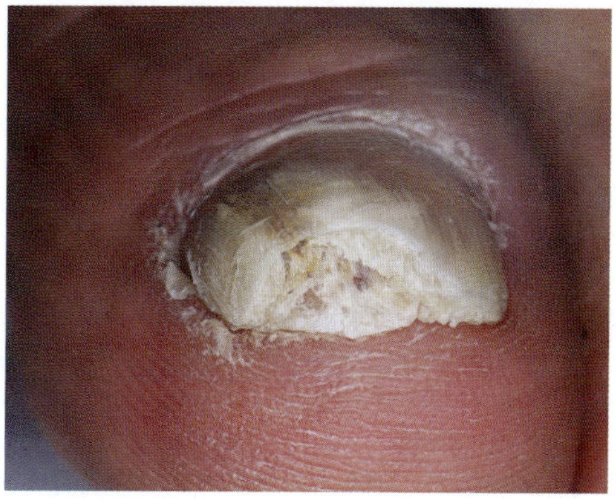

Fig. 8.67 Onychomycosis and Lifting of the Nail Plate. (From Hordinsky MK, Sawaya ME, Scher RK: *Atlas of hair and nails*, Philadelphia, 2000, Churchill Livingstone.)

single lesion resembling tinea corporis. After several days, the generalized eruption appears. Papulosquamous plaques appear over the trunk and rarely on the face and distal extremities. Although patients may complain of mild itching, they feel pretty well. The full-blown picture develops slowly over 5 to 10 days and lasts approximately 3 to 6 weeks. Slight hyperkeratosis of the epidermis with moderate dermal perivascular infiltration occurs. Fig. 8.68 shows a herald patch, and the characteristic lesions of pityriasis rosea, and Fig. 8.69 illustrates a cross-sectional view. Notice the delicate scale at the border of the annular lesion. Secondary syphilis may manifest with a similar eruption. It is, therefore, essential to order a serologic test for syphilis in any individual with pityriasis rosea.

Herpes Zoster

Herpes zoster, or shingles, is an intraepidermal vesicular eruption in a dermatomal distribution. Bullae and multinucleated giant cells are present in the epidermis, with perivascular

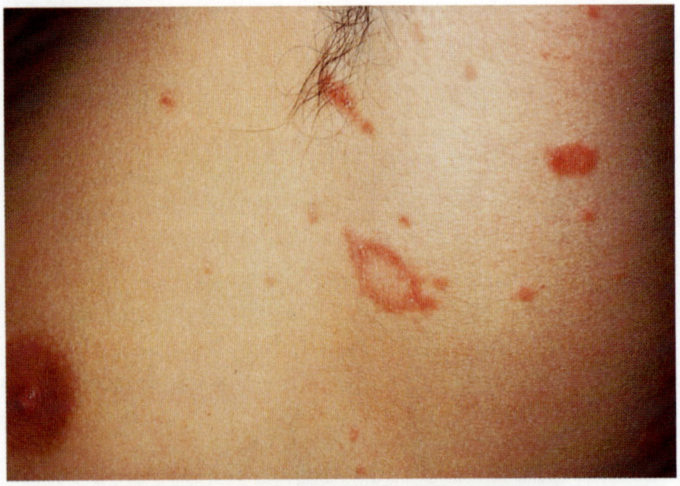

Fig. 8.68 Pityriasis Rosea. Note the herald patch.

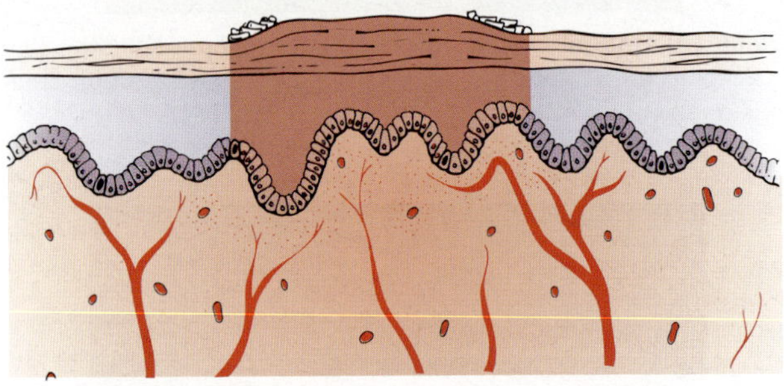

Fig. 8.69 Cross-Section Through a Lesion of Pityriasis Rosea.

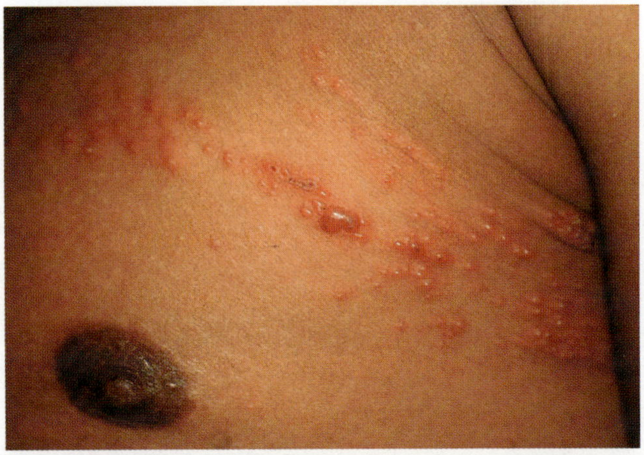

A

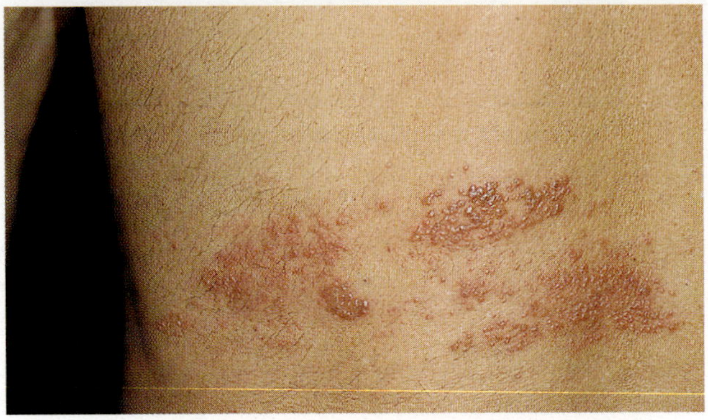

B

Fig. 8.70 (A and B) Herpes zoster lesions in T3 distribution. (From Callen JP, Paller AS, Greer KE, et al: *Color atlas of dermatology*, ed 2, Philadelphia, 2000, WB Saunders.)

inflammation of the dermis. The activation of the varicella-zoster virus causes the condition. Groups of vesicles and bullae on erythematous bases are present along the distribution of peripheral nerves. Severe pain often precedes the eruption. Fig. 8.70 shows herpes zoster lesions along the T3 distribution in two patients. Usually, the distribution occurs along the spinal or cranial nerves, but it can become generalized, as pictured in Fig. 8.71; Fig. 8.72 illustrates a cross-section. Fig. 8.73 is a close-up photograph of the typical vesicles on an erythematous base in a dermatomal distribution.

Herpesvirus

Herpesvirus infections are frequently encountered in patients with HIV infection; approximately 25% to 50% of these patients have some form of herpetic disease during their illness. Herpesvirus infections are thought to predict future progression from HIV infection to AIDS; the rate of this association with progression is 23% at 2 years and up to 73% at 6 years. When $CD4^+$ T-cell counts fall to fewer than 100 cells/mm^3, the likelihood of a herpesvirus infection approaches 95%. Herpes zoster infections may be severe and fulminant in immunocompromised patients, such as in the patient shown in Fig. 10.62.

Acne

Acne is a pustular disease affecting the hair follicles and sebaceous glands. Pustules, papules, and comedones are the primary lesions in this condition. There are collections of intradermal

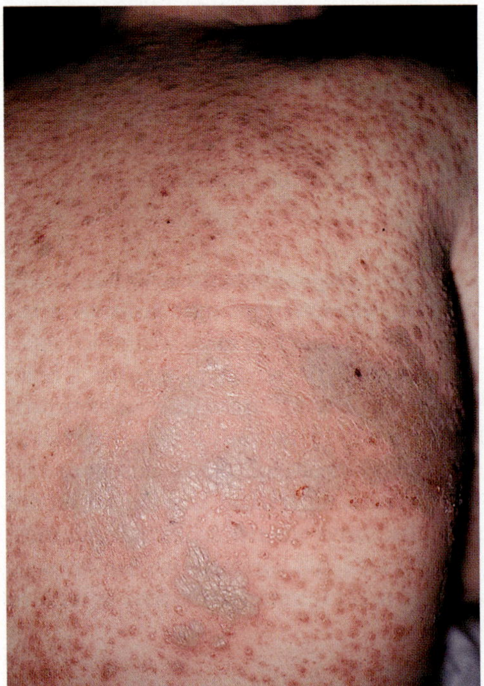

Fig. 8.71 Herpes Zoster, Generalized. (From Callen JP, Paller AS, Greer KE, et al: *Color atlas of dermatology*, ed 2, Philadelphia, 2000, WB Saunders.)

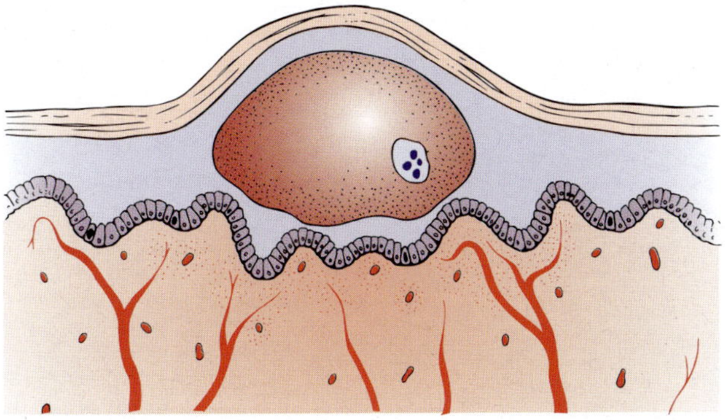

Fig. 8.72 Cross-Section Through One of the Vesicles in Herpes Zoster. Note the large epidermal bullae with the classic multinuclear cells.

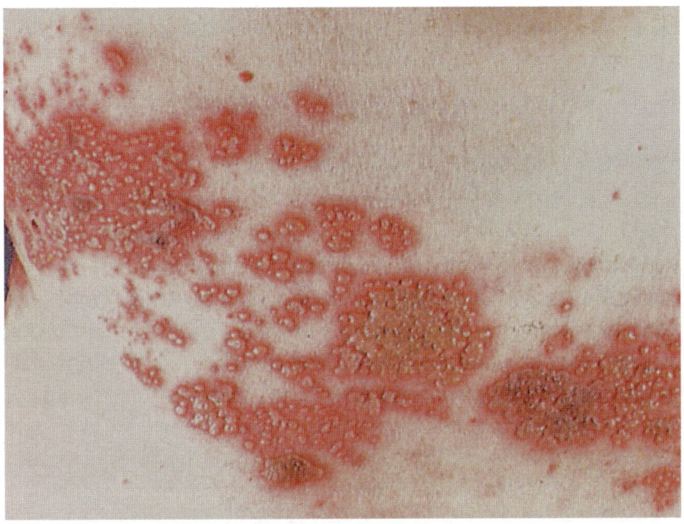

Fig. 8.73 Herpes Zoster Vesicle. (From Friedman-Kien AE, Cockerell CJ (eds): *Color atlas of AIDS*, ed 2, Philadelphia, 1996, WB Saunders.)

and intrafollicular neutrophils. Within the dermis, the hair follicle is occluded by a collection of keratin, sebum, and inflammatory cells. In addition, the hair follicle often ruptures into the dermis due to increasing pressure, which leads to further dermal inflammation (Figs. 8.74 to 8.77).

Tinea Versicolor

Tinea versicolor is a common superficial, noninflammatory, noncontagious fungal skin infection of young adults, most often during the summer. Pregnancy, warm climate, corticosteroids, and debilitation are predisposing factors. Persons older than 40 years are rarely affected. The lesion consists of fine, scaly patches that coalesce as they enlarge. The hypopigmented lesions are frequently seen on seborrheic areas of the body: the neck; the upper trunk; the upper arms; the shoulders; and, on occasion, the groin. The lesions are usually asymptomatic but may be mildly pruritic. Fig. 8.78 shows a patient's back with the classic hypopigmented patches of tinea versicolor. Fig. 8.79 shows another patient with tinea versicolor.

Ganglion Cyst

A *ganglion cyst,* also known as a *Bible cyst,* is a chronic, painless lesion on the dorsum of the wrist or ankle. It results from the

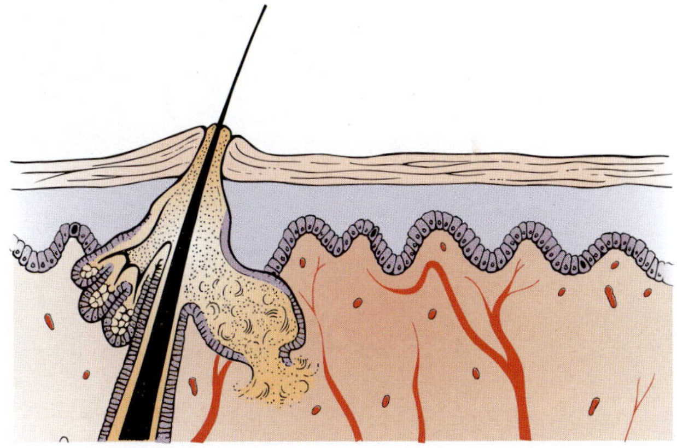

Fig. 8.74 Cross-Section Through an Area of Acne. Note the rupturing of the sebaceous gland in the dermis as a result of a plugged hair follicle, which results in dermal inflammation.

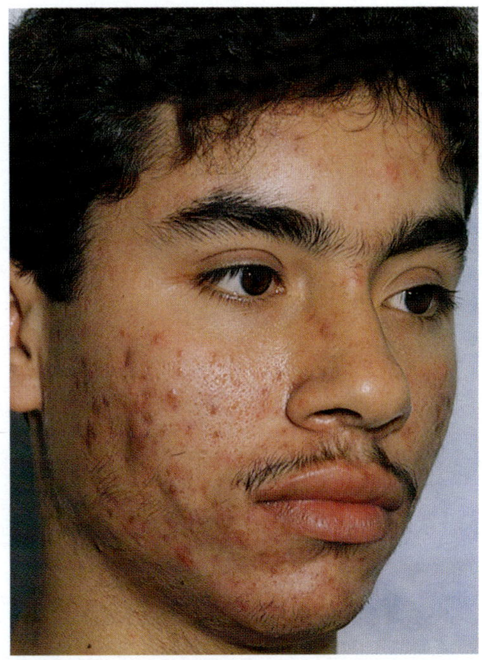

Fig. 8.75 Acne.

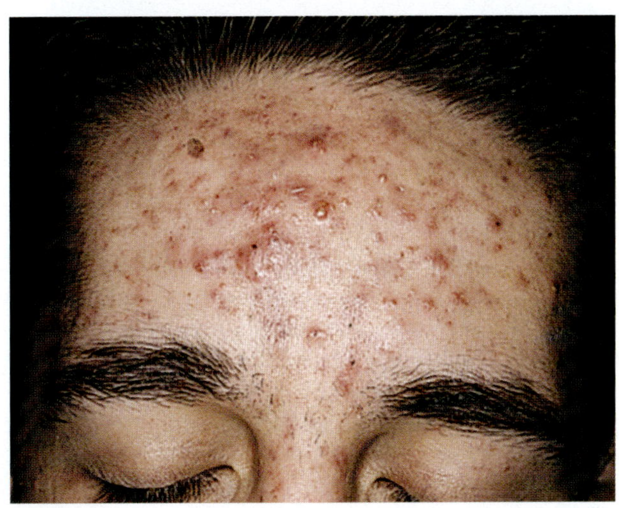

Fig. 8.76 Acne. (From Callen JP, Paller AS, Greer KE, et al: *Color atlas of dermatology*, ed 2, Philadelphia, 2000, WB Saunders.)

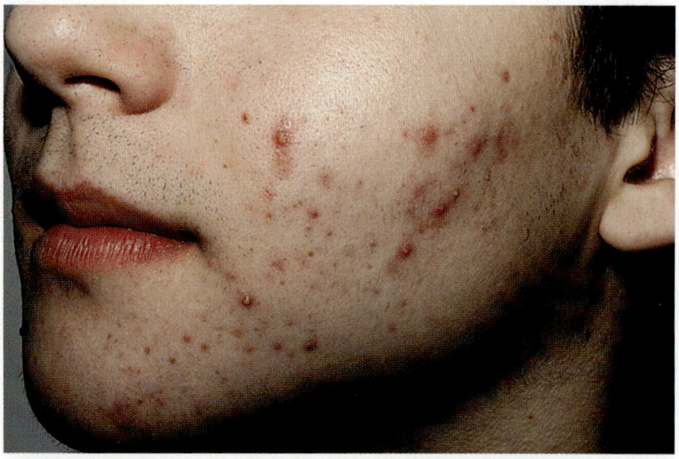

Fig. 8.77 Acne. (From Callen JP, Paller AS, Greer KE, et al: *Color atlas of dermatology*, ed 2, Philadelphia, 2000, WB Saunders.)

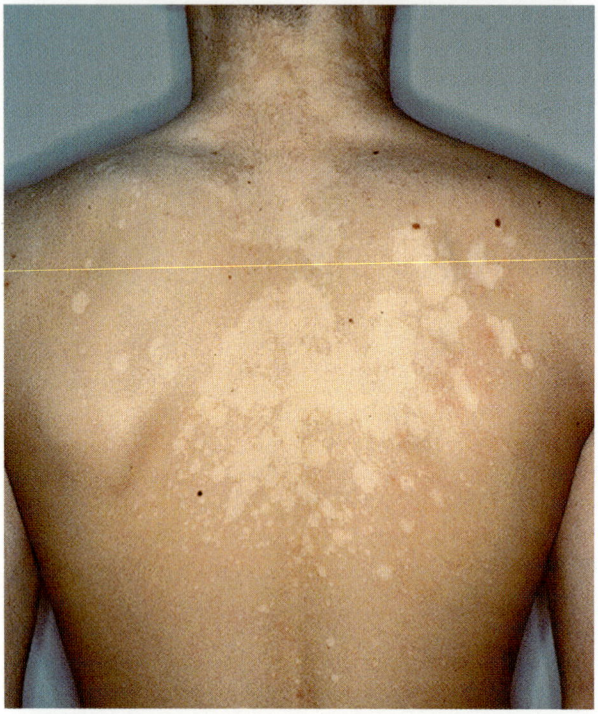

Fig. 8.78 Tinea Versicolor. (From Callen JP, Greer KE, Hood AF, et al: *Color atlas of dermatology*, Philadelphia, 1993, WB Saunders.)

synovial fluid leakage through the joint capsule's tendon sheath. This fluid eventually becomes encapsulated, and a cyst results. The term *Bible cyst* is derived from a standard treatment of hitting the cyst with a Bible or similarly large book. Striking the ganglion cyst with a hefty tome is usually sufficient to rupture the cyst, and reaccumulation is uncommon. Ganglion cysts are more common in females, and 70% occur in people between 20 and 40. Rarely, ganglion cysts can occur in children younger than 10 years. Multiple small cysts can give the appearance of more than one cyst, but a common stalk within the deeper tissue usually connects them. This type of cyst is not harmful and accounts for approximately half of all soft tissue tumors of the hand. Fig. 8.80 shows a large ganglion cyst of the wrist, the typical location.

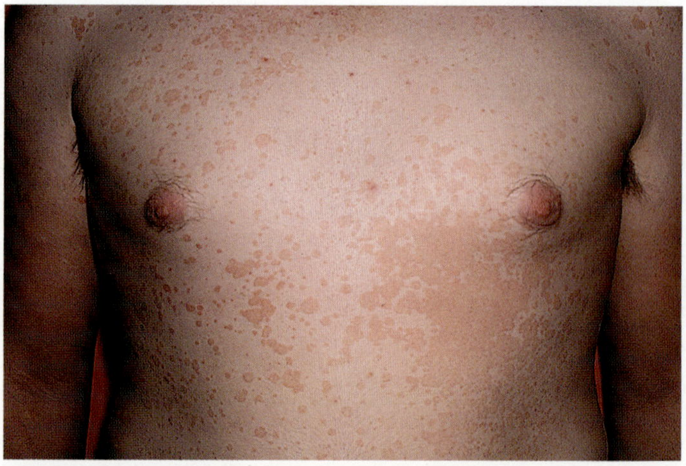

Fig. 8.79 Tinea Versicolor. (From Callen JP, Paller AS, Greer KE, et al: *Color atlas of dermatology*, ed 2, Philadelphia, 2000, WB Saunders.)

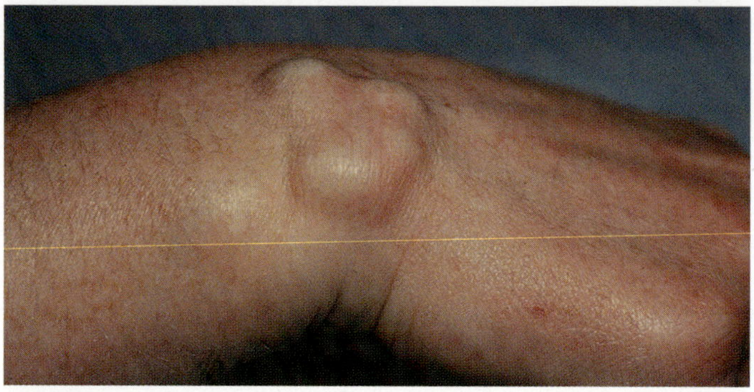

Fig. 8.80 Ganglion Cyst. (From Callen JP, Greer KE, Hood AF, et al: *Color atlas of dermatology*, Philadelphia, 1993, WB Saunders.)

Spider Angioma

A *spider angioma* is a typical pale red lesion, usually less than 2 cm in diameter, with a pulsating central arteriole, often raised, surrounded by erythema and radiating "legs." If pressure is exerted on the main body, the spider's legs blanching occurs. These benign lesions are commonly seen on the face, neck, arms, and upper trunk but rarely on the lower extremities. Although seen in normal individuals, spider angiomas are found more commonly in pregnant females and in patients with liver disease or vitamin B deficiency. These angiomas frequently become more evident during a female's menstrual cycle. Fig. 8.81 shows a spider angioma on the face of a young female. Notice the central arteriole with the peripheral blush.

Vitiligo

Vitiligo consists of patches of lightened skin resulting from the destruction of the pigment-producing cells (melanocytes); this condition is often autoimmune. It can also be hereditary or related to a trigger effect such as sunburn, stress, or exposure to a toxic substance. Vitiligo is a large macule that is depigmented. The epidermis manifests a complete absence of pigment, whereas the dermis is normal. Vitiligo can occur in any area,

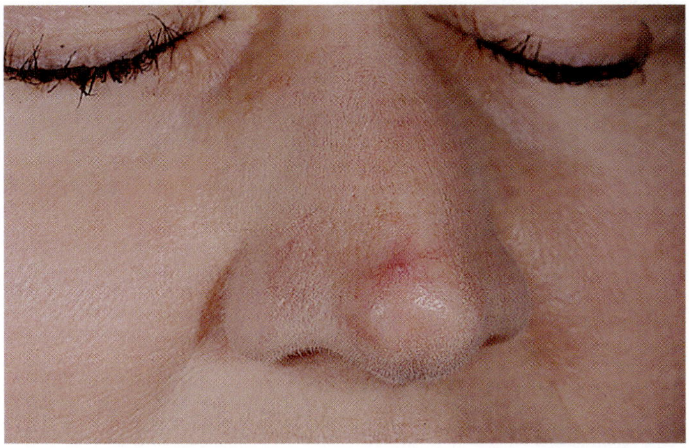

Fig. 8.81 Spider Angioma. (From Callen JP, Paller AS, Greer KE, et al: *Color atlas of dermatology*, ed 2, Philadelphia, 2000, WB Saunders.)

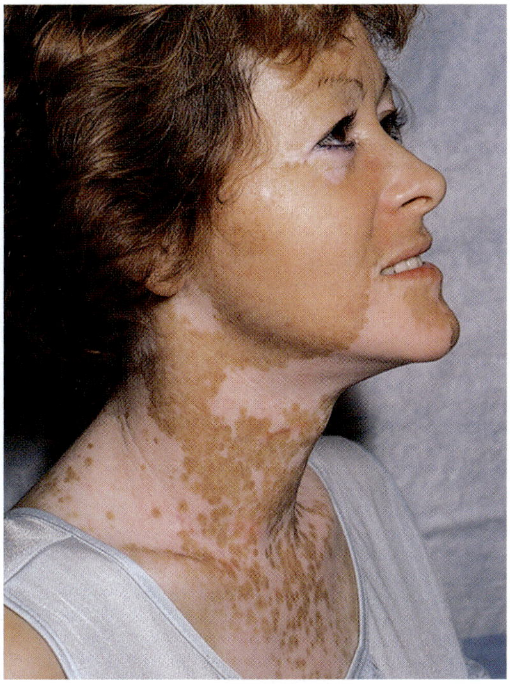

Fig. 8.82 Vitiligo.

but it is commonly found on the neck, knees, elbows, and back of the hands. Fig. 8.82 shows extensive vitiligo on the face and neck; a cross-section is shown in Fig. 8.83. Diffuse vitiligo is pictured in the patient shown in Fig. 8.84.

Urticaria

Urticaria is a common condition. The primary lesion is the wheal or hive. In urticaria, the epidermis is normal. The dermis demonstrates papillary edema. Inflammatory cells may be found surrounding dilated blood vessels. Itching is a common concern. There are several mechanisms for developing urticaria, including immunologic and nonimmunologic causes. Regardless of the reason, the common factor is the release of substances, such as histamine, that change vascular permeability and produce dermal edema. Fig. 8.85 shows urticaria, and Fig. 8.86 depicts the cross-section.

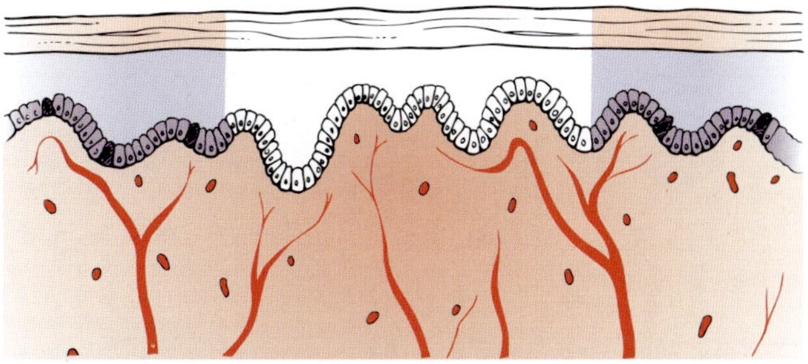

Fig. 8.83 Cross-Section Through an Area of Vitiligo. Note the absence of melanocytes and skin pigment.

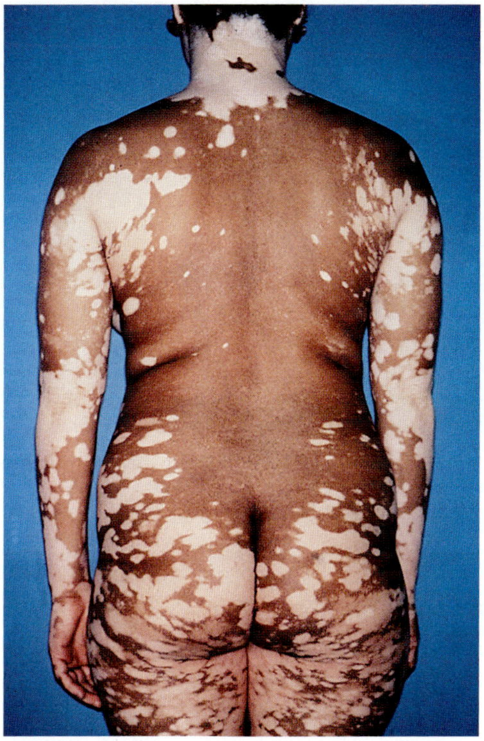

Fig. 8.84 Diffuse Vitiligo. (From Callen JP, Paller AS, Greer KE, et al: *Color atlas of dermatology*, ed 2, Philadelphia, 2000, WB Saunders.)

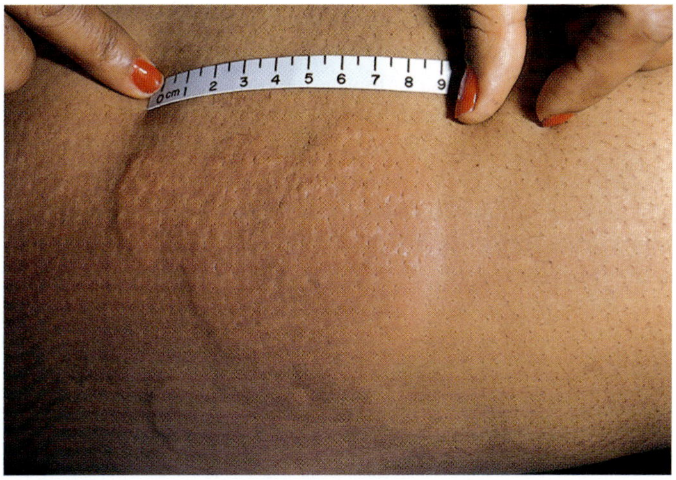

Fig. 8.85 Urticaria.

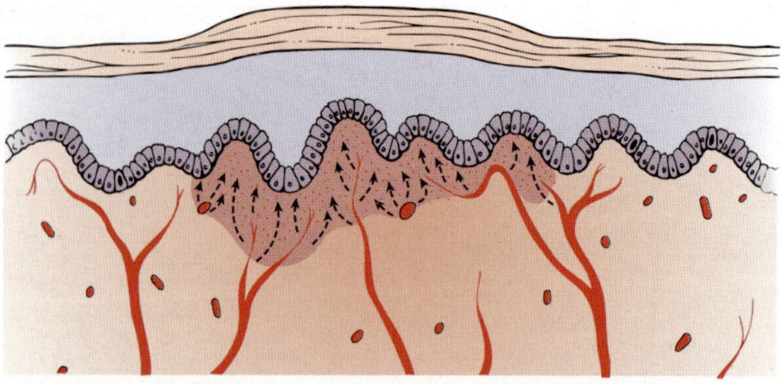

Fig. 8.86 Cross-Section Through an Area of Urticaria.

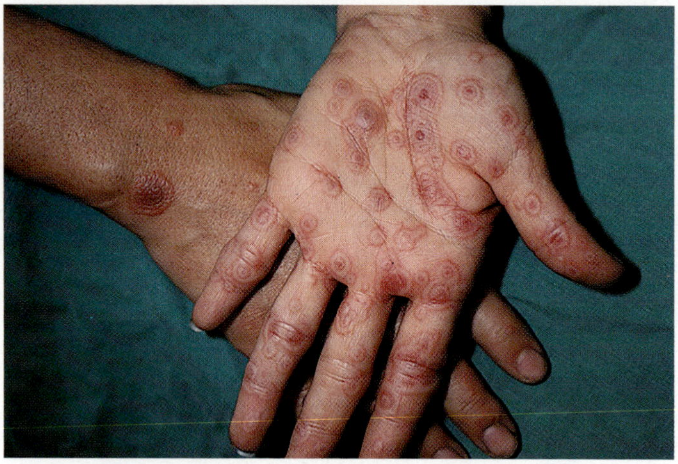

Fig. 8.87 Target Lesions on Palms and Hands in a Patient With Erythema Multiforme. (From Callen JP, Paller AS, Greer KE, et al: *Color atlas of dermatology*, ed 2, Philadelphia, 2000, WB Saunders.)

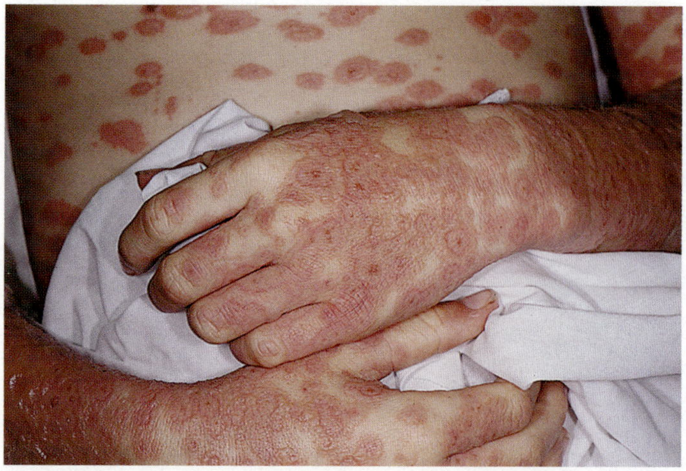

Fig. 8.88 Erythema Multiforme. (From Callen JP, Paller AS, Greer KE, et al: *Color atlas of dermatology*, ed 2, Philadelphia, 2000, WB Saunders.)

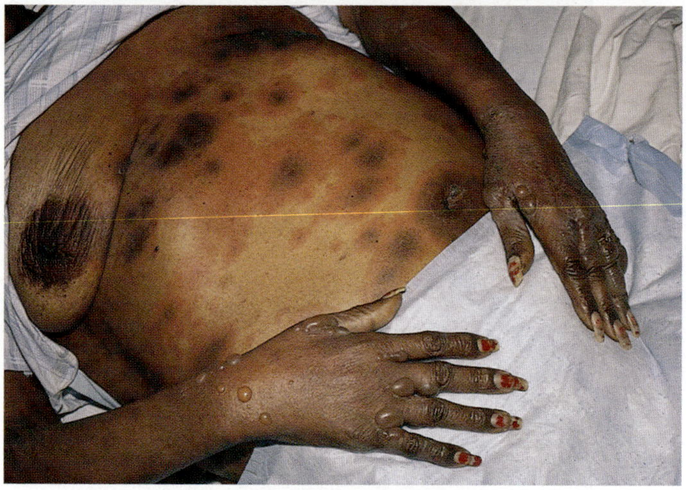

Fig. 8.89 Erythema Multiforme.

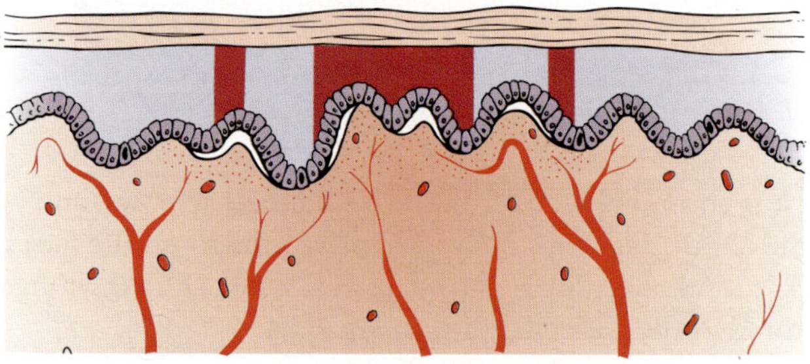

Fig. 8.90 Cross-Section Through an Area of Erythema Multiforme. Note the separation of the epidermis from the dermis.

Erythema Multiforme

Erythema multiforme is an immunologic reaction in the skin triggered by various causative agents, including viruses, bacteria, drugs, and x-radiation. In many cases, the agent cannot be identified. As the name implies, the condition includes a variety of lesions: papules, bullae, plaques, and "target lesions." Target lesions are diagnostic lesions and have three zones of color: A central, tense bulla, or dark area, is surrounded by a zone of relative pallor that is rimmed by a thin area of erythema. Typically, target lesions are seen on the palms and soles (Fig. 8.87). The epidermis is usually normal. The dermis has a subepidermal separation with inflammatory cells in the papillary dermis. Penicillin and sulfonamides are the drugs most commonly implicated as the cause of this condition. The most severe form of erythema multiforme—*Stevens-Johnson syndrome*—involves the mucous membranes. The classic skin lesions of erythema multiforme are shown in Figs. 8.88 and 8.89; Fig. 8.90 illustrates a cross-sectional view.

Scabies

Scabies is a common, intensely pruritic skin disorder caused by a mite, *Sarcoptes scabiei* var. *hominis*. The female mite burrows into the skin's stratum corneum and lays her eggs. A month or longer may pass before the symptom of generalized pruritus develops. The physical diagnostic sign is the burrow, a serpiginous, palpable track approximately 1 cm long that may end in a papule, nodule, or tiny vesicle. The adult female mite is present in the burrow. The *extremely pruritic rash* of scabies has a predilection for the web spaces of the fingers, toes, and groin. The buttocks are also frequently involved, as are the genitals of males and the nipples of females. A generalized papular or urticarial eruption may ensue after localized scabies infection. The presence of papules on the genitalia in a patient with intense pruritus

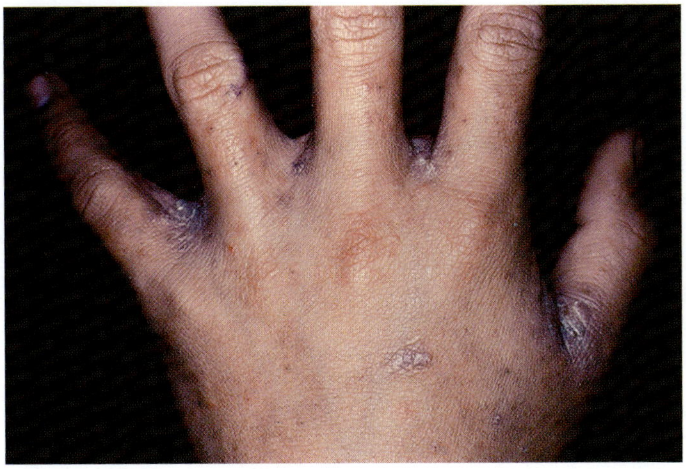

Fig. 8.91 Scabies.

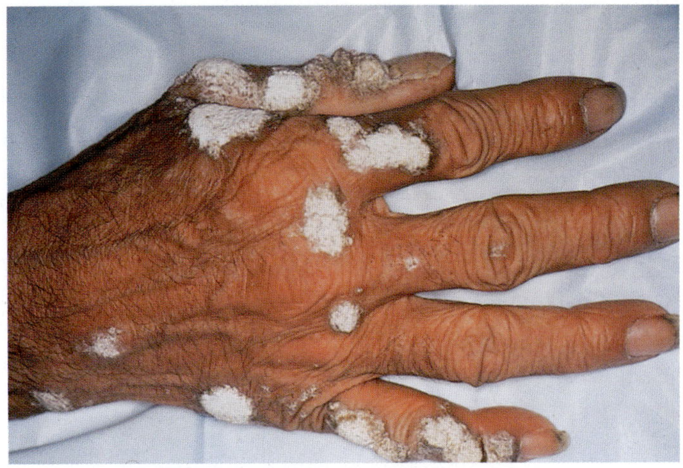

Fig. 8.92 Norwegian Scabies. (From Lebwohl MG, ed: *Atlas of the skin and systemic disease*, New York, 1995, Churchill Livingstone.)

should raise a strong suspicion of scabies. Outbreaks of scabies are common in population groups where HIV infection is prevalent. Fig. 8.91 shows the hand of a patient with scabies. Notice the classic eruption between the fingers. Fig. 18.16 shows another patient with scabies; the papular rash in the groin and on the penis is seen.

Norwegian scabies, also known as *crusted scabies,* is a rare, highly infectious form of scabies often seen in immunosuppressed patients, especially patients who are HIV positive, have lymphoma, who are cognitively impaired, or who are taking immunosuppressing medications. Unlike classical scabies, Norwegian scabies presents thick, exuding hyperkeratotic crusts with *less or no itching.* The dorsal aspects of the hands, the feet, and the extensor surfaces of the elbows and knees are commonly involved. In Norwegian scabies, there appears to be a problem with the immune response to the mites, allowing for the infestation of an individual with hundreds of thousands to millions of mites. The life cycle of the ectoparasite *Sarcoptes* is the same in classic and Norwegian scabies, but the incubation periods of the two vary broadly. In a previously unexposed person, symptoms of classic scabies take 4 to 6 weeks to appear, but in Norwegian scabies, they appear much faster, in 2 weeks at most. In addition, the number of mites present on the host body in the two cases differ significantly; compared with fewer than 20 mites in the case of classical scabies, Norwegian scabies, as mentioned, is associated with millions of mites in extreme cases. Fig. 8.92 shows the hand of a patient with Norwegian scabies. There have been many cases of Norwegian scabies in homeless AIDS patients reported, and this particular population is considered to be very susceptible to infection by the *Sarcoptes* mite. Neglected personal hygiene and impaired immune system lead to the development of highly contagious Norwegian scabies infection, which spreads to other individuals with a low immune state. Fig. 8.93 shows the diffuse lesions of Norwegian scabies in a homeless AIDS patient.

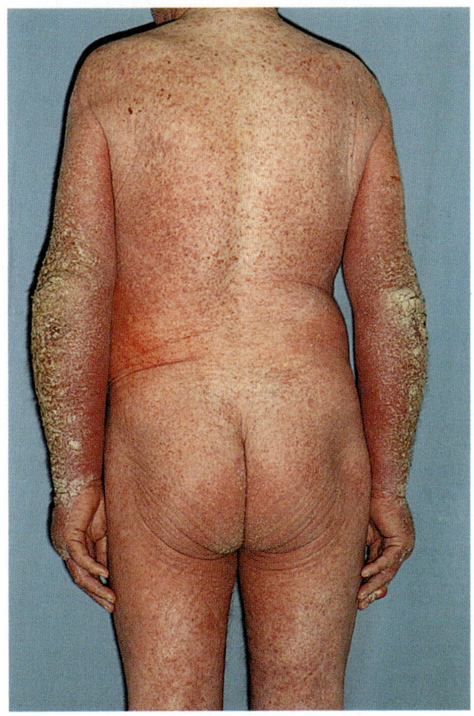

Fig. 8.93 Norwegian Scabies. (From Callen JP, Paller AS, Greer KE, et al: *Color atlas of dermatology*, ed 2, Philadelphia, 2000, WB Saunders.)

Pyoderma Gangrenosum

Pyoderma gangrenosum is an uncommon, ulcerative, cutaneous condition consisting of large, tender, necrotic ulcers having a violaceous, overhanging edge with a purulent base. Pyoderma gangrenosum occurs in approximately 1 in 100,000 persons annually in the United States. The exact cause is unknown. Although pyoderma gangrenosum affects both sexes, a slight female predominance may exist.

The disease may affect all ages, but it predominantly occurs in the fourth and fifth decades of life. The lesions are most frequently seen on the lower legs but can also be seen on the dorsal surface of the hands, the extensor parts of the forearms, or the face. It is associated with systemic diseases in at least 50% of affected patients. Although most often associated with inflammatory bowel disease, this condition is also associated with rheumatoid arthritis, various blood dyscrasias (especially

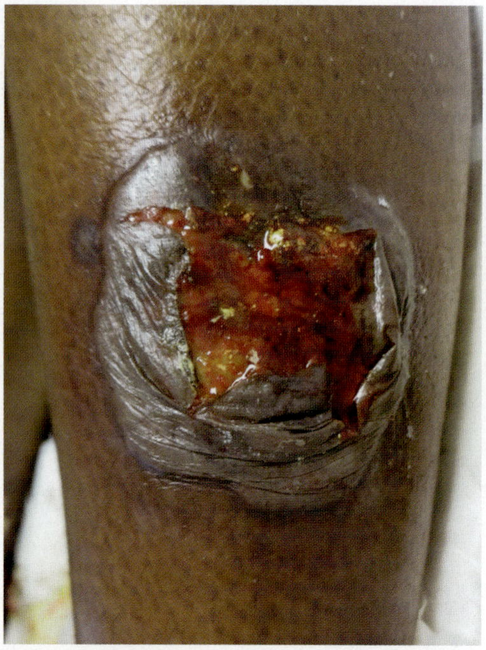

Fig. 8.94 Pyoderma Gangrenosum. (From Micheletti RB, Elston DM, James WD, et al: *Andrews' diseases of the skin clinical atlas*, ed 2, Philadelphia, 2023, Elsevier.)

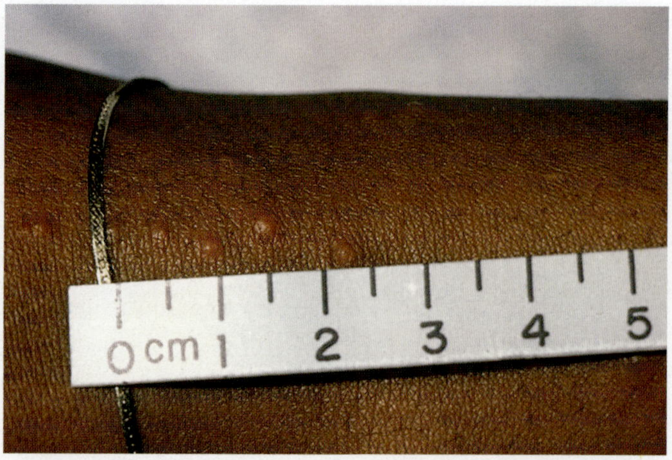

Fig. 8.95 Bedbug Bites.

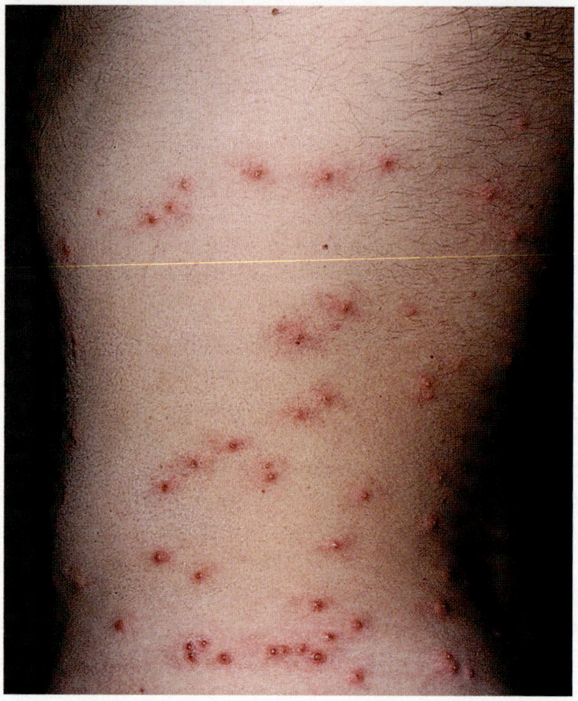

Fig. 8.96 Bedbug Bites. (From Callen JP, Paller AS, Greer KE, et al: *Color atlas of dermatology*, ed 2, Philadelphia, 2000, WB Saunders.)

multiple myeloma), chronic active hepatitis, systemic lupus erythematosus, and acute leukemias. However, approximately 10% of all patients with ulcerative colitis have cutaneous manifestations, especially pyoderma gangrenosum. The skin lesions of pyoderma gangrenosum are closely linked to bowel disease; exacerbations of bowel symptoms are associated with the extension of existing lesions or the development of new ones. Removal of the diseased bowel often leads to improvement in the cutaneous manifestations. Fig. 8.94 shows the classic shin lesions of pyoderma gangrenosum in a patient with Crohn disease. See also Fig. 17.5, which shows another patient with an exacerbation of ulcerative colitis and pyoderma gangrenosum of the shin.

Insect Bites

Insect bites are common and should always be considered when a patient complains of a pruritic rash. Papules, vesicles, and wheals amid excoriations suggest the diagnosis. Papules in a grouped or linear arrangement on an arm or face suggest *bedbug bites.* These insects, which live in crevices in furniture, shun the light and feed at night on exposed areas of the body. They bite and then move around, only to bite again. Fig. 8.95 shows the linear papules on the arm of a patient bitten by bedbugs. Fig. 8.96 shows another patient with persistent erythematous papules due to bedbug bites. *Flea bites* were the cause of the pruritic eruption on the feet of the patient shown in Fig. 8.97. Notice the excoriations. The lower legs and feet are common sites for flea bites. Local reactions to bites from toxic bugs look the same: redness, swelling, itching, and pain. Most *spider bites* are harmless, but occasionally, spider bites can cause severe allergic reactions. Bites by the venomous black widow and brown recluse spiders can be very dangerous to people. Fig. 8.98 shows the face of a female bitten under her left eye by a spider, possibly a jumping spider. The patient pulled the spider off her face and suffered immediate pain, itching, and edema lasting more than 4 days. The jumping spider is the most common biting spider in the United States. People are caught by surprise and scared when they see the spider jump, especially if it jumps toward them. Bites from a jumping spider are painful and itchy and cause redness and significant swelling. Other symptoms may include painful muscles and joints, headache, fever, chills, nausea, and vomiting. The symptoms usually last approximately 1 to 4 days.

Kaposi Sarcoma

Kaposi sarcoma (KS) is a neoplasm characterized by dark blue–purple macules, papules, nodules, and plaques. The *classic form*

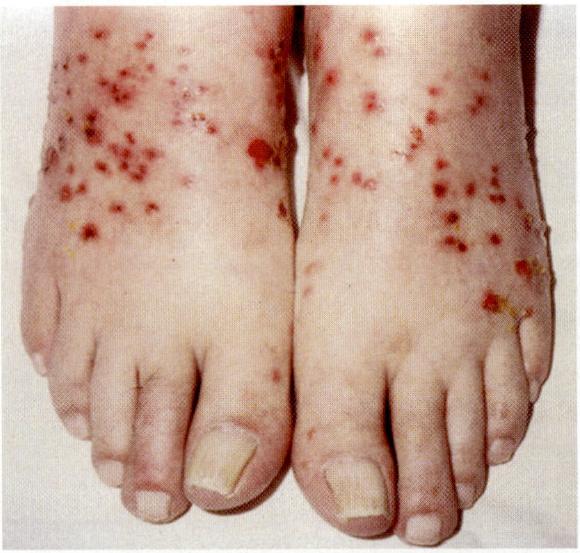

Fig. 8.97 Flea Bites. (From Callen JP, Greer KE, Hood AF, et al: *Color atlas of dermatology*, Philadelphia, 1993, WB Saunders.)

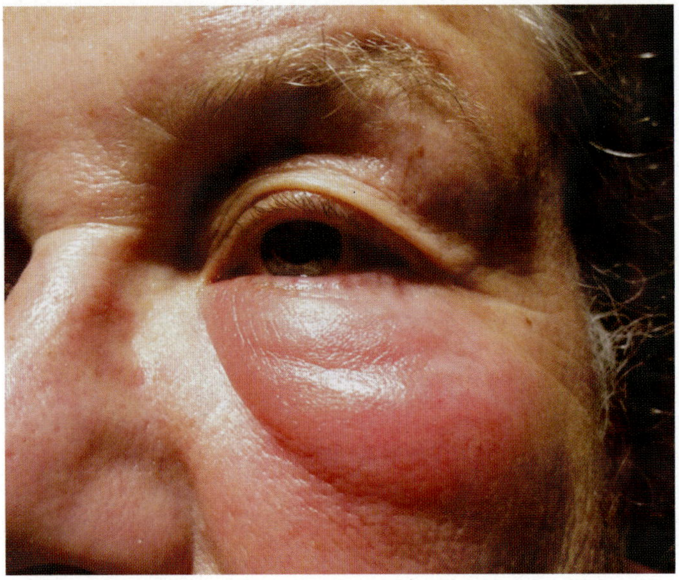

Fig. 8.98 Spider Bite to Lower Eyelid.

of the disease is a rare, slow-growing neoplasm occurring mainly on the lower extremities of older males of Mediterranean or Jewish Eastern European descent, especially the ankles, and soles. The male-to-female ratio is 10:1 to 15:1, and most patients are aged 60 to 80. Fig. 8.99 shows a large, reddish-colored plaque, which was slowly growing, on the sole of a 60-year-old male of Eastern European origin. Some patients with classic KS may develop another type of cancer before the KS lesions appear or even later in life. Most often, this second cancer is non-Hodgkin lymphoma.

Currently, the most common type of KS in the United States is *epidemic* or *AIDS-related KS*. This type of KS develops in people who are infected with HIV. A person infected with HIV does not necessarily have AIDS. The virus can be present in the body for a long time, typically many years, before causing major

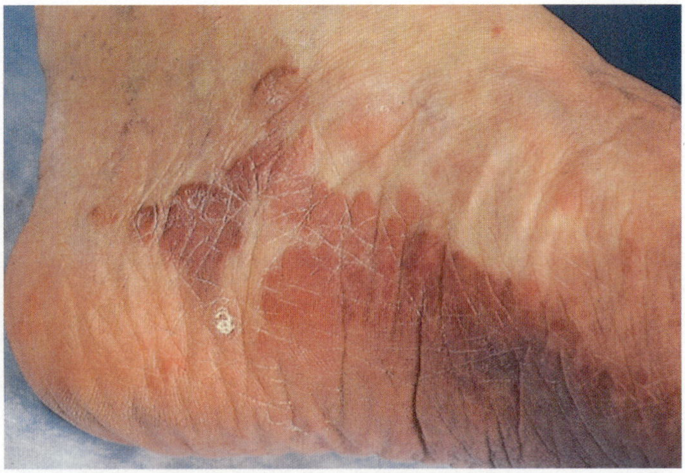

Fig. 8.99 Kaposi Sarcoma: A Classic Plaque. (From Friedman-Kien AE, Cockerell CJ (eds): *Color atlas of AIDS*, ed 2, Philadelphia, 1996, WB Saunders.)

illness. The disease known as AIDS begins when the virus has seriously damaged the immune system, which results in certain types of infections and other medical complications, including KS. When HIV damages the immune system, people infected with a particular virus (the KS herpesvirus) are more likely to develop KS. The risk of developing KS is closely linked to the CD4 count. The CD4 count is a measure of the effect of HIV on the immune system. The lower the CD4 count, the more likely the patient will develop KS. KS is considered an "AIDS-defining" illness, meaning that when KS occurs in someone infected with HIV, that person officially has AIDS (and is not just HIV positive).

Approximately 35% of patients with AIDS who acquired the disease by sexual contact are affected, as opposed to about 5% of patients whose infection was acquired from intravenous drug use. Overall, 24% of all patients with AIDS develop this rapidly progressive form of the disease, also known as the epidemic AIDS-related form. The widely disseminated lesions are present on the legs, trunk, arms, neck, and head. They start as light-colored papules or nodules and coalesce into larger, darker lesions. Unlike the classic form, the AIDS-related epidemic is commonly associated with visceral involvement, frequent oral lesions, and lymphadenopathy. In addition, this type of KS is different from other cancers in that lesions may begin in more than one place in the body simultaneously. The average length of patient survival from the onset of the disease is 18 months. The skin lesions of epidemic AIDS-related KS are shown in Fig. 8.100. Fig. 8.100A shows the typical lesions on the arm and chest; Fig. 8.100B shows the widely disseminated plaque lesions varying in color from dark red to violet; Fig. 8.100C shows a violaceous lesion on the lateral aspect of the lower eyelid; Fig. 8.100D shows a large confluent plaque of KS on the hard palate; and Fig. 8.100E shows a purplish-red, nodular lesion of KS on the gingiva and an infiltrative, violaceous lesion of the nose.

Fig. 8.101 demonstrates the rapidity of the growth of epidemic AIDS-related KS. The initial manifestation (Fig. 8.101A)

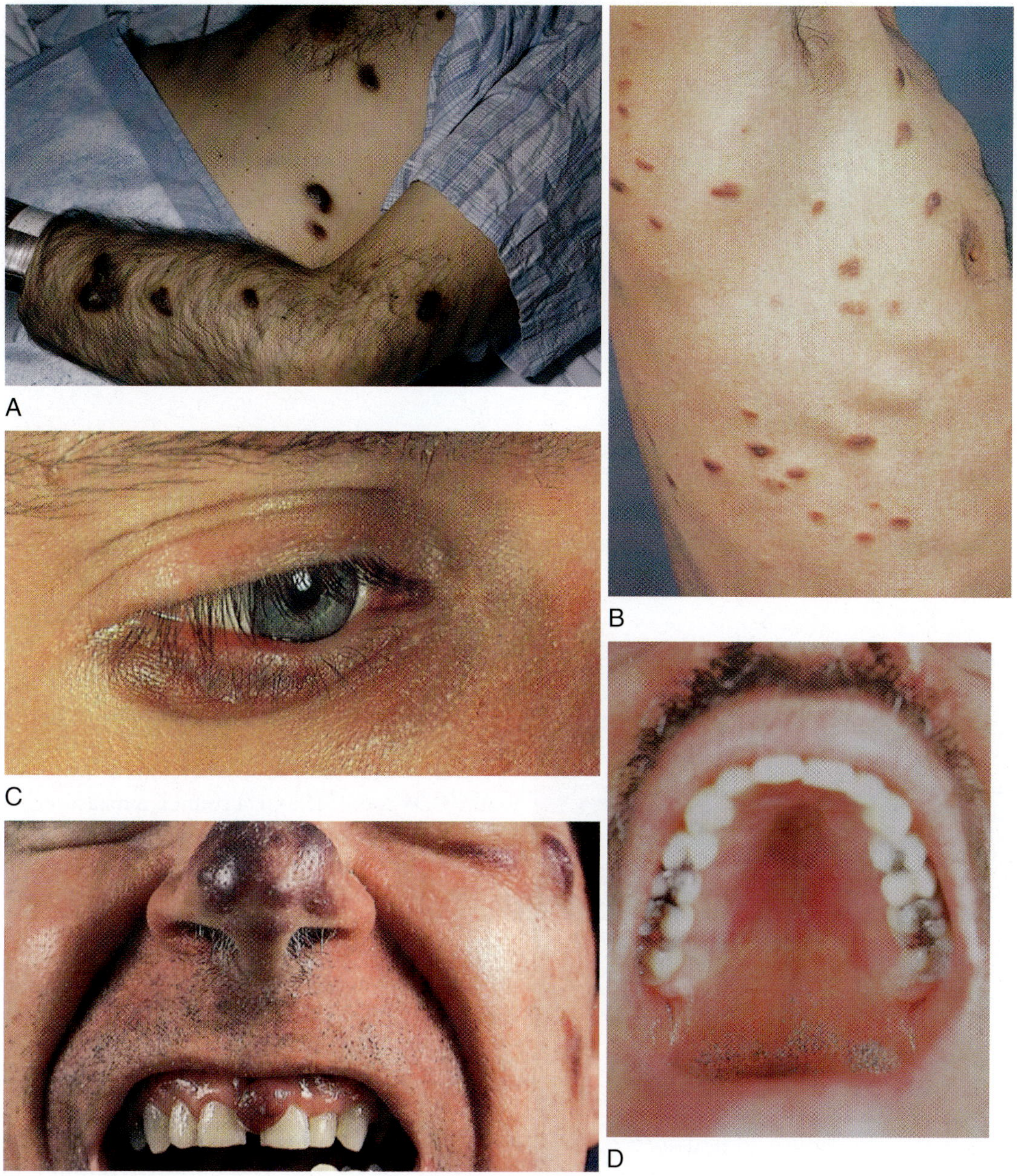

A B C D E

Fig. 8.100 Kaposi Sarcoma: Epidemic Human Immunodeficiency Virus Associated. (A and B) Plaque lesions. (C) Violaceous lesion affecting the lateral lower eyelid. (D) Confluent plaque on the hard palate. (E) Nodular lesion on the gingiva and the nose. (B to E, From Friedman-Kien AE, Cockerell CJ (eds): *Color atlas of AIDS*, ed 2, Philadelphia, 1996, WB Saunders.)

on the back of a 36-year-old male was only a few macular lesions of KS; a follow-up photograph, taken only 6 months later, shows the widely disseminated, purplish plaques of KS (Fig. 8.101B).

KS lesions are frequently seen on the feet. Fig. 8.102 shows a patient's foot who presented with this lesion between his fourth and fifth toes. A biopsy of the lesion confirmed the diagnosis of KS. This was the patient's first manifestation of AIDS. Fig. 8.103 shows the plantar arch of another patient who presented with painful nodules. Again, a biopsy confirmed the diagnosis of KS. KS of the heel is pictured in another patient in Fig. 8.104.

Mpox

Mpox, which was previously known as *monkeypox*, is an uncommon illness that results from being infected with the mpox virus. The virus that causes mpox is part of the same family of viruses as the variola virus, which is responsible for causing smallpox. The symptoms of mpox are like those of smallpox but are typically milder. Mpox, unlike smallpox, usually does not result in death.

The first recorded human case of mpox was in 1970. Prior to the outbreak in 2022, mpox had been reported in several central and western African countries. Almost all cases of mpox

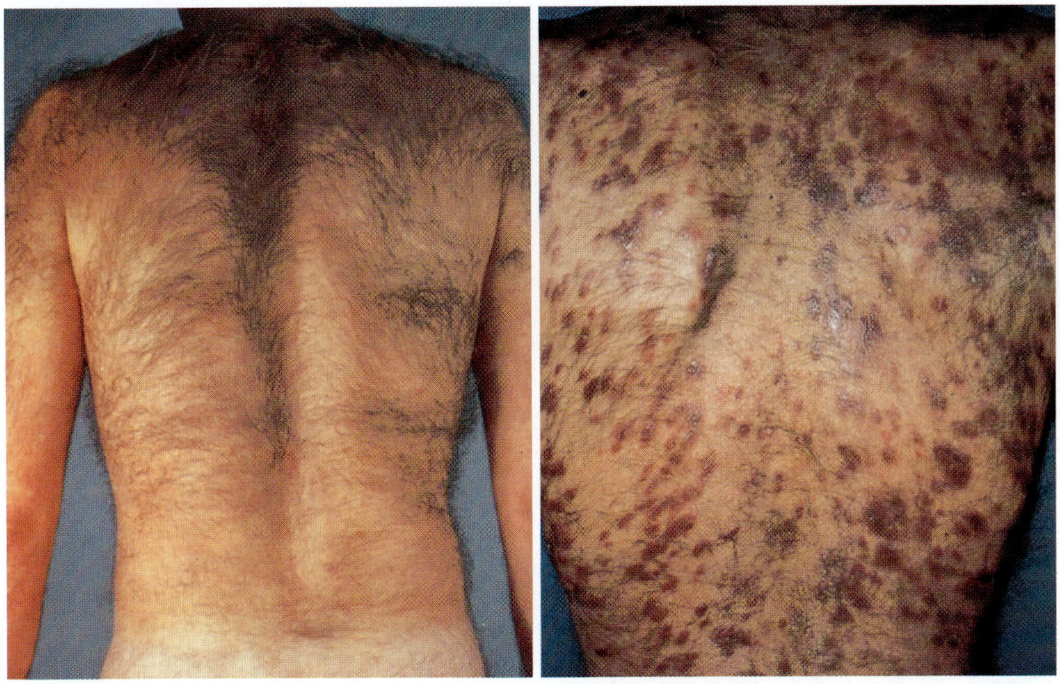

A B

Fig. 8.101 (A) Early lesions of Kaposi sarcoma on the back. (B) Follow-up photograph, 6 months later, showing the rapid development of purplish plaques of Kaposi sarcoma. (From Friedman-Kien AE, Cockerell CJ (eds): *Color atlas of AIDS*, ed 2, Philadelphia, 1996, WB Saunders.)

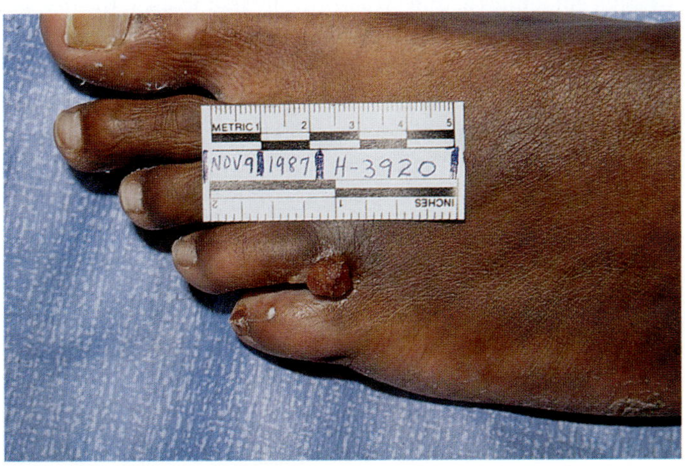

Fig. 8.102 Kaposi Sarcoma Between the Toes.

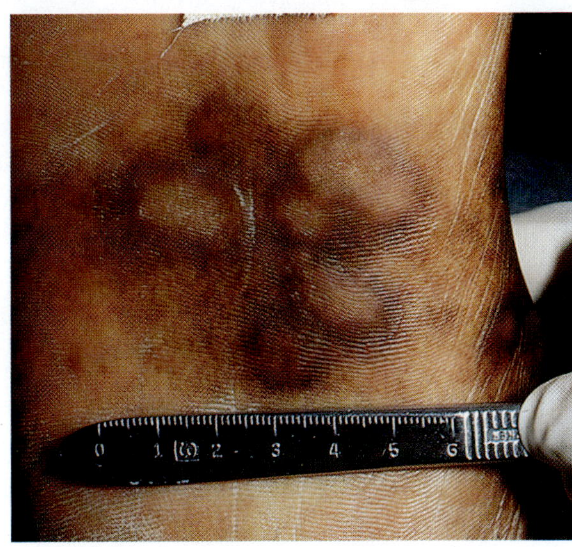

Fig. 8.103 Kaposi Sarcoma on the Plantar Arch of the Foot.

outside of Africa were previously linked to international travel to countries where the disease was common or through imported animals. However, in May 2022, an unprecedented global outbreak of mpox was detected, with cases rapidly increasing in the United States and peaking in August 2022. As of the end of October 2023, there were 32,782 cases and 60 deaths due to mpox in the United States, and globally, there were 95,912 cases. It is worth noting that individuals living with HIV are disproportionately affected by the current outbreak of mpox.

Symptoms of mpox include a skin rash or mucosal lesions lasting 2 to 4 weeks, fever, headache, muscle aches, back pain, fatigue, and swollen lymph nodes. The rash may be anywhere on the body (Fig. 8.105A), including the penis, testicles, labia, vagina, and anus. See Fig. 8.105B. The rash starts as a small, red macule, which, over the time of 3 to 4 days, develops into papules with a diameter of 3 to 4 mm. After 4 to 5 days, the papules then develop into vesicles with a diameter of 2 to 5 mm. The pustules last for 5 to 8 days before umbilication (Fig. 8.105C) and crusting. The incubation period is 3 to 17 days. During this time, a person does not have symptoms and may feel fine. A person with mpox can spread it to others from when symptoms start until the rash has fully healed and a fresh layer of skin has formed.

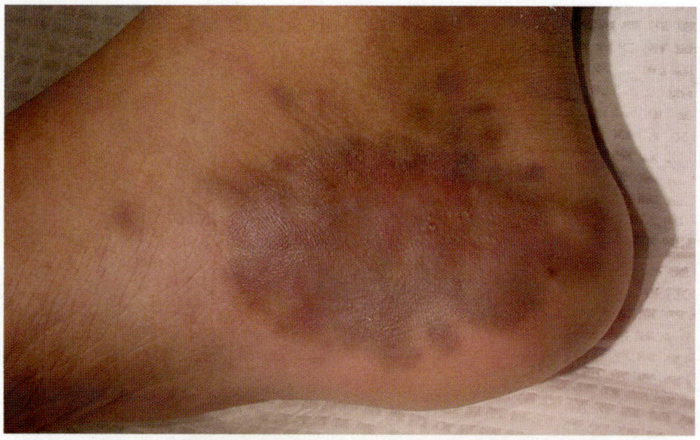

Fig. 8.104 Kaposi Sarcoma on the Heel of the Foot.

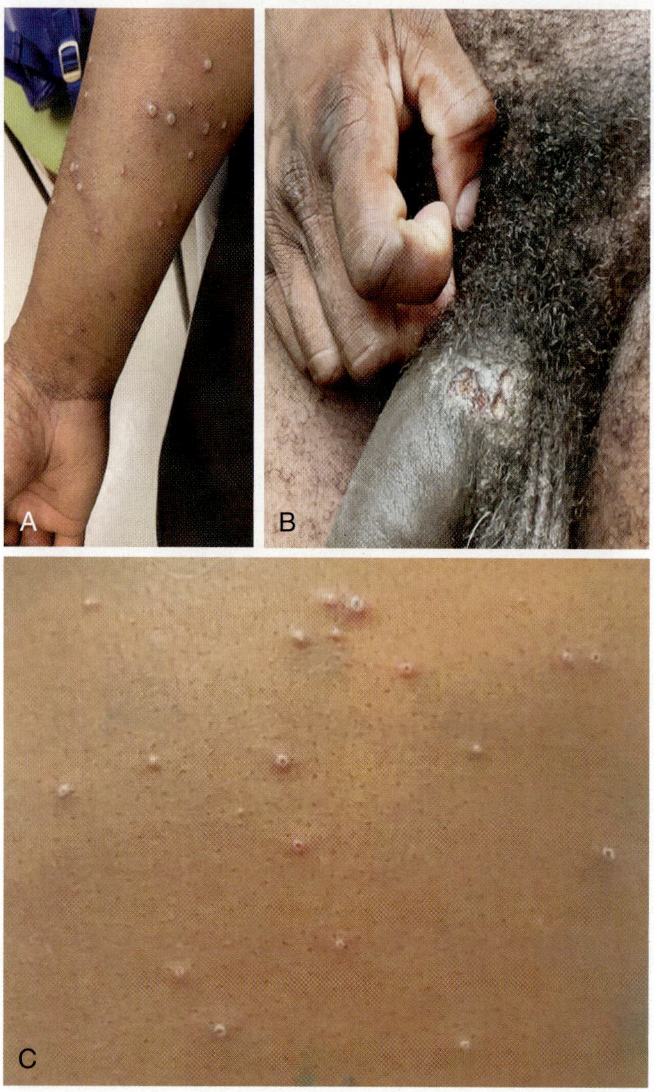

Fig. 8.105 Mpox lesions. (Courtesy of Richard Silvera, MD, MPH.)

Mpox can spread to anyone through close, personal, skin-to-skin contact, including direct contact with mpox rash and scabs from a person with mpox, as well as contact with their saliva, upper respiratory secretions, and areas around the anus, rectum, or vagina. This direct contact can happen during intimate contact, including oral, anal, or vaginal sex, or touching the genitals or anus of a person with mpox as well as with hugging, massage, and kissing. The diagnosis of monkeypox frequently requires laboratory confirmation.

Studies have revealed that individuals with weakened immune systems, either due to medication or medical conditions, are at a higher risk of severe illness and death caused by mpox. Individuals living with HIV that is not well controlled or not being treated are more susceptible to developing severe symptoms. It is unclear if having HIV increases the chances of contracting the mpox virus upon exposure. However, it is a known fact that individuals with advanced or untreated HIV (i.e., immunocompromised individuals) are at an increased risk of severe mpox and death if they contract the virus. Limited data suggests that individuals with HIV, especially those with low CD4 counts (<350 cells/mL) or who are not virally suppressed, have a higher likelihood of being hospitalized and potentially dying if they contract mpox compared to those without HIV. Therefore, the Centers for Disease Control and Prevention (CDC) strongly recommends that all people living with HIV get vaccinated against mpox. Vaccination is an important tool in stopping the spread of mpox. The CDC recommends that individuals at risk have the two-dose vaccine before attending any gathering where mpox may be present.

The current association of HIV and mpox is known as a *syndemic.* A syndemic is the aggregation of concurrent or sequential epidemics acting synergistically that worsen the disease burden. The CDC defines syndemics simply as "synergistically interacting epidemics." One medical example of a syndemic was the 1918–1919 influenza pandemic, which involved interactions between diseases caused by two different kinds of pathogens: viruses and bacteria. The current association of HIV and mpox is a syndemic. Syndemics consider not only health disorders that occur in communities but also the fact that the diseases may be worsened by their socioeconomic and environmental milieu, such as substance misuse (e.g., alcohol, smoking, etc.), aging, or poverty, as examples.

Scleroderma

Scleroderma, also known as *progressive systemic sclerosis,* is an autoimmune, connective tissue disease that involves changes in the skin, blood vessels, muscles, and internal organs characterized by skin hardening. There is a broad spectrum of disease manifestations of scleroderma, ranging from limited skin lesions associated with *c*alcinosis, *R*aynaud phenomenon, *e*sophageal motility problems, *s*clerodactyly, and *t*elangiectasia (referred to as the *CREST variant*) to full encasement of the body by diffuse sclerosis. The cause of scleroderma is unknown. People with this condition have a buildup of collagen in the skin and other organs. This buildup leads to the symptoms of the disease. The disease usually affects people 30 to 50 years old. Females get scleroderma more often than males. Some people with scleroderma have a history of being around silica dust and polyvinyl chloride, but most do not. Vascular changes occur with visceral involvement and involve the microvessels and small arteries. The onset of the disease is often heralded by the development of the Raynaud phenomenon, which is discussed in Chapter 15, The Peripheral Vascular System.

The cutaneous manifestations of scleroderma involve tightening of the skin, especially on the face and hands, due to tendon contractures, and flexion of the fingers results. The fingers of a patient with scleroderma are shown in Fig. 8.106; notice that the skin is bound tightly and obscures the superficial vasculature. Skin lines are absent. Fig. 8.107 shows the face of the same patient. Notice the tightening and wrinkling of the skin around her mouth and the fixed, expressionless countenance due to the flattening of the nasolabial folds. The patient had great difficulty in opening her mouth. The skin around the mouth has many furrows radiating outward, creating a mouse-like appearance known as *mauskopf.*

Calcification of the soft tissues can produce a stony-hard tissue and range from a small area of involvement to massive calcium deposits. Fig. 8.108A shows the Raynaud phenomenon and calcinosis cutis in a patient with the CREST syndrome. Note the telangiectases of the fingertips. Fig. 8.108B shows calcinosis cutis of the heel in the same patient. The distal finger pad commonly assumes a tapered appearance, with a tuft of scarred tissue between the fingertip and the nail bed. Ulceration can also occur, which can lead to osteomyelitis. Fig. 8.109 shows the plantar view of the hallux in the same patient with CREST syndrome; note the characteristic tapering of the digit and pterygium inversus (growth of soft tissue along the ventral aspect of the nail plate).

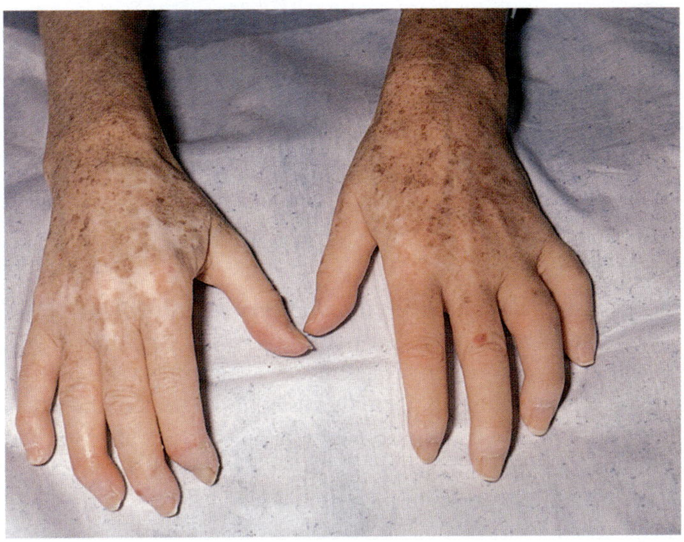

Fig. 8.106 Scleroderma: Hands.

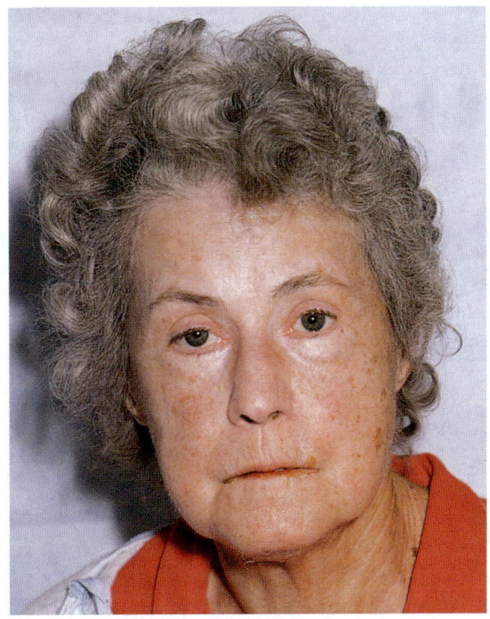

Fig. 8.107 Scleroderma: Face.

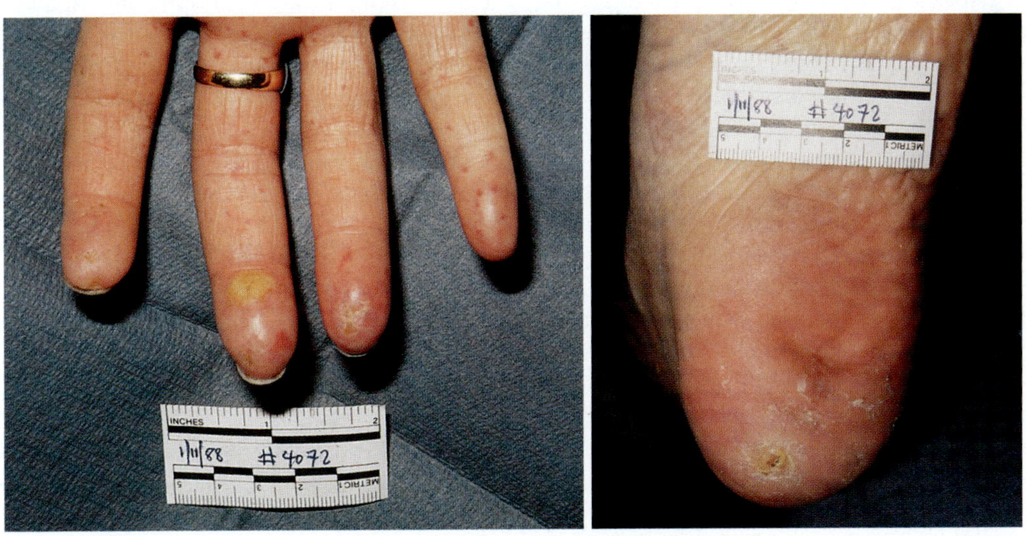

A B

Fig. 8.108 **C**alcinosis, **R**aynaud phenomenon, **e**sophageal motility problems, **s**clerodactyly, and **t**elangiectasia (CREST) syndrome. (A) Telangiectases of the fingertips. (B) Calcinosis cutis of the heel.

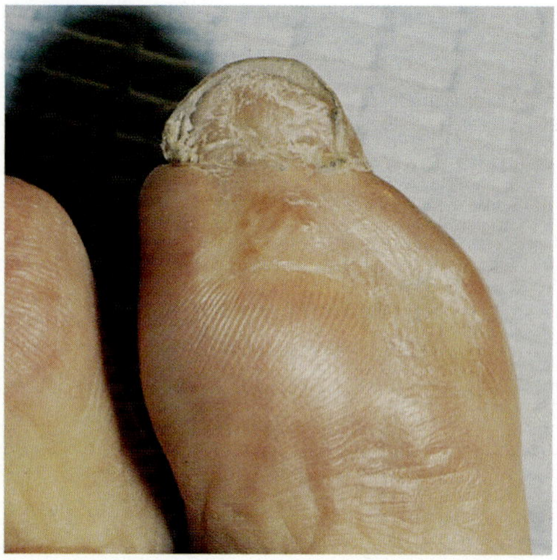

Fig. 8.109 **C**alcinosis, **R**aynaud phenomenon, **e**sophageal motility problems, **s**clerodactyly, and **t**elangiectasia (CREST) syndrome. With tapered digit and pterygium inversus. (From Kosinski MA, Stewart D: Nail changes associated with systemic disease and vascular insufficiency, *Clin Podiatr Med Surg* 6:295–318, 1989.)

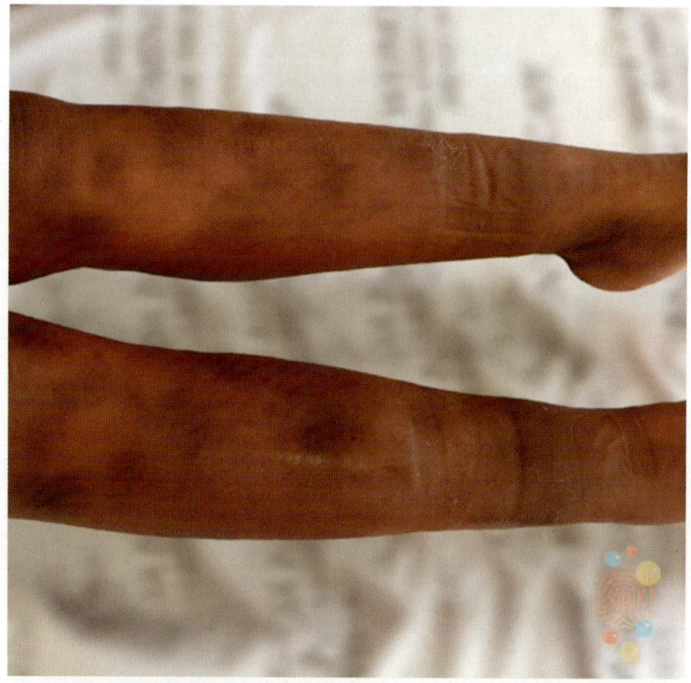

Fig. 8.110 Erythema Nodosum. (From Drake M, Armbruster A, Oxenham GP, et al: *Medicine in a day: Revision notes for medical exams, finals, UKMLA and foundation years,* Glasgow, UK, 2023, Elsevier Ltd.)

Erythema Nodosum

The hallmark of *erythema nodosum,* an inflammatory disorder, is tender, erythematous, subcutaneous nodules that typically are located symmetrically on the shins. Erythema nodosum does not ulcerate and usually resolves without atrophy or scarring. Most direct and indirect evidence supports the involvement of type IV delayed hypersensitivity response to numerous antigens. In approximately 55% of cases, the cause of erythema nodosum is unknown, but it has been associated with various diseases, including infections. It is commonly associated with streptococcal infections in approximately 28% to 48% of all cases and has been associated with chlamydia, histoplasmosis, coccidioidomycosis, mycobacteria, and mycoplasma. In addition to the association with infections, erythema nodosum is associated with sarcoidosis (11% to 25% of all cases); inflammatory bowel disease (1% to 4% of all cases); pregnancy (2% to 5% of all cases); medications (3% to 10% of all cases) such as sulfonamides, oral contraceptives, and bromides; vaccinations; and cancer. Erythema nodosum may also occur on the buttocks, calves, ankles, thighs, and arms. The lesions begin as flat, firm, hot, red, painful lumps approximately an inch across. Within a few days, they may become purplish, then fade to a brownish, flat patch over several weeks. Patients, primarily young females, seek medical attention after the appearance of these extremely painful lesions, which range in size from 1 cm to several centimeters in diameter. The lesions can then coalesce and spread over the entire leg. The lesions of erythema nodosum begin to regress after 1 to 2 weeks. As they disappear, they undergo a series of characteristic color changes: bright erythema to shades of purple, yellow, and green. Fig. 8.110 shows the early lesions of erythema nodosum in a 33-year-old female in whom sarcoidosis was diagnosed three months later.

Lichen Planus

Lichen planus is a relatively common skin disorder of unknown cause. The primary lesion is a polygonal, shiny, flat-topped papule with a violaceous hue. The pruritic lesions can be seen on any part of the body but have a predilection for the front of the wrists and forearms, the backs of the hands, the ankles, the shins, the genitalia, and the lumbar areas. The lesions range in size from 2 mm to more than 1 cm. Fig. 8.111A shows the characteristic rash on the arm. Fine reticulated scales are visible (see Fig. 8.111B). In 50% of all patients with lichen planus, oral lesions consist of a white, lacy network on the buccal mucosa. On occasion, involvement of the mouth may be the only manifestation of lichen planus. The patient usually experiences severe pain as the lesions ulcerate. Fig. 12.15 depicts lichen planus of the buccal mucosa. Lichen planus may also involve the genitalia. Fig. 8.112 shows lichen planus of the penis. Note the reticular markings on the penis. Fig. 18.10 depicts another case of lichen planus of the penis. Note again the fine reticular markings.

Seborrheic Dermatitis

Seborrheic dermatitis is a papulosquamous disorder associated with epidermal hyperplasia and scaling. The lesions have a greasy-looking scale in a seborrheic distribution: scalp, eyebrows, nasolabial fold, perioral area, midchest, and groin. Seborrheic dermatitis is one of the most common skin conditions associated with HIV infection; it is estimated that 85% of patients infected with HIV have this skin lesion at some time. In some patients, the development of seborrheic dermatitis is the first sign of HIV infection. Fig. 8.113 shows the typical greasy scales of seborrheic dermatitis on the face.

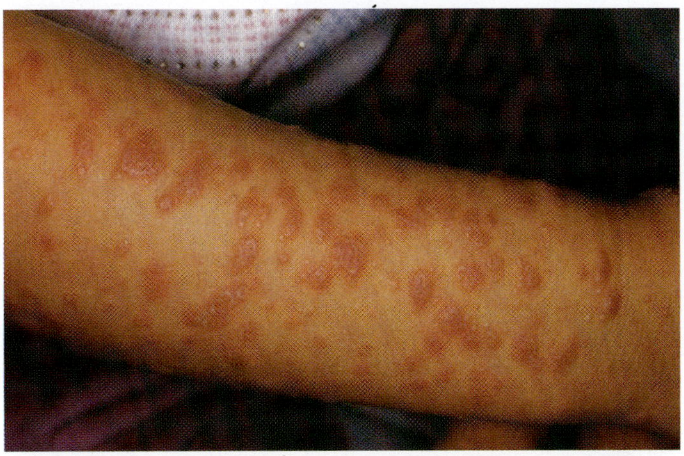

A

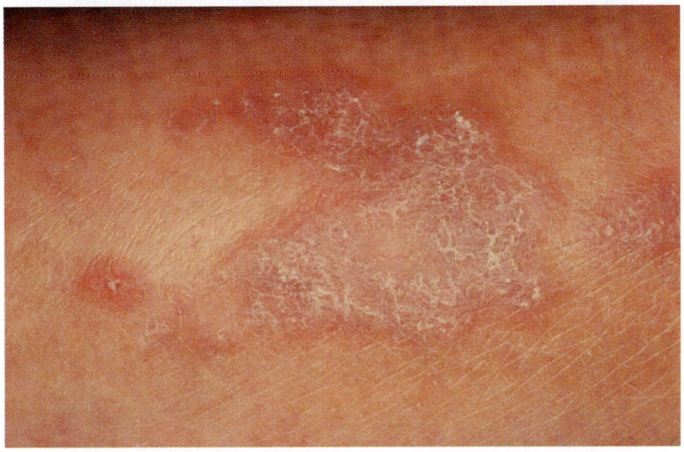

B

Fig. 8.111 (A) and (B) Lichen planus. Notice the fine, reticulated white scales. (From Callen JP, Greer KE, Hood AF, et al: *Color atlas of dermatology*, Philadelphia, 1993, WB Saunders.)

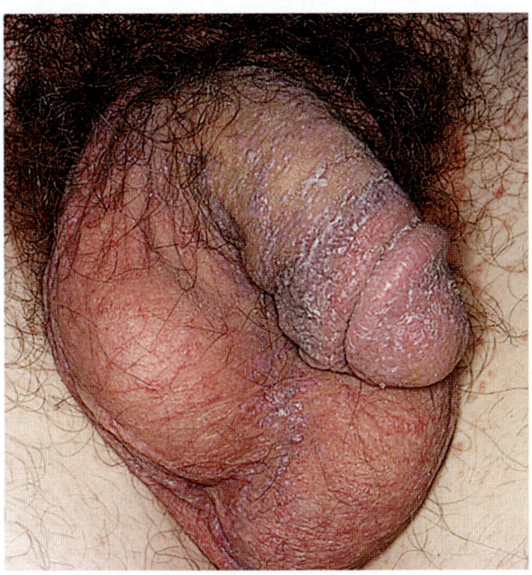

Fig. 8.112 Lichen Planus of the Penis. (From Callen JP, Paller AS, Greer KE, et al: *Color atlas of dermatology*, ed 2, Philadelphia, 2000, WB Saunders.)

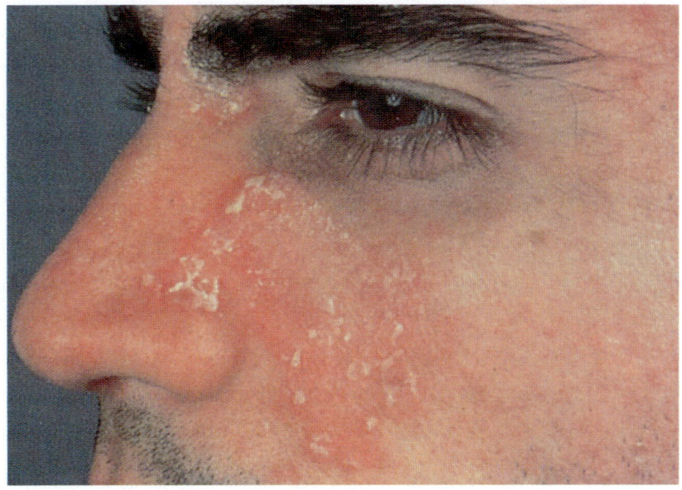

Fig. 8.113 Seborrheic Dermatitis. (From Callen JP, Greer KE, Hood AF, et al: *Color atlas of dermatology*, Philadelphia, 1993, WB Saunders.)

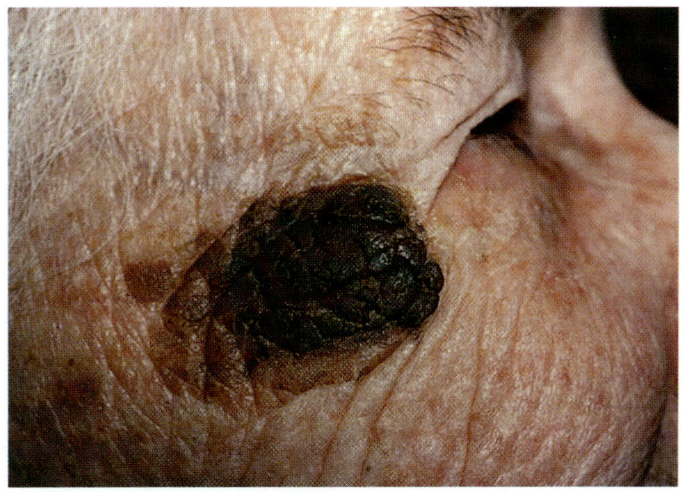

Fig. 8.114 Seborrheic Keratosis.

Seborrheic Warts

Seborrheic warts are common, benign skin tumors seen in light-skinned individuals; they occur more frequently with advancing age. Also known as *seborrheic keratosis* (Fig. 8.114), seborrheic warts may be solitary or have multiple lesions. They occur in any area of the body exposed to ultraviolet light. The lesions are well-defined and raised and have a fissured surface. The lesions result from a failure of keratinocytes to mature normally, which produces an accumulation of immature cells in the epidermis. Fig. 8.115 is a close-up photograph of the characteristic appearance of a seborrheic wart. Sometimes the lesions may be pedunculated. A similar condition known as *dermatosis papulosis nigra* is seen in African Americans.

Cutaneous Horn

A *cutaneous horn* is discussed in Chapter 10, "The Eye" (see Figs. 10.22 and 10.23). The tag sticks out of the skin and may have a short, narrow stalk connecting it to the skin's surface. It

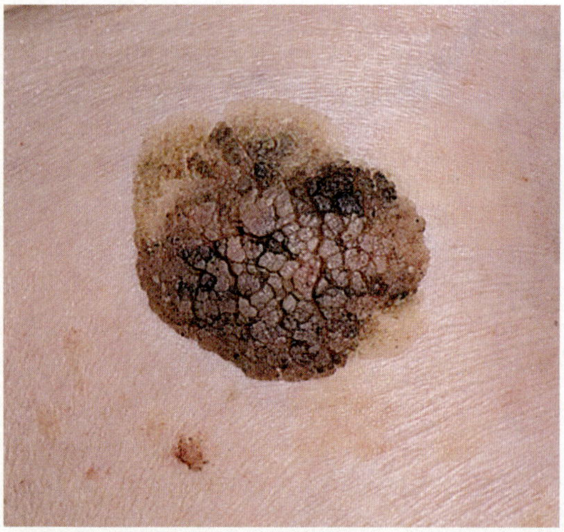

Fig. 8.115 Seborrheic Wart, Close-Up. (From Callen JP, Paller AS, Greer KE, et al: *Color atlas of dermatology*, ed 2, Philadelphia, 2000, WB Saunders.)

is usually small but may be half an inch long. The tag is usually the same color as the skin or a little darker. It is generally painless and does not grow or change. However, it may be irritated from rubbing by clothing or other materials.

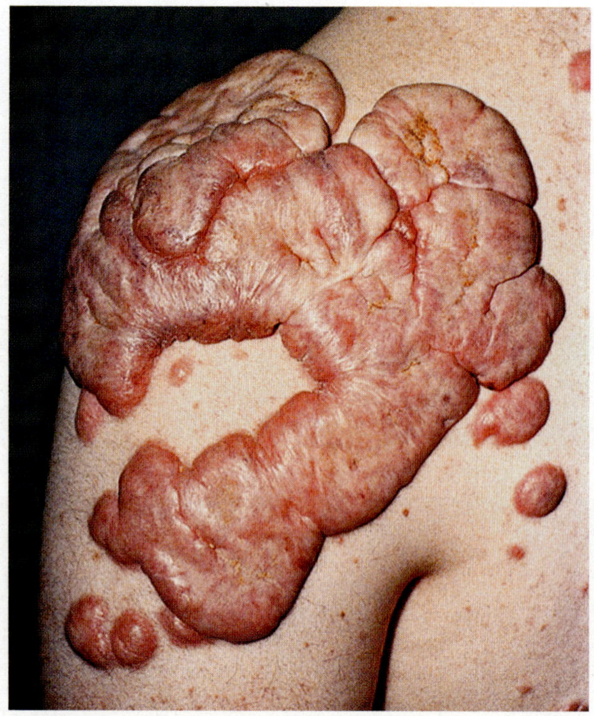

Fig. 8.116 Keloid. (From Callen JP, Greer KE, Hood AF, et al: *Color atlas of dermatology*, Philadelphia, 1993, WB Saunders.)

Keloid

A *keloid* is a hyperproliferative response of fibrous tissue to injury, inflammation, or infection. It has a smooth appearance with a shiny surface and is raised and firm to palpation. It more commonly develops in dark-skinned individuals. Keloids can grow in any place where an abrasion has occurred. They can result from pimples, insect bites, scratching, burns, or other skin trauma. Keloid scars can also commonly develop after surgery. They are more common in some sites, such as the central chest, the back and shoulders, and the ear lobes. Keloids can also occur after body piercings. The most common spots are earlobes, arms, and over the collarbone. The lesion characteristically spreads beyond the site of the initiating factor. Fig. 8.116 shows an extensive keloid on the shoulder.

Nevi

Nevi are common, localized skin abnormalities that may be present at birth or appear within the first few decades of life. Sometimes called "moles," nevi may arise from almost any area of the skin. They are well-defined, with a smooth surface and a round shape (Fig. 8.117). Hair may sometimes project from the surface. A *strawberry nevus* is a vascular tumor or hemangioma that occurs shortly after birth and is red and raised. These proliferate and are often seen on the face of a child. They may bleed and ulcerate. Fortunately, most strawberry nevi involute by the time the child is 6 or 7 years of age. Fig. 24.50 shows a hemangioma in a child.

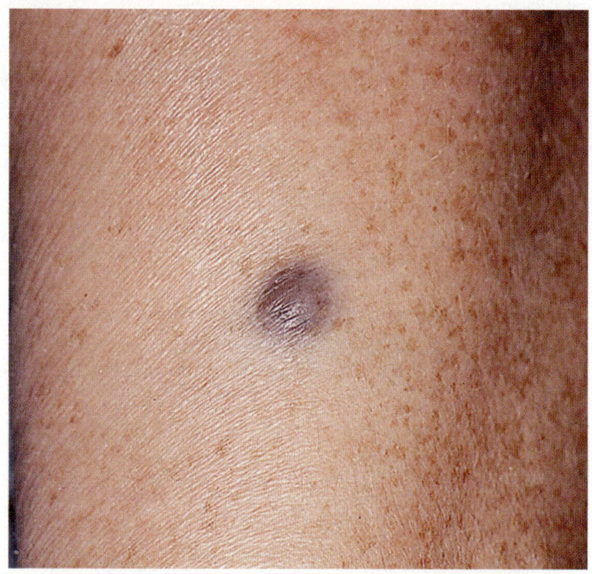

Fig. 8.117 Blue Nevus. (From Callen JP, Paller AS, Greer KE, et al: *Color atlas of dermatology*, ed 2, Philadelphia, 2000, WB Saunders.)

Pemphigus Vulgaris, Pemphigus Vegetans, and Bullous Pemphigoid

Blistering, or vesiculobullous, skin diseases are rare but essential to recognize. *Pemphigus vulgaris, pemphigus vegetans,* and *bullous pemphigoid* are autoimmune diseases that affect skin and mucosal surfaces. Pemphigus vulgaris is a vesiculobullous disease of middle age, seen more commonly in Jewish people. The lesions are superficial, flaccid blisters that break easily, leaving the skin denuded and eroded. This is often termed the *Nikolsky sign*. This sign is said to be present when a slight rubbing of the skin produces exfoliation of the outermost layer; it is almost always present in drug reactions like Stevens-Johnson syndrome and scalded skin syndrome. Likewise, a pencil eraser

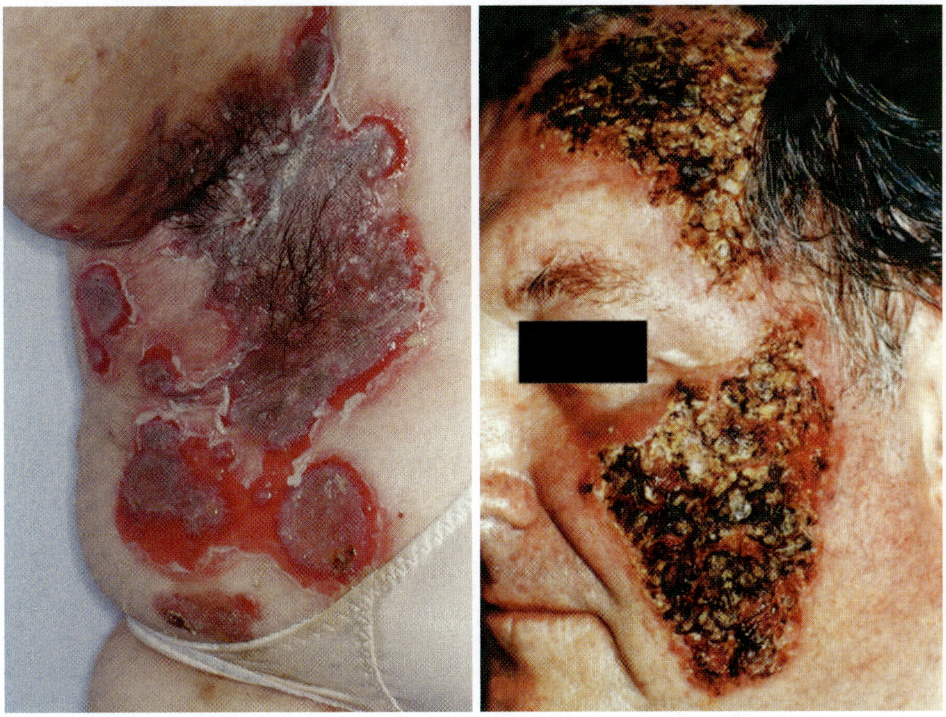

A B

Fig. 8.118 (A and B) Pemphigus vulgaris. (B) A vegetative form sometimes called *pemphigus vegetans*. (From Callen JP, Greer KE, Hood AF, et al: *Color atlas of dermatology*, Philadelphia, 1993, WB Saunders.)

or finger applied to the skin will slip the top layers of the skin away from the underlying layers: a positive Nikolsky sign. The broken bullae of pemphigus vulgaris may crust but do not heal spontaneously. These lesions are nonpruritic but are painful. The disease is caused by the production of antibodies to the intercellular junctions of the epidermis. The defective junctions lead to the formation of traumatic fissures and bullae. Fig. 8.118A shows pemphigus vulgaris and broken bullae. Fig. 8.118B shows pemphigus vegetans. The lesions may be present on any area of the skin, especially the trunk, umbilicus, intertriginous areas, and scalp. The lesions are frequently found in the mucous membranes of the oral cavity, pharynx, and genitalia. Fig. 8.119 shows pemphigus vegetans of the lips.

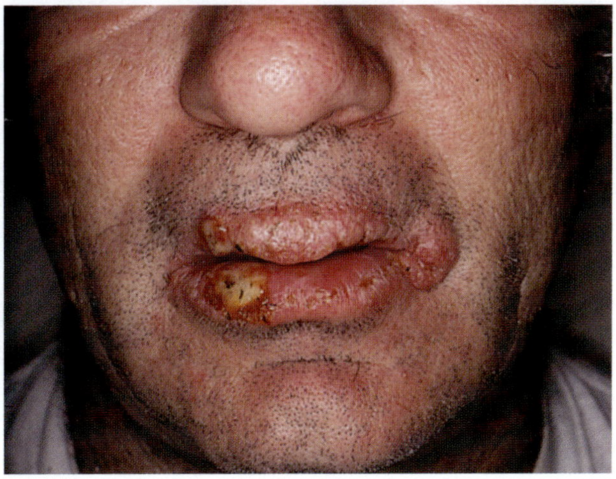

Fig. 8.119 Pemphigus Vegetans of the Lips. (From Callen JP, Paller AS, Greer KE, et al: *Color atlas of dermatology*, ed 2, Philadelphia, 2000, WB Saunders.)

Bullous pemphigoid is a blistering disorder seen more frequently in older adult patients. It is more common than pemphigus vulgaris. No racial predilection exists, and the disease is less severe than pemphigus. The lesions are intensely pruritic, tense bullae, often on an erythematous base, and are symmetric on the limbs, inner aspects of the arms, thighs, and trunk. Oral and mucosal lesions are rarer than those of pemphigus. Nikolsky sign is negative in bullous pemphigoid. Fig. 8.120 depicts generalized bullous pemphigoid. Figs. 8.121A and B show the tense bullae, which help to differentiate this disease from pemphigus.

Atopic Dermatitis

Atopic dermatitis, a form of eczema, is a common disease associated with other atopic disorders such as asthma and allergic rhinitis. It is characterized by itchy, dry, inflamed skin. The symptoms of atopic dermatitis often begin at a young age. Infants and young children may have eczematous patches on the face, scalp, and extensor surfaces of the extremities. These patches may erode and ooze. Scaling erythematous plaques often develop. As the child ages, atopic dermatitis involves flexural areas such as the neck, antecubital fossae, and popliteal fossae. The pruritic lesions result in excoriations; thickening and lichenification of the skin with increased skin markings are common. Oozing, weeping, and excoriated plaques in the adult may become generalized. Although the pathogenesis of atopic dermatitis is unknown, many patients have elevated levels of

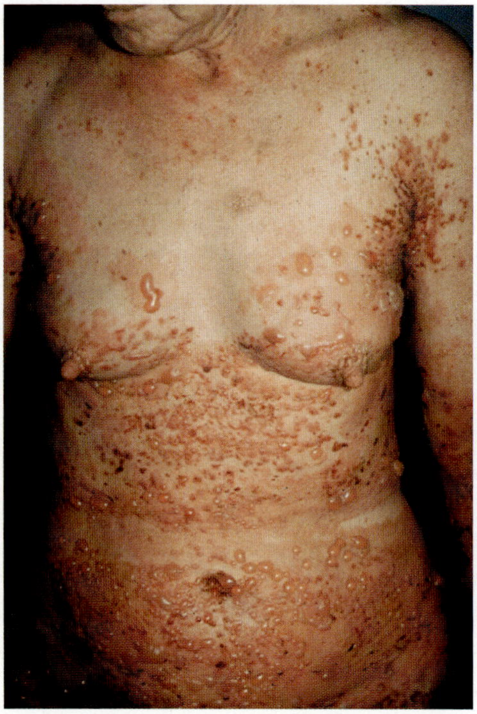

Fig. 8.120 Bullous Pemphigoid. (From Jordon RE: *Atlas of bullous disease*, Philadelphia, 2000, Churchill Livingstone.)

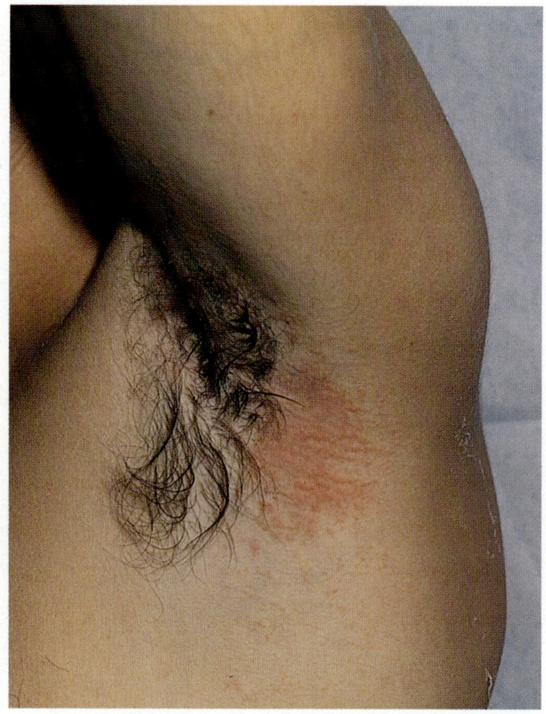

Fig. 8.122 Atopic Dermatitis.

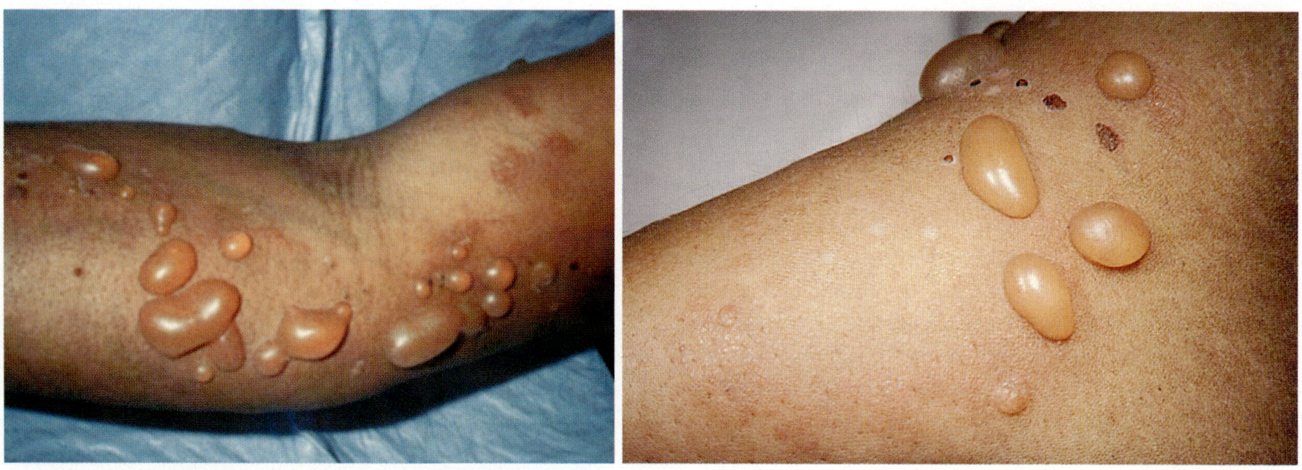

A B

Fig. 8.121 (A and B) Bullous pemphigoid; close-up of tense bullae. (A, From Callen JP, Greer KE, Hood AF, et al: *Color atlas of dermatology*, Philadelphia, 1993, WB Saunders. B, From Callen JP, Greer KE, Hood AF, et al: *Color atlas of dermatology*, Philadelphia, 1993, WB Saunders.)

serum immunoglobulin E. Since the 1970s, the incidence of atopic dermatitis has increased from 4% to 12%; the reasons are unclear. Immune dysregulation appears to play an essential role in atopic dermatitis. Up to 50% of children with atopic dermatitis may have evidence of food sensitivity. Emotional stressors do not cause atopic dermatitis but do exacerbate the symptoms. Fig. 8.122 shows classic lesions of atopic dermatitis in the axilla. Fig. 8.123 shows atopic dermatitis in another patient. Notice the oozing lesions and excoriations.

Lyme Disease

Lyme disease is an infection caused by the spirochete *Borrelia burgdorferi* transmitted by the usually asymptomatic bite of certain ticks of the genus *Ixodes*. Lyme borreliosis occurs in northeastern, mid-Atlantic, north central, and far western regions of the United States; Lyme disease was first described in the United States in Old Lyme, Connecticut, in 1975.

Early localized Lyme disease (stage 1) symptoms begin days or weeks after being bitten by the tick. The early systemic

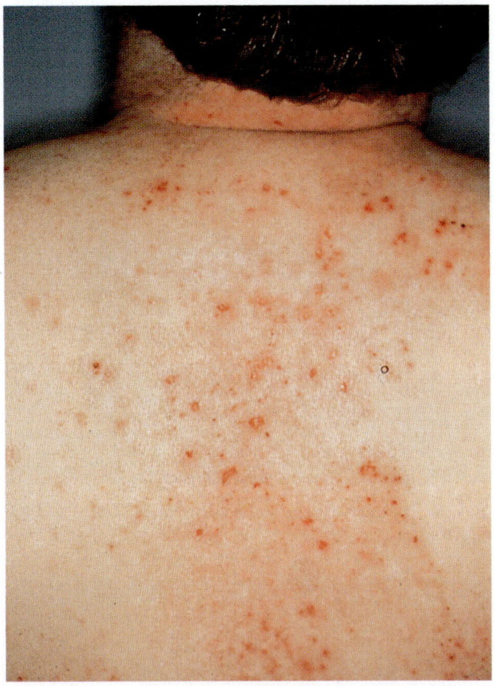

Fig. 8.123 Atopic Dermatitis. (From Lebwohl MG, ed: *Atlas of the skin and systemic disease*, New York, 1995, Churchill Livingstone.)

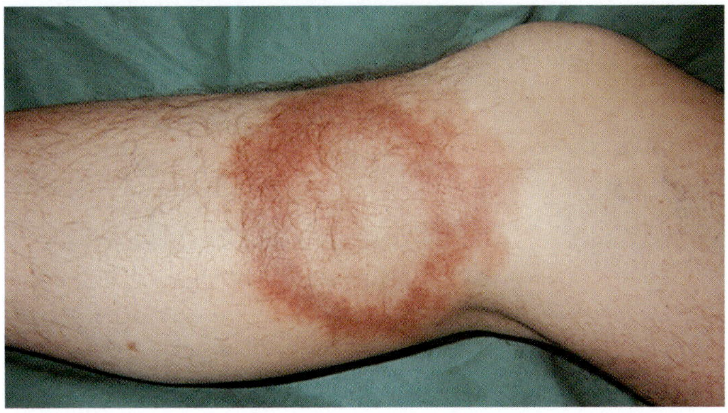

Fig. 8.124 Erythema Migrans of Lyme Disease. (From Callen JP, Paller AS, Greer KE, et al: *Color atlas of dermatology*, ed 2, Philadelphia, 2000, WB Saunders.)

symptoms are similar to the flu and may include fatigue (54%), myalgia (44%), arthralgia (44%), headache (42%), fever and chills (39%), and stiff neck (35%). The most common sign is regional lymphadenopathy (23%). Symptoms may come and go.

Erythema migrans is the clinical, distinctive dermatologic hallmark of Lyme disease. It is an active lesion, and the appearance can change dramatically over days. The rash is recognized in 90% of patients with objective evidence of *B. burgdorferi* infection. The erythema begins as a red macule or papule at the tick bite site 7 to 10 days earlier. The rash expands as an annular erythematous plaque as the spirochetes spread centrifugally through the skin. Central clearing may or may not be present. Local symptoms of pruritus or tenderness are hardly noticeable. Figs. 8.124 and 8.125 show the classic erythema migrans of Lyme disease. Note the central lesion in Fig. 8.125, which was the area of the tick bite.

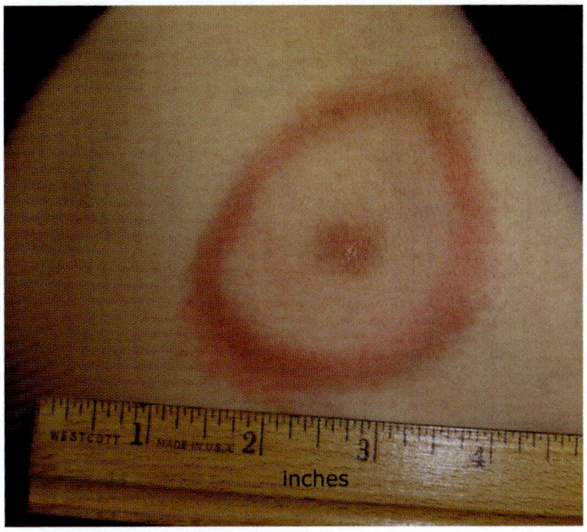

Fig. 8.125 Erythema Migrans of Lyme Disease: Site of the Tick Bite.

Early disseminated Lyme disease (stage 2) symptoms may occur weeks to months after the initial tick bite. They may include paralysis or weakness in the muscles of the face, muscle pain and pain or swelling in the knees and other large joints, and cardiac symptoms, including chest pain and palpitations. Late disseminated Lyme disease (stage 3) symptoms can occur months or years after the initial infection. The most common symptoms are muscle and joint pain. Other symptoms may include abnormal muscle movement, weakness, numbness and tingling, and speech problems.

Some of the more critical risk factors for Lyme disease include:

- Doing outside activities that increase tick exposure (e.g., gardening, hunting, or hiking) in an area where Lyme disease is known to occur
- Having a pet that may carry ticks home
- Walking in high grasses

Despite these risk factors:

- In most cases, a tick must be attached to your body for 24 to 36 hours to spread the bacteria to your blood.
- Blacklegged ticks can be so small that they are almost impossible to see. As a result, many people with Lyme disease never even saw a tick on their body.
- Most people who are bitten by a tick do *not* get Lyme disease.

AIDS

As indicated in this chapter, there are many cutaneous manifestations of AIDS. Three of these common lesions are shown on the face of a patient with AIDS in Fig. 8.126. The umbilicated, white papules on and around the lips, nose, and cheek are molluscum contagiosum lesions. The verrucous papule on the upper lip is a wart. Finally, the violaceous lesions of KS are present on the lips and chin.

Diabetes

Approximately 30% of patients with diabetes mellitus have disease-related dermatologic problems. Neurotrophic foot ulcers are prevalent in diabetic patients. Fig. 8.127 shows bilateral

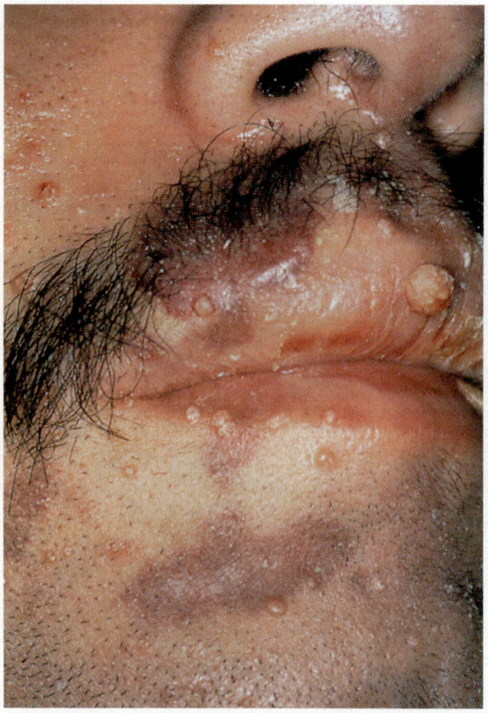

Fig. 8.126 Cutaneous Manifestations of Acquired Immune Deficiency Syndrome.

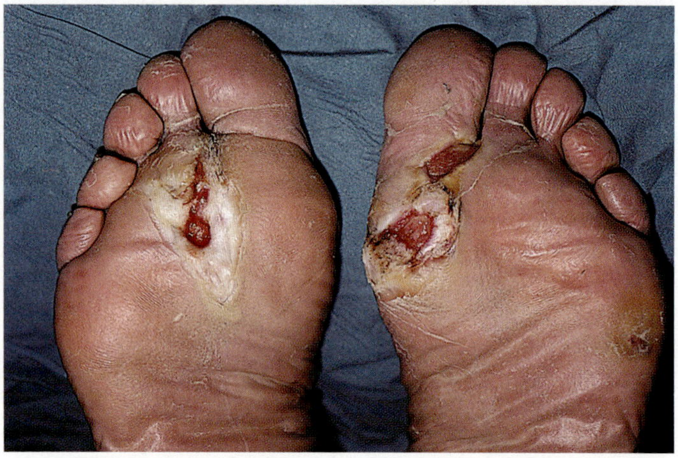

Fig. 8.127 Diabetic Neurotrophic Foot Ulcers. (From Callen JP, Paller AS, Greer KE, et al: *Color atlas of dermatology*, ed 2, Philadelphia, 2000, WB Saunders.)

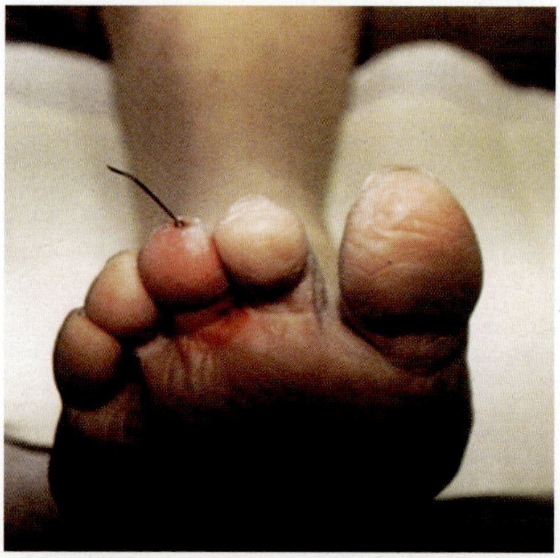

Fig. 8.128 Foreign Body in the Toe of a Diabetic Patient.

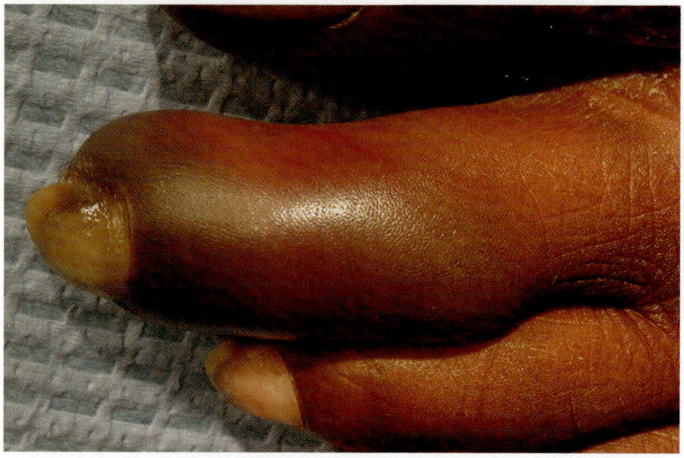

Fig. 8.129 Bullous Diabeticorum.

neurotrophic ulcers. Painless plantar ulcers heal slowly after apparently minor trauma. The "diabetic foot" is characterized by chronic sensorimotor neuropathy, autonomic neuropathy, and poor peripheral circulation. Sensorimotor neuropathy results in a loss of normal sensation, which prevents the detection of traumatic events. See also Fig. 15.17, which depicts diabetic dry gangrene of the big and fourth toes; Fig. 15.18, which depicts a patient with the classic lesion of necrobiosis lipoidica diabeticorum; and Fig. 15.19, which is a close-up photograph of the same skin lesion in another patient. It is common for diabetic patients, owing to the decreased sensitivity in their feet, to present with foreign bodies in their toes or feet. Fig. 8.128 shows a foreign body protruding from the tip of the right third toe of a diabetic patient. This patient had dropped a needle on the carpet and later stepped on the needle, which penetrated the toe. Only after noticing it visually did the patient seek medical attention.

Bullosis diabeticorum (Fig. 8.129) is a relatively uncommon, noninflammatory, blistering condition of unknown origin in patients with long-standing diabetes. The tense bullae develop on normal-appearing skin in acral areas (feet, lower legs, and hands). It has been associated with insulin-dependent diabetes mellitus and non–insulin-dependent (type 2) diabetes. Intraepidermal and subepidermal blisters occur spontaneously, usually without trauma, and heal within 2 to 6 weeks. Treatment consists of aspiration of the bullae and topical antibiotics.

Tuberous Sclerosis

Tuberous sclerosis is a dominantly inherited hamartomatous disorder characterized by intellectual disability, seizures, and eye and skin lesions. The classic triad of symptoms is mental retardation, seizures, and adenoma sebaceum. *Adenoma sebaceum* occurs near the nasolabial folds and over the cheeks. These lesions are facial angiofibromas. Other common skin lesions are periungual and subungual fibromas. Fig. 8.130A shows a patient's foot with tuberous sclerosis and periungual fibromas. Fig. 8.130B shows the foot of another patient with tuberous sclerosis and subungual fibromas.

Cutaneous Larva Migrans

Cutaneous larva migrans is caused by animal hookworms, commonly the dog parasites *Ancylostoma braziliense* or *Ancylostoma caninum.* The creeping eruption occurs when the skin comes in direct and prolonged contact with the hookworm larva contained in the feces of dogs, cats, or humans. Moist areas visited by the infected animals, such as beaches or exposed soil covered by porches, are common sites for acquiring infection. The clinical appearance is that of a raised, serpiginous, erythematous, pruritic eruption, and it represents the paths of migration within the epidermis. The parasite cannot invade the dermis because the organism lacks collagenase and cannot disrupt the basement membrane. The lesions migrate approximately 1 to 2 cm per day and may evolve into bullae. The topical application of thiabendazole is the treatment, although the infection is usually self-limited. Fig. 8.131 shows the sole of a foot of an infected 31-year-old male after a beach vacation in Jamaica.

Anthrax, Smallpox, and Plague

On September 11, 2001, the country and world changed. As a result of the events of that day and the events afterward, everyone must be aware of the possibility of terrorist activity.

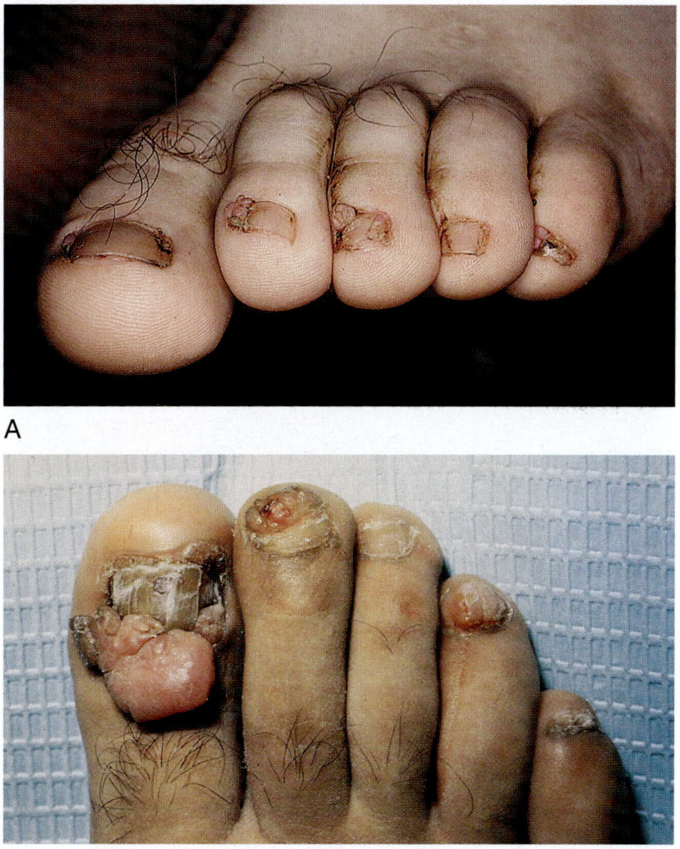

A

B

Fig. 8.130 (A and B) The feet of two patients with tuberous sclerosis and periungual fibromas. (A, From Callen JP, Paller AS, Greer KE, et al: *Color atlas of dermatology*, ed 2, Philadelphia, 2000, WB Saunders. B, From Nzuzi SM: Common nail disorders, *Clin Podiatr Med Surg* 6:273, 1989.)

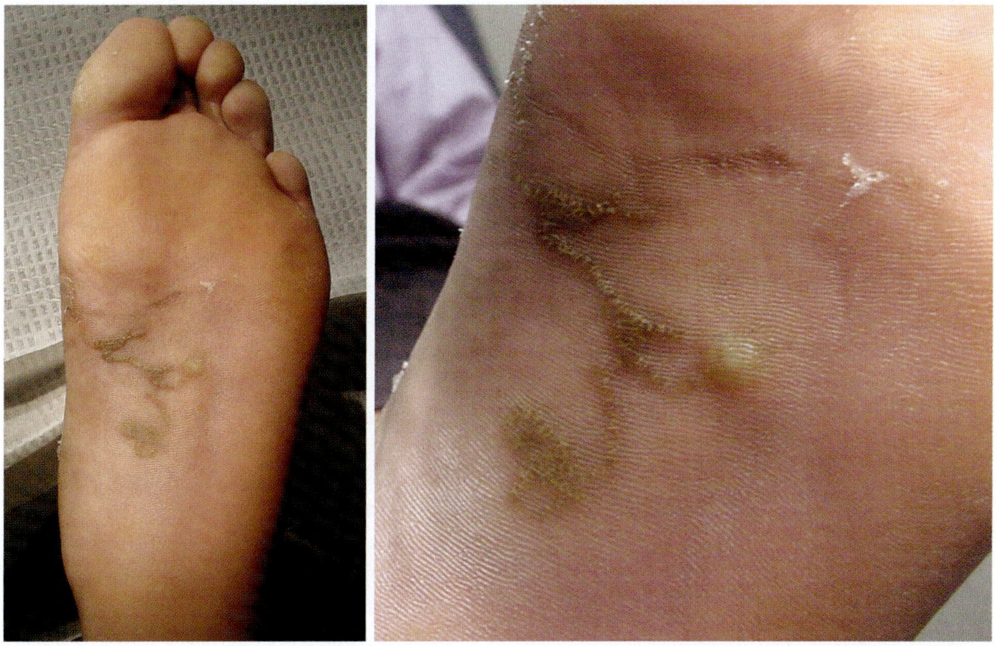

A B

Fig. 8.131 Cutaneous Larva Migrans. (A) Sole of foot. (B) Close-up photograph of lesion.

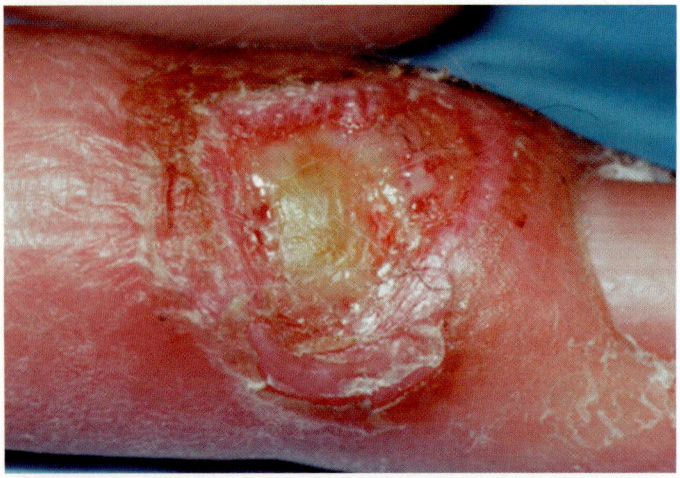

Fig. 8.132 Anthrax (Intention Exposure Secondary to Bioterrorism), Partially Treated Finger.

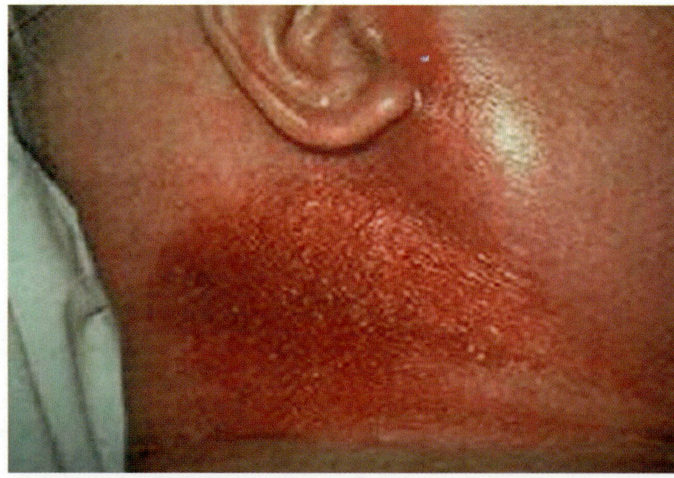

Fig. 8.133 Anthrax. Note the early lesion and marked edema. (Photographs courtesy of the Centers for Disease Control and Prevention [CDC].)

Healthcare workers must be alert to illness patterns caused by possible acts of terrorism.[h]

Several biological agents associated with possible terrorist attacks have dermatologic signs: anthrax, smallpox, and plague.

Anthrax (from the Greek *anthrax*, meaning "coal") is a disease caused by the spore-forming *Bacillus anthracis.* Anthrax occurs in three forms: cutaneous (95%), inhalational (5%), and gastrointestinal and oropharyngeal (extremely rare). In the most common cutaneous form, typically several days after exposure, a raised, inflamed, painless, pruritic papule appears and develops over one day. The papule enlarges to approximately 1 to 3 cm, and vesicles may develop around the lesion (Fig. 8.132). Extensive edema of the area is common (Fig. 8.133). Adjacent lymph nodes become swollen and may become tender. The vesicles enlarge and rupture to form an ulcer, including a tough, adherent, black scab, or eschar, forming in the developing lesion's center (Fig. 8.134). In 1 to 2 weeks, the lesion dries with the separation of the eschar, leaving a permanent scar. The mortality rate ranges from 20% if the disease is untreated to very low if treated.

The inhalation, or pulmonary, form of anthrax usually occurs 1 to 60 days after exposure, although more extended incubation periods can follow milder degrees of exposure. During the initial stage of the disease, nonspecific, influenza-like symptoms are common: myalgias, cough, low-grade fever, nonproductive cough, malaise, nausea, vomiting, chills, sweating, headache, and shortness of breath. Usually, there follows a period of 1 to 3 days of improvement and then the rapid progression of high fever, severe respiratory distress, and cardiovascular collapse, often leading to shock and death within 24 to 36 hours. Massive mediastinal adenopathy usually occurs.

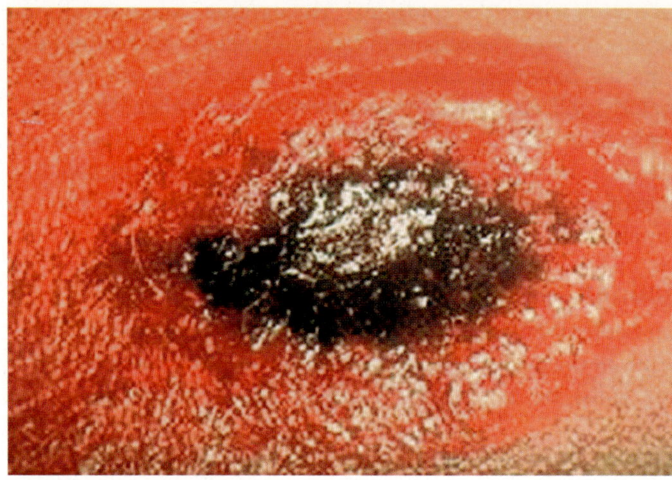

Fig. 8.134 Anthrax. Note the black eschar. (Photographs courtesy of the CDC).

Person-to-person spread is not a significant risk because the primary lesions are in the mediastinal lymph nodes and surrounding tissue. The mortality rate is 90% to 100% among untreated patients but 30% to 50% if patients are treated, depending on how quickly antibiotic treatment is initiated. *B. anthracis* is susceptible to common antibiotics, including ciprofloxacin, penicillin G, or tetracyclines.

Smallpox is a severe, highly contagious, febrile viral disease caused by a DNA virus of the *Orthopoxvirus* genus. These viruses are among the largest and most complex of all viruses. There is an incubation period of 10 to 12 days after exposure. The illness begins with the symptoms of fever, fatigue, and myalgias. A distinctive erythematous, vesicular rash, centrifugal in distribution, then develops over the next 1 to 2 days, with the lesions appearing early on the face (Fig. 8.135) and arms, with relative sparing of the trunk. As the disease progresses, lesions appear on the trunk. The lesions are uniform in their stage of development and are often umbilicated (Fig. 8.136). After approximately 2 weeks, the lesions form crusts, which fall away after 3 to 4 weeks. The case fatality rate is 30% to 40% or more.

[h]If you suspect an incident of biologic, chemical, or radiologic terrorism, contact your local state department of health immediately, as well as the Hotline for the Bioterrorism Preparedness and Response Program of the Centers for Disease Control and Prevention at 770-488-7100 or at www.cdc.gov.

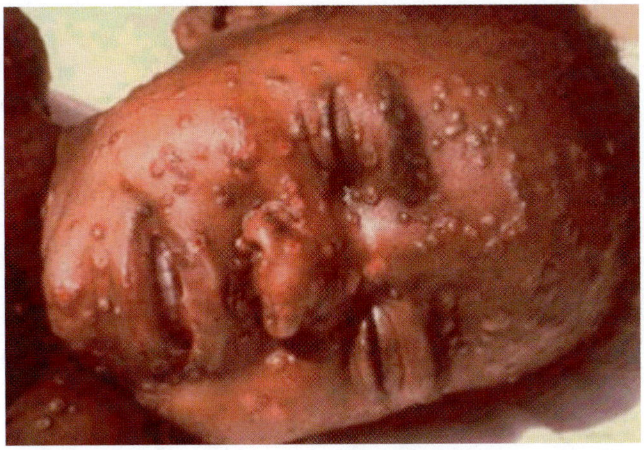

Fig. 8.135 Smallpox. Note the uniform stage of development of the vesicles. (Photo courtesy of Public Health Image Library [PHIL] ID #3. Source: CDC/Cheryl Tyron.)

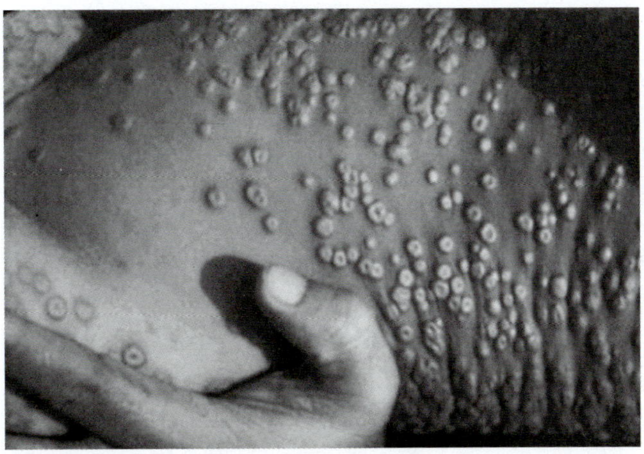

A

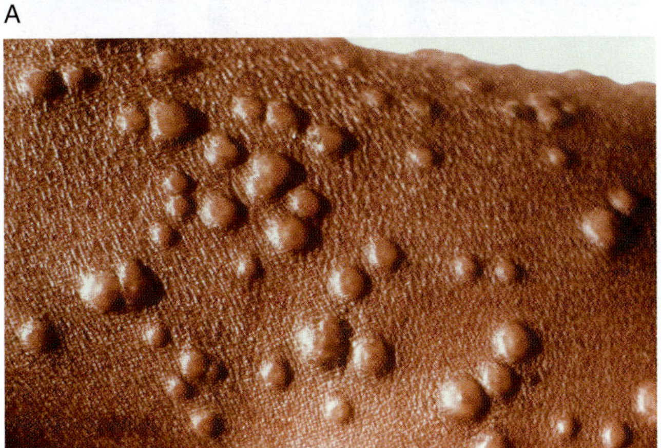

B

Fig. 8.136 Smallpox. A, Note the umbilicated lesions on the trunk. (A, Courtesy of Public Health Image Library [PHIL] ID #284. Source: CDC/James; B, Courtesy of Centers for Disease Control and Prevention, Paul B. Dean, Public Health Image Library #16056)

The last naturally occurring case of smallpox was in 1977 in Somalia. In 1980 the World Health Organization declared that smallpox was eradicated worldwide due to a global vaccination program. Although smallpox was long feared as one of the most devastating infectious diseases, its potential for devastation nowadays is far greater than ever before. In a now highly susceptible, mobile population that is medically ignorant of this infection once considered eradicated, smallpox could spread widely and rapidly throughout the world. The presence of even one case would constitute an international health emergency.

Plague is caused by a gram-negative, non–spore-forming bacillus, *Yersinia pestis.* Natural human infection usually follows the bite of an infected flea and is less commonly caused by droplets spread from a person or cat with pneumonic plague. Plague occurs in three forms: bubonic, pneumonic, and septicemic. In the case of pneumonic plague, after an incubation period of 1 to 6 days, there is the fulminant onset of high fever, chills, extreme malaise, headache, and myalgias. Within 24 hours, a cough with hemoptysis occurs. Dyspnea rapidly develops, and respiratory and cardiovascular collapse ensues. The mortality rate is 100% if the disease is untreated and could be as high as 50% even with treatment.

In the bubonic form of plague, sudden flu-like symptoms develop after an incubation period of 2 to 8 days. At approximately the same time, the patient notices the presence of an oval, elevated, 1- to 10-cm, firm, nonfluctuant mass associated with intense pain in the enlarged regional lymph nodes, known as a *bubo.* Gangrene of the extremities is one of the common manifestations of plague, accounting for the name of the "Black Death" throughout the ages. The mortality rate is 50% to 60% if the disease is untreated. Treatment for all forms of plague is streptomycin, doxycycline, or ciprofloxacin.

Skin Self-Examination

All patients should be instructed to perform routing skin self-examinations. In addition, the Skin Cancer Foundation recommends that everyone practice monthly head-to-toe self-examination of their skin. The examination can be accessed at: http://www.skincancer.org/skin-cancer-information/early-detection/step-by-step-self-examination.

Recommended monthly skin self-examination.

To summarize the examination, instruct your patient to:

- First, examine your body front and back in the mirror, then look at your right and left sides with your arms raised.
- Bend your elbows and carefully examine your forearms, upper underarms, and palms.
- Look at the backs of your legs and feet, the spaces between your toes, and the soles of your feet.
- Examine the back of your neck and your scalp with a hand mirror. Part your hair for a closer look.
- Finally, using a hand mirror, check your back and buttocks.

The typical distribution of lesions in six common skin disorders is shown in Fig. 8.137.

Table 8.1 describes the differential diagnosis of common maculopapular diseases. Table 8.2 lists the differentiation of some common eczematous disorders and gives some characteristics based on the history and body location. Table 8.3 provides information for a differential diagnosis of vesiculobullous diseases. Table 8.4 classifies some of the common benign tumors by color. Table 8.5 lists some of the common allergens associated with contact dermatitis. Finally, Table 8.6 lists the essential differences between chickenpox and smallpox.

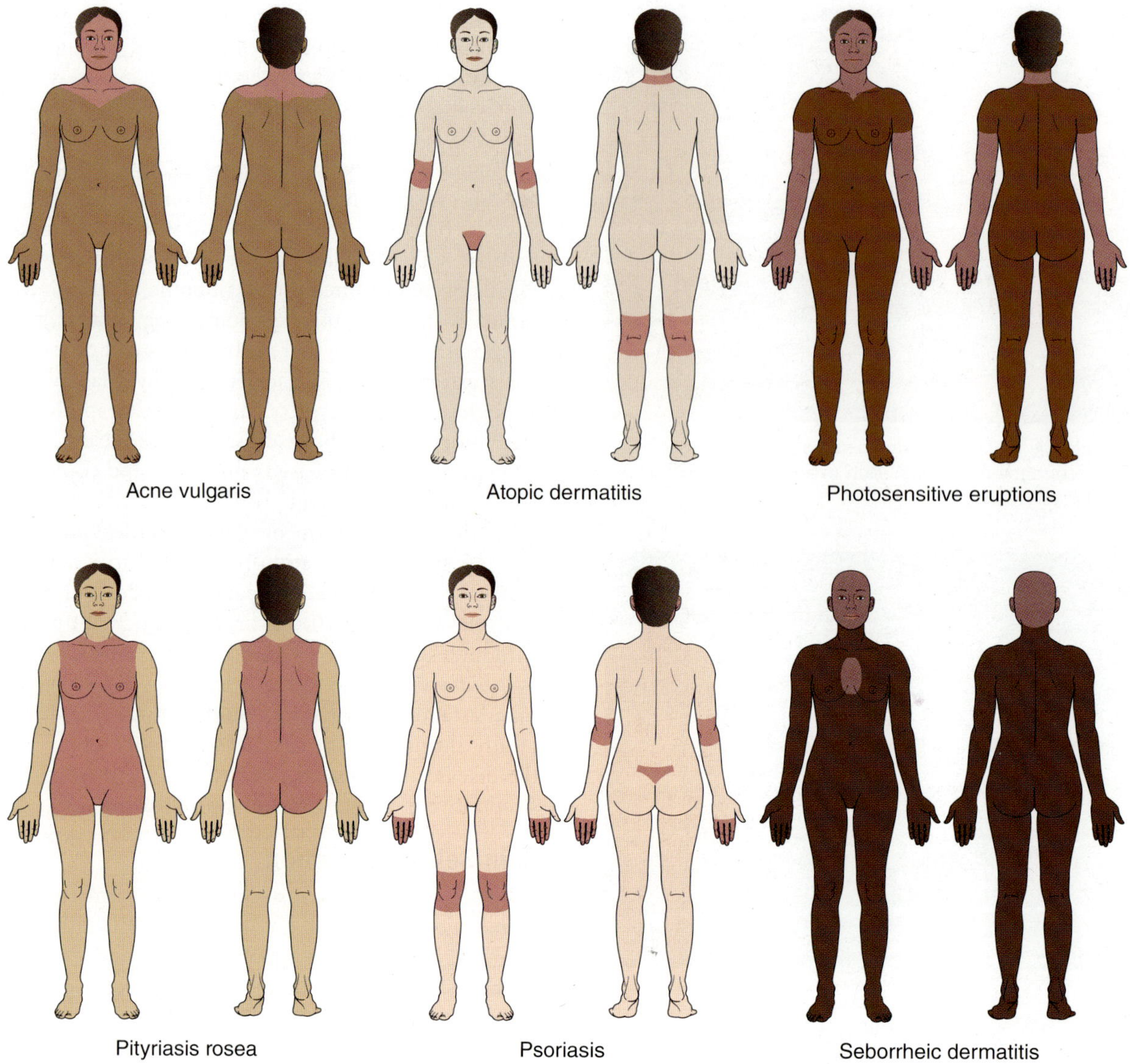

Fig. 8.137 Typical Distributions of Common Skin Conditions.

TABLE 8.1 Common Maculopapular Diseases

Characteristic	Psoriasis (See Figs. 8.14, 8.53, 8.54, 8.56, 8.57, and 18.8)	Pityriasis Rosea (See Fig. 8.68)	Tinea Versicolor (See Figs. 8.78 and 8.79)	Lichen Planus (See Figs. 8.111, 8.112, 12.15, and 18.10)	Seborrheic Dermatitis (See Fig. 8.113)
Color	Dull red	Pinkish-yellow	Reddish-brown	Violaceous	Pinkish-yellow
Scale	Abundant	Fine, adherent	Fine	Shiny, adherent	Greasy
Induration	1+	0	0	1+	1+
Face lesions	Rare	Rare	Occasional	Rare	Common
Oral lesions	0	0	0	2+	0
Nail lesions	4+	0	0	Rare	0

0, Rarely seen; *1+*, occasionally seen; *2+*, frequently seen; *4+*, nearly always associated.

TABLE 8.2 Common Eczematous Diseases

Characteristic	Contact Dermatitis (See Fig. 8.51)	Atopic Dermatitis (See Figs. 8.122, 8.123, 24.21 and 24.22)	Neurodermatitis	Stasis Dermatitis (See Figs. 15.2 and 15.3)
History	Acute, localized to specific area	History in patient or family member of asthma, hay fever, or eczema	Chronic, in same areas, associated with anxiety	Varicosities, past history of thrombophlebitis or cellulitis
Location	Areas of exposure to allergen	Eyelids, groin, flexural areas	Head, lower legs, arms	Lower legs

TABLE 8.3 Vesiculobullous Diseases

Characteristic	Pemphigus Vulgaris (See Figs. 8.118 and 8.119)	Dermatitis Herpetiformis	Epidermolysis Bullosa[a]	Bullous Pemphigoid (See Figs. 8.120 and 8.121)
Age of patient	40–60 years	Children and adults	Infants and children	60–70 years
Initial site	Oral mucosa	Scalp, trunk	Extremities	Extremities
Lesions	Normal skin at margins	Erythematous base	Bullae produced by trauma	Normal skin at margins
Sites	Mouth, abdomen, scalp, groin	Knees, sacrum, back, elbows	Hands, knees, elbows, mouth, toes	Trunk, extremities
Groupings	0	4+	1+	0
Weight loss	Marked	None	None	Minimal
Duration	1 or more years	Several years	Normal lifetime	Months to years
Pruritus	0	4+	0	±
Oral pain	4+	0	±	±
Palms and soles involved	No	No	Yes	Yes
Typical lesion	Flaccid bullae	Grouped vesicles	Flaccid vesicles	Tense bullae

[a]Refers to a group of inherited diseases that causes fragile, blistering skin. The blisters may occur in response to minor trauma.
0, Rarely seen; *1+*, occasionally seen; *4+*, nearly always associated; ±, sometimes present.

TABLE 8.4 Common Benign Tumors by Color

Color	Benign Tumor
Skin color	Warts (see Figs. 8.26, 8.27, and 8.115) Cysts Keloids (see Fig. 8.116) Nevi (see Figs. 8.117 and 24.2)
Pink or red	Hemangiomas (see Figs. 24.50 and 24.11) Keloids (see Fig. 8.116)
Brown	Seborrheic keratoses (see Fig. 8.114) Nevi (see Figs. 8.117 and 24.2) Lentigines (see Fig. 25.1) Dermatofibromas (see Fig. 8.50)
Tannish-yellow	Xanthomata (see Figs. 14.12 to 14.15) Xanthelasma (see Fig. 14.18) Warts (see Fig. 8.26) Keloids (see Fig. 8.116)
Dark blue or black	Seborrheic keratoses (see Fig. 8.114) Hemangiomas (see Figs. 24.50 and 24.51) Blue nevi (see Fig. 8.117) Dermatofibromas (see Fig. 8.50)

TABLE 8.5 Allergens Associated with Contact Dermatitis

Location	Possible Allergen
Scalp	Hair dyes Shampoos Tonics
Eyelids	Eye makeup Hair sprays
Neck	Aftershave lotions Perfumes Soaps Washing agents Nickel jewelry
Trunk	Clothing Washing agents
Axillae	Deodorants Soaps
Genitalia	Soaps Contraceptives Deodorants Washing agents
Feet	Shoes Sneakers Deodorants Socks Washing agents
Hands	Nickel jewelry Soaps Dyes Plants

TABLE 8.6 Important Differences Between Chickenpox and Smallpox

Characteristics	Chickenpox (See Fig. 24.59)	Smallpox (See Figs. 8.135 and 8.136)
Onset of symptoms	Begin with rash	Begin 2–4 days before rash
Rash	Evenly distributed all over body	More dense on face, head, arms, and legs (centrifugal distribution)
Presence on palms and soles	Almost never	Common
Development into other lesions	Rapidly into vesicles (less than 24 hours)	Slowly into pustules (7–14 days)
Time frame of lesions	New lesions form and scab at different times	Lesions form and go through their stages at the same time
Nature of lesions	Pruritic but relatively soft	Painful and hard
Patient appears extremely ill and moribund	Rarely	Commonly

USEFUL VOCABULARY

Listed here are the specific roots that are important to understand the terminology related to skin diseases.

Root	Pertaining to	Example	Definition
kerat(o)-	horny	***kerat***oma	Horny growth
derm(a)-	skin	***derma***titis	Inflammation of the skin
trich(o)-	hair	***trich***oid	Resembling hair
seb(o)-	sebum	***sebo***rrhea	Excess flow of sebum
hidr(o)-	sweat	***hidr***adenitis	Inflammation of sweat glands
onych(o)-	nails	***onycho***mycosis	Disease of the nails caused by fungus

WRITING UP THE PHYSICAL EXAMINATION

Listed here are examples of the write-up for the examination of the skin.

- Oval plaques with well-defined borders and silvery scales are symmetrically present on the elbows, knees, scalp, and gluteal cleft. The plaques on the scalp are along the hairline. The scales are large. Examination of the nails reveals pitting of the nail plates. The hair is of normal texture.
- There is an annular lesion 3 to 4 cm in diameter on the right forearm. Scale is present on the narrow (1- to 2-mm), raised, erythematous border. The central area is slightly hypopigmented. The hair and nails are unremarkable.
- There is a linear bullous eruption along the lateral aspect of the left leg. The eruption consists of bright red, edematous papules and bullae. There are no lesions on the palms or soles or in the mouth.
- A wide variety of lesions are seen on the face, shoulders, and back. The predominant lesions are pustules on an inflammatory base. Many pustules are present, and several have become confluent over the chin and forehead. Open and closed comedones are on the face, especially along the nasolabial folds. Inflammatory papules are present on the lower cheeks and chin. Large abscesses and ulcerated cysts are present over the upper shoulder areas. Numerous scars are present over the face and upper back.
- A diffuse erythematous maculopapular rash is present on the trunk. Some excoriations are present over the shoulders and chest. The hair and nails are unremarkable.
- Examination of the skin reveals several types of lesions. The main lesions are small papules in the antecubital and popliteal fossae. The papules in some areas have become confluent, and plaques are present. On the dorsum of the feet, eczema is present with erythema, weeping, crusting, and scaling. Lichenification of the anogenital area, especially the scrotum, is present.
- The skin is slightly cool and dry. Scattered lentigines are present over the trunk. The hair is very fine and soft. There is a loss of the lateral one-third of the eyebrows. No nail abnormalities are present.

REVIEW QUESTIONS

1. **A 56-year-old male laborer visited his podiatrist for nail clipping. The podiatrist noticed the following nail on the right second toe that may be:**

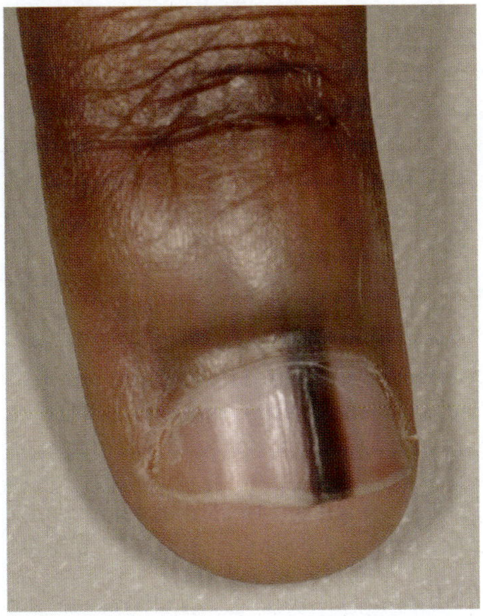

A. Splinter hemorrhage
B. Beau's line
C. Basal cell carcinoma
D. Acral lentiginous melanoma
E. Lindsay's nail

2. **A sexually active 38-year-old female experiencing frequent urination visited the emergency room of a nearby hospital. During a physical examination, she was observed to have distinct, waxy, red patches with noticeable blood vessels on both shins. Which of the following statements is true?**

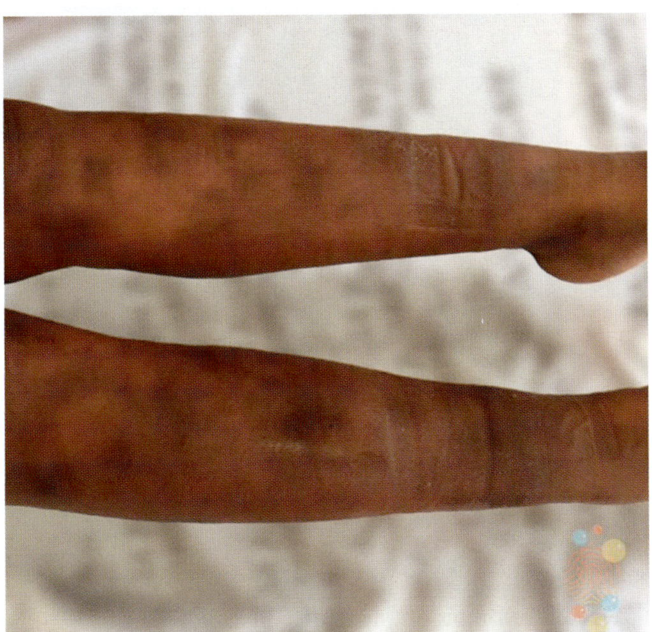

A. These lesions are painful.
B. These lesions are painless.
C. These lesions indicate a sexually transmitted disease.
D. These lesions indicate a gastrointestinal condition.
E. These lesions generally resolve in 2 to 3 weeks.

3. **Urticaria is a common pruritic skin condition. Skin mast cells are the main effector cells in the pathogenesis of chronic spontaneous urticaria, but the underlying causes of their activation are unknown. The primary lesions are:**

A. Papules
B. Vesicles
C. Wheals
D. Bullae
E. Pustules

4. **A 40-year-old male with AIDS is shown below. What is the most likely diagnosis of the lesions shown?**

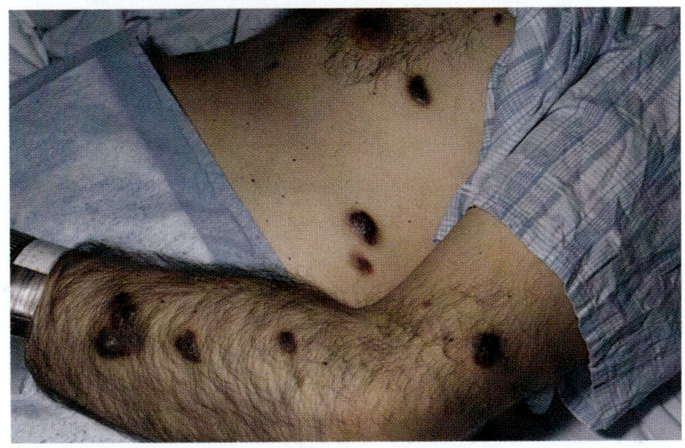

A. Kaposi sarcoma
B. Molluscum contagiosum
C. Venereal warts
D. Basal cell carcinomas
E. Lentigo malignant melanomas

5. **The fingernail shown in this image may be from a person with a deficiency in:**

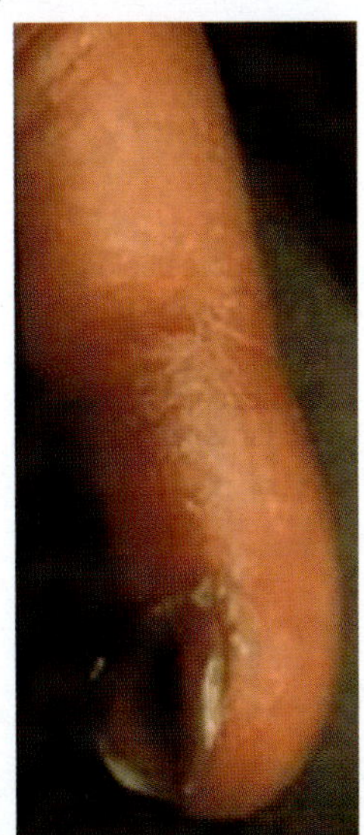

A. B_{12}
B. Folate
C. Iron
D. Magnesium
E. Zinc

6. The lesion on the shin of this 50-year-old male may represent a disease of the:

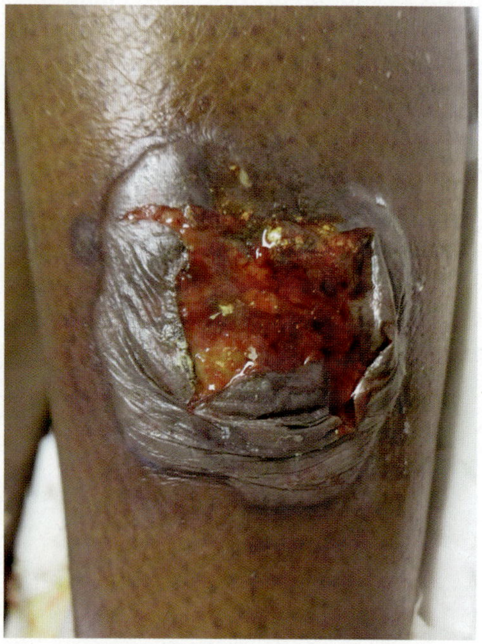

A. Pancreas
B. Colon
C. Gall bladder
D. Lungs
E. Kidney

7. The lesions on the knees of this 36-year-old female are commonly seen in:

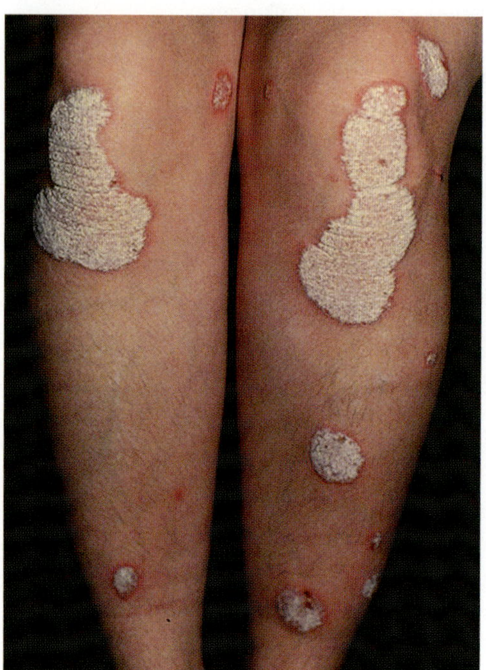

A. Kaposi sarcoma
B. Contact dermatitis
C. Syphilis
D. Psoriasis
E. Drug reactions

8. The acute linear versicular-bullous eruption shown in the referenced picture on the calf of a 28-year-old female is most likely the result from:

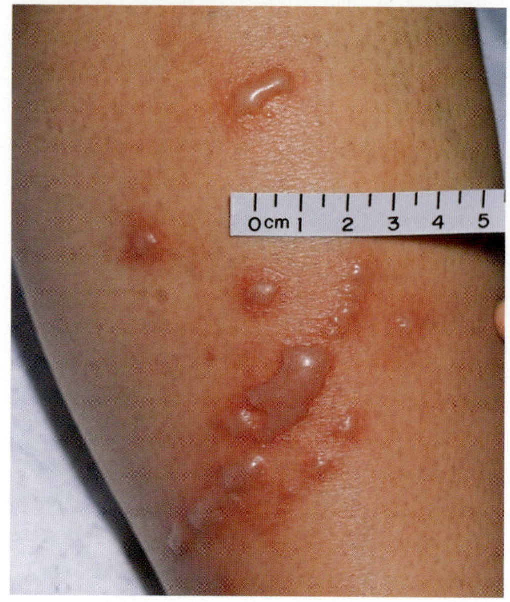

A. Bedbug bites
B. Syphilis
C. Poison oak (contact dermatitis)
D. Flea bites
E. Psoriasis

9. Which of the following statements below is *incorrect* regarding the foot of the patient shown below?

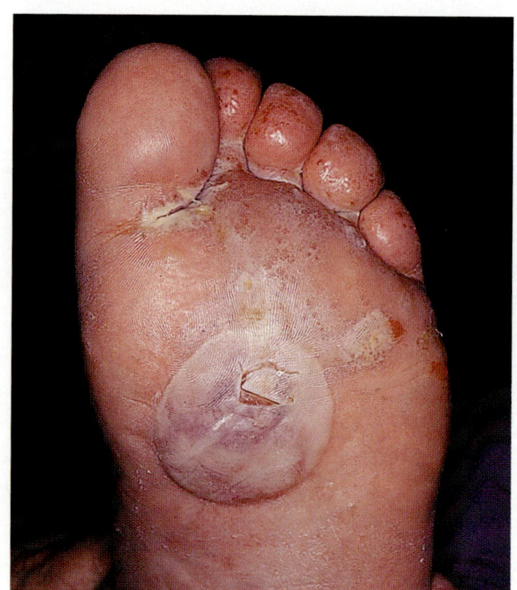

A. It is a common fungal infection.
B. *Trichophyton* and *Epidermophyton* are often responsible for it.

C. The lesions are nonpruritic.
D. The condition produces a scaling, erythematous patch, often with a reddened, raised border.
E. The name of this condition denotes the area of the body involved.

10. **Which of the following statements is true regarding this intensely pruritic and contagious condition?**

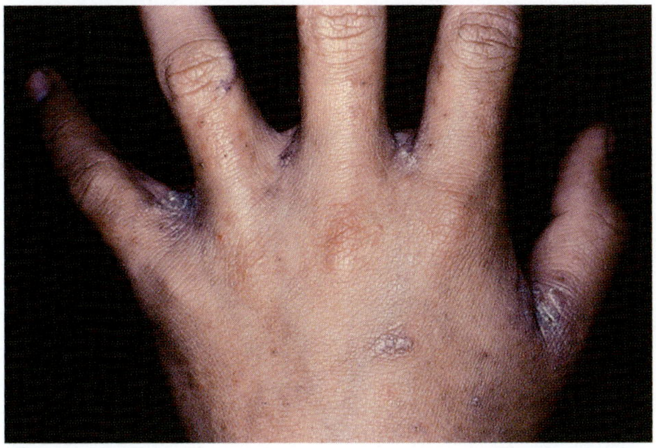

A. Has a predilection for the web spaces of the fingers and toes, as well as the groin
B. Rarely involves the buttocks or the genitals of males or the nipples of females
C. Is rare in population groups in which HIV is prevalent
D. Is associated with pustules and vesicles
E. Is caused by a virus

REFERENCES

Available online.

BIBLIOGRAPHY

Available online.

9

The Head and Neck

Mark H. Swartz

A lady, aged twenty, became affected with some symptoms which were supposed to be hysterical… After she had been in this nervous state about three months it was observed that her pulse had become singularly rapid… She next complained of weakness on exertion and began to look pale and thin… It was observed that the eyes assumed a singular appearance, for the eyeballs were apparently enlarged. In a few months… a tumour, of a horseshoe shape, appeared on the front of the throat and exactly in the situation of the thyroid gland.

Robert James Graves (1796–1853)

VIDEOS

9.1 Palpating the cranium and lymph nodes of the head and neck
9.2 Palpating the thyroid gland
9.3 Palpating for supraclavicular nodes

GENERAL CONSIDERATIONS

The appearance of the head and face, and their contours and texture, often provides the first insight into the nature of illness. Sunken cheeks, wasting of the temporal muscles, and flushing of the face are important visible clues of systemic illness. In addition, some facial appearances are pathognomonic of disease. The pale, puffy face of nephritis, the startled expression of hyperthyroidism, and the immobile stare of parkinsonism are examples of classic facies.

The appearance of the patient's face may also provide information regarding psychological makeup: is the person happy, sad, angry, or anxious?

Thyroid disease takes many forms. The World Health Organization (WHO) estimates that more than 200 million people in the world have enlarged thyroid glands, a condition known as *goiter.* Asians first described goiter around 1500 BCE. However, even at that time, they recognized that seaweed in the diet tended to make goiters smaller. Iodine was not discovered until the 19th century. Still, it is now believed that those goiters were related to an iodine deficiency that was partially corrected by the iodine in the seaweed.

The ancient Greeks and Romans recognized that when a thin thread tied around the neck of a newly married female broke, she was pregnant. This was caused by an increase in the size of the thyroid during pregnancy.

Almost one-third of the world's population lives in areas of iodine deficiency.[1] In areas where the daily iodine intake is less than 50 μg,[a] goiter is usually endemic, and when the daily intake falls less than 25 μg, congenital hypothyroidism is seen. The prevalence of goiter in areas of severe iodine deficiency can be as high as 80%. Populations at particular risk tend to be remote and live in mountainous areas in Southeast Asia, Latin America, and Central Africa.

In iodine-replete areas, most persons with thyroid disorders have autoimmune diseases, ranging from primary atrophic hypothyroidism, Hashimoto thyroiditis, to thyrotoxicosis caused by Graves disease.

Thyroid cancer is the most common endocrine cancer, and its incidence has increased by approximately 3% per 100,000 people yearly. The thyroid is the seventh leading site of new cancers in females. According to the American Cancer Society, in 2023, there were 43,720 new cases of thyroid cancer (31,180 in females and 12,540 in males). There were about 2120 deaths from thyroid cancer (1150 females and 970 males) in 2023. Worldwide, an estimated 586,202 people were diagnosed with thyroid cancer in 2020. Risk factors include radiation exposure related to medical treatment during childhood.

The 5-year survival rate for all thyroid cancer patients is 98% in the United States. Survival, however, varies markedly by stage, age of diagnosis, and disease subtype. The 5-year survival rate approaches 100% for localized papillary, follicular, and medullary thyroid cancer; for localized anaplastic thyroid cancer, the 5-year survival is 39%. If thyroid cancer has spread to nearby tissues or organs and/or the regional lymph nodes, it is called regional thyroid cancer. The 5-year regional survival rate for regional papillary thyroid cancer is 99%. For regional follicular thyroid cancer, the rate is 98%, and for regional medullary thyroid cancer, the rate is 92%. For regional anaplastic

[a]The daily recommended dietary allowance for iodine is 150 μg for adults, 220 μg for pregnant females, and 290 μg for breastfeeding females.

thyroid cancer, the 5-year survival is 11%. Medullary and anaplastic thyroid cancers, which comprise about 3% of all thyroid cancers, are the most likely to spread and have the lowest survival rates.

The chance of being diagnosed with thyroid cancer has risen in recent years; it is the most rapidly increasing cancer in the United States, tripling in the past 3 decades. Much of this rise appears to be the result of the increased use of thyroid ultrasound, which can detect small thyroid nodules that might not otherwise have been found in the past. Thyroid cancer is often diagnosed at a younger age compared with other cancers in adults. White people are 70% more likely to be diagnosed with the disease than Black people, who have the lowest incidence rate of the disease.

Head and neck cancer accounts for about 4% of all cancers in the United States. In 2023, 66,920 people (49,190 males and 17,730 females) developed head and neck cancer. While younger people can develop the disease, most people are older than 50 when diagnosed. There were 15,400 deaths (11,210 males and 4190 females) from head and neck cancer in 2023. Worldwide, an estimated 562,328 people were diagnosed with head and neck cancer in 2020.

Head and neck cancer includes cancers of the mouth, nose, sinuses, salivary glands, throat, and lymph nodes in the neck. Most begin in the moist tissues that line the mouth, nose, and throat. Symptoms include a lump or sore in the mouth that does not heal, a persistent sore throat, trouble swallowing, or a change or hoarseness in the voice. Using tobacco or alcohol increases the risk of developing head and neck cancer. In fact, 85% of all head and neck cancers are linked to tobacco use. Tobacco use includes smoking cigarettes, cigars, and pipes; chewing tobacco; and using snuff. It is the single largest risk factor for head and neck cancer. Eighty-five percent (85%) of head and neck cancers are linked to tobacco use. However, if found early, these cancers may be curable. Treatment can include surgery, radiation therapy, chemotherapy, or a combination, but these treatments may affect eating, speaking, or even breathing.

Chewing areca nuts (known as *betel nuts*) is another well-known risk factor for head and neck squamous cell carcinoma.[2] The WHO classifies betel nut as a carcinogen. Many studies have shown a clear link between betel nut use and cancer of the mouth and esophagus. The areca nut is the fruit of the areca palm tree *(Areca catechu)*, which grows in much of the tropical Pacific, Southeast and South Asia, and parts of East Africa. Betel nut chewing is a unique problem in India and other Southeast Asian countries, especially Taiwan. The nut is commonly chewed after being ground up or sliced and wrapped in leaves of the *Piper betle* vine coated with lime. Habitual chewing of the nut stains the lips and teeth red… a telltale sign of chewing betel nuts!

Betel nut has a long history in Southeast Asia and the Pacific Basin. Its use can be traced back as far as 2000 years in these areas. A habit passed down through generations, chewing betel nut is a time-honored custom for 10% to 20% of the world's population. Today, the WHO estimates that around 600 million people use some form of betel nut. It is one of the most popular psychoactive substances in the world, in fourth place after nicotine, alcohol, and caffeine. But while betel nut is an important cultural and social tradition in many countries, growing evidence points to serious health effects from regular use.

The reasons for betel nut consumption are for its psychostimulating effects, which cause a euphoric feeling and heightened alertness, for sweetening the breath, as a digestive, or as a cultural practice often during religious ceremonies. The nut is a highly addictive substance with a severity score resembling that of amphetamines.[3] In Taiwan, betel nuts are often chewed by truck and bus drivers who work long hours and need to stay awake while driving at night.

STRUCTURE AND PHYSIOLOGY

The Head

The skull is composed of 22 bones, 14 in the face alone. This bony structure acts as a support and protection for the softer tissues within.

The *facial skeleton* comprises the mandible, the maxilla, and the nasal, palatine, lacrimal, and vomer bones. The unpaired *mandible* forms the lower jaw. The *maxilla* is an irregular bone and forms the upper jaw on each side. The *nasal bones* form the bridge of the nose. The other bones are not relevant to this discussion.

The prominent bones of the *cranial skeleton* include the frontal, temporal, parietal, and occipital bones. The *frontal bones* form the forehead. The *temporal bones* form the anterolateral walls of the brain. The *mastoid process*, part of the temporal bone, is particularly important in ear disease and is discussed in Chapter 11, The Ear and Nose. The *parietal bones* form the top and posterolateral portions of the skull. The *occipital bones* form the posterior part of the skull. The bones of the face and skull are shown in Fig. 9.1.

The principal muscle of the mouth is the *orbicularis oris*. This single muscle surrounds the lips, and numerous other facial muscles insert into it. The action of the orbicularis oris is to close the lips.

The *orbicularis oculi* muscle surrounds the eye. Its function is to close the eyelids. Chapter 10, The Eye, further discusses this muscle and its action.

The *platysma* is a thin, superficial muscle of the neck, crossing the outer border of the mandible and extending over the lower anterior portion of the face. The main action of the platysma is to pull the mandible downward and backward, which results in a mournful facial expression.

The muscles of mastication include the masseter, pterygoid, and temporalis. These muscles insert on the mandible and effect chewing. The *masseter* is strong and thick and is one of the most powerful muscles of the face. The action of the masseter is to close the jaw by elevating and drawing the mandible backward. Tension in the masseter may be felt by clenching the jaw. Although essential to jaw function, the other muscles of mastication are not clinically relevant to physical diagnosis and are not discussed here. The locations of these muscles are shown in Fig. 9.2.

The *trigeminal*, or fifth cranial, nerve carries sensory fibers from the face, oral cavity, and teeth and carries efferent motor

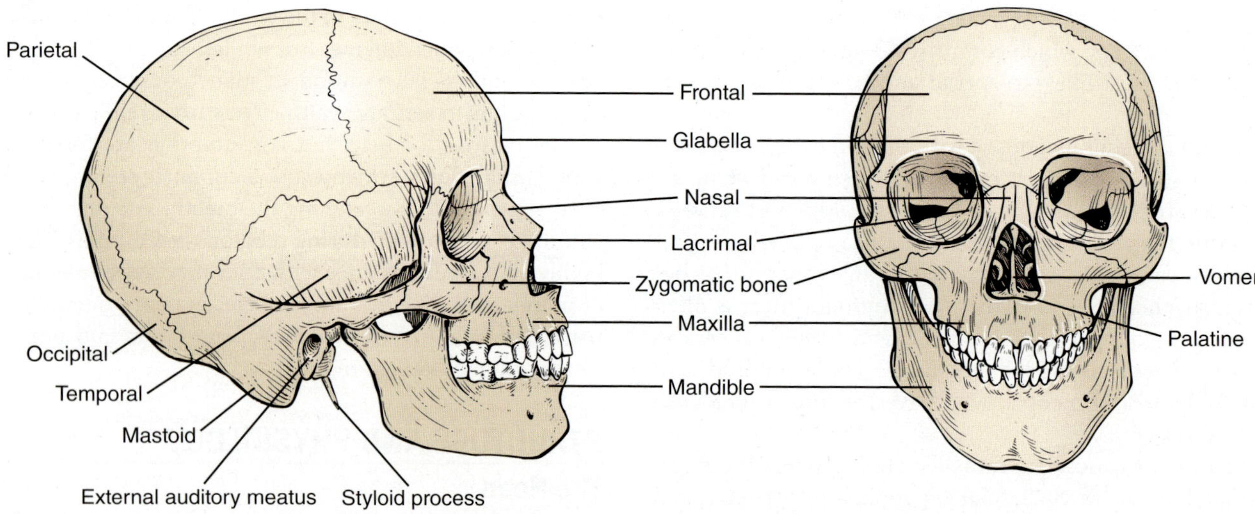

Fig. 9.1 Bones of the Face and Skull.

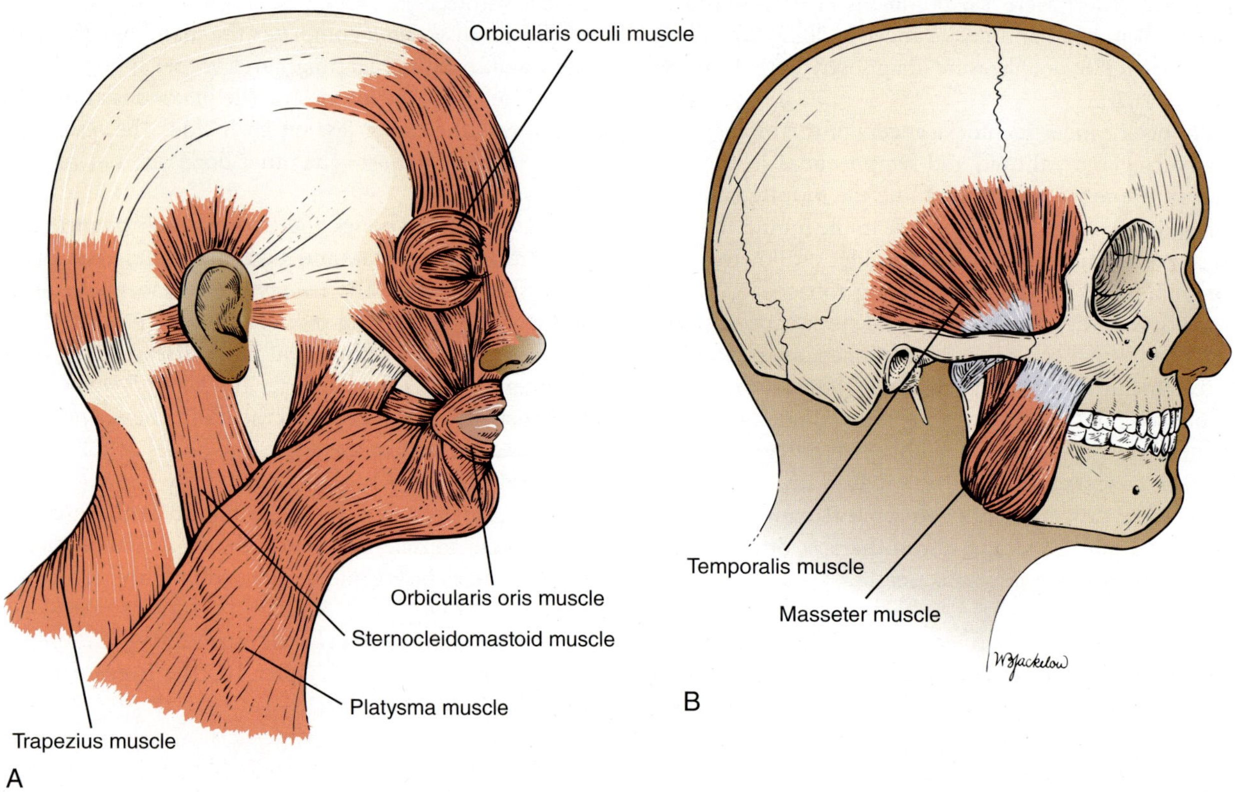

Fig. 9.2 Muscles of the Face and Skull. (A) The more superficial muscles. (B) The underlying muscles.

fibers to the muscles of mastication. The principal divisions of this nerve are discussed in subsequent chapters.

The Neck

The neck is divided by the sternocleidomastoid muscle into the *anterior*, or *medial*, *triangle* and the *posterior*, or *lateral*, *triangle*. These are illustrated in Fig. 9.3.

The *sternocleidomastoid* is a strong muscle that raises the sternum during respiration. The sternocleidomastoid has two heads: the *sternal* head arises from the manubrium sterni, and the *clavicular* head originates on the sternal end of the clavicle. The two heads unite and insert on the lateral aspect of the mastoid process. The spinal accessory, or eleventh cranial, nerve innervates the sternocleidomastoid.

Anterior to the sternocleidomastoid muscle is the *anterior triangle*. The other boundaries of the anterior triangle are the clavicle (inferiorly) and the midline (anteriorly). The anterior triangle contains the thyroid gland, larynx, pharynx, lymph nodes, submandibular salivary gland, and fat.

The *thyroid gland* envelops the upper trachea and consists of two lobes connected by an isthmus. It is the largest endocrine gland in the body. As seen from the front, the thyroid is butterfly

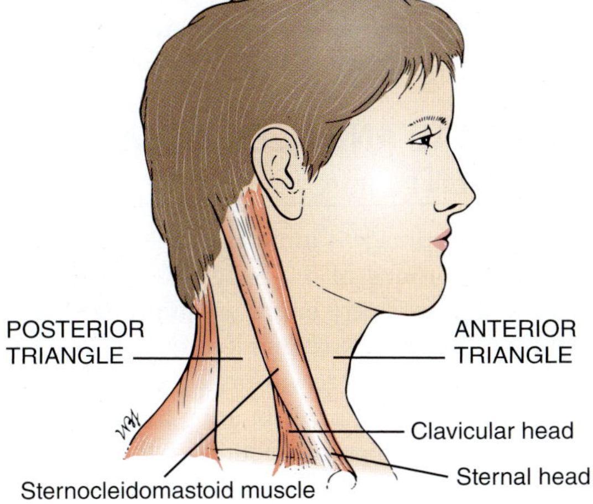

Fig. 9.3 Boundaries of the Triangles of the Neck.

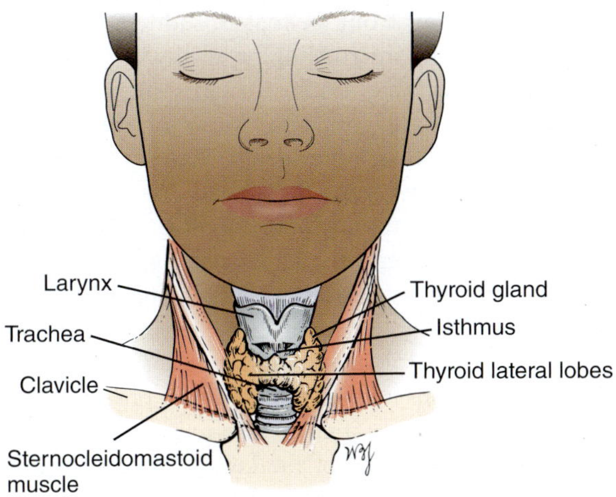

Fig. 9.4 Thyroid Gland.

shaped and wraps around the anterior and lateral portions of the larynx and trachea, as shown in Fig. 9.4.

The thyroid isthmus lies across the trachea just below the cricoid cartilage of the larynx. The lateral lobes extend along both sides of the larynx, reaching the middle of the thyroid cartilage of the larynx. On occasion, the thyroid gland may extend downward and enlarge within the thorax, producing a substernal goiter. The function of the thyroid gland is to produce thyroid hormone in accordance with the needs of the body.

The pharynx and larynx are discussed in Chapter 12, The Oral Cavity and Pharynx.

The sternocleidomastoid muscle overlies the *carotid sheath.* The carotid sheath lies lateral to the larynx. This sheath contains the common carotid artery, the internal jugular vein, and the vagus nerve.

Posterior to the sternocleidomastoid is the *posterior triangle.* This is bounded by the trapezius muscle posteriorly and by the clavicle inferiorly. The posterior triangle also contains lymph nodes.

It has been estimated that the neck contains more than 75 lymph nodes on each side. The chains of these lymph nodes are named for their location. Starting posteriorly, they are the *occipital, posterior auricular, posterior cervical, superficial and*

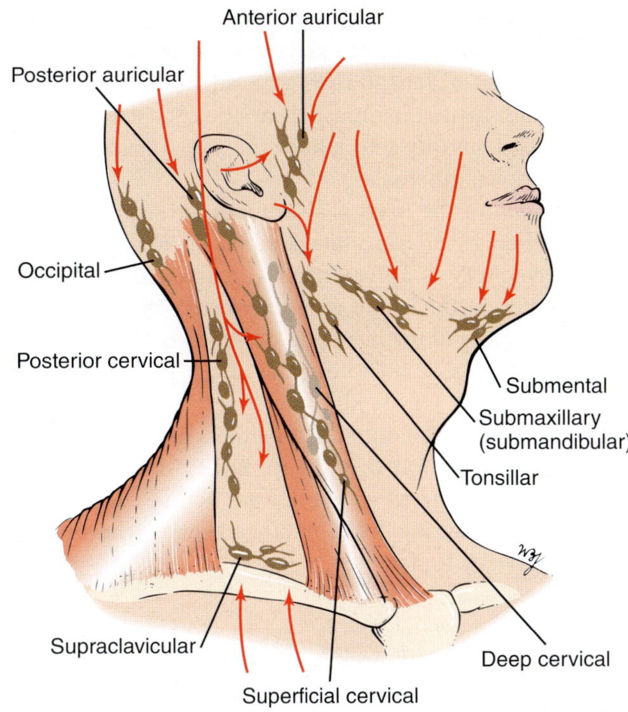

Fig. 9.5 Lymph Nodes of the Neck and Their Drainage.

deep cervical (adjacent to the sternocleidomastoid muscle), *tonsillar, submaxillary* (or *submandibular*), *submental* (at the tip of the jaw in the midline), *anterior auricular,* and *supraclavicular* (above the clavicle) chains. Knowledge of lymphatic drainage is essential because the presence of an enlarged lymph node may signal disease in the area draining into it. The main groups of lymph nodes and their drainage areas are shown in Fig. 9.5.

Review of Specific Symptoms

The most common symptoms related to the neck are as follows:

- Neck mass
- Neck stiffness

Neck Mass

The most common symptom is a lump or swelling in the neck. Once a patient describes a neck lump, ask the following questions:

"When did you first notice the lump?"
"Does it hurt?"
"Does the lump change in size?"
"Have you had any ear infections? Infections in your mouth?"
"Has there been hoarseness associated with the mass?"
"Is there a family history of thyroid cancer?"
"Is there a history of prior neck or thyroid gland radiation?"

If there is associated pain with a mass in the neck, an acute infection is likely. Masses present for only a few days are commonly inflammatory, whereas those present for months are more likely to be neoplastic. A mass that has been present for months to years without any change in size often turns out to be a benign or congenital lesion. Blockage of a salivary gland duct may produce a mass that fluctuates in size while the patient eats.

The patient's age is relevant in assessing a neck mass. A lump in the neck of a patient younger than 20 years of age may be an enlarged tonsillar lymph node or a congenital mass. If the mass is in the midline, it will most likely be a thyroglossal cyst.[b]

From the ages of 20 to 40 years, thyroid disease is more common, although lymphoma must always be considered. When a patient is older than 40, a neck mass must be considered malignant until proven otherwise.

The *location* of the mass is also important. Midline masses tend to be benign or congenital lesions, such as thyroglossal cysts or dermoid cysts. Lateral masses are frequently neoplastic. Masses located in the lateral upper neck may be metastatic lesions from tumors of the head and neck. In contrast, masses in the lateral lower neck may be metastatic from tumors of the breast and stomach. One benign lateral neck mass is a branchial cleft cyst, which may manifest as a painless neck mass near the anterior upper third border of the sternocleidomastoid muscle.

Hoarseness associated with a thyroid nodule suggests vocal cord paralysis resulting from impingement of the recurrent laryngeal nerve by tumor.

Neck Stiffness

If a patient reports a stiff neck, ask the following questions:

"How long have you had the stiff neck?"

"Have you done any strenuous activity recently?"

"Are you aware of sleeping differently before the stiff neck occurred?"

"Do you have a headache associated with the stiff neck?"

"Do you have a fever?"

"Have you had recent nausea or vomiting?"

"Does light bother you?"

"Have you noted unusual sleepiness?"

"Have you had recent chest pain or chest discomfort?"

A stiff neck is typically characterized by soreness and difficulty moving the neck, especially when turning the head to the side. A stiff neck may also be accompanied by a headache, neck pain, shoulder pain, or arm pain and, in severe cases, may cause the individual to turn the entire body as opposed to the neck when trying to look sideways or backward. However, by far, the most common cause of a stiff neck is a muscle sprain or muscle strain, particularly to the levator scapula muscle. Located at the back and side of the neck, the levator scapula muscle connects the cervical spine (the neck) with the shoulder. This muscle is controlled by the third and fourth cervical nerves (C3, C4).

The levator scapula muscle may be strained or sprained throughout the course of many everyday activities, such as sleeping in a position that strains the neck muscles, sports injuries, rapid swimming, poor posture, stress, or holding the neck in an abnormal position for an extended period.

The sudden occurrence of a stiff neck, high fever, nausea, vomiting, sleepiness, or headache should raise suspicion of possible meningeal irritation. Any time a stiff neck is accompanied by a fever, it is advisable to seek medical evaluation.

[b]A thyroglossal cyst may arise anywhere along the route of the thyroid gland's descent from the foramen cecum of the tongue to its adult location in the neck. See Fig. 24.35.

Neck pain may be associated with referred pain from the chest. Patients with angina or a myocardial infarction may report neck pain or stiffness.

EFFECT OF HEAD AND NECK DISEASE ON THE PATIENT

The concept of body image is important. The head and neck are the most visible portions of the body. The shape of the eyes, mouth, face, and nose is very important to people. Many dislike their body image and want to change it through cosmetic surgery. Others require cosmetic surgery to repair alterations caused by trauma. Still others suffer from disfiguring head and neck cancer and need to undergo surgical procedures for the removal of these lesions. Many of these procedures are mutilating.

Distortion of the body image, especially on the head and neck, can have a devastating effect on the patient. The most common reaction to head and neck disease is depression. Many affected patients suffer from feelings of sadness and hopelessness. They look in the mirror hoping they will see themselves with a more acceptable body image someday. Recurrent thoughts of suicide are common. Many of these depressed patients turn to alcohol or other drugs.

On occasion, patients who have undergone cosmetic surgery are dissatisfied with the results. Many of these patients are trying to escape feelings of inferiority and social maladjustment. They may have had only minor defects, but they viewed those defects as a major source of their interpersonal problems. Cosmetic surgery is a way to change their image to improve their social maladjustment. Some individuals may even blame their physicians for "destroying" their faces. Even after further revisions, these patients may never be satisfied. One of the keys to successful cosmetic surgery is the proper psychological evaluation of patients.

PHYSICAL EXAMINATION

No special equipment is needed for the examination of the head and neck. It is performed with the patient seated, facing the examiner. The examination consists of the following steps:

- Inspection
- Auscultation for carotid bruits (discussed in Chapter 15, The Peripheral Vascular System)
- Palpation

Inspection

Inspect the position of the head. Does the patient hold the head erect? Is there any asymmetry in the facial structure? Is the head in proportion to the rest of the body?

Inspect the scalp for lesions. Describe the hair.

Are any masses present? If so, describe their size, consistency, and symmetry. Figure 24.35 depicts a child with a midline *thyroglossal duct cyst.* The cyst is smooth, firm, and midline. The thyroglossal duct cyst moves upward when the patient is asked to swallow or stick out the tongue.

The thyroid gland in an embryo starts as a small group of cells at the very back of the base of the tongue (the posterior one-third of the tongue). The furthest point backward is where the thyroid begins to develop. From here, in the earliest weeks of gestation, the thyroid cells begin a journey downward along the midline of the neck until they arrive low in the neck just above the sternum. These cells then grow into the butterfly-shaped gland that we recognize as the thyroid gland. The tube-like path these cells took to reach their final destination then closes. If it doesn't close in its entirety, it may leave an open space that may fill up with fluid or thick mucus-like material. This fluid-filled sac is called a *thyroglossal duct cyst*.

Thyroglossal duct cysts usually make themselves known early in life, either in childhood or young adulthood. They are usually round or oval soft masses found in the midline of the neck (or a little to the left of the midline) just above the larynx.

Most commonly, thyroglossal duct cysts are approximately the size of a ping-pong ball but can get much larger. If they become infected, the skin may turn red and become tender; sometimes these cysts will spontaneously rupture through the skin, and the fluid and pus within will drip down the neck. Therefore, avoiding infection is one of the primary reasons to remove these cysts.

One must always determine whether the thyroglossal duct cyst contains any thyroid tissue. The reason the presence of thyroid tissue is significant is twofold. First, in a rare patient, it may be that the thyroid tissue in a thyroglossal duct cyst is the entire thyroid gland that did not make its normal descent to its correct anatomic location lower down in the neck. For this reason, it is essential to make sure the patient has a normal thyroid gland as well as the cyst. Second, thyroid cancer can exist in thyroid tissue within a thyroglossal duct cyst.

Inspect the eyes for proptosis (a forward displacement, or bulging, of the eyeball). Proptosis may be caused by thyroid dysfunction or a mass in the orbit.

Inspect the neck for areas of asymmetry. Ask the patient to extend the neck so that it can be inspected for scars, asymmetry, or masses. The normal thyroid is barely visible. Ask the patient to swallow while you observe any upward motion of the thyroid with swallowing. A diffusely enlarged thyroid gland often causes generalized enlargement of the neck. A patient with diffuse thyromegaly is pictured in Fig. 9.6. This patient has Graves disease with bilateral proptosis.

Is nodularity of the neck present? Nodular neck masses caused by a multinodular goiter are pictured in Fig. 9.7.

Is superficial venous distention present? Evaluating venous distention in the neck is important because it may be associated with a goiter.

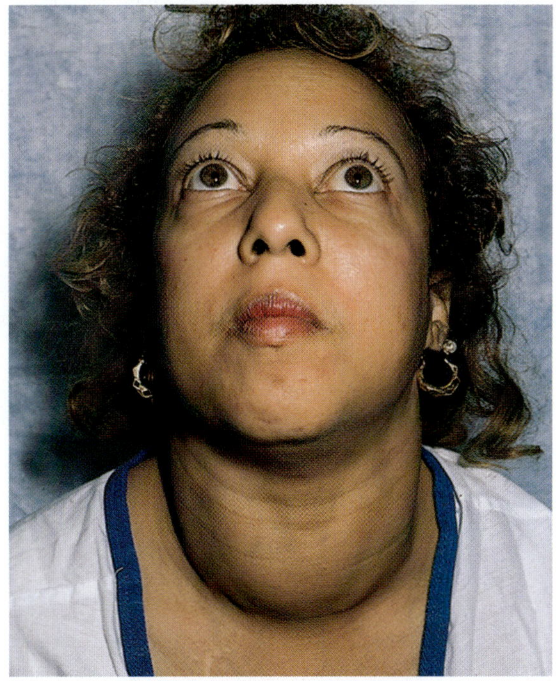

Fig. 9.6 Graves Disease.

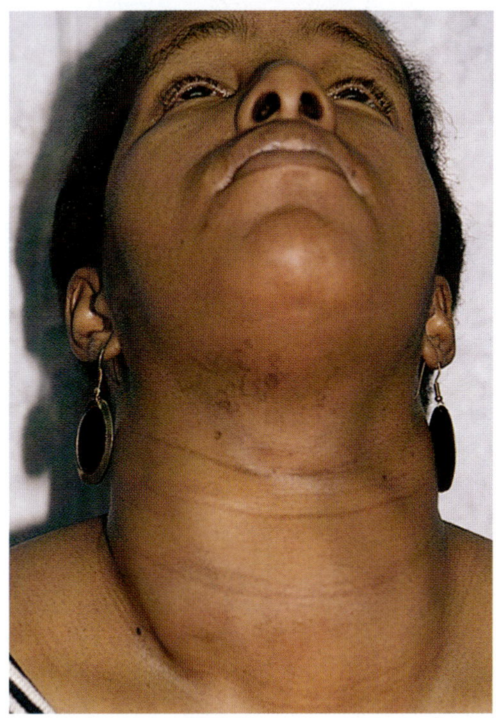

Fig. 9.7 Multinodular Goiter.

Palpation

Palpate the Head and Neck

See Video 9.1: Palpating the cranium and lymph nodes of the head and neck.

To confirm the information gathered by inspection, palpation is necessary. The examiner must cradle the patient's head in their hands with a slight flexion, as shown in Fig. 9.8.

When examining the cranium, it is important to check for any areas of tenderness or lumps. The examiner should use their fingertips to gently roll over the skull in circular motions to feel for any concave areas or areas of tenderness.

To assess the lymph nodes in the head and neck, begin by examining the occipital region. Move your hands toward the posterior auricular area, which is located above the mastoid process, then proceed down to the posterior triangle to check for the posterior cervical lymph node chain. Along the sternocleidomastoid muscle, feel for the superficial cervical chain, then hook around the muscle to check for the deep cervical chain. Continue to the anterior triangle region and up to the

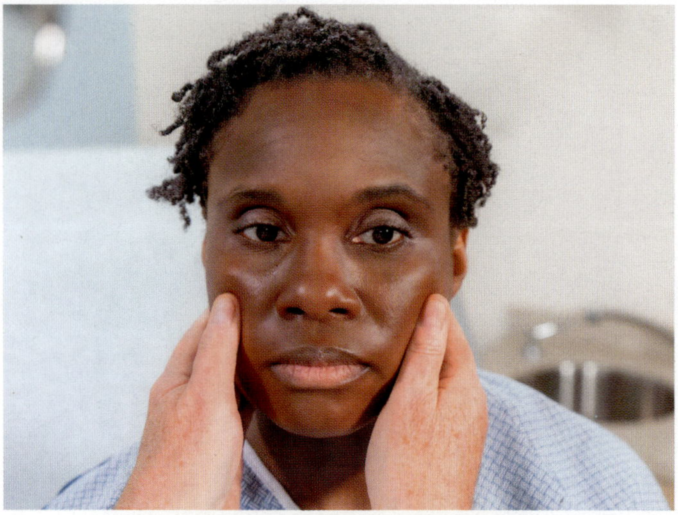

Fig. 9.8 Palpation of the Head and Neck.

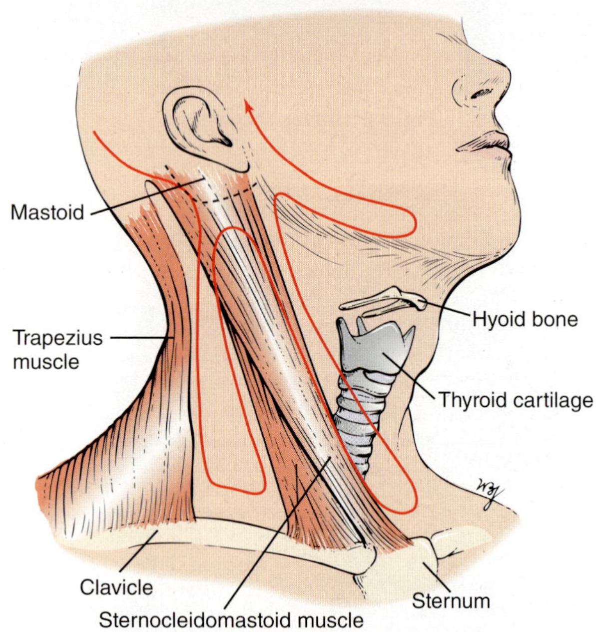

Fig. 9.9 Suggested Approach for Palpation of the Lymph Nodes of the Neck.

jaw margin to evaluate the tonsillar group. Follow the jawline to palpate the submaxillary (or submandibular) chain, then examine the submental nodes at the tip of the jaw. Finally, evaluate the anterior auricular chain in front of the ear. This sequence of examination is illustrated in Fig. 9.9.

Enlarged posterior auricular and posterior cervical nodes are pictured in Fig. 9.10.

Swollen, often tender, nodes may indicate inflammation, while solid and fixed nodes are more likely to be a sign of malignancy.

Palpate the Thyroid Gland

See Video 9.2: Palpating the thyroid gland.

To conduct a proper thyroid exam, it's crucial to have a good grasp of the anatomy. Start by placing your finger on the tip of the chin and sliding it down the center. The first hard structure

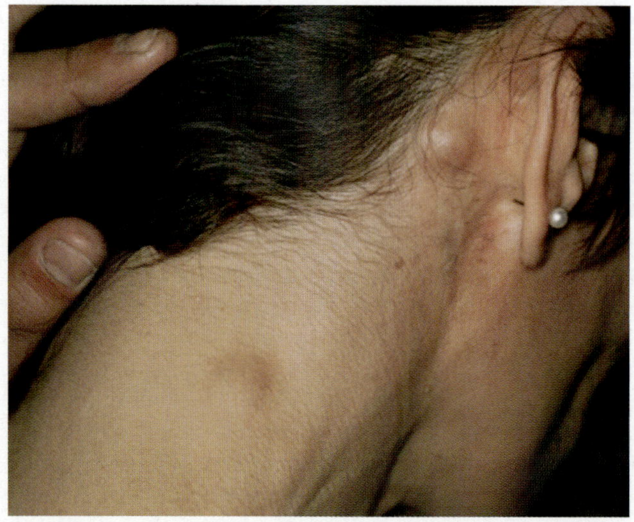

Fig. 9.10 Posterior Auricular and Posterior Cervical Adenopathy.

you'll feel is the top of the thyroid cartilage. Keep going down until you reach the cricothyroid membrane notch, followed by the first two tracheal rings. It's important to note that the thyroid gland is not situated directly over the thyroid cartilage.

When examining the thyroid gland, there are two approaches: anterior and posterior. The anterior approach requires the patient and examiner to sit face to face. The neck should be observed to check for any enlargement of the thyroid gland. To relax the neck muscles, place one hand at the back of the neck and slightly tilt the head to the side. Using the right hand, palpate the left lobe with three fingers while the head is turned to the right. Push the front edge of the sternocleidomastoid muscle backward while sliding your fingers over the thyroid gland. It is helpful to have the patient move their neck slightly during the palpation process. Repeat this process for the other side (Fig. 9.11). After evaluating the left lobe, displace the larynx to the left and evaluate the right lobe by reversing the hand positions.

For the posterior approach, stand behind the patient and encircle their neck with your hands. Place your fingers on the first two tracheal rings and move your hands slightly to the sides to cover the wings of the gland. Ask the patient to swallow and observe if there is any uneven movement in your hands. The patient may be given water to drink to facilitate swallowing.

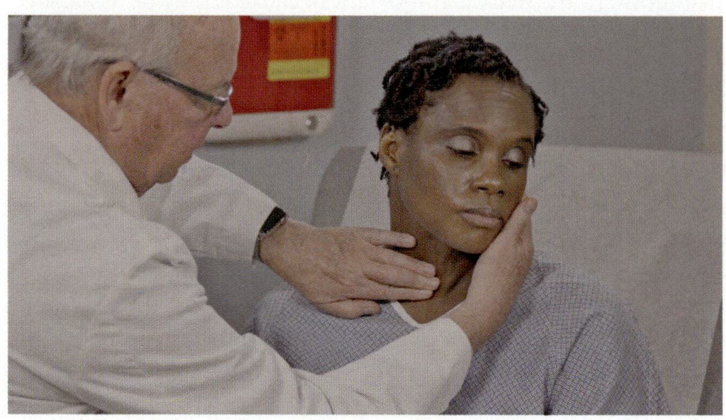

Fig. 9.11 Anterior Approach for Palpation of the Thyroid Gland.

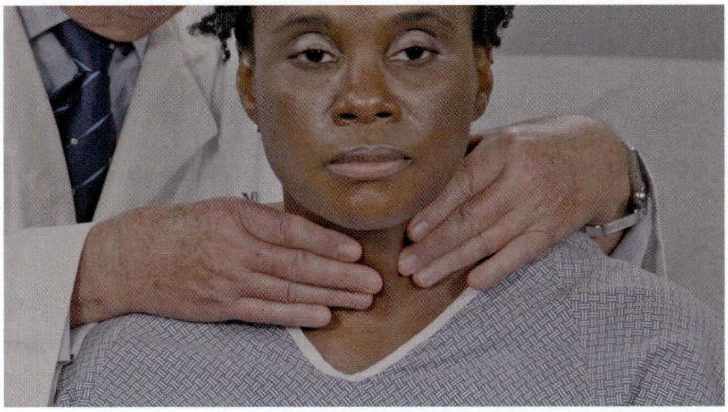

Fig. 9.12 Posterior Approach for Palpation of the Thyroid Gland.

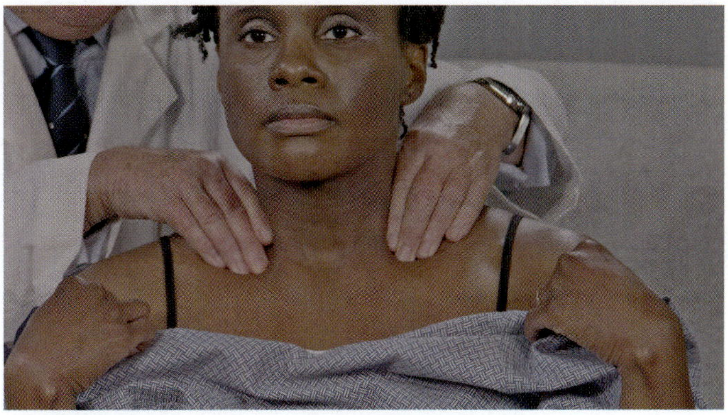

Fig. 9.13 Technique for Palpation of the Supraclavicular Lymph Nodes.

The posterior approach is shown in Fig. 9.12. Next, use one hand to gently move the trachea and thyroid sideways while feeling the thyroid lobe with your other hand. Repeat this procedure on the other side.

Although both the anterior and posterior approaches of palpation are usually performed, the examiner can rarely feel the thyroid gland in its normal state.

The consistency of the gland should be evaluated. The normal thyroid gland has a consistency of muscle tissue. Unusual *hardness* may be associated with malignancy or scarring. Softness, or sponginess, is often observed with a toxic goiter. *Tenderness* of the thyroid gland is associated with acute infections or hemorrhage into the gland.

If the thyroid is enlarged, it should also be examined by auscultation. The bell of the stethoscope is placed over the lobes of the thyroid while the examiner listens for the presence of a bruit (a murmur heard when there is increased turbulence in a vessel). The finding of a systolic or to-and-fro[c] *thyroid bruit*, mainly if heard over the superior pole, indicates an abnormally large blood flow and is highly suggestive of a *toxic goiter*.

Palpate for Supraclavicular Nodes

See Video 9.3: Palpating for supraclavicular nodes.

Palpation for supraclavicular nodes concludes the examination of the head and neck. The examiner stands behind the patient and places their fingers into the medial supraclavicular fossae, which is located deep to the clavicle and next to the sternocleidomastoid muscles. The patient is instructed to take a deep breath while the examiner applies pressure with the pads of their fingers deeply behind the clavicles. Any enlarged supraclavicular nodes are felt as the patient inhales and pushes any nodes up while the healthcare professional pushes down. Fig. 9.13 provides a visual demonstration of this technique.

The examination of the trachea is discussed in Chapter 13, The Chest. The examination of the carotid arterial and jugular venous pulsations is discussed in Chapter 14, The Heart.

CLINICOPATHOLOGIC CORRELATIONS

Although iodine deficiency is still a worldwide cause of thyroid enlargement, other important causes of goiter are infection, autoimmune disease, cancer, and isolated nodules. An enlarged thyroid may be associated with *hyperthyroidism*, *hypothyroidism*, or a *simple* or *multinodular* goiter of normal function.

As mentioned earlier in this chapter, the thyroid may enlarge and expand into the chest cavity. If the thyroid is large enough, it may impair venous outflow from the head and neck and may even be responsible for airway or vascular compromise. *Pemberton's sign* is helpful in detecting latent obstruction in the thoracic inlet. To determine whether the sign is present, the patient is asked to elevate both arms until they touch the sides of the head. Pemberton's sign is present when facial suffusion with dilation of the cervical veins develops within a few seconds. After 1 to 2 minutes, the face may even become cyanotic. Fig. 9.14 shows a patient with a positive Pemberton's sign. The patient is a 62-year-old male with an anterior neck mass, the existence of which was known for 25 years. The upper border of the thyroid was palpable on examination, but the lower pole descended below the clavicle and was not detectable.

As indicated in the quotation at the beginning of this chapter, hyperthyroidism may manifest with various generalized symptoms and signs. It has been said, "To know thyroid disease is to know medicine," because there are so many generalized effects of thyroid hormone excess. Table 9.1 lists the variety of clinical symptoms related to thyroid hormone excess.

A nervous, perspiring patient with a stare and bulging eyes offers an unmistakable combination of physical signs associated with hyperthyroidism. The diffuse toxic goiter, known as Graves disease, is the most common type of hyperthyroidism. Symptomatic Graves disease has an incidence of 1 per 1000 females in multinational studies. This disease can occur at any age and in all races. Graves disease is viewed as an autoimmune disorder provoked by the elaboration of a thyroid-stimulating immunoglobulin. The many clinical manifestations of Graves disease are truly multisystemic and include the following:

- Warm, moist skin
- Hand tremor
- Erythema
- Easy fatigability
- Hyperhidrosis (increased sweating)
- Anxiety
- Insomnia
- Alopecia (hair loss)

[c]Refers to two separate murmurs, systolic and diastolic.

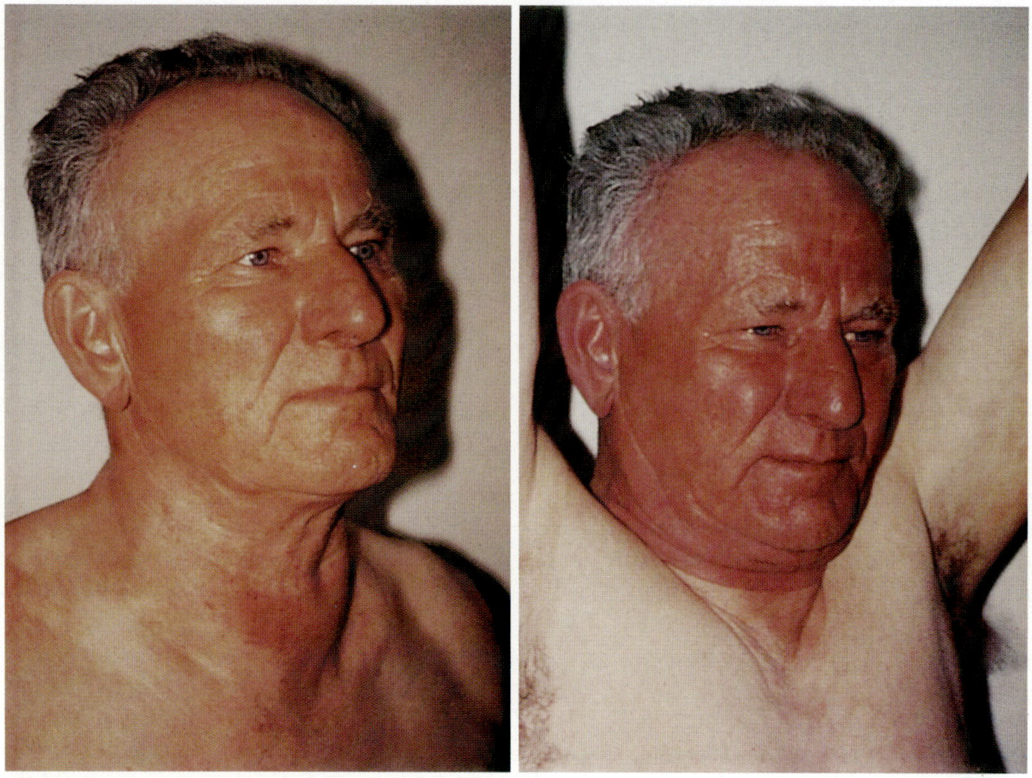

A B

Fig. 9.14 (A and B) Pemberton's sign. (From Wallace C, Siminoski K: The Pemberton sign, *Ann Intern Med* 125:568, 1996.)

TABLE 9.1 Symptoms of Hyperthyroidism

Organ System	Symptom
General	Preference for the cold Weight loss with good appetite
Eyes	Prominence of eyeballs[a] Puffiness of eyelids Double vision Decreased motility
Neck	Goiter
Cardiac	Palpitations Peripheral edema[b]
Gastrointestinal	Increased numbers of bowel movements
Genitourinary	Polyuria Decreased fertility
Neuromuscular	Fatigue Weakness Tremulousness
Emotional	Nervousness Irritability
Dermatologic	Hair thinning Increased perspiration Change in skin texture Change in pigmentation

[a]Appears to result from mucopolysaccharide deposition behind the orbit.
[b]Appears to result from excessive mucopolysaccharide deposition under the skin, especially in the legs.

- Hyperpigmentation
- Nail growth changes
- Palpitations
- Proptosis
- Lid retraction
- Gastroesophageal reflux
- Weight loss
- Increased bowel motility
- Amenorrhea
- Decreased libido
- Heat intolerance

Graves disease occasionally manifests with unilateral proptosis, as shown in Fig. 9.15. This patient presented with proptosis and was treated for Graves disease 20 years before this photograph was taken. As is common, the proptosis never disappeared.

Sometimes hyperthyroidism is caused by a single hot nodule.[d]

Toxic adenomatous goiter, also known as *Plummer disease*, accounts for fewer than 10% of all cases of hyperthyroidism.

[d]The terms *hot* and *cold* are descriptions of nodules seen on a thyroid scan and are used to indicate whether a nodule accumulates more or less radioactive iodine than the surrounding thyroid tissue. A hot nodule is functioning thyroid tissue and has a greater iodine uptake than the surrounding tissue. A cold nodule is nonfunctioning and fails to take up the radioactive tracer.

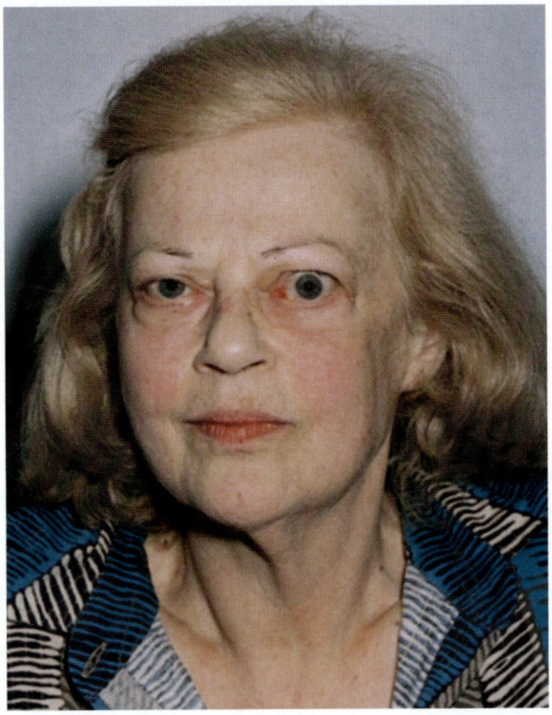

Fig. 9.15 Graves Disease: Unilateral Proptosis.

Hyperthyroidism may be caused by a single, autonomously functioning thyroid adenoma. The adenoma is usually papillary and is unrelated to any autoimmune process. Hyperfunction may also occur in multiple nodules. The distinctive features of hyperthyroidism caused by Graves and Plummer diseases are summarized in Table 9.2.

Approximately 5% of the population has a single thyroid nodule larger than 1 cm in diameter. Although most (90% to 95%) of these nodules are benign and necessitate no therapy, all should be investigated for malignancy. They develop from thyroid follicular cells and can be found in normal-sized thyroid glands and goiters. The history and physical examination can provide some clues as to the nature of the lump. Table 9.3 summarizes some of the essential characteristics of benign and malignant nodules.

Many patients with thyroid cancer, especially in the early stages, do not experience any symptoms. As the cancer grows, symptoms may include a lump or nodule in the neck, hoarseness, difficulty speaking, difficulty swallowing, pain in the neck or throat, and swollen lymph nodes. Many symptoms and signs of thyroid disease have been evaluated for their sensitivity and specificity. Most of these findings are specific but are too insensitive to be helpful. Table 9.4 summarizes the characteristics that are significant when a thyroid nodule is evaluated for malignancy. A palpable, hard nodule and a fixed mass are the most useful signs.

There are several types of thyroid cancer: papillary, follicular, medullary, and anaplastic. *Papillary* and *follicular carcinomas* are well differentiated and represent 80% to 90% of all thyroid cancers. Both types begin in the follicular cells of the thyroid. *Papillary thyroid carcinomas* are the most common (80% to 90% of all thyroid cancers). They typically grow very slowly. Usually they occur in only one lobe of the thyroid gland, but approximately 10% to 20% of the time, both lobes are involved. Even

TABLE 9.2 Distinctive Features of Graves Disease and Plummer Disease

Feature	Graves Disease (Toxic Diffuse Goiter; See Figs. 9.6 and 9.15)	Plummer Disease (Toxic Adenomatous Goiter; See Fig. 9.7)
Age at onset	40 years	40 years
Onset	Acute	Insidious
Goiter	Diffuse	Nodular
Signs and symptoms	Clear-cut	Vague
Myopathy (muscle disease)	Present	Absent
Heart involvement	Sinus tachycardia Atrial fibrillation (occasional)	Atrial fibrillation (frequent) Congestive heart failure
Ophthalmopathy	Exophthalmos Vision changes Motility abnormalities Chemosis (conjunctival edema) (see Fig. 10.44)	Eyelid lag Eyelid retraction

TABLE 9.3 Characteristics of Benign and Malignant Thyroid Nodules

Characteristic	Benign Nodule	Malignant Nodule
Age at onset	Adulthood	Adulthood
Predominant gender	Female	Male
Patient history	Symptoms present	Previous x-ray treatment to head or neck
Family history	Benign thyroid diseases	None
Speed of enlargement	Slow	Rapid
Change in voice	Absent	Present
Number of nodules	More than one	One
Lymph nodes	Absent	Present
Remainder of thyroid	Abnormal	Normal

TABLE 9.4 Characteristics of Thyroid Nodules Suspect for Cancer

Characteristic	Sensitivity (%)	Specificity (%)
Palpable, hard nodule	42	89
Fixed mass	31	94
Local symptoms	3	97
Dysphagia	10	93
Unilateral adenopathy	5	96
Nodule found on routine examination	50	56
Family history of goiter	17	79

Data from Kendall LW, Condon RE: Prediction of malignancy in solitary thyroid nodules, *Lancet* 1(7605):1071–1073, 1969; Haff RC, et al: Factors increasing the probability of malignancy in thyroid nodules, *Am J Surg* 131:707, 1976.

though papillary thyroid cancer is slow growing, it often spreads early to the lymph nodes in the neck. *Follicular thyroid cancer* is much less common than papillary thyroid cancer, making up approximately 5% to 10% of all thyroid cancers. It tends to occur in older individuals, which is more common in countries where people do not get enough iodine in their diet. If there is early detection, these cancers can be treated successfully. *Medullary thyroid carcinoma* (MTC) accounts for only 5% to 10% of all thyroid cancers. MTC is the only thyroid cancer that develops from the C cells, not the follicular cells, of the thyroid gland. There are two types of MTC: sporadic and familial.

Occasionally, MTC is associated with tumors of certain other organs (adrenal and parathyroid glands) and is called multiple endocrine neoplasia (MEN) syndromes. Tumors from MEN may be benign or cancerous. The MEN syndromes are a group of rare inherited conditions that typically run in families. These syndromes can affect multiple organ systems and increase a person's cancer risk. There are several types of MEN. The two most common types are MEN type 1 (MEN1) and MEN type 2 (MEN2). People with MEN1 develop tumors or excessive growth of two or more endocrine glands. These tumors are typically benign. The most frequently affected glands are parathyroid, pituitary, and pancreas. Females with MEN1 are at an increased risk of developing breast cancer. There are two subtypes of MEN2: MEN 2A is associated with medullary thyroid cancer, pheochromocytomas, and parathyroid gland tumors; MEN 2B is rare and lacks parathyroid gland tumors. Genetic studies should be performed on individuals with MTC. *Anaplastic thyroid carcinoma* is the least common of all thyroid cancers, accounting for 1% to 2%. It is also, however, the most aggressive type and therefore the most difficult to control and treat.

A heavy, puffy-faced, lethargic patient with dry skin, sparse hair, and a hoarse voice provides the classic picture of hypothyroidism. Hypothyroidism develops insidiously. Often the only concern is a tired or "run-down" feeling. The careful interviewer and examiner must be alert with any patient, especially one older than 60 years, who has these symptoms. Patients with hypothyroidism commonly have *hung*, or delayed, reflexes. Measurement of the relaxation time of the Achilles tendon reflex has long been used to monitor the effects of treatment in patients with hypothyroidism. However, it is useless as a screening technique because there may be many false-negative or false-positive results.

Table 9.5 lists some of the major symptoms and signs of hypothyroidism.

TABLE 9.5 Symptoms and Signs of Hypothyroidism

System	Symptom	Sign
General	Weight gain with regular diet Feeling chilly while other people are warm	Obesity
Gastrointestinal	Constipation	Enlarged tongue
Cardiovascular	Fatigue	Hypotension Bradycardia
Nervous	Speech disorders Short attention span Tremor	Hyporeflexia Defective abstract reasoning Spasticity Tremor Depressed affect
Musculoskeletal	Lethargy Thickened, dry skin Hair loss Brittle nails Leg cramps Puffy eyelids Puffy cheeks	Hypotonia Puffy facies
Reproductive	Heavier menses Decreased fertility	

USEFUL VOCABULARY

Listed here are the specific roots that are important for understanding the terminology related to head and neck diseases.

Root	Pertaining to	Example	Definition
capit-	head	***capit***ate	Head-shaped
cephal(o)-	head	***cephal***ometry	Measurement of the head
cleido-	clavicle	***cleido***mastoid	Pertaining to the clavicle and mastoid process
cranio-	skull	***cranio***malacia	Abnormal softening of the skull
occipito-	back portion of the skull	***occipito***parietal	Pertaining to the occipital and parietal bones
odont(o)-	tooth; teeth	***odont***orrhagia	Hemorrhage that follows tooth extraction
thyro-	thyroid gland	***thyro***megaly	Enlargement of the thyroid gland

WRITING UP THE PHYSICAL EXAMINATION

Listed here are examples of the write-up for examining the head, neck, and thyroid.

- The head is normocephalic without evidence of trauma. The neck is supple, with full range of motion. No adenopathy is present in the neck. The thyroid is nontender and not enlarged. No thyroid nodules are felt.
- The head is normocephalic and atraumatic. There is a 2-cm, rubbery, nontender mass in the superficial cervical chain on the left side. The mass is freely mobile and not fixed to the skin or underlying muscle. Another 4-cm, rubbery, nontender mass is felt in the right supraclavicular fossa. The thyroid is unremarkable.
- There is frontal bossing of the head with prominence of the cheekbones. There is no evidence of trauma. The neck is supple, with no adenopathy present. There is a 2-cm, soft, painless thyroid nodule felt 3 cm from the midline in the upper portion of the right lobe (at approximately the 10 o'clock position). The nodule is not fixed to the overlying skin or muscles.

REVIEW QUESTIONS

1. **The female patient shown in the photo below might be expected to have the following symptoms *except*:**

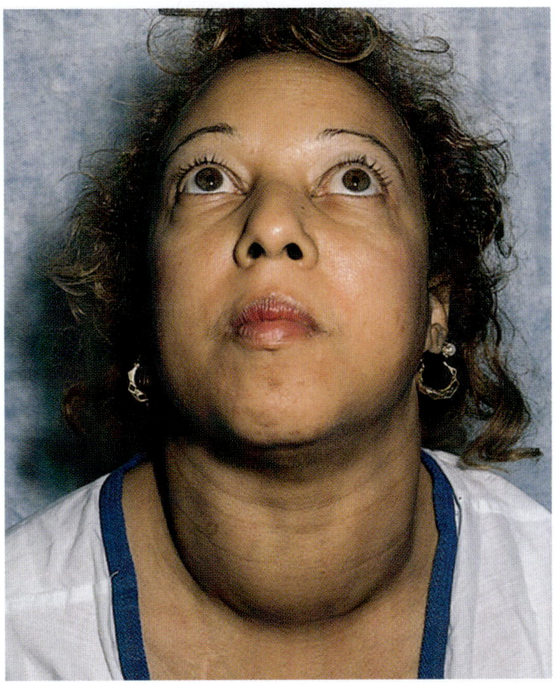

   A. Anxiety
   B. Easy fatigability
   C. Amenorrhea
   D. Palpitations
   E. Constipation

2. **A 62-year-old male has a 20-pack-year smoking history and a 15-pound weight loss over the past 3–4 months. On physical examination, the patient is found to have an isolated left supraclavicular node. This finding is most likely related to:**
   A. Lung cancer
   B. Esophageal cancer
   C. Gastric cancer
   D. Colon cancer
   E. Pancreatic cancer

3. **Which statement about the thyroid gland is *incorrect?***
   A. It envelops the upper trachea.
   B. It is the largest gland in the body.
   C. The thyroid isthmus lies across the trachea just above the cricoid cartilage.
   D. The thyroid may, on occasion, extend into the thorax.
   E. The normal thyroid gland has a consistency of muscle tissue.

4. **Cancers of the oral pharynx are increasing. Which of the following statements is *incorrect*?**
   A. Thyroid cancer is the most common endocrine cancer.
   B. Risk factors for thyroid cancer include radiation exposure related to medical therapy in childhood.
   C. Most people who develop head and neck cancer are older than 50 when diagnosed.
   D. Chewing betel nuts is one of the most important risk factors for head and neck cancers.
   E. One of the primary reasons for chewing betel nuts is due to their reputed aphrodisiac properties.

5. **Which statement about neck masses is *incorrect*?**
   A. If there is associated pain, an acute infection is likely.
   B. Masses that have been present for only a couple of days are commonly inflammatory.
   C. A mass that has been present for months to years without any change often turns out to be neoplastic.
   D. Blockage of a salivary gland may produce a mass that fluctuates in size when the patient eats.
   E. A round, soft, midline mass is generally thyroid in etiology.

6. **The lymph nodes shown in the patient below are:**

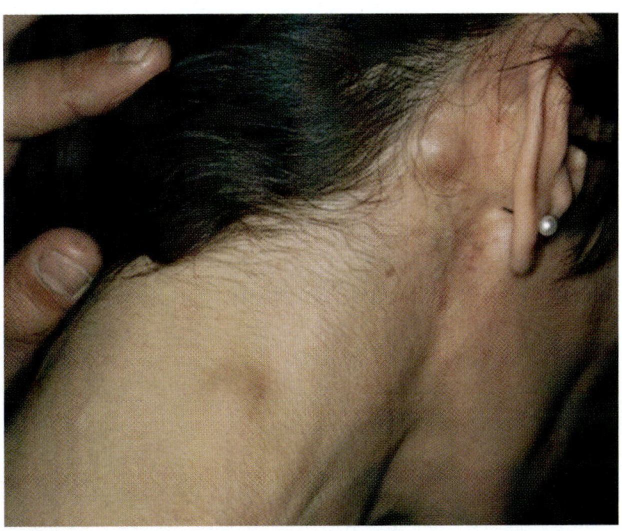

A. Anterior auricular
B. Tonsillar
C. Submental
D. Superficial cervical
E. Posterior cervical

7. Some of the signs of hypothyroidism include all of the following *except*:
A. Obesity
B. Hypertension
C. Bradycardia
D. Hyporeflexia
E. Puffy facies

8. Which of the following is a characteristic of a benign thyroid nodule?
A. Male predominant gender
B. No family history
C. Slow speed of enlargement
D. Change in voice
E. Presence of lymph nodes

9. Which of the following is a characteristic of Plummer disease (toxic adenomatous goiter)?
A. Acute onset
B. Nodular goiter
C. Myopathy present
D. Sinus tachycardia
E. Vision changes

10. Which of the following symptoms should *not* raise the suspicion of meningitis?
A. Stiff neck
B. High fever
C. Nausea
D. Sleepiness
E. Palpitations

REFERENCES

Available online.

BIBLIOGRAPHY

Available online.

10

The Eye

Mark H. Swartz and Vivian Hirshaut

Who would believe that so small a space could contain the images of all the universe?
O mighty process!

Leonardo da Vinci (1452–1519)

VIDEOS

Video 10.1	Assessing visual acuity (CN II–optic)
Video 10.2	Assessing visual fields
Video 10.3	Assessing ocular movements (eye alignment) and pupillary light reflex
Video 10.4	Evaluating the cardinal positions of gaze (CN III–oculomotor; CN IV–trochlear; CN VI–abducens)
Video 10.5	Examining the external eye structures
Video 10.6	Using the ophthalmoscope
Video 10.7	Inspecting the optic disc and retinal vessels
Video 10.8	Full video: Examination of the eye

HISTORICAL AND GENERAL CONSIDERATIONS

The eyes are the windows to the world. Most of the sensory input to the brain comes from the eyes. For centuries, the eye has been considered the person's essence, representing the "I." In mythology and the writings of ancient times, the eye is an organ associated with mystical powers.

The eye has long been associated with mythical gods. In ancient Egypt, the eye symbolized the Great Mother Goddess Maat, goddess of law, morality, and justice. The Egyptians believed that Maat held the universe together. The Eye of Maat later became known as the Eye of Horus. The Eye of Horus was supposed to protect against all evil and ensure success. The "evil eye" from the myth of Medusa was an expression of envy and greed. To this day, people wear talismans to ward off the "evil eye."

Another interesting association is the subconscious linking of "eyeball" with male genitalia. Blindness can symbolize castration because testicles and eyeballs have the same shape and are important in developing a sense of identity. This linking goes back to the legend of Oedipus, who pierced his eyeballs when he discovered that he had been married to his mother and had killed his father. This can be thought of as an act of self-castration, as well as a means of cutting oneself off from all worldly relationships. Throughout literature, the blinding of an individual was frequently a form of punishment for lust. The age-old notion that masturbation causes blindness further reinforces this close association of these organs.

Tumors in the eye are uncommon and are usually metastatic from breast, lung, bowel, or prostate cancer. Two types of primary tumors arise within the eye: retinoblastoma in children and melanoma in adults. Retinoblastoma is a cancer of the retina. This most common childhood eye cancer usually strikes children under the age of 5 years, affecting 500 to 600 children in the United States annually. In nearly a third of the cases, retinoblastoma occurs in both eyes. While symptoms are not evident early in the disease, increasing pain and vision loss eventually signal the problem. Malignant melanoma occurs most frequently in adults 60 to 65 years of age, arising from uncontrolled growth of melanocytes. There are 1500 to 2000 new cases diagnosed annually in the United States.

STRUCTURE AND PHYSIOLOGY

The external landmarks of the eye are shown in Fig. 10.1, and the cross-sectional anatomy of the eye is shown in Fig. 10.2.

The *eyelids* and *eyelashes* protect the eyes. The eyelids cover the globe and lubricate its surface. The *meibomian glands,* which are modified sebaceous glands in the eyelids, secrete *meibum*, an oily lubricating substance that retards evaporation of the tear film. The openings of these glands are at the eyelid margins. This is illustrated in Fig. 10.28B and seen in Fig. 10.28C.

The *orbicularis oculi muscle* encircles the lids and is responsible for their closure. This muscle group is the reason we have such expressive eyes. This muscle is supplied by the facial, or seventh cranial, nerve. The *levator palpebrae muscle* elevates the lids and is innervated by the oculomotor, or third cranial, nerve. Müller's muscle is a small part of the levator muscle with sympathetic innervation.

The globe has six *extraocular muscles* that control its motion. There are four rectus and two oblique muscles: the medial rectus, the lateral rectus, the superior rectus, the inferior rectus, the superior oblique, and the inferior oblique muscles. These six extraocular muscles are shown in Fig. 10.3.

The extraocular muscles work in a parallel, conjugate manner to maintain single binocular vision. When the head is turned to look left, for example, the *left lateral rectus* and the

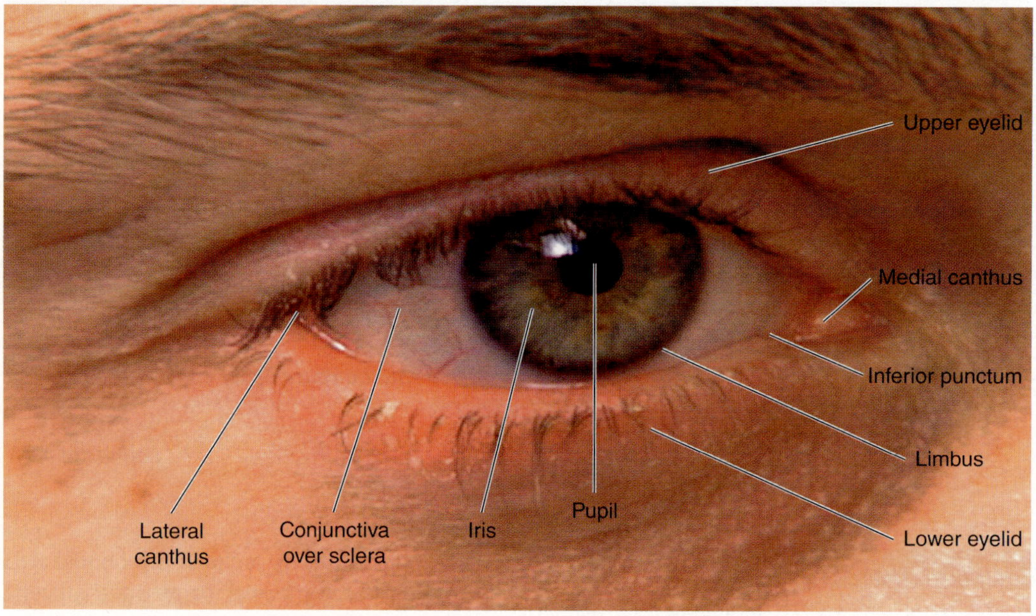

Fig. 10.1 External Landmarks of the Eye.

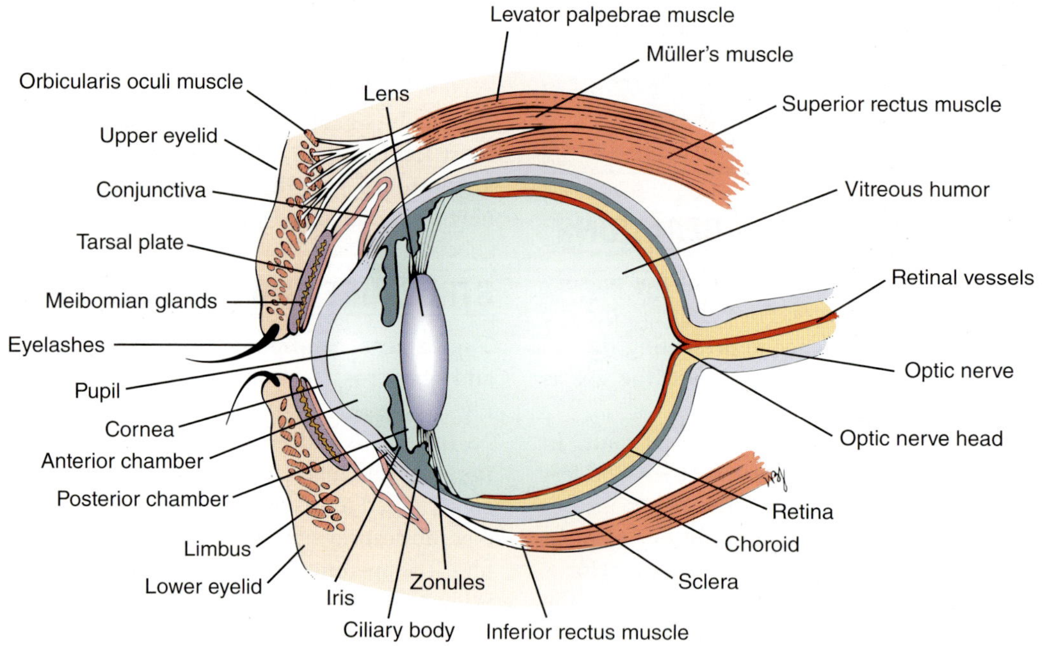

Fig. 10.2 Cross-Sectional Anatomy of the Eye.

right medial rectus contract to turn the eyes to the left. The actions and innervations of the extraocular muscles are listed in Table 10.1, and the extraocular movements are illustrated in Fig. 10.4.

The *lateral rectus muscle,* innervated by the *abducens nerve,* turns the eye laterally (*abducts* the eye), as do both oblique muscles. An easy way to remember the innervations is the formula $\mathbf{LR_6SO_4}$, meaning that the lateral rectus is innervated by cranial nerve VI (abducens), and the superior oblique is innervated by cranial nerve IV (trochlear); all the other muscles are innervated by cranial nerve III (oculomotor).

The *conjunctiva* is a thin, vascular, transparent mucous membrane that lines the lids of the anterior portion of the globe. The *palpebral* portion covers the inner surface of the lids, whereas the *bulbar* portion covers the sclera up to the *limbus,* which is the corneal-scleral junction. The conjunctiva contains many tiny blood vessels, which, when dilated, produce the appearance of a "red" eye. There is little nervous innervation to the conjunctiva.

The *lacrimal apparatus* comprises the lacrimal gland, accessory tear glands, canaliculi, tear sac, and nasolacrimal duct. These are shown in Fig. 10.5.

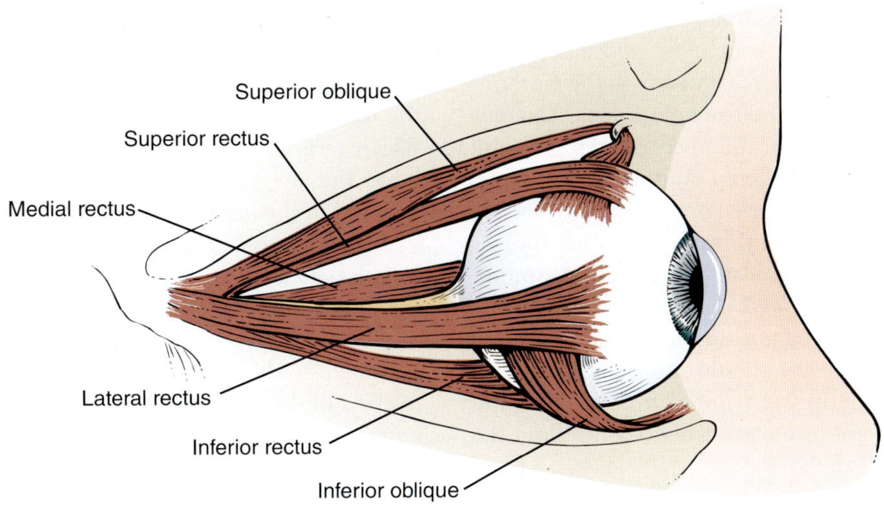

Fig. 10.3 The Extraocular Muscles.

TABLE 10.1 Actions and Innervations of the Extraocular Muscles

Muscle	Action	Cranial Nerve Innervation
Medial rectus	Adduction (eye moves nasally)	Oculomotor (III)
Lateral rectus	Abduction (eye moves temporally [away from the nose])	Abducens (VI)
Inferior rectus	Depression (eye moves down) Extorsion (the 12 o'clock position on the cornea rotates temporally) Adduction	Oculomotor (III)
Superior rectus	Elevation (eye moves up) Intorsion (the 12 o'clock position on the cornea rotates nasally) Adduction	Oculomotor (III)
Superior oblique	Intorsion Depression Abduction	Trochlear (IV)
Inferior oblique	Extorsion Elevation Abduction	Oculomotor (III)

Remember "LR_6SO_4." This mnemonic means that the lateral rectus (LR) muscle is innervated by the sixth cranial nerve, and the superior oblique (SO) muscle is innervated by the fourth cranial nerve. All the other muscles are innervated by the third cranial nerve.

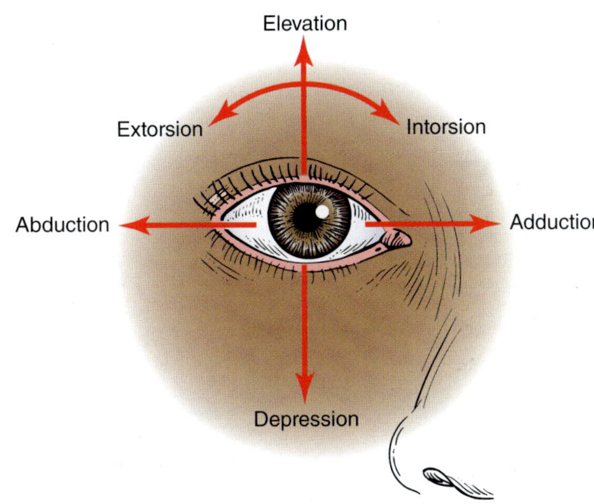

Fig. 10.4 Extraocular Movements.

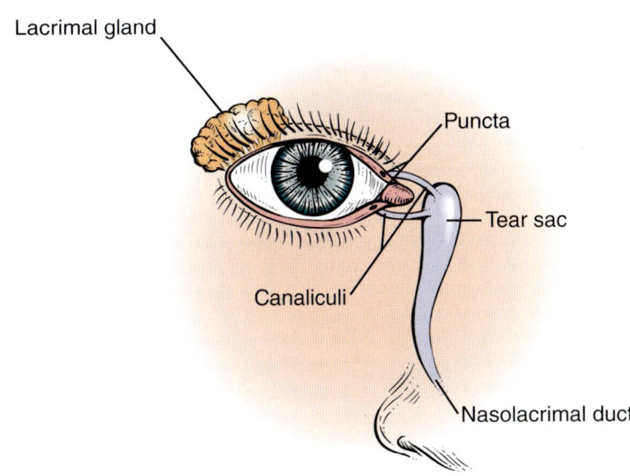

Fig. 10.5 The Lacrimal Apparatus.

The *lacrimal gland* produces watery tears and is located above and slightly lateral to the globe. Secretion occurs mainly as reflex tearing or crying. Tears drain through the *puncta* on the lids and into the superior and inferior *canaliculi.* These canaliculi join and enter the *tear sac,* located at the medial *canthus* of the eye. The *nasolacrimal duct* drains tears from the sac to the nose. Of the lacrimal apparatus, only the *puncta* are visible on routine examination.

The *sclera* is the white, fibrous, outer coat of the globe visible just beneath the conjunctiva. The extraocular muscles insert onto the sclera.

The *cornea* is a smooth, transparent, avascular tissue that covers the iris and joins with the sclera and conjunctival reflection at the limbus. The cornea functions as a protective window, allowing light to pass into the eye. The cornea is richly innervated by the trigeminal, or fifth cranial, nerve and therefore exquisitely sensitive to touch and pain.

The *anterior chamber,* or space between the cornea anteriorly and the iris posteriorly, is filled with clear *aqueous humor.* Aqueous humor is produced by the *ciliary body* in the *posterior chamber,* the area behind the iris, and front of the lens. Aqueous humor circulates from the posterior chamber through the pupil into the anterior chamber and is filtered out through the *canal of Schlemm,* from where it eventually enters the venous system. This filtration regulates pressure within the eye. The *angle* is formed by the juncture of the cornea and the iris at the limbus. A section through the eye at this level is shown in Fig. 10.6.

The *iris* is the circular, colored portion of the eye. The pupil is the small, round aperture in the middle of the iris. Because it is optically empty in the healthy eye, it appears black. The pupil functions much like the aperture of a camera, controlling the amount of light that enters the eye.

When a light is shined on one eye, both pupils constrict consensually. This constriction is the *pupillary light reflex.* A brief review of the neuroanatomy is in order to understand this reflex. Fig. 10.7 illustrates the pathways of the pupillary light reflex.

The optic, or second cranial, nerves comprise 80% *visual* and 20% afferent *pupillary* fibers. The optic nerves leave both retinas and travel a short course to where they join each other. This joining is the *optic chiasm.* At the optic chiasm, the nasal fibers cross and join the uncrossed fibers of the other side, forming the *optic tract.* The visual fibers continue in the optic tract to the *lateral geniculate body,* where synapses occur, the axons of which terminate in the primary visual cortex of the occipital lobe. The afferent pupillary fibers bypass the geniculate body and end in the *midbrain's superior colliculus and pretectal area.*

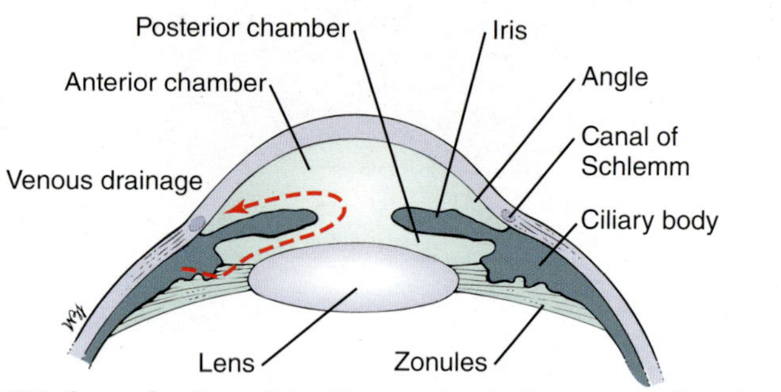

Fig. 10.6 Cross Section of the Normal-Angle Structures, Showing the Flow of Aqueous Humor.

Light impulses to the eye cause the retina to transmit nerve impulses to the optic nerve, the optic tract, the midbrain, and the visual cortex of the occipital lobes. This is the *afferent limb* of the light reflex. In the midbrain, the pupillary fibers diverge and are relayed by crossed fibers to the opposite *Edinger-Westphal* nucleus of the oculomotor, or third cranial, nerve. Some fibers remain on the same side. The third cranial nerve is the *efferent limb,* which goes via the ciliary body to the sphincter muscle of the iris to cause it to contract. The *direct effect* is the constriction of the pupil of the eye on which the light is shined (the *ipsilateral eye*). The *consensual effect* is the simultaneous constriction of the opposite pupil (the *contralateral eye*).

The *near reflex* occurs when the subject looks at a nearby target. The three parts of the near reflex are *accommodation, convergence,* and *pupillary constriction. Accommodation* is defined as the near focusing of the eye, which is affected by increasing the power of the lens by contraction of the ciliary muscle, innervated by the third cranial nerve.

There is also autonomic innervation of the eyes. Sympathetic and parasympathetic fibers supply the iris. When the sympathetic fibers are stimulated, the pupil dilates, and the eyelid elevates. Think of the cat stalking its prey, pupils dilated, ready to pounce in the dark. The cat needs all the light it can get. The reflex is purely sympathetic. When the parasympathetic fibers in the oculomotor nerve are stimulated, pupillary constriction occurs. When we sleep, our bodies are in a parasympathetic mode, and our pupils are constricted.

The lens is positioned just behind the iris and is a colorless, biconvex structure that alters its shape to focus the image on the

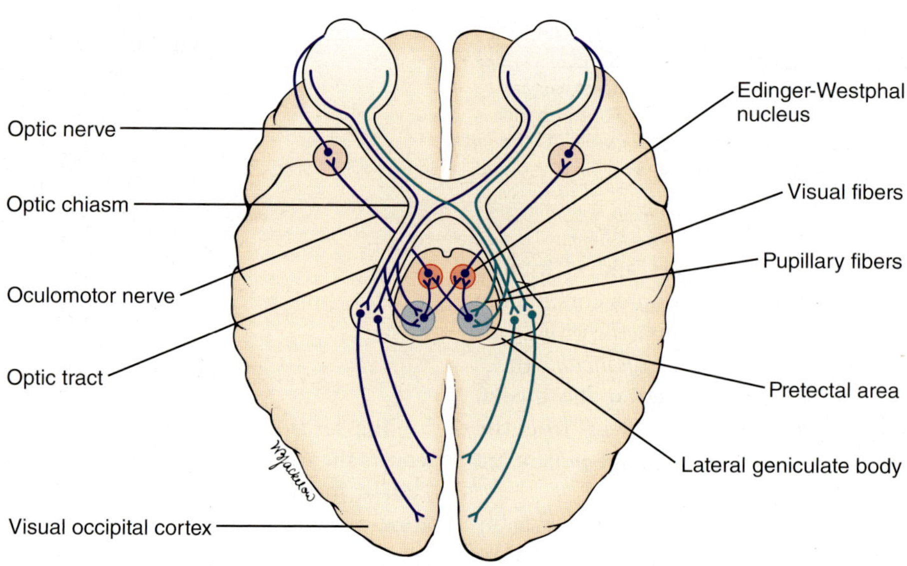

Fig. 10.7 The Pupillary Light Reflex.

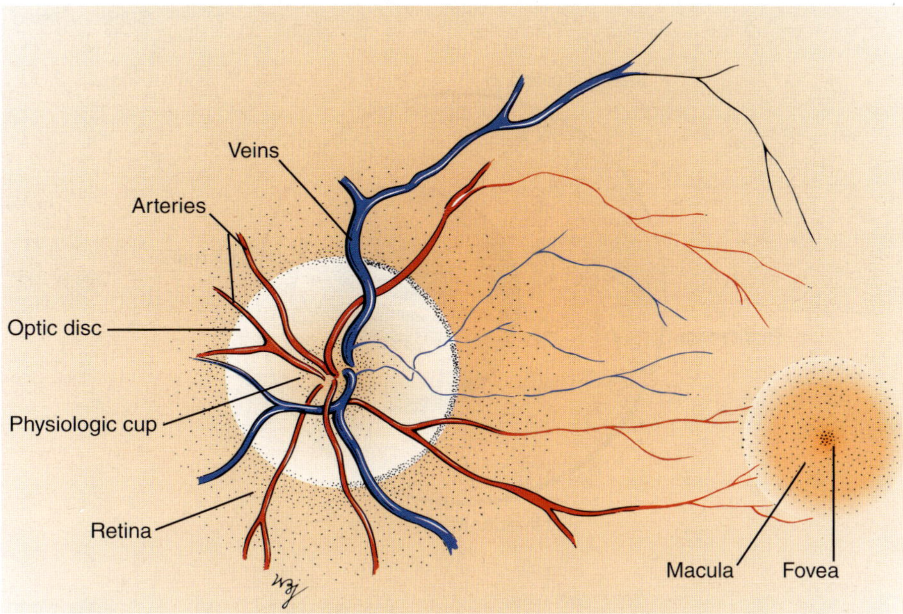

Fig. 10.8 The Retina of the Left Eye.

retina. This shape is controlled by the ciliary body muscles, which contract and are linked to the zonules of the lens.

The vitreous humor is a clear, gel-like substance that is located behind the lens and in front of the retina in the eye, occupying 80% of its volume. It is made up of collagen, hyaluronic acid, and water and is not connected to any blood vessels. The vitreous humor is surrounded by the posterior lens capsule in the front and the retina at the back.

As people age, they may experience eye **floaters.** These are spots in the field of vision that can appear as black or gray specks, strings, flies, or cobwebs. Eye floaters move around when the eyes move and appear to disappear when one tries to look at them directly. Floaters are tiny shadows that can be cast on the retina when the vitreous collagen fibers aggregate.

The *choroid* is the middle vascular layer of the globe between the sclera and the retina. It acts as a source of nourishment, as well as a heat sink, serving to remove the extreme heat produced by the light energy entering the eye. Bruch's membrane separates the choroid from the retina. Superficial to Bruch's membrane (closer to the retina) is the retinal pigment epithelium (RPE). The RPE is a monolayer of cells between Bruch's membrane and the retina. Some of the critical functions of the RPE are to absorb light passing through the retina and to regenerate the visual pigments.

The *retina* is the innermost layer, or "camera film," of the eye. The retina is attached firmly to the underlying choroid at the optic nerve posteriorly and at the ora serrata anteriorly. Between these two points, the retina is in contact with the choroid but not attached. The ora serrata is the junction of the retina and ciliary body. The retina is only 0.4 mm in thickness and is thinnest in the region of the macula. Histologically, the retina is made up of 10 distinct layers. The retina senses light through the rods and cones in its outer layer (closest to the RPE), performs initial signal processing in its middle layer, and encodes and transmits the data in its inner nerve fiber layer. The nerve fiber layer is the layer closest to the vitreous. These axons are unmyelinated until they penetrate the sclera at the optic disc to form the optic nerve.

Within the retina are several important structures: the optic disc, the retinal vessels, and the macula. Fig. 10.8 illustrates the retina of the left eye.

The *optic disc* is located at the nasal aspect of the posterior pole of the retina. This is the head of the optic nerve, from where the nerve fibers of the retina exit the eye. The optic disc is 1.5 mm in diameter and is ovoid. It is lighter than the surrounding retina and appears yellowish-pink due to myelination of the optic nerve. The disc margins are sharp, with some normal blurring of the nasal portion. African-American patients may have pigmentation at the margins. The *physiologic cup* is the center of the disc, where the retinal vessels penetrate. This slight depression typically occupies approximately 30% of the disc diameter.

The *retinal vessels* emerge from the disc and arborize on the retinal surface. The arteries are brighter red and thinner than the veins. An artery-to-vein ratio of 2:3 is average.

The *macula* is a small, round area, approximately the size of the disc, located 3.5 mm temporal to and 0.5 mm inferior to the disc. The macula is easily seen because it is devoid of retinal vessels. In the center of the macula is the *fovea,* a depressed area composed only of *cones.* Cones provide detailed vision and color perception.

The remaining areas of the retina contain mostly *rods,* which compose the other neurosensory element of the retina. The rods are responsible for motion detection and night vision. Remember that the image on the retina is upside down and reversed left to right; the right world is projected onto the left half of the retina, and the left is projected onto the right half. An image in the superior world strikes the inferior part of the retina, and an inferiorly positioned image strikes the superior part. This concept is illustrated in Fig. 10.9. The image is ultimately

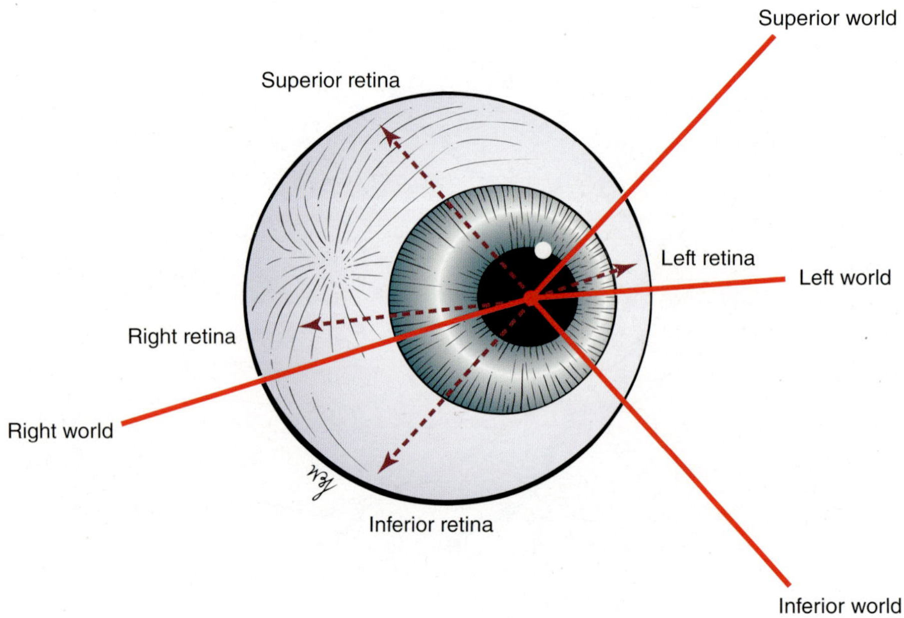

Fig. 10.9 How Images Strike the Retina.

reversed up and down and left to right by the time the image has reached the visual cortex.

There is little pigment in the iris at birth, which is why many infants are born with blue eyes. By 6 months of age, the pigmentation is complete. The lens is more spherical at birth than in later life. Most infants are born hyperopic (farsighted) because the eye is small, and the image falls posterior to the retina (see Fig. 10.89). By 3 months after birth, the medullation process of the optic nerve is completed. As the child grows, hyperopia increases until the age of 8 years and then gradually decreases. After age 8, myopia (nearsightedness) appears to increase.

Many changes occur with advancing age. First, there is the gradual loss of elasticity of the skin around the eyes, which may lead to droopy eyelids, known as *ptosis*. The cornea may show infiltration of cholesterol deposits around the limbus, known as an *arcus senilis*. The lens consistency changes from plastic to rigid, making it progressively more difficult to change its shape to focus on near objects. This condition is called *presbyopia*. The lens may undergo changes resulting from metabolic disorders that cause its opacification; this condition is called a *cataract*. The vitreous humor may develop condensations called *floaters*. The retinal arteries may develop *atherosclerosis*, with resultant retinal ischemia or infarction.

REVIEW OF SPECIFIC SYMPTOMS

The major symptoms of eye disease are the following:

- Vision loss
- Eye pain
- Diplopia (double vision)
- Tearing and dryness
- Discharge
- Redness

Vision Loss

When a patient complains of loss of vision, the following two questions must be asked:

"Did the loss of vision occur suddenly or gradually?"
"Is the eye painful?"

It is important to determine how severe the vision loss is and whether or not there is any pain associated with it. A sudden and painless loss of vision may be caused by a retinal vascular occlusion or a retinal detachment, while sudden and painful loss of vision may be a result of acute narrow-angle glaucoma. Chronic simple glaucoma and cataracts often cause gradual and painless loss of vision.

Eye Pain

Eye pain may result from a variety of causes. Ask the patient the following questions:

"Can you describe the pain?"
"Did the pain come on suddenly?"
"Does the light bother your eye?"
"Do you have pain when you blink?"
"Do you have the sensation of something in the eye?"
"Do you have headaches?"
"Do you have pain on movement of the eye?"
"Do you have pain over the brow on the same side?"
"Do you wear contact lenses?"

Pain may be experienced as "burning," "aching," "throbbing," "tenderness," or pain behind the eye. Each of these descriptions may have a range of causes. It is essential to determine whether the patient has the sensation of a foreign body in the eye. Pain in the eye while blinking occurs in corneal abrasions and with foreign bodies in the eye. *Photophobia* is eye pain associated with light, as seen in inflammations of the *uveal tract* (i.e., iris, ciliary body, or choroid). Inflammations of the conjunctiva, *conjunctivitis,* produce a gritty sensation. Diseases of the cornea are associated with significant pain because the cornea is so richly innervated. Headaches and eye pain are common in acute narrow-angle glaucoma. Pain on motion of the eye occurs in optic neuritis. Eye pain associated with brow or temporal pain may indicate temporal arteritis (see Chapter 25, The Geriatric Patient). Contact lens wearers may have corneal irritation and may complain of eye pain.

Diplopia

Diplopia, or double vision, is a common complaint. Diplopia results from a faulty alignment of the eyes. Usually, when the eyes fixate on an object, the object is seen clearly, even though the two retinal images are not precisely superimposed. These slightly different images, however, are fused by the brain; it is this fusion that produces *binocular vision,* or the perception of depth. When the eyes are misaligned, the two images fall on different parts of the retinas, with only one falling normally on the fovea. The field of vision of the deviated eye is different so that its image is not projected on its fovea; therefore, this second image is different and not superimposable. The patient may close one eye to relieve this distressing situation. In addition, the patient may use a compensatory head posture to relieve the double vision (see Fig. 10.152). Elevation or depression of the patient's chin is used to overcome a vertical deviation. Tilting of the head is often used to counteract the torsional and vertical deviation. Suggested questions for the patient with diplopia are listed in Chapter 21, The Nervous System.

Tearing and Dryness

Excessive tearing of the eyes is a common complaint. Abnormal tearing may be caused by the overproduction of tears or an obstruction of outflow. The eye depends on the flow of tears to provide constant moisture and lubrication to maintain vision and comfort. Tears are a combination of water for moisture; oils for lubrication; mucus for even spreading of the tears; and antibodies and particular proteins for resistance to infection. These components are secreted by special glands located around the eye. Thus, tears provide lubrication, reduce the risk of eye infection, wash away foreign matter in the eye, and keep the eyes' surface smooth and clear.

When there is an imbalance in this tear system, a person may experience dry eyes. Nearly 55 million Americans 50 years and older are estimated to have dry eye, with only 17% being diagnosed with the condition. The prevalence of dry eyes has been estimated to be up to 30% in persons equal to or older than 50 years, and it is expected to increase as the population ages. Based on data from the National Health and Wellness Survey, 6.8% of the United States adult population (approximately 16.4 million people) has been diagnosed with dry eye disease. The prevalence increases with age (2.7% in those 18 to 34 years old vs. 18.6% in those equal to or older than 75 years) and is higher in females than males (8.8% vs. 4.5%). It is not affected by race, education, or location of residence.

The most common form of dry eyes is due to an inadequate amount of the water layer of tears. This condition, called *keratoconjunctivitis sicca,* is called the *dry eye syndrome.*

Patients suffering from the dry eye syndrome often experience the following:

- Dryness
- Eye pain
- Stinging or burning sensation
- Stringy discharge from the eye
- Light sensitivity
- Heavy eyelids
- Foreign body sensation
- Sand in the eye; a gritty feeling
- Itching
- Redness
- Blurring of vision
- Decreased tolerance of reading, working on the computer, or any activity that requires sustained visual attention

There are many causes of the dry eye syndrome. These include:

Age: Dry eye is a part of the natural aging process. The majority of people older than age 50 experience some symptoms of dry eyes.

Gender: Women are more likely to develop dry eyes because of hormonal changes and menopause.

Medications: Certain medicines, including antihistamines, decongestants, statins, beta-blockers, diuretics, analgesics, and antidepressants, can cause dry eyes.

Medical conditions: Persons with rheumatoid arthritis, systemic lupus erythematosus, progressive systemic sclerosis, diabetes, and thyroid problems may develop dry eyes. Patients who have suffered from Stevens-Johnson syndrome (also known as erythema multiforme) may develop severe dry eyes. Also, problems with inflammation of the eyelids (blepharitis), inflammation of the surfaces of the eye, or the inward or outward turning of eyelids (entropion or ectropion, respectively) can cause dry eyes.

Environmental conditions: Exposure to pollutants such as smoke, exhaust, smog, and arid and windy conditions can increase tear evaporation, resulting in dry eye symptoms. Failure to blink regularly, such as staring at a computer screen for long periods, can also contribute to the dry eye syndrome. Excessive alcohol consumption is also associated with the dry eye syndrome.

Other factors: Long-term use of contact lenses can be a factor in developing dry eyes. Refractive eye surgeries, such as laser-assisted in situ keratomileusis (LASIK),[a] can cause decreased tear production and dry eyes.

Sometimes, a person with a dry eye will have excess tears running down the cheeks, which may seem confusing. This happens when the eye isn't getting enough lubrication. The eye sends a distress signal through the nervous system for more lubrication. In response, the eye is flooded with tears to

[a]LASIK, commonly referred to as *laser eye surgery,* is a procedure for the correction of refractive errors such as myopia, hyperopia, and astigmatism (see Fig. 10.89). LASIK surgery requires the use of an excimer laser, or microkeratome, to reshape the eye's cornea to improve visual acuity. In most patients, LASIK surgery provides a permanent alternative to wearing eyeglasses or contact lenses.

TABLE 10.2 Differential Diagnosis for Red Eye

Manifestation	Acute Conjunctivitis[a]	Acute Iritis (Fig. 10.67)	Narrow-Angle Glaucoma	Corneal Abrasion
History	Sudden onset Exposure to conjunctivitis	Fairly sudden onset Often recurrent	Rapid onset Sometimes history of attack Highest incidence among Jews, Swedes, and the Inuit	Trauma Pain
Vision	Normal	Impaired if untreated	Rapidly lost if untreated[b]	Can be affected if central
Pain	Gritty feeling	Photophobia	Severe	Exquisite
Bilaterality	Frequent	Occasional	Occasional	Usually unilateral
Vomiting	Absent	Absent	Common	Absent
Cornea	Clear (epidemic keratoconjunctivitis has corneal deposits)	Variable	"Steamy" (like looking through a steamy window)	Irregular light reflex
Pupil	Normal, reactive	Sluggishly reactive Sometimes irregular in shape	Partially dilated, oval, nonreactive	Normal, reactive
Iris	Normal	Normal[c]	Difficult to see, owing to corneal edema	Shadow of corneal defect may be projected on the iris with penlight
Ocular discharge	Mucopurulent or watery	Watery	Watery	Watery or mucopurulent
Systemic effect	None	Few	Many	None
Prognosis	Self-limited	Poor if untreated	Poor if untreated	Good if not infected

[a]Can be viral, bacterial, or allergic.
[b]Seeing "rainbow" can be an early symptom during an acute attack.
[c]Slit-lamp examination revealing cells in anterior chamber is diagnostic. See Fig. 10.92.

compensate for the underlying dryness. However, these tears are primarily watery and do not have the lubricating qualities or the rich composition of normal tears. As a result, they wash debris away but do not adequately coat the eye surface.

Discharge

Discharge from the eye can be watery, mucoid, or purulent. A watery or mucoid discharge is often associated with allergic or viral conditions, whereas a purulent discharge occurs in association with bacterial infections. Most of the time, eye discharge is harmless. However, sometimes it can be an indication of a more severe condition. For example, pollen, gusty winds, dry eyes, or an eyelash can cause an irritation that will also lead to discharge. Other causes of eye discharge can be associated with medical conditions such as conjunctivitis or, more serious, corneal ulcers.

Redness

The symptom of the red eye is widespread. The interviewer should ask the following questions:
"Have you had any injury to the eye?"
"Does anyone else in the family have a red eye?"
"Have you had any recent coughing spells? Vomiting?"
"Have you had any associated eye pain?"
"Does light bother your eyes?"
"Is there any associated discharge?"
"Do you wear contact lenses?"

The eye may appear bloodshot. Redness may result from trauma, infection, allergy, or sudden increased pressure in the eye. Severe coughing spells, Valsalva maneuver for any reason, or recurrent vomiting may cause a patient to have a subconjunctival hemorrhage. A family member or friend with viral conjunctivitis may be the source of a patient's red eye. The combination of eye pain and red eye may indicate acute narrow-angle glaucoma or an inflammatory condition known as *scleritis* or *episcleritis*. Table 10.2 summarizes the differential diagnosis for the red eye. Uveitis, inflammation of the uveal tract associated with a red eye, can manifest with light sensitivity. Patients wearing contact lenses may suffer from corneal irritation and eye redness.

General Suggestions

It is important to determine the medications that a patient is taking because many drugs have deleterious effects on the eye. For example, some antimalarial, antituberculous, antiglaucoma, and anti-inflammatory drugs can cause eye disorders. In addition, a thorough family history reveals familial disease tendencies such as glaucoma, cataracts, retinal degeneration, strabismus, or corneal dystrophies.

There are many specific symptoms related to eye disease. First, Table 10.3 lists some common visual eye symptoms and their associated disease states. Next, Table 10.4 lists some common nonvisual but *painful* conditions and their associated disease states. Finally, Table 10.5 lists some common nonvisual, *painless* eye symptoms and their disease states.

EFFECT OF BLINDNESS ON THE PATIENT

The loss of sight is a terrifying experience. The sighted person lives mainly in a visual and auditory world illuminated by lights

TABLE 10.3 Common Visual Eye Symptoms and Disease States

Visual Symptom	Possible Causes
Loss of vision	Optic neuritis
	Detached retina
	Retinal hemorrhage
	Central retinal vascular occlusion
	Central nervous system disease
Spots	No pathologic significance[a]
Flashes	Migraine
	Retinal detachment
	Posterior vitreous detachment
Loss of visual field or presence of shadows or curtains	Retinal detachment
	Retinal hemorrhage
Glare, photophobia	Iritis (inflammation of the iris)
	Meningitis (inflammation of the meninges)
Distortion of vision	Retinal detachment
	Macular edema
Difficulty seeing in dim light	Myopia
	Vitamin A deficiency
	Retinal degeneration
Colored halos around lights	Acute narrow-angle glaucoma
	Opacities in lens or cornea
Colored vision changes	Cataracts
	Drugs (digitalis increases yellow vision)
Double vision	Extraocular muscle paresis or paralysis

[a]May precede a retinal detachment or may be associated with ingestion of fertility drugs.

TABLE 10.4 Common Nonvisual, Painful Eye Symptoms and Disease States

Nonvisual, Painful Symptom	Possible Causes
Foreign body sensation	Foreign body
	Corneal abrasion
Burning sensation	Uncorrected refractive error
	Conjunctivitis
	Sjögren syndrome
Throbbing, aching	Acute iritis (inflammation of the iris)
	Sinusitis (inflammation of the sinuses)
Tenderness	Eyelid inflammation
	Conjunctivitis
	Iritis
Headache	Refractive errors
	Migraine
	Sinusitis
Drawing sensation	Uncorrected refractive errors

TABLE 10.5 Common Nonvisual, Painless Eye Symptoms and Disease States

Nonvisual, Painless Symptom	Possible Causes
Itching	Dry eyes
	Eye fatigue
	Allergies
Tearing	Emotional states
	Hypersecretion of tears
	Blockage of drainage
Dryness	Sjögren syndrome
	Decreased secretion as a result of aging
Sandiness, grittiness	Conjunctivitis
Fullness of eyes	Proptosis (bulging of the eyeball)
	Aging-related changes in the lids
Twitching	Fibrillation of orbicularis oculi
Eyelid heaviness	Fatigue
	Eyelid edema
Dizziness	Refractive error
	Cerebellar disease
	Vestibular disease
Excessive blinking	Local irritation
	Facial tic
Eyelids sticking together	Inflammatory disease of eyelids or conjunctivae

and colors. When blindness occurs, the person loses not only the ability to see but also the perceptual center of their world. This center must now be replaced by hearing and touch. Because light is often equated with life, the inability to see light is associated with death. The newly blinded patient must take a new place in society. They can no longer read ordinary books, can no longer receive visual stimuli, and cannot appreciate the world of visual communication. This can result in a reactive depression. The healthcare professional must show genuine concern for blind patients and try to understand their feelings of discouragement and despair.

The person who is blind from birth or early childhood has little or no conception of the visual world. Having never been able to see, this patient has no visual frame of reference.

On occasion, a blind individual recovers sight as a result of a surgical procedure later in life. Many difficulties may arise owing to the reorganization of the patient's perception. Their frame of reference has been shifted from touch to sight. Surprisingly, many of these patients become depressed after attaining vision. Facial expressions mean nothing because only with experience can people understand them. The following quote from a case history by Gregory and Wallace illustrates the response of such an individual: "He suffered one of the greatest hardships (blindness), and yet he lived with energy and enthusiasm. When his handicap was apparently swept away, as by a miracle, he lost his peace and self-respect."

Similarly, a patient with normal vision may develop psychosomatic eye problems due to anxiety. Loss of vision also can accompany panic disorders. Such individuals can have partial or complete vision loss in one or both eyes. Supportive care of the primary problem usually results in the return of vision.

In multiple sclerosis, one of the presenting symptoms may be the sudden onset of blindness caused by optic neuritis. This blindness in most cases reverses entirely in approximately six weeks. This is a very frightening experience for a typically young patient.

PHYSICAL EXAMINATION

The equipment necessary for examining the eye is as follows: an ophthalmoscope, a penlight, a pocket visual acuity card, and a 3 × 5 inch (7.6 × 12.7 cm) card.

The physical examination of the eye includes the following:

- Visual acuity
- Visual fields
- Ocular movements
- External and internal eye structures
- Ophthalmoscopic examination

Visual Acuity

See Video 10.1.

Visual acuity is expressed as a ratio, such as 20/20. The first number is the distance in feet from which the patient reads the chart. The second number is the distance in feet at which a person with normal vision can read the same line on the chart. Another way of describing visual acuity is as follows: if a person has 20/20 vision, that person has 20/20 or 100% vision because 20 divided by 20 equals 1, or 100% of normal vision. The abbreviation *OD* refers to the right eye (oculus dexter); *OS* refers to the left eye (oculus sinister); and *OU* refers to both eyes (oculus uterque).

Using the Standard Snellen Eye Chart

The most commonly used eye chart is known as the Snellen eye chart. It usually shows 11 rows of capital letters. The first line has one very large letter. Each row after that has increasing numbers of letters that are smaller in size.

The patient is positioned 20 feet away from the chart. If the patient wears glasses for distance, they should wear them for the examination. The patient is asked to cover one eye with the palm[b] or *an index card* and read the smallest line possible. If the best they can see is the 20/200 line, the patient's vision in that eye is 20/200; this means that at 20 feet, the patient can see what a person with normal vision can see at 200 feet. This can also be explained as 10% of normal vision in that eye. If patients at 20 feet cannot see the 20/200 line, they are moved closer until the letters are recognizable. If the patient can read these letters at 5 feet, the patient's visual acuity in that eye is 5/200.

Using a Pocket Visual Acuity Card

A pocket visual acuity card is helpful if the standard Snellen eye chart is unavailable. This is viewed at 14 inches (35.6 cm). The patient is again asked to read the smallest line possible. If neither eye chart is available, any printed material may be used. The examiner should remember that most patients older than 40 years require reading glasses. Although visual acuity cannot be quantified, the examiner can determine whether the patient has any vision. In such a case, the patient is asked to cover an eye and read the smallest line on a printed page.

[b]Always ask a patient to cover the eye with the palm. When fingers cover the eye, a patient may peek between the fingers to see the chart.

Evaluation of Patients With Poor Vision

Patients with poor vision who cannot read any lines of print should be tested for finger-counting ability. This crude measurement of visual acuity is obtained by the examiner's holding up fingers in front of one of the patient's eyes with the other eye covered. The patient is then asked how many fingers are seen. If the patient is still unable to see, the next step would be to evaluate whether they have any light perception. This is performed by covering one eye and directing a light at the other eye. Finally, the examiner asks the patient whether they can see when the light is on or off. *No light perception* (NLP) is the term used when a person cannot perceive light.

Evaluation of Patients Who Cannot Read

For individuals who cannot read, such as young children or illiterate patients, using the letter "E" in different sizes and directions is helpful. The examiner asks the patient to point in the letter's direction: up, down, right, or left. A vision testing chart using simple pictures of houses, flowers, and other objects can be used alternatively with young children or people who cannot read.

Visual Fields

See Video 10.2.

Visual field testing is helpful in determining lesions of the visual pathway. Many techniques are used for this purpose. First, the examiner should learn to perform the technique known as *confrontation visual field testing*. In this technique, the examiner compares their peripheral vision with the patient's.

Assess Fields by Confrontation Visual Field Testing

The examiner stands or sits 3 to 4 feet in front of and at eye level with the patient. The patient is asked to close their right eye while the examiner closes their left eye, each fixating on the other's nose. The examiner holds up fists with the palms facing the examiner. The examiner then shows one or two fingers (second or second and third fingers) on each hand simultaneously and asks the patient how many fingers together they see. The hands are moved from the upper to the lower quadrants, and the examination is repeated. One hand should be in the nasal half, while the other is in the temporal half of the visual fields. The test is then repeated with the other eye of the patient and the examiner. The fingers should be seen by both patient and examiner simultaneously. To position the patient to better advantage, the hands are held up slightly closer to the examiner. This provides a wider field for the patient. If the examiner can see the fingers, the patient should be able to see them unless they have a visual field deficit. This technique for examining the patient's left eye is shown in Fig. 10.10.

Because lesions along the visual pathway develop insidiously, the patient may only be aware of changes in visual fields late in the course of the disease. Therefore, confrontation fields,

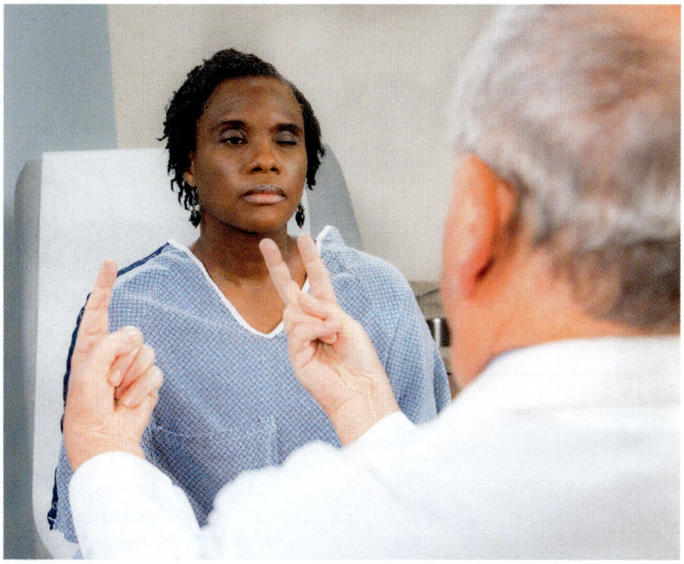

A

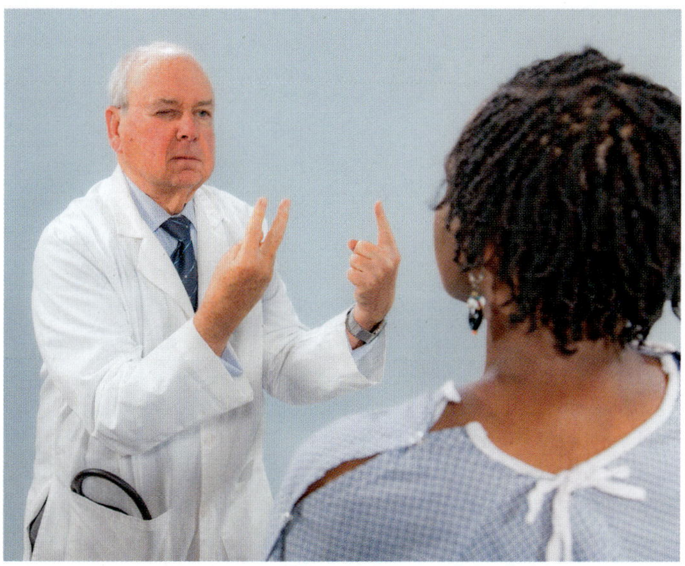

B

Fig. 10.10 Confrontation Visual Field Testing. (A) View of the patient during examination of the lower fields of the patient's right eye. (B) Position of the examiner during examination of the lower fields of the patient's right eye.

performed by the internist, may provide the first objective evidence that the patient has a lesion involving the visual pathway. An area of depressed vision is called a *scotoma.*

The normal central vision extends approximately 30 degrees in all directions of central fixation. The *blind spot* is the physiologic scotoma located about 15 to 20 degrees temporal to central fixation, corresponding to the optic nerve head. No sensory elements like rods or cones are located on the nerve head.

Assess Visual Field Abnormalities

Pathologic scotomata may be appreciated on visual field testing. Scotomata may result from primary ocular diseases, such as glaucoma, or lesions in the central nervous system, such as tumors. Fig. 10.11 illustrates some of the common defects.

Total vision loss in one eye constitutes a *blind* eye, resulting from a disease of the eye or a lesion of its optic nerve.

Hemianopsia refers to the absence of half of a visual field. A defect in both temporal fields is termed *bitemporal hemianopsia.* It results from a lesion involving the optic nerves at the level of the optic chiasm. Pituitary tumors are common causes.

A *homonymous hemianopsia* results from damage to the optic tract, optic radiation, or occipital cortex. The term *homonymous* indicates that the visual loss is in similar fields. For example, a patient with a left homonymous hemianopsia cannot see the left half of the fields of both eyes. This defect occurs with damage to the right optic tract. Homonymous hemianopsia is the most common form of field loss and occurs frequently in stroke patients.

A *quadrantanopsia* is a field loss in one quadrant, also known as a "pie in the sky" lesion. For example, a patient with a left upper homonymous quadrantanopsia has damage to the right lower optic radiations or the right lower occipital region.

Tunnel vision is the loss of peripheral vision with retention of central vision, resulting in a constricted circular tunnel-like field of vision. It may occur in advanced glaucoma. Total blindness may also occur with glaucoma if untreated.

Visual fields enlarge with increasing testing distance, unlike *hysterical blindness,* in which the field size typically remains the same at all times, regardless of the testing distance.

Assess Optokinetic Nystagmus

On occasion, a patient may feign blindness. They may be trying to qualify for disability insurance or some other issue of secondary gain. Alternatively, they may have psychologic problems. A helpful test for ruling out such malingering involves *optokinetic nystagmus* (*OKN*). OKN is the rapid alternating motion of the eyes that occurs when the eyes try to fixate on a moving target. For example, observe a person's eyes riding a train as it enters the station. The eyes move rapidly back and forth as the person tries to fixate on a station sign. OKN indicates physiologic continuity of the optic pathways from the retina to the occipital cortex. OKN may be elicited in the examining room by having the patient fixate on the numbers on a tape measure while you rapidly pull out the tape. Because OKN is involuntary, a positive response[c] provides excellent verification that the patient is feigning blindness.

Ocular Movements

See Video: 10.3.

The contraction and relaxation of the extraocular muscles affect ocular movements. This results in simultaneous movement of the eyes up or down or from side to side and convergence.

Assess Eye Alignment

Alignment of the eyes is seen by observing the location of reflected light on the cornea. The penlight should be held directly

[c]*Positive response* means that the eyes are trying to fixate on the target, indicating that vision is present.

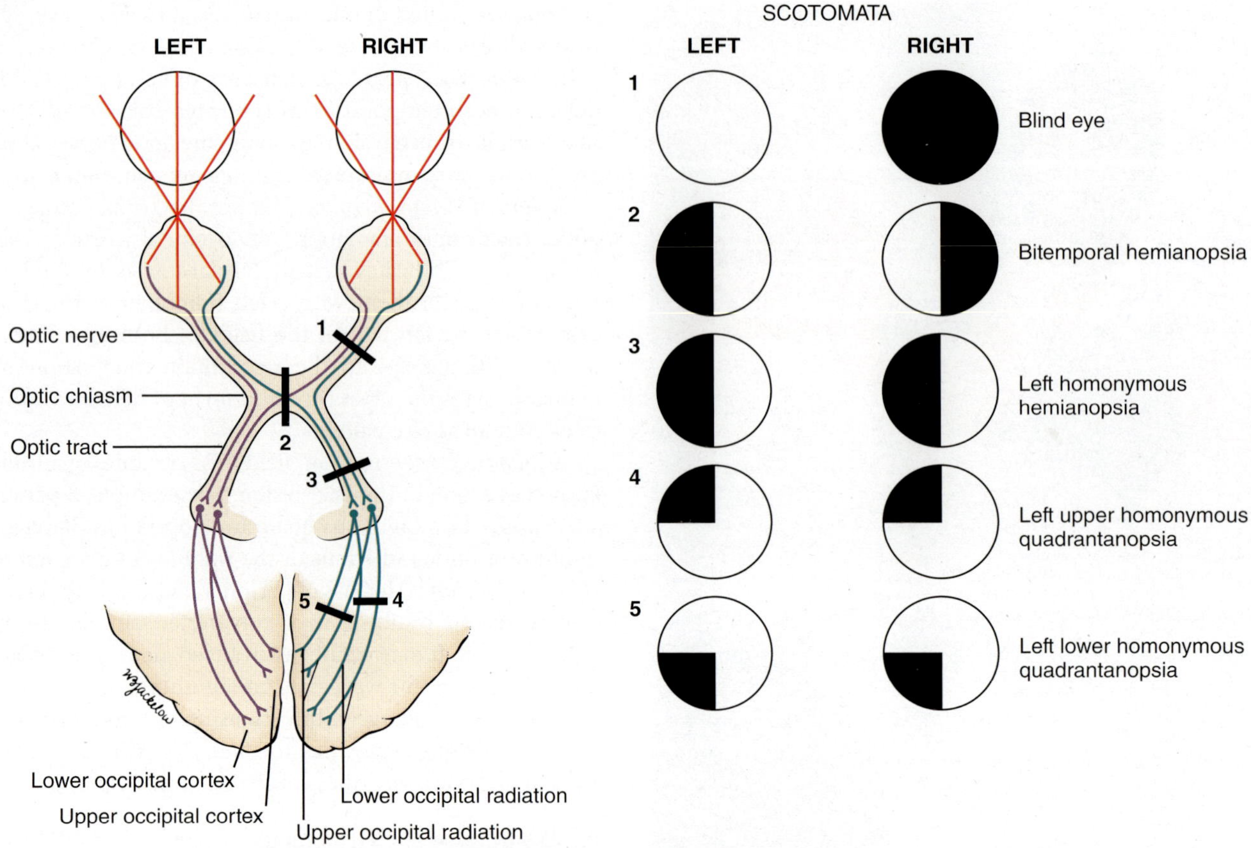

Fig. 10.11 Visual Field Defects.

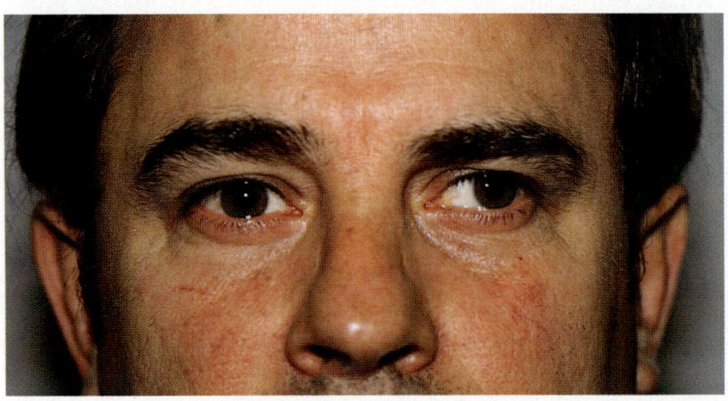

Fig. 10.12 Left Exotropia.

in front of the patient. If the patient is looking now at the pen-light, the light reflex should be in the center of each pupil. If the light falls in the pupillary center of one eye but is displaced away from the pupillary center in the other eye, *deviation* of the eye may exist.

The condition of a deviated or crossed eye is called *strabismus* or tropia. Strabismus is the nonalignment of the eyes in such a way that the object being observed is not projected simultaneously on the fovea of each eye. *Esotropia* is the deviation of an eye nasally; *exotropia* is the deviation of an eye temporally; *hypertropia* is the deviation upward. An *alternating tropia* is a term used to describe the condition in which either eye deviates. Fig. 10.12 shows a patient with a left exotropia.

Perform the Cover Test

The cover test helps determine whether the eyes are aligned (if a deviated eye is present). The patient is instructed to look at a distant target. One eye is covered with a 3 × 5 inch (7.6 × 12.7 cm) card. The examiner should observe the uncovered eye. If the uncovered eye moves to take up fixation of the distant point, that eye was not straight before the other eye was covered. If the eye did not move, it was straight. The test is then repeated with the other eye.

Evaluate the Six Diagnostic Cardinal Positions of Gaze

See Video 10.4.

An important cause of a deviated eye is a *paretic* (weak) or paralyzed extraocular muscle or muscles. Paralysis of these muscles is detected by examination of the *six diagnostic cardinal positions of gaze.*

Because the rotational actions of the oblique and vertical rectus muscles cannot be easily assessed, the eye must be moved into six diagnostic gaze positions that best isolate the vertical movements of these muscles to test their innervations. First, the oblique muscles are tested in adduction to maximize their vertical action. In contrast, the vertical rectus muscles are tested in abduction; in these positions, the superior rectus acts now as a pure elevator and the inferior rectus as a pure depressor. **These diagnostic cardinal positions of gaze are the *testing* positions for the muscles, and the abduction and adduction testing movements are different from the normal actions of the muscles, as indicated in Table 10.1.**

Hold the patient's chin steady with your left hand, and ask the patient to follow your right hand as it traces a large H in the air. Hold your right index finger approximately 15 to 18 inches (38 to 46 cm) from the patient's nose. From the midline, move your finger about 12 inches (30 cm) to the patient's left and pause; then up about 8 inches (20 cm) and pause, as shown in Fig. 10.13; down approximately 16 inches (40 cm) and pause; up about 8 inches (20 cm); and then slowly back to the midline. Switch your hands, holding the patient's chin with your right hand. Cross the midline and repeat the finger movements on the other side. These are the six diagnostic cardinal positions of gaze. Observe the movement of both eyes, which should follow the finger smoothly. Look for the parallel movements of the eyes in all directions.

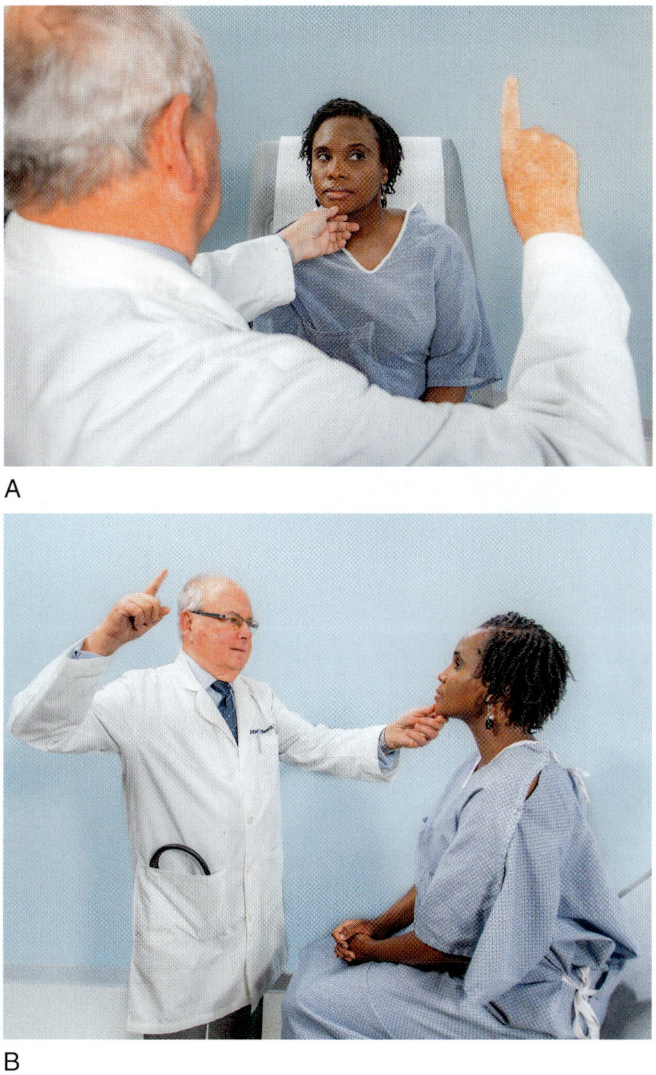

Fig. 10.13 (A) and (B) Technique for testing ocular motility.

On occasion, when looking to the extreme side, the eyes develop a rhythmic motion called *end-point nystagmus.* First, there is a quick motion in the gaze's direction, followed by a slow return. This test differentiates end-point nystagmus from pathologic nystagmus, in which the rapid movement is always in the same direction, regardless of gaze.

Lid lag is present if the eye and eyelid do not move together.

The six diagnostic cardinal positions of gaze, with the related muscles, are illustrated in Fig. 10.14, and Table 10.6 summarizes the abnormalities in ocular motility caused by paretic muscles.

The brain may interpret the images projected on the retina in one of three ways: fusion, diplopia, or suppression. Fusion and diplopia have already been discussed. In children, strabismus leads to diplopia, which leads to confusion, suppression of the image, and *amblyopia.* Amblyopia is the loss of visual acuity secondary to suppression. Amblyopia is reversible until the retinas are fully developed, at approximately the age of 7 years. Amblyopia is a phenomenon that occurs only in children. For example, an adult who acquires strabismus secondary to a stroke cannot suppress the deviated eye's image and will experience intolerable diplopia.

Evaluate the Pupillary Light Reflex

See Video 10.3.

TABLE 10.6 Paretic Muscles Causing Abnormal Ocular Motility

Paretic Muscle	Position to Which Eye Will Not Turn
Medial rectus	Nasal
Inferior oblique	Up and nasal
Superior oblique	Down and nasal
Lateral rectus	Temporal
Superior rectus	Up and temporal
Inferior rectus	Down and temporal

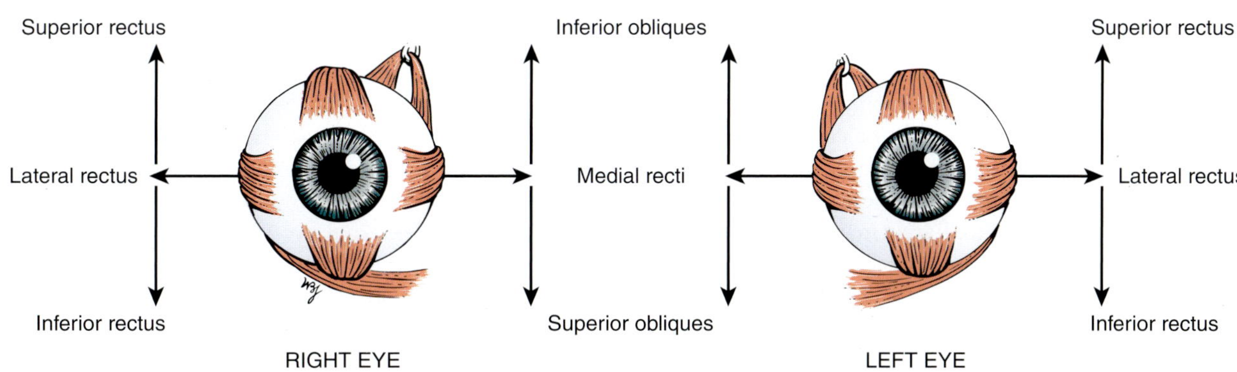

Fig. 10.14 Diagnostic Positions of Gaze.

Ask the patient to look in the distance while you shine a bright light in the patient's eye. The light source should come from the side, with the patient's nose acting as a barrier to light to the other eye. Observe both the direct and consensual pupillary responses. Then repeat the test on the other eye.

The *swinging light test* is a modification for testing the pupillary light reflex. This test reveals differences in the response to afferent stimuli of the two eyes. The patient fixates on a distant target while the examiner rapidly swings a light from one eye to the other, observing for constriction of the pupils. In some conditions, there is a paradoxical dilation of the pupil on which the light is shined. This condition, a *Marcus Gunn defect* or *relative afferent pupillary defect* (*RAPD*), is associated with an afferent limb defect in the eye being illuminated.

The most extreme example of an eye displaying the Marcus Gunn, or RAPD, phenomenon is a blind eye. When light is shined into the blind eye, there is neither a direct nor a consensual response. When the light is moved to the other eye, there is a direct and consensual response because both afferent and efferent pathways are normal. When the light is swung back to the blind eye, no impulses are received by the retina (afferent), and the pupil of the blind eye no longer remains constricted; it therefore dilates. There are different degrees of severity of Marcus Gunn pupils, depending on the involvement of the optic nerve.

Evaluate the Near Reflex

The near reflex is tested by having the patient look first at some distant target and then at a target approximately 5 inches (13 cm) away from their nose. When the patient focuses on the near target, the eyes should converge, and the pupils should constrict.

External and Internal Eye Structures

See Video 10.5.

The examination of the external and internal eye structures includes the following:

- Orbits and eyelids
- Lacrimal apparatus
- Conjunctiva
- Sclera
- Cornea
- Pupils
- Iris
- Anterior chamber
- Lens

Inspect the Orbits and Eyelids

Are the globes present in the orbits? Removing the entire globe, known as *enucleation*, from the orbit may be caused by trauma, surgery (as in the case of a ruptured globe), or self-induced injury by a psychotic person. For example, the *enucleation* of the left eye is pictured in Fig. 10.15. Rarely may one see a patient with *anophthalmos*, the congenital absence of an eye. This can be caused by genetic abnormalities and environmental influence from gestational infections, which are typically viral.

Examine the eyelids for evidence of drooping, infection, erythema, swelling, crusting, masses, or other abnormalities. Then, have the patient open and close the eyelids. The motion should be smooth and symmetric. Do the eyes close completely?

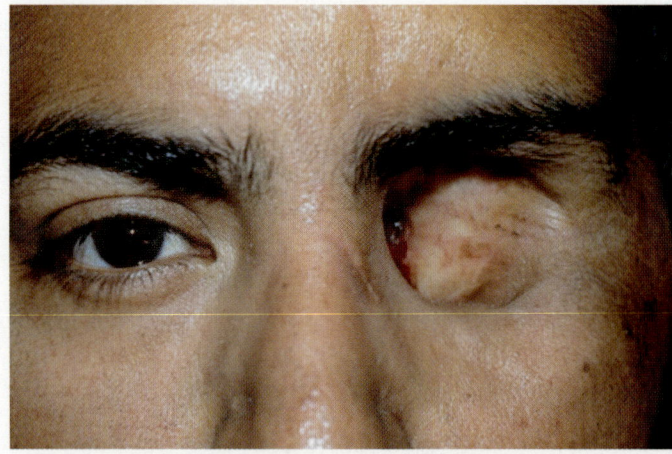

Fig. 10.15 Enucleation of Left Eye.

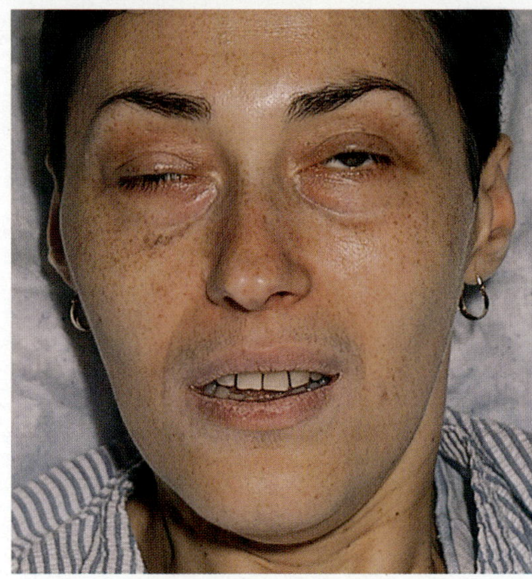

Fig. 10.16 Bilateral Ptosis.

Note the position of the eyelids. When the eye is open, the upper eyelid typically covers only the upper margin of the iris. When the eye is closed, the eyelids should approximate each other completely. The space between the upper and lower lids is the *palpebral fissure*. Drooping of the eyelid is known as *blepharoptosis* or *ptosis*. Fig. 10.16 depicts marked bilateral ptosis, causing the palpebral fissure's narrowing resulting from a muscle-weakening disorder, myasthenia gravis.

Fig. 10.17 shows a patient with *Kearns-Sayre syndrome*, also known as *chronic progressive external ophthalmoplegia*. This autosomal-dominant condition has a slowly progressive, symmetric ptosis and symmetric external ophthalmoplegia (weakness of the external eye muscles). The syndrome also is associated with retinal pigmentary degeneration and cardiac conduction defects such as complete heart block. In addition, affected patients are frequently of short stature and may be deaf. In the patient shown in Fig. 10.17, notice the arching of the brows to lift the eyelids to reduce the ptosis.

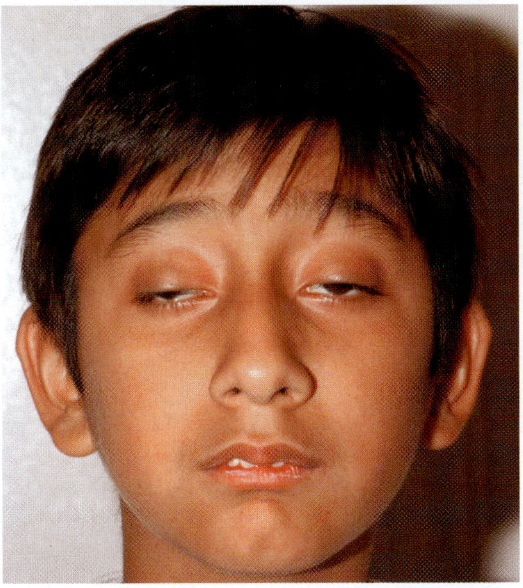

Fig. 10.17 Kearns-Sayre Syndrome.

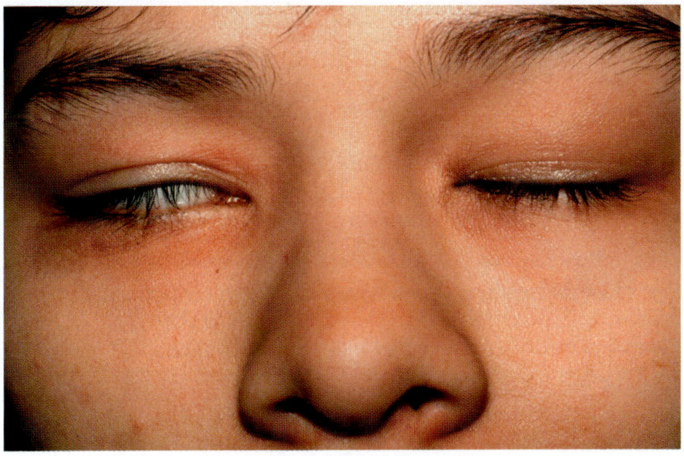

Fig. 10.18 Lagophthalmos.

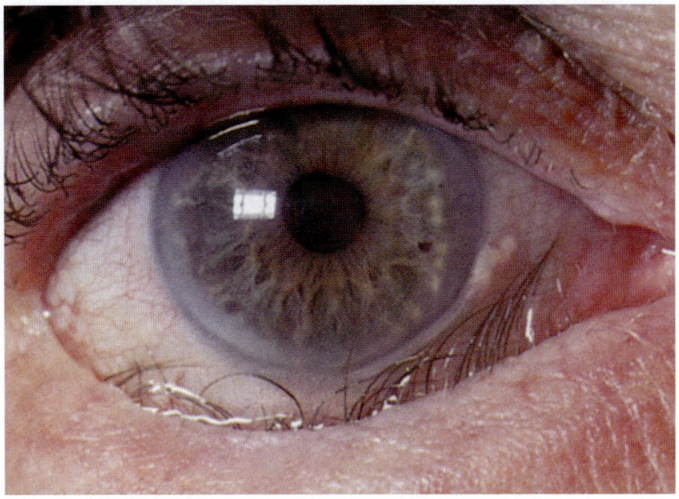

Fig. 10.19 Entropion. (From Kanski JJ, Nischal KK: Ophthalmology: clinical signs and differential diagnosis, St. Louis, 2000, Mosby.)

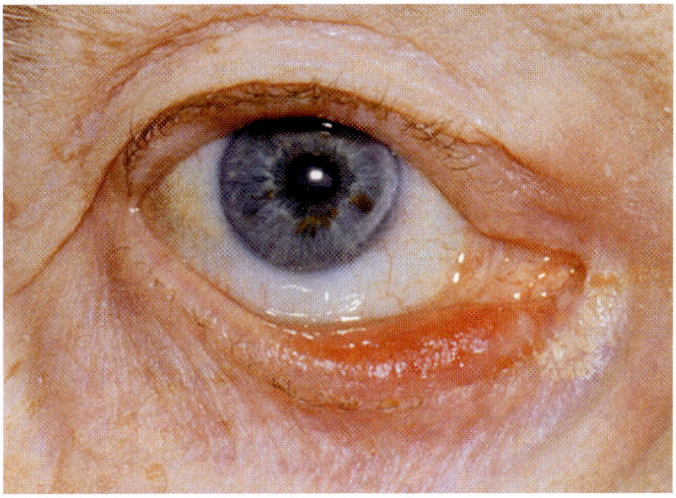

Fig. 10.20 Ectropion. (Courtesy of Christina Ryu, MD, and Alexis Cullen, CRA, Henry Ford Health System, Detroit, MI.)

Lagophthalmos is a condition pictured in Fig. 10.18, in which there is an inability to close the eyelids completely. It is seen in thyroid disease secondary to orbital infiltration caused by inflammation, as a result of autonomic stimulation, or as a consequence of ocular surgery. The name comes from the Greek word *lagos,* meaning "hare," an animal believed to sleep with its eyes open.

Fig. 10.19 shows a patient with entropion. Entropion is a turning inward of the lid margin so that the eyelashes abrade the cornea and globe. An *ectropion* is a turning outward of the eyelid margin. An ectropion is pictured in Fig. 10.20. Both entropion and ectropion may be seen as involutional changes associated with aging and may be related to the dry eye syndrome.

A common benign lesion of the eyelid is a marginal intradermal nevus, shown in Fig. 10.21. Such lesions are well differentiated, and hairs commonly grow from them. However, one associated problem is that these hairs may scratch the cornea, causing corneal abrasions like those caused by entropion.

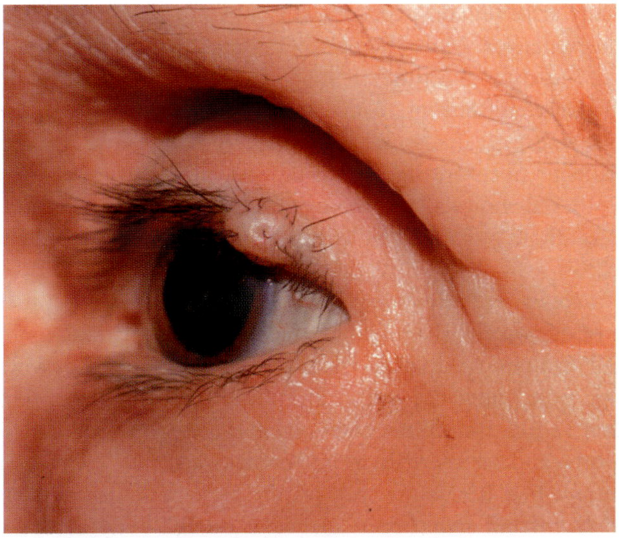

Fig. 10.21 Marginal Nevus of Upper Eyelid.

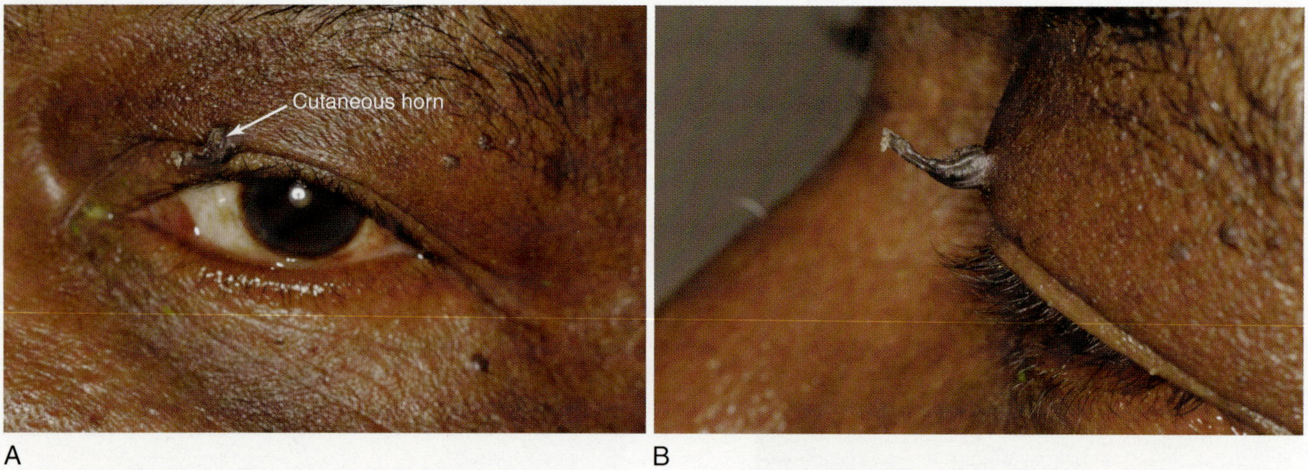

Fig. 10.22 Cutaneous Horn. (A) Patient's left eye with horn on medial aspect of upper eyelid. (B) Close-up of lesion.

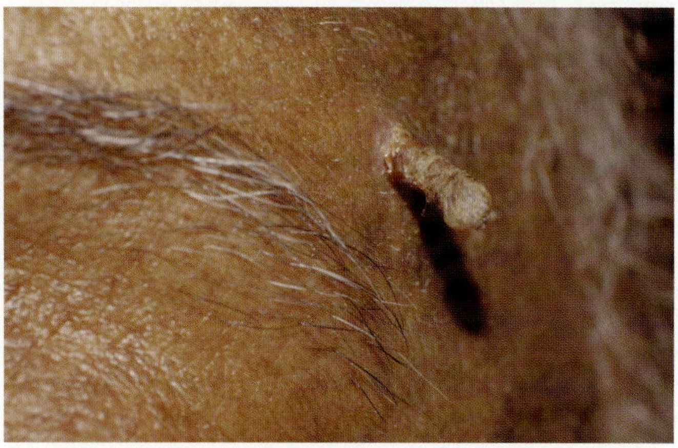

Fig. 10.23 Cutaneous Horn Over Left Eyebrow.

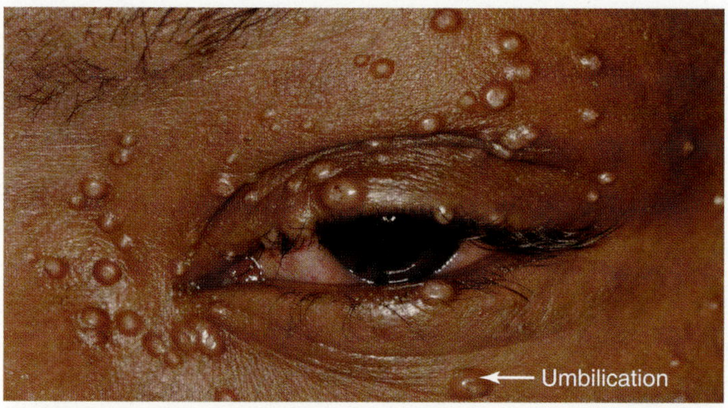

Fig. 10.24 Molluscum Contagiosum. Note the umbilicated (dimpled) lesions; one example is indicated. (Courtesy Christina Ryu, MD, and Steve Oglivy, CRA, Henry Ford Health System, Detroit, MI.)

A *cutaneous horn* is a clinical diagnosis referring to a conical projection above the skin's surface that resembles a small horn. The base of the horn may be flat, nodular, or crateriform. The horn is composed of compacted keratin. Cutaneous horns usually arise on sun-exposed skin but can occur even in sun-protected areas. More than half of all cutaneous horns are benign. No clinical features reliably distinguish between benign and malignant lesions. Tenderness at the base and lesions of larger size favor malignancy. Fig. 10.22A shows a patient with a cutaneous horn on the medial aspect of the left upper eyelid. Fig. 10.22B shows a close-up of the cutaneous horn. Fig. 10.23 shows another patient with a cutaneous horn above her left eyebrow.

Molluscum contagiosum is a viral infection caused by a member of the poxvirus family that causes raised, pearl-like, umbilicated (dimpled) papules on the skin. In most people, the growths range from about the size of a pinhead to as large as a pencil eraser (2 to 5 mm in diameter). This is a common infection in children and occurs when a child comes into direct contact with a lesion. It is frequently seen on the face, neck, armpit, arms, and hands but may occur anywhere on the body except the palms and soles. The virus can spread through contact with contaminated objects, such as towels, clothing, or toys. The virus also spreads through sexual contact. Early lesions on the genitalia (see Figs. 18.36 and 18.37) may be mistaken for herpes or warts but unlike herpes, these lesions are painless. Persons with an impaired immune system, such as patients with acquired immune deficiency syndrome (AIDS), may have significantly more severe cases of molluscum contagiosum. Fig. 10.24 shows a patient with molluscum contagiosum around the eye. Note the umbilicated lesions in this figure and in Fig. 18.37.

A common ocular occurrence of aging is herniation of the orbital fat, caused by progressive thinning of the orbital septum, allowing orbital fat to move forward, and resulting in puffy areas around the globe. Fig. 10.25 shows an example of herniated orbital fat. Note the unrelated old corneal scars and the arcus senilis, discussed later in this chapter.

Fig. 10.26 depicts a small hemangioma of the lower eyelid. *Sturge-Weber syndrome* is a congenital condition recognizable by a characteristic port wine stain, or *nevus flammeus,* on one side of the face that follows the distribution of one or more of the divisions of the trigeminal nerve. Hemangiomas may develop on the episclera, iris, ciliary body, and choroid. Unilateral glaucoma frequently develops on the affected side if the eye has

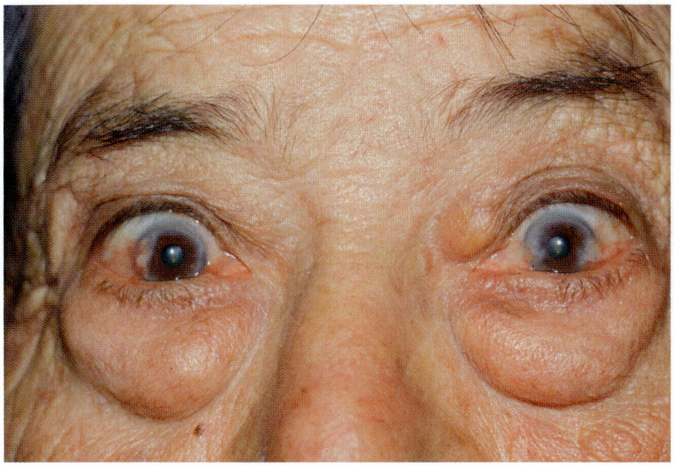

Fig. 10.25 Herniated Orbital Fat.

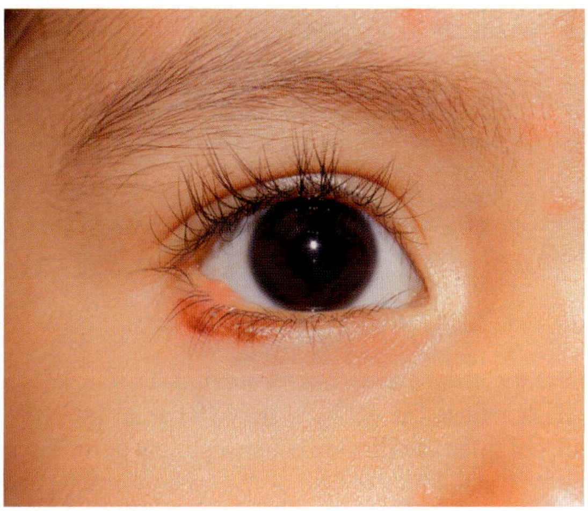

Fig. 10.26 Hemangioma of Lower Eyelid.

extensive involvement with a uveal hemangioma. Therefore, these patients should be screened for glaucoma early. Fig. 10.27 shows a patient with Sturge-Weber syndrome. Notice the sharply demarcated patch of the hemangioma with the involvement of the ophthalmic and maxillary divisions of the left trigeminal nerve. The lesion does not blanch on pressure and tends to darken with age from red to purple.

A *chalazion* is a granulomatous reaction to inspissated secretions of the meibomian glands in the eyelid. It is caused by a blocked duct in one of the glands. These glands are aligned vertically in the eyelids perpendicular to the lid margin. The openings of these glands are located on the eyelid margin directly behind the eyelashes. The glands, approximately 30 in the upper lid and 20 in the lower lid, produce a thin, oily fluid that lubricates the eye. A chalazion may appear as a localized mass on the eyelid near the orifice of the gland, painful at first but usually painless when chronic. Fig. 10.28A shows a patient with a chalazion; Fig. 10.28B illustrates the position of the meibomian glands on the lids. Fig. 10.28C shows a surface illumination view of normal meibomian glands. Fig. 10.29 shows a patient with bilateral chalazions. A chalazion will often disappear without treatment within a month or so. The initial

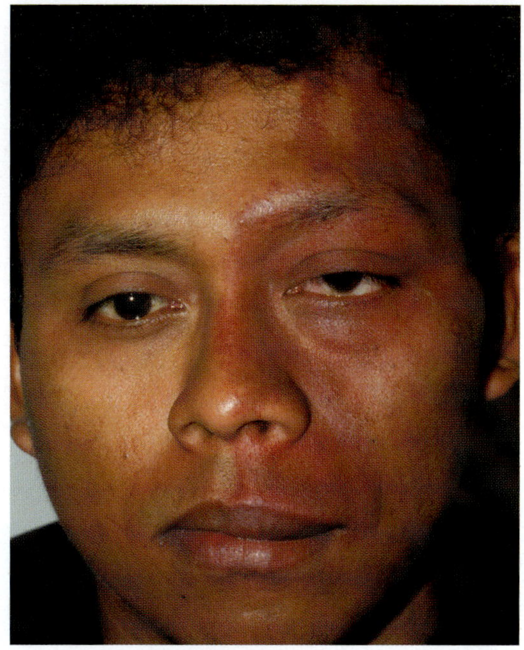

Fig. 10.27 Sturge-Weber Syndrome.

treatment is to place very hot, but not burning,[d] compresses over the eyelid for 10 to 15 minutes at least four times a day. This tends to soften the hardened oils blocking the duct and promote drainage and healing. Fig. 10.30A shows another patient with a chalazion; Fig. 10.30B shows the same patient with the lid everted. Note the chalazion distorting the lid margin and the granuloma formed on the lower inner eyelid at the proximal end of the meibomian gland.

In *herpes zoster ophthalmicus,* rows of vesicles, ulcers, and crusted scabs are scattered along the course of one or more of the branches of the ophthalmic division of the trigeminal nerve. The vesicles contain clear fluid. These rupture, leaving ulcers that can become infected secondarily and form crusts. The eyelids become edematous and red. Pain can be excruciating. Ophthalmoplegia secondary to involvement of the extraocular muscles may also occur. Fig. 10.31 shows a patient with AIDS and herpes zoster ophthalmicus at different stages of evolution (fresh and crusted vesicles) in the ophthalmic division of the trigeminal nerve. Treatment with antivirals will dramatically reduce the symptoms.

Is orbital discoloration present? One type of orbital pigmentation known as *raccoon eyes* is an important sign of a basilar skull fracture. This discoloration is caused by extravasated blood from the fracture of the base of the brain. This is a vital sign to recognize, especially in an unconscious patient, when a history is unavailable. Fig. 10.32 shows a patient with a basilar skull fracture—notice also the subconjunctival hemorrhages on the lateral aspects.

Inspect the eyelids for *xanthelasma.* Although not specific for hypercholesterolemia, these asymptomatic, sharply demarcated

[d]Tell the patient to apply hot compresses to the closed eye using the hottest water they can stand, without burning the face.

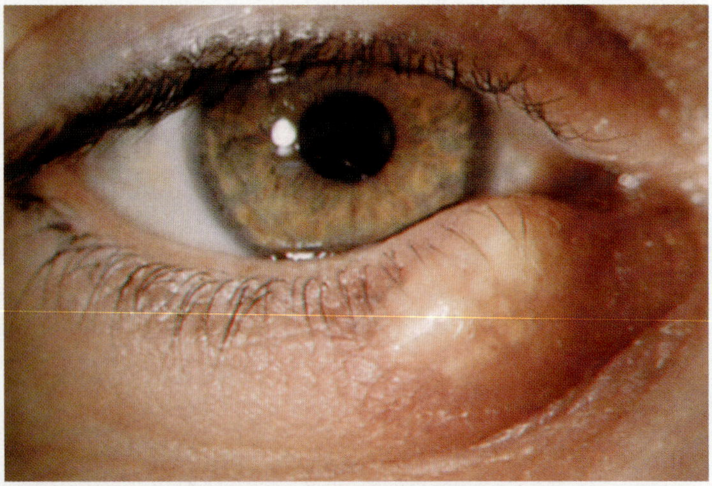

A

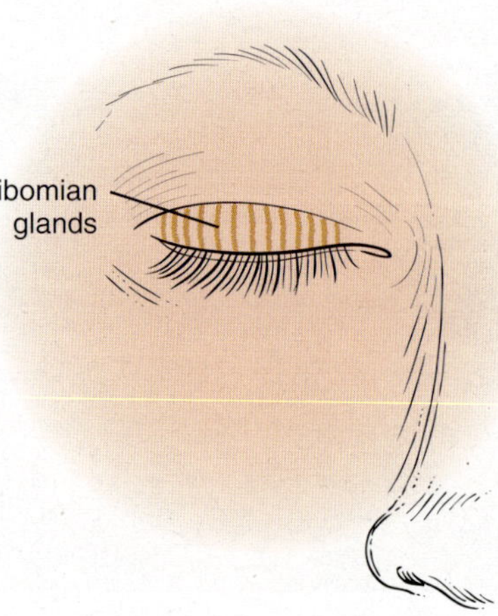

B

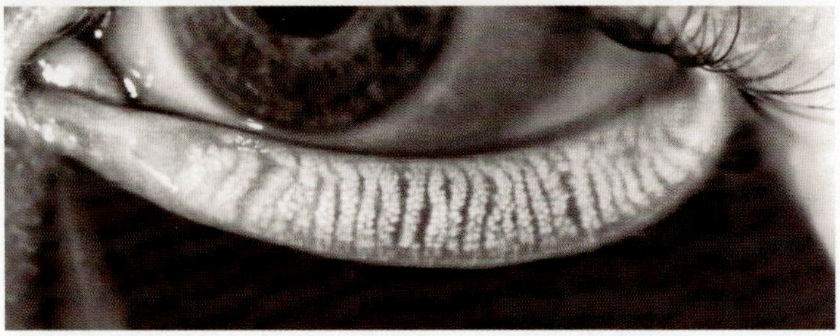

C

Fig. 10.28 (A) Chalazion. (B) This illustration shows the position of the meibomian glands on the eyelids. (C) Surface Illumination view of normal meibomian glands. (A and B, From Kanski JJ, Nischal KK: *Ophthalmology: clinical signs and differential diagnosis*, St. Louis, 2000, Mosby; C, Photo courtesy of TearScience. 5151 McCrimmon Parkway, Suite 250, Morrisville, NC 27560. Image captured using Dynamic Meibomian Imaging (DMI).)

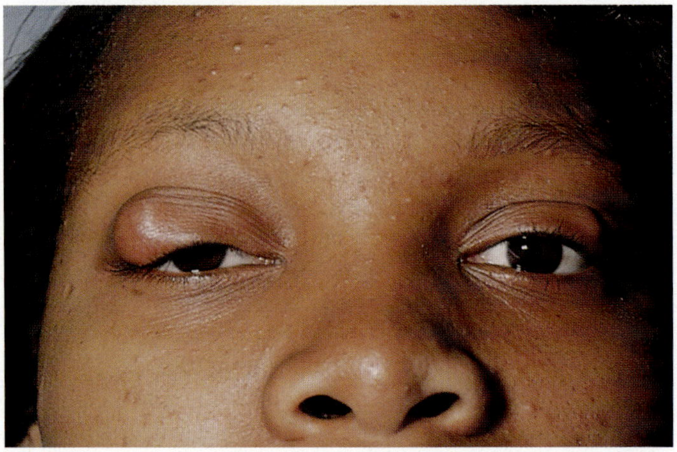

Fig. 10.29 Bilateral Chalazions.

yellowish papules and plaques are commonly associated with lipid deposition in the periorbital skin. Xanthelasma occurs most commonly near the inner canthus of the eyelid, more often on the upper lid than the lower lid. The prevalence is estimated at 4%, with an incidence of 1.1% in females and 0.3% in males. The age of onset can range from 15 to 73 years, although typical peaks are seen in the fourth and fifth decades. In about half of the cases, it can be associated with underlying hyperlipidemia, and a presentation before 40 years of age should prompt screening to rule out underlying inherited disorders of lipoprotein metabolism. Xanthelasma on the upper lid and lower periorbital area is shown in Fig. 10.33.

A *stye,* or *acute external hordeolum,* is a localized abscess in an eyelash follicle caused by a staphylococcal infection. It is a painful, red infection that looks like a pimple pointing on the lid margin where the hair follicle of the eyelash or cilia is situated. Fig. 10.34 depicts a stye. *Blepharitis* is a chronic inflammation of the eyelid margins. The most common form is associated with small white scales around the lid margin and the eyelashes, which stick together and may fall out. There are several annoying symptoms: itching, tearing, and redness. The condition is frequently associated with seborrheic dermatitis and acne rosacea. Fig. 10.35 shows a patient with blepharitis.

Malignant tumors of the eyelids are not uncommon. Characteristics suggesting malignancy include:

- Telangiectasia
- Alteration of the normal architecture (e.g., loss of eyelashes)
- Neither painful nor tender
- Irregular pigmentary changes

Carcinoma of the eyelids has the highest incidence of any malignant ocular tumor. Males are more commonly affected than females; the average age at onset is 50 to 60 years. Of all eyelid carcinomas, 95% are of the basal cell type. The location of basal cell carcinomas is on the lower eyelid (50% to 60%), medial canthus (25% to 30%), upper eyelid (15%), and lateral canthus (5%). Fig. 10.36 shows a *basal cell carcinoma* of the lower lid. The lesion grows slowly and painlessly, eventually forming the typical rodent ulcer with a raised border and an indurated base. The tumor erodes the surrounding area, creating the ulcer. Note the raised border of the lesion in Fig. 10.36.

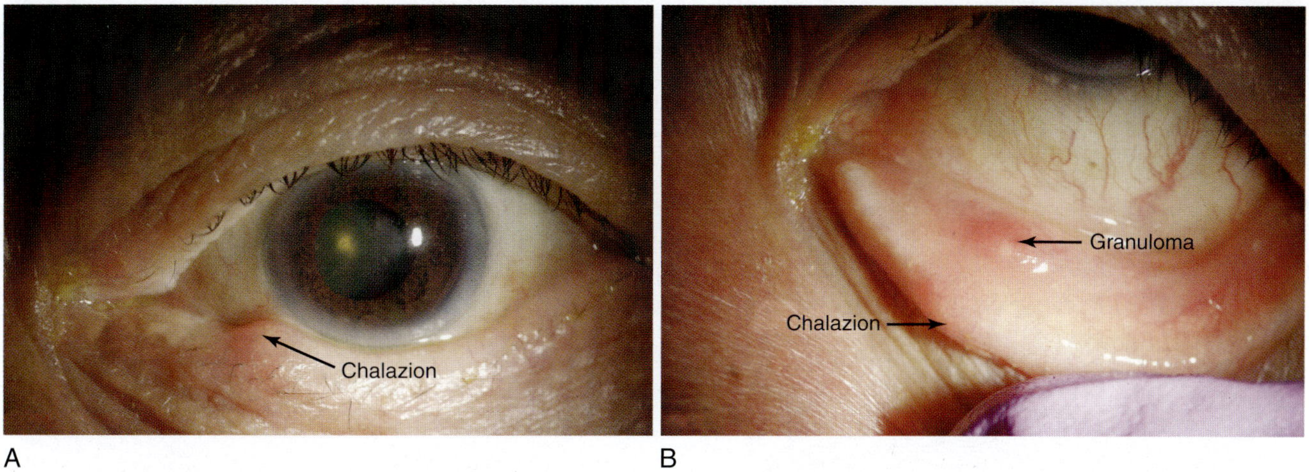

Fig. 10.30 Chalazion. (A) Note the lesion on the lower eyelid. (B) Close-up of the lesion with the eyelid everted. Note the chalazion distorting the lid margin and the granuloma formed on the lower inner eyelid at the proximal end of the meibomian gland. (Courtesy Christina Ryu, MD, Bradley Stern, CRA, Henry Ford Health System, Detroit, MI.)

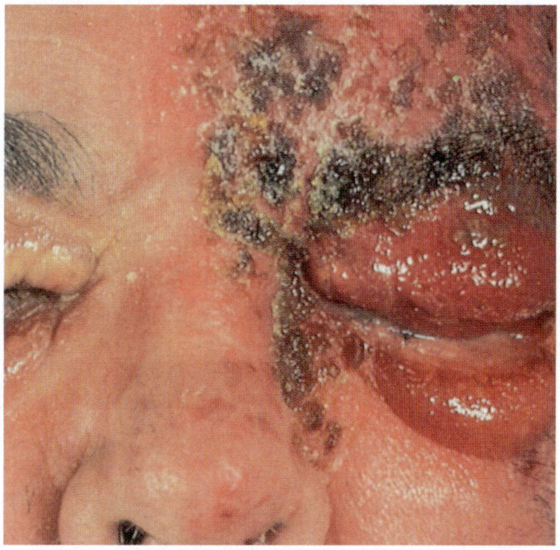

Fig. 10.31 Herpes Zoster Ophthalmicus. (From Friedman-Kien AE, Cockerell CJ, editors. *Color atlas of AIDS*, ed 2, Philadelphia, 1996, WB Saunders.)

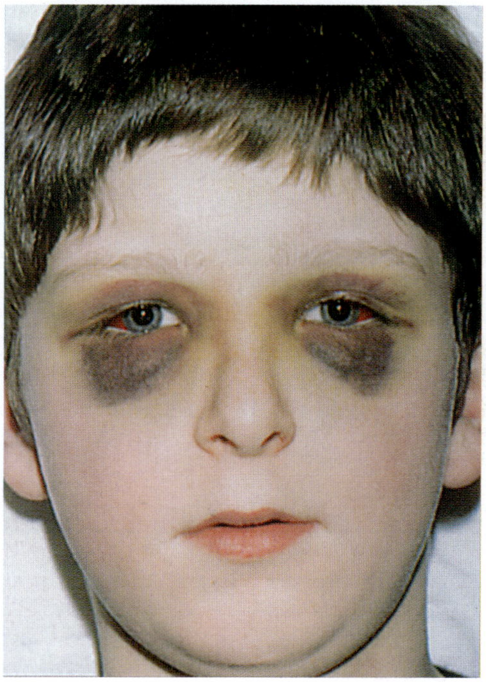

Fig. 10.32 Raccoon Eyes Secondary to a Basilar Skull Fracture. (From Mir MA: *Atlas of clinical diagnosis*, London, 1995, WB Saunders.)

The remaining 5% consists of meibomian gland carcinomas and squamous cell carcinomas. *Meibomian gland carcinoma* is the second most common eyelid malignancy after basal cell carcinoma. These tumors are slowly growing, which may initially look benign and masquerade as more benign conditions like a chalazion and a papilloma. Unfortunately, this often leads to inappropriate management with resultant increased morbidity and mortality rates.

Squamous cell carcinomas are 40 times less common than basal cell carcinomas, tend to be on the upper eyelid, and grow faster than basal cell carcinomas. Early ulceration is common. Squamous *cell carcinoma* of the eyelid is shown in Fig. 10.37. The base and edges of the ulcer are hard and hyperemic.

Malignant melanomas are less than 1% of all malignant tumors of the eyelid. A malignant melanoma of the eyelid is distinguished from an eyelid nevus in that it can be variably pigmented, change color, bleed, and grow. The most common location of eyelid melanomas is the lower eyelid, which is approximately 2.6 times more likely to occur than the upper eyelid.

An ophthalmologist should evaluate all pigmented tumors of the eyelid.

The most common ocular manifestation of AIDS affecting the eyelids is lesions of Kaposi sarcoma. The initial manifestation may be subtle and mistaken for blepharitis or a chalazion. Refer to Figure 8.100C, which shows a patient with AIDS and Kaposi sarcoma of the eyelid.

Inspect the Lacrimal Apparatus

The lacrimal apparatus has little to be seen, except the punctum. If tearing, also known as *epiphora*, is present, there may be some

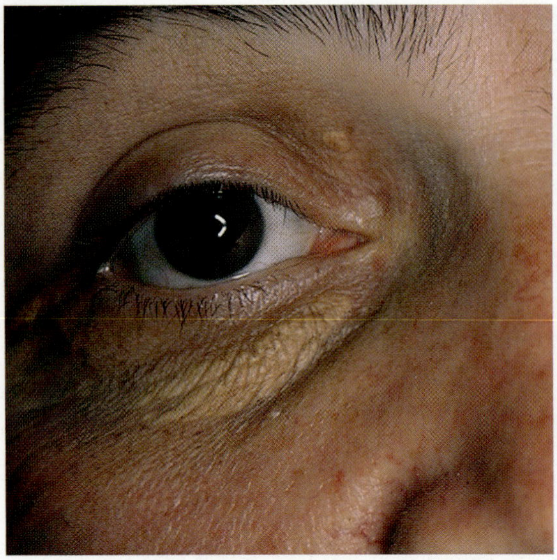

Fig. 10.33 Xanthelasma.

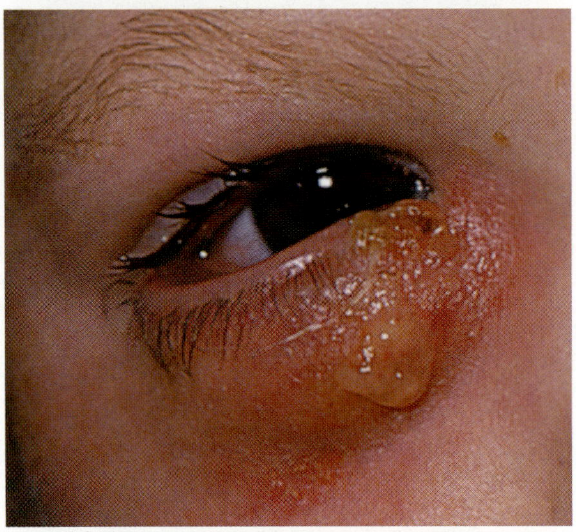

Fig. 10.34 Stye. (From Kanski JJ, Nischal KK: *Ophthalmology: clinical signs and differential diagnosis*, St. Louis, 2000, Mosby.)

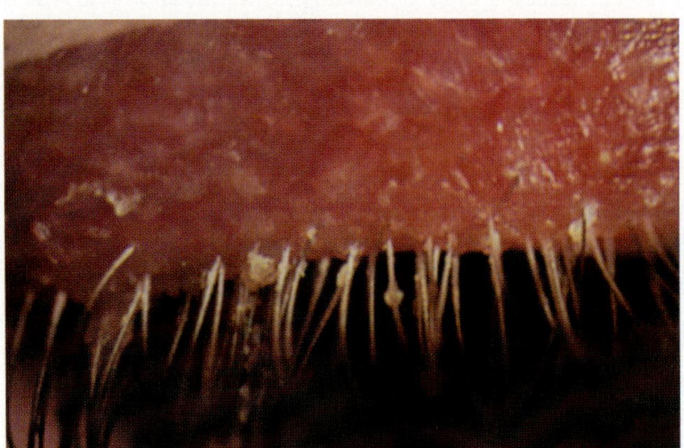

Fig. 10.35 Blepharitis. (From Kanski JJ, Nischal KK: *Ophthalmology: clinical signs and differential diagnosis*, St. Louis, 2000, Mosby.)

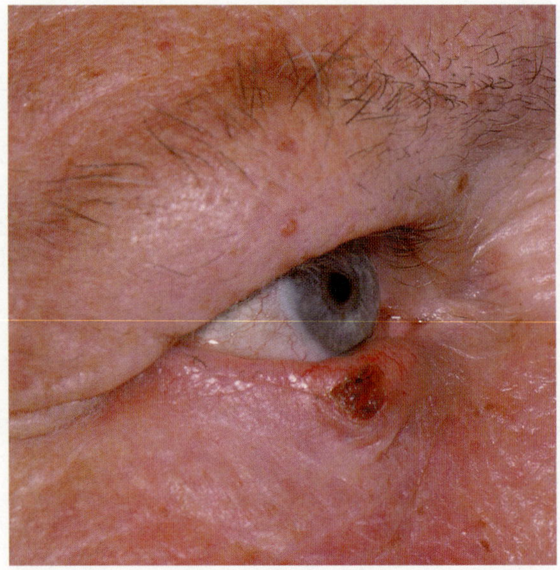

Fig. 10.36 Basal Cell Carcinoma of the Eyelid. (From Kanski JJ, Nischal KK: *Ophthalmology: clinical signs and differential diagnosis*, London, 2002, Mosby.)

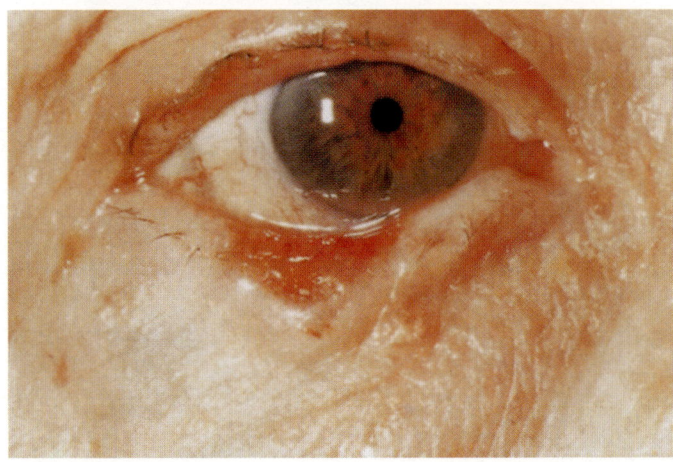

Fig. 10.37 Squamous Cell Carcinoma of the Eyelid. (From Kanski JJ, Nischal KK: *Ophthalmology: clinical signs and differential diagnosis*, London, 2002, Mosby.)

obstruction to flow through the punctum. If excessive moisture is present, gently check for a nasolacrimal duct blockage by pressing the lacrimal sac against the inner orbital rim. If a backup is present, material may be expressed through the punctum. Fig. 10.38 shows massive lacrimal gland enlargement as a result of sarcoidosis.

Fig. 10.39 shows marked bilateral proptosis of the globe in a hyperthyroid patient. Note the massive lacrimal gland enlargement.

Dacryocystitis describes the inflammation of the lower lacrimal passages, usually seen in infants or older individuals. The causes include congenital anomalies, infection, and lacrimal duct stenosis. Chronic dacryocystitis, seen in Fig. 10.40, is a common disorder and almost always arises secondary to ductal obstruction.

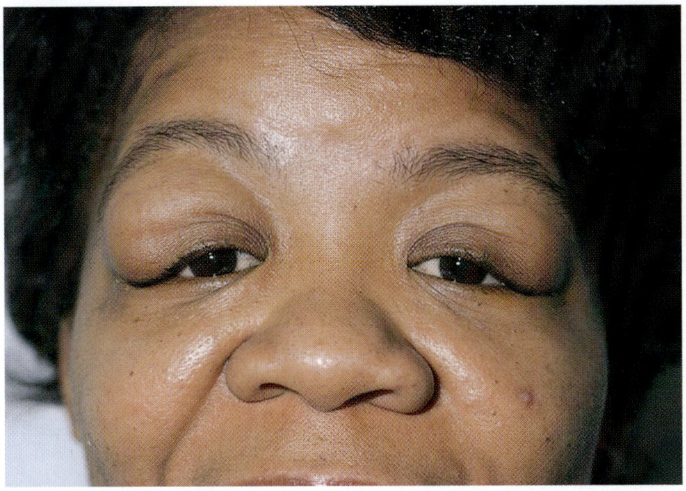

Fig. 10.38 Bilateral Lacrimal Gland Enlargement. Note the classic sigmoid shape of the eyelids.

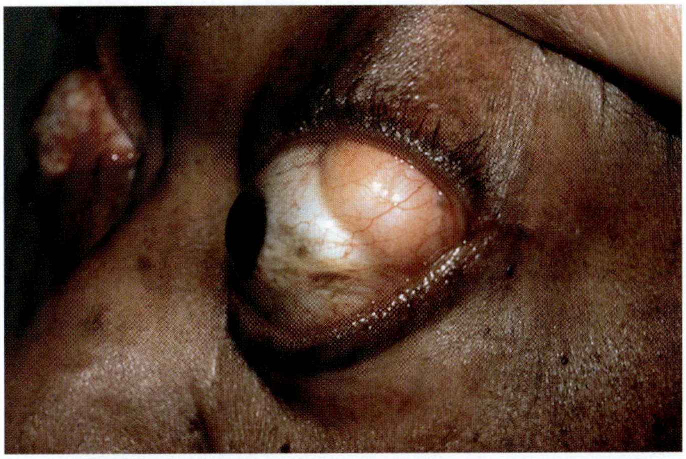

Fig. 10.39 Hyperthyroidism. Note proptosis and lacrimal gland enlargement.

Inspect the Conjunctiva

The conjunctivae should be examined for signs of inflammation (i.e., injection caused by dilatation of its blood vessels), pallor, unusual pigmentation, swelling, masses, and hemorrhage.

The tarsal conjunctiva may be seen by everting the eyelid. Ask the patient to keep the eyes open and look downward. Grasp gently some of the eyelashes of the upper lid. Pull the eyelid away from the globe, and press the tip of an applicator stick against the upper border of the tarsal plate. Then quickly turn the tarsal plate over the applicator stick, using it as a fulcrum. Your thumb can hold the everted lid, and the applicator stick can be removed. After inspecting the tarsal conjunctiva, have the patient look up to return the lid to its normal position.

The normal conjunctiva is transparent. Note the number of blood vessels. Typically, only a small number of vessels are seen. Ask the patient to look up while pulling down the lower eyelids. Compare the vascularity in the two eyes.

Conjunctivitis is the most common of all eye diseases in the Western Hemisphere. The causes are numerous: bacterial, viral, chlamydial, fungal, parasitic, spirochetal, allergic, traumatic, chemical, and idiopathic. Bacterial conjunctivitis is the most frequent type and is self-limited, lasting 10 to 14 days. Fig. 10.41 shows *acute hemorrhagic conjunctivitis.* This highly contagious ocular infection, often bilateral, is caused by enteroviruses (members of the picornavirus family), *Pneumococcus* organisms, and *Haemophilus influenzae. Giant papillary conjunctivitis* is an ocular syndrome consisting of excessive secretion of conjunctival mucus, itching, and the development of giant papillae (1 mm or more in diameter) on the tarsal conjunctiva. This syndrome occurs mainly in patients who wear soft contact lenses but can occur in patients with ocular prostheses or other foreign bodies in the eye. Fig. 10.42 shows a patient with giant papillary conjunctivitis.

Fig. 10.43 shows an extensive *subconjunctival hemorrhage.* This common condition may occur spontaneously in any age group, usually in only one eye. The patient may become

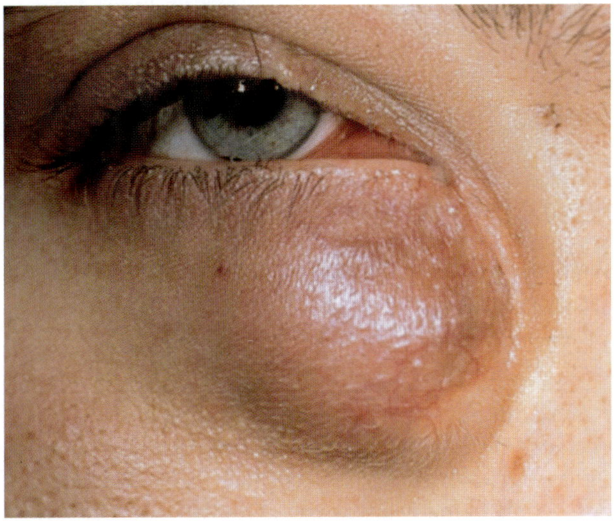

Fig. 10.40 Chronic Dacryocystitis.

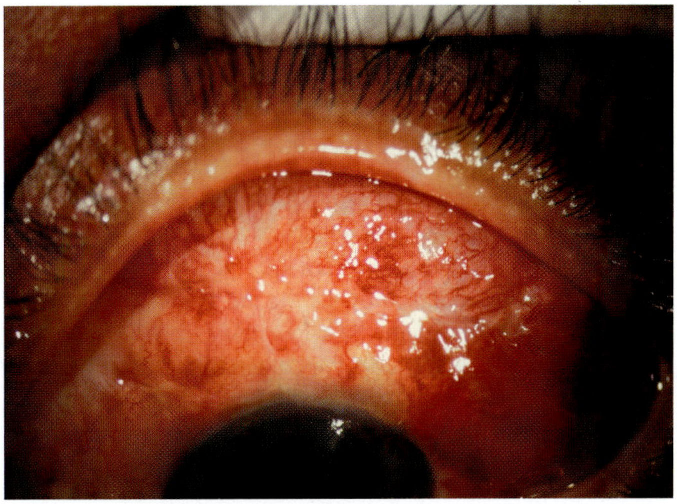

Fig. 10.41 Acute Hemorrhagic Conjunctivitis.

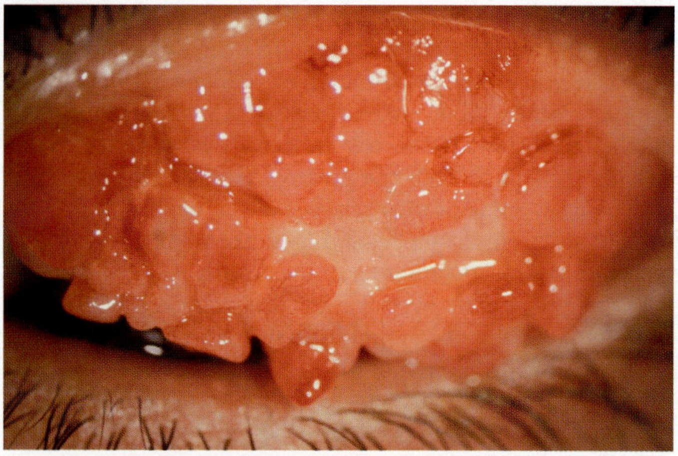

Fig. 10.42 Giant Papillary Conjunctivitis.

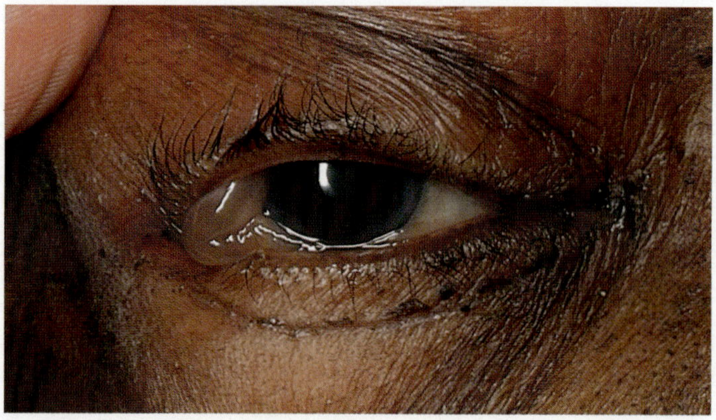

Fig. 10.44 Chemosis. Note the presence of fluid in the subconjunctival space.

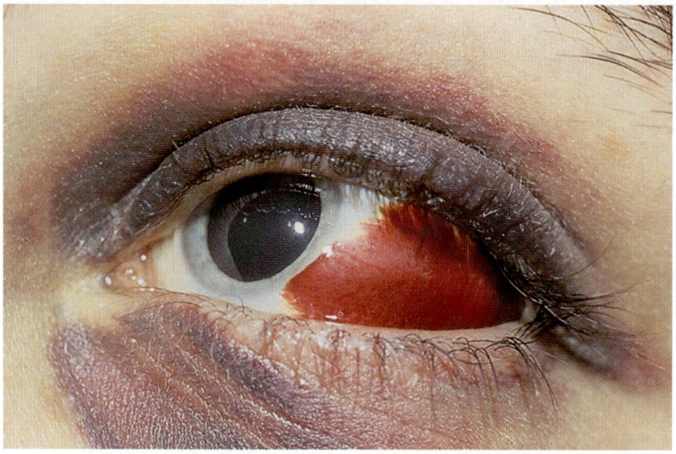

Fig. 10.43 Subconjunctival Hemorrhage.

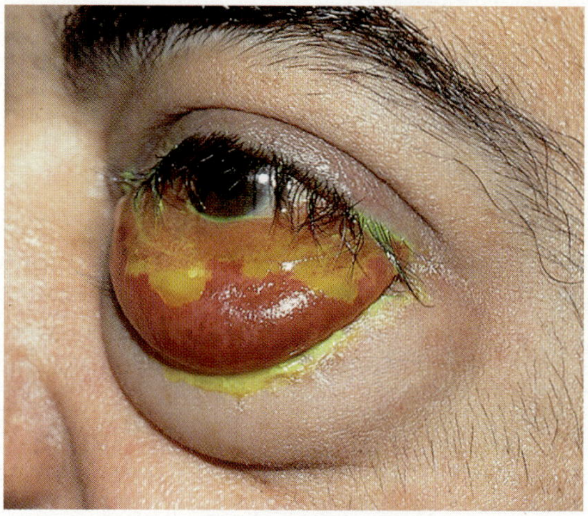

Fig. 10.45 Hemorrhagic Chemosis.

alarmed because of its sudden appearance and bright red color. The hemorrhage is usually caused by a rupture of a small conjunctival vessel after severe coughing, sneezing, or a sustained Valsalva maneuver. Occasionally, a subconjunctival hemorrhage may occur due to elevated blood pressure. There is no treatment, and the hemorrhage resolves within 1 to 2 weeks.

The conjunctiva is attached to the episclera by loose connections. This potential space can quickly be filled with fluids such as blood or serum. *Chemosis* is the presence of fluid in this space. Trauma, allergies, and chronic exposure, as seen in the proptosis of hyperthyroidism and neurologic deficits, are important causes of chemosis. Fig. 10.44 shows chemosis secondary to hay fever. An example of hemorrhagic chemosis is pictured in Fig. 10.45. The patient, a 42-year-old male, had a 7-year history of progressive proptosis secondary to a melanoma.

Two common benign growths on the conjunctiva are the pinguecula and pterygium. A *pinguecula* is a whitish-yellow triangular nodular growth on the bulbar conjunctiva adjacent to the corneal-scleral junction (limbus), as seen in Fig. 10.46; it does not cross onto the cornea. A *pterygium* is a more vascular growth on the bulbar conjunctiva that begins at the medial canthus and extends beyond the corneal-scleral junction to the cornea. This triangle-shaped fibrovascular connective tissue may cause astigmatism or decreased vision if it extends toward or occludes the pupillary margin. The cause of pterygium is thought to be chronic dry eyes because its frequency is higher among people living near the equator. Fig. 10.47A shows a pterygium; Fig. 10.47B is a close-up photograph of a pterygium in

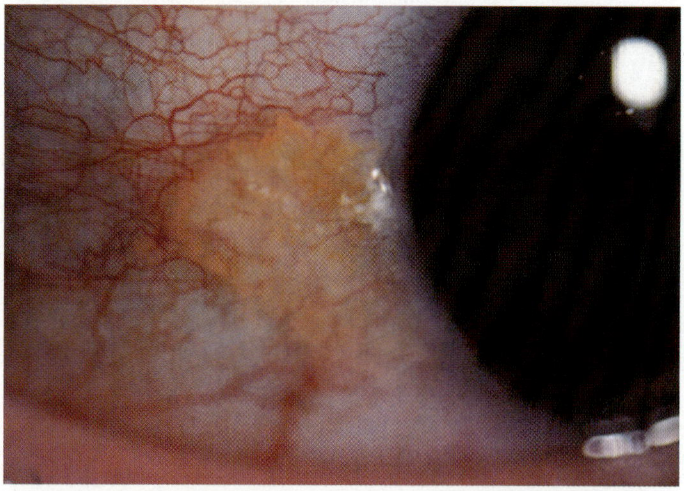

Fig. 10.46 Pinguecula. (From Kanski JJ, Nischal KK: *Ophthalmology: clinical signs and differential diagnosis*, St. Louis, 2000, Mosby.)

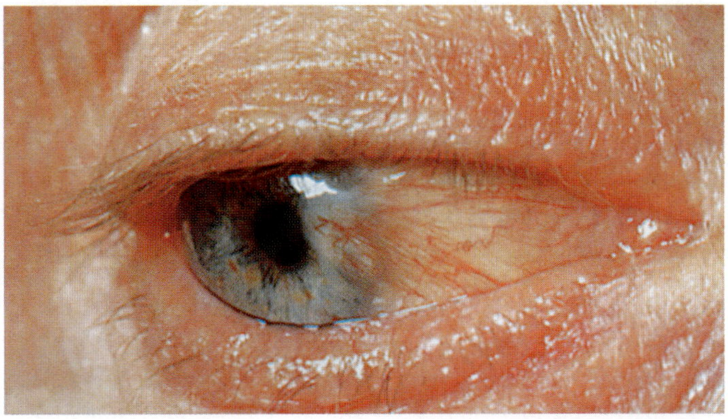

A

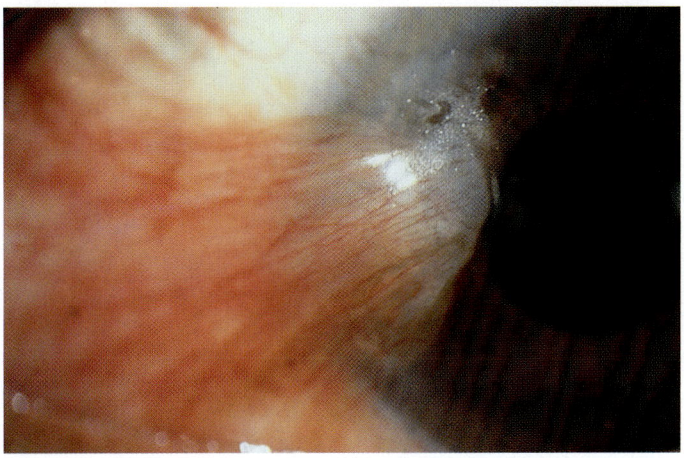

B

Fig. 10.47 (A) and (B) Pterygium. (B) A close-up view. (A, From Mir MA: *Atlas of clinical diagnosis*, London, 1995, WB Saunders.)

another patient. Notice the vascularity and how all the blood vessels reach a point at the pterygium's head (or apex). It is postulated that a pterygium is the eyes' reaction to constant dry, hot winds, thereby "protecting" itself.

Primary acquired melanosis is a unilateral condition in which melanotic pigmentation develops in the conjunctival or corneal epithelium. It starts insidiously during middle age. A biopsy is often needed to rule out a malignant melanoma. Fig. 10.48 shows primary acquired melanosis. Primary acquired melanosis of the plica semilunaris in another patient is seen in Fig. 10.49.

A benign pigmented tumor of the conjunctiva may be a *conjunctival nevus.* This is a solitary, well-defined, slightly elevated lesion. Nevi have a predilection for the limbus, plica semilunaris, caruncle, and lid margin. Most nevi are tan or brown, and many have zones of clearing known as *lacunae.* Fig. 10.50 shows a patient with a conjunctival nevus.

A *dermolipoma of the conjunctiva* is a common congenital tumor, often bilateral, that usually appears as a smoothly rounded growth in the superotemporal quadrant of the bulbar conjunctiva near the lateral canthus. They may contain a variety of histologically aberrant tissues, including epidermal appendages, connective tissue, skin, fat, sweat gland, lacrimal gland, muscle, teeth, cartilage, bone, vascular structures, and neurologic tissue. Fig. 10.51A shows bilateral dermolipomas of the conjunctiva. A close-up of the lesion in the right eye is shown in Fig. 10.51B. The yellowish color is secondary to the increased fatty deposits in the lesion. Fine hairs often protrude from its surface, best seen with a slit lamp. Treatment is usually not indicated.

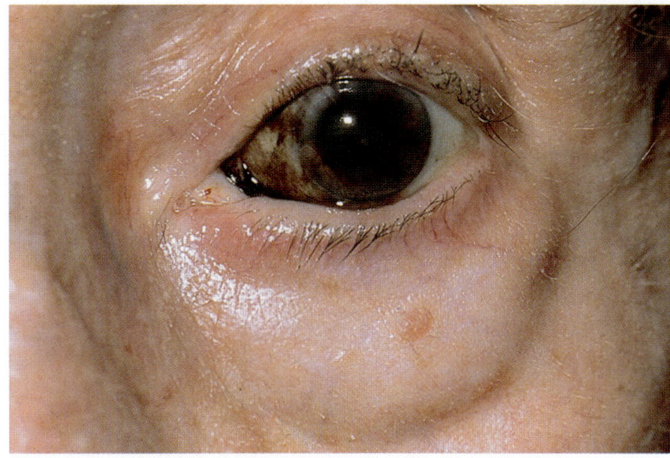

Fig. 10.48 Primary Acquired Melanosis.

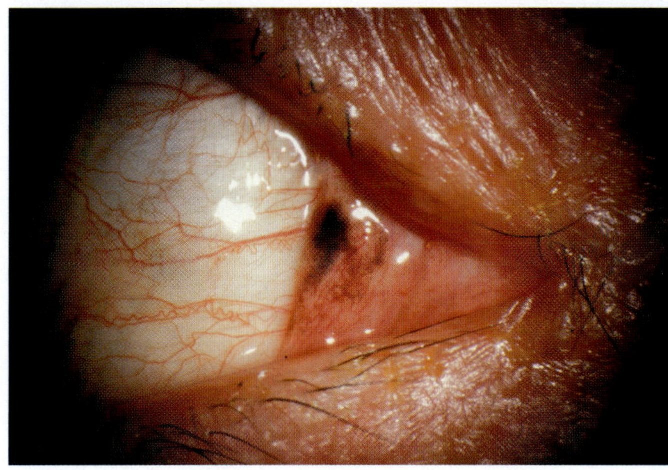

Fig. 10.49 Primary Acquired Melanosis.

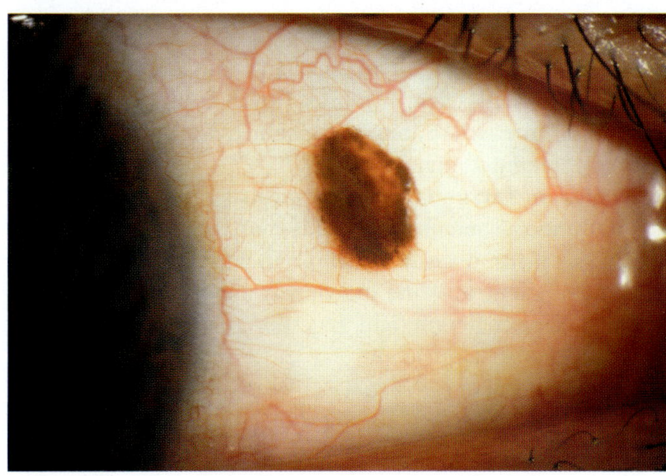

Fig. 10.50 Conjunctival Nevus.

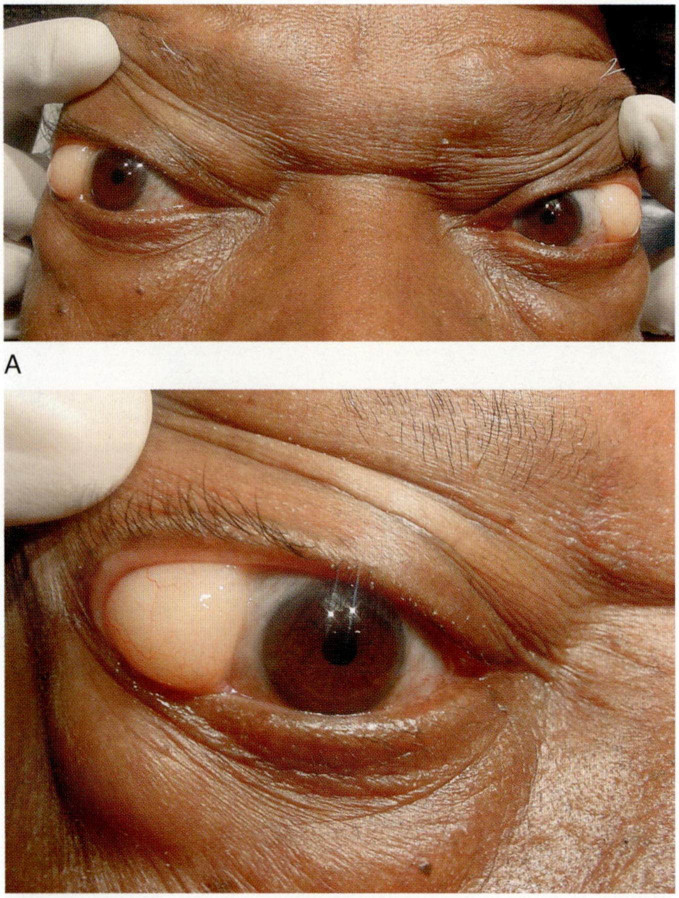

A

B

Fig. 10.51 **Dermolipoma of the Conjunctiva.** (A) Bilateral view. (B) A close-up view of the lesion in the right eye. (From Kanski JJ, Nischal KK: *Ophthalmology: clinical signs and differential diagnosis*, St. Louis, 2000, Mosby.)

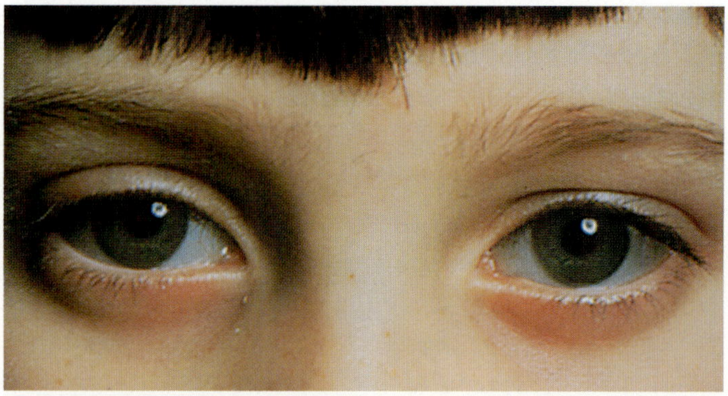

Fig. 10.52 **Blue Sclerae Secondary to Osteogenesis Imperfecta.** (From Mir MA: *Atlas of clinical diagnosis*, London, 1995, WB Saunders.)

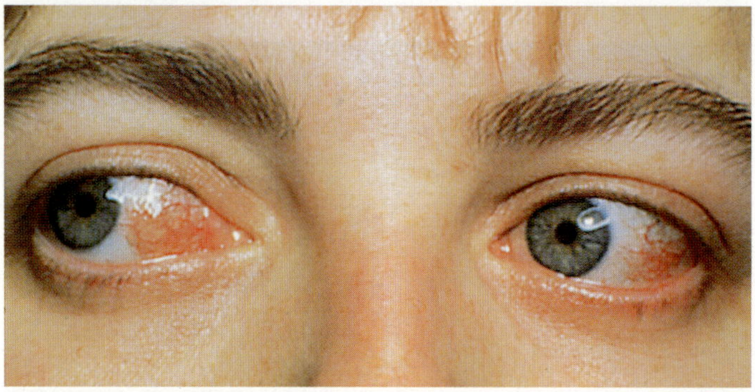

Fig. 10.53 **Episcleritis.** (From Mir MA: *Atlas of clinical diagnosis*, London, 1995, WB Saunders.)

Inspect the Sclera

The sclera is examined for nodules, hyperemia, and discoloration. The normal sclera is white. However, in dark-skinned individuals, the sclera may be slightly brownish in color because of pigment migration.

Jaundice, or *icterus,* is a yellowish discoloration of the sclera, skin, and mucous membranes and is caused by the retention of bilirubin or its products of metabolism. Jaundice is more easily seen in the sclera of white individuals and may be missed in people of color or in dim light. Ingestion of too many carotene-containing foods, *carotenoids,* may cause yellowing of the skin but not of the sclera (see Fig. 17.4). Many foods are associated with high levels of carotenoids; these include carrots, sweet potatoes, tomatoes, asparagus, yellow corn, cheese, mustard, oranges, papayas, peaches, pineapple, pumpkin, and many more.

The sclera may appear bluish, usually in infants or pathologically in *osteogenesis imperfecta*. Osteogenesis imperfecta is a group of hereditary disorders with bone fragility. Individuals with these disorders may suffer bone fractures after mild trauma. The autosomal dominant form is most widely recognized. In this form, the sclerae are very thin and have a blue hue because the uveal pigment shows through the sclera. Deafness is also seen in this form of the disorder. Fig. 10.52 shows blue sclerae in a patient with osteogenesis imperfecta.

Episcleritis is a benign, usually painless, commonly recurring disorder, frequently affecting both eyes of young adults, more commonly females. It is a noninfectious inflammation that is subconjunctival and yet superficial to the underlying sclera. The affected area may be either flat and diffuse or localized and nodular (1 to 4 mm in diameter). Although the cause in most cases is unclear, episcleritis also occurs in patients with inflammatory bowel disease, herpes zoster, collagen vascular disease, gout, syphilis, and rheumatoid arthritis. Fig. 10.53 shows the classic features of episcleritis.

Scleritis is a painful, often bilateral, recurrent disorder that is less common than episcleritis, affects older age groups, and occurs in females more often than males. There is inflammation of the sclera with possible involvement of the cornea, uveal tract (i.e., iris, choroid, and ciliary body), or retina. Photophobia is common. Scleritis is usually related to a systemic disorder. It occurs much more commonly in patients with connective tissue disorders. It may be diffuse or localized and nodular. Nodular scleritis is marked by dark localized blue patches in the anterior portion of the sclera; these are seen because the choroid is visible through the translucent sclera. The condition may resolve spontaneously. Fig. 10.54 shows nodular scleritis.

Scleromalacia perforans is an uncommon, painless scleral condition characterized by the appearance of one or more dehiscences in the sclera in the absence of inflammatory changes.

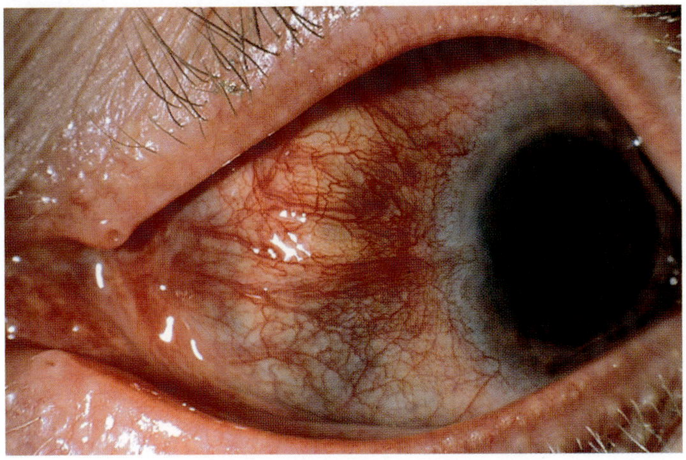

Fig. 10.54 Nodular Scleritis.

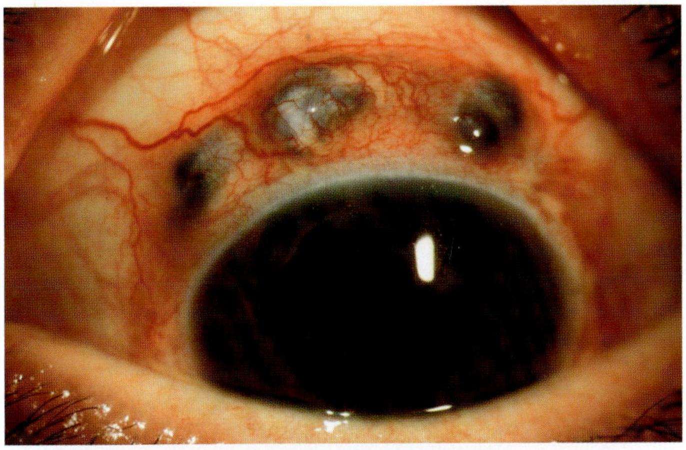

Fig. 10.55 Scleromalacia Perforans.

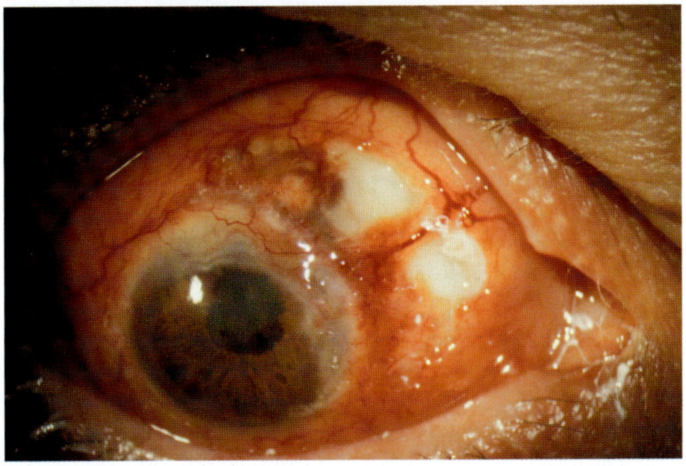

Fig. 10.56 Scleromalacia Perforans. Note the anterior synechiae.

This necrotizing scleritis without inflammation is classically seen in patients with long-standing rheumatoid arthritis. The underlying uvea is often visible and may bulge out, as shown in Fig. 10.55. Another example of scleromalacia perforans is shown in Fig. 10.56. Notice the thinning of the sclera, the underlying dark uvea, and the irregular border of the iris. Anterior synechiae are present, holding the iris down to the lens and causing the scalloped appearance of the iris. There is corneal disease as well.

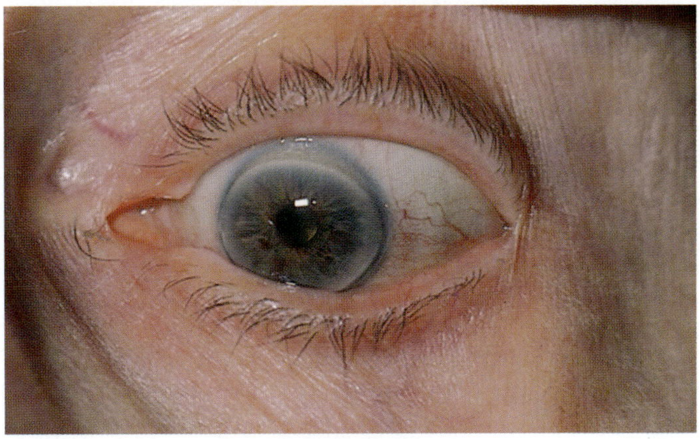

Fig. 10.57 Arcus Senilis.

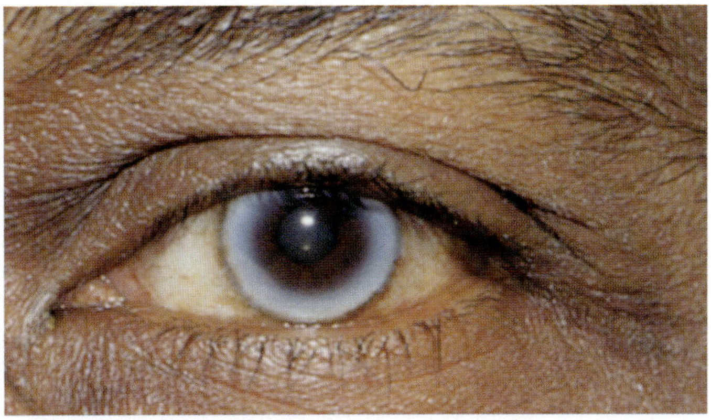

Fig. 10.58 Arcus Senilis. (From Kanski JJ, Nischal KK: *Ophthalmology: clinical signs and differential diagnosis*, St. Louis, 2000, Mosby.)

Inspect the Cornea

The cornea should be clear and without cloudiness, ulceration, or opacities.

A whitish ring at the perimeter of the cornea is probably an *arcus senilis.* In patients older than 40 years, this white, gray, or blue opaque ring or arc at the corneal margin (peripheral corneal opacity) is usually a normal phenomenon. Nearly 100% of people over 80 years old will have an arcus. Around 60% of people over 60 will have this condition, which is more likely to occur in males. Although many false-positive findings exist, patients younger than 40 should be evaluated for hypercholesterolemia. An arcus senilis is seen in Figs. 10.57 and 10.58.

A Kayser-Fleischer ring is an abnormal golden to greenish-brown ring near the limbus, most evident superiorly and inferiorly. This ring is a specific and sensitive sign of *Wilson disease,* which is hepatolenticular degeneration as a result of an inherited disorder of copper metabolism. Approximately 95% of patients with Wilson disease who present with neurologic signs will have a Keyser-Fleischer ring. This ring is caused by the deposition of copper in Descemet's membrane of the

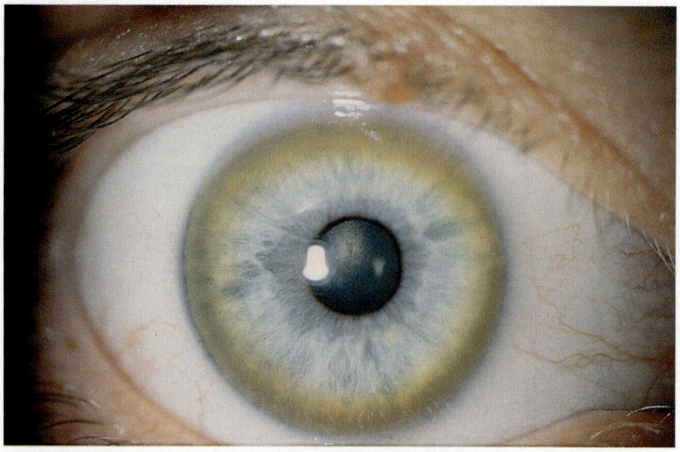

Fig. 10.59 Kayser-Fleischer Ring. (From Kanski JJ, Nischal KK: *Ophthalmology: clinical signs and differential diagnosis*, London, 2002, Mosby.)

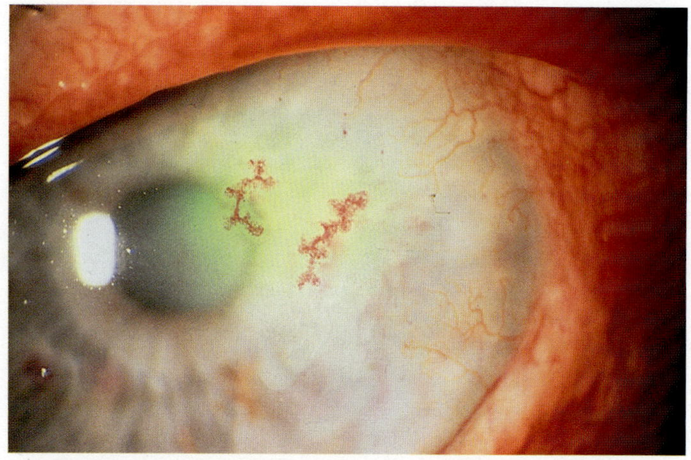

Fig. 10.61 Herpes Simplex Virus–Related Keratitis. The eye has been stained with rose bengal.

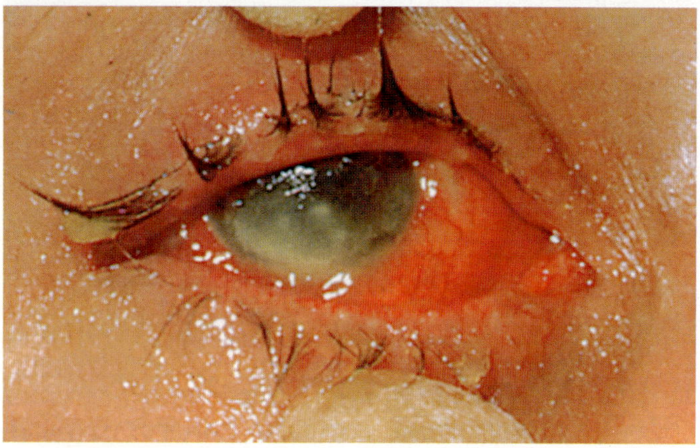

Fig. 10.60 Corneal Ulceration. Note the pus in the anterior chamber. (From Mir MA: *Atlas of clinical diagnosis*, London, 1995, WB Saunders.)

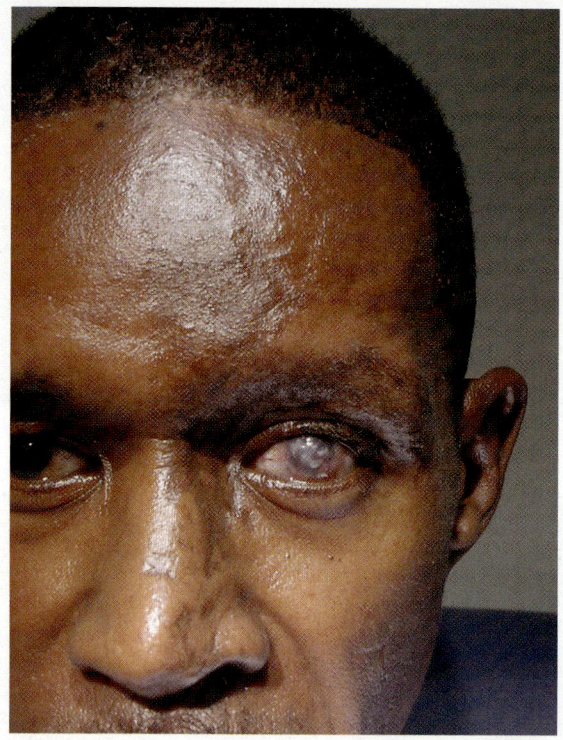

Fig. 10.62 Corneal Scarring Secondary to Previous Herpes Zoster Infection.

peripheral cornea. Fig. 10.59 shows a Kayser-Fleischer ring. Notice that the ring is most prominent in the vertical meridian.

Corneal ulcers are extremely painful lesions caused by loss of substance from the cornea by progressive erosion and necrosis of tissue. Various agents, including bacteria, viruses, fungi, and hypersensitivity reactions may cause these ulcers. *Pneumococcus* organisms are common bacteria associated with corneal ulceration. *Pseudomonas* infection is less common but is associated with a rapid spread and corneal perforation. Herpes simplex virus (HSV) is another common cause of corneal ulceration and is the most common cause of corneal-related blindness. It is almost always unilateral and may affect any age group. The keratitis (inflammation of the cornea) is commonly accompanied by conjunctival hyperemia, tearing, and photophobia. Recurrent attacks may be less painful to painless as generalized corneal anesthesia develops. Patients with AIDS or other immunosuppressive conditions are susceptible to this recurring infection. Fig. 10.60 shows a corneal ulceration secondary to HSV infection. Marked blepharospasm is common with corneal ulceration. The most common characteristic of HSV-related keratitis is the dendritic ulcer on the cornea. This ulcer results from active viral replication in the corneal epithelial cells. Fig. 10.61 shows HSV-related keratitis. The eye has been stained with rose Bengal. The devitalized, swollen cells laden with the replicating virus stain brightly with this substance. Fig. 10.62 shows corneal scarring in another patient due to a previous herpes zoster infection. Note the discrete areas of infiltrates in the cornea, as well as the darkening of the skin on the ipsilateral side from the nose to the forehead.

Keratoconus is an acquired abnormality of the shape of the cornea. It has a gradual onset. It is usually bilateral but asymmetric. It is estimated to occur in 1 per 20,000 individuals. The cornea protrudes as a cone, with the apex becoming thin and scarred. Affected patients experience slow visual deterioration.

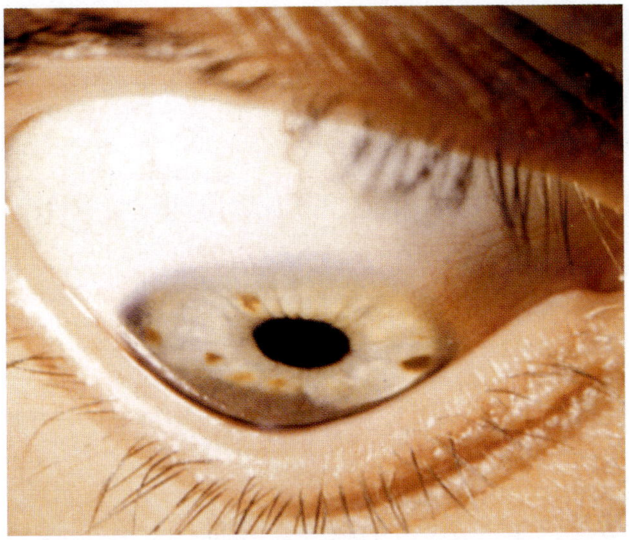

Fig. 10.63 Keratoconus Munson's Sign. (From Kanski JJ, Nischal KK: *Ophthalmology: clinical signs and differential diagnosis*, St. Louis, 2000, Mosby.)

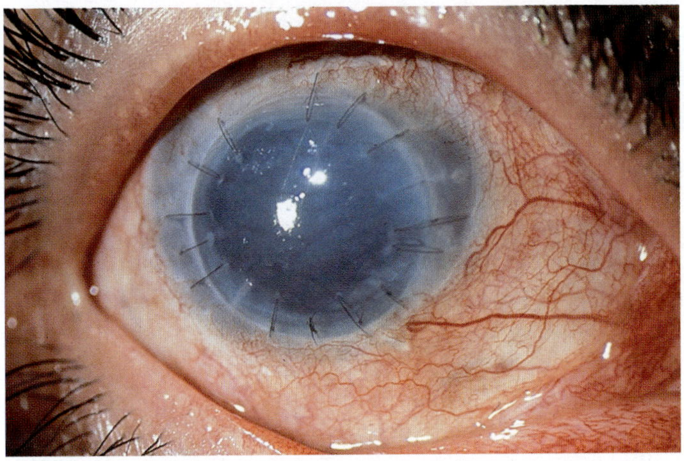

Fig. 10.64 Corneal Transplant.

When the patient is asked to look downward, the cone can become quite apparent, deforming the lower lid to a pointed shape, as seen in Fig. 10.63. This is known as *Munson's sign.*

Patients with keratoconus or corneal scarring from other causes may require corneal transplantation. A recent corneal transplant is shown in a patient in Fig. 10.64. Note the sutures and the mild edema. In recent years, a new treatment, corneal cross-linking, has been developed to prevent the need for corneal transplantation; corneal cross-linking causes the cornea to harden, and the cornea can then be reshaped with laser correction.

Dermolipomas of the corneal limbus are benign congenital tumors that contain tissue not found commonly at that site. They appear most frequently at the inferior temporal quadrant of the corneal limbus. However, they may occasionally present entirely within the cornea or confined to the conjunctiva (see Fig. 10.51). As mentioned previously, they may contain a variety of histologically aberrant tissues. Malignant degeneration is extremely rare. Fig. 10.65 shows a patient with a dermolipoma

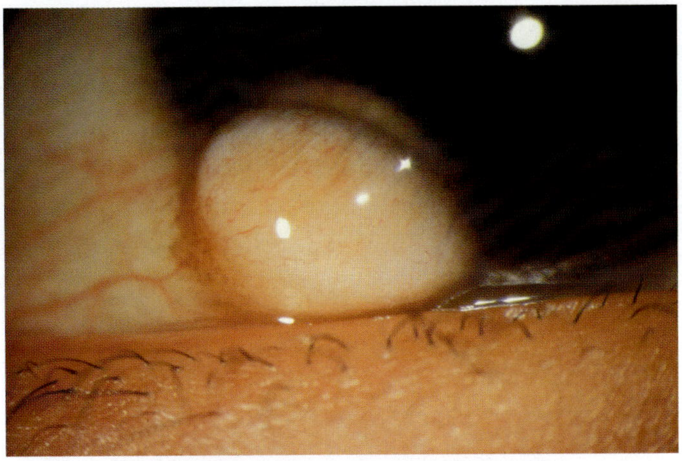

Fig. 10.65 Dermolipoma of Corneal Limbus.

of the corneal limbus. It is a smoothly rounded, yellowish, benign growth.

Inspect the Pupils

The pupils should be equal in size, round, and reactive to light and accommodation. In approximately 5% of normal individuals, pupillary size is not equal; this is called *anisocoria.* Anisocoria may be an indication of neurologic disease. Pupillary enlargement, or *mydriasis,* is associated with ingesting sympathomimetic agents or administering dilating drops. A sluggish, mid-dilated pupil may be present with acute angle-closure glaucoma. Pupillary constriction, or *miosis,* occurs with ingestion of parasympathomimetic drugs, with inflammation of the iris, and drug treatment for glaucoma. Many medications can cause anisocoria. It is, therefore, essential to ascertain whether the patient has used any eyedrops or has taken any medications.

Pupillary abnormalities may be markers of neurologic disease. The *Argyll Robertson pupil* is a pupil constricted 1 to 2 mm that reacts to accommodation but is nonreactive to light. It occurs in association with neurosyphilis. *Horner syndrome* is sympathetic paralysis of the eye caused by interruption of the cervical sympathetic chain. In addition to miosis and ptosis, anhidrosis[e] is also present. A benign condition known as *Adie tonic pupil* is a pupil dilated 3 to 6 mm that constricts little in response to light and accommodation. This pupil is often associated with diminished to absent deep tendon reflexes in the extremities. It occurs more commonly in females 25 to 45, and the cause is unknown. There are no serious clinical implications. Table 10.7 lists the features of these significant pupillary abnormalities.

Inspect the Iris

The iris is evaluated for its shape, color, presence of nodules, and vascularity. Normally, iris blood vessels cannot be seen unless the eye is observed with magnification.

[e]Absence of sweating in this syndrome is related to interruption of the sympathetic chain. The amount of sweating is assessed by examination of the forehead or the axilla of the affected side.

TABLE 10.7 Pupillary Abnormalities

Feature	Adie Tonic Pupil	Argyll Robertson Pupil	Horner Syndrome
Laterality	Often unilateral	Bilateral	Unilateral
Reaction to light	Minimally reactive	Nonreactive	Reactive
Accommodation	Sluggishly reactive	Reactive	Reactive
Pupillary size	Mydriatic	Miotic	Miotic
Other signs	Absent or diminished tendon reflexes	Absent knee-jerk reflexes	Slight ptosis[a] Anhidrosis

[a]The ptosis is slight owing to interruption of the sympathetic chain innervating only the Müller's muscle portion of the levator palpebrae. The rest of the levator palpebrae functions normally; thus ptosis is not severe.

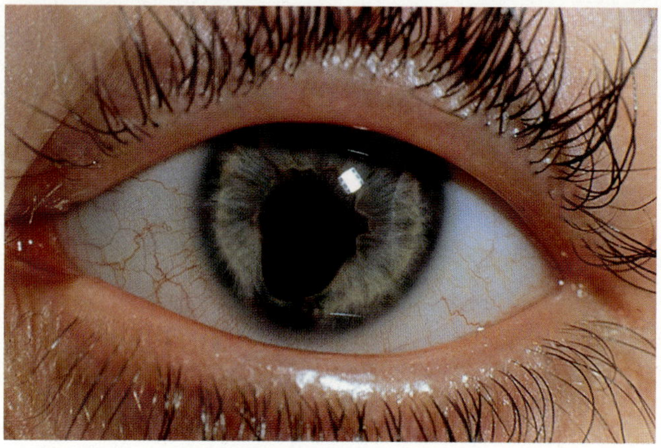

Fig. 10.66 Iris Coloboma.

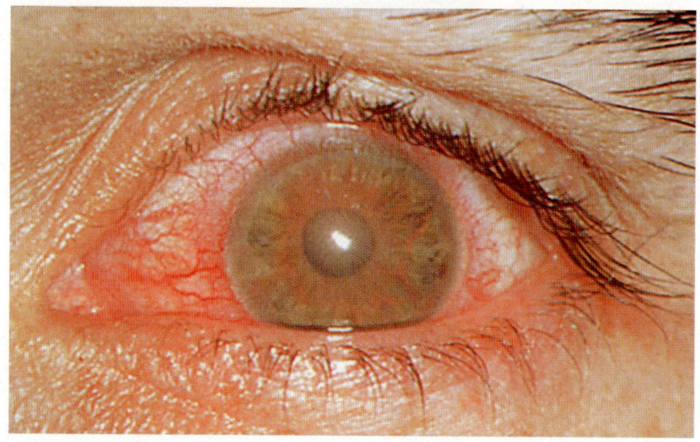

Fig. 10.67 Acute Iritis. (From Mir MA: *Atlas of clinical diagnosis*, London, 1995, WB Saunders.)

An *iris coloboma* is a notch or gap in the iris. It results from the failure of fusion of the embryonic tissue. The typical iris coloboma is usually part of a choroidal coloboma, an autosomal dominant trait. It is often bilateral, is generally located inferiorly, and involves the iris, choroid, or overlying retina (see Fig. 10.146). Visual acuity may be normal if the macula and optic nerve head are spared. Fig. 10.66 shows a patient with an iris coloboma involving the ciliary body and the choroid.

Inflammation of the iris, known as *iritis* or *iridocyclitis,* is associated with severe pain, photophobia, tearing, decreased vision, and circumcorneal congestion. This congestion is caused by injection of the deep episcleral vessels (ciliary flush). The dilation of the iris vessels leads to the transudation of protein into the aqueous humor and deposition of inflammatory cells on the corneal endothelium, known as *keratic precipitates.* As a result of this deposition, the iris becomes blurred and loses its distinctive radial appearance (a "muddy iris"). There are many causes of iritis, including exogenous infection from perforating injuries; secondary infection from the cornea, sclera, or retina; endogenous infection such as tuberculosis, gonorrhea, syphilis, and viral and mycotic infections; and systemic diseases such as rheumatoid arthritis, systemic lupus erythematosus, Reiter disease, Behçet syndrome, and relapsing polychondritis. Fig. 10.67 shows the classic features of an extremely severe case of acute iritis. Note the severe hyperemia, especially around the limbus. In addition, the view of the anterior chamber is hazy due to keratic precipitates. Most of the time, iritis is not visible to the naked eye and requires examination using the slit lamp, since these findings are often not obvious.

As a result of the inflammatory reaction of the iris, the iris may adhere to the cornea, forming anterior *synechiae*; posterior synechiae are adhesions between the iris and lens. Glaucoma is a well-known sequela of iritis and synechiae formation. Visualization of synechiae requires slit lamp examination.

Inspect the Anterior Chamber

Is the anterior chamber clear? If not, is it filled with pus or blood? Fig. 10.68A shows pus in the anterior chamber, known as a *hypopyon,* in a patient with HSV keratitis. Another example of hypopyon together with severe conjunctival injection is demonstrated in Fig. 10.68B.

Is there blood in the anterior chamber? This condition, known as a *hyphema,* is illustrated in Fig. 10.69. Note the subconjunctival hemorrhage also in the patient in Fig. 10.69A. A hyphema can occur due to significant blunt trauma to that eye causing bleeding within the eyeball. This bleeding comes from the anterior chamber angle or the iris, so pupillary abnormalities are common. A hyphema can occur spontaneously also, not related to trauma. The presence of neovascularization of the iris, as seen in severe diabetes mellitus or after a central retinal vein occlusion (CRVO), predisposes to a spontaneous hyphema. Note the meniscus of the blood in Fig. 10.69B. Fig. 10.70 depicts an example of a "candy cane" hyphema resulting from neovascularization of the iris due to a CRVO. The photograph shows blood breakdown products intermingled with fresh blood.

Assess the *depth of the anterior chamber.* By shining a light obliquely across the eye, you can estimate the depth of the

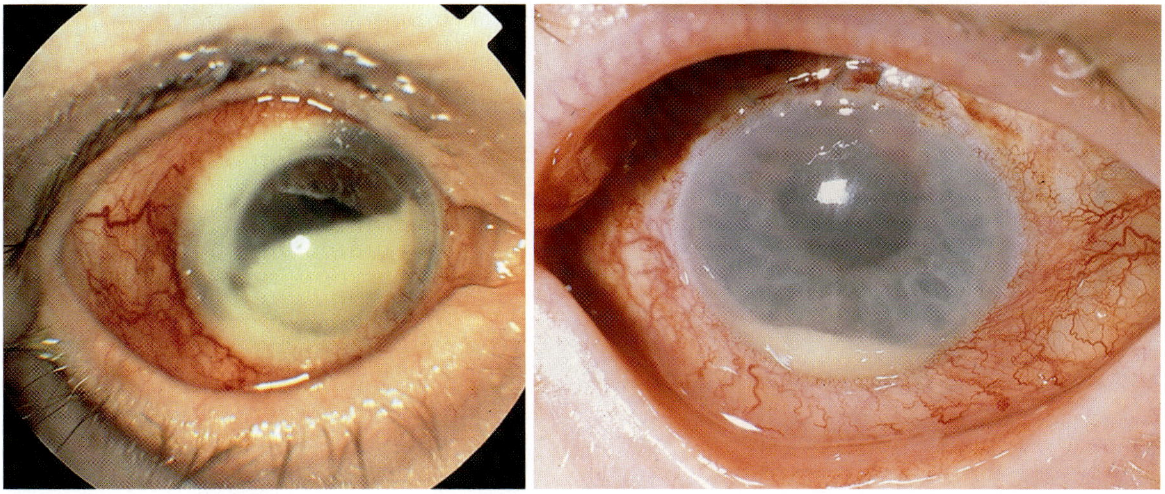

A B

Fig. 10.68 (A) and (B) Two examples of hypopyon. Note the conjunctival injection.

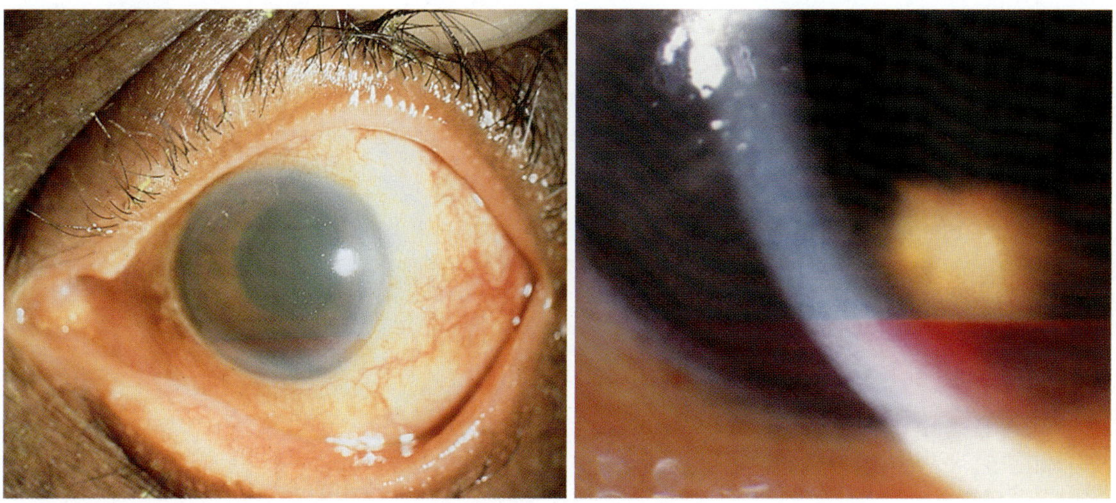

A B

Fig. 10.69 (A) and (B) Two examples of hyphema. (B, From Kanski JJ, Nischal KK: *Ophthalmology: clinical signs and differential diagnosis*, St. Louis, 2000, Mosby.)

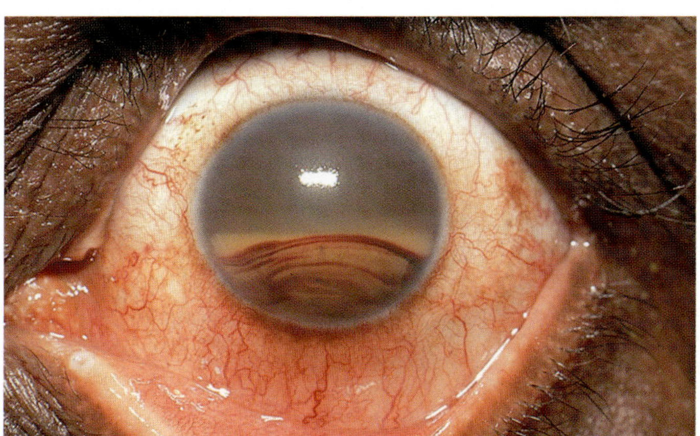

Fig. 10.70 "Candy Cane" Hyphema.

chamber. For example, if a crescentic shadow on the far portion of the iris is visible, the anterior chamber may be shallow. *Shadowing of the anterior chamber* refers to the decreased space between the iris and the cornea. The technique for estimating the depth of the anterior chamber is illustrated in Fig. 10.71.

The presence of a shallow anterior chamber predisposes an individual to a condition called *narrow-angle glaucoma.* The term *glaucoma* refers to a symptom complex that occurs in a variety of disease states. The characteristic finding in all types of glaucoma is increased intraocular pressure. The *Schiotz tonometer,* a small, portable instrument, can assess intraocular pressure quantitatively. There is more sophisticated equipment available to measure intraocular pressure. Palpation of the globe to determine intraocular pressure is a technique of low sensitivity. If performed incorrectly, palpation may be deleterious,

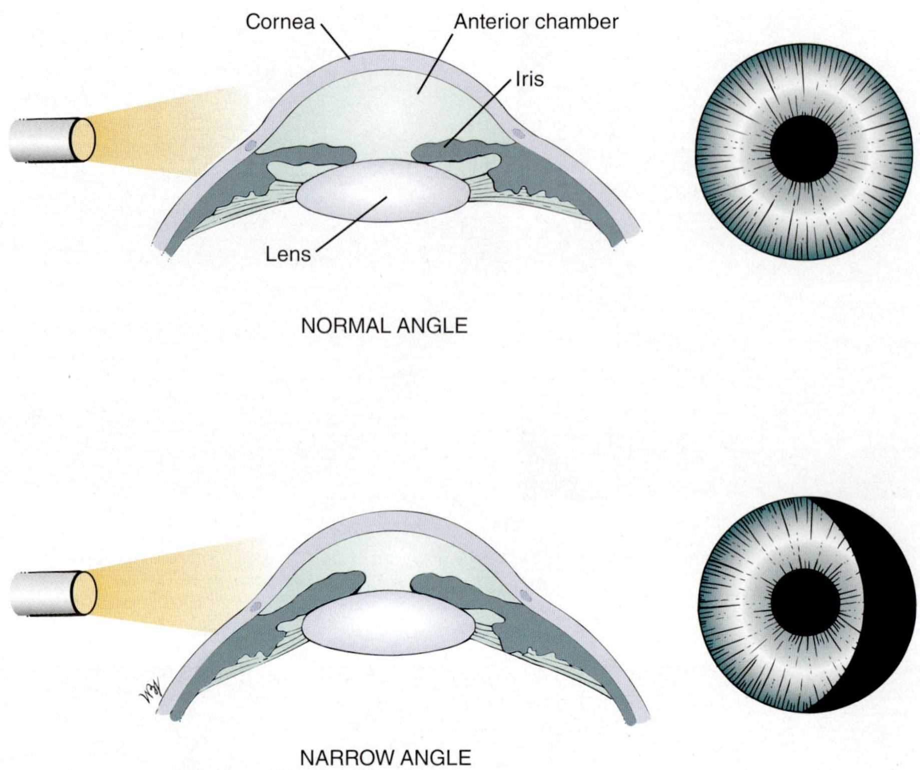

Fig. 10.71 Assessing the Depth of the Anterior Chamber.

because a retinal detachment may result. If the patient has had recent trauma to the eye, palpation of the globe may result in the extrusion of ocular content in the case of a ruptured globe. **Therefore palpation of the eye should never be performed.**

Inspect the Lens

With oblique lighting, inspect the lens. Is the lens clear? Note any opacity that may be visible through the pupil.

The most commonly observed abnormality of the lens is opacification; the most common cause of opacification is aging. Slow, gradual vision loss is the symptom. Other causes include hereditary diseases, such as Down syndrome and cretinism; ocular diseases, such as high myopia, iritis, and retinal dystrophy; systemic diseases, such as diabetes and hypoparathyroidism; medications, such as steroids; and trauma, such as a penetrating eye wound.

A *cataract* is any opacification of the lens that causes reduced visual acuity and interferes with the patient's everyday life. Fig. 10.72A shows a dense cataract of the left eye. Note the leukocoria[f] related to the cataract. Fig. 10.72B shows a dense nuclear or central cataract of the left eye in another patient. Fig. 10.73 is a close-up view of a dense nuclear cataract with anterior cortical spokes (opacification of the anterior cortex of the lens). The red reflex, described in the following section, "Ophthalmoscopic Examination," is absent in all of these patients in the affected eye.

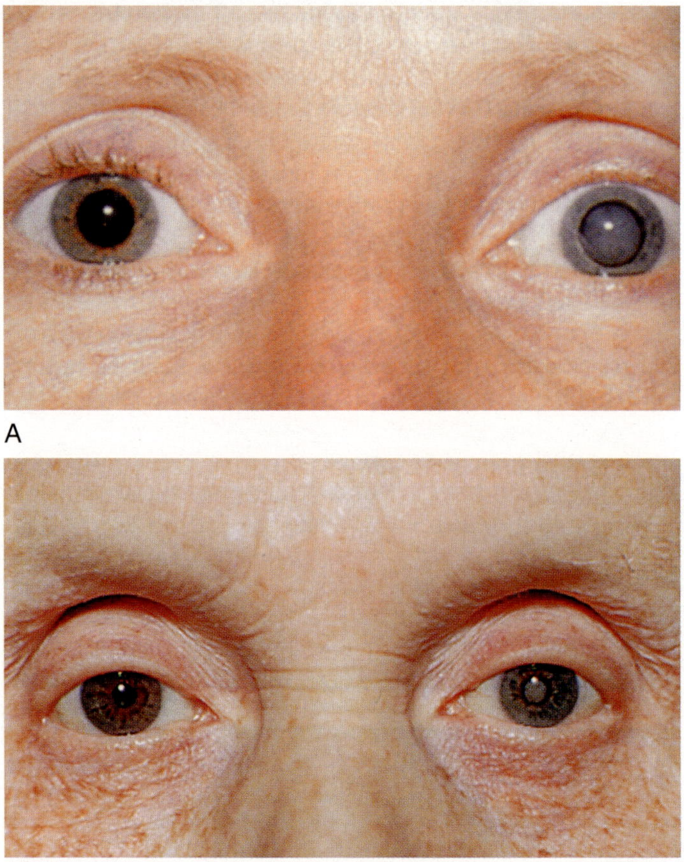

Fig. 10.72 (A) and (B) Cataract of the left eye. (B, From Mir MA: *Atlas of clinical diagnosis*, London, 1995, WB Saunders.)

[f] A white pupil.

Is the lens in the normal position, or is it dislocated? The lens may be dislocated anteriorly, pressing the iris against the posterior cornea and blocking aqueous humor outflow, or it may be dislocated posteriorly. Secondary glaucoma may result. Marfan syndrome is an autosomal dominant condition, often with incomplete expression, with increased length of the long bones; ocular complications include dislocation, or subluxation, of the lens, usually superiorly and nasally. Fig. 10.74 shows a subluxated lens secondary to Marfan syndrome. This is the pupil of the patient's left eye. Note the lower edge of the lens and the attached zonules that are apparent from the 3 to 7 o'clock positions (white lines). The red behind these lines is the red reflex of the retina in the background.

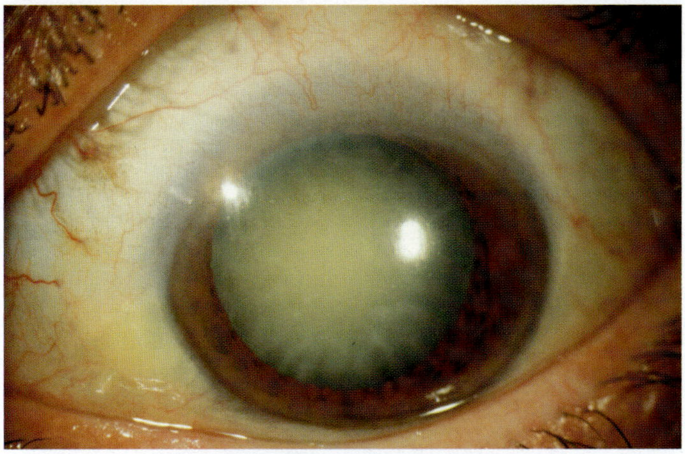

Fig. 10.73 Dense Nuclear Cataract.

Patients now receive intraocular lens implants after cataract surgery. Fig. 10.75 shows a dislocated intraocular lens implant. Note the dislocated wire attachment.

Ophthalmoscopic Examination

The Ophthalmoscope

Before the examination of the optic fundus is discussed, a few words about the ophthalmoscope are in order. The ophthalmoscope is an instrument with a mirror optical system for viewing the interior anatomy of the eye. There are two dials on the ophthalmoscope: one adjusts the light apertures and filters, and the other changes the lenses to correct the refractive errors of both the examiner and the patient.

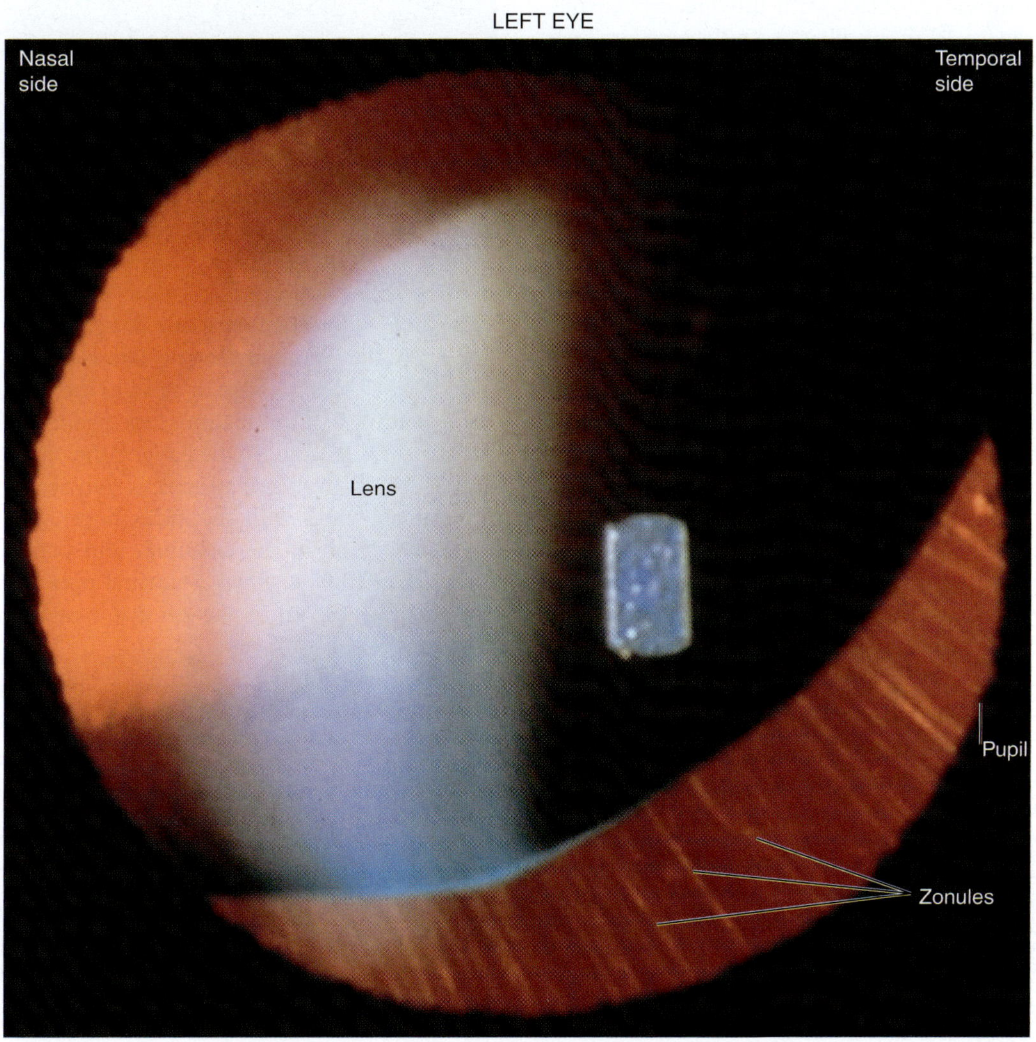

Fig. 10.74 Subluxated Lens (Left Eye) in Marfan Syndrome.

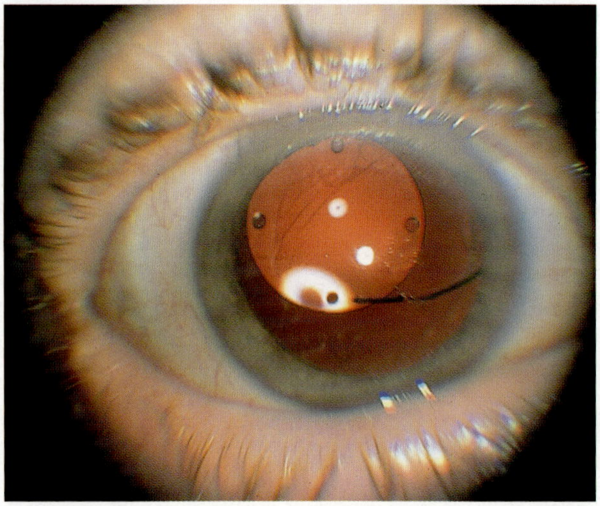

Fig. 10.75 Dislocated Intraocular Lens Implant.

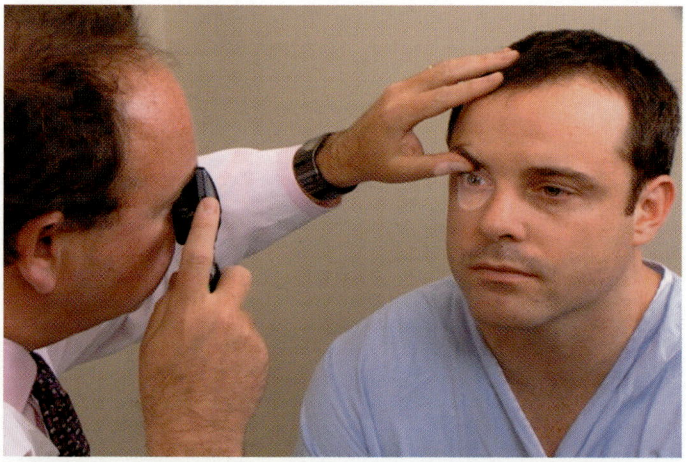

Fig. 10.76 Correct position for holding the ophthalmoscope and patient's eye.

The most important apertures and filters are the *small* aperture, the *large* aperture, and the *red-free* (*green*) filter. The small aperture is for an undilated pupil; the large aperture is for a dilated pupil; and the red-free filter excludes rays of red light and is designed to visualize blood vessels (see Fig. 10.107; note that the blood vessels are grayish-black with this green (red-free) filter) and hemorrhages. With this filter, the retina appears gray, the disc appears white, the macula appears yellow, and blood appears black.

Using the Ophthalmoscope

See Video 10.6.

Hold the ophthalmoscope in your *right* hand in front of your *right* eye to examine the patient's *right* eye. Ask the patient to look straight ahead and fixate on a distant target. If you or the patient wear glasses, remove them for better visualization of the retina. The ophthalmoscope light is turned on, and the aperture is switched to the small aperture. Start with the lens diopter[g] dial set to 0 if you do not use glasses. The myopic examiner should start with "minus" lenses, which are indicated by red numbers; the hyperopic examiner needs "plus" lenses, which are indicated by black numbers. Your index finger remains on the dial to enable easy focusing.

Place the ophthalmoscope against your forehead while your left thumb gently elevates the patient's right upper eyelid gently against the superior orbital rim. The ophthalmoscope and your head should function as one unit. While looking through the ophthalmoscope, approach the patient at eye level from about 15 inches (38 cm) away at an angle of approximately 15 to 20 degrees lateral from the center, as shown in Fig. 10.76. The light should shine on the pupil. A red glow, the *red reflex*, can be seen in the pupil if the light path is not obstructed by an opaque lens. Note any opacity in the cornea or lens. Because the macula is temporal to the optic disc, by shining the light 15 to 20 degrees lateral from center, no direct light will fall on the macula, and the patient will not find the light beam uncomfortable.

[g]A unit of optical power of a lens to cause light rays to diverge or converge.

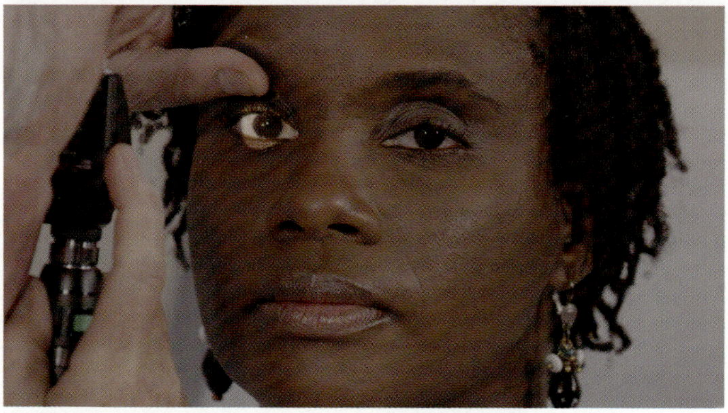

Fig. 10.77 Correct Position for Examining the Retina.

Moving in toward the patient along the same 15- to 20-degree line with the ophthalmoscope allows you to see the retinal blood vessels. Next, move in close to the patient, bringing your hand holding the ophthalmoscope against the patient's cheek. As contact is made with the patient, the optic disc or vessels are visible. You bring these structures into sharp focus by rotating the diopter wheel with the index finger. Fig. 10.77 shows the correct position of the examiner and patient for viewing the retina; Fig. 10.78A shows a normal optic fundus in the right eye and Fig. 10.78B in the left eye. Notice that the macula is temporal to the optic disc.

After the right eye is examined, hold the ophthalmoscope in your *left* hand and use your *left* eye to examine the patient's *left* eye.

Careful assessment of the optic fundus is essential for several reasons. The optic fundus is the only area where the blood vessels can be seen *in vivo*; it can provide an excellent picture of the state of the vasculature of other organs. In addition, the optic fundus is frequently involved with manifestations of systemic disease such as AIDS, infective endocarditis, hypertension, and diabetes; a thorough evaluation of the fundus can provide valuable clues to their diagnosis. Finally, because the eye is an extension of the central nervous system, evaluation of the optic fundus can provide information about many neurologic disorders.

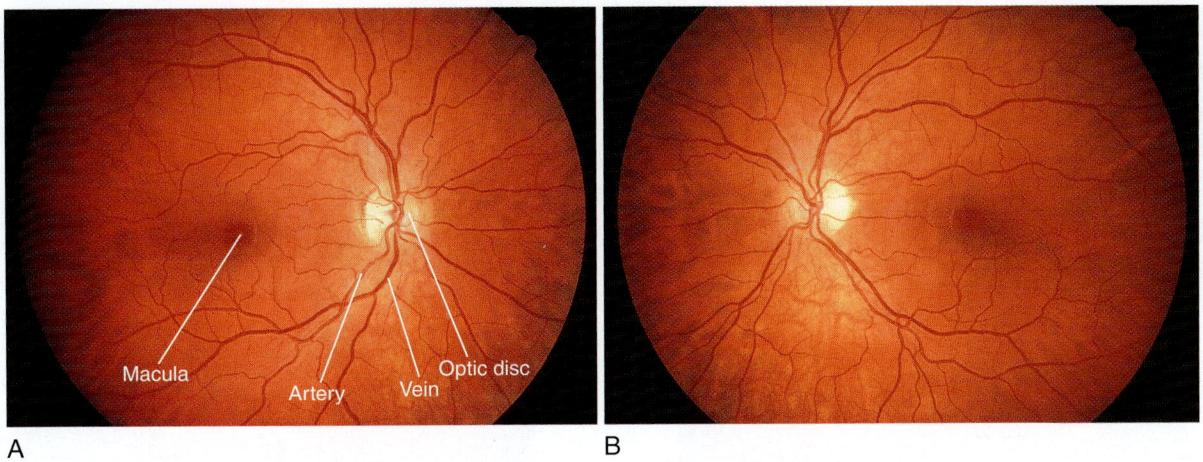

Fig. 10.78 Photograph of the retinas of the right (A) and left (B) eyes.

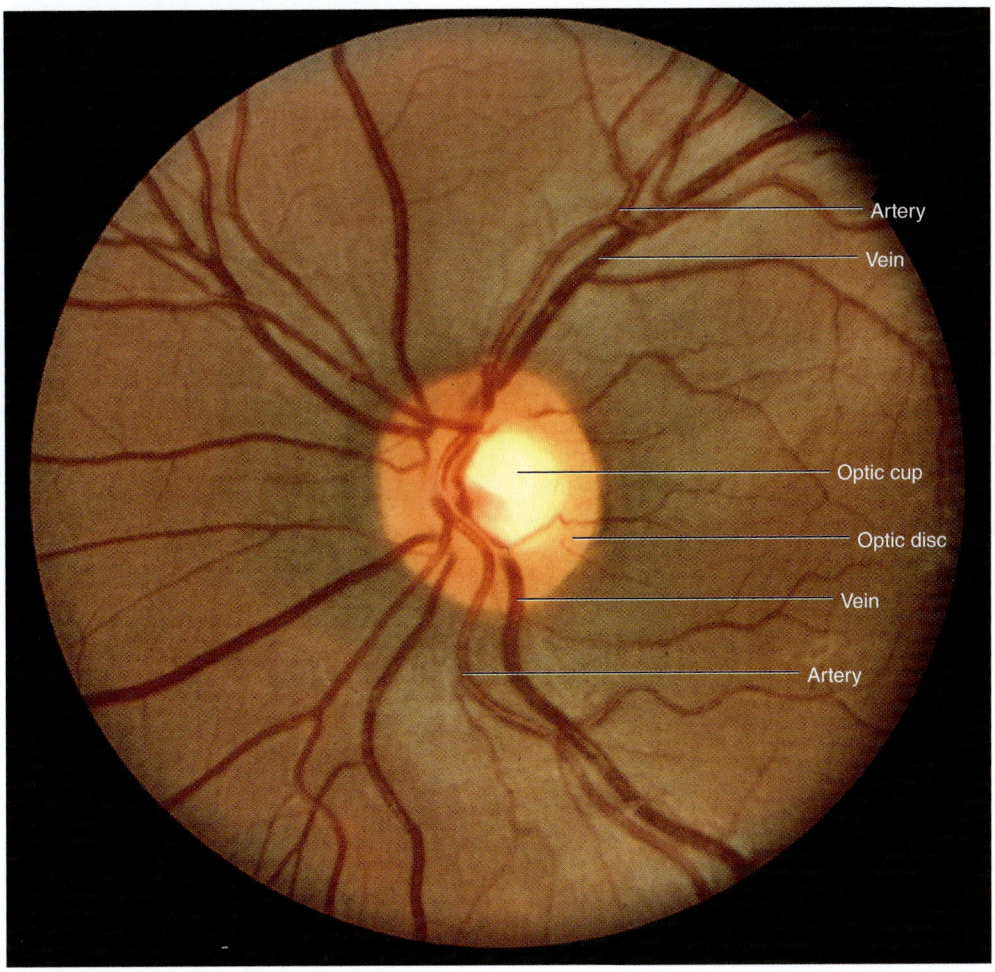

Fig. 10.79 Normal Optic Disc, Left Eye.

The optic fundus must be assessed methodically, starting at the optic disc, tracing the retinal vessels emerging from it, inspecting the macula, and evaluating the rest of the retina.

Inspect the Optic Disc

See Video 10.7.

The optic disc is the most conspicuous landmark of the retina (Fig. 10.79). The optic disc is the intraocular portion of the optic nerve and is seen with the ophthalmoscope. First, its *margins, color,* and *cup-disc ratio* should be determined. The disc should be round or slightly oval, with the long axis usually vertical and with sharp borders. The nasal border is typically

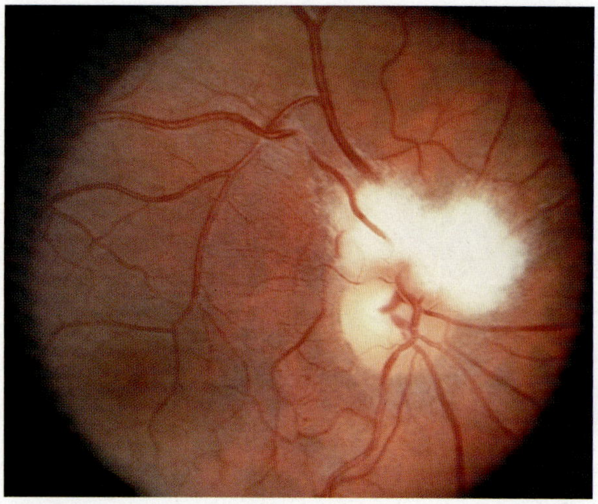

Fig. 10.80 Retina With Myelinated Nerve Fibers.

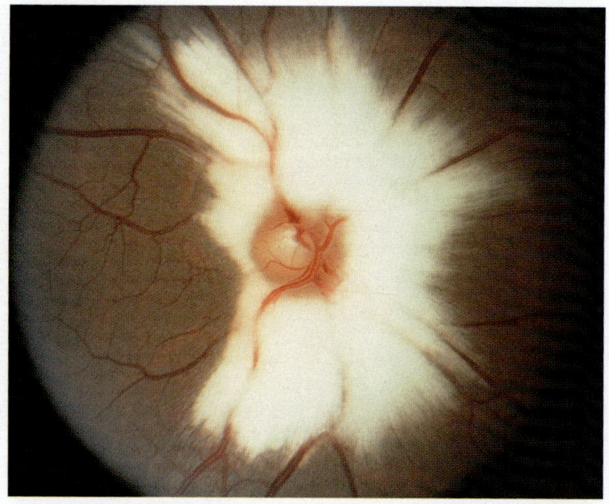

Fig. 10.81 Myelinated Nerve Fibers at the Optic Disc.

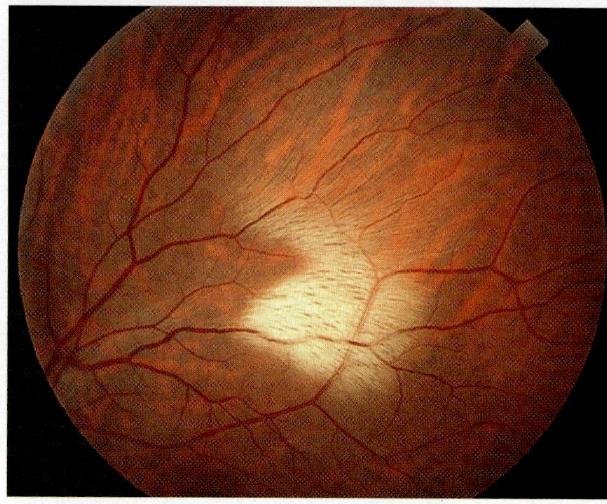

Fig. 10.82 Myelinated Nerve Fibers at Peripheral Retina.

slightly blurred. The disc is pinkish in light-skinned individuals and yellowish-orange in darker-skinned individuals. The relative pallor of the optic disc is caused by the reflection of light from the myelin sheaths of the optic nerve. In the center of the normal optic disc, there is a funnel-shaped depression known as the *physiologic cup.* The cup is the central portion of the disc, lighter in color, and penetrated by the retinal vessels. The normal ratio of the cup diameter to the disc diameter varies from 0.1 to 0.5. The examiner should check the cup-disc ratio in both eyes for symmetry. Asymmetry of the physiologic cups is not typical, and the patient should be evaluated for possible early glaucoma.

The benign condition of *myelinated,* or *medullated, nerve fibers* is seen in 0.3% to 0.6% of all individuals. In this condition, the nerve fiber layer continues to myelinate into the retina. The fibers appear as white patches with feathery borders that radiate from the optic disc and obscure the retinal vessels over which they pass. The condition can be seen soon after birth, does not change, and usually causes no visual impairment. Fig. 10.80 shows the retina of a patient with myelinated nerve fibers. Another dramatic example of myelinated nerve fibers at the disc is shown in Fig. 10.81. Fig. 10.82 shows myelinated nerve fibers in the peripheral retina.

An *optic pit* is a congenital anomaly of the optic disc. It is a slight depression, located temporally in 75% of cases, in the optic nerve and is usually gray or yellow. In 85% of cases, it is unilateral. Fig. 10.83A shows an optic pit. Retinal tears and detachment can occur in 50% of patients with an optic pit, as shown in Fig. 10.83B; this patient has an optic pit and a retinal tear involving the macula of the left eye.

Inspect the Retinal Vessels

See Video 10.7.

The retinal vessels are evaluated as they arborize over the retina. The central retinal artery enters the globe through the physiologic cup. It divides within the cup and again on the surface, giving rise to four main branches that supply the optic fundus's superior and inferior temporal and nasal quadrants. The arteries are two-thirds to four-fifths the diameter of the veins and have a prominent *light reflex.* This light reflex is a reflection of the ophthalmoscope's light on the arterial wall and usually is approximately one-fourth the diameter of the column of blood. The veins exhibit spontaneous pulsations in 85% of patients. This can best be demonstrated as the retinal vein enters the optic nerve, where it can be seen on end.

As all the vessels course away from the disc, they appear to narrow. The crossing of the arteries and veins occurs within two disc diameters from the disc.

The normal vessel wall is invisible with its thin light reflex. In hypertension, the vessel may have focal or generalized areas of narrowing or spasm, causing the light reflex to be narrowed. With time, the vessel wall becomes thickened and sclerotic, and the light reflex widens to over half of the blood column's diameter. The light reflex develops an orange metallic appearance called *copper wiring* (Fig. 10.84A). When such an artery crosses over a vein, there appears to be a discontinuity of the venous column due to the widened, but invisible, arterial wall. This is termed *arteriovenous nicking* (see Figs. 10.84B and C). It has been postulated that because the artery and vein share a common sheath, the artery's thicker walls push against those of the

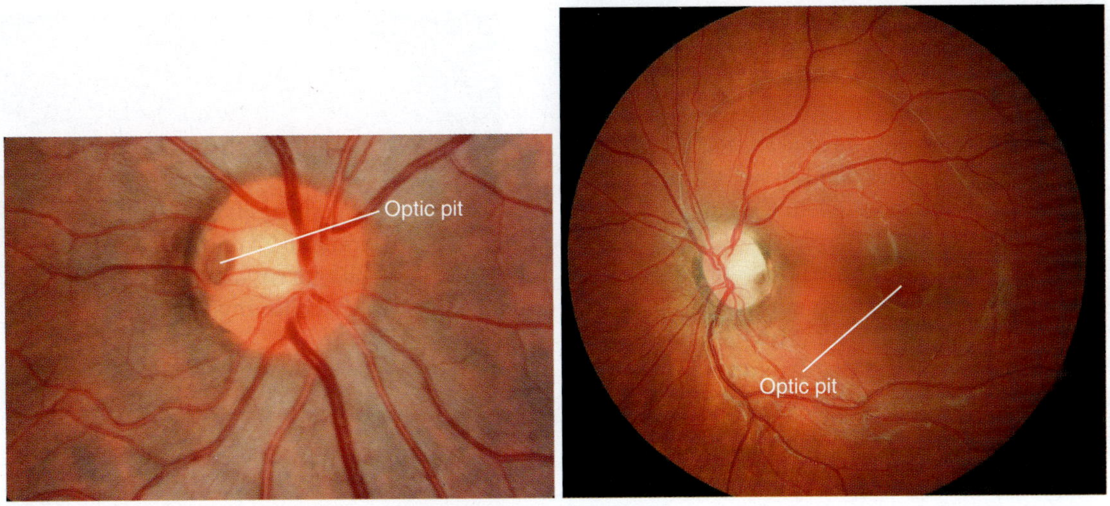

A B

Fig. 10.83 (A) Optic pit, right eye. (B) Optic pit and a retinal tear, left eye, in another patient.

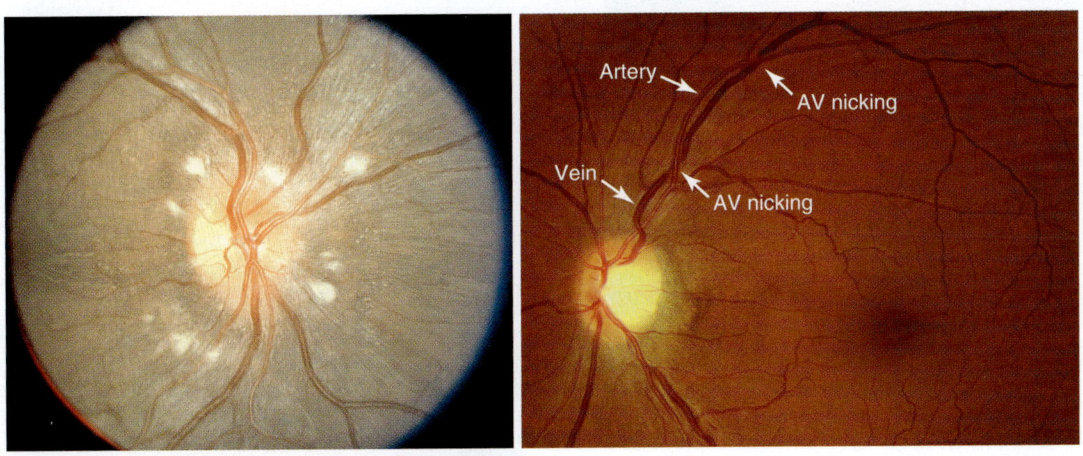

A B

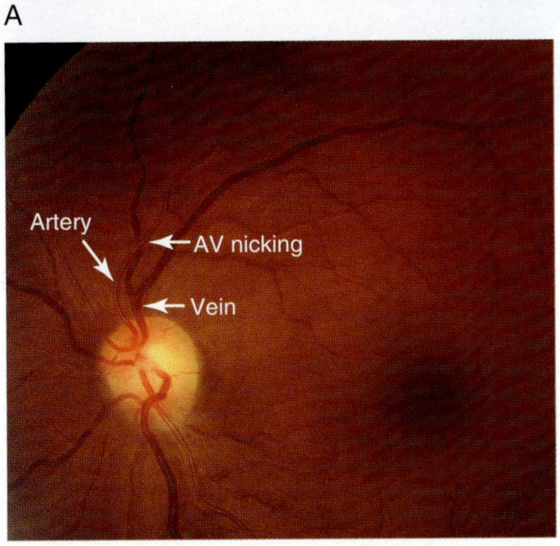

C

Fig. 10.84 Hypertension. (A) Note the "copper wiring" of the arteries and the numerous cotton-wool spots, which are exudates caused by infarctions of the nerve fiber layer. (B) Notice the two areas of arteriovenous *(AV)* nicking in this patient's left eye. (C) A close-up of the retina of another patient showing AV nicking and marked copper wiring of the arterial wall. (B, Courtesy Christina Ryu, MD, and Alexis Cullen, CRA, Henry Ford Health System, Detroit, MI. C, Courtesy Christina Ryu, MD, Jim Thomas, CRA, Henry Ford Health System, Detroit, MI.)

vein forcing the vein to collapse. This makes the vein form an hourglass shape (nicking) around the artery.

Follow the vessels in all four directions: superior temporal, superior nasal, inferior nasal, and inferior temporal. Remember to move your head and the ophthalmoscope as one unit.

Inspect the Macula

The macula is seen when the ophthalmoscope is kept level with the disc and moved temporally approximately 1.5 to 2 disc diameters. This appears as an avascular area with a pinpoint reflective center, the fovea. If the examiner has difficulty seeing

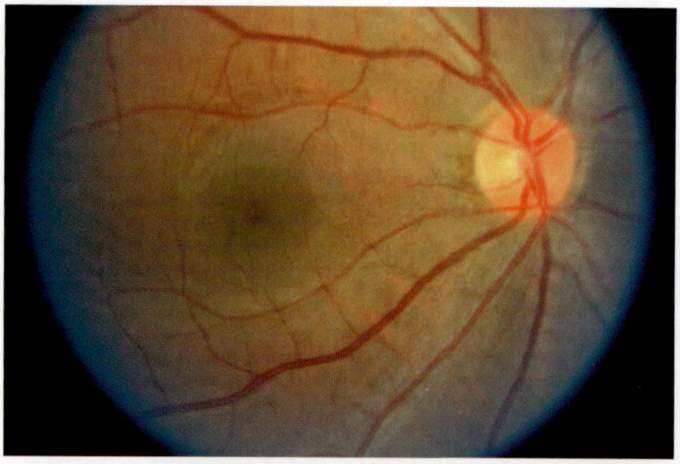

Fig. 10.85 Normal Macula, Right Eye.

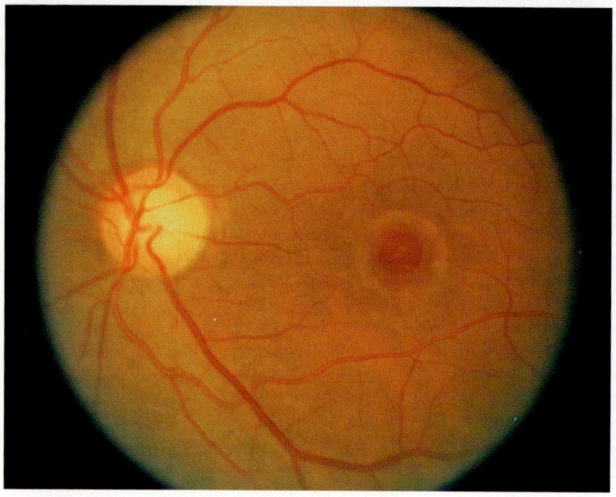

Fig. 10.86 Macular Hole.

the macula, the patient can be instructed to look directly into the light; the fovea is visible. The red-free filter is also helpful in locating the macula. Fig. 10.85 shows a normal macula of the right eye.

Fig. 10.86 shows a patient with a macular hole of the left eye; notice the punched-out appearance at the macula. Macular holes can be seen in patients with high myopia. Macular holes can cause blurred and distorted central vision.

Describe Any Retinal Lesions

When a lesion is seen, its color and shape are important in determining its cause. Is it red, black, gray, or whitish? Red lesions are usually hemorrhages. They can be located best by using the ophthalmoscope's green (red-free) filter. Linear, or *flame-shaped,* hemorrhages occur in the nerve fiber layer of the retina (Fig. 10.87), whereas round hemorrhages are located in deeper intraretinal layers. Are the borders of the lesions sharp or blurred?

A common benign retinal finding is *congenital hypertrophy of the retinal pigment epithelium* (*RPE*). This appears as a round, dramatically dark pigmented lesion, often one to several disc

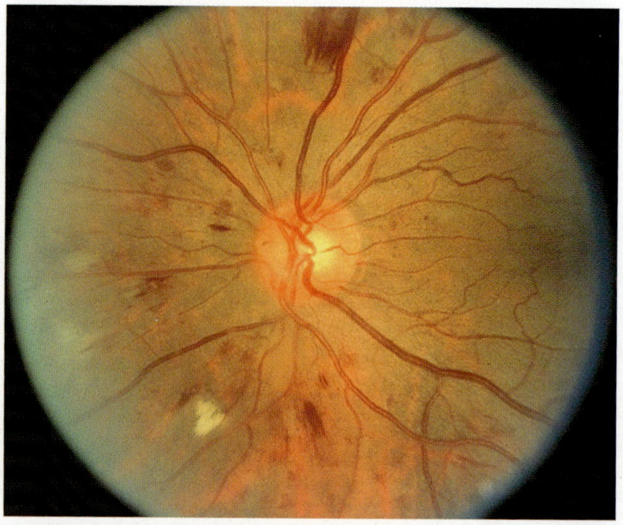

Fig. 10.87 Flame-Shaped Hemorrhages and a Cotton-Wool Spot in a Patient With Hypertension.

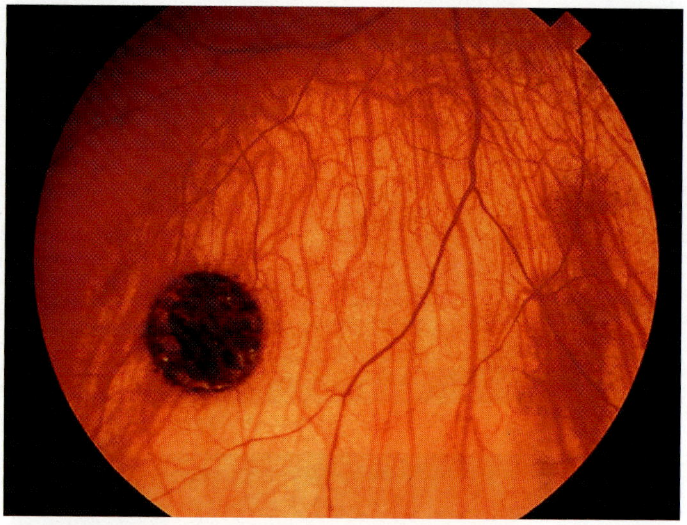

Fig. 10.88 Congenital Hypertrophy of the Retinal Pigment Epithelium.

diameters in size. The surface is flat, and the edges are very sharp. Several small, punched-out holes are commonly present within. The retinal vessels appear normal. This asymptomatic lesion is usually unilateral; it may occur in any position in the retina. Nevertheless, its recognition is essential and should not be misdiagnosed as a malignant melanoma. Fig. 10.88 shows a retina with congenital hypertrophy of the RPE.

Black lesions shaped like bone spicules are associated with retinitis pigmentosa (RP). In this condition, melanin tends to unsheathe the retinal vessels (see Fig. 10.148 and a discussion of this condition at the end of this chapter). A doughnut-shaped lesion is often found in chronic inactive toxoplasmosis chorioretinitis (see Fig. 10.133). A pigmented, raised, disc-shaped lesion suggests melanoma (see Fig. 10.145). Diffuse spotting of the retina is often a degenerative state. Flat, *gray* lesions are usually benign choroidal nevi (see Fig. 10.144).

TABLE 10.8 Differentiation of Whitish Lesions of the Fundus

Feature	Cotton-Wool Spots (See Figs. 10.84A and 10.87)	Fatty Exudates (See Figs. 10.108 and 10.109)[a]	Drusen (See Fig. 10.125)[b]	Chorioretinitis (See Figs. 10.131 to 10.141)
Cause[c]	Hypertension Diabetic retinopathy Acquired immune deficiency syndrome Lupus erythematosus Dermatomyositis Papilledema	Diabetes mellitus Retinal venous occlusion Hypertensive retinotherapy	Can be normal with aging Age-related macular degeneration	Toxoplasmosis Sarcoidosis Cytomegalovirus
Border	Fuzzy	Well defined	Well defined, nonpigmented	Often large with ragged edge, heavily pigmented
Shape	Irregular	Small, irregular	Round, well circumscribed	Very variable
Patterns	Variable	Often clustered in circles or stars	Variable; symmetrical in both eyes	Variable
Comments	Caused by an ischemic infarct of the nerve fiber layer of the retina; obscures retinal blood vessels; usually several in number	In deep retinal layer	Often confused with fatty exudates; deep to retinal blood vessels	Acute with white exudate; healed lesion with pigmented scar (toxoplasmosis)

[a]Also known as *edema residues*.
[b]Also known as *colloid bodies*.
[c]The diseases noted do not constitute a complete etiologic list. Only the most common causes are indicated.

White lesions may appear soft, as in cotton-wool spots, or dense, as in drusen. Soft, *cotton-wool spots* or exudations are caused by retinal nerve fiber layer microinfarcts (see Figs. 10.84A and 10.87). Infarcted retinal ganglion cell axons extrude their axoplasm and form these yellowish-white spots. These spots are commonly arrayed around the optic disc and along the temporal vascular arcades. Cotton-wool spots are frequently associated with hypertension or diabetes. *Drusen* appear in normal aging but may also be found in other pathologic conditions, as is discussed later in this chapter (see Figs. 10.124 to 10.126). The differentiation of white lesions of the retina is summarized in Table 10.8 and is discussed later in this chapter under "Clinicopathologic Correlations."

Difficulties in Using the Ophthalmoscope

Frequently, difficulties arise in the use of the ophthalmoscope. These include the following:

- A small pupil
- Extraneous light
- Improper use of the ophthalmoscope
- Myopia in the patient
- Cataract in the patient

The use of mydriatic drops to better visualize the retina is important. However, many medical students fear that these drops will precipitate an attack of narrow-angle glaucoma. It is clear from the data that more retinal findings are missed by not dilating the pupils than when the drops precipitate such an attack, which occurs in less than 0.1% of patients. If, by some chance, this reaction occurs, the patients are in the best possible facility for treatment.

The examiner should use one drop of tropicamide 1% (Mydriacyl®) in each eye. Care should be taken to place the drop on the inside of the lower lid by pulling the lower eyelid away from the eye to make a space. The patient should be told that the drop will sting slightly and make everything appear much brighter, especially if it is a sunny day. Often a drop of proparacaine hydrochloride 0.5% is instilled beforehand to cut down on the sting of the tropicamide. The duration of the mydriatic action depends primarily on the patient's sensitivity to the medication: a more heavily pigmented iris requires more time to achieve mydriasis. The cycloplegic[h] action lasts for approximately 3 to 4 hours. These drops should not be used in patients wearing contact lenses; patients need to remove the lenses first. Atropine should be avoided because its effect lasts for up to 2 weeks. The large aperture of the ophthalmoscope is used when the pupil is dilated. Record in the chart that the patient's pupil or pupils were dilated and which medications were used.

The room should be darkened as much as possible for the most accessible evaluation of the retina. Another common problem is corneal reflection. Often, light is reflected from the cornea, which makes the examination more difficult. Again, use of the small aperture or a polarizing filter, which many ophthalmoscopes include, may be helpful.

Patients with myopia provide the most problems for the novice examiner. In myopic eyes, the retinal image is enlarged, making it difficult sometimes to visualize the retina adequately. If the patient is severely myopic, it may be necessary for the patient to wear corrective lenses while being examined.

A mature, or advanced, cataract may not allow adequate visualization of the retina.

[h]Producing loss of accommodation by causing paralysis of the ciliary muscle.

CLINICOPATHOLOGIC CORRELATIONS

There are many ophthalmoscopic conditions with which the examiner should be familiar. An image is normally focused directly on the retina. A refractive error is present when the image is not focused on the retina. Lenses are used to correct refractive errors. The absence of a refractive error is called *emmetropia.* Refractive errors are extremely common. Listed here are the common refractive errors and their causes:

Hyperopia (*hypermetropia* or *farsightedness*): Light is focused posterior to the retina.

Myopia (also known as *nearsightedness*): Light is focused anterior to the retina.

Astigmatism: Light is not uniformly focused in all directions. Astigmatism is commonly a result of a cornea that is not perfectly spherical.

Presbyopia: Near vision decreases progressively due to a decrease in the eye's ability to accommodate. Presbyopia occurs after age of 40 years.

Fig. 10.89 illustrates normal (emmetropic), hyperopic (hypermetropic), myopic, and astigmatic eyes.

Cataracts (see Figs. 10.72 and 10.73) are the most common cause of blindness in the world. A cataract is a type of degenerative eye disease. More than 22 million Americans have cataracts. By age 80, more than half of all people in the United States will either have a cataract or have had cataract surgery. One of the first symptoms that patients with cataracts experience is a "mistiness" of vision. Affected patients typically give a history in which vision has become "like looking through a dirty window." As the lenticular opacity increases with time, visual acuity diminishes in association with glare in bright light. This effect results from pupillary constriction limiting the light rays passing through the central portion of the lens, where the opacity is often most dense.

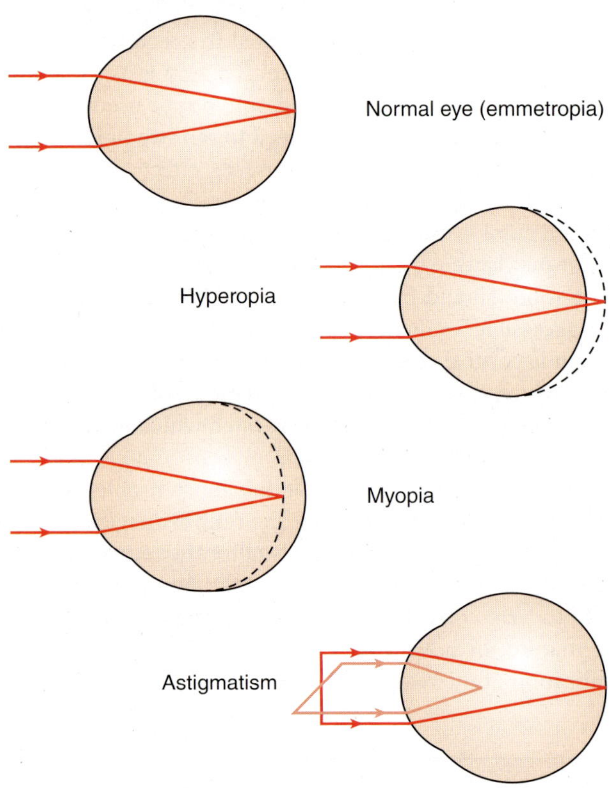

Fig. 10.89 Common Refractive Errors.

Narrow-angle glaucoma results from an obstruction to the drainage of aqueous humor at the canal of Schlemm. Patients with narrow-angle glaucoma have periodic attacks of acute elevation of intraocular pressure caused by intermittent obstruction. This is associated with pain, seeing halos, and poor vision. These glaucoma attacks commonly occur in a darkened room when pupillary dilation occurs. When the pupil is dilated in a person with a narrow angle, the redundant iris folds at its base cause the increased obstruction and decreased drainage.

In contrast, *primary open-angle,* or *chronic simple, glaucoma* is associated with an open angle and is the second most common cause of blindness worldwide. There are many causes for primary open-angle glaucoma, which induces slowly progressive blindness. The most important diagnostic difference from narrow-angle glaucoma is that in chronic simple glaucoma, pain is absent. Patients have reduced outflow of aqueous humor through the trabecular meshwork and into the canal of Schlemm, which results in elevated intraocular pressure. As a result, progressive cupping of the optic nerve (i.e., loss of nerve substance) occurs, accompanied by changes in the visual field. Other newer technologies[i] are available to help the ophthalmologist evaluate the progression of glaucoma. Although primary open-angle glaucoma is usually bilateral, its asymmetric onset results in a difference in optic cup size between the two eyes, one of the most characteristic early signs (Fig. 10.90). Vision is increasingly impaired as progressive atrophy of the optic nerve continues, owing to the increased intraocular pressure. Late in the disease, only a tiny area on the nasal aspect of the nerve head may remain. Fig. 10.91 shows a close-up of the optic disc of a patient with 50% to 60% cupping of the optic nerve head. Table 10.9 lists the major characteristics of both types of glaucoma.

Acute eye inflammations are common. They may be associated with local or systemic disease. Therefore, the differential diagnosis of the red eye is essential. The presence of pain, visual loss, and irregularities of the pupils are important signs signifying a serious, potentially blinding disorder. Fig. 10.92 shows a patient with a red eye. Table 10.2 provides an approach to the diagnosis of the red eye.

Diabetic retinopathy is the leading cause of blindness in Americans aged 20 to 75 years, responsible for 4.8% of visual impairment worldwide. It is estimated that more than 12 million Americans have diabetes. Diabetic retinopathy is a highly specific vascular complication of type 1 and type 2 diabetes mellitus and is directly related to the duration and management of the disease. By 25 years after the onset of diabetes, nearly all patients

[i]These technologies include Heidelberg retinal tomography (HRT) and optical coherence tomography (OCT). HRT is a scanning laser ophthalmoscope capable of acquiring and analyzing three-dimensional images of the optic nerve head and peripapillary retina. OCT is an imaging modality analogous to ultrasound.

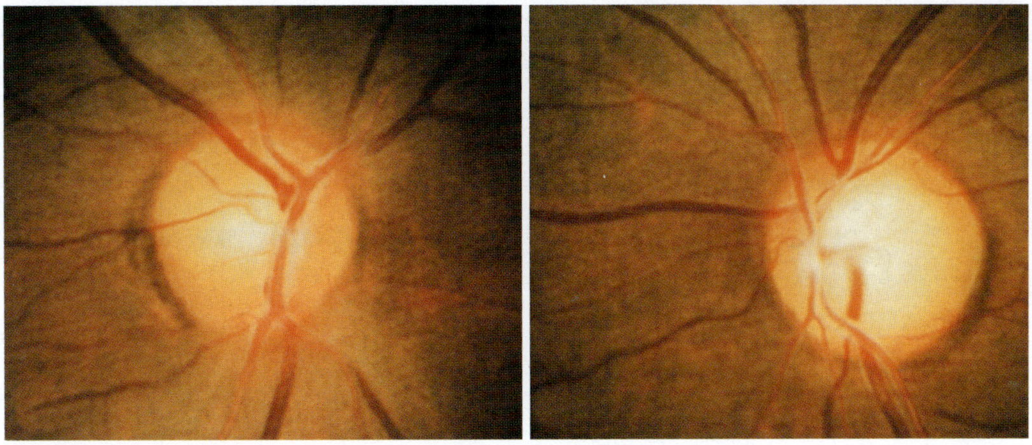

A B

Fig. 10.90 (A) and (B) Optic cup asymmetry in glaucoma. The cup-disc ratio is approximately 30% in (A) *(right eye)* and 70% in (B) *(left eye)*.

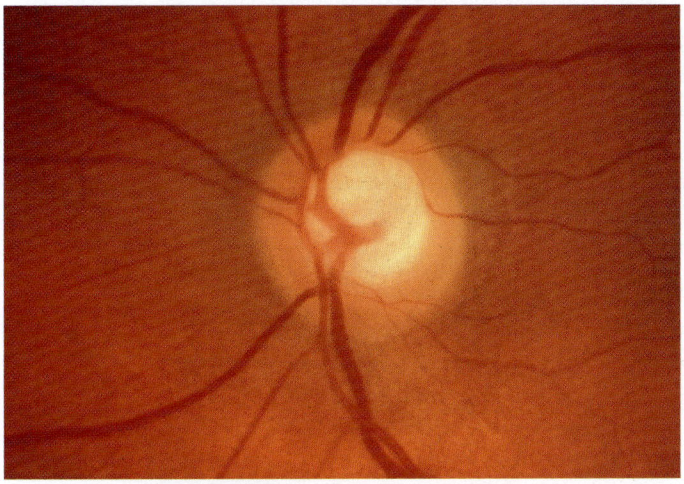

Fig. 10.91 Glaucomatous Cupping of the Optic Nerve Head. The cup-to-disc ratio is approximately 50% to 60%.

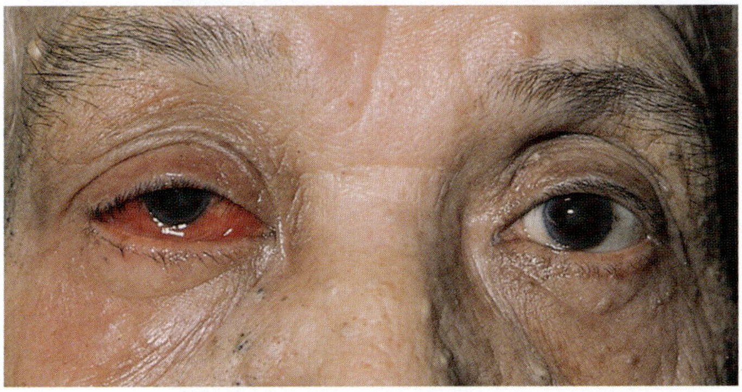

Fig. 10.92 Red Eye.

with type 1 diabetes and 65% of patients with type 2 diabetes have some degree of retinopathy.

The retinal findings of diabetic retinopathy result from retinal microangiopathy, which causes increased vascular permeability that results in macular edema and decreased vision. In addition, vascular occlusive changes result in fibrovascular proliferation, hemorrhage, and scarring. The early changes of nonproliferative retinopathy are capillary microaneurysms, dilatation and tortuosity of vessels, and nonperfusion of areas of the retina. As the disease progresses to proliferative retinopathy, retinal neovascularization appears either at the optic disc (neovascularization of the disc [NVD]) or elsewhere in the retina (neovascularization elsewhere in the retina [NVE]). Neovascularization may further diminish vision by vitreous hemorrhage or traction detachment of the retina.

Nonproliferative, or *background, retinopathy* is the first stage of diabetic retinopathy. An early sign is the development of microaneurysms. These usually have smooth borders and round shapes. In addition, intraretinal hemorrhages result from the rupture of the microaneurysms, capillaries, and venules. The location of the hemorrhage within the retinal layers governs the shape of the hemorrhage: hemorrhages in the nerve fiber layer typically are flame-shaped with feathery borders, whereas hemorrhages in the deep areas of the retina have a fuzzy, blot-shaped appearance. Exudates may appear as clusters, streaks, or rings around the macula. These exudates result from leakage through the abnormally permeable capillary walls. Commonly, these microaneurysms, hemorrhages, and exudates occur near the macula. The retinal findings in a patient with nonproliferative diabetic retinopathy are shown in Fig. 10.93. Note the hemorrhages and exudates. Fig. 10.94 shows the marked tortuosity of the vessels in another patient with background retinopathy. Fig. 10.95 shows the flame-shaped hemorrhages and exudates characteristic of nonproliferative diabetic retinopathy. Fig. 10.96 shows circinate retinopathy in a diabetic patient.

Proliferative diabetic retinopathy is characterized by neovascularization: that is, new blood vessels that arise from the retinal and optic disc vessels. Neovascularization appears as a fine network, known as tufts, of blood vessels that seem to bud off other vessels. NVD is shown in Fig. 10.97; NVE is shown in Fig. 10.98. These vessels proliferate along the retinal surface and into the vitreous humor, often with fibrous band components. The vessels often adhere to the posterior vitreous, and preretinal hemorrhages occur due to vitreoretinal separation pulling on the fragile vessels. The blood resulting from a preretinal hemorrhage

TABLE 10.9 Characteristics of Glaucoma

Feature	Primary Open-Angle Glaucoma	Narrow-Angle Glaucoma
Occurrence	85% of all glaucoma cases	15% of all glaucoma cases
Cause	Unclear[a]	Closed angle prevents aqueous drainage
Age at onset	Variable	50–85 years
Anterior chamber	Usually normal	Shallow
Chamber angle	Normal	Narrow
Symptoms	Usually none Decreased vision, late	Headache Seeing halos around lights Sudden onset of severe eye pain Vomiting during attack
Cupping of disc	Progressive if not treated (see Figs. 10.90 and 10.91)	After one or more untreated attacks
Visual fields	Peripheral fields are involved early Central involvement is a very late sign	Involvement is a late sign
Ocular pressure	Progressively higher if not medically controlled Late: high	Early: detected with provocative tests only
Other signs		Fixed, partially dilated pupil Conjunctival injection "Steamy" cornea[b]
Treatment	Medical Laser surgery	Surgical
Prognosis	Good if recognized early Very dependent on patient compliance	Good

[a]Thought to be a defect in the trabecular network ultrastructure.
[b]Like looking through a steamy window.

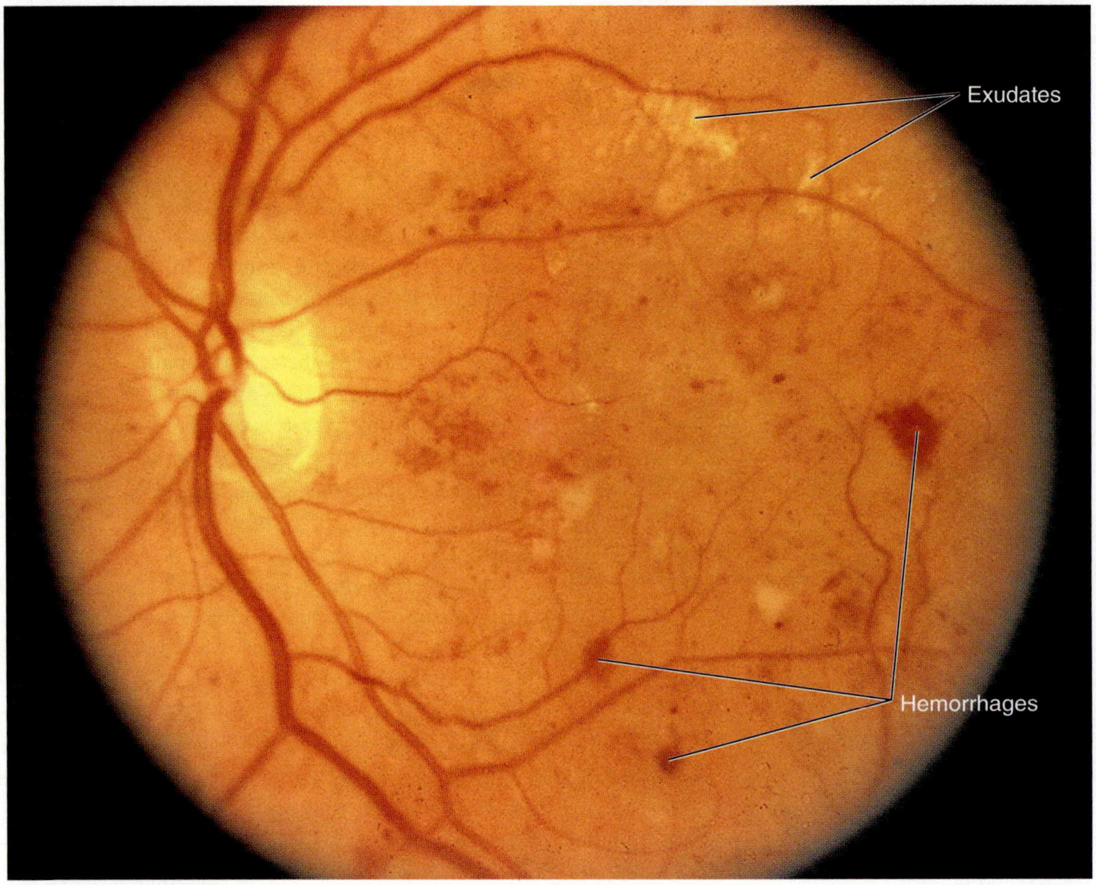

Fig. 10.93 Nonproliferative Diabetic Retinopathy.

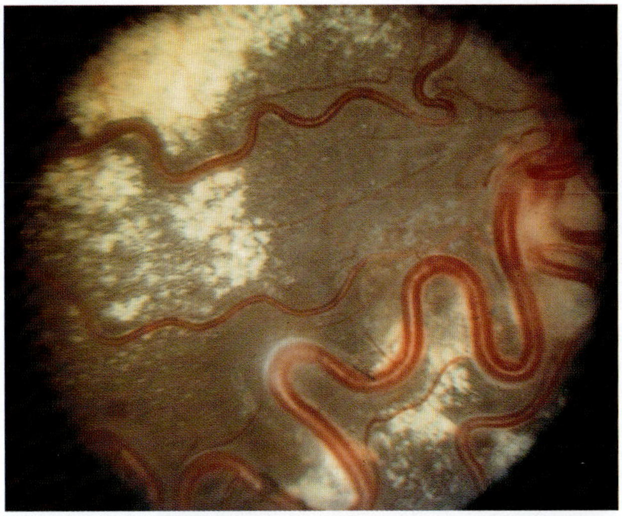

Fig. 10.94 Nonproliferative Diabetic Retinopathy. Note the markedly tortuous vessels.

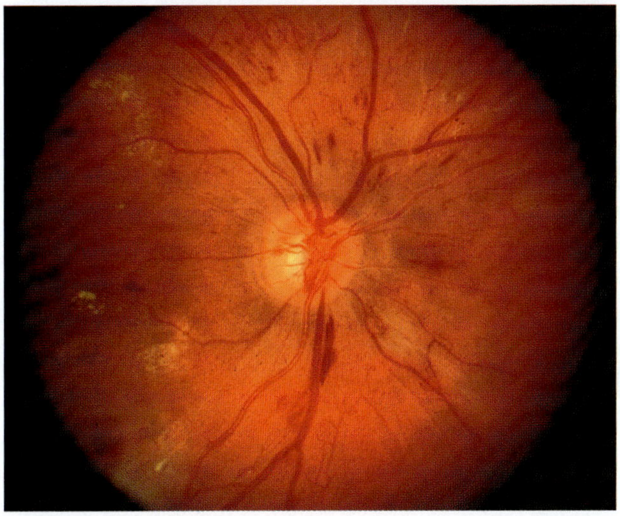

Fig. 10.95 Nonproliferative Diabetic Retinopathy. Note the flame-shaped hemorrhages.

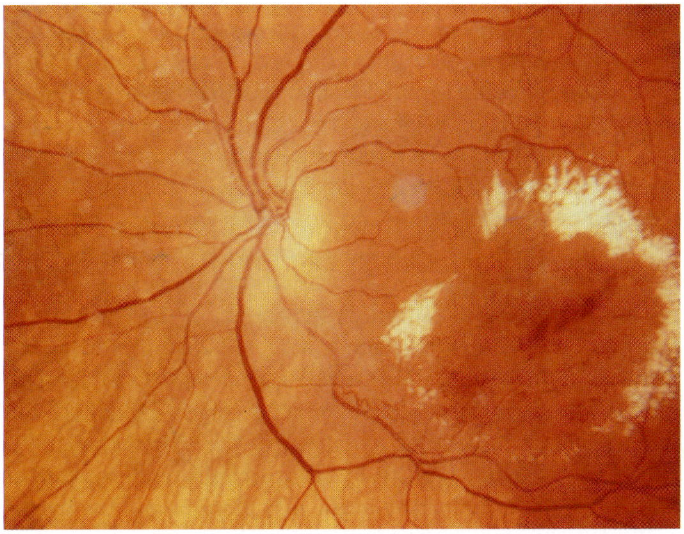

Fig. 10.96 Nonproliferative Retinopathy, Circinate Retinopathy. Note the ring of exudates around or near the macula, as well as the hemorrhages at the macula. (From Kanski JJ, Nischal KK: *Ophthalmology: clinical signs and differential diagnosis*, St. Louis, 2000, Mosby.)

is trapped in the potential space between the retina and the vitreous humor (under the inner limiting membrane), forming a classic boat-shaped hemorrhage (Fig. 10.99). Further pulling on the retina can progress to retinal tears and tractional retinal detachments. Figs. 10.100 to 10.102 show vitreous strands in patients with proliferative diabetic retinopathy. Fig. 10.102 shows vitreous traction and a macular hole. Note the light-colored area surrounding the macula.

Fig. 10.103 shows a patient with proliferative diabetic retinopathy with NVE, NVD, preretinal hemorrhage, and a fatty exudative maculopathy.

The therapy for proliferative retinopathy is panretinal photocoagulation (PRP), to cause regression of the neovascularization. Figs. 10.104 and 10.105 show proliferative retinopathy and the laser burns of PRP. Note the PRP-treated areas that appear as round, punched-out spots with pigmentation in the center or margins. The treated areas first appear white or yellow, but within several weeks, pigmentation occurs. The laser burns are brought up to the vascular arcades and up to one disc diameter from the optic disc. Vitrectomy is also indicated for tractional detachments. The final stages of diabetic retinopathy, *involutional* or *burned-out retinopathy,* show a tangle of new vessels, hemorrhages, traction, and fibrosis.

The role of *vascular endothelial growth factor* (*VEGF*) in the growth of both regular and abnormal blood vessels was identified in the 1980s, and agents that could block the angiogenic cascade first came on the scene for cancer treatments in the early 1990s. VEGF is a signal protein produced by cells that stimulates vasculogenesis and angiogenesis. It is part of the system that restores the oxygen supply to tissues when blood circulation is inadequate. The normal function of VEGF is to create new blood vessels during embryonic development, new blood vessels after injury, and new vessels (collateral circulation) to bypass blocked vessels. However, when VEGF is overexpressed, it can contribute to disease.

VEGF is an essential mediator in diabetic retinopathy and wet age-related macular degeneration (AMD). The microcirculatory problems in the retina of people with diabetes can cause retinal ischemia, which results in the release of VEGF. VEGF may then cause the creation of new blood vessels in the retina and elsewhere in the eye, heralding diabetic changes that may threaten sight. Researchers have found a new treatment paradigm for the abnormal growth of blood vessels in the eye and the exudation of fluid (wet AMD) from otherwise normal blood vessels: anti-VEGF agents. The use of these agents, such as bevacizumab (Avastin®), ranibizumab (Lucentis®), and aflibercept (Eylea®) has been shown not only to slow vision loss or maintain current visual acuity but also to offer the potential of improving and even restoring functional vision.

Hypertension also produces significant characteristic retinal features. Systemic hypertension may be reflected in the retina in terms of irregularities in arteriolar size, tortuosity of the retinal arteries, retinal edema, and changes in the arteriovenous crossings. Progressive hypertensive changes may include arteriolar narrowing with increasing areas of retinal ischemia, evident by the development of cotton-wool exudates, hemorrhages, retinal edema, and papilledema. Fig. 10.106 shows the retinal changes in a patient with hypertension. Notice in

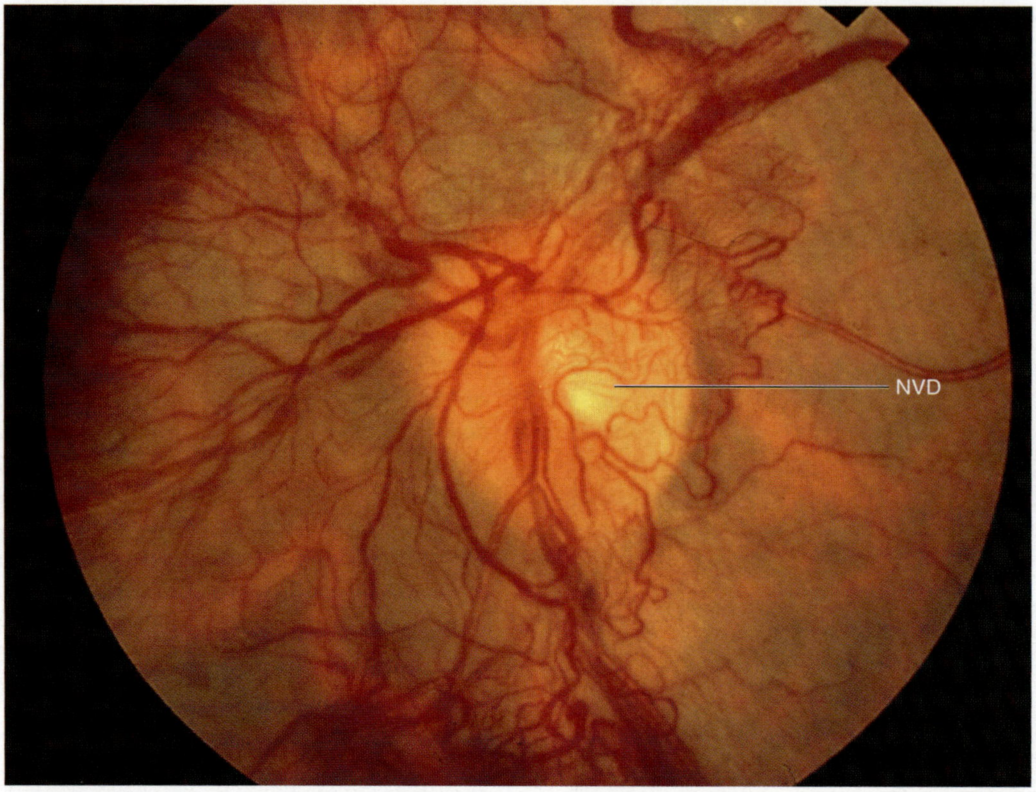

Fig. 10.97 Proliferative Diabetic Retinopathy. Note the neovascularization of the disc. *NVD,* Neovascularization of the disc.

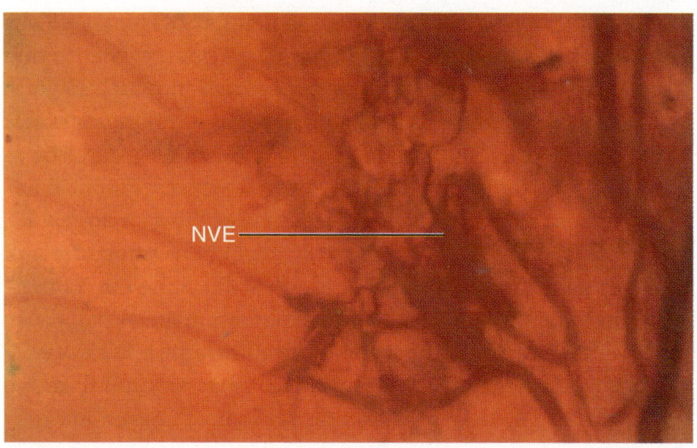

Fig. 10.98 Proliferative Diabetic Retinopathy. Note the neovascularization elsewhere in the retina. *NVE,* Neovascularization elsewhere in the retina. (From Kanski JJ, Nischal KK: *Ophthalmology: clinical signs and differential diagnosis,* St. Louis, 2000, Mosby.)

Fig. 10.107 the tortuosity of the retinal vessels in another patient with hypertension; a green (red-free) filter is used to enhance the visualization of the vessels. Cotton-wool spots and flame-shaped retinal hemorrhages in another patient with hypertension are shown in Fig. 10.87. As the arterial walls thicken due to sustained hypertension, the arteries lose their transparency, and noticeable changes are seen at the crossings of the arteries and veins. Veins appear to disappear abruptly on either side of an artery. Some of the arteries develop a burnishing of the red reflex.

Macular exudates are also common in hypertension (Fig. 10.108). These are well-defined, whitish-yellow intraretinal collections of lipids secondary to vascular leakage. A *macular star* is an accumulation of edema residues arranged in a stellate pattern around the macula. Macular stars are commonly seen in patients with hypertension, papilledema, papillitis, and *central retinal venous occlusion.* A macular star is shown in Fig. 10.109. Arteriolar dilations may also develop. These are known as arteriolar *macroaneurysms* and are prone to leak blood and serous fluid. A hemorrhage from a macroaneurysm is shown in Fig. 10.110.

Increased intracranial pressure, frequently secondary to a space-occupying intracranial lesion, produces a classic picture of *papilledema.* Papilledema is a swelling of the optic disc. The increased pressure is believed to be transmitted to the optic nerve sheath, causing axoplasmic flow stasis in the disc. This, in turn causes axonal swelling and secondary vascular congestion. The most characteristic finding is blurring of the optic disc and its margins. This occurs in association with the loss of spontaneous retinal venous pulsation, hyperemia of the disc, loss of the optic cup, hemorrhages and exudates of the disc, and dilated tortuous retinal veins. Despite these changes, vision remains remarkably normal in the early or acute stages. Fig. 10.111 is a photograph and a labeled schematic of the retinal changes in chronic papilledema. Fig. 10.112 shows papilledema in another patient. Notice the blurring of the disc margins and the hyperemia of the disc. Fig. 10.113 shows papilledema in yet another patient; notice the flame-shaped hemorrhages and the hyperemia of the disc. There are other causes of a blurred disc

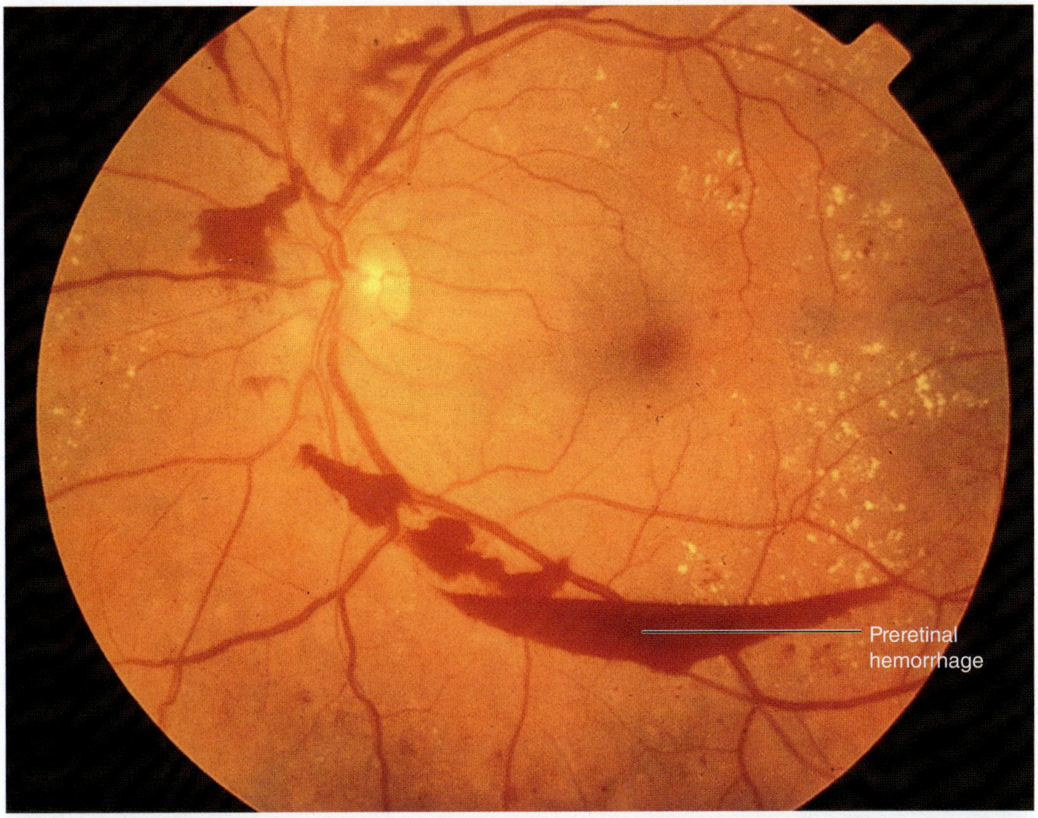

A

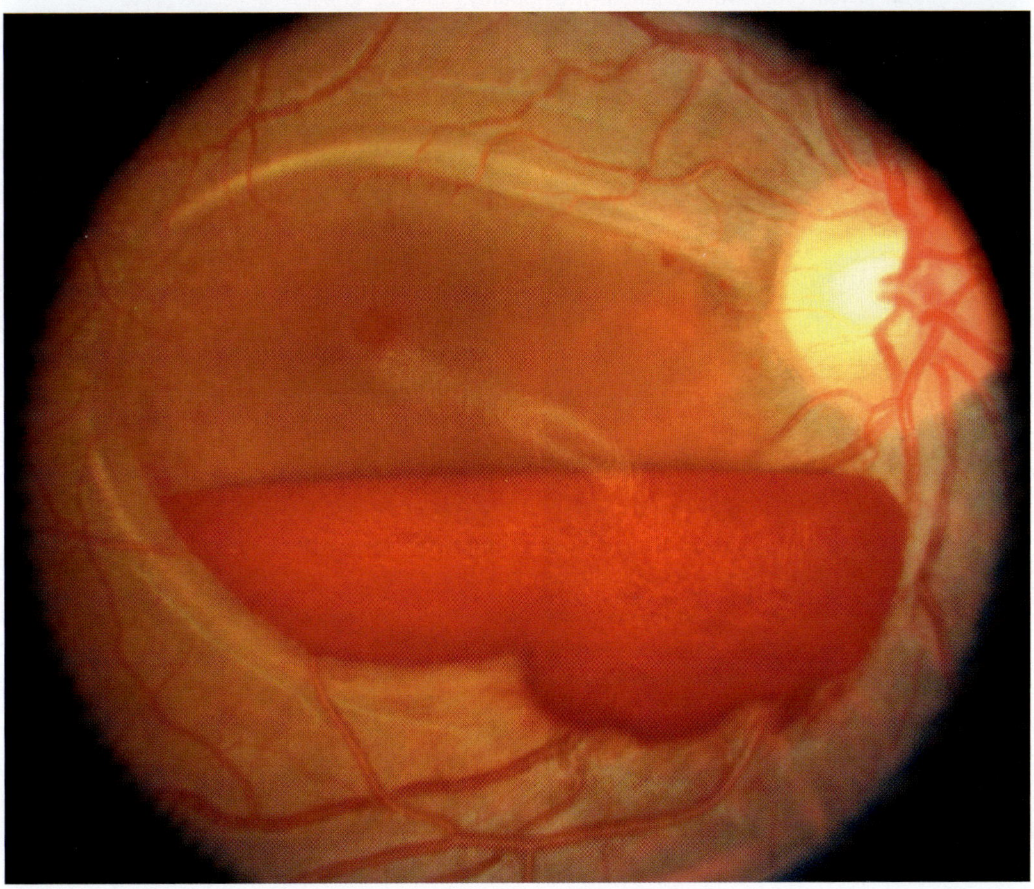

B

Fig. 10.99 (A) and (B) Proliferative diabetic retinopathy. Note the preretinal hemorrhage.

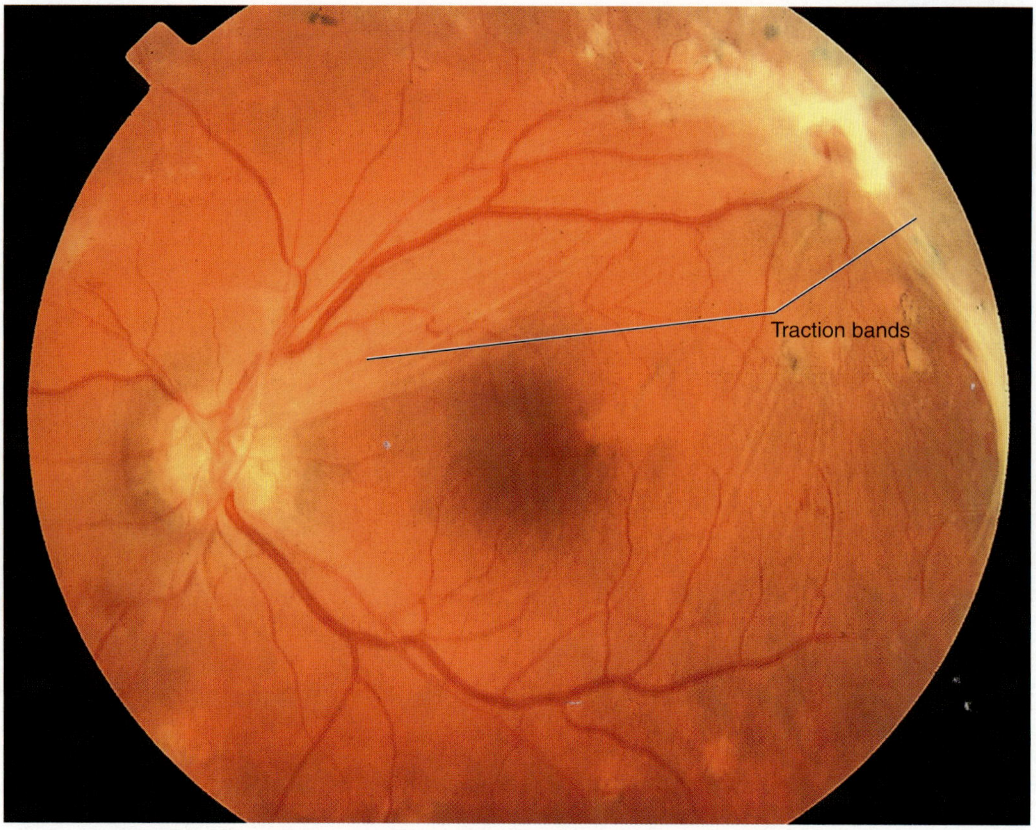

Fig. 10.100 **Proliferative Diabetic Retinopathy.** Note the vitreoretinal fibrous bands.

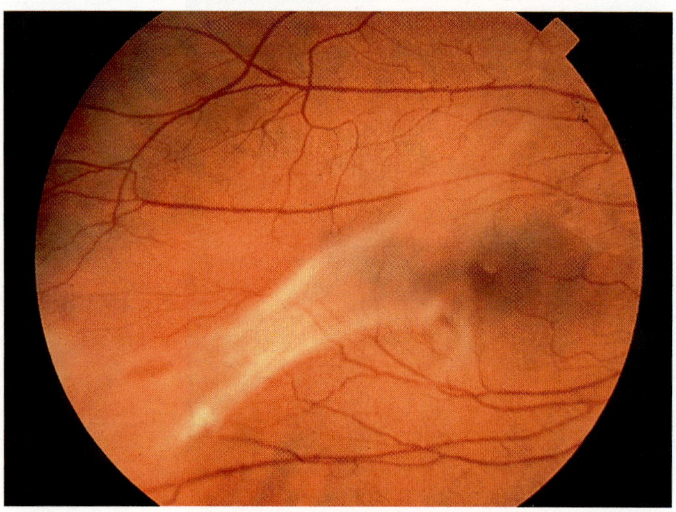

Fig. 10.101 **Proliferative Diabetic Retinopathy.** Note the vitreoretinal fibrous bands.

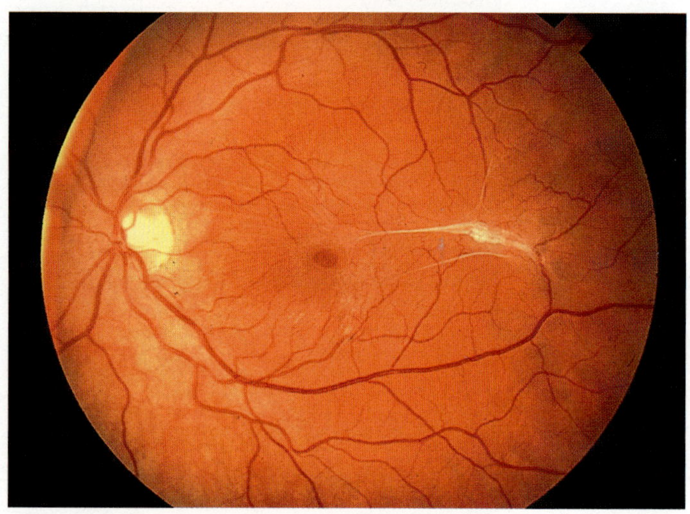

Fig. 10.102 **Proliferative Diabetic Retinopathy.** Note the vitreoretinal fibrous bands and macular hole.

margin. Table 10.10 provides a differential diagnosis of blurred disc margins.

Blood dyscrasias are frequently diagnosed from the examination of the retina. Fig. 10.114 shows the retina of a patient with leukemia. Notice the multiple hemorrhages, perivascular infiltrates of the retinal arterioles, and *Roth spots.* These spots have a clear white center and are surrounded by hemorrhage; they are believed to be areas of emboli and retinal infarcts. The white center usually represents fibrin-platelet plugs. Roth spots are also seen in infective endocarditis, diabetes, hypertensive retinopathy, and human immunodeficiency virus (HIV) retinitis.

Occlusive disorders of the retinal circulation are dramatic. A *central retinal artery occlusion* (*CRAO*) is usually caused by an embolus from the heart or from a large artery. It results in sudden, painless loss of vision in one eye. The pupillary direct light

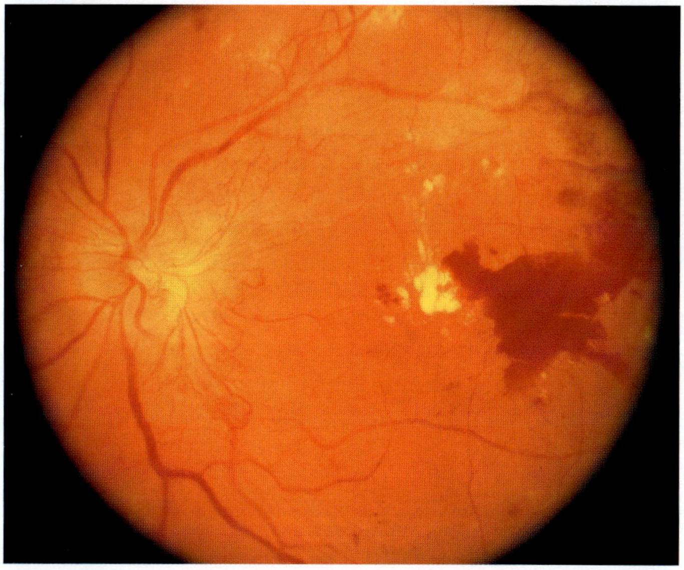

Fig. 10.103 Diabetic retinopathy with neovascularization of the disc, neovascularization elsewhere in the retina, preretinal hemorrhage, and fatty macular exudates.

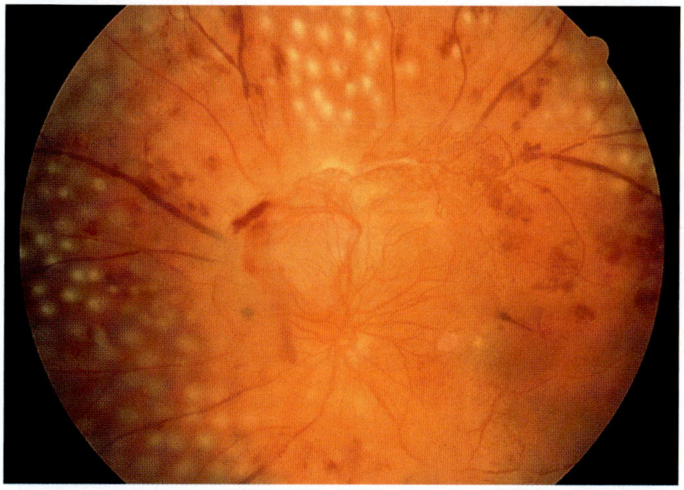

Fig. 10.104 Proliferative Diabetic Retinopathy. Note the lesions of panretinal photocoagulation.

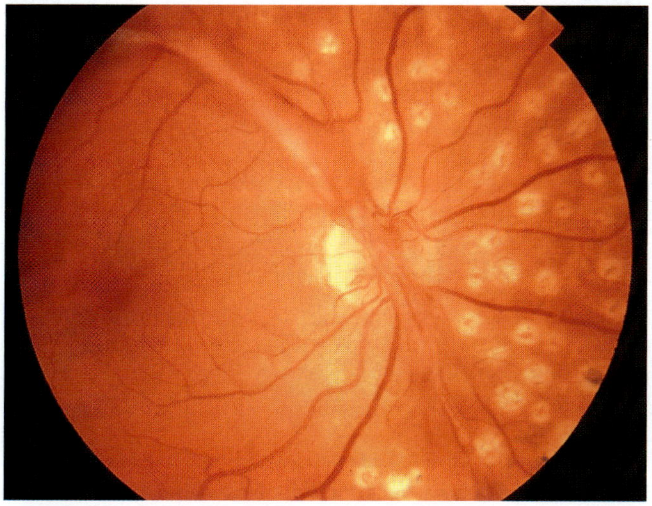

Fig. 10.105 Proliferative Diabetic Retinopathy. Note the lesions of panretinal photocoagulation.

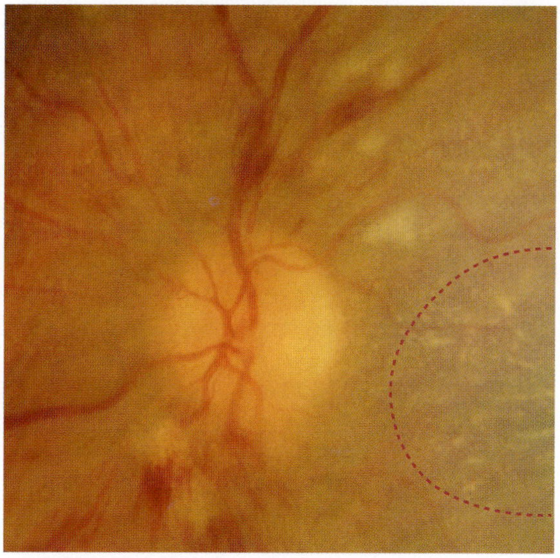

Fig. 10.106 Retinal Changes in a Patient With Long-Standing Hypertension. Note the cotton-wool spots and flame-shaped hemorrhages. Part of a macular star is seen on the bottom right. (From Kanski JJ, Nischal KK: *Ophthalmology: clinical signs and differential diagnosis*, St. Louis, 2000, Mosby.)

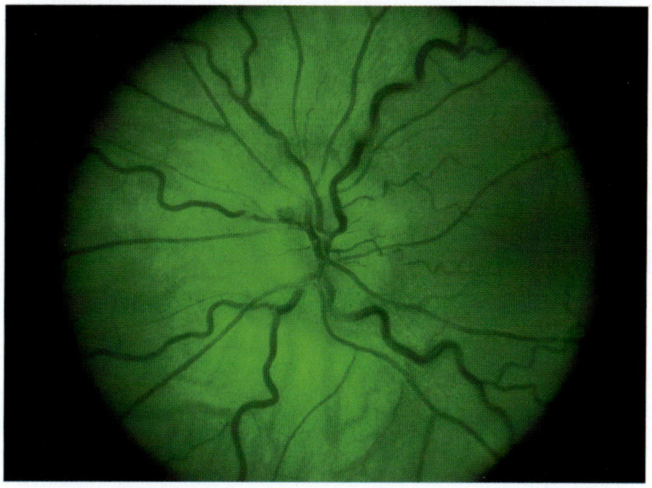

Fig. 10.107 Hypertensive Retinopathy. Note the markedly tortuous vessels seen through the red-free *(green)* filter.

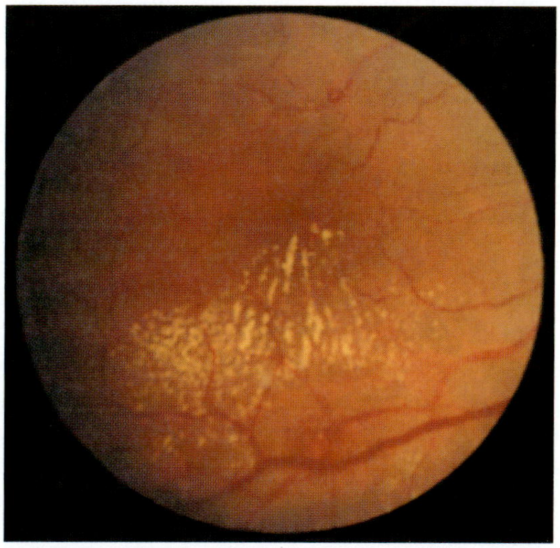

Fig. 10.108 Macular Exudates in a Patient With Hypertension.

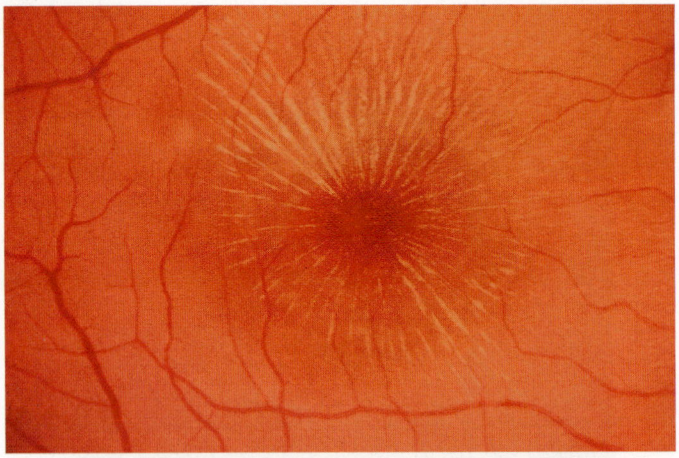

Fig. 10.109 Macular Star in Hypertensive Retinopathy.

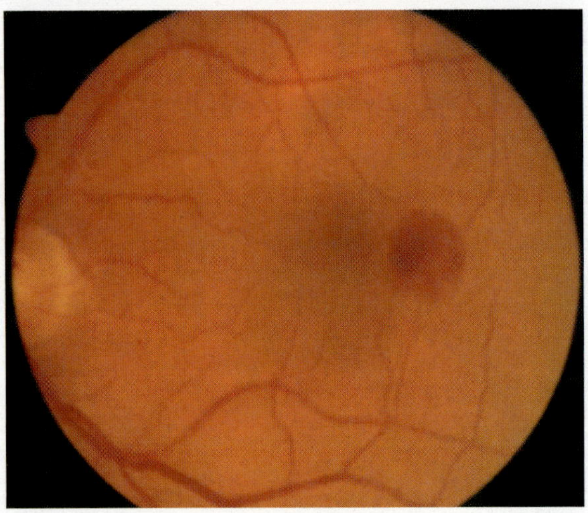

Fig. 10.110 Macroaneurysms in Hypertensive Retinopathy. Note the hemorrhage lateral to the macula.

reflex is lost, and spontaneous venous pulsations are absent. Within minutes, the retina becomes pale and milky white with narrowed arteries, and a cherry-red spot appears at the macula. This cherry-red spot appears because in the foveal area, the retina is thin, allowing visibility of the underlying choroidal circulation that is obscured elsewhere by retinal edema. This is a true ocular emergency because the retina may be lost if it is not treated within 45 minutes. Fig. 10.115 shows the left retina of a patient with a CRAO. Notice the pale retina with the cherry-red spot at the macula. Figs. 10.116A and B show the retinas of two patients with a CRAO with cilioretinal artery sparing. The cilioretinal arteries are present in 40% of normal individuals. They are derived from the posterior ciliary circulation and usually emerge from the temporal aspect of the disc to supply a small portion of the retina. Occasionally, this artery may supply enough circulation to the macula, sparing central vision. Notice the area of retina spared due to perfusion by the cilioretinal artery in both images. Fig. 10.116B shows the patent cilioretinal artery. Fig. 10.117 shows a CRAO in another patient. In this example, the retina is also pale (ischemic and edematous), but the area of the cherry-red spot at the macula is

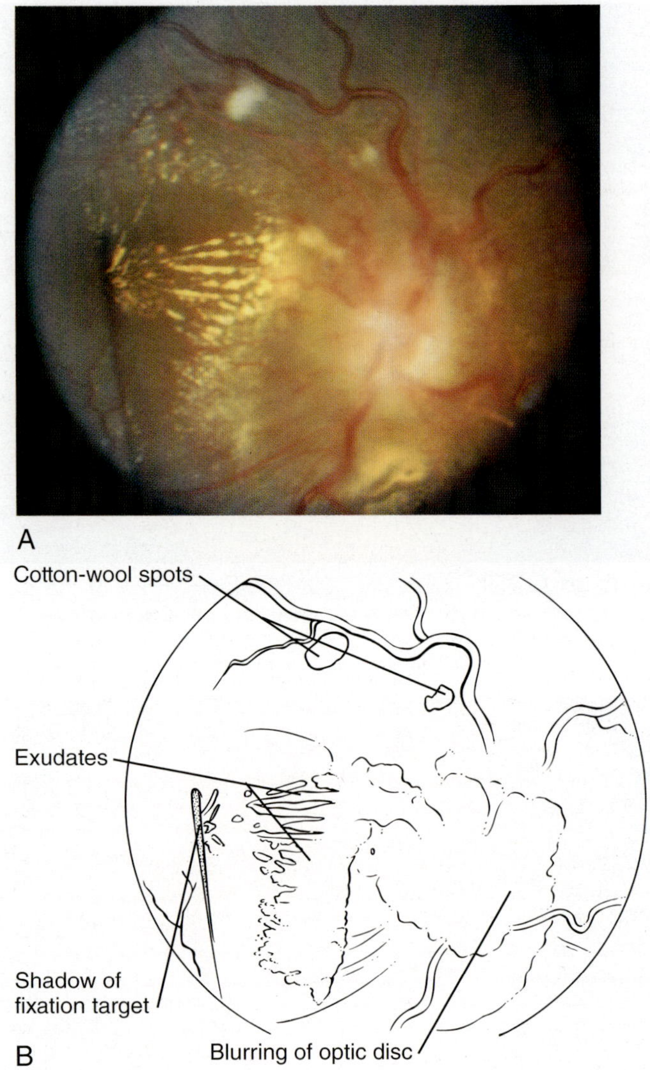

Fig. 10.111 Photograph (A) and schematic (B) showing the retinal changes in papilledema.

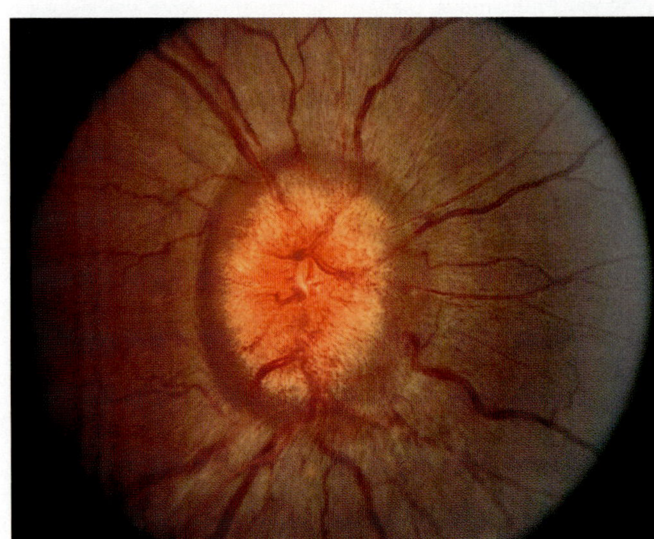

Fig. 10.112 Papilledema. Note the hyperemia and blurring of the disc margins.

TABLE 10.10 Differentiation of Blurred Disc Margins

Feature	Papilledema[a] (See Figs. 10.111 to 10.113)	Papillitis[b]	Drusen (See Fig. 10.123)	Myelinated Nerve Fibers[c] (See Figs. 10.80 to 10.82)	Central Retinal Vein Occlusion (See Fig. 10.121)
Visual acuity	Normal	Decreased	Normal	Normal	Decreased
Venous pulsations	Absent	Variable	Present	Present	Usually absent
Pain	Headache	Eye movement pain	No	No	No
Light reaction	Present	Marcus Gunn (see text)	Present	Present	Present
Hemorrhage	Present	Present	Uncommon	No	Marked
Visual fields	Enlarged blind spot	Central scotoma	Enlarged blind spot	Scotomata correspond to areas of myelination	Variable
Laterality	Bilateral	Unilateral	Bilateral	Seldom bilateral	Unilateral

[a]Edema of the optic disc resulting from increased intracranial pressure.
[b]Inflammation of the optic disc.
[c]Myelination of the optic nerve ends at the optic disc. When it continues into the retina, white, flame-shaped areas obscure the disc margins.

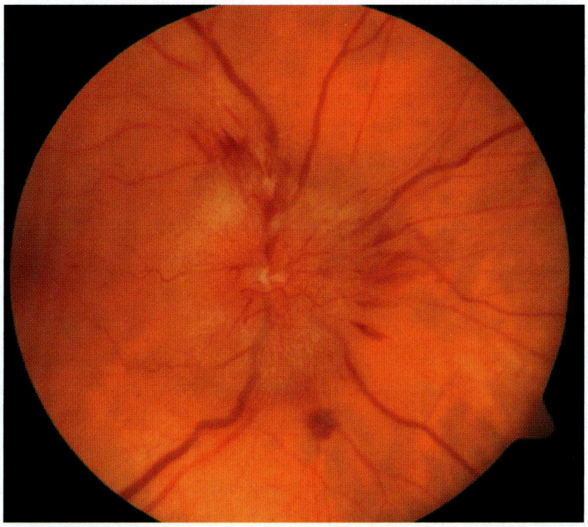

Fig. 10.113 **Papilledema.** Note the hyperemia of the disc, the blurring of the disc margins, and the flame-shaped hemorrhages.

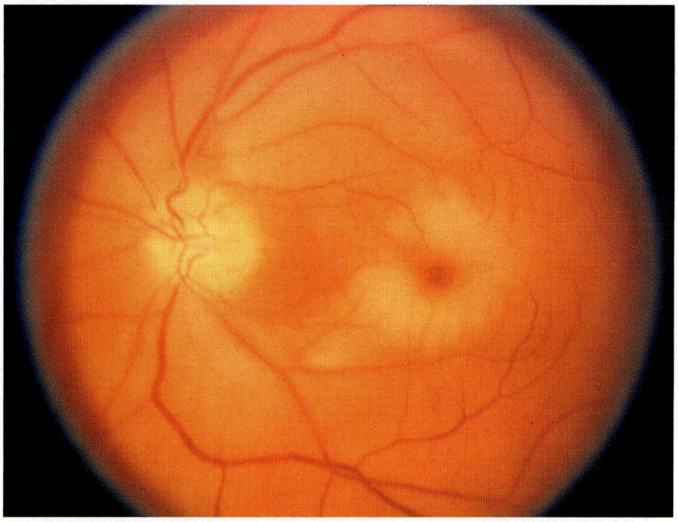

Fig. 10.115 Central Retinal Artery Occlusion.

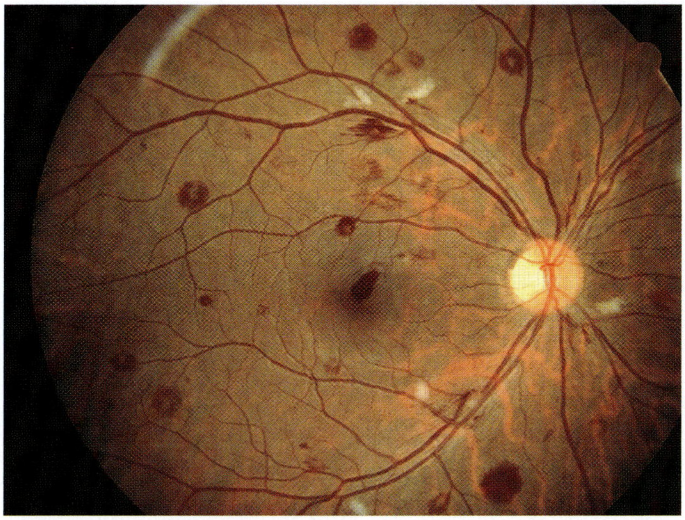

Fig. 10.114 **Leukemia-Related Retinitis.** Note the multiple hemorrhages, perivascular infiltrates, and Roth spots.

heavily pigmented. This is the finding in dark-skinned individuals with a CRAO.

Hollenhorst plaques are cholesterol emboli found at the bifurcation of the retinal arteries. The source of these emboli is usually the heart or the carotid arteries. These plaques are typically unilateral and occur in older adults with advanced atherosclerosis. Symptoms of fleeting alterations of vision may accompany these emboli. Figs. 10.118A and B show classic examples of a Hollenhorst plaque in two different patients. Fig. 10.119 shows a *branch retinal artery occlusion* (BRAO). Note the area of the ischemic retina and the cotton-wool spots and adjacent flame-shaped hemorrhage. Fig. 10.120 shows a BRAO in another patient involving the left retina's superior portion. Note the superior pallor representing the ischemic retina.

Venous occlusion is one of the most common retinal vascular disorders. A central retinal venous occlusion (CRVO) occurs deep within the nerve head. The patient experiences painless loss of vision in that eye. The fundus exhibits venous dilation

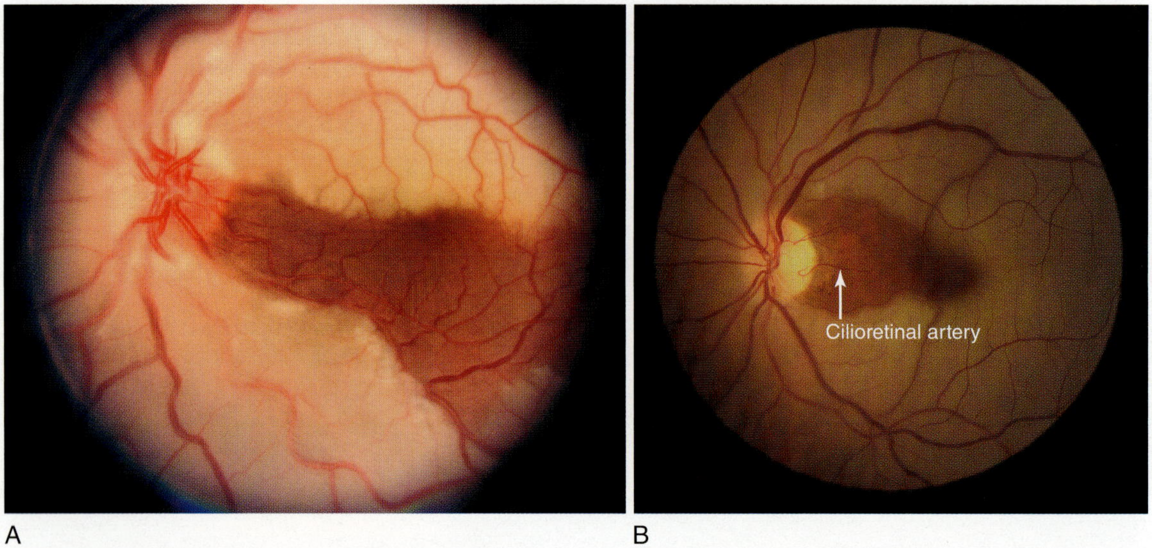

Fig. 10.116 (A) and (B) Two examples of central retinal artery occlusion with cilioretinal artery sparing. Note the patent cilioretinal artery in (B). (B, Courtesy of Beth Snodgrass, CRA, Byers Eye Institute at Stanford, Palo Alto, CA.)

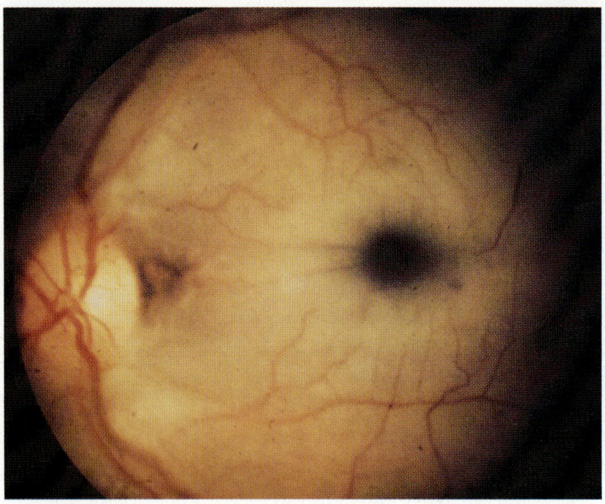

Fig. 10.117 Pigmented Central Retinal Artery Occlusion in a Person of Color.

and tortuosity, blurred optic disc and margins caused by edema, flame-shaped hemorrhages in all quadrants, cotton-wool spots, and often an extensive hemorrhage at the macula. The fundus in a CRVO has been described as a "pizza thrown against a wall." The patients are usually from 70 to 80 years of age. The causes of CRVO are many: hypertension, glaucoma, atherosclerosis, diabetes, or hyperviscosity syndromes. Fig. 10.121 shows the retina of a patient with a CRVO. Notice the dark, engorged, tortuous, dusky-colored retinal veins. A branch retinal vein occlusion (BRVO) occurs at a site of retinal arteriovenous crossing. BRVO is commonly associated with systemic hypertension, although any systemic disease associated with hypercoagulability may predispose to BRVO. Distal to the occlusion site, the retinal vein becomes engorged and tortuous with associated capillary dysfunction that leads to intraretinal edema and hemorrhage. Fig. 10.122 shows two examples of the retinas of patients with a BRVO. Anti-VEGF therapy is currently being used with good results in these patients.

Drusen of the optic disc are acellular, calcified hyaline deposits in the substance of the optic nerve that occurs secondary to axonal degeneration. The disc margins are irregular or blurred. Drusen are found to be bilateral in 70% of affected patients, and the condition is transmitted as an irregular dominant trait with incomplete penetrance. Drusen occur almost exclusively in white individuals. Fig. 10.123 shows optic disc drusen. Notice the scalloped appearance of the optic nerve border. Because of the irregular disc border, optic disc drusen sometimes can be confused with papilledema. However, the *absence* of optic disc hyperemia, exudates, and venous congestion, as well as a normal optic cup, differentiates drusen from papilledema.

Optic disc drusen should not be confused with *retinal drusen.* Diffuse retinal drusen, as shown in Fig. 10.124, are not age-related phenomena and are benign. On the other hand, hard and soft retinal drusen at the level of the RPE located near the macula are part of the disorder known as *age-related macular degeneration.* AMD is the most common cause of central visual loss in patients older than 60 in the United States. It is usually bilateral but may be asymmetric. Retinal drusen are yellowish-white, round lesions that may vary in size and are frequently concentrated at the posterior pole. Fig. 10.125 shows the retina of a patient with AMD and subfoveal choroidal neovascularization. The neovascularization appears as the gray pigmentation around the drusen at the macula. This gray area represents new blood vessels from the choroid between it and the RPE. Fig. 10.126 is a close-up photograph of macular drusen in another patient. The growing vessels leak blood, lipids, and serum under the sensory retinal layer, stimulating the formation of a fibrous scar, further damaging the sensory retinal layers. Studies have implicated VEGF in the pathogenesis of AMD. This growth factor is naturally expressed in the retina, with high levels concentrated in the RPE. In the normal eye, VEGF may play a protective role in maintaining adequate blood flow to RPE and photoreceptors. Studies have indicated that a reduction of choroidal blood flow and oxidative stress may stimulate the initial overexpression of VEGF in the RPE and retina. This stimulates proliferation and permeability, promoting angiogenesis, increased vascular permeability, and the breakdown of the blood-retinal barrier, which are hallmarks of choroidal

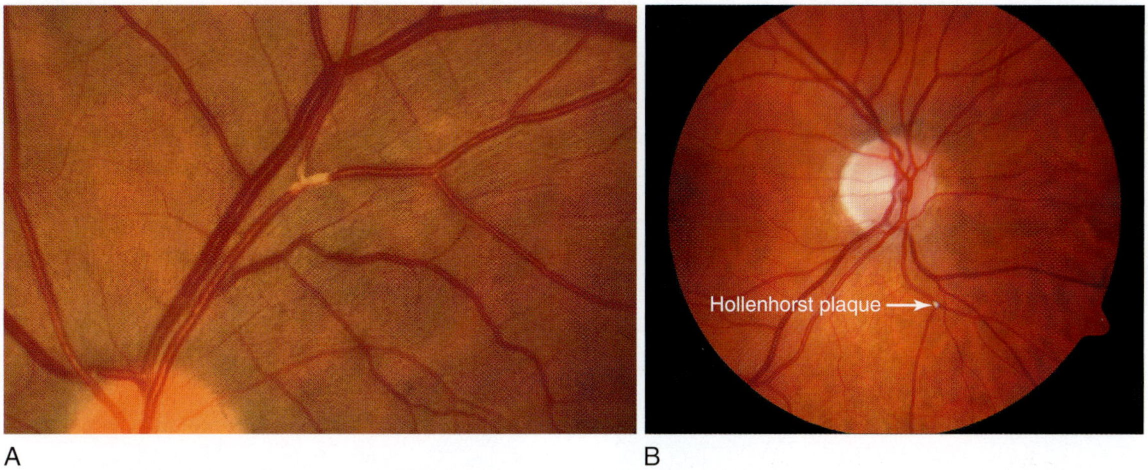

Fig. 10.118 (A) and (B) Two examples of a Hollenhorst plaque. (B, Courtesy Beth Snodgrass, CRA, Byers Eye Institute at Stanford, Palo Alto, CA.)

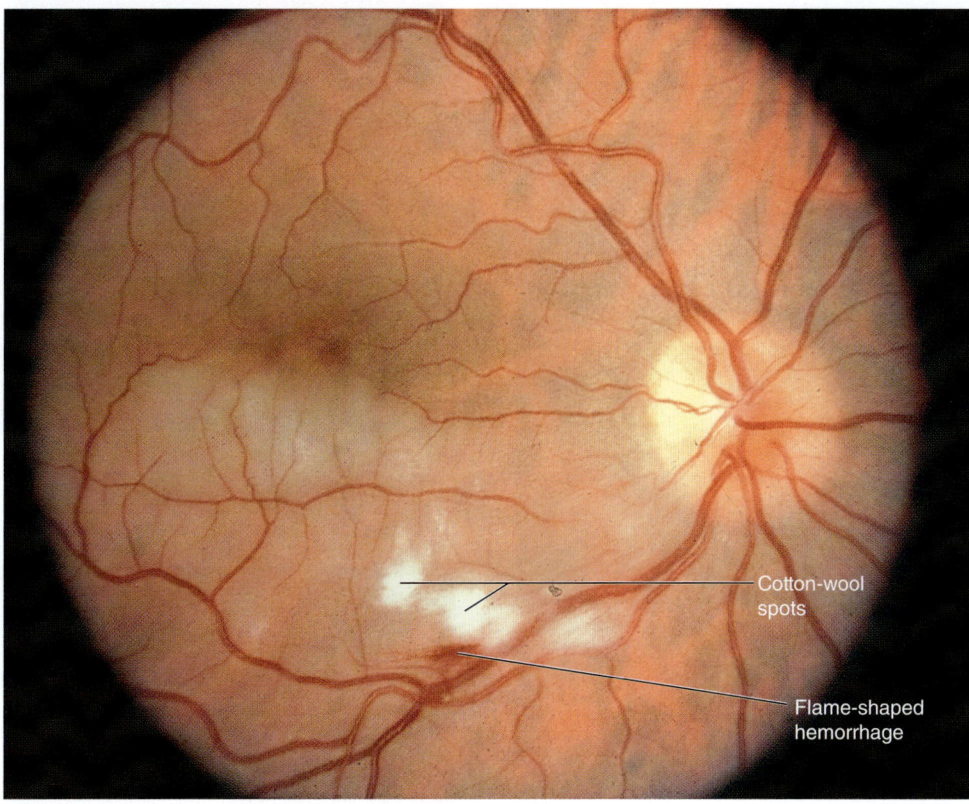

Fig. 10.119 Branch Retinal Artery Occlusion.

neovascularization and AMD. Anti-VEGF agents, discussed previously in this chapter, are efficacious in patients with wet AMD. Fig. 10.127 shows a patient's retina with long-standing AMD; note that the macula has been destroyed, and only a scar exists.

Optic atrophy is a reduction in size and substance of the optic nerve caused by the loss of axons and myelin sheaths. Optic atrophy may result from a lesion anywhere in the anterior visual pathway between the retina and the lateral geniculate body. The ophthalmoscopic hallmark of optic atrophy is optic disc pallor. The patient may have a loss of visual acuity, narrowed visual fields, deficit in color vision, or an afferent pupillary defect. The pallor of the disc is caused by the loss of its capillary network and by glial tissue formation. Fig. 10.128 shows the right retina of a patient with optic atrophy. Note the pallor of the temporal aspect of the disc.

Anterior ischemic optic neuropathy (*AION*) is the most common cause of *acute optic neuropathy* in older age groups. It can be nonarteritic or arteritic, the latter being associated with *giant cell arteritis*[j] (*GCA*). AION is characterized by visual loss associated

[j]The diagnosis of GCA is made definitively by biopsy of the temporal artery. If the diagnosis of temporal arteritis is confirmed, steroid therapy must be initiated immediately to avoid blindness. See also Chapter 25, The Geriatric Patient.

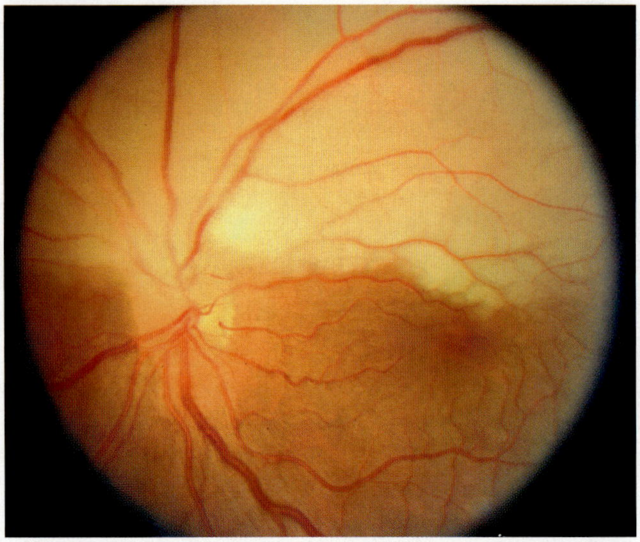

Fig. 10.120 Branch Retinal Artery Occlusion. Note the pallor of the superior left retina, resulting from occlusion of the artery supplying this area.

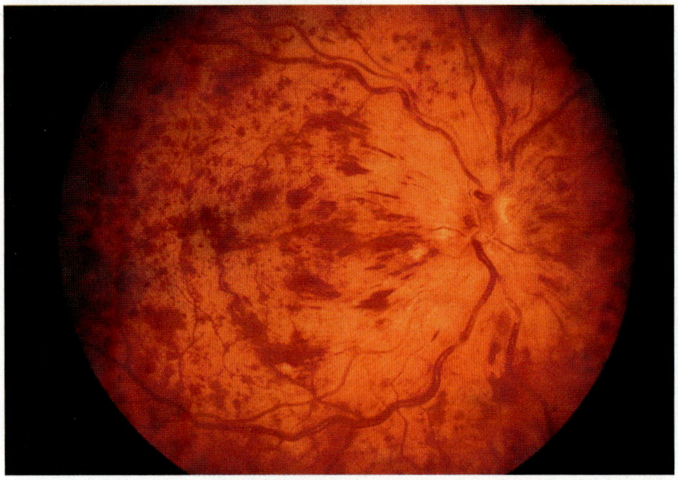

Fig. 10.121 Central Retinal Vein Occlusion.

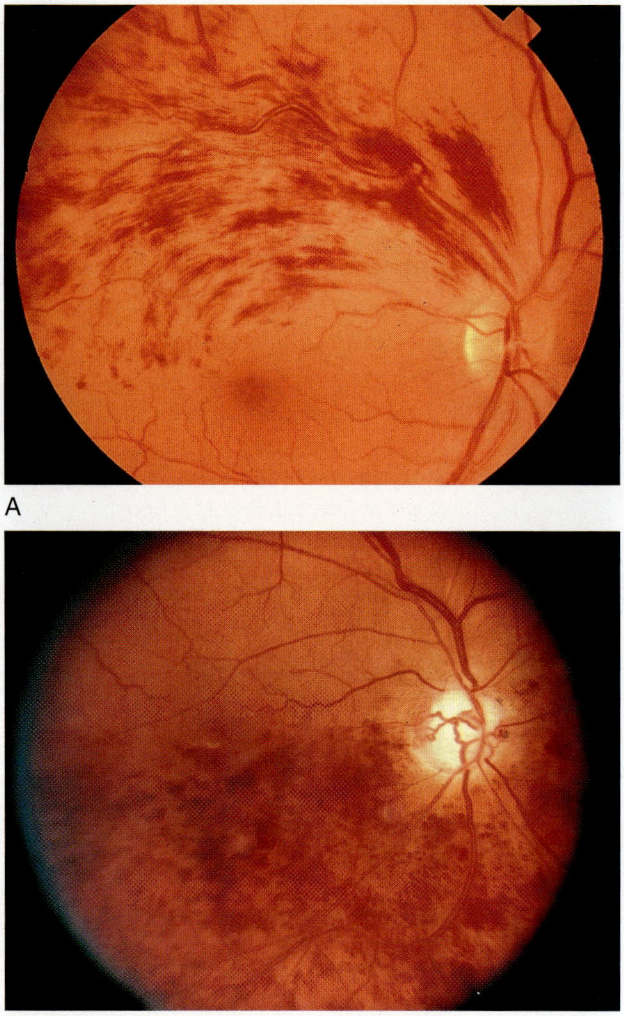

A

B

Fig. 10.122 (A) and (B) Two examples of branch retinal vein occlusions.

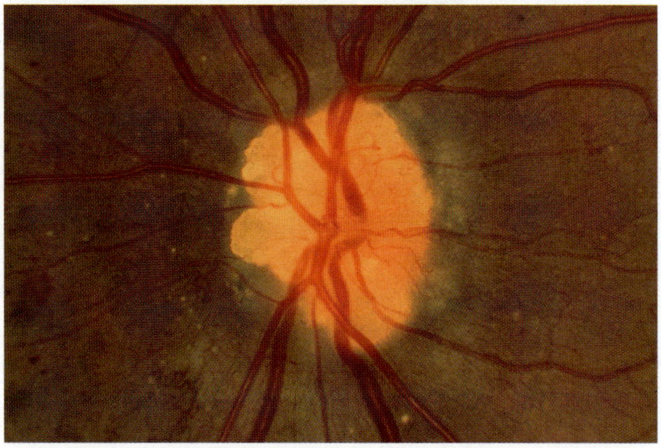

Fig. 10.123 Optic Disc Drusen.

with *pale* optic disc swelling, occasionally with flame hemorrhages on the swollen disc, and sometimes with nearby cotton-wool exudates. Fig. 10.129A shows a patient with AION secondary to GCA (arteritic); note the presence of *pale* papilledema caused by ischemia to the optic nerve. This is in sharp contrast to papilledema caused by increased intracranial pressure, which causes the disc to become hyperemic and pinkish-red. In both types of AION, visual loss is often sudden or occurs over a few days at most and is usually permanent; with high-dose steroid treatment, some recovery from arteritic AION may occur within the first weeks or months. Continuously monitor the erythrocyte sedimentation rate in patients with arteritic AION and titrate the steroid dose based on the results. As the edema resorbs, optic atrophy becomes visible, as shown in the same patient 2 months later (see Fig. 10.129B). Fig. 10.130 shows a different patient with nonarteritic AION. Note the pale papilledema and the infarct on the nerve fiber layer again. Control of blood pressure in the nonarteritic type is of paramount importance.

Chorioretinitis is an inflammatory process that originates in the choroid and subsequently spreads to involve the retina. Most inflammatory changes in the choroid are of endogenous origin, including tuberculosis, syphilis, Q fever, HIV, herpes zoster, cytomegalovirus (CMV), measles, sarcoidosis, histoplasmosis, *Aspergillus* infection, *Candida* infection, cryptococcosis, coccidioidomycosis, toxoplasmosis, *Toxocara* infection, and onchocerciasis. In acute chorioretinitis, blurred vision results from vitreous haze, and the patient sees light flashes and multiple floating spots. Loss of vision may occur if the macula is involved. In chronic chorioretinitis, there is clumping of pigment around the lesions, which are whitish owing to the presence of scar tissue and the underlying sclera that is visible because the retina and choroid have been destroyed.

Toxoplasmosis, caused by the organism *Toxoplasma gondii,* is most frequently a congenital condition transmitted to the fetus from the mother during the first trimester of pregnancy. The early lesions heal once the organisms become encysted; only retinochoroidal scarring is seen on routine ophthalmoscopy. The condition may recur with the liberation of the encysted organisms, and further retinal damage can result. The visual prognosis depends on the location of the lesion. Fig. 10.131

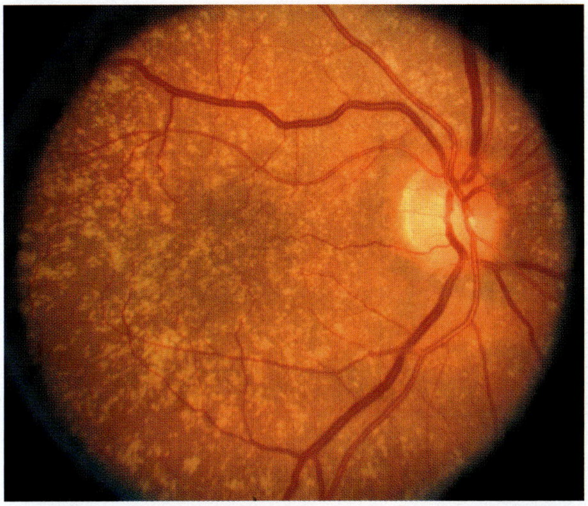

Fig. 10.124 Diffuse Retinal Drusen That Are Not Age Related.

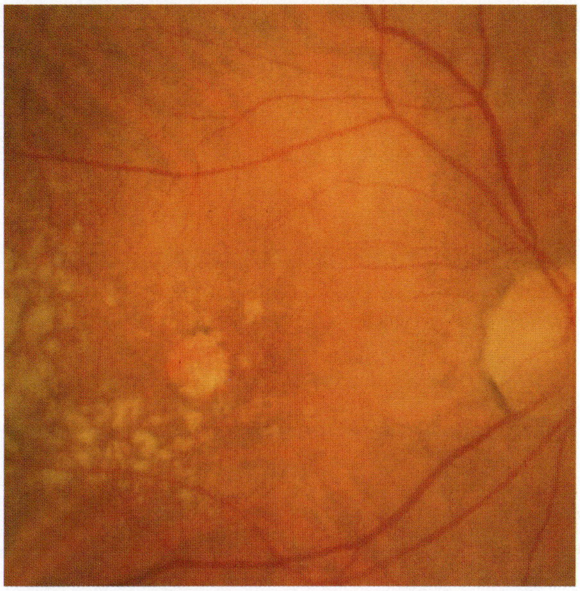

Fig. 10.126 Close-Up Photograph of Macular Drusen. (From Kanski JJ, Nischal KK: *Ophthalmology: clinical signs and differential diagnosis,* St. Louis, 2000, Mosby.)

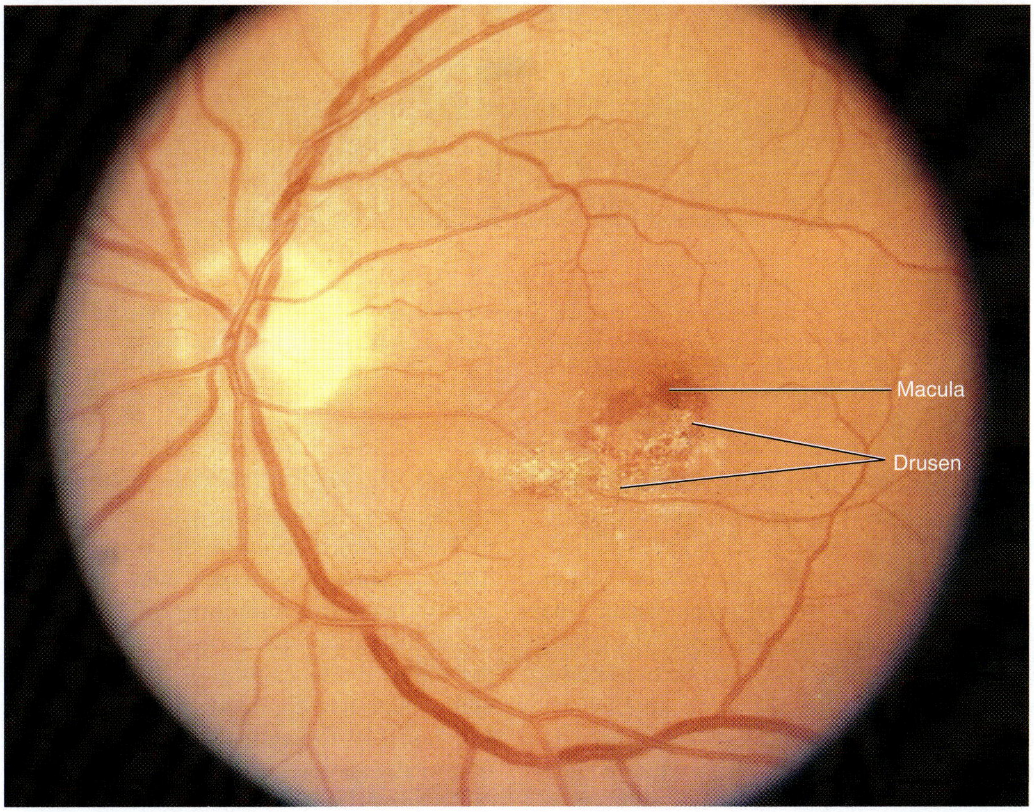

Fig. 10.125 Age-Related Macular Degeneration and Subfoveal Choroidal Neovascularization.

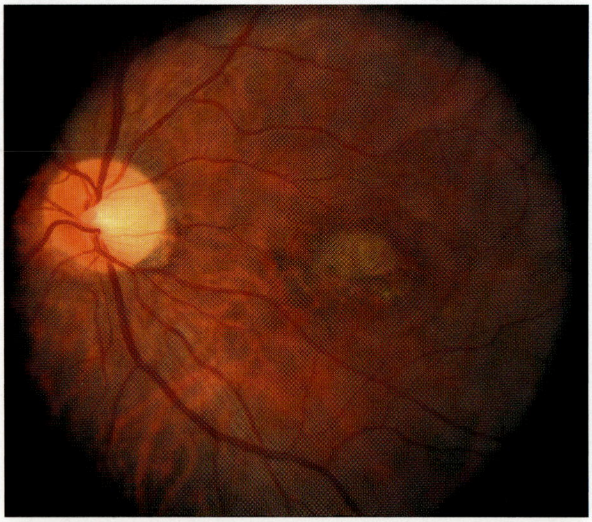

Fig. 10.127 **Age-Related Macular Degeneration, Late Stage.** Note the gray scar at the macular area.

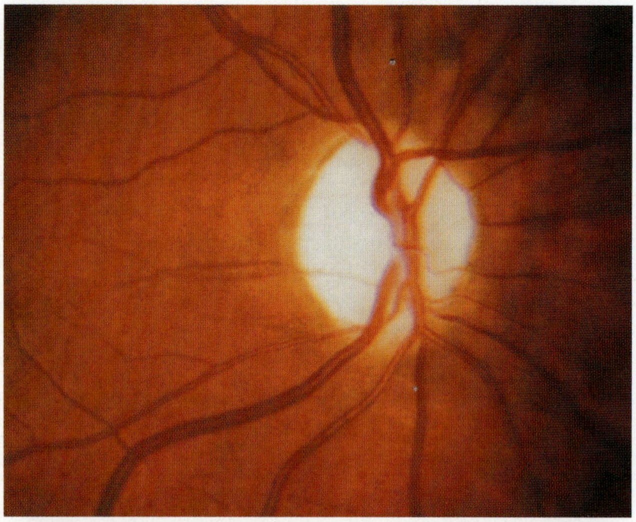

Fig. 10.128 **Right Retina With Optic Atrophy.** Note the marked pallor of the temporal aspect of the disc. (From Kanski JJ, Nischal KK: *Ophthalmology: clinical signs and differential diagnosis*, St. Louis, 2000, Mosby.)

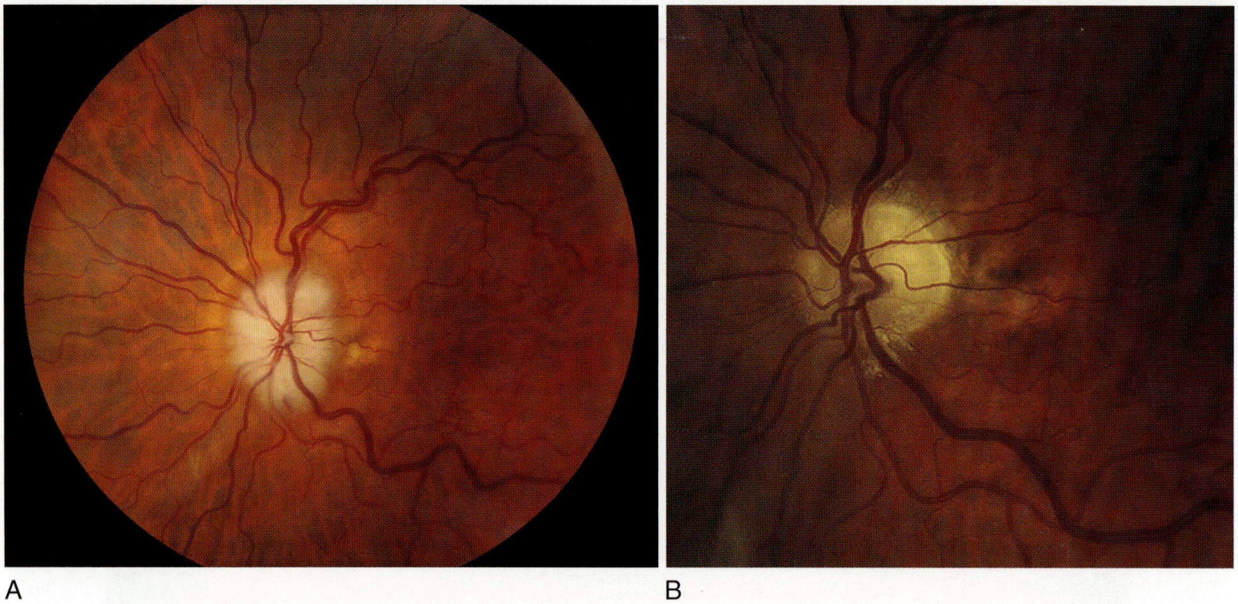

Fig. 10.129 **Anterior Ischemic Optic Neuropathy—*Arteritic*.** (A) Note the pale papilledema secondary to the inflammation caused by giant cell arteritis, which interferes with circulation. (B) The same patient 2 months later showing optic atrophy. Note the marked pallor of the disc as the edema has been resorbed. (Courtesy Christina Ryu, MD, and Steve Oglivy, CRA, Henry Ford Health System, Detroit, MI.)

shows the retina of the right eye of a patient with AIDS and acute toxoplasmosis chorioretinitis. The acute lesions are round with an overlying yellow-white haze as a result of vitreitis; these acute lesions have been described as looking like a "headlight in fog." Notice the multifocal areas of retinal involvement. This patient had similar multifocal lesions in the left eye. The multifocal areas and bilaterality are typical of acute toxoplasmosis retinitis in patients with AIDS. Fig. 10.132 shows another patient with acute toxoplasmosis; notice the dense "fog" caused by the active vitreitis. Fig. 10.133 shows a retina of another patient with a healed, inactive lesion of toxoplasmosis chorioretinitis at the macula. Fig. 10.134 shows another patient with diffuse retinal scars secondary to inactive toxoplasmosis.

The *presumed ocular histoplasmosis syndrome* (POHS) has a distinct retinal appearance characterized by small atrophic areas in the retina. A dimorphic yeast, *Histoplasma capsulatum*, causes histoplasmosis. It exists in humans in the yeast form and the soil as the mold form. It is endemic in the soil along the Ohio and Mississippi River valleys and in Maryland, Florida, and Texas. Histoplasmosis enters the body through the inhalation of the spores. Infection may be asymptomatic, or it may cause a mild flulike syndrome. Dissemination throughout the

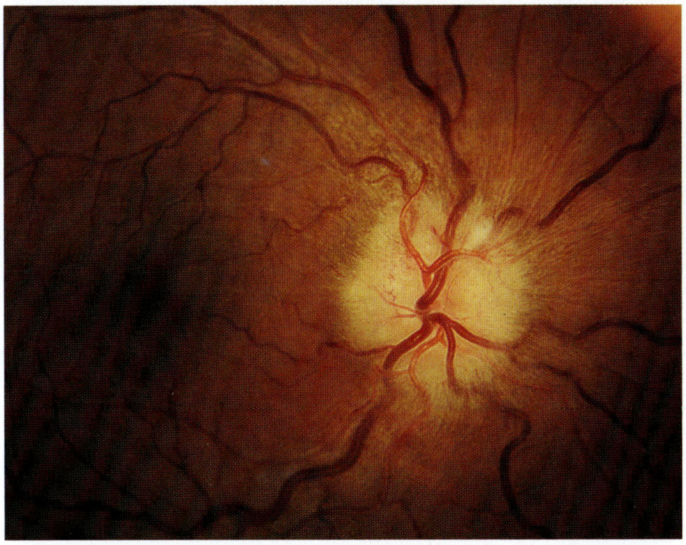

Fig. 10.130 Anterior Ischemic Optic Neuropathy—*Nonarteritic*. Note the pale papilledema and the white infarct on the nerve fiber layer. (Courtesy Christina Ryu, MD, Bradley Stern, CRA, Henry Ford Health System, Detroit, MI.)

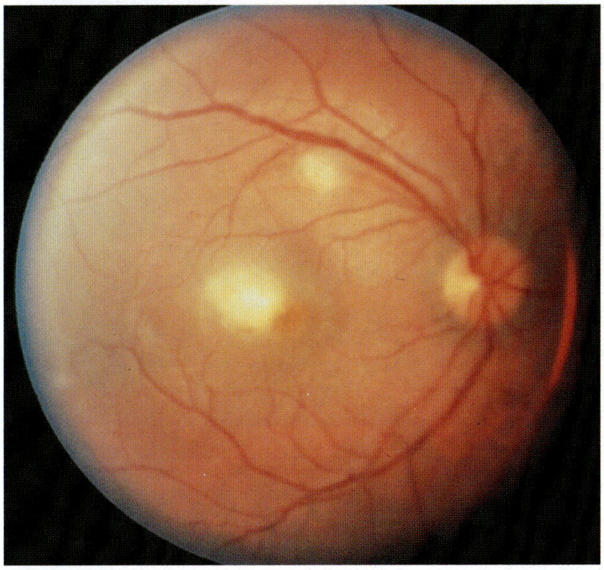

Fig. 10.131 Acute Toxoplasmosis Chorioretinitis in a Patient With Acquired Immune Deficiency Syndrome.

body may occur. Histoplasmosis infections in immunocompromised patients may cause a fulminating, life-threatening systemic infection. In POHS, a ring of pigmented atrophic scarring surrounds the optic nerve. The macula may also be affected. POHS is so named because the organism has never been isolated from the choroid of individuals who have been ill with histoplasmosis and have developed retinal lesions. Fig. 10.135 shows the classic lesion of POHS.

CMV chorioretinitis is the most common ocular opportunistic infection in patients with AIDS. Autopsy studies have shown that more than 95% of viral chorioretinitis in patients with AIDS is a result of CMV infection. CMV chorioretinitis is progressive and often preterminal. It appears that the patient with

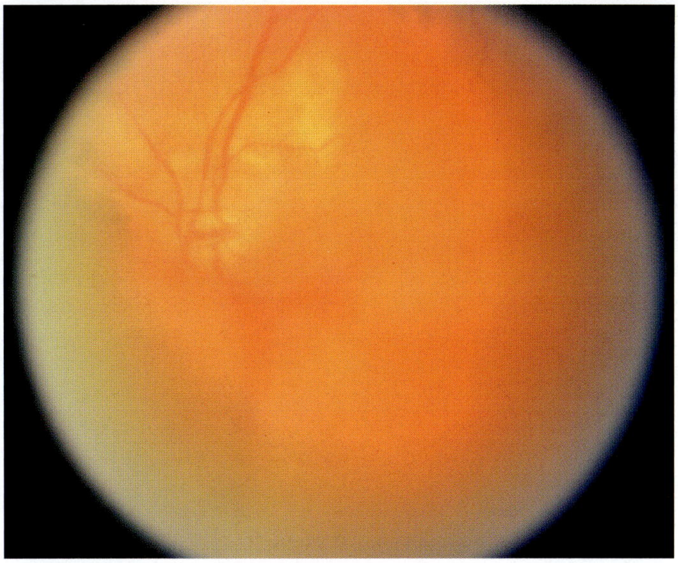

Fig. 10.132 Active Vitreitis Secondary to Acute Toxoplasmosis.

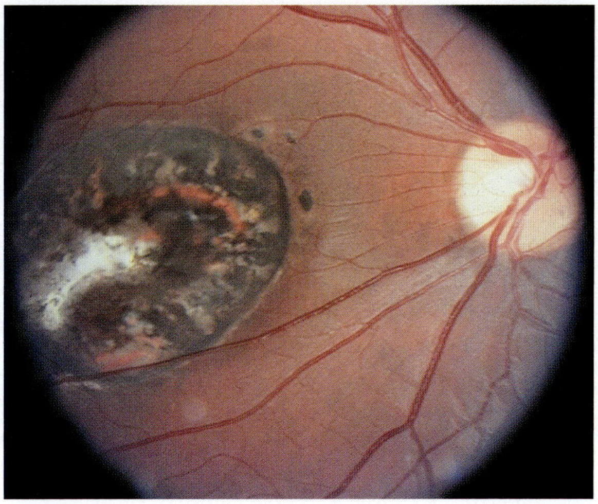

Fig. 10.133 Chronic (Inactive) Toxoplasmosis Chorioretinitis Scar.

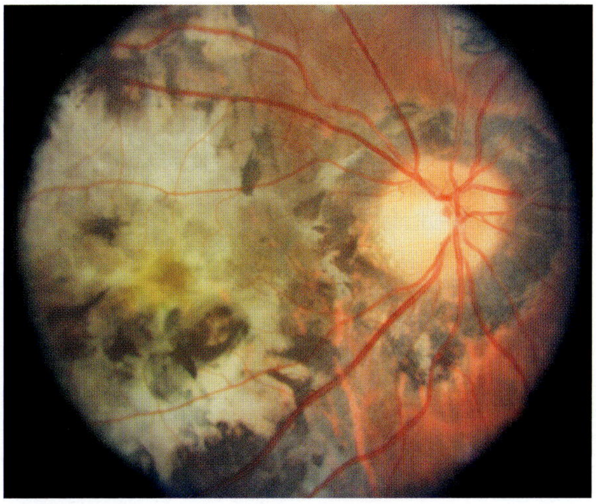

Fig. 10.134 Inactive Toxoplasmosis Chorioretinitis. Note the diffuse retinal scars.

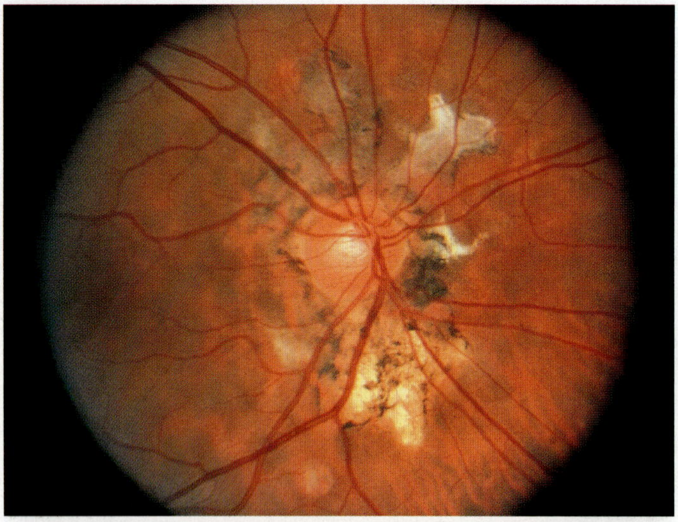

Fig. 10.135 Presumed Ocular Histoplasmosis Syndrome.

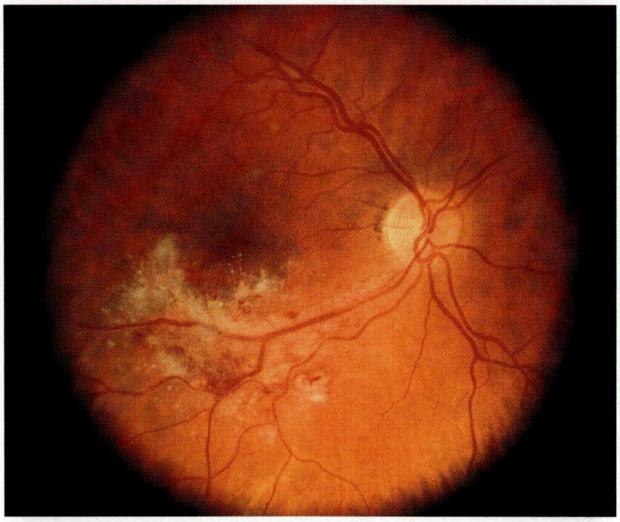

Fig. 10.136 Cytomegalovirus Retinitis in a Patient With Acquired Immune Deficiency Syndrome, Right Retina.

AIDS is at most significant risk for CMV retinitis when the $CD4^+$ T-cell count is less than $40/mm^3$. Fig. 10.136 depicts retinal necrosis and vasculitis in a patient with AIDS and CMV chorioretinitis. Fig. 10.137 shows the retina of the left eye of a patient with CMV chorioretinitis. Notice the marked retinal necrosis extending from the optic nerve superiorly and temporally. Fig. 10.138 shows the retina of the right eye of another patient with CMV retinitis. There is extensive necrotizing optic neuritis with retinal necrosis and retinal vasculitis. Notice the white sheathing of the retinal vessels (especially superiorly off the disc), which is typical of vasculitis. Fig. 10.139 shows the left eye of another patient with active CMV retinitis; notice the retinal vessel sheathing and extensive necrotizing optic neuritis. Fig. 10.140 shows the retina of a patient with burned-out CMV retinitis. Notice the sclerosed retinal arteries and the paucity of vessels. The patient was blind as a result of the CMV infection.

Fig. 10.141A shows the left retina of a patient with HIV chorioretinitis. Notice the cotton-wool spots and the extremely large flame-shaped hemorrhage. Fig. 10.141B shows another

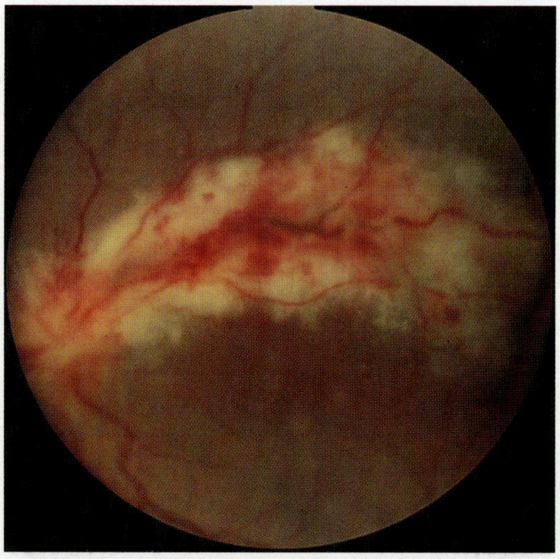

Fig. 10.137 Cytomegalovirus Chorioretinitis, Left Retina.

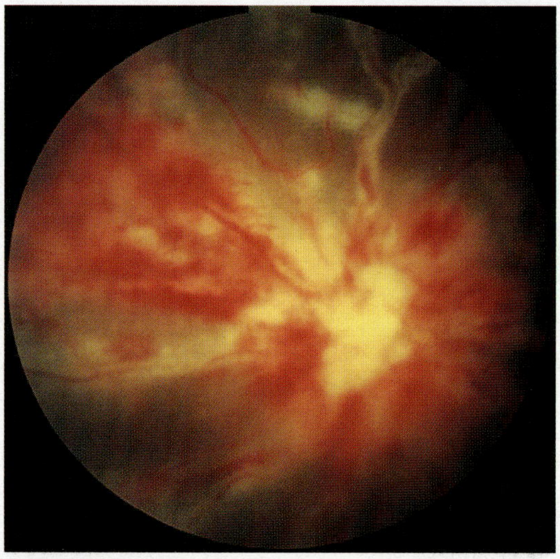

Fig. 10.138 Cytomegalovirus Chorioretinitis, Right Retina.

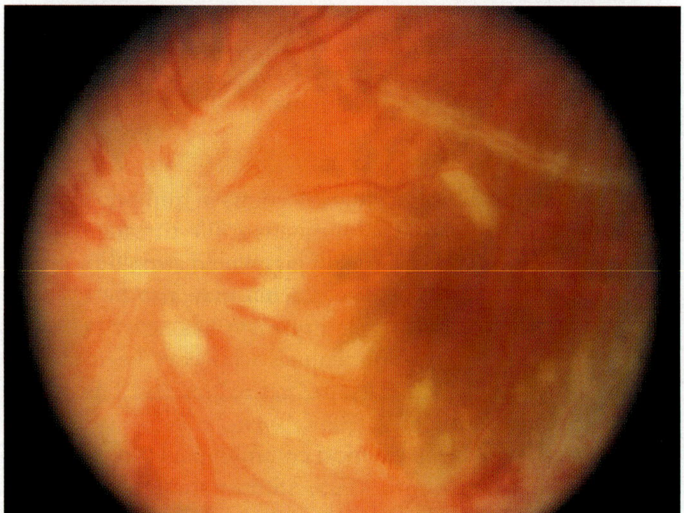

Fig. 10.139 Active Cytomegalovirus Retinitis. Note the retinal sheathing, retinal vasculitis, and the necrotizing optic neuritis.

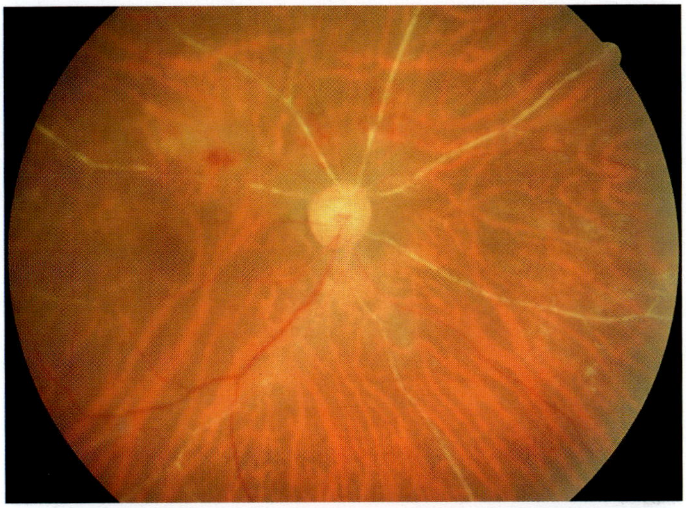

Fig. 10.140 Burned-Out Cytomegalovirus Retinitis.

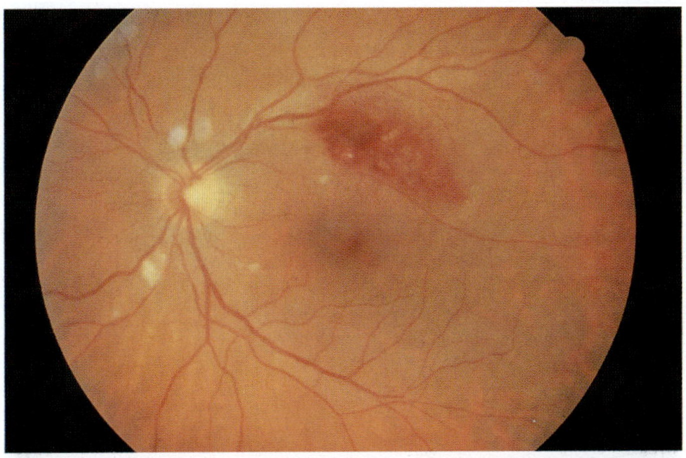

A

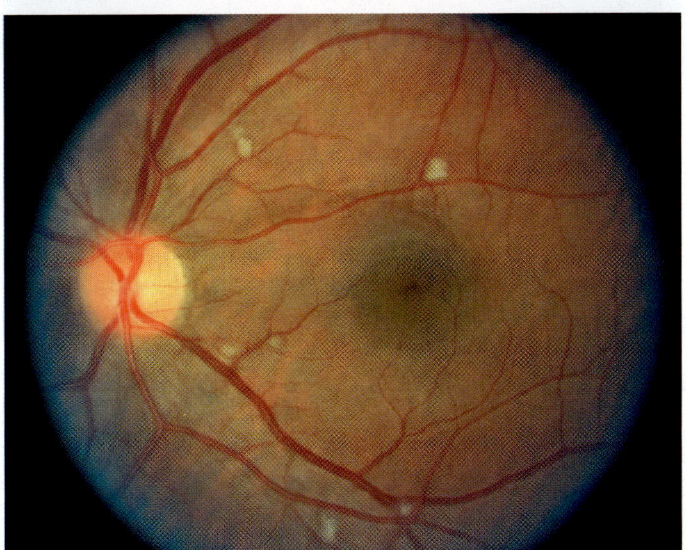

B

Fig. 10.141 (A) Human immunodeficiency virus (HIV) chorioretinitis. Note the large flame-shaped hemorrhage and the cotton-wool spots. (B) Another patient with HIV chorioretinitis. Note the many cotton-wool spots.

patient with HIV chorioretinitis infection. Again, notice the many cotton-wool spots. Roth spots are commonly seen in patients with HIV chorioretinitis. Fig. 10.114 shows examples of Roth spots in a patient with leukemia.

There are several important tumors of the ocular fundus. *Retinoblastoma* is the most common malignant tumor of the sensory retina. It has been estimated to occur in 1 per 18,000 live births. The cancer is generally found in children younger than 6; it is most commonly diagnosed in children aged 1 to 2 years. It can be sporadic or familial, with an autosomal dominant mode of inheritance. The abnormal gene has been localized to the long arm of chromosome 13. Persons who inherit the gene are more likely to have bilateral retinoblastomas than those without the gene. Children with retinoblastomas present with leukocoria or a white pupil. Fig. 10.142 shows a photograph of a child with leukocoria of the left eye. Leukocoria is present because most of the globe contains a large white tumor, which is often lobulated. Fig. 10.143 shows the right and left retinas of a child with bilateral retinoblastomas. Note the large tumor mass in the left retina.

The two most important tumors of the choroid are the choroidal nevus and the choroidal melanoma. The *choroidal nevus* is the most common fundus tumor. It is commonly a flat, slate-gray lesion with a slightly ill-defined border. Fig. 10.144 shows a choroidal nevus. A nevus must be differentiated from a choroidal melanoma. Choroidal *melanoma* is the most common primary intraocular malignancy. It occurs in approximately 6 per 1 million people per year. It has no sex predisposition and is usually nonfamilial. It is rare in African Americans and is most common in white persons. Unlike the choroidal nevus, the choroidal melanoma has depth and is frequently dome-shaped or mushroom-shaped. Fig. 10.145 shows the retina of a patient with a choroidal melanoma.

Colobomas of the retina and choroid are congenital defects in these tissues caused by failure of the embryonic fissure to fuse correctly. Colobomas appear as large white areas in which the retina or choroid is absent, and thus the white sclera is seen. In addition, retinal vessels may cross into the lesion. Typically, colobomas are seen in the inferior aspect of the fundus because the embryonic fissure is inferonasal in the developing eye. Fig. 10.146 shows the classic features of a coloboma. See also Fig. 10.66, which shows an iris coloboma.

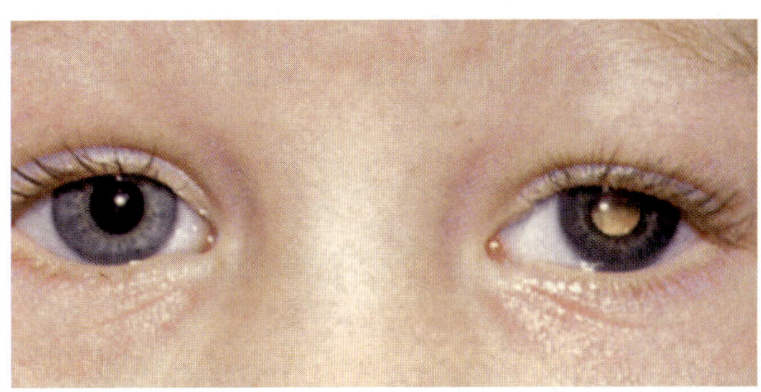

Fig. 10.142 Leukocoria. (From Kanski JJ, Nischal KK: *Ophthalmology: clinical signs and differential diagnosis*, St. Louis, 2000, Mosby.)

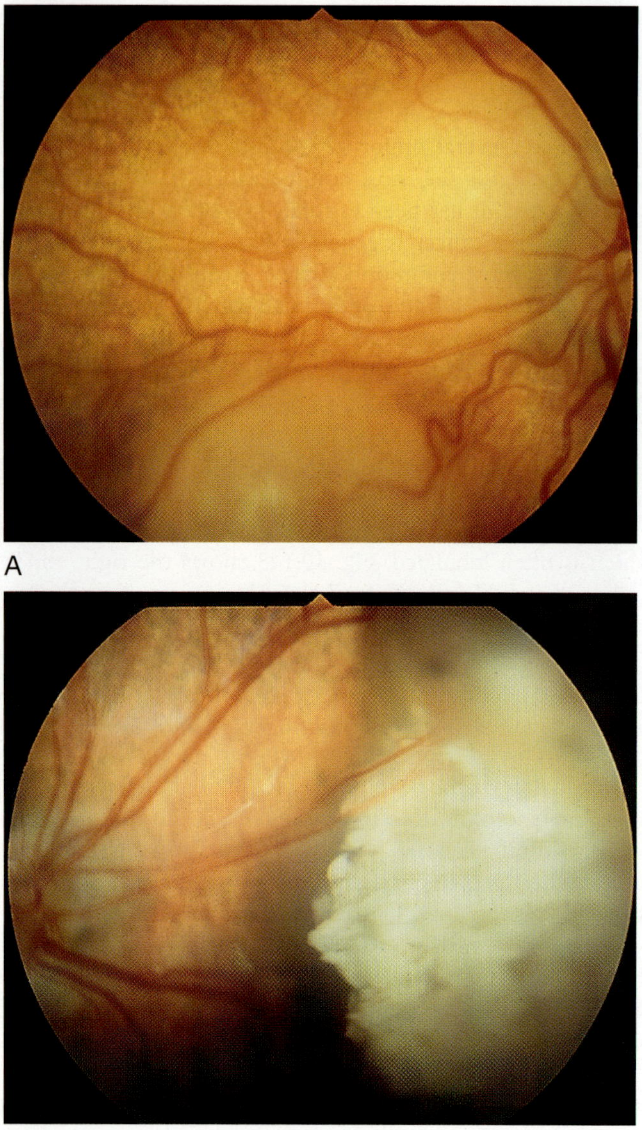

A

B

Fig. 10.143 Retinoblastoma. (A) Right retina. (B) Left retina.

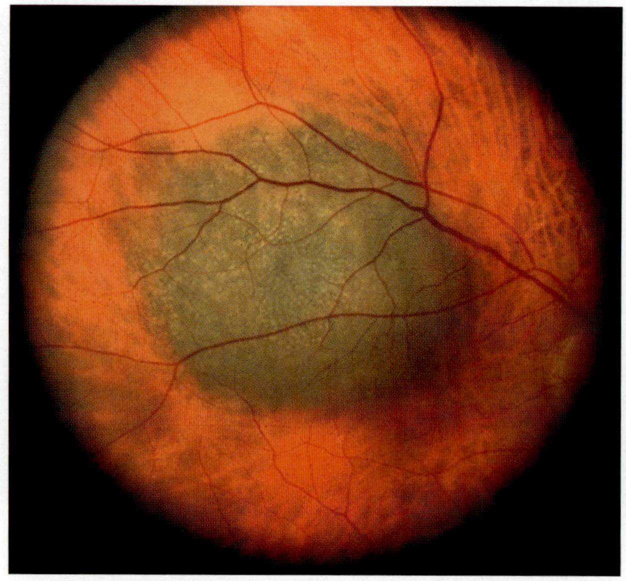

Fig. 10.145 Choroidal Malignant Melanoma.

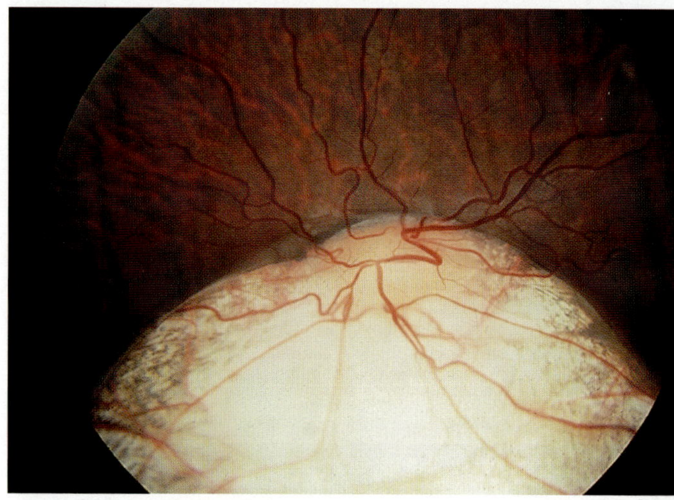

Fig. 10.146 Retinal Coloboma.

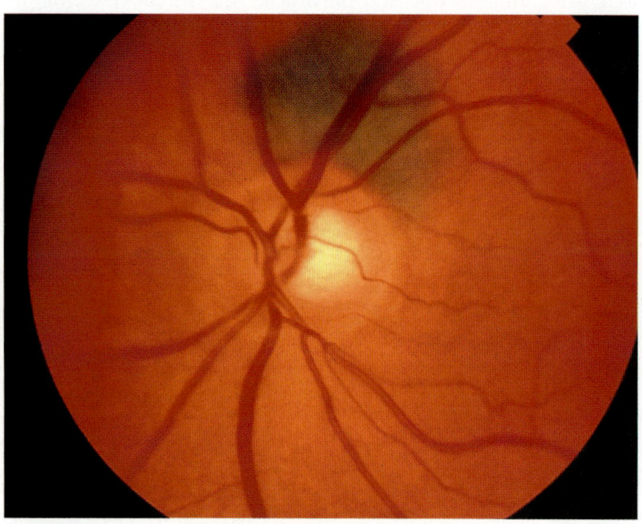

Fig. 10.144 Choroidal Nevus.

Retinal tears and detachments are painless. Seeing floaters or flashes is a warning sign that someone may have retinal tears. The signs of retinal tears and detachment include vision reduction and a shadow or curtain in the peripheral vision. Typically, the shadow will move toward the center of vision over hours, days, or weeks. The patient may also experience a shower of floaters that cloud the vision. Acute retinal tears with or without flashes and floaters pose a risk because fluid can enter through the tear under the retina and lift the retina off, causing a retinal detachment. Fig. 10.147 shows a giant retinal tear. A large area of bare choroid is visible through the break.

Retinitis pigmentosa (*RP*) is a very rare, genetically determined degenerative disease of the retina with an onset seen between the ages of 6 and 12 years. It is more common in boys than girls and almost always bilateral. An estimated 100,000 people in the United States have RP, mainly caused by gene

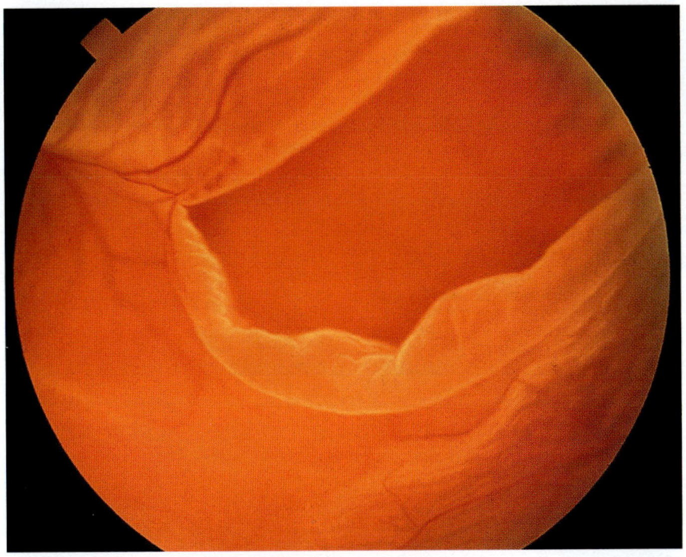

Fig. 10.147 Retinal Tear.

mutations inherited from one or both parents. Mutated genes give the wrong instructions to photoreceptor cells, instructing them to make an incorrect protein or too little or too much protein. Many different gene mutations exist in RP. Night blindness is the first symptom, followed by a gradually progressive constriction of the peripheral fields and, eventually blurred vision. Evaluation of the retina reveals the very characteristic picture of black "bone spicule" pigmentary changes, particularly in the midperipheral retina. Macular degeneration occurs in the late stages. No treatment is available, but recent studies have shown that proper vitamin A supplementation can postpone blindness by up to 10 years in some individuals. Fig. 10.148A is the classic picture of RP. A close-up photograph of the "bone spicules" is seen in Fig. 10.148B.

A *staphyloma* is an outward bulging of the sclera and protrusion of intraocular contents at a point where the sclera is too thin to support the ocular structure. When present in the posterior pole, as shown in Fig. 10.149, it is associated with degenerative high myopia. Macular holes, retinal tears, and retinal detachment are common. Staphylomas may be congenital or occur after trauma or chronic inflammation that has weakened the scleral wall. In most cases, no therapy is available. In severe cases, the staphyloma gradually enlarges, and enucleation may be necessary.

Abnormalities of gaze are not uncommon. *Ophthalmoplegia* is paralysis of the eye muscles. Lesions causing this paralysis may be acute, chronic, or progressive. The abnormalities of this condition are demonstrated in Fig. 10.150. When the patient is asked to look straight ahead, the right eye is abducted. Notice the ptosis of the right eyelid. When the patient is asked to look to the far right, both eyes move normally, although the right ptosis is well seen. When the patient is asked to look to the far left, the right eye cannot cross the midline. This patient has acute oculomotor paralysis secondary to a fungal lesion near the nucleus of the third cranial nerve.

When the patient shown in Fig. 10.151 is asked to look straight ahead, or to the right, both eyes move smoothly

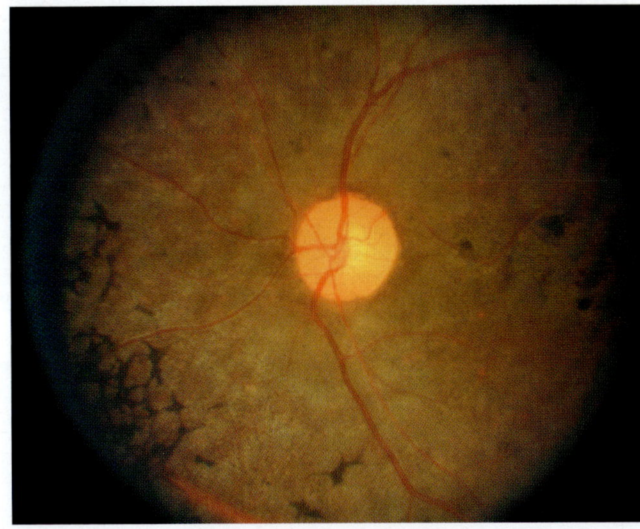

A

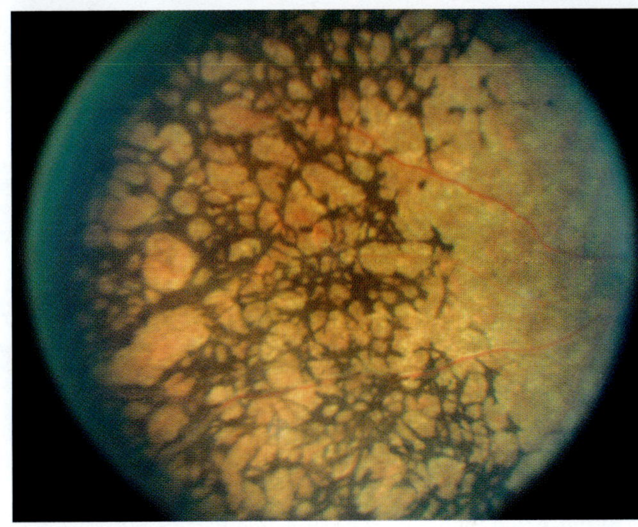

B

Fig. 10.148 (A) Retinitis pigmentosa. Note the black "bone spicules" in the midperipheral retina. (B) Close-up photograph of the "bone spicules."

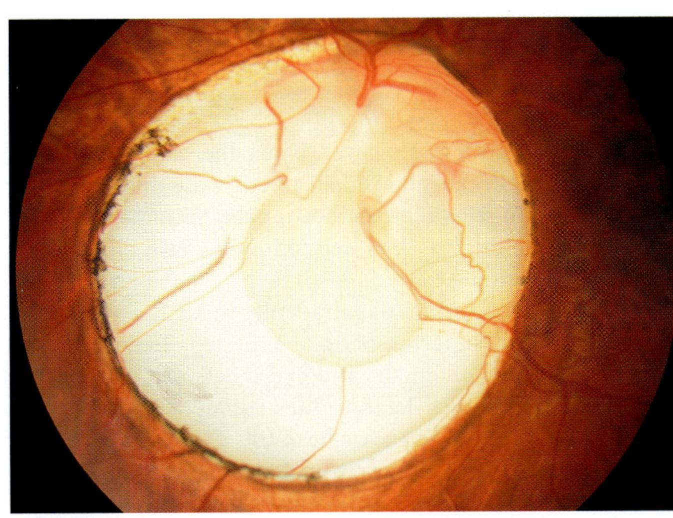

Fig. 10.149 Staphyloma.

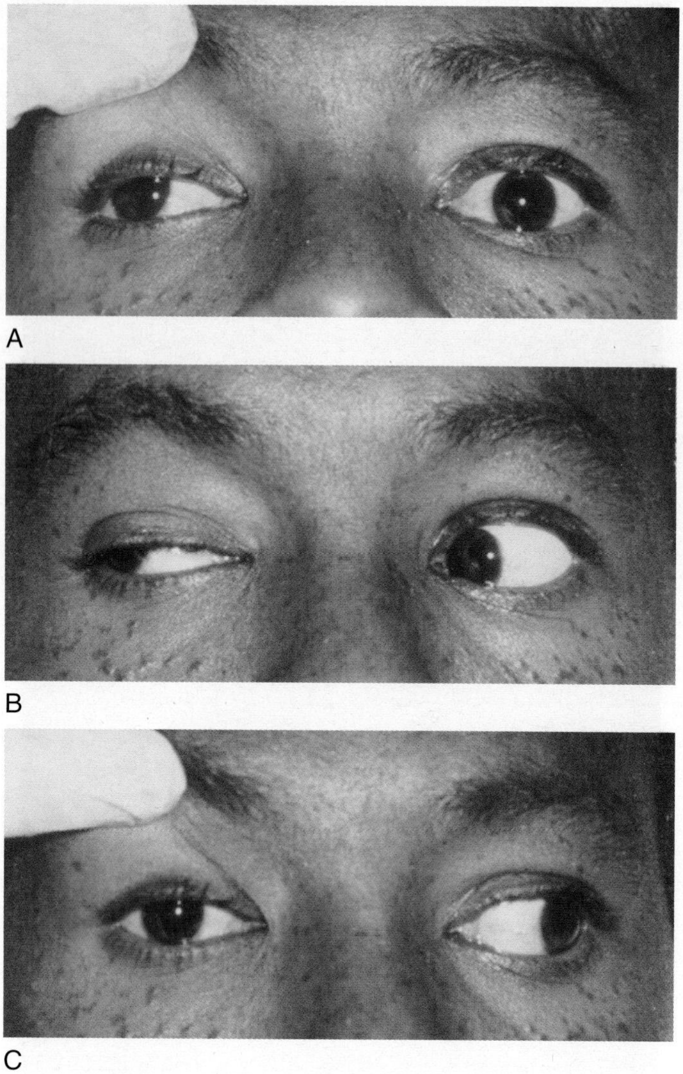

Fig. 10.150 Acute Right Oculomotor Nerve Paralysis. (A) When the patient is asked to look straight ahead, the right eye is turned laterally (note the position of the corneal light reflexes). The right palpebral fissure is markedly narrowed, requiring the eyelid to be elevated to visualize the position of the eye. (B) When the patient is asked to look to the far right, both eyes are able to move in that direction. Note the marked ptosis of the right eyelid. (C) When the patient is asked to look to the far left, the right eye cannot cross the midline.

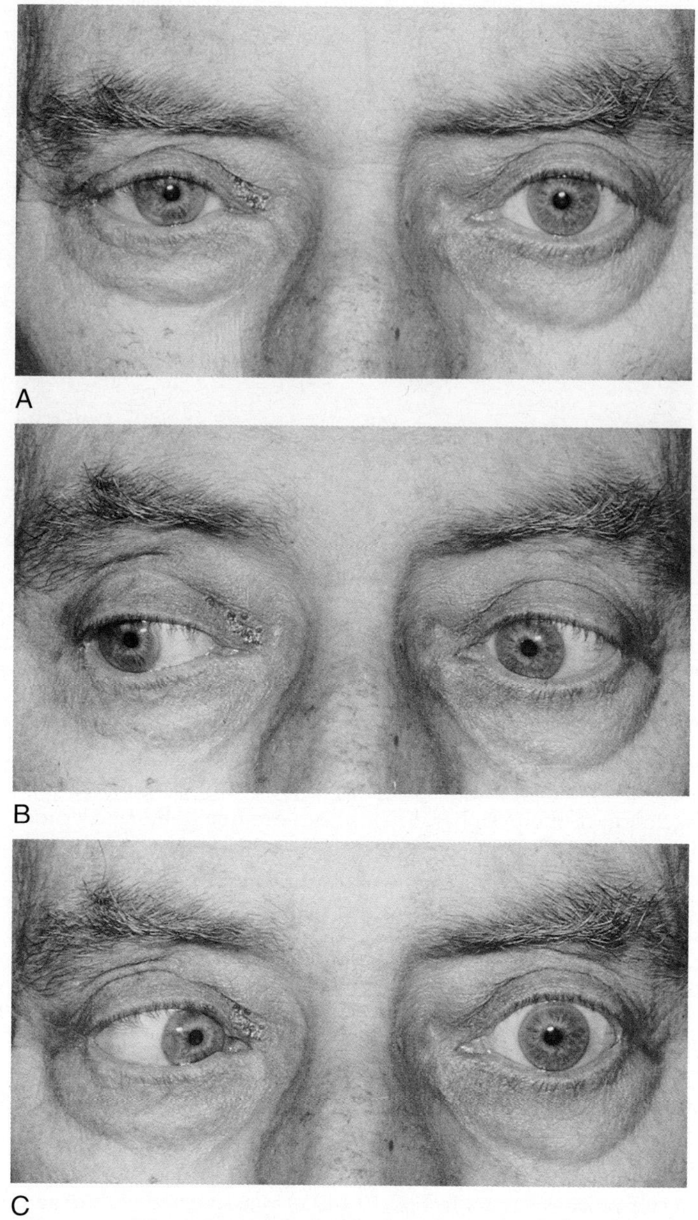

Fig. 10.151 Acute Left Abducens Paralysis. (A) When the patient is asked to look straight ahead, both eyes are straight. (B) When the patient is asked to look to the right, both eyes turn normally. (C) When the patient is asked to look to the left, the left eye cannot cross the midline; this indicates left abducens palsy.

in the correct motion. However, when the patient is asked to look to the left, the left eye fails to cross the midline. Diplopia occurred due to a left abducens palsy secondary to carcinomatous meningitis. Another common cause of diplopia is diabetes mellitus.

Head tilt may be a sign of extraocular muscle weakness. A weakness of the superior oblique muscle, often resulting from birth trauma secondary to forceps delivery, may not be recognized until much later in life. Diplopia may develop associated with a characteristic head tilt. The head is habitually held in such a position as to avoid horizontal, vertical, or torsional diplopia. Fig. 10.152 illustrates the classic head tilts associated with paralysis of the oblique muscles. With a *superior oblique palsy* (see Figs. 10.152A and B), the face is turned, and the head is tilted to the uninvolved side; the chin is depressed. With an *inferior oblique palsy* (see Figs. 10.152C and D), the face is turned to the uninvolved side, the head is tilted to the involved side, and the chin is elevated. Head tilt also may be seen in paralysis of the vertical rectus muscles.

The retinal findings of common diseases are summarized in Table 10.11. Many common diseases display their disorders at the macula of the retina. Table 10.12 provides differentiation of some of these lesions.

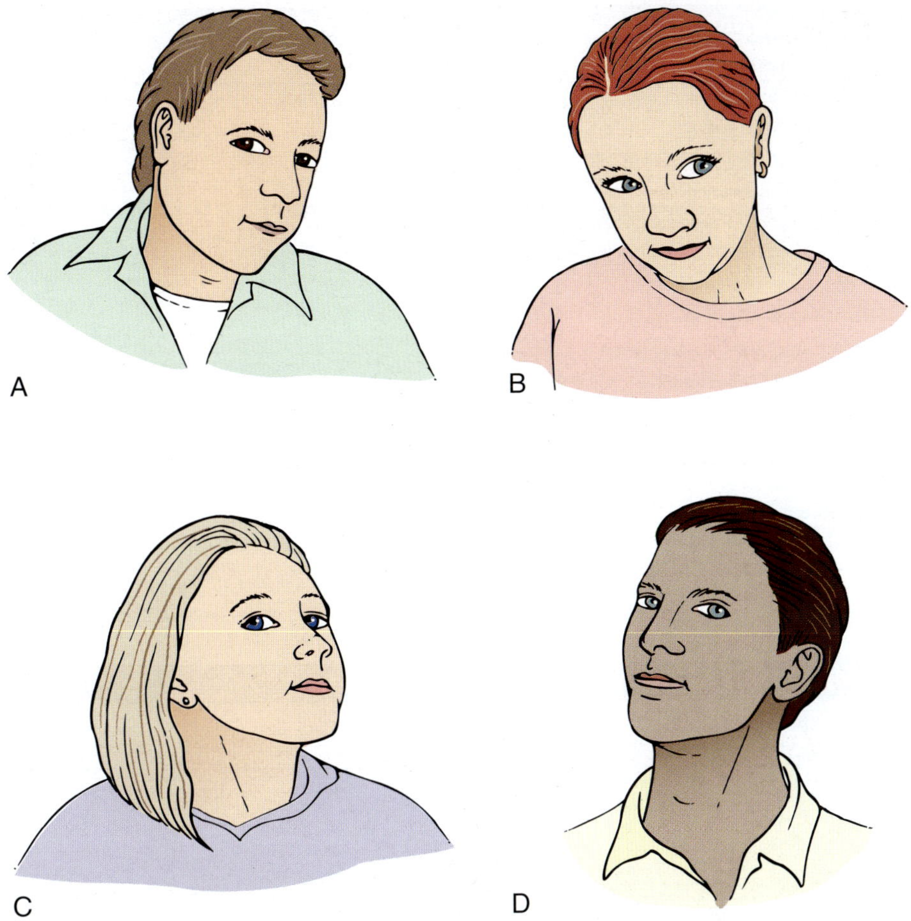

Fig. 10.152 Classic Head-Tilt Positions in Patients With Palsies of the Oblique Muscles. (A) Right superior oblique. (B) Left superior oblique. (C) Right inferior oblique. (D) Left inferior oblique.

TABLE 10.11 Retinal Characteristics of Common Diseases

Condition	Primary Findings	Distribution	Secondary Findings
Diabetes (see Figs. 10.93–10.105)	Microaneurysms Neovascularization Retinitis proliferans[a]	Posterior pole	Hard exudates[b] Deep hemorrhages Retinal venous occlusions Vitreous hemorrhages
Hypertension (see Figs. 10.84, 10.87, and 10.106–10.110)	Arteriolar narrowing "Copper wiring" Flame hemorrhages Arteriovenous nicking	Posterior pole	Hard exudates Deep hemorrhages Retinal venous occlusions Vitreous hemorrhages
Papilledema (see Figs. 10.111–10.113)	Hyperemia of the disc Venous enlargement Retinal hemorrhages Disc elevation Loss of spontaneous venous pulsations Cotton-wool spots	On or near disc	Hard exudates Optic atrophy, late
Retinal vein occlusion (see Figs. 10.121 and 10.122)	Hemorrhages Neovascularization	Confined to area drained by affected vein	Exudates
Retinal arterial occlusion (see Figs. 10.115–10.120)	Pallor of retina Decreased width of artery Embolus possibly visible	Confined to area supplied	Optic atrophy, late

Continued

TABLE 10.11 Retinal Characteristics of Common Diseases—cont'd

Condition	Primary Findings	Distribution	Secondary Findings
Arteriolar sclerosis	Widening of light reflex "Copper wiring" Arteriovenous nicking	Throughout retina	Decrease in retinal pigment
Blood dyscrasias (see Fig. 10.114)	Diffuse hemorrhages Venous dilation common Roth spots (hemorrhagic lesions with white centers)		
Sickle cell disease	Sharp cutoff of arterioles Arteriovenous anastomoses Neovascularization in "sea fan" formations (resembling the marine organism with a similar pattern)	Peripheral retina	Vitreous hemorrhages Retinal detachments

[a]A growth of a light-colored sheet of opaque connective tissue over the inner surface of the retina. Neovascularization of the tissue with tortuous vessels is seen. These vessels bleed easily.
[b]*Exudate* is the term used for small intraretinal lesions caused by retinal disturbances in a variety of disorders.

TABLE 10.12 Differentiation of Common Macular Lesions

Feature	Macular Degeneration (See Figs. 10.125 and 10.127)	Macular Star (See Fig. 10.109)	Circinate Retinopathy (See Fig. 10.96)
Appearance	Pigmentary mottling, often with hemorrhage	Whitish exudate that radiates around macula	Broken ring-shaped whitish exudate around macula
Etiologic factors		Hypertension Papilledema Papillitis Central retinal vein occlusion	Diabetes Central retinal vein occlusion

USEFUL VOCABULARY

Listed here are the specific roots that are important for understanding the terminology related to eye diseases.

Root	Pertaining to	Example	Definition
blepharo-	eyelid	***blepharo***plasty	Surgical repair of eyelid
choroi-	choroid	***choroi***ditis	Inflammation of the choroid
-cor- (or -kor-)	pupil	aniso***cor***ia	Unequal pupils
cyclo-	ciliary body	***cyclo***plegia	Paralysis of accommodation
dacryo-	tear	***dacryo***cystitis	Inflammation of the lacrimal sac
-duction	to lead	ab***duction***	Turning outward
irid-	iris	***irid***ectomy	Surgical excision of part of the iris
kerato-	cornea	***kerato***pathy	Disease of the cornea
lacri-	tears	***lacri***mal	Pertaining to the tears
nyct-	night	***nyct***alopia	Night blindness
-ocul-	eye	intra***ocul***ar	Within the eye
ophthalm-	eye	***ophthalm***oscope	Instrument for visualizing the retina
-opsia	vision	hemian***opsia***	Blindness in half of the visual field
-phak(os)-	lens	a***phak***ia	Without a lens
photo-	light	***photo***sensitive	Sensitive to light
presby-	old	***presby***opia	Impairment of vision as a result of increasing age
tars-	eyelid structure	***tars***orrhaphy	Surgical suturing of the lid
-trop-	turn	eso***trop***ia	Eye turning inward

WRITING UP THE PHYSICAL EXAMINATION

Listed here are examples of the write-up for the examination of the eye.

- Visual acuity is OD 20/20 and OS 20/30 according to the standard Snellen chart. The visual fields by confrontation field testing are normal. Examination of the external structures of the eyes is normal. The pupils are equal, round, and reactive to light and accommodation.[1] The EOMs are normal. On ophthalmoscopic examination, the disc margins are sharp. A normal cup-disc ratio is present. The vasculature is normal.
- Visual acuity is OD 20/60 and OS 20/20 according to the pocket visual acuity card. Examination of the eyes reveals marked conjunctival injection on the right with a dilated pupil on the same side. The pupils are round and are reactive to light. The visual fields by confrontation field testing are normal. The optic disc margins are sharp, and the vascularity of both retinas appears normal.
- The patient is able to read the newspaper without corrective lenses. The EOMs are normal. The left pupil is miotic and is 2 mm smaller than the right pupil. A mild ptosis of the left upper lid is present. Both pupils react to light directly and consensually. Confrontation fields are within normal limits. Funduscopic examination is within normal limits.
- The visual acuity with corrected lenses appears normal. There is a paralysis of abduction of the left eye, accompanied by diplopia on attempted left lateral gaze. The pupils are equal, round, and reactive to light. The optic disc margins are sharp. The vasculature is normal.
- There is decreased visual acuity in both eyes. The patient has difficulty reading ¼-inch (6.35-mm) print in the newspaper at approximately 6 inches (15 cm) with his right eye. There is OS NLP. The examination of the external eye is normal. The EOMs are intact. The left optic disc margin is slightly blurred on its nasal aspect. The cup-disc ratio is normal. There are multiple, soft, cotton-wool exudates seen bilaterally. A large, flame-shaped hemorrhage is seen in the right eye at the 2 o'clock position. Arteriovenous nicking is present bilaterally.
- The visual acuity is OD 20/40 and OS 20/100 according to the pocket visual acuity card. A bitemporal hemianopsia is present by confrontation field testing. EOMs are normal. Ophthalmoscopic examination reveals blurring of both optic discs with loss of spontaneous venous pulsations. A flame-shaped hemorrhage is present in the right eye one disc diameter at the 10 o'clock position.

[1]Often abbreviated as PERRLA, although accommodation cannot really be tested. EOM, Extraocular movement; NLP, no light perception; OD, oculus dexter (right eye); OS, oculus sinister (left eye).

FULL VIDEO

- Video 10.8 Full video: Examination of the eye

REVIEW QUESTIONS

1. **Regarding the characteristics of narrow-angle glaucoma, which statement is most correct?**
   - **A.** 45% of all glaucoma cases are narrow-angle glaucoma.
   - **B.** The anterior chamber is usually normal in narrow-angle glaucoma.
   - **C.** Visual fields are involved early in narrow-angle glaucoma.
   - **D.** There is a sudden onset of symptoms with narrow-angle glaucoma.
   - **E.** Treatment of narrow-angle glaucoma is the same as the treatment for simple glaucoma.
2. **The 29-year-old female referenced in the picture below should have which laboratory test(s) drawn?**

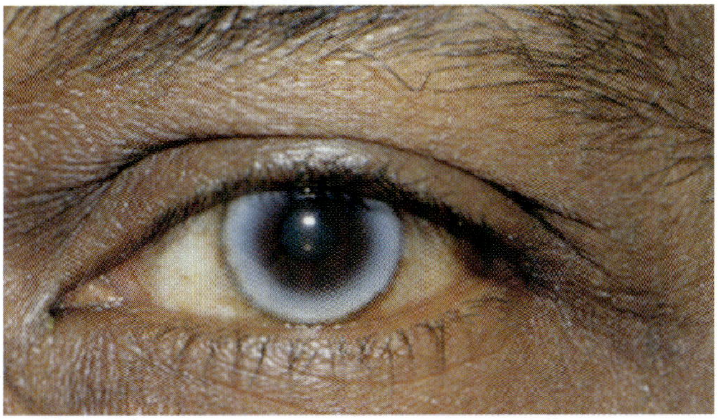

   - **A.** Total bilirubin (liver function)
   - **B.** Creatinine (kidney function)
   - **C.** Total cholesterol (lipid metabolism)
   - **D.** None, as it is a normal finding
3. **The 60-year-old-male probably has which of the following symptoms?**

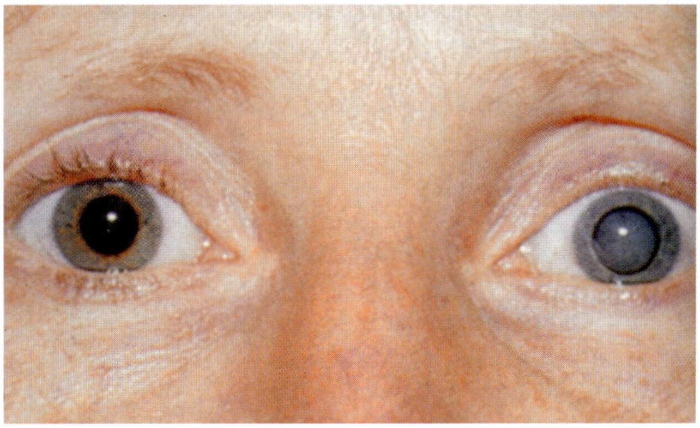

   - **A.** Left eye, tearing
   - **B.** Left eye, decreased vision
   - **C.** Left eye, afferent pupillary defect
   - **D.** Right eye, efferent pupillary defect
   - **E.** Right eye, tearing

4. The eye lesion on the lower lid shown in the referenced picture is on a 65-year-old male. Notice the raised margins. Which statement below is most correct?

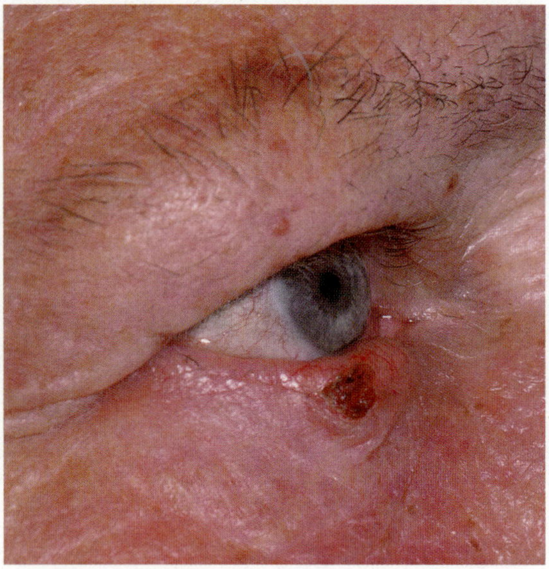

A. The lesion grows by direct invasion.
B. The lesion metastasizes frequently.
C. The lesion is highly malignant.
D. The lesion is often painful.
E. The lesion is more common in females.

5. The photo taken below with a specialized technique shows glands in the upper tarsus of a 45-year-old female. Which statement below is most correct?

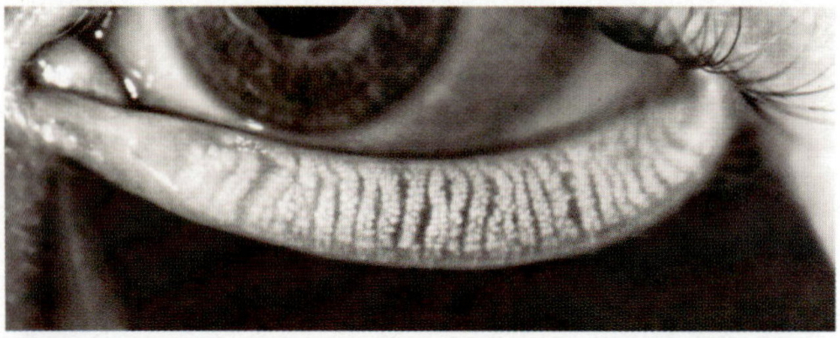

A. These glands produce a watery secretion when a patient cries.
B. These glands produce an oily secretion to lubricate the cornea.
C. These glands develop after puberty.
D. These glands are abnormal.
E. Inspissated secretions of these glands is caused by herpes zoster.

6. Which of the muscle actions is correct?
A. Medial rectus – abduction of eye
B. Lateral rectus – adduction of eye
C. Inferior rectus – abduction of eye
D. Superior rectus – abduction of eye
E. Superior oblique – abduction of eye

7. Which of the statements about the optic disc is correct?
A. It is located at the nasal aspect of the posterior pole.
B. The optic disc is ovoid, 2.5–3.0 mm in diameter.
C. It is darker in color than the surrounding retina.
D. The physiologic cup occupies approximately 50% of the disc diameter.
E. Asian patients may have pigmentation at the disc margins.

8. Which of the statements about the macula is *incorrect*?
A. It is a small, round area approximately the size of the disc.
B. It is located 3.5 mm temporal to the disc.
C. It is devoid of retinal vessels.
D. It is composed only of rods.
E. Detailed vision and color perception is related to cones.

9. Which of the statements about the subconjunctival hemorrhage seen in the patient below is *incorrect*?

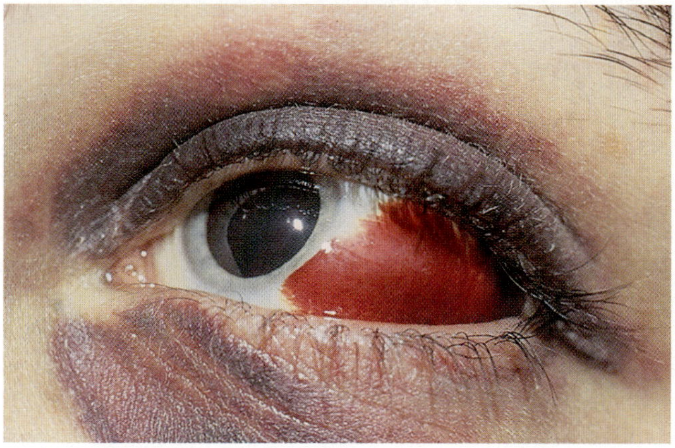

A. It is a common, benign condition.
B. It is often seen in both eyes.
C. It is caused commonly after a bout of severe coughing.
D. It can be seen after sneezing or a sustained Valsalva maneuver.
E. It may occur because of elevated blood pressure.

10. Which of the statements about pupillary abnormalities is correct?
A. Adie tonic pupil is often bilateral.
B. An Argyll Robertson pupil is reactive to light.
C. Horner syndrome produces a pupil that is miotic.
D. Adie tonic pupil is miotic.
E. Horner syndrome produces a pupil that is unreactive to accommodation.

BIBLIOGRAPHY

Available online.

11

The Ear and Nose

Mark H. Swartz

Yet it was not possible for me to say to people, "Speak louder, shout, for I am deaf." ... Alas! how could I declare the weakness of a sense which in me ought to be more acute than in others—a sense which formerly I possessed in highest perfection, a perfection such as few in my profession enjoy, or ever have enjoyed.

Ludwig van Beethoven (1770–1827)

VIDEOS

Video 11.1	Examining the external ear
Video 11.2	Palpating the external ear
Video 11.3	Testing auditory acuity
Video 11.4	Performing the Rinne test
Video 11.5	Performing the Weber test
Video 11.6	Using the otoscope
Video 11.7	Inspecting the nose
Video 11.8	Inspecting the frontal, ethmoid, and maxillary sinuses
Video 11.9	Full video: Examination of the ear, sinuses, and nose

GENERAL CONSIDERATIONS

Most people are fortunate to hear music, noise, and, above all, speech. Sometimes "silence is golden," but silence can be golden only when a person can choose not to hear.

Typically, children have the physical ability to speak, but they need to learn how to do it. Their ears and brain work together to process sounds, which they then imitate. If they can't hear sounds, they can't copy them, and this prevents them from developing their language skills. Without hearing sounds, they won't be able to form words, sentences, or speech.

Tinnitus, or ringing in the ears, is often accompanied by some level of hearing loss. It is uncommon to experience tinnitus without any noticeable hearing loss. However, individuals who are born deaf do not typically report experiencing tinnitus.

STRUCTURE AND PHYSIOLOGY

The Ear

The ear can be divided into the following four parts:

1. External ear
2. Middle ear
3. Inner ear
4. Nervous innervation

A cross-section through the ear is illustrated in Fig. 11.1.

The *external ear* consists of the *pinna* and the *external auditory canal.* The pinna is composed of elastic cartilage and skin. Fig. 11.2 illustrates the parts of the pinna.

The external auditory canal is approximately 1 inch in length. Its outer third is cartilaginous, and its inner two-thirds are composed of bone. Within the cartilaginous portion are hair follicles; pilosebaceous glands; and *ceruminous,* or wax-producing, glands. Secretions of these ceruminous glands, debris, and desquamated keratin are "earwax." The glands secrete their product around the base of the hairs, as depicted in Fig. 11.3. Fig. 11.4 shows earwax in the external ear canal. Earwax color and consistency depend on the type of cerumen secreted, the amount of keratin present, and the presence of debris. The soft, brown form shown here is the most common type. The cartilaginous portion of the ear is continuous with the pinna. The canal curves slightly, being directed forward and downward. The innervation to most of the external canal is through the trigeminal, or fifth cranial, nerve. The innermost portion of the canal is innervated by the vagus, or tenth cranial nerve.[a]

The *middle ear,* or tympanic cavity, consists of connections to the *mastoid antrum,* to its connecting air cells, and, through the *eustachian tube,* to the nasopharynx. The function of the eustachian tube is to provide an air passage from the nasopharynx to the ear to equalize pressure on both sides of the tympanic membrane. The eustachian tube is usually closed but opens during swallowing and yawning.

The *tympanic membrane* forms the lateral boundary of the middle ear. The medial border is formed by the *cochlea.* The tympanic membrane is gray, with blood vessels at its periphery. It is composed of two parts: the *pars flaccida* and the *pars tensa.* The pars flaccida is the upper, smaller portion of the tympanic membrane. The pars tensa comprises the remainder of the membrane. The handle of the malleus is a prominent landmark and divides the pars tensa into the *anterior* and *posterior folds.*

[a]On occasion, coughing may result when the distal external canal is cleaned. This cough reflex is mediated through the vagus nerve.

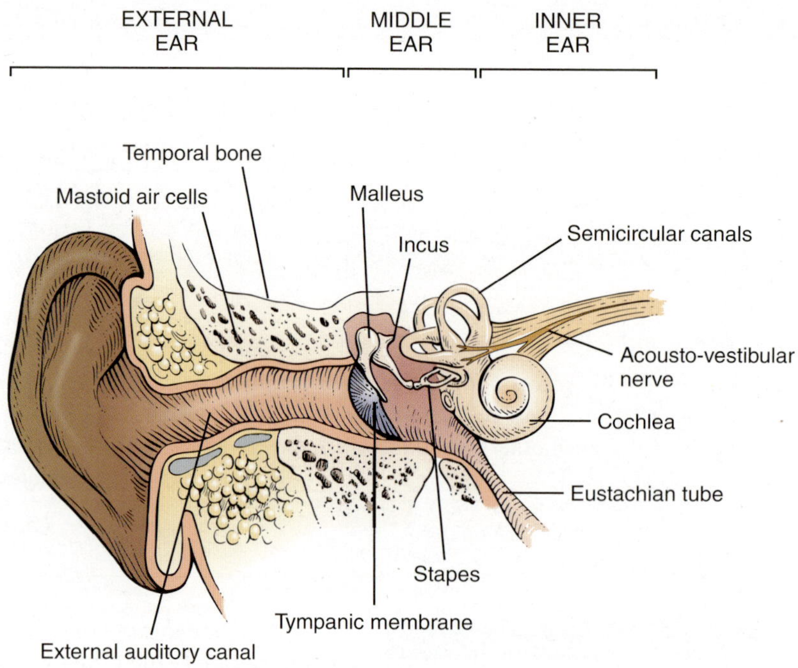

Fig. 11.1 Cross-Sectional View Through the Ear.

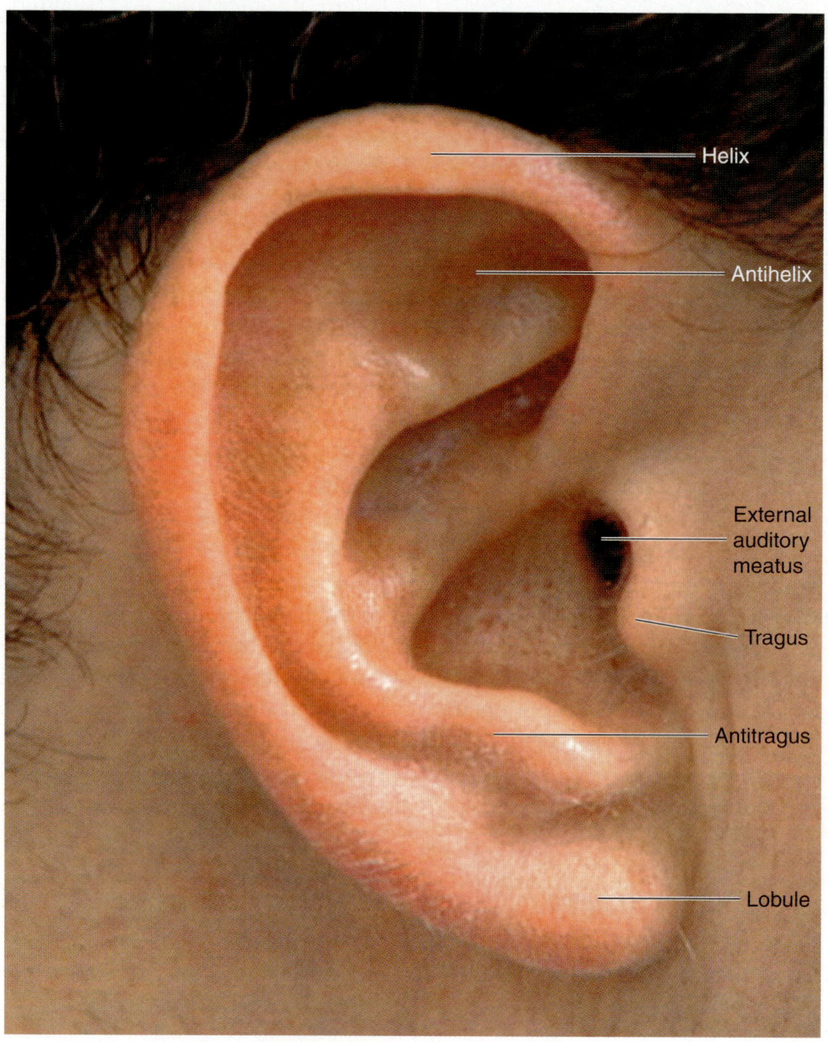

Fig. 11.2 Landmarks of the Pinna.

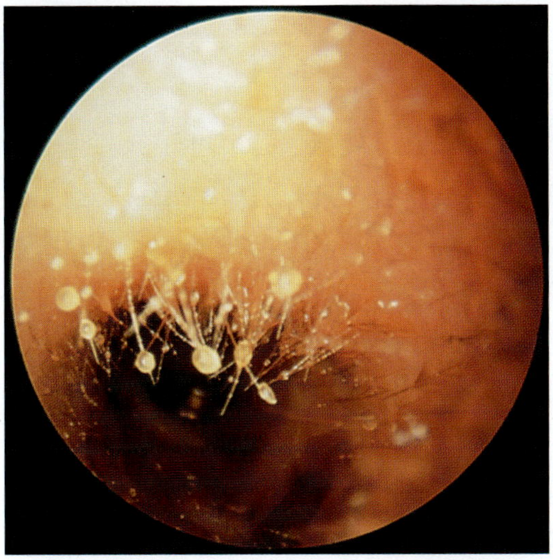

Fig. 11.3 Earwax on the Base of Hairs.

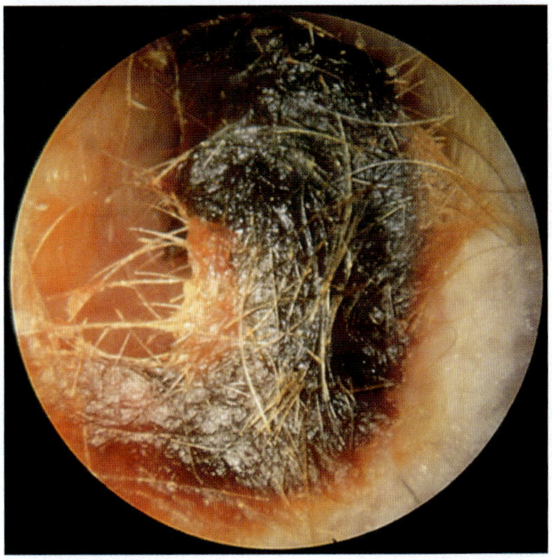

Fig. 11.4 Earwax in the External Ear Canal.

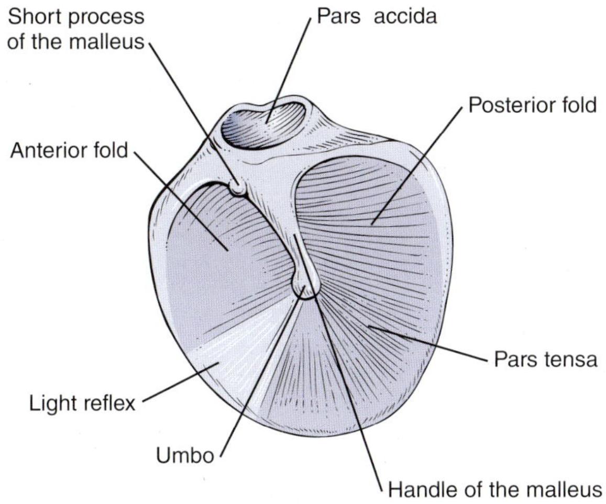

Fig. 11.5 Landmarks of the Left Tympanic Membrane.

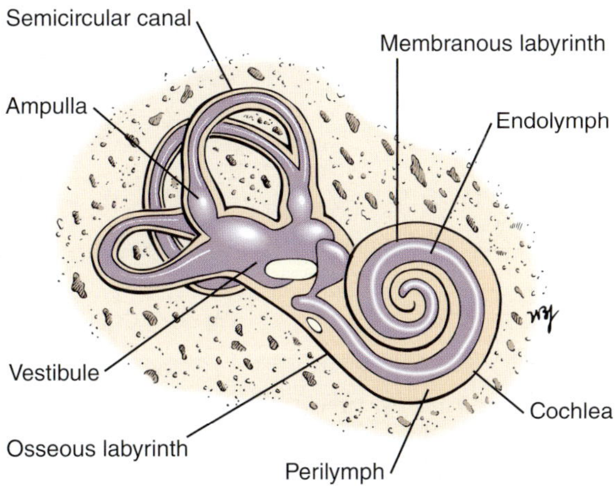

Fig. 11.6 Cross-Sectional View Through the Cochlea.

The tympanic membrane is set slightly at an angle to the external canal. The inferior portion is more medial than the superior portion. Fig. 11.5 illustrates the left tympanic membrane.

Sound is conducted from the tympanic membrane to the inner ear by three *auditory ossicles:* the *malleus,* the *incus,* and the *stapes.* The malleus is the largest ossicle. At its upper end is the *short process,* which appears as a tiny knob. The *handle* (long process) of the malleus, or *manubrium,* extends downward to its tip, called the *umbo.* The short process and the handle of the malleus attach directly to the tympanic membrane. At the other end of the malleus is its head, which articulates with the incus. The incus then articulates with the head of the stapes, the footplate of which attaches to the *oval window* of the inner ear.

The middle ear also contains two muscles: the *tensor tympani* and the *stapedius.* The tensor tympani muscle attaches to the malleus, and the stapedius muscle attaches to the neck of the stapes. The trigeminal nerve innervates the tensor tympani muscle, and the stapedius muscle is innervated by the facial, or seventh cranial, nerve. Both muscles contract in response to high-intensity sound.

The facial nerve passes through the middle ear and provides, in addition to the nerve to the stapedius muscle, the *chorda tympani* nerve. The chorda tympani nerve travels through the middle ear between the incus and the malleus and exits near the temporomandibular joint. It carries taste sensation from the anterior two-thirds of the tongue.

The *inner ear* is the end-organ for hearing and equilibrium. It is situated in the petrous portion of the temporal bone and consists of the three *semicircular canals,* the *vestibule,* and the *cochlea.* Each of these structures is made up of three parts: the *osseous labyrinth,* the *membranous labyrinth,* and the *space between.* The osseous labyrinth is the outer bone casing. The inner membranous labyrinth is within the osseous labyrinth and contains a fluid called *endolymph* and the sensory structures. Finally, the space between these two labyrinths is filled with another fluid called *perilymph.* A cross-section through this area is illustrated in Fig. 11.6.

The three semicircular canals are directed posteriorly, superiorly, and horizontally. Each canal has a dilated end, the *ampulla,* the sensory end-organ for balance.

The cochlea is a snail shell-shaped structure composed of 2¾ turns. Within its membranous labyrinth is the end-organ

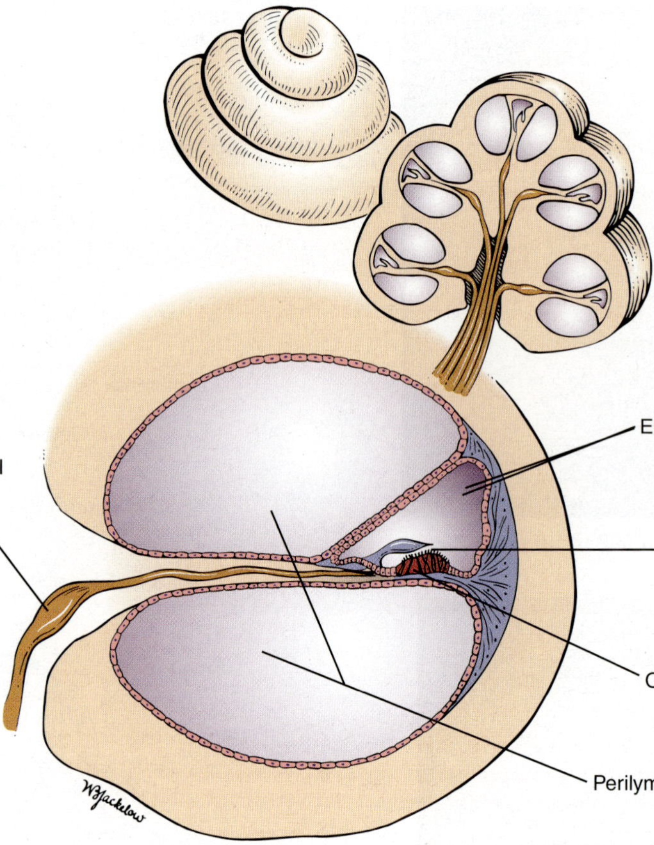

Fig. 11.7 Cross-Sectional View Through the Cochlear Duct.

for hearing. The *acoustic,* or eighth cranial, nerve consists of the *vestibular* and *cochlear* divisions. These connect to the semicircular canals and cochlea, respectively. They join and pass through the internal auditory meatus to the brainstem.

Sound waves stimulate the afferent fibers by bone conduction (BC) or *air conduction (AC).* BC is directly through the bones of the skull. AC is through the external auditory canal, tympanic membrane, and ossicles to the oval window. Most hearing is mediated by AC.

Sound waves set up vibrations that enter the external canal and are transmitted to the ossicles, which vibrate. This vibration causes an inward motion of the stapes footplate and deforms the oval window. Waves are created in the perilymphatic fluid of the labyrinth. These fluid motion changes are transmitted in a wavelike manner to the endolymphatic fluid, which distorts the *hair cells* of the *organ of Corti.* These hair cells convert the mechanical force into an electrochemical signal propagated down the acoustic nerve and interpreted as sound. It has been estimated that more than 30,000 of these afferent hair fibers constitute the auditory division. After many synapses, the impulse reaches the temporal cortex, where the appreciation of the sound occurs. A cross-section through the cochlear duct is shown in Fig. 11.7.

The sense of *balance* is achieved by visual, vestibular, and proprioceptive[b] senses. The loss of one of these senses frequently goes unnoticed. The vestibular apparatus is the most important. Motion within the endolymphatic fluid stimulates the hair cells in the ampulla of the semicircular canals. Electric impulses are transmitted to the vestibular portion of the eighth cranial nerve. Synapses occur in the vestibular and oculomotor nuclei, which send efferent fibers to the extraocular and skeletal muscles. This produces a deviation of the eyes with rapid compensatory motions to maintain gaze and increased tone in the skeletal muscles.

Any alteration in the endolymphatic mechanism may affect the control of the eyes. *Nystagmus* is an involuntary, rapid back-and-forth eye motion, which can be horizontal, vertical, rotatory, or mixed. The direction of the quick component determines the direction of the nystagmus. Abnormalities of the labyrinth tend to produce *horizontal* nystagmus, brainstem disorders often have *vertical* nystagmus, and retinal lesions may produce *ocular* nystagmus, which is slow and produces an irregular, searching quality to the eyes.

The Nose

The external nasal skeleton comprises the *nasal bones,* part of the *maxilla,* and the *cartilage.* The upper third of the skeleton is composed of nasal bones, which articulate with the maxilla and frontal bones. The lower two-thirds are made of cartilage.

The internal portion of the nose consists of two cavities divided by the *nasal septum,* which forms the medial wall of the nasal cavity. Projecting from the lateral wall are three *turbinates,* or *conchae.* The *inferior turbinate* is the largest and

[b]Sensory stimulation from within the tissues of the body about their movement or position.

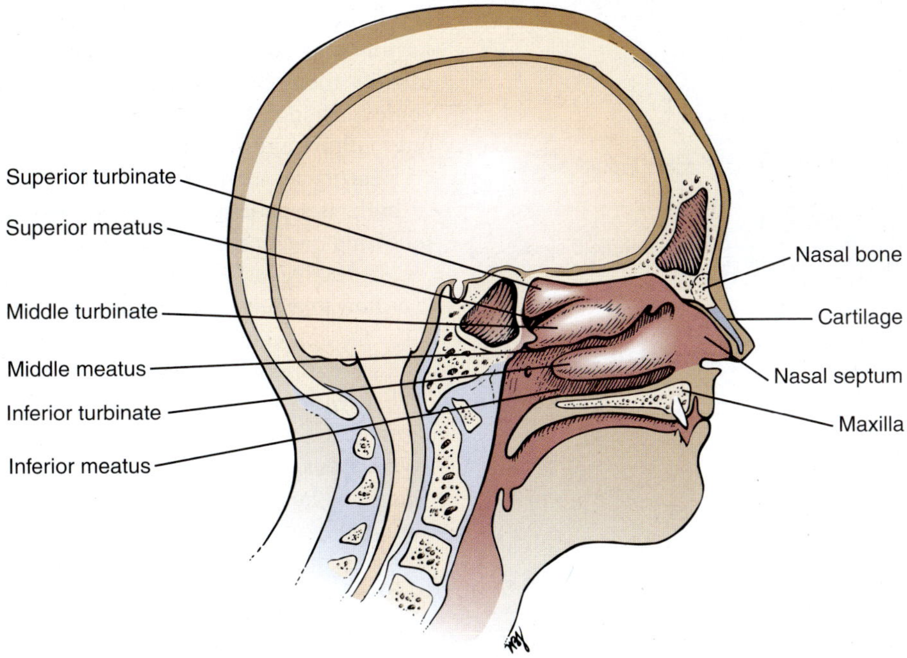

Fig. 11.8 Lateral Wall of the Nose.

contains semi-erectile tissue. Inferior to each turbinate are openings to the *paranasal sinuses*; each opening is known as a *meatus.* Each meatus is named for the turbinate above it. The *nasolacrimal duct* empties into the *inferior meatus.* The *middle meatus,* below the *middle turbinate,* contains the openings of the *frontal, maxillary,* and *anterior ethmoid sinuses.* The posterior ethmoid sinus drains into the *superior meatus.* The *olfactory region* is located high in the nose between the nasal septum and the *superior turbinate.* Fig. 11.8 illustrates the lateral wall of the nose.

The blood supply to the nose is derived from the internal and external carotid arteries. The turbinates are vascular and contain large vascular spaces. The blood vessels of the anterior nasal septum meet at an area approximately 1 inch (2.54 cm) from the mucocutaneous junction, known as *Little's area.* This is the area usually responsible for *epistaxis* or nosebleed. The blood vessels are under autonomic nervous system control. If there is an excess of *sympathetic* stimulation, the blood vessels constrict, and the vascular spaces in the turbinates shrink. If there is an increase in *parasympathetic* tone, the blood pools in the turbinates, resulting in their swelling, obstruction to airflow, and elaboration of a watery discharge.

The nerve supply to the internal area of the nose is from branches of the trigeminal nerve. The olfactory, or first cranial, nerve supply the olfactory epithelium. Moist air with the dissolved odorous particles acts as a stimulus. The nerve fibers from this area pierce the *cribriform plate* to the olfactory bulb in the brain. In humans, the olfactory receptors' ability to discern a stimulus diminishes rapidly with exposure.

The main functions of the nose are to provide the following:

- An airway
- Olfaction
- Humidification of inspired air
- Warming of inspired air
- Filtering of inspired air

The inspired air flows above and below the middle turbinate. This produces eddy currents that serve to protect the olfactory epithelium in the superior portion of the nose. The nasal mucosa produces mucus, increasing relative humidity to nearly 100%. This prevents the epithelium from drying out and helps prevent possible infection. The air, by its circulation around the conchae, is warmed to nearly body temperature by the time it enters the nasopharynx. The mucus and the nasal hairs, or *vibrissae,* prevent particulate matter from entering the distal respiratory tract. The mucous blanket is swept posteriorly by the *cilia* and is swallowed. The mucus also contains immunoglobulins and enzymes, which serve as a line of defense.

The four *paranasal sinuses* of the head—the maxillary, the ethmoid, the frontal, and the sphenoid—are air-filled cavities lined with mucous membranes. The *maxillary sinus* is the largest and is bounded by the eye, the cheek, the nasal cavity, and the hard palate. The *ethmoid sinuses* are multiple and are present in the *ethmoid bone,* which lies medial to the orbit and extends to the pituitary fossa. The *frontal sinus* is located above the ethmoid sinuses and is bounded by the forehead, the orbit, and the anterior cranial fossa. Behind the ethmoid sinuses is the *sphenoid sinus.* The paranasal sinuses have no known functions. The maxillary, frontal, and ethmoid sinuses and their connections to the nose are illustrated in Fig. 11.9.

REVIEW OF SPECIFIC SYMPTOMS

The Ear

The major symptoms of ear disease are the following:

- Hearing loss
- Vertigo

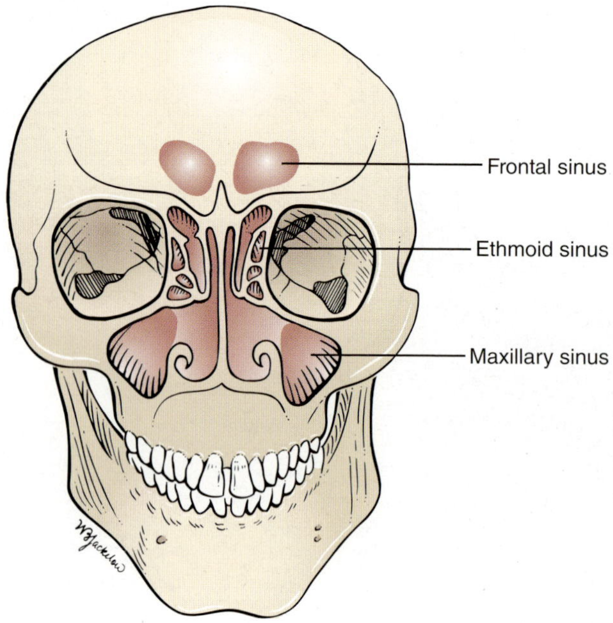

Fig. 11.9 Nasal Sinuses.

- Tinnitus
- Otorrhea
- Otalgia
- Itching

Hearing Loss

The terms "hearing impaired," "hard of hearing," "deaf," and "deafened" are often confusing in terms of their definitions and appropriate usage.

People with varying degrees of hearing loss, including those who are deaf or hard of hearing, are often called "hearing impaired." However, some individuals prefer to be identified as "deaf" or "hard of hearing" as they perceive the terms to be more optimistic than "hearing impaired," which can suggest a deficiency or an inadequacy that diminishes a person's wholeness.

The term "deaf" is typically used to describe a significant loss of hearing that dramatically affects a person's ability to hear. On the other hand, "hard of hearing" is used when a person has some remaining hearing and can benefit from using a hearing aid or frequency modulated (FM) system to help understand speech. "Deafened" usually refers to a person who becomes deaf as an adult and, therefore, faces different challenges than those of someone who became deaf at birth or as a child.

Deaf, deafened, and hard of hearing individuals may use hearing aids, cochlear implants, and other assistive listening devices to boost available hearing. In addition, they may read lips, use sign language, sign language interpreters, and captioning. People who are deaf or hard of hearing often have speech that is difficult to understand due to the inability to hear their own voice.

The terms "deaf-mute" or "deaf-dumb" are no longer acceptable. This 19th-century terminology is offensive today. Being deaf and Deaf are not the same thing. The word deaf (not capitalized) is the terminology used to describe the audiologic condition of hearing loss. The word Deaf (capitalized) is the terminology used by deaf people who are culturally deaf and identify themselves as members of a Deaf community. In this context, being Deaf is associated with considerable pride in one's culture and society.

Hearing loss can occur gradually or suddenly in one ear or both. If a patient has hearing loss, it's important to ask the following questions:

"Is the hearing loss in one ear?"
"For how long have you been aware of hearing loss?"
"Was the loss sudden?"
"Is there a family history of hearing loss?"
"What type of work do you do?" and *"What other work have you done?"*
"What types of hobbies do you have?"
"Have you noticed that you can hear better when it's noisy?"
"What kind of medications are you currently taking?"
"Do you know if you have ever been given an antibiotic called streptomycin or gentamicin?"

Occupational history is essential to ascertain. Patients with otosclerosis[c] can often hear better in a noisy environment. It's common knowledge that certain drugs can lead to sudden loss of hearing in both ears. Salicylates and diuretics like furosemide and ethacrynic acid may cause temporary hearing loss if taken in high doses. Antibiotics like streptomycin and gentamicin can harm the hair cells in the organ of Corti, leading to permanent hearing loss. Additionally, the anticancer drug cisplatin has been associated with severe ototoxicity.

There are two main types of hearing loss: *conductive* and *sensorineural*. Any condition that interferes with or blocks the transmission of sound waves from the external ear to the inner ear may result in conductive hearing loss. Blockage may occur due to cerumen (earwax), foreign bodies, infection, or congenital abnormalities. Often the position of the cerumen is more critical than the amount present. Not infrequently, a small amount of cerumen lying against the tympanic membrane can produce significant hearing loss. Blockage by foreign bodies occurs primarily in 2- to 5-year-old children. Once children discover the external canal, they may experiment and place beads or other objects inside. Fig. 11.10 shows a clear plastic bead in the external canal of a young child. Effusions from infections in the middle ear represent one of the most common causes of conductive deafness among children 4 to 15 years of age. The fluid impedes the transmission of sound impulses by the tympanic membrane and the ossicles. Otosclerosis is the leading cause of conductive hearing loss in individuals 15 to 50 years of age. Except for otosclerosis, conditions causing conductive hearing loss produce alterations in the appearance of the tympanic membrane.

Hearing loss that is caused by a disease process in the inner ear structures or auditory nerve is known as sensorineural hearing loss. Some cases of deafness may be present at birth or develop later in life. Approximately 50% of deafness in children

[c]Otosclerosis is the formation of new bone in the labyrinth, causing progressive fixation of the footplate of the stapes to the oval window.

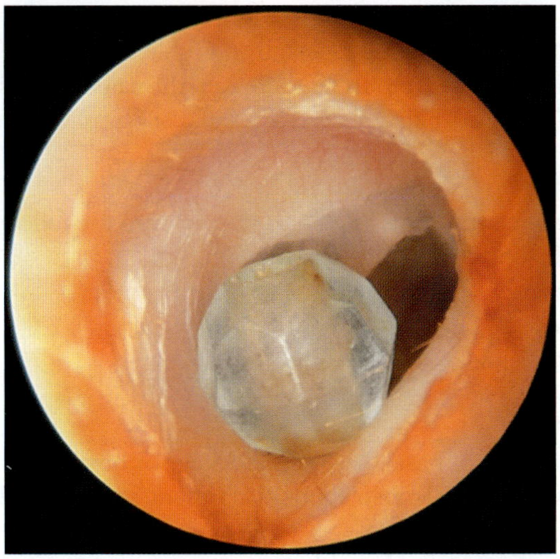

Fig. 11.10 Clear Plastic Bead in the External Ear Canal.

is caused by congenital factors. In most cases of congenital sensorineural hearing loss, there are no other congenital abnormalities present. In some cases, individuals may experience deafness along with other issues, particularly related to kidney function. Sensorineural deafness caused by abnormal development of the cochlea in the fetus is often a result of rubella infection during pregnancy. Sensorineural hearing loss can be acquired and onset may be delayed, and it may have a genetic component or not. There are many factors that can cause this type of deafness, such as viral infections, ototoxic drugs, and various syndromes. Additionally, systemic diseases, tumors, and exposure to noise can also contribute to this type of hearing loss.

The way a patient speaks can often indicate the type of deafness they have. This is because a person's voice is affected by how they hear themselves. For example, if a patient has conductive hearing loss, they hear their voice better through BC than through AC, which can make them think their voice is too loud and speak softly. On the other hand, if a patient has sensorineural hearing loss, they hear less through both AC and BC, causing them to speak louder.

Vertigo

Vertigo is a feeling of spinning or turning even when not moving. It is often linked with decreased vestibular function, which can cause unsteadiness when walking. If a patient is experiencing vertigo, it is essential to answer the following questions:

"How long have you had this sensation?"
"Have you had repeated attacks?"
"How long does an attack last? Seconds? Minutes? Hours? Days?"
"Is the onset of an attack abrupt?"
"Was the sensation brought on by, or worsened by, changes in position?"
"Does the spinning sensation get worse during an attack?"
"Are there any positions that make you feel better?"
"During an attack, have you had double vision? Loss of strength? Decreased hearing? A disturbance of gait? Nausea? Vomiting? Ringing in your ears?"
"What kind of medications are you currently taking?"
"Do you know if you have ever been given an antibiotic called streptomycin or gentamicin?"

Vertigo may result from otologic, neurologic, psychologic, or iatrogenic causes. *Ménière disease* causes severe paroxysmal vertigo as a result of labyrinthine lesions. The vertigo has an abrupt onset and may last several hours. It is often associated with nausea, vomiting, headache, a ringing sensation in the ear, and decreased hearing. The auditory abnormalities frequently antedate vertigo. Vertigo associated with an acoustic neuroma is usually mild. Some antibiotics, such as gentamicin, streptomycin, and kanamycin, are vestibulotoxic and cause vertigo. The neurologic causes of vertigo are discussed further in Chapter 21, The Nervous System.

Benign paroxysmal positional vertigo (BPPV) is one of the most common causes of vertigo. A person with BPPV experiences a sudden spinning sensation whenever they move their head. BPPV is a condition that causes brief episodes of dizziness ranging from mild to intense. The dizziness is usually brought on by specific changes in the position of the head such as tipping it up or down, lying down, or turning over or sitting up in bed. Symptoms of BPPV may be intermittent and typically last for less than a minute. Episodes of BPPV can disappear for some time and then recur. BPPV can cause inconvenience, but it is usually not a serious issue, except when it raises the risk of falling.

BPPV occurs when tiny calcium carbonate particles, called otoconia, become stuck in the semicircular canals. Normally, these particles are found in your utricle, a vestibular organ near the canals. Loose otoconia in the utricle can result from injury, infection, or aging. When the head changes position, the otoconia move around and push against the cilia in the semicircular canals. The cilia then transmit information about balance to your brain. Vertigo develops when these rolling otoconia stimulate the cilia.

The *Epley maneuver*, also known as the canalith repositioning procedure, is a method to remove the otoconia trapped in the ear's semicircular canal.[1,2] This technique requires a sequence of movements of the head that are intended to alleviate symptoms of vertigo. After undergoing the procedure, many individuals experience immediate relief from BPPV symptoms. Yet, in some individuals, it may be required to repeat the maneuvers to alleviate symptoms further.

Tinnitus

Tinnitus is the sensation of hearing sound, such as buzzing or ringing, in the absence of environmental input. It is often associated with conductive or sensorineural hearing loss. Usually the description of the type of tinnitus (e.g., "ringing" or "buzzing") is of little help in determining its cause. The most common causes are inner ear disease, such as Ménière disease, noise trauma, ototoxic drugs, and otosclerosis. On occasion, patients describe *pulsatile tinnitus*. This type of tinnitus beats at the same rate as the heart and may be a symptom of a head or neck vascular tumor. See Table 11.1 for a list of common causes of tinnitus.

TABLE 11.1 Common Causes of Tinnitus

Location	Pulsatile/Clicking Sensation	Nonpulsatile
External ear	Otitis externa Bullous myringitis Foreign body	Cerumen Tympanic membrane perforation Foreign body
Middle ear	Otitis media Vascular anomalies Neoplasm Eustachian tube dysfunction	Otosclerosis Serous otitis media
Inner ear	Vascular anomalies	Cochlear otosclerosis Ménière disease Labyrinthitis Noise trauma Drug toxicity Presbycusis
Central nervous system	Vascular anomalies Hypertension	Syphilis Degenerative disease Cerebral atherosclerosis

Otorrhea

Otorrhea, or discharge from the ear, usually indicates acute or chronic infection. For any patient complaining of an ear discharge, ask the following:

"Can you describe the discharge?"
"Have you had similar episodes?"
"Do you experience dizziness?"
"Do you have ear pain?"
"Have you had a recent ear or throat infection?"
"Have you had any change in your hearing?"
"Have you used ear drops?"
"Have you been swimming recently?"
"Have you had any recent head or ear injury?"

A bloody discharge may be associated with carcinoma or trauma. A clear, watery discharge may indicate a leakage of cerebrospinal fluid. Determine how long the discharge has been present, its color, its smell, and its relationship to itching, pain, or trauma.

Otalgia

Otalgia, or ear pain, may be related to inflammatory conditions in or around the ear, or it may be *referred*[d] from distant anatomic sites in the head and neck. External otitis and otitis media are infections of the external and middle ear, respectively, and are common causes of locally produced pain. Pain from the teeth, pharynx, and cervical spine is commonly referred to the ear. Inflammation, trauma, and neoplasms anywhere along the course of the trigeminal, facial, glossopharyngeal, and vagus cranial nerves or cervical nerves C2 or C3 may be responsible for referred pain in the ipsilateral ear.

[d]Referred pain is felt in an area that is separate from the area that is actually the source of the pain. For example, pain from gallbladder disease is frequently felt in the right shoulder. Chapter 17, The Abdomen, discusses further aspects of referred pain.

Itching

Itching in the ear can be caused by a problem with the external ear or a discharge from the middle ear. The cause may also be a systemic disease, like diabetes, hepatitis, or lymphoma.

The Nose

The specific symptoms related to the nose are the following:

- Obstruction
- Discharge
- Bleeding
- Loss of smell

Obstruction

The main sign of nasal disease is blockage or obstruction. If the symptom of nasal obstruction is present, ask the following questions:

"Is the obstruction on one side?"
"Have you ever had an injury to your nose?"
"How long has the obstruction been present?"
"Do you have any allergies?"
"Does the obstruction worsen with stress?"
"Is there a history of nasal polyps?"
"Is the obstruction associated with other symptoms?"
"Is there a seasonal change in your symptoms?" If so, *"Which season is the worst?"*

Rhinitis, which is inflammation of the nasal mucosa, can have allergic or nonallergic causes. *Allergic rhinitis* is congestion of the nasal mucosa triggered by an allergen such as pollen. The main symptoms include nasal obstruction, sneezing, and a clear, watery nasal discharge. It is helpful to try to determine the allergen. Weeds pollinate in the spring and fall, trees in the spring, and grasses in the summer. Nonseasonal allergic rhinitis may result from animal dander, mold, or dust. *Nonallergic rhinitis* produces the same symptoms but is nonseasonal and is not triggered by allergens. An example of nonallergic rhinitis is vasomotor rhinitis. Vasomotor rhinitis occurs at stressful times and results in venous engorgement of the conchae, causing obstruction. There are many other causes of vasomotor rhinitis, such as nasal spray abuse (also known as *rhinitis medicamentosa*), pregnancy, and hypothyroidism.

Nasal polyps, typically affecting both sides of the nose, can cause blockage and are a frequent reason for anosmia, or the inability to detect smells.

Nasal obstruction may be responsible for symptoms referable to other organs. Eye tearing may result from obstruction of the nasolacrimal duct beneath the inferior turbinate. Sinus symptoms may result from obstruction to their drainage. Ear pain or a "clogged" sensation is commonly associated with eustachian tube obstruction.

Discharge

Nasal discharge can be unilateral or bilateral. It usually accompanies nasal obstruction. The discharge may be characterized as follows:

- Thin and watery
- Thick and purulent
- Bloody
- Foul-smelling

Excess mucus production due to a viral infection or allergic condition can cause a thin and watery discharge, while a bacterial infection can cause a thick and purulent nasal discharge. Bloody discharge can be caused by various factors, including neoplasms, trauma, and opportunistic infections like mucormycosis (a fungal disease). A bad-smelling discharge can indicate the presence of foreign objects in the nose, chronic sinusitis, or even cancer. A clear, watery discharge that is increased by bending the head forward or coughing suggests cerebrospinal fluid leakage.

Bleeding

Epistaxis, which is also known as nasal bleeding, typically occurs when the superficial mucosal vessels in Little's area rupture spontaneously or due to trauma. To exclude other causes, the healthcare professional must determine whether the epistaxis is related to trauma or to a bleeding disorder. It may also result from chronic sinusitis or malignancy within the sinuses. Nose-picking is the most frequent cause of epistaxis. Cocaine abuse is another significant factor that can lead to this condition.

Loss of Smell

There are various factors that can cause anosmia, which is the loss of smell. These include colds, allergies, sinus infections, viral infections like the flu or COVID-19, nasal polyps, blockages, tumors, or a deviated septum. An individual with anosmia may find that food tastes bland and it's difficult to distinguish between different foods. The extent of the loss of smell can be partial (hyposmia) or complete (anosmia), and the duration can be temporary or permanent, depending on the cause.

A notable symptom of COVID-19 is the loss of smell, which can persist for several weeks, months, or even years after the illness has ended. Research indicates that this symptom may be a stronger predictor of the disease than fever or cough. However, it is not yet fully understood why patients with COVID-19 experience this loss of smell. The upper nasal cavity appears to be the most susceptible area to SARS-CoV-2 infection, the virus that leads to COVID-19.

Sinus Disease Symptoms

Sinus disease symptoms can be similar to those of nasal disease. These symptoms include fever, cough, malaise, nasal congestion, maxillary toothache, purulent nasal discharge, headache, and slight relief with decongestants. If a patient experiences pain, particularly when bending forward, it may indicate sinus disease. Pain from localized sinus disease is usually felt overlying the affected sinus. Sphenoid sinus disease is the only exception, as it is felt diffusely. Maxillary sinus pain is felt behind the eye and near the second premolar and first and second molar teeth. Frontal sinus pain is localized above the eye. Ethmoid sinus pain is usually periorbital. Sometimes sinus pain can be referred to another area. In addition to pain, ocular abnormalities may also be present with diseases of the sinuses.

The accuracy of sinusitis symptoms and signs has been assessed. The symptoms with the highest sensitivity were colored nasal discharge, cough, and sneezing, with percentages of 72%, 70%, and 70%, respectively. However, these symptoms were not very specific. Sinusitis is often associated with maxillary toothache, which has a high specificity rate of 93%. However, only 11% of patients actually report experiencing this symptom. Nevertheless, it holds the highest positive likelihood ratio at 2.5. The conclusion was that the combination of maxillary toothache, poor response to decongestants, colored nasal discharge, and abnormality in sinus transillumination (discussed later in this chapter) was the strongest predictor of sinusitis in primary care populations. If all these symptoms were present in one patient, the positive likelihood ratio was 6.4, and the patient probably had sinusitis; if none were present, sinusitis was ruled out.

Table 11.2 summarizes the location of pain associated with sinus disease. Table 11.3 lists other clinical signs and symptoms associated with sinus disease.

TABLE 11.2 Location of Pain Associated With Sinus Disease

Sinus Involved	Local Pain	Referred Pain
Maxillary	Behind eye Cheek Nose Upper teeth Upper lip	Teeth Retrobulbar
Ethmoid	Periorbital Retronasal Retrobulbar	Occipital Upper cervical
Frontal	Supraorbital Frontal	Bitemporal and occipital headache

TABLE 11.3 Clinical Signs and Symptoms in Sinus Disease

Sinus Involved	Signs and Symptoms
Maxillary	Ocular abnormalities Diplopia Proptosis Epiphora (tearing) Nasal obstruction and rhinorrhea Epistaxis Loosening of teeth
Ethmoid	Orbital swelling Nasal obstruction and purulent rhinorrhea Ocular abnormalities Proptosis Diplopia Tenderness over inner canthus of eye
Frontal	Nasal obstruction and rhinorrhea Tenderness over frontal sinus Pus in middle meatus Signs of meningitis

EFFECT OF DEAFNESS ON THE PATIENT

The ear is responsible for hearing and is a crucial component of communication. If there are issues with the external ear's reception of sound waves or the transmission of electric impulses to the brain, it can lead to misinterpretation of language.

It is believed that more than 15 million Americans are experiencing hearing loss that affects their ability to comprehend speech. Out of these individuals, 7.2 million are dealing with hearing difficulties in both ears. While individuals over 70 make up 30% of the deaf population, there are more than 250,000 deaf children below the age of 3. The rate of hearing loss has significantly increased since the late 1970s.

To comprehend how deafness impacts a person, it's crucial to consider their age when it started, the degree of hearing loss, how fast it occurred, and if there is any remaining hearing. Those who experience gradual or sudden hearing loss often face feelings of sorrow and depression. Take, for instance, the distress conveyed through the quote by Beethoven mentioned at the start of this chapter.

Deafness can have psychologic effects such as paranoia, depression, withdrawal, irritability, and anxiety. While not confirmed, there is a tendency for deaf people to experience more paranoia. Furthermore, many deaf individuals are often suspicious of conversations happening around them.

Severe hearing loss often leads to depression and withdrawal, as illustrated by the following quote from Beethoven:

> *"Oh you men who think that I am malevolent, stubborn, or misanthropic, how greatly do you wrong me. You do not know the secret cause which makes me seem that way to you. ... For me there can be no relaxation with my fellow men, no refined conversations, no mutual exchange of ideas. I must live alone, like one who has been banished. ... What a humiliation for me when someone standing next to me heard a flute in the distance, and I heard nothing ... a little more of that and I would have ended my life—it was only my art that held me back."*

People who are hearing impaired often struggle with social identity issues and are often left out of social groups they were previously a part of. Individuals who use sign language may face difficulty socializing with those who do not know sign language. It may be necessary to make changes to one's work or career. Wearing a hearing aid can make someone feel even more isolated from others due to the negative social perception surrounding it. Some patients may choose not to wear a hearing aid due to the fear of being stigmatized.

Children who are deaf face more significant challenges in their development. Their inability to hear affects their personality, early experiences, attitudes, and relationships with others. They miss out on comforting sounds that help shape their character, and they cannot pick up on verbal cues of affection from their parents. Additionally, they cannot be warned of potential danger by hearing warning signs.

Psychologic problems, social inadequacy, and educational retardation are common among deaf children. The worse the handicap is, the worse the psychologic and educational implications are.

A young hearing-impaired child who delays language development may be diagnosed as developmentally disabled. In general, children who are congenitally deaf or have severe hearing impairment before 3 years of age suffer the most. As the type of lesion causing deafness progresses from the periphery inward, the deleterious effects increase.

PHYSICAL EXAMINATION

To examine the ear and nose, you will need specific equipment such as an otoscope, a penlight, a 512-Hz tuning fork, and a choice of specula. Additionally, you may choose to use a nasal illuminator attachment for the otoscope and a nasal speculum, but these are not necessary.

The physical examination of the ear and the nose is performed with the examiner seated in front of the patient.

The Ear

If the patient has symptoms referable to one ear, examine the uninvolved ear first. The physical examination of the ear includes the following:

- External examination
- Auditory acuity testing
- Otoscopic examination

External Examination

See Video 11.1.

Inspect the pinna and postauricular skin. Note the position, size, and shape of the pinna. The pinna should be positioned centrally and proportionately to the face and head. Note any obvious abnormalities or surgical scars.

Inspect the external ear structures. A small dimple in front of the tragus is usually a remnant of the first branchial arch.

Inspect the external ear for deformities, nodules, inflammation, or lesions. The presence of *tophi* is a highly specific but nonsensitive sign of gout. Tophi are deposits of uric acid crystals. They appear as hard nodules in the helix or antihelix. In rare cases, a white discharge may be seen in association with them. A "cauliflower ear" is a pinna that is gnarled due to repeated trauma. Fig. 11.11 shows a squamous cell carcinoma and a malignant melanoma of one lobule.

Inspect for discharge. If discharge is present, note its characteristics, such as color, consistency, and clarity.

Palpate the external ear structures. See Video 11.2.

Palpate the pinna for tenderness, swelling, or nodules. If pain is elicited by pulling up and down on the pinna or pressing in on the tragus, an external canal infection is probably present.

Inspect the posterior auricular region for scars or swelling. Apply pressure to the mastoid tip, which should be painless. Tenderness may indicate a suppurative process of the mastoid bone.

Auditory Acuity Testing

See Video 11.3.

The next step in the physical examination is to test for auditory acuity. The examiner can easily test for gross hearing loss by covering one external canal by pressing the tragus inward

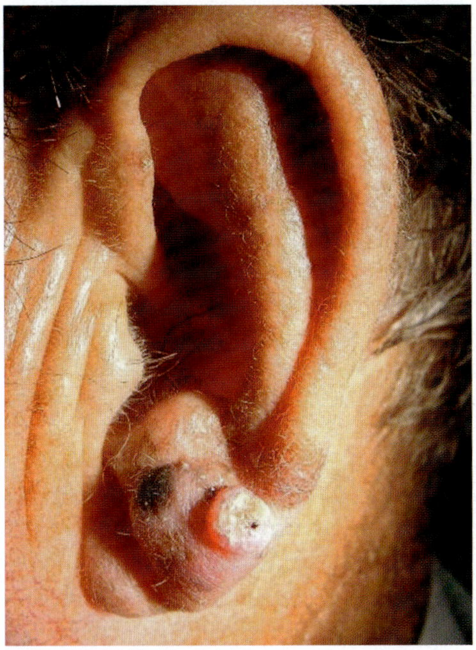

Fig. 11.11 Squamous Cell Carcinoma *(on the Right)* and Malignant Melanoma *(on the Left)* of the Lobule.

and speaking softly into the other ear. To prevent the patient from lip reading, the examiner should stand behind the patient. Then, the examiner should whisper words like "park," "dark," or "daydream" in one ear and check if the patient can hear them. This process should be repeated with the other ear. Alternatively, the examiner can whisper three letters or numbers, such as "A, 7, F" while standing approximately 2 feet behind the patient and asking the patient to repeat the sequence. If the patient answers correctly, hearing should be considered within normal limits. Studies have shown that the normal test practically excludes significant hearing loss. An abnormal whispered hearing test has a sensitivity of 90% to 99% and a specificity of 80% to 87%.

Another test, known as the *finger rub test,* has the highest specificity for hearing loss.[3] The inability to hear a vigorous finger rub is pathognomonic for a hearing loss. In contrast, hearing a faint finger rub indicates normal hearing on the side examined. To perform the finger rub test, the examiner stands with hands outstretched directly in front of the patient, whose eyes are closed. The examiner tests one ear at a time by rubbing fingers together. The patient is instructed to raise their hand on the side where the rubbing occurred.

Tuning fork testing for hearing loss is more accurate and should be performed regardless of the whisper test results. Although several tuning fork frequencies are available, the best for evaluating hearing is the 512-Hz fork.[e]

A tuning fork is held by its stem, and the tines are briskly struck against the palm of the hand. It should never be struck

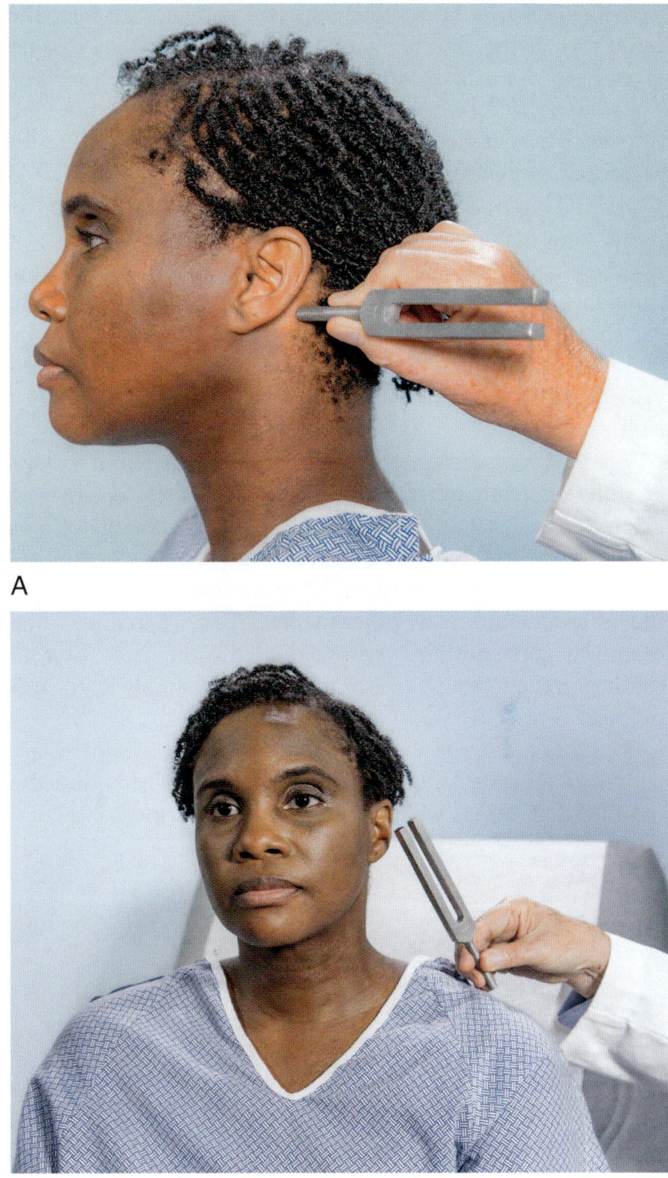

A

B

Fig. 11.12 The Rinne Test. (A) The 512-Hz tuning fork is first placed on the mastoid process. (B) When the sound can no longer be heard, the tuning fork is placed in front of the external auditory meatus. Normally, air conduction (AC) is better than bone conduction (BC); that is, AC > BC.

on a solid wooden or metal object. The two tuning fork tests to assess hearing are the Rinne and Weber tests.

The Rinne test. See Video 11.4.

In the Rinne test, air conduction (AC) is compared with bone conduction (BC). Each ear is tested separately. Strike or pluck a 512-Hz tuning fork and place its handle on the mastoid tip near the external auditory meatus. Ask the patient whether they hear the sound and indicate when they no longer hear it. When the patient can no longer hear the sound, place the tines of the vibrating tuning fork in front of the external auditory meatus of the same ear, and ask the patient whether they can still hear the sound. The tines of the vibrating tuning fork should not touch any hair because the patient may have a hearing impairment but still feel the vibration. The Rinne test is demonstrated in Fig. 11.12.

[e]Different examiners prefer tuning forks of different frequencies for determining auditory acuity. A tuning fork of too high a frequency yields a tone that fades too quickly.

Normally, AC is better than BC, and patients can hear the tuning fork at the external auditory meatus after they can no longer hear it on the mastoid tip; this is a *Rinne positive* test result (AC > BC). In patients with a conductive hearing loss, however, BC is better than AC: a *Rinne negative* test result (BC > AC). Patients with sensorineural deafness have impaired AC *and* BC but maintain the normal response (AC > BC). The middle ear amplifies the sound in both positions.

If there is total deafness in one ear, the patient may hear the tuning fork even when it is placed on the mastoid process of the deaf ear. This results from the transmission of vibrations by bone across the skull to the opposite side, where they are sensed by the healthy ear. This is termed a *false-negative Rinne* test result.

Note that the words *positive* and *negative* are used in a manner different from other usage in medical tests. Positive or negative means that a certain parameter that was evaluated was present or not. In this case, that parameter refers to whether AC is better than BC. Thus a "positive" result indicates the healthy state, in contrast to many other medical tests. Therefore, when presenting your findings, to avoid confusion, it is best to avoid using the term *positive* or *negative,* and simply state your findings.

The Weber test. See Video 11.5.

In the Weber test, BC is compared in both ears, and the examiner determines whether monaural impairment is neural or conductive in origin. Stand in front of the patient and place a vibrating 512-Hz tuning fork firmly against the center of the patient's forehead. Ask the patient to indicate whether they hear or feel the sound in the right ear, in the left ear, or in the middle of the forehead. Hearing the sound, or feeling the vibration, in the middle is the normal response. If the sound is not heard in the middle, the sound is said to be *lateralized,* and thus a hearing loss is present. Sound is lateralized to the *affected* side in conductive deafness. Try it on yourself. Occlude your right ear and place a vibrating tuning fork in the center of your forehead. Where do you hear it? On the *right*. You have created a conductive hearing loss on the right by blocking the right canal; the sound is lateralized to the right side. The Weber test is illustrated in Fig. 11.13.

The reason behind the Weber test effect is due to the influence of background noise. Normally, there is a significant amount of background noise that reaches the ear through AC, which can make it difficult to hear the tuning fork via BC. However, in an ear with conductive hearing loss, the AC is reduced, leading to less masking effect. Consequently, the affected ear can hear and feel the vibrating tuning fork better than the normal ear.

In patients with unilateral sensorineural deafness, the sound is not heard on the affected side but is heard by, or localized to, the *unaffected* ear.

To test the reliability of the patient's responses, it is occasionally useful to strike the tuning fork against the palm of the hand

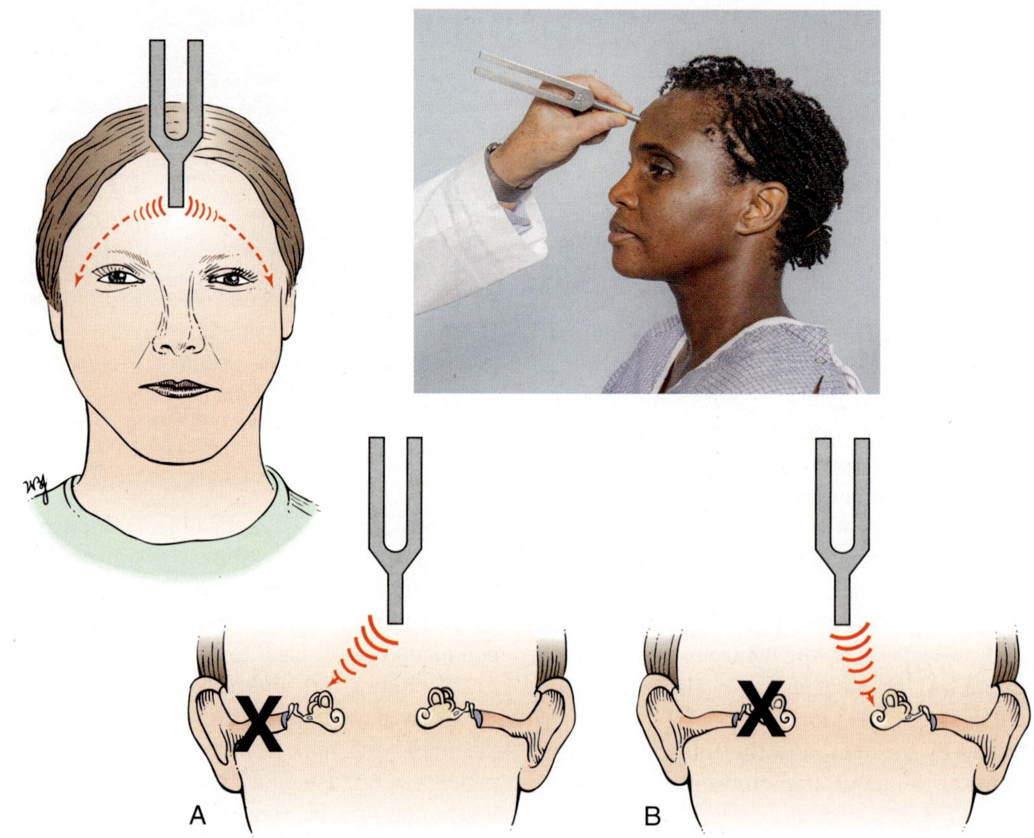

Fig. 11.13 The Weber Test. When a vibrating 512-Hz tuning fork is placed on the center of the forehead, the normal response is for the sound to be heard in the center, without lateralization to either side. (A) In the presence of a conductive hearing loss, the sound is heard on the side of the conductive loss. (B) In the presence of a sensorineural loss, the sound is heard better on the opposite (unaffected) side.

and hold it briefly to silence it. The Rinne and Weber tests are then carried out as indicated, using the silent tuning fork. This serves as a good control.

In summary, consider the examples in Box 11.1.

It is important to remember that both the Rinne and Weber tests are screening tests and do not replace formal audiometry hearing tests.

Otoscopic Examination

To examine the ear, an otoscope is used which has a halogen light source and a 360-degree ring of light-conducting fibers within its shell. This allows the observer to see the inner structures of the ear. The otoscope is usually powered by a 3.5-V power supply and a bright quartz halogen bulb. Polypropylene specula, which can be reused or disposed of, are designed to slip over the tip of the instrument. A rubber squeeze bulb can be used with most otoscopic heads for pneumatic otoscopy, as explained later in this chapter. Take care in the use of the otoscope. The most effective way to visualize the structure does not involve wedging the speculum into the canal. To get the best view of the anatomy, it's important to be gentle.

Choose the correct speculum size: small enough to prevent discomfort to the patient and large enough to provide an adequate beam of light. Usually a tip 4 to 6 mm in diameter is used for adults, 3 to 4 mm in diameter for children, and 2 mm in diameter for infants.

The Techniques

See Video 11.6.

BOX 11.1 Weber Test Examples

Example 1

Rinne: *Right ear:* AC > BC (Rinne positive—*normal*); *left ear:* AC > BC (Rinne positive—*normal*)

Weber: Lateralization to the left ear

Diagnosis: Right sensorineural deafness

Example 2

Rinne: *Right ear:* AC > BC (Rinne positive—*normal*); *left ear:* BC > AC (Rinne negative—*abnormal*)

Weber: Lateralization to the left ear

Diagnosis: Left conductive deafness

	Weber No Lateralization	Weber Lateralizes to Left	Weber Lateralizes to Right
Rinne Both Ears AC > BC	Normal	Right SN	Left SN
Rinne Left BC > AC		Left CD	Left SCL
Rinne Right BC > AC		Right SCL	Right CD
Rinne Both Ears BC > AC	Both ears CD	Left CD Right SCL	Right CD Left SCL

AC, Air conduction; *BC,* bone conduction; *CD,* conductive deafness; *SCL,* combined loss (sensorineural and conductive); *SN,* sensorineural deafness.

To examine the patient's right ear, the examiner holds the otoscope in the right hand. To make the examination more comfortable for the patient and improve visualization, the examiner straightens the canal by pulling the pinna up, out, and back with their left hand. The straighter the canal, the easier it is to visualize.

To straighten the canal of a child's ear, gently pull down and back on the pinna.

The patient is asked to turn their head to the side slightly so that the examiner can examine the ear more comfortably. The otoscope may be held in either of two positions. The first, and preferred, position involves holding the otoscope like a pencil, between the thumb and index finger, in a downward position with the ulnar aspect of the examiner's hand braced against the side of the patient's face. This position provides a buffer against sudden movement by the patient. By holding the end of the otoscope handle, the examiner then angles the speculum into the external canal. This technique at first feels more cumbersome than the alternative technique, but it is safer, especially for children. This technique is shown in Fig. 11.14.

To perform the second position, the otoscope should be held upwards while inserting the speculum into the canal. Although this technique may feel more comfortable, sudden movements by the patient can result in pain and injury. This technique is shown in Fig. 11.15.

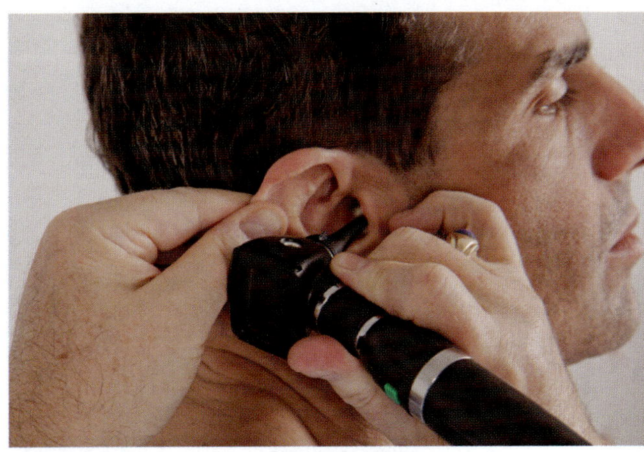

Fig. 11.14 Technique for Otoscopic Examination. Notice that the ear is pulled up, out, and back.

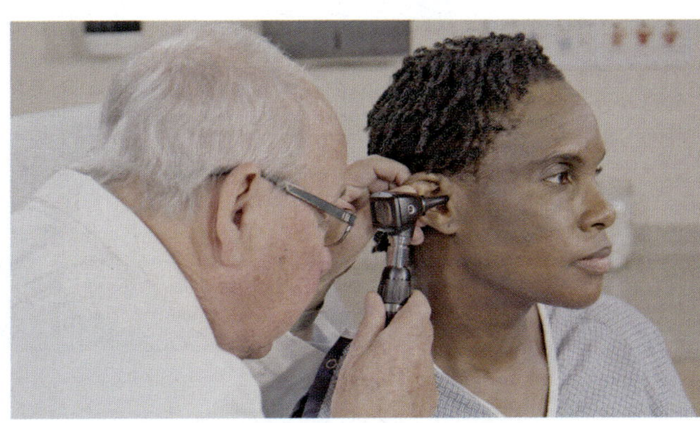

Fig. 11.15 Alternative Technique for Otoscopic Examination. The ear is pulled up, out, and back.

Inspect the external canal. Gently insert the speculum and inspect the external canal. The external auditory canal is 24 mm long in the adult and is the only skin-lined, blind-ended canal in the body. The canal follows a tortuous course from the external meatus to the tympanic membrane. The techniques previously described are used to straighten the canal. There should be no evidence of redness, swelling, or tenderness, which indicates inflammation. The walls of the canal should be free of foreign bodies, scaliness, and discharge. If a foreign body is seen, pay particular attention when inspecting the opposite ear canal, the nose, and other accessible body orifices.

Any cerumen should be left as is, unless it interferes with the visualization of the rest of the canal and tympanic membrane. Removal of cerumen is best left to an experienced examiner because any manipulation may result in trauma or abrasions. Fig. 11.16 depicts an external ear canal with a large hematoma secondary to aggressive use of a cotton-tipped applicator stick. Notice the tympanic membrane in the background.

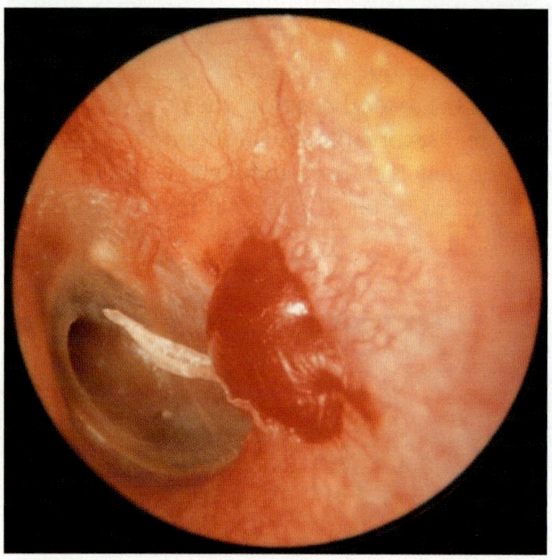

Fig. 11.16 External Ear Canal With Large Hematoma.

If a discharge is present, look for the site of origin.

Inspect the tympanic membrane. When the speculum is moved downward and forward into the canal, the examiner should be able to see the tympanic membrane. It should look like a complete, oval-shaped, partially clear, and pearly gray membrane at the canal's end. The lower four-fifths of the tympanic membrane are called the *pars tensa*; the upper fifth, the *pars flaccida*. The handle of the malleus should be seen near the center of the pars tensa. From the lower end of the handle, there is frequently a bright triangular cone of light reflected from the pars tensa. This is called the *light reflex,* which is directed anteroinferiorly. The pars flaccida, the short process of the malleus, and the anterior and posterior folds should be identified. A normal tympanic membrane is pictured in Fig. 11.17A, and the important landmarks are identified in Fig. 11.17B.

It is not reliable to determine whether an ear is normal or diseased based on the presence or absence of the light reflex. The light reflex is not a sensitive indicator of disease. Both normal and abnormal tympanic membranes can have or lack a light reflex equally.

Describe the color, integrity, transparency, position, and landmarks of the tympanic membrane.

Normally, healthy tympanic membranes have a pearly gray appearance. However, when they are diseased, they can become dull and change in color to red or yellow. Is the eardrum injected? *Injection* refers to the dilation of blood vessels, making them more apparent. The blood vessels should be visible only around the perimeter of the membrane. Dense white plaques on the tympanic membrane may be caused by *tympanosclerosis,* which is caused by deposition of hyaline material and calcification within the layers of the tympanic membrane. This condition is commonly (in 50% to 60% of cases) secondary to the insertion of ventilation tubes. The classic horseshoe shape of

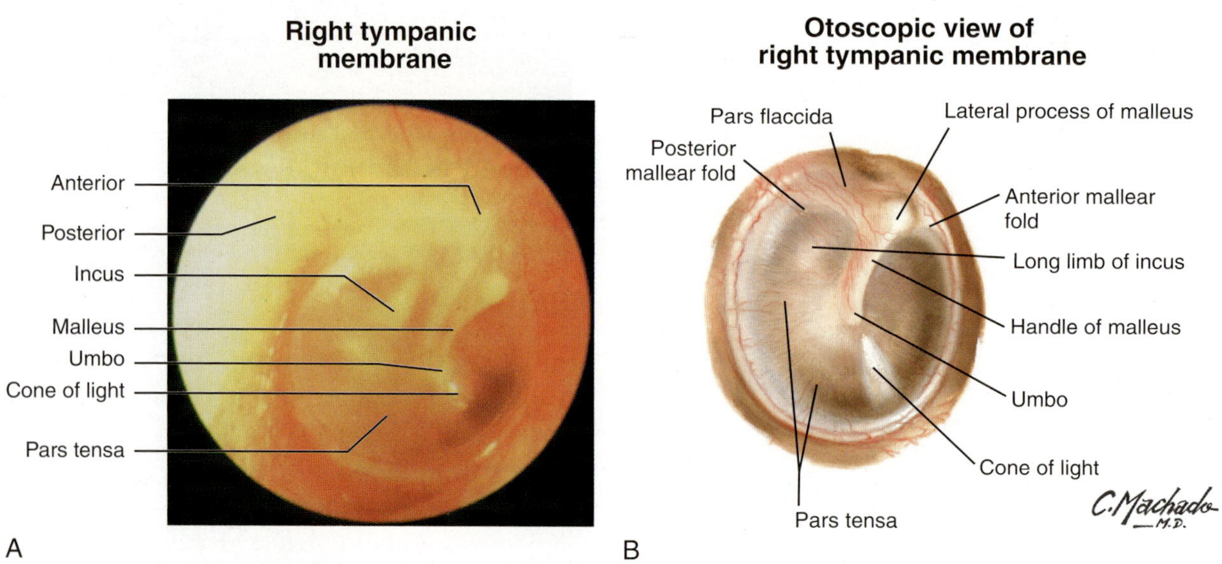

Fig. 11.17 Photograph (A) and labeled schematic (B) illustrating a normal right tympanic membrane. (B reused with permission from Netter FH: *Netter atlas of human anatomy: classic regional approach*, ed 8, Philadelphia, 2023, Elsevier.)

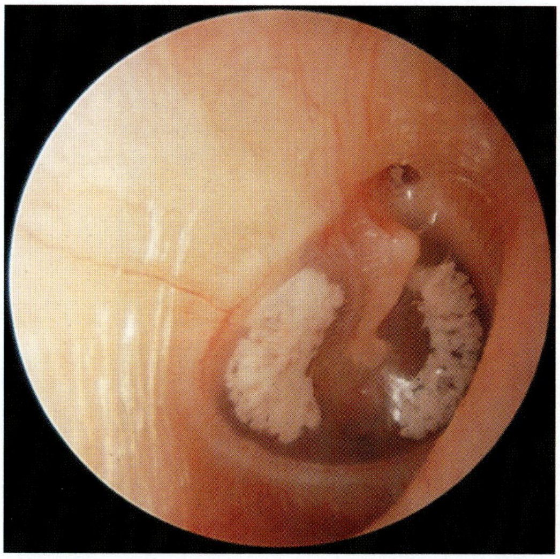

Fig. 11.18 Tympanosclerosis.

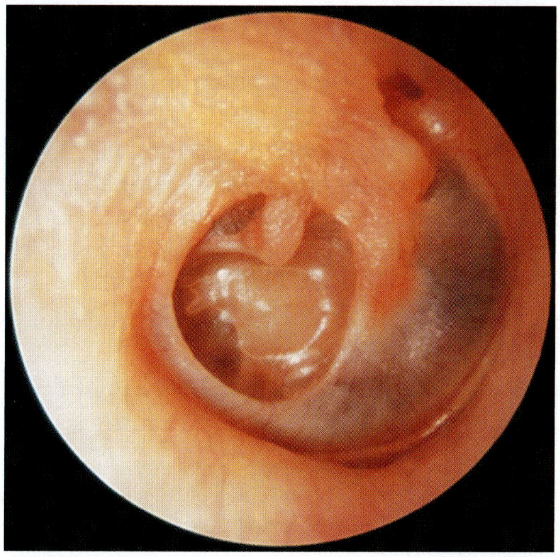

Fig. 11.19 Retraction Pocket.

tympanosclerosis is seen in the tympanic membrane shown in Fig. 11.18. Despite the size of these lesions, they usually do not impair hearing and are rarely of clinical importance. If the lesion extends into the middle ear, however, conductive deafness may result.

Is the tympanic membrane bulging or retracted? Bulging of the membrane may indicate fluid or pus in the middle ear. No bubbles or fluid should be seen behind the tympanic membrane in the middle ear. A tympanic membrane becomes retracted when intratympanic cavity pressures are reduced—for example, when the eustachian tube is obstructed. Fig. 11.19 depicts a "retraction pocket" just above the lateral process of the malleus, a condition known as *attic retraction.* On occasion, the entire tympanic membrane may become retracted onto the ossicles of the middle ear. The ossicles may become eroded, with the development of a conductive hearing loss.

If the tympanic membrane is perforated, describe the characteristics. Perforation of the tympanic membrane can occur after trauma or infection.

The normal position of the tympanic membrane is oblique to the external canal. The superior margin is closer to the examiner's eye. This is frequently better seen in infants than in adults.

In the normal ear, the handle of the malleus attached to the tympanic membrane is the primary landmark. Frequently, the long process of the incus may be seen posterior to the malleus. The chorda tympani nerve, which supplies innervation to the anterior two thirds of the tongue and stimulates taste there, is frequently visible in the upper posterior quadrant; it passes horizontally across the middle ear behind the tympanic membrane between the long process of the incus and the handle of the malleus. Keratin patches appear as multiple, discrete white patches on the tympanic membrane of all normal membranes; if illumination is not adequate, however, they may not be visualized. In the presence of a retracted tympanic membrane, the malleus is seen in sharp outline.

There are many differences in the color, shape, and contour of the tympanic membrane, which can be recognized only with experience.

After examining the right ear, examine the *left* ear by holding the otoscope in the *left* hand and straightening the canal with the *right* hand.

Determine the mobility of the tympanic membrane. To determine if there is a middle ear infection, healthcare professionals will perform a pneumatic otoscopy. This involves using a speculum that fits comfortably into the external ear canal to create a closed air chamber between the canal and the inside of the otoscopic head. A rubber squeeze bulb is then attached to the otoscopic head. By squeezing the bulb, the examiner can increase the air pressure in the canal. Pneumatic otoscopy must be performed gently, and the patient should be informed that they may experience a blowing noise during the procedure. When one squeezes the bulb to increase the pressure in the otoscopic head, the normal tympanic membrane will promptly move inward. When a person's eustachian tube is blocked, their eardrum may move slowly inward. When there is fluid in the middle ear, the movement is significantly reduced or absent. The reduction of movement of the tympanic membrane increases the probability of middle ear infection by as much as 40%. This simple technique can provide invaluable assistance in the early diagnosis of many middle ear problems.

The Nose

The examination of the nose consists of the following:

- External examination
- Internal examination

External Examination

Inspect the nose. See Video 11.7.

The external examination consists of inspection of the nose for any *swelling, trauma,* or *congenital anomalies.* Is the nose straight? Does a deviation involve the upper bony portion or the lower cartilaginous portion?

Inspect the external nares. Are they symmetric?

To test the patency of each nostril, gently place a finger across one nostril and ask the patient to sniff. Make sure not to apply aggressive pressure that could compress the other nostril.

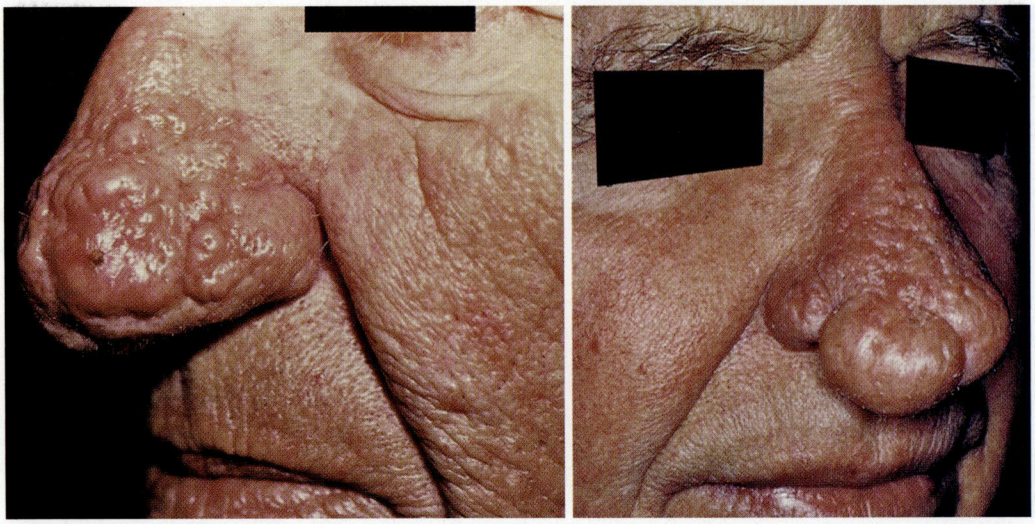

Fig. 11.20 **Rhinophyma.** (From Callen JP, Greer KE, Hood AF, et al: *Color atlas of dermatology*, Philadelphia, 1993, WB Saunders.)

Any swelling or deformity should be palpated for pain and firmness.

Rhinophyma is a condition where the sebaceous glands of the nose hypertrophy, causing overgrowth of the soft tissue. It is more prevalent in males than in females. The patient pictured in Fig. 11.20 also has *acne rosacea,* which is a common associated condition consisting of papules, pustules, and erythema of the face. The cause is unknown. The rash is worsened by hot drinks, highly spiced food, and alcohol.

Palpate the sinuses. See Video 11.8.

Palpation over the frontal and maxillary sinuses may reveal tenderness that is indicative of sinusitis.

Internal Examination

The key to the internal examination is proper positioning of the head. Ask the patient to hold their back. Place your left hand firmly on top of the patient's head and use your left thumb to elevate the tip of the patient's nose. In this manner, change the position of the patient's head to visualize the intranasal structures. Use a light source to illuminate the internal structures. This technique is shown in Fig. 11.21.

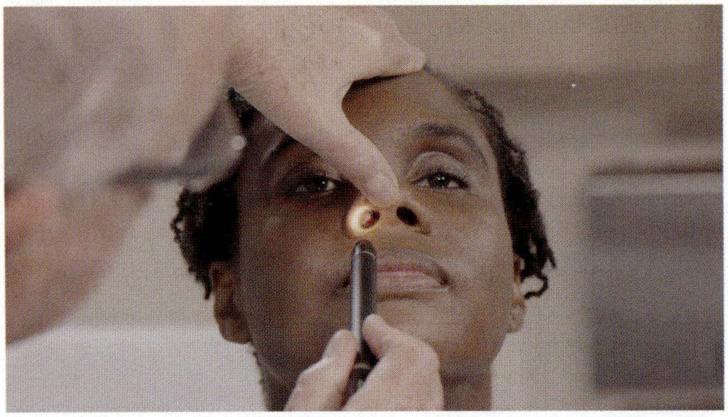

Fig. 11.21 Inspection of the Internal Structures of the Nose.

Inspect the position of the septum to the lateral cartilages on each side. Examine the vestibule for inflammation and the anterior septum for deviation or perforation. Evaluate the *color* of the nasal mucous membrane. Normal nasal mucous membranes are dull red and moist and have a smooth, clean surface. Nasal mucosa is usually darker in color than oral mucosa. Inspect for exudate, swelling, bleeding, and trauma. If epistaxis has occurred, examine Little's area for vascular engorgement or crusting.

Is a discharge present? If so, describe it as purulent, watery, cloudy, or bloody. Is crusting present? Are any masses or polyps present?

Tip the patient's head farther back and check the posterior septum for deviation or perforation. Note the size and color of the inferior turbinates. The two inferior turbinates are rarely symmetric.

Inspect the size, color, and mucosal condition of the middle turbinates. Are polyps present? Most polyps are found in the middle meatus.

It's best to avoid using an otoscopic speculum to examine the inside of the nostrils as it can cause damage to the nasal septum due to its small size.

Use a nasal illuminator. If a nasal illuminator is used, the examiner's left thumb is placed on the tip of the patient's nose while the palm of the examiner's hand steadies the patient's head. The patient's neck is slightly extended as the tip of the speculum of the illuminator is inserted into the nostril. After one nostril is evaluated, the illuminator is placed in the other nostril. The technique of using a nasal illuminator is shown in Fig. 11.22.

Use a nasal speculum. When using a nasal speculum, the examiner should hold the instrument in their left hand and insert it into the patient's nostril with the blades facing up and down in a vertical position. The speculum should not rest on the nasal septum. The blades are inserted approximately 1 cm into the vestibule, and the patient's neck should be slightly

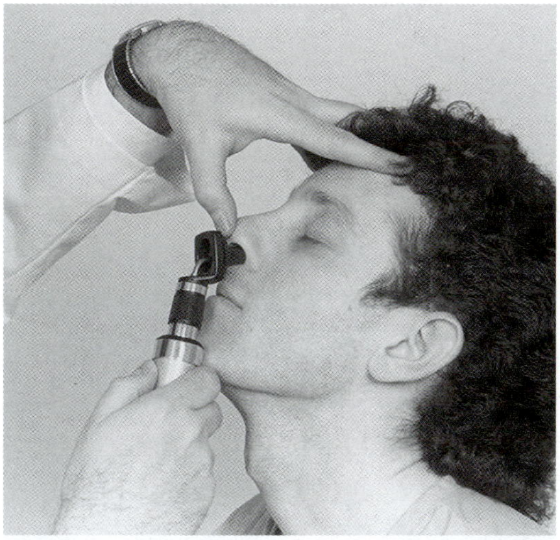

Fig. 11.22 Using a Nasal Illuminator to Inspect the Internal Structures of the Nose. Never use an otoscopic speculum to evaluate the nasal structures.

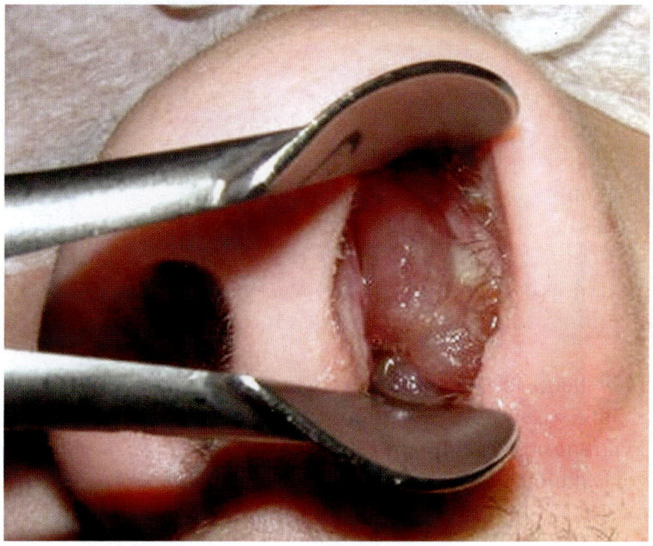

Fig. 11.23 Nasal Polyps.

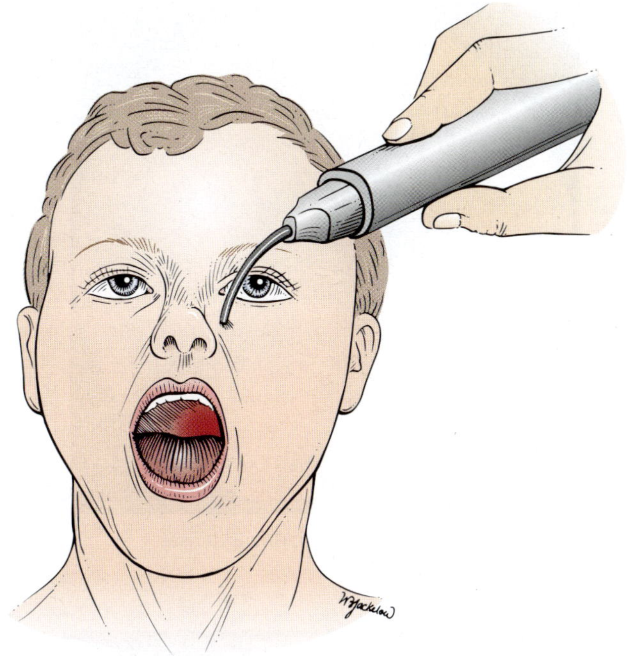

Fig. 11.24 Transillumination of the Maxillary Sinus. Note the red glow seen on the hard palate.

extended. The examiner's left index finger is placed on the ala of the patient's nose to anchor the upper blade of the speculum while the examiner's right hand steadies the patient's head. The right hand is used to change the head position for better visibility of the internal structures. After one nostril has been examined, the speculum, still being held in the examiner's left hand, is introduced into the patient's other nostril. Fig. 11.23 shows a patient with nasal polyps, visible by means of the nasal speculum.

Transilluminate the sinuses. If a patient has symptoms referable to sinus problems, transillumination of the sinuses is performed. This examination is performed in a darkened room, and a bright light source is placed in the patient's mouth on one side of the hard palate. The light is transmitted through the maxillary sinus cavity and is seen as a crescent-shaped dull glow under the eye. The other side is then examined. Normally, the glow on each side is equal. If one sinus contains fluid, a mass, or mucosal thickening, there is a decrease in the glow, indicating loss of aeration on that side. An alternative method of examining the maxillary sinus is to direct a light downward from under the medial aspect of the eye. The patient is asked to open the mouth, and the glow is observed in the hard palate. This technique is illustrated in Fig. 11.24. The frontal sinus can be examined in a similar manner by directing the light upward under the medial aspect of the eyebrow and observing the glow above the eye.

The ethmoid and sphenoid sinuses cannot be examined by transillumination.

The patient-to-patient variability of sinus transillumination is tremendous. In the absence of sinus symptoms, these differences in transillumination are nonspecific.

CLINICOPATHOLOGIC CORRELATIONS

The organs of the ear and nose are vulnerable to various types of diseases, such as infectious, inflammatory, traumatic, and neoplastic. This section focuses on some of the frequently occurring ear infections.

Acute otitis externa is a common inflammatory condition of the external ear canal, most often caused by *Pseudomonas aeruginosa.* The prominent symptom is severe ear pain (otalgia) accentuated by manipulation of the pinna and especially by pressure on the tragus. Edema of the external ear canal, erythema, and a yellowish-green discharge are prominent signs of this disease. Commonly, the canal is so tender and swollen that adequate visualization of the entire canal and tympanic membrane is impossible. Swimmer's ear is a type of otitis externa where the protective cerumen is lost, leading to chronic irritation and maceration caused by water and bacteria. Itching is a

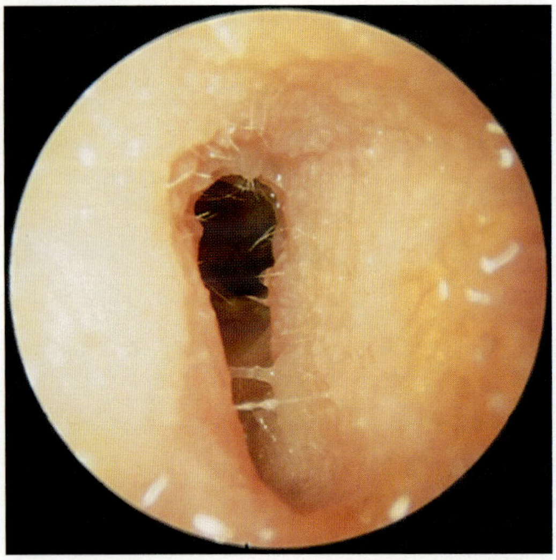

Fig. 11.25 Acute Otitis Externa.

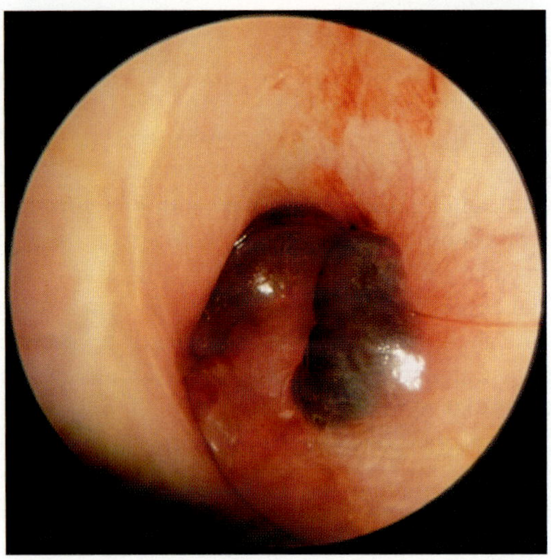

Fig. 11.26 Bullous Myringitis.

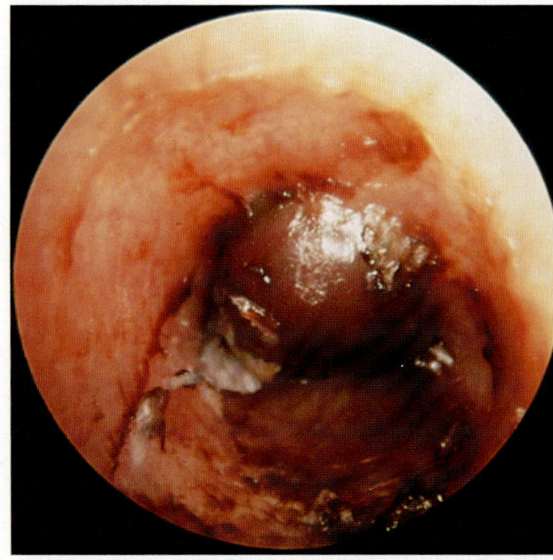

Fig. 11.27 Bullous Myringitis.

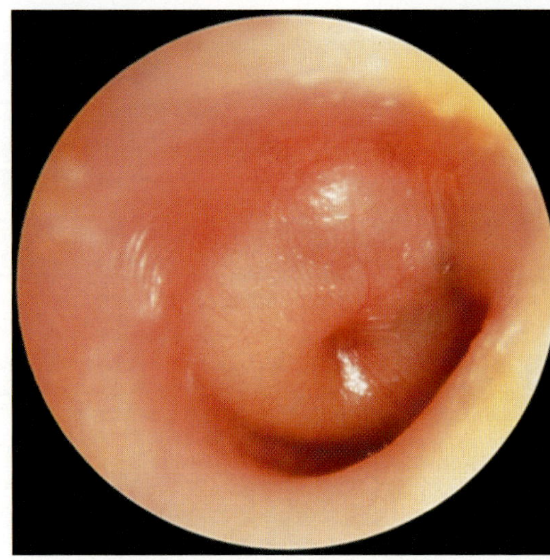

Fig. 11.28 Acute Otitis Media.

common precursor of otalgia. Fig. 11.25 shows the external ear canal of a patient with acute otitis externa. Notice the follicular appearance of the canal, which resulted from epithelial swelling. As the condition progresses, the lumen may be occluded, producing conductive deafness.

Bullous myringitis is a localized form of external otitis, commonly associated with an acute viral upper respiratory infection. Severe otalgia is present, caused by bullous, often hemorrhagic, lesions on the skin in the deep external ear canal and on the tympanic membrane. A blood-tinged discharge may also occur. Fortunately, bullous myringitis is a self-limited condition. Fig. 11.26 shows the tympanic membrane of a patient with bullous myringitis. Notice the blood-filled bullae on the membrane. Fig. 11.27 shows the left ear of another patient with bullous myringitis. Notice the huge bulla filled with serosanguineous fluid arising from the floor of the bony external auditory canal. The bulla is so large that it obscures the tympanic membrane from view.

Acute otitis media is a bacterial infection of the middle ear, occurring most commonly in children. Up to 50% of all children experience an attack of acute otitis media before they reach 1 year of age, and 75% of children are affected before their second birthdays. After 5 years of age, the incidence declines rapidly. Affected patients suffer ear pain and have constitutional symptoms of fever and malaise, often associated with gastrointestinal problems and a conductive hearing loss. In contrast to external otitis, in which pulling on the auricle and tragus causes pain, no pain is elicited when these maneuvers are performed on a patient with acute otitis media. The tympanic membrane becomes injected, and the entire membrane is a fiery red. A mucopurulent exudate in the middle ear causes the membrane to bulge outward. In most cases, antibiotic therapy resolves the condition and restores normal hearing. Fig. 11.28 shows the tympanic membrane of a young child with the classic features of acute otitis media. Notice the erythema, resulting from the acute inflammation, and the cloudiness and bulging of the tympanic membrane resulting from the middle ear exudate.

Spontaneous rupture of the tympanic membrane may result from the increased pressure, with discharge of the mucopurulent exudate into the external ear canal. If this occurs, *advanced acute otitis media* is said to be present. Fig. 11.29 illustrates perforation of a tympanic membrane as a result of otitis media.

Perforations may be *central* or *marginal* and may result from either otitis media or trauma. A central perforation does not involve the margin or annulus of the tympanic membrane; a marginal perforation involves the margin. Marginal perforations are more serious because they predispose the patient to the development of a *cholesteatoma,* which is a chronic condition of the middle ear. A marginal perforation allows squamous epithelium from the external canal to grow into the middle ear. As these cells invade, they desquamate, and debris accumulates in the middle ear, forming a cholesteatoma. Slow enlargement of the cholesteatoma leads to erosion of the ossicles and expansion into the mastoid antrum. Fig. 11.30 illustrates a cholesteatoma.

A congenital cholesteatoma of the right anterior middle ear is pictured in Fig. 11.31. It is smooth and white, medial to a normal tympanic membrane. Fig. 11.32 depicts chronic tympanic membrane perforation of the right ear. Notice the smooth epithelium-covered margin of chronic perforation, as well as patches of tympanosclerosis.

Serous otitis media occurs primarily in adults with viral upper respiratory infections or during sudden atmospheric pressure changes. In the presence of a blocked eustachian tube, air becomes trapped within. The tiny blood vessels in the middle ear absorb much of the air, producing a vacuum that draws in or retracts the tympanic membrane. The sensation of "plugged ears" occurs. If the pressure is not relieved, this vacuum draws serous, nonpurulent fluid from the blood vessels into the middle ear. The tympanic membrane appears yellowish-orange as a result of the amber-colored fluid, and the landmarks are clearly seen as the membrane is retracted against these structures. Partial obstruction of the eustachian tube produces air bubbles or an air-fluid level in the middle ear. Fig. 11.33 shows the tympanic membrane of a patient with serous otitis media.

Recurrent middle ear infections and tympanic membrane rupture may lead to *chronic otitis media.* Chronic infections may produce a foul-smelling discharge, which is the main symptom of chronic otitis media; pain is usually not present.

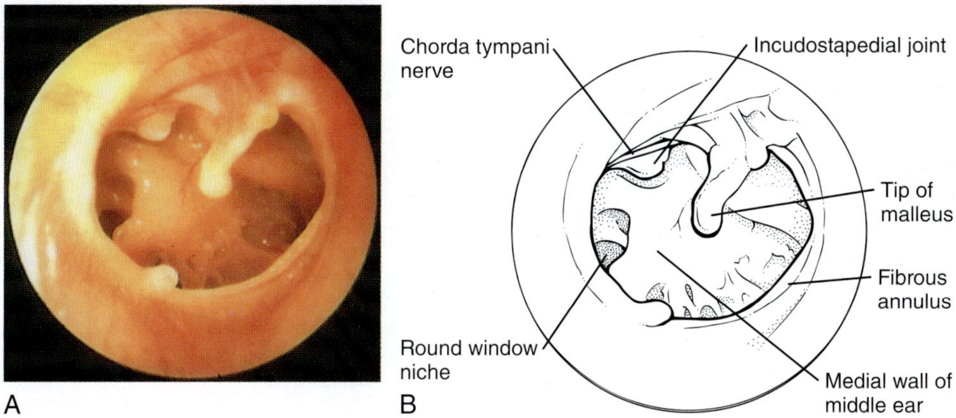

Fig. 11.29 Photograph (A) and labeled schematic (B) illustrating a central perforation of the right tympanic membrane.

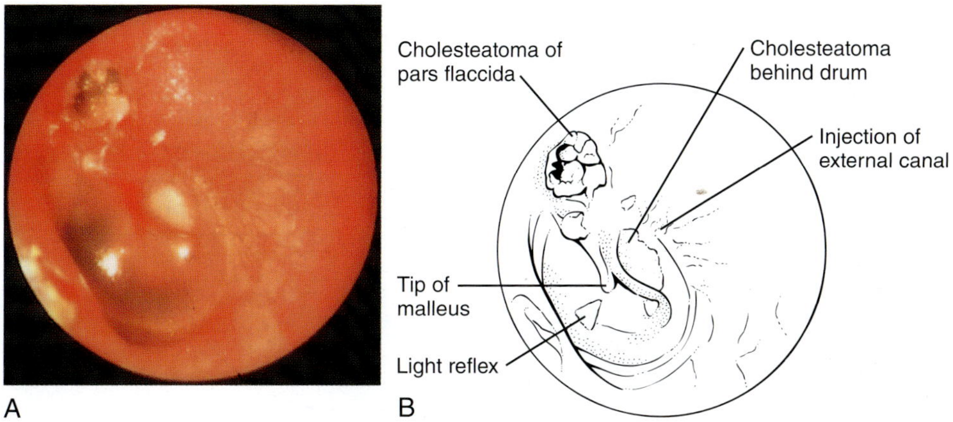

Fig. 11.30 Photograph (A) and labeled schematic (B) illustrating a cholesteatoma of the left ear that resulted from a marginal perforation of the tympanic membrane. Note the injection of the distal external canal.

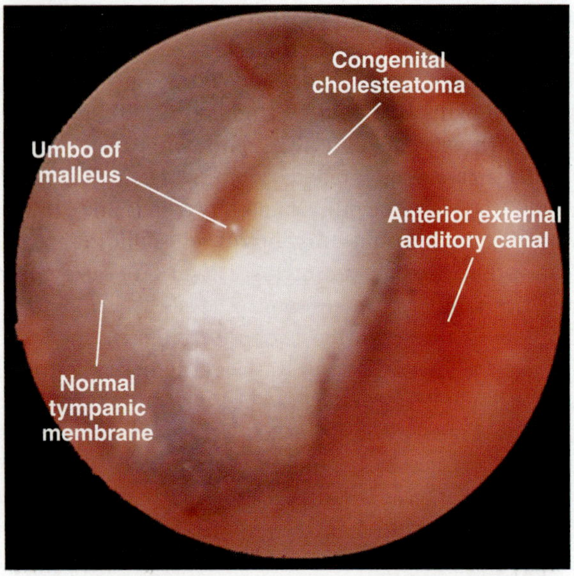

Fig. 11.31 Congenital Cholesteatoma.

Erosion of the ossicles with formation of scar tissue may occur, causing a conductive hearing loss.

Fig. 11.34 shows the right tympanic membrane in an adult patient with chronic eustachian tube dysfunction. An early pars flaccida retraction pocket is seen. These retraction pockets result from chronic negative pressure within the middle ear and may progress to form an acquired cholesteatoma. A pressure-equalizing tube, called a *tympanostomy tube,* or T-tube, has been placed to eliminate the negative middle ear pressure. Fig. 11.35 shows the right tympanic membrane in another patient with long-standing eustachian tube dysfunction whose middle ear is ventilated with a long-term T-tube. Resolving mild otitis externa is seen, with canal skin erythema and desquamation of the epithelium.

Table 11.4 summarizes the comparative features of conductive and sensorineural hearing loss.

Table 11.5 enumerates the common causes of deafness. Table 11.6 differentiates acute otitis externa from acute otitis media.

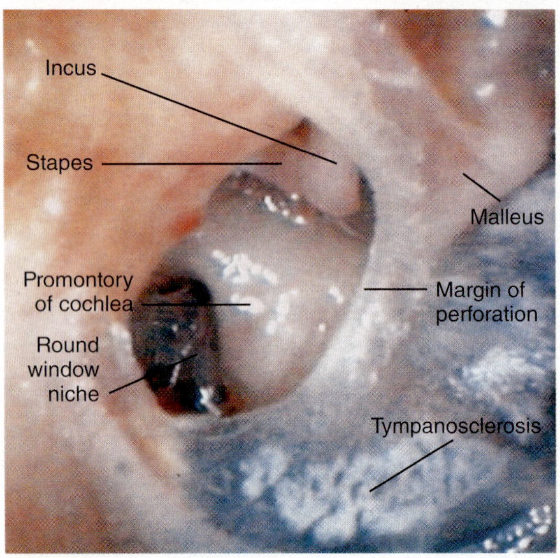

Fig. 11.32 Chronic Tympanic Membrane Perforation.

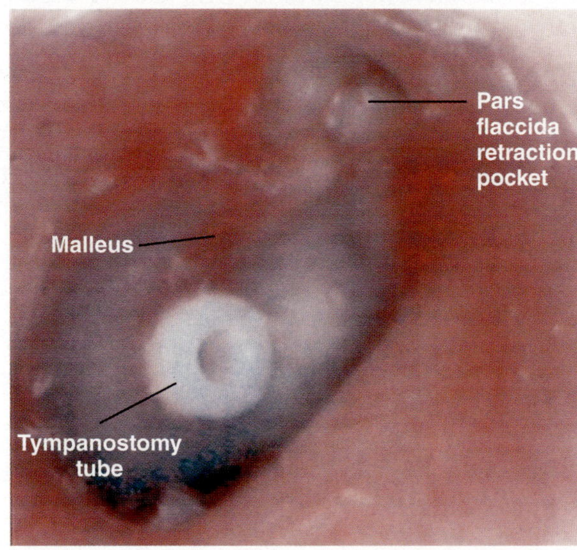

Fig. 11.34 Chronic Eustachian Tube Dysfunction.

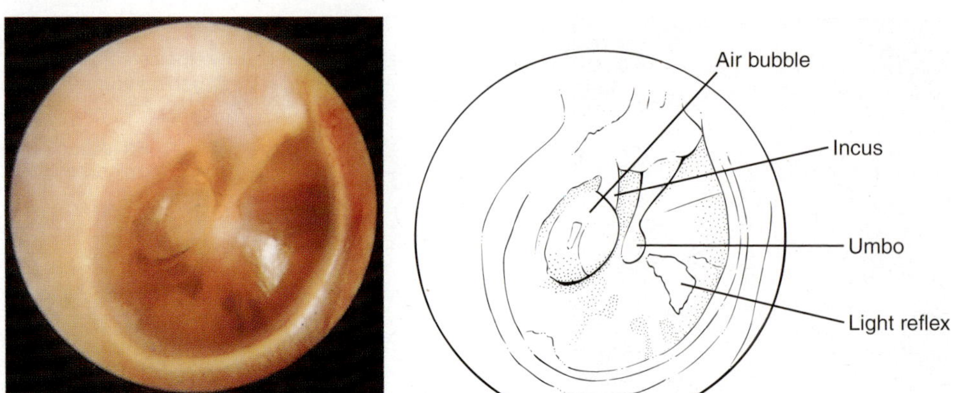

A B

Fig. 11.33 Photograph (A) and labeled schematic (B) illustrating serous otitis media of the right ear. Note the air bubble in the middle ear behind the tympanic membrane.

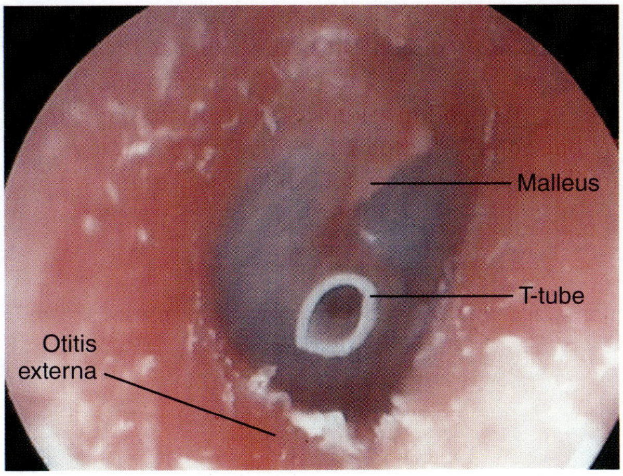

Fig. 11.35 Tympanic Membrane Ventilated With Tympanostomy Tube *(T-tube)*.

TABLE 11.5 Common Causes of Loss of Hearing

Patient	Conductive Deafness	Sensorineural Deafness
Child	Congenital Acute otitis media Chronic otitis media Cerumen Trauma	Congenital Mumps labyrinthitis Maternal rubella during first trimester Birth trauma Congenital syphilis
Adult	Serous otitis media Chronic otitis media Otitis externa Cerumen Eustachian tube blockage Viral myringitis Cholesteatoma Otosclerosis	Delayed-onset congenital Ménière disease Ototoxic drugs Viral labyrinthitis Acoustic neuroma Presbycusis (age-related deafness)

TABLE 11.4 Comparative Features of Conductive and Sensorineural Hearing Loss

Feature	Conductive Hearing Loss	Sensorineural Hearing Loss
Pathologic process	External canal Middle ear	Cochlea Cochlear nerve Brainstem
Loudness of speech	Softer than normal	Louder than normal
External canal	May be abnormal	Normal
Tympanic membrane	Usually abnormal	Normal
Rinne test result	BC>AC	AC>BC
Weber test result	Heard on "deaf" side	Heard on better side (only in severe unilateral loss)

TABLE 11.6 Differentiation of Acute Otitis Externa From Acute Otitis Media

Signs and Symptoms	Acute Otitis Externa (See Fig. 11.25)	Acute Otitis Media (See Fig. 11.28)
Pressure on tragus	Painful	Painless
Lymphadenopathy	Frequent	Absent
External canal	Edematous	Normal
Season	Summer	Winter
Tympanic membrane	Normal	Fluid behind eardrum, possible perforation
Fever	Yes	Yes
Hearing	Slight loss or normal	Decreased

USEFUL VOCABULARY

Listed here are the specific roots that are important to understand the terminology related to diseases of the ear and nose.

Root	Pertaining to	Example	Definition
audio-	to hear	***audio***meter	Device to measure hearing
aur-	ear	***aur***icle	Portion of the external ear not contained within the head
-cusis	hearing	presby***cusis***	Progressive decrease in hearing with age
-lalia	speech	echo***lalia***	Meaningless repetition by a patient of words addressed to them
myringo-	tympanic membrane	***myringo***tomy	Surgical incision of the tympanic membrane
ot(o)-	ear	***ot***itis	Inflammation of the ear
phon-	sound; the sound of a voice	***phon***asthenia	Weakness of the voice
rhino-	nose	***rhino***plasty	Plastic surgery of the nose
tympan(o)-	middle ear	***tympano***tomy	Surgical puncture of the tympanic membrane

WRITING UP THE PHYSICAL EXAMINATION

Listed here are examples of the write-up for the examinations of the ear and nose.

- The external ear appears normal without evidence of inflammation or lesions. The patient has no difficulty hearing the whispered word. The Weber test result is midline. Rinne test result: AC > BC. The external canals are normal as are the tympanic membranes. There is no injection of the external canals or the tympanic membranes. No discharge is present.
- A 1-cm, round, hard, painless mass is present on the right pinna. The patient has no problem with hearing. The Weber test result shows no lateralization. The external canals and tympanic membranes are normal.
- The external structures of the ears are within normal limits. There is a hearing loss in the left ear. The Weber test result lateralizes to the left ear. The left tympanic membrane appears opaque. The ossicles are not seen on the left. The right tympanic membrane appears normal. The ossicles appear normal on the right.
- The nose is not deviated. No swellings are seen. The anterior septum appears pink without discharge or vascular engorgement. The septum is midline. No sinus tenderness is present.
- The nose appears deviated to the right. The nasal mucous membranes are bright red and moist. A whitish-yellow discharge is present on a deviated septum to the right. The sinuses are not tender.

AC, Air conduction; *BC*, bone conduction.

FULL VIDEO

- Video 11.9 Full video: Examination of the ear, sinuses, and nose

REVIEW QUESTIONS

1. **Which of the following statements about the ear canal condition shown below is correct?**

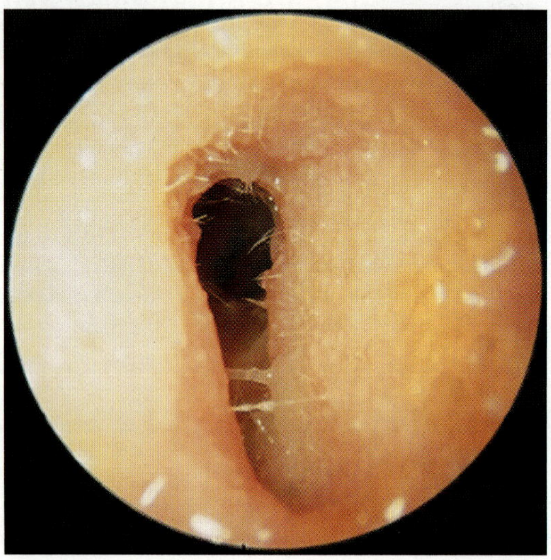

   A. It is very painful when the pinna and tragus are moved.
   B. It is usually bilateral.
   C. It is infectious.
   D. It persists for years, even with treatment.
   E. It is caused by coliform bacteria.

2. **The following statements compare the main types of hearing loss. Which statement is *incorrect?***
   A. Conductive hearing loss occurs in the external canal and middle ear.
   B. In sensorineural hearing loss, speech is softer than normal.
   C. In conductive hearing loss, the tympanic membrane is usually abnormal.
   D. In sensorineural hearing loss, the pathologic process is in the cochlea, cochlear nerve, or brainstem.
   E. The Weber test is heard best on the side of the conductive hearing loss.

3. **Which of the following have been associated with hearing loss?**
   A. Gestational rubella
   B. Diuretics (e.g., ethacrynic acid)
   C. Antibiotics (e.g., gentamicin)
   D. Salicylates
   E. All of these conditions

4. **Which of the following statements about ear symptoms is *incorrect?***
   A. Tinnitus is the sensation of hearing sounds like buzzing or ringing.
   B. Otorrhea is a discharge from the ear and usually indicates acute or chronic infection.
   C. Otalgia is ear pain almost always related to chronic diseases of the external ear.
   D. Vertigo may result from otologic, neurologic, or psychologic causes.
   E. Itching of the ear may result from diabetes, hepatitis, or lymphoma.

5. **Which of the following statements about the tympanic membrane shown below is correct?**

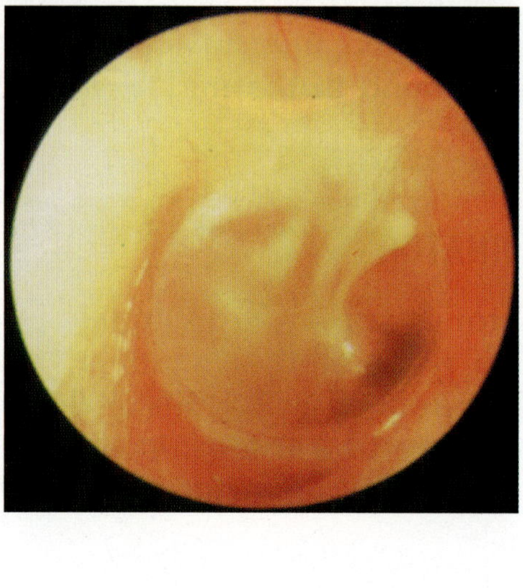

A. Injection over the ossicle indicates infection.
B. The stapes is clearly visible.
C. This is the tympanic membrane of the right ear.
D. There is tympanic membrane perforation.
E. The light reflex indicates an abnormality of the middle ear.

6. Which of the following statements about hearing tests is *incorrect?*
A. The whisper test has a high sensitivity of 90% to 99%.
B. The best tuning fork for testing hearing is the 512-Hz fork.
C. In the Rinne test, BC>AC is the normal (positive) response.
D. In the Weber test, no lateralization (louder in one ear) is the normal response.
E. If there is total deafness in one ear, the patient may hear the tuning fork even when placed on the mastoid process of the deaf ear (the Rinne test).

7. To examine an adult patient's ear, the healthcare professional must do which of the following maneuvers to straighten the external canal?
A. Pull the pinna down, out, and forward.
B. Pull the pinna down, and back.
C. Pull the pinna up, out, and back.
D. Pull the pinna up, out, and forward.
E. Don't pull the pinna at all.

8. The photograph below shows which of the following conditions?

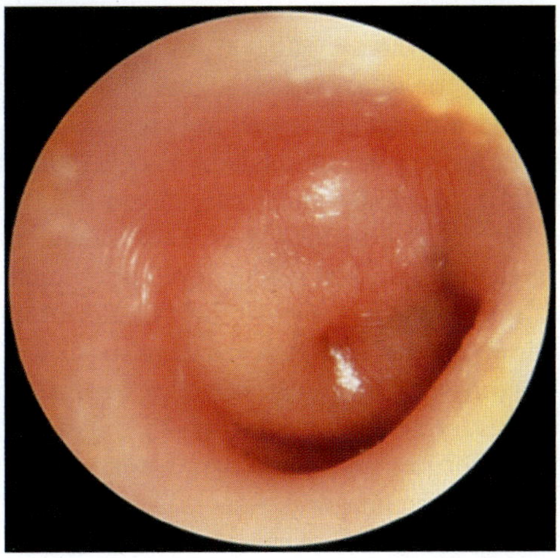

A. Acute otitis externa
B. Acute serous otitis
C. Acute otitis media
D. Bullous myringitis
E. Acute tympanic membrane perforation

9. Common causes of deafness in an adult include:
A. Cholesteatoma
B. Ménière disease
C. Cerumen
D. Acoustic neuroma
E. All of the above

10. Which of the following *matches* of involved sinus and their signs and symptoms is *incorrect?*
A. Maxillary – Ocular abnormalities
B. Ethmoid – Orbital swelling
C. Frontal – Nasal obstruction and rhinorrhea
D. Maxillary – Epistaxis
E. Ethmoid – Pus in the middle meatus

REFERENCES

Available online.

BIBLIOGRAPHY

Available online.

12

The Oral Cavity and Pharynx

Mark H. Swartz

Look to thy mouth; diseases enter here.

George Herbert (1593–1632)

VIDEOS

Video 12.1	Examining the oral cavity
Video 12.2	Palpating the tongue
Video 12.3	Palpating the floor of the mouth
Video 12.4	Full Video: Examination of the oral cavity
See also,	
Video 21.5	Testing Cranial Nerve IX (Glossopharyngeal) and Cranial Nerve X (Vagus)
Video 21.7	Cranial Nerve XII (Hypoglossal)

GENERAL CONSIDERATIONS

From infancy, people use their mouths and oral cavity to express various emotions, providing both gratification and sensory pleasure.

Did you know that around 20% of visits to primary healthcare professionals are due to oral cavity and throat issues? One of the common symptoms patients present with is throat pain, which can be acute and come with fever or difficulty in swallowing. It's important to note that a sore throat may be a sign of a local or systemic problem.

Research suggests that more than 90% of individuals with HIV experience oral symptoms related to the disease. As the immune system weakens, the likelihood of developing oral lesions also increases. These findings highlight the significance of monitoring and addressing oral health in HIV patients.

Oral cancer is the largest group of those cancers that fall into the head and neck cancer category. In 2023, an estimated 54,540 adults (39,290 males and 15,250 females) in the United States were diagnosed with oral or oropharyngeal cancer. Worldwide, an estimated 476,125 people were diagnosed with oral or oropharyngeal cancer in 2020. The rates of these two cancers are more than twice as high in males as in females.

Oral cavity and oropharyngeal cancers occur most often on the tongue, the tonsils, the oropharynx, the gums, and the floor of the mouth. The remainder of the cancers are found in the lips and the minor salivary glands.

The oral cancer incidence rates for people of color have decreased significantly over the past three decades for both sexes, especially males. Oral cancer incidence rates are higher for White males than Hispanic and Black males. Together, oral and oropharyngeal cancers are the eighth-most common cancer among males. The average age of diagnosis is 64. These types of cancer can be diagnosed at any age, with about 20% of cases occurring in people younger than 55. The incidence of oral cancer increases more rapidly after age 50, particularly for adults aged 65.

Cancer rates differ between countries. Hungary and France have higher rates than the United States, while Mexico and Japan have lower rates.

In general, 10.5 out of 100,000 adults may develop oral cancer. However, the rates are still higher among Hispanic and African American males compared to White males.[1]

Oral cancer is often detected late in its development, leading to a high death rate. This cancer can spread to other areas or invade local structures, making it especially dangerous. Additionally, there is an increased risk of developing second primary tumors, with patients who survive their first encounter having up to a 20 times greater risk of developing another cancer.

When diagnosed with oral or pharynx cancer, around 84% of individuals survive for 1 year after all stages of treatment. The percentage of patients who survive for 5 years is 64.8%. Although there are various oral cancers, squamous cell carcinomas account for about 90% of cases.

There are two distinct etiologic factors by which most people develop oral cancer. One is through the use of tobacco and alcohol. The second is human papillomavirus (HPV). Recent studies have shown that the incidence is increasing for oral cancers associated with HPV type 16 infection among White males younger than 50 years of age. In addition, a small percentage of people (<7%) develop oral cancers from no currently identified cause. See *Clinicopathologic Correlations* at the end of this chapter for further information about HPV and oral cancer.

The underlying reason for lingual cancer, which affects the tongue, is uncertain. However, it frequently develops in individuals who use tobacco products such as cigarettes, cigars, e-cigarettes, pipes, and smokeless tobacco, as well as those who drink alcohol (particularly in combination with tobacco use) or chew betel nuts. While betel nut chewing is not prevalent in the United States, it is a widespread custom in many regions worldwide, mainly in Taiwan and India (see Fig. 12.51). HPV infection is linked to cancer in the oropharynx, including the tonsil and the base of the tongue.

In the year 2024, the United States reported 12,650 new cases of laryngeal cancer, resulting in 3880 deaths. Males accounted for 3120 of the deaths while females accounted for 760. Laryngeal cancer usually starts in the glottis (vocal cords) in about 60% of cases and the supraglottic area in around 35%. The remaining cases occur in the subglottis or involve more than one area. Smoking and excessive alcohol consumption are strongly linked to the development of squamous cell cancers in the larynx. While quitting smoking reduces the risk of laryngeal cancer, it remains higher than that of nonsmokers even years after quitting. Supraglottic cancers often cause a sore throat, difficulty swallowing, ear pain, changes in voice quality, or swollen neck nodes. Hoarseness is usually the first sign of early vocal cord cancer. Laryngeal cancer survival rates in the United States vary depending on different factors like cancer stage, age, general health, and treatment effectiveness. However, the 5-year relative survival rate is 61%.

Healthcare professionals recognized the symptoms of obstructive sleep apnea (OSA) syndrome for a long time but didn't understand the underlying cause. The term "Pickwickian syndrome," used to describe the syndrome, was named by the renowned physician Sir William Osler in the early 20th century, who was likely a fan of Charles Dickens. In Dickens's novel *The Pickwick Papers*, the character of Joe, described as "the fat boy," is actually an accurate clinical representation of an adult with OSA syndrome. Initially, the medical literature on OSA or sleep-disordered breathing (SDB) focused on extremely severe cases where patients experienced significant hypoxemia, hypercapnia, and heart failure. We now recognize that SDB is linked to cardiovascular disease, stroke, hypertension, and other morbidity.

Sleep apnea is a common sleep disorder that causes frequent pauses in breathing during sleep. These breathing pauses typically last between 10 to 20 seconds and can happen from 5 to 100 times per hour. Most people with sleep apnea experience symptoms such as loud snoring and daytime sleepiness.

The two main types of sleep apnea are OSA and central sleep apnea (CSA). In OSA, the most common form of sleep apnea, narrowing of the airway during sleep leads to breathing disruptions. It occurs when the muscles that support the soft tissues in the upper airway relax during sleep and block the normal flow of air in and out of the nose and mouth, and, thus, snoring results. CSA is a much less common type of sleep apnea that involves the central nervous system. It occurs when the brain temporarily stops sending signals to the muscles that control breathing and is often caused by an underlying health condition. People with CSA seldom snore. These two types of breathing interruptions reduce sleep quality and, if left untreated, can lead to potentially serious health consequences. A recent study showed accelerated vascular aging in individuals with a high risk of OSA.[2]

The Wisconsin Sleep Cohort Study (WSC)[3] was established in 1988 and was a prospective population-based study of the natural history of SDB. The WSC is an ongoing longitudinal study of the causes, consequences, and natural history of sleep disorders, particularly sleep apnea, now in its 35th year. The prevalence of moderate or severe SDB is estimated at least 6% of American adults, with 17% having mild to moderate SDB. It is also estimated that, in middle age, 9% of females and 24% of males are affected, undiagnosed, and untreated. At least 75% of cases of severe SDB remain undiagnosed.

Mortality follow-up of the WSC indicated that severe SDB is significantly associated with a threefold increased all-cause mortality risk independent of age, sex, body mass index (BMI), and other potential confounders. The costs of untreated sleep apnea reach further than just health issues. In the United States, the economic burden of undiagnosed sleep apnea is nearly $150 billion per year.[4]

Many healthcare professional visits for oral problems are associated with psychiatric disturbances. Psychosomatic disease symptoms often center on the mouth. Patients with psychosomatic disease may have concerns of "burning" or "dryness" of the mouth or tongue. *Bruxism,* or grinding of the teeth other than for chewing, occurs especially during sleep. This overuse of the muscles of mastication has often been interpreted as a manifestation of rage or aggression that is not overtly displayed; it may also be an infantile response to reduce psychic tension.

Although it might be thought that the oral cavity is examined only by dentists, other healthcare professionals must have competency in evaluating this important region of the body. All healthcare professionals must recognize oral signs of chronic, systemic health issues, including lympho- and myeloproliferative disorders, eating disorders, HIV, and anemia. Poor oral health can contribute to many systemic health issues, including heart disease, diabetes, stroke, and preterm labor. The healthcare professional must be able to accomplish the following:

1. Appraise oral hygiene.
2. Recognize dental caries and periodontal disease.
3. Recognize the presence of oral lesions and disorders of the regional lymph nodes, salivary glands, and bony structures.
4. Recognize oral manifestations of systemic disease.
5. Recognize systemic problems caused by oral disease and procedures.
6. Assess physical findings concerning the range and smoothness of jaw motion.
7. Identify dental appliances.
8. Know when a dental consultation is required or should be postponed because of a medical problem.

STRUCTURE AND PHYSIOLOGIC CHARACTERISTICS

The Oral Cavity

The oral cavity consists of the following structures:

- Buccal mucosa
- Lips
- Tongue
- Hard and soft palates
- Teeth
- Salivary glands

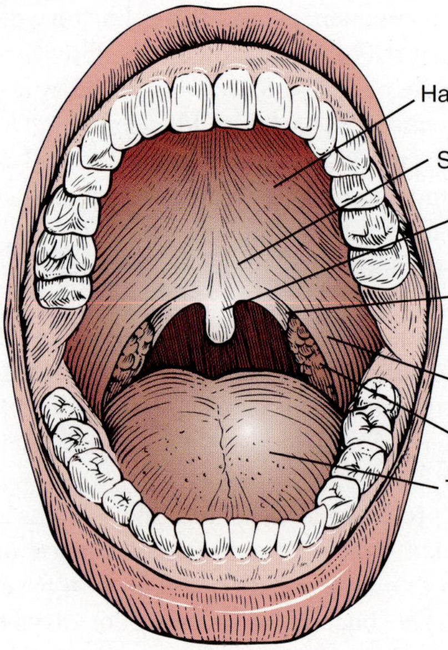

Fig. 12.1 The Oral Cavity.

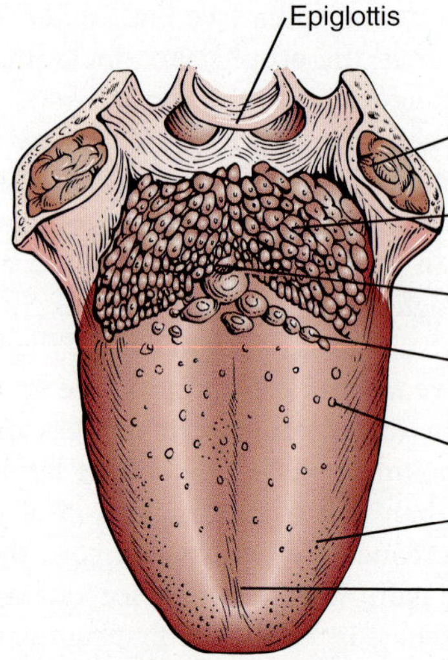

Fig. 12.2 The Tongue Viewed From Above.

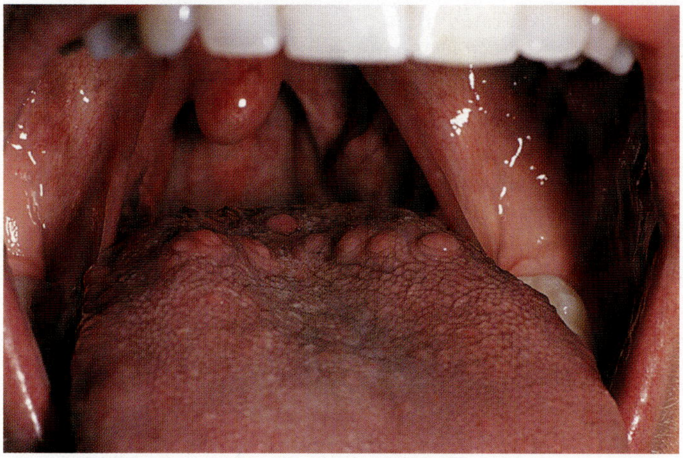

Fig. 12.3 Circumvallate Papillae. (From Eisen D, Lynch DP: *The mouth: diagnosis and treatment*, St. Louis, 1998, Mosby.)

The oral cavity extends from the inner surface of the teeth to the oral pharynx. The hard and soft palates form the roof of the mouth. The soft palate terminates posteriorly at the *uvula.* The *tongue* lies on the floor of the mouth. The tonsils lie at the most posterior aspect of the oral cavity, between the anterior and posterior *pillars.* The oral cavity is illustrated in Fig. 12.1.

The *buccal mucosa* is a mucous membrane that is continuous with the gingivae and lines the insides of the cheeks. The *linea alba,* or bite line, is a pale or white line along the line of dental occlusion. It may be slightly raised and show impressions of the teeth.

Lips are red due to the increased number of vascular dermal papillae and the thinness of the epidermis in this area. An increase in desaturated hemoglobin, *cyanosis,* is manifested as blue lips. The familiar blue discoloration of the lips in a cold environment is related to the decreased blood supply and increased oxygen extraction.

The tongue lies on the floor of the mouth and is attached to the *hyoid bone.* It is the main organ of taste, aids in speech, and serves an essential function in mastication. The body of the tongue contains intrinsic and extrinsic muscles and contains the strongest muscle of the body. The hypoglossal, or twelfth cranial, nerve supplies the tongue.

The dorsum of the tongue has a convex surface with a *median sulcus.* Fig. 12.2 shows the tongue viewed from above. At the posterior portion of the sulcus is the *foramen cecum,* which marks the area of the origin of the *thyroid gland.* Behind the foramen cecum are mucin-secreting glands and an aggregate of lymphatic tissue called the *lingual tonsils.* The texture of the tongue is rough as a result of the presence of papillae, the largest of which are the *circumvallate papillae* (Fig. 12.3). There are approximately 10 of these round papillae, which are located just in front of the foramen cecum and divide the tongue into the anterior two-thirds and the posterior one-third. *Filiform papillae* are the most common papillae and are present over the surface of the anterior portion of the tongue. The *fungiform papillae* are located at the tip and sides of the tongue. These papillae can be recognized from their red color and broad surface.

The *taste buds* are located on the sides of the circumvallate and fungiform papillae. Taste is perceived from the anterior two-thirds of the tongue by the *chorda tympani* nerve, a division of the facial nerve. The *glossopharyngeal,* or ninth cranial nerve, perceives taste sensation from the posterior third of the tongue. There are four basic taste sensations: sweet, salty, sour, and bitter. Sweetness is detected at the tip of the tongue. Saltiness is sensed at the lateral margins of the tongue. Sourness and bitterness are perceived at the posterior aspect of the tongue and are carried by the glossopharyngeal nerve.

When the tongue is elevated, a mucosal attachment, the *frenulum,* may be seen underneath the tongue in the midline connecting the tongue to the floor of the mouth.

The *hard palate* is a concave bone structure. The anterior portion has raised folds or *rugae.* Fig. 12.4 shows the palatal rugae. The *soft palate* is a muscular, flexible area posterior to the hard palate. The posterior margin ends at the *uvula.* The uvula aids in closing off the nasopharynx during swallowing.

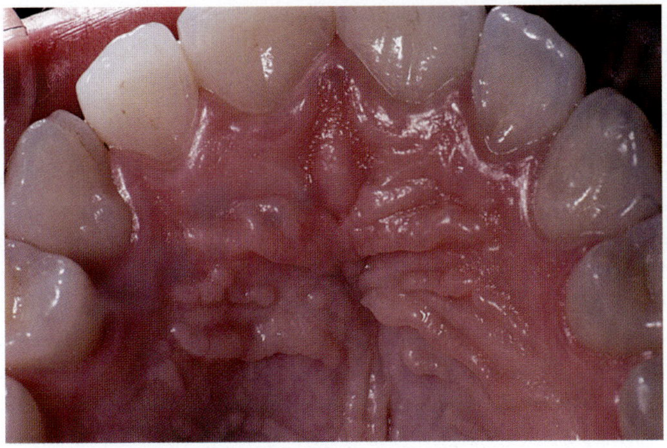

Fig. 12.4 Palatal Rugae. (From Eisen D, Lynch DP: *The mouth: diagnosis and treatment*, St. Louis, 1998, Mosby.)

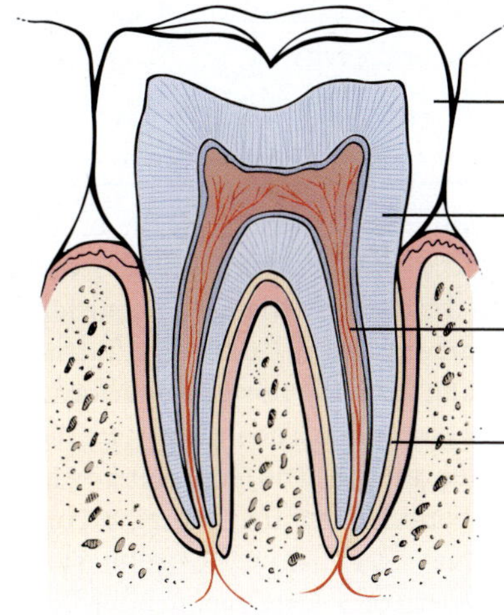

Fig. 12.5 Cross-Sectional View Through a Molar Tooth.

Teeth are composed of several tissues: enamel, dentin, pulp, and cementum. *Enamel* covers the tooth and is the most highly calcified tissue in the body. The bulk of the tooth is the *dentin.* Under the dentin is the *pulp,* which contains branches of the trigeminal, or fifth cranial, nerve and blood vessels. Finally, the *cementum* covers the tooth's root and attaches it to the bone. Fig. 12.5 shows a cross-section through a molar tooth.

The *primary dentition,* or the deciduous teeth, consists of 20 teeth that erupt from 6 to 30 months. The primary dentition per jaw quadrant consists of two incisors, one canine, and two premolars. These teeth are shed from the ages of 6 to 13 years. The *secondary dentition,* or the permanent teeth, consists of 32 teeth that erupt from 6 to 22 years old. The secondary dentition per jaw quadrant consists of two incisors, one canine, two premolars, and three molars. Fig. 12.6 illustrates the primary and secondary dentition, and Fig. 24.33 summarizes the chronology of dentition.

Although not part of the oral cavity, the *salivary glands* are considered part of the mouth. There are three major salivary glands: the parotid, the submandibular, and the sublingual glands. The *parotid gland* is the largest of the salivary glands. It lies anterior to the ear on the side of the face. The facial, or seventh cranial, nerve courses through the gland. The duct of the parotid gland, the *Stensen duct,* enters the oral cavity through a small papilla opposite the upper first or second molar tooth. The *submandibular gland* is the second largest salivary gland. It is located below and in front of the angle of the mandible. The duct of the submandibular gland, the *Wharton duct,* terminates in a papilla on either side of the frenulum at the base of the tongue. The *sublingual gland* is the smallest of the major salivary glands. It is located on the floor of the mouth, beneath the tongue. There are numerous ducts of the sublingual gland, some of which open into the Wharton duct. In addition to these

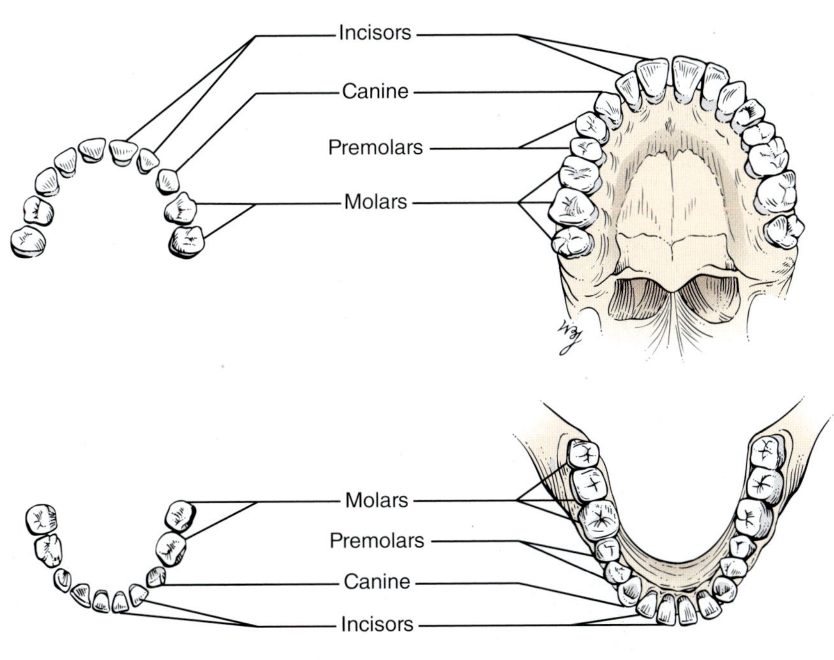

Fig. 12.6 Primary Dentition *(left)* and Secondary Dentition *(right).*

major salivary glands, hundreds of very small salivary glands are located throughout the oral cavity.

THE PHARYNX

The pharynx is divided into the nasopharynx, the oropharynx, and the hypopharynx. The *nasopharynx* lies above the soft palate and is posterior to the nasal cavities. On its posterolateral wall is the opening of the *eustachian tube.* The *adenoids* are pharyngeal tonsils and hang from the posterosuperior wall near the opening of the eustachian tube. The *oropharynx* lies below the soft palate, behind the mouth, and superior to the hyoid bone. Posteriorly, it is bounded by the superior constrictor muscle and the cervical vertebrae. Below the oropharynx is the area known as the *hypopharynx* (or *laryngopharynx*). The hypopharynx is surrounded by three constrictor muscles innervated by the glossopharyngeal and vagus nerves. The hypopharynx ends at the level of the cricoid cartilage, where it communicates with the esophagus through the upper esophageal sphincter. Fig. 12.7 illustrates the functional parts of the pharynx.

The muscular walls of the pharynx are formed by the constrictor muscles, which function during swallowing. The blood supply is derived from the external carotid artery.

Lymphatic tissue is abundant in the pharynx. The lymphoid tissue consists of the *palatine tonsils,* the *adenoids,* and the *lingual tonsils.* These tissues form the *Waldeyer ring.* The palatine tonsils lie between the anterior and posterior pillars in the tonsillar fossa. The palatine tonsils are almond-shaped and vary considerably in size. The adenoids lie on the posterior wall of the nasopharynx, and the lingual tonsils are located at the base of the tongue. The upper portion of the pharynx drains to the retropharyngeal nodes, and the lower part drains to the deep cervical lymph nodes.

The functions of the pharynx are as follows:

- Enable swallowing
- Enable speech
- Provide an airway

Swallowing, or *deglutition,* is divided into three stages. The voluntary stage occurs when the tongue forces a food bolus past the tonsils to the posterior pharyngeal wall. The second stage is involuntary constriction by the pharyngeal muscles, propelling the bolus from the pharynx to the esophagus. The third stage is also involuntary, in which the esophageal muscles push the bolus into the stomach. The larynx is first raised and then closed during the first two stages of swallowing. The eustachian tubes open during swallowing when the nasopharynx closes.

The pharynx also acts as a structure of resonation and articulation. *Resonation* refers to the vibration of a structure. *Articulation* is the change in the shape of a structure to produce speech. Contracting the pharyngeal muscles causes a change in the acoustic quality of speech. Changes in the size and shape of the pharynx affect resonance. The soft palate affects resonance by opening and closing the partition between the oral and nasal cavities. If closure is incomplete, nasal speech results.

THE LARYNX

The larynx is located at the superior margin of the trachea and below the hyoid bone, which is located at the base of the tongue. The larynx is at the level of the fourth to sixth cervical vertebrae. The larynx guards against the entrance of solids and liquids into the trachea and is the organ of voice production.

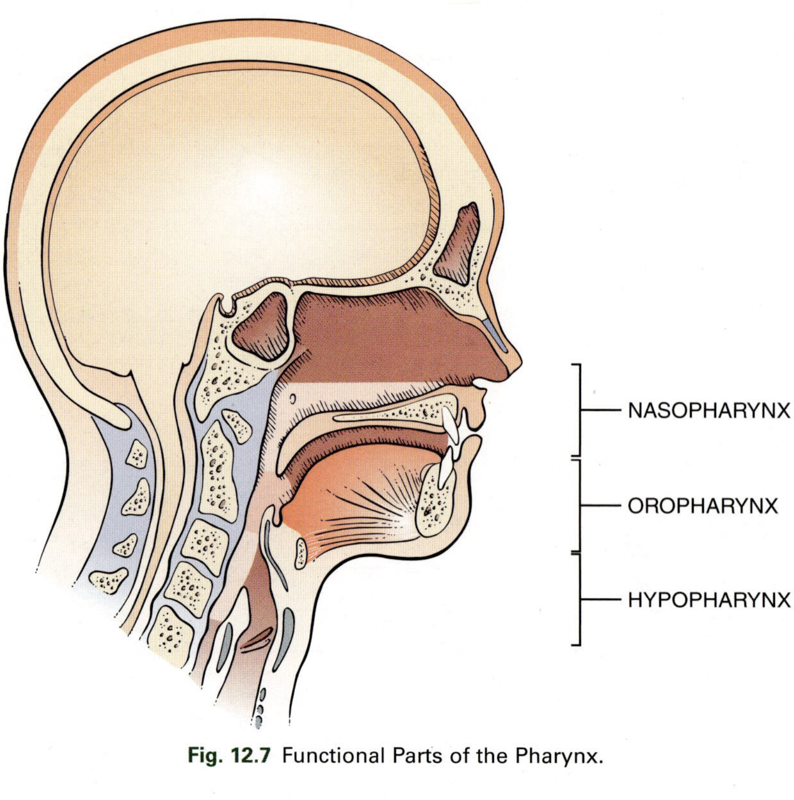

Fig. 12.7 Functional Parts of the Pharynx.

The *epiglottis* is attached above the larynx. The function of the epiglottis is generally believed to protect the airway during swallowing.

The body of the larynx consists of a series of cartilaginous structures: the thyroid, the cricoid, and the arytenoid cartilages. The *thyroid cartilage* forms the bulk of the structure of the larynx and produces the prominence in the neck known as *Adam's apple.* Toward the top of the thyroid cartilage is the *thyroid notch.* Farther down on the thyroid cartilage, there is a space, the *cricothyroid space,* and *membrane* that separates the thyroid cartilage from the cricoid cartilage. The *cricoid cartilage* articulates with the cricothyroid membrane superiorly and the trachea inferiorly. It is the only complete ring of cartilage in the larynx. The paired *arytenoid cartilages* provide an essential area for attachment of the vocal cords. A diagram of the thyroid and cricoid cartilages onto the neck is illustrated in Fig. 12.8, and the laryngeal skeleton is illustrated in Fig. 12.9.

The *vocal cords* vibrate to generate speech. Sound is produced by the rapid vibration of the vocal cords excited by the exhaled stream of air. The vocal cords are brought together, and the action of various laryngeal muscles changes their tension. The nerve supply to the larynx is derived from the superior and recurrent laryngeal branches of the *vagus* or the tenth cranial nerve. The pharynx and oronasal cavity modify voice produced at the larynx.

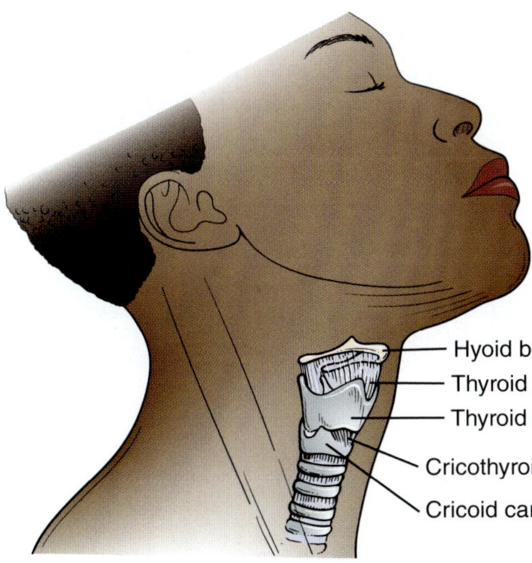

Fig. 12.8 Laryngeal Cartilages.

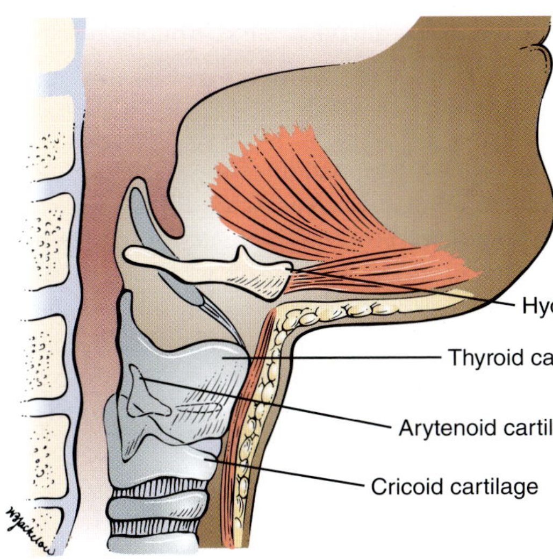

Fig. 12.9 Laryngeal Skeleton.

REVIEW OF SPECIFIC SYMPTOMS

The Oral Cavity

All patients should be asked the following:

"When did you last see a dentist?"

"What did the dentist do?"

"Do your gums bleed?"

"Have you any pain, sores, or masses on your lips or mouth that do not heal?"

"Have you had any problems after the extraction of a tooth?"

(If the patient wears dentures) *"Have you noticed any change in the way your dentures fit?"*

Cancers of the oral cavity are most often found in people who are older than 45 years of age. Cancer of the lip is more common in males than in females and is more likely to develop in people with light-colored skin who have spent extensive time in the sun. Cancer of the oral cavity is more common in people who chew tobacco or smoke pipes. A possible sign of cancer of the mouth or gums is when dentures no longer fit well.

The most important symptoms of disease of the oral cavity are as follows:

- Pain
- Ulceration
- Bleeding
- Mass
- Halitosis (bad breath)
- Xerostomia (dry mouth)

Pain

When a patient has a concern of oral pain, it is essential to ask the following:

"Where is the pain?"

"Describe the pain."

"Do you feel the pain anywhere else?"

"How long has the pain been present?"

"What brings the pain on?"

"What makes it better? Worse?"

"When you have the pain, do you have other symptoms?"

Tooth pain may be a symptom of underlying gingival disease. Therefore, a history of dental procedures and recent work should be documented.

Pain in the teeth may sometimes be referred from the chest. Patients with angina may be concerned with pain in their teeth associated with exertion. Careful and thoughtful questioning is indicated.

Ulceration

Oral ulcerative lesions are common and may manifest local or systemic immunogenic, infectious, malignant, or traumatic diseases. The patient's history is important because it indicates whether the lesions are acute or chronic, single or multiple, and primary or recurrent.

Oral pain is frequently related to ulceration of the lips or tongue. Cancer is not the most common cause of oral cavity ulceration, but it must always be considered. When a patient has a concern of ulceration, ask the following questions:

"Have you had a lesion like this before?"
"Are there multiple lesions?"
"How long have the lesions been present?"
"Are there lesions anywhere else on the body, such as in the vagina? In the urethra? In the anus?"
"Are the lesions painful?"
"Do you smoke?" If so, *"How much?"*
"Do you drink alcohol?"
"Do you have a history of venereal disease?"

The examiner should ask about a patient's sexual habits. These questions were discussed in Chapter 1, The Interviewer's Questions. Smoking and drinking alcohol predispose an individual to precancerous lesions of the mouth, such as leukoplakia and erythroplakia.

Bleeding

Bleeding may result from a primary hematologic disorder or local inflammation or neoplasm. Many medications may also cause or predispose a patient to bleeding. Therefore, always ask whether the patient is taking any medications.

Mass

If a patient has a concern of, or on physical examination is found to have, an intraoral mass or a mass in the region of a salivary gland, determine its duration and whether the mass is painful. A painless mass is usually a sign of a tumor.

Are there associated symptoms such as excessive salivation, known as *ptyalism,* or dryness of the mouth, known as *xerostomia*? Is dysphagia (difficulty in swallowing) present?

Halitosis

Halitosis affects approximately 50% of all adults. Fortunately, only in a small percentage does the problem persist the entire day. Unfortunately, others tell most individuals with halitosis that they have bad breath, although they may be unaware of the problem. In some cases, the odor in the mouth is so objectionable that it can compromise the patient's social and professional life.

The source of bad breath is in the oral cavity in 90% of cases; the other 10% have disorders in the nasal passages or lungs or systemic disease. It is questionable whether the gastrointestinal tract is a source of halitosis.

It is believed that halitosis is caused by volatile sulfur and other compounds exhaled during speech and respiration. These compounds are produced by putrefactive, gram-negative anaerobic bacteria colonizing on the posterior dorsum of the tongue, in periodontal pockets, and around some dental restorations and prostheses. The volatile sulfur compounds are generated by the bacterial metabolism of sulfur-containing amino acids. Xerostomia increases the level of volatile sulfur compounds.

Patients with systemic diseases such as diabetes mellitus, cirrhosis, uremia, and cancer; infections of the perioral regions; and trimethylaminuria (fish odor syndrome) can suffer from bad breath. Therefore, these conditions must be considered in the absence of oral and sinonasal disease.

Treatment of halitosis should be directed toward the underlying cause. Once it has been determined that the source of the bad breath is the oral region, the patient should be instructed in procedures of good oral hygiene, including proper tooth brushing, flossing, and, most important, cleaning of the posterior dorsum of the tongue with a unique scraping device or toothbrush. Appropriate mouthwash may also be used. These procedures must be performed at least twice daily to remove the bacteria and accumulated metabolic products.

Xerostomia

Xerostomia, or dry mouth, is a common symptom of reduced or absent salivary secretion. It is most common in females and aging populations. It is frequently observed as a side effect of various medications, including antihistamines, decongestants, tricyclic antidepressants, antihypertensives, and anticholinergic drugs. It may also occur with mouth breathing, neurologic disorders, radiation therapy to the head and neck, HIV infection, and autoimmune disorders. The saliva is thick, and the oral mucosal surfaces are dry; the tongue is commonly fissured and atrophic. The dry environment predisposes to candidiasis and dental caries.

The Pharynx

The most common symptoms of disease of the pharynx include the following:

- Nasal obstruction
- Pain
- Dysphagia
- Deafness
- Snoring

Nasal Obstruction

Nasal obstruction can result from enlarged adenoids or tumor formation in the nasopharynx. It is essential to determine whether the patient has allergies, sinus trouble, or sustained nasal trauma.

Pain

Pain can result from inflammation of the tonsils or posterior pharynx or a tumor in this area. Acute throat pain may be caused by inflammatory processes or injury. A foreign body in the pharynx often produces severe pain worsened by swallowing. Often, throat pain may be referred to the ipsilateral ear. Chronic throat pain may be caused by inflammatory processes and by neoplasms. Enlarged thyroid lobes or diffuse thyroid enlargement may cause throat pain associated with dysphagia. Hysteria is another cause of chronic throat pain.

Dysphagia

Dysphagia is difficulty in swallowing. Determine the site of obstruction. Does the dysphagia occur with liquids, solids, or tablets? Questions related to tonsillar infections are relevant because enlarged tonsils may interfere with swallowing. It is prudent to ask whether *regurgitation* of food occurs; this results from an abnormal pharyngeal pouch. The patient may say that the "food gets stuck." This is often associated with significant disease.

Deafness

A tumor at the distal end of the eustachian tube in the nasopharynx can produce *conductive deafness*. Benign masses such as hypertrophied adenoids may be responsible. Nasopharyngeal malignancies may also be the cause of conductive deafness. In addition, serous effusions in the middle ear space often cause eustachian tube dysfunction.

Snoring

Snoring is a common concern. As discussed earlier in this chapter, OSA is a critical problem often associated with heavy snoring. Sleep apnea, a form of SDB, is a severe and potentially life-threatening condition suffered by more than 20 million Americans.

Ask the following questions:

"Have you been told that you snore?"
"How often do you snore?"
"Does your snoring bother other people?"
"Have breathing pauses been noticed?"
"Are you tired after sleeping?"
"Are you tired during the daytime?"
"Have you ever fallen asleep while driving?"
"Do you have high blood pressure?"
"Is your body mass index greater than 28?"
"Are you 50 years old or older?"
"Are you a male with a neck circumference greater than 17 inches (43 centimeters) or a female with a neck circumference greater than 16 inches (41 centimeters)?"
"During usual sleep, have you noticed or been told that you toss and turn frequently?"
"Have you noticed or been told that you kick or jerk your legs repeatedly?"
"During the time you are usually awake (daytime and evening), how often do you become irresistibly sleepy or fall asleep in the following situations:

- *After a meal*
- *Reading or watching TV*
- *Sitting and talking to someone*
- *At work*
- *While a passenger in a vehicle*
- *While driving a vehicle"*

"About how many times per night do you wake up?"
"Do you have difficulty falling asleep at night?"
"How many hours do you sleep?"

SDB also deprives the person of oxygen, which can lead to morning headaches or a decline in mental functioning. It is also linked to high blood pressure, irregular heartbeats, and an increased risk of heart attacks and stroke. In addition, patients with severe, untreated SDB are two to three times more likely to have automobile accidents than the general population. In some high-risk individuals, SDB may even lead to sudden death from respiratory arrest during sleep, heart attacks, or strokes.

Snoring, sleepiness, and tiredness are suggestive symptoms of SDB.

To diagnose SDB, healthcare professionals may order a sleep study such as a polysomnogram (PSG). For a PSG, the patient usually stays overnight at a sleep center. This study records brain activity, eye movements, heart rate, blood pressure, oxygen saturation, nasal air movement, snoring, and chest movements. The chest movements show whether the patient is making an effort to breathe. If the PSG shows that the patient has SDB, a continuous positive airway pressure (CPAP) machine may be recommended. CPAP is a treatment that uses mild air pressure to keep the airways open.

Refer to Chapter 13, The Chest, for more information on SDB.

The Larynx

Dysphonia

The primary symptom of laryngeal disease is a change in the voice, especially the development of dysphonia or hoarseness. Ask the following questions:

"How long have you had the hoarseness?"
"What seems to make it better? Worse?"
"Is there any time of day when it is worse?"
"Have you had any surgery necessitating general anesthesia?"
"Have you had any injury to your neck?"

Determine whether the patient is or was a smoker. Recent onset of hoarseness may result from impingement on the recurrent laryngeal nerve as it hooks around the left bronchus. This may be caused by a tumor or by an enlarged left atrium. Voice overuse or vocal cord neoplasms are other causes of hoarseness. Procedures involving general anesthesia necessitate using an endotracheal tube, which could potentially damage a vocal cord and cause hoarseness.

EFFECT OF A VOICE DISORDER ON THE PATIENT

Phonation is the process of sound production by the interaction of airflow through the glottis and the opening and closing of the vocal cords of the larynx. Voice loudness is proportional to the air pressure below the glottis; pitch is related to this pressure and the vocal cords' length. Therefore, voice quality may change when there is interference with the vocal cords or pharyngeal cavity vibration (i.e., resonance).

A voice disorder may be related to an enlarged vocal cord, a laryngeal mass, or a neurologic or psychologic problem. A voice disorder is defined as the presence of a voice that is different in pitch, quality, loudness, or flexibility compared to the voices of other persons of similar age, sex, and ethnic group. An abnormal voice may be a symptom or sign of illness, and its cause should be determined.

In a study of a school-aged population, voice disorders were found in up to 23% of children. Most of these disorders were related to voice abuse, not organic problems. In another study, 7% of males and 5% of females from 18 to 82 years of age were found to have voice disorders. Again, most of these disorders were related to organic problems.

Many patients with organic speech disorders are rejected by other people. Their speech may be high-pitched or nasal and a cause of embarrassment. Their self-esteem is low. Others reject them because their voice patterns are objectionable.

As a voice disorder affects a person, they can use their voice to influence others. How a person speaks—the quality, pitch, loudness, stress patterns, and rate—reflects their personality. Psychogenic voice disorders are functional disorders that are manifestations of psychologic imbalance. Voice is a helpful indicator of *affective disorders like* depression, manic states, mood swings, and *schizophrenia.*

PHYSICAL EXAMINATION

Examining the oral cavity requires a penlight, gauze pads, gloves, applicator sticks, and tongue depressors.

The Oral Cavity

See Video 12.1.

The physical examination of the oral cavity includes inspection and palpation of the following structures:

- Lips
- Buccal mucosa
- Gingivae
- Teeth
- Tongue
- Floor of the mouth
- Hard and soft palates
- Salivary glands
- Twelfth cranial nerve

Sit or stand directly in front of the patient, who should be seated. The patient's face should be well illuminated. Work systematically from front to back so that no areas are omitted. Put on a pair of gloves when palpating any structure in the mouth. When any lesion is found, note its consistency and tenderness. If the patient is wearing dentures, ask them to remove them. Inspect the face and mouth for asymmetries and abnormalities.

Evaluate the patient's breath. Is there any distinctive odor on the patient's breath? This may suggest poor oral hygiene or systemic disease. A fetid odor may be caused by extensive caries or periodontal disease.

Have the patient open their mouth. If the mouth can be opened beyond 35 mm, subluxation of the jaw may be present. Deviation of the jaw is suggestive of a neuromuscular or temporomandibular joint problem.

Inspect the Lips

Inspect the lips for localized or generalized swellings, and assess the patient's ability to open the mouth.

Assess the *color* of the lips. Is cyanosis present? Are there any lesions on the lips? If a lesion is detected, palpate it to characterize its texture and consistency. Fig. 12.10 depicts a patient's mouth with multiple herpetic ulcers, commonly known as *cold sores* or herpes simplex labialis, on the lips and external nares. Fig. 12.11 depicts multiple telangiectatic lesions on the tongue secondary to *Osler-Weber-Rendu syndrome.* In this syndrome, multiple telangiectases are present throughout the gastrointestinal tract. These may bleed insidiously, causing anemia. Fig. 12.12 depicts the classic brown pigmentary changes on the lips of a patient with *Peutz-Jeghers syndrome.* This autosomal dominant disorder is characterized by generalized gastrointestinal hamartomatous polyposis and mucocutaneous pigmentation.

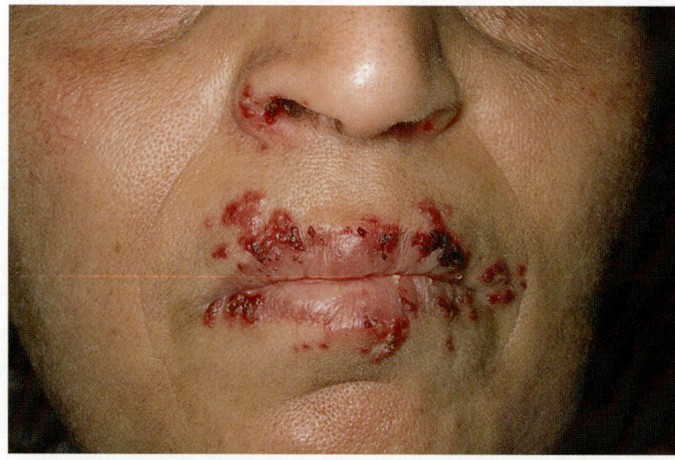

Fig. 12.10 Herpes Simplex Labialis.

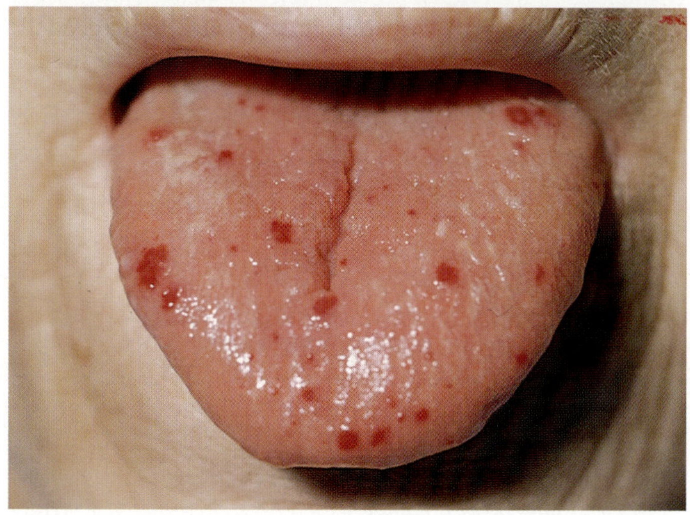

Fig. 12.11 Osler-Weber-Rendu Syndrome. Note the telangiectatic lesions.

A *mucocele* of the lip is a common bluish, cystic-appearing, painless, translucent, traumatically induced lesion. Mucoceles, which occur mainly on the lower lip, range in size from several millimeters to several centimeters and arise from obstruction or rupture of the minor salivary gland. When ruptured, a mucocele releases a clear, thick fluid. Fig. 12.13 depicts a mucocele of the lower lip.

Inspect the Buccal Mucosa

The patient should be asked to open their mouth widely. The mouth should be illuminated with a light source. The buccal mucosa must be evaluated for any lesions or color changes, and the buccal cavity must be inspected for any evidence of

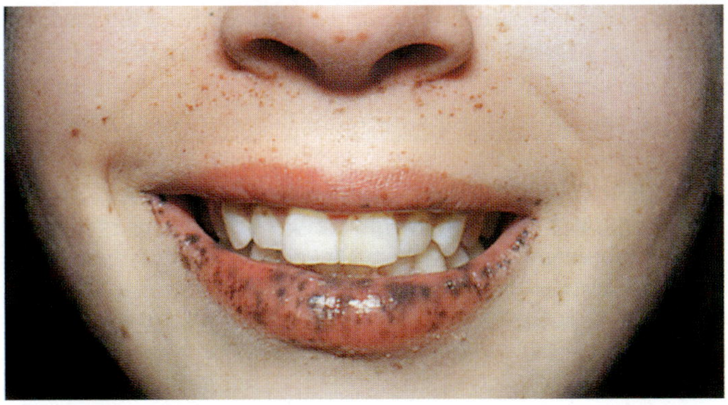

Fig. 12.12 Peutz-Jeghers Syndrome. Note the pigmentary changes. (From Cohen BA: *Atlas of pediatric dermatology*, London, 1993, Wolfe Publishing.)

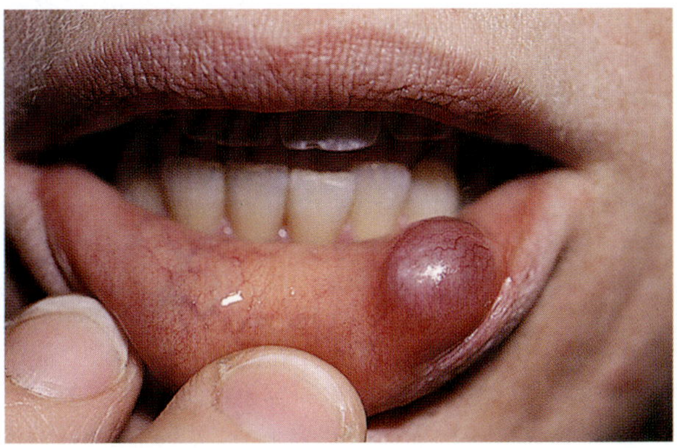

Fig. 12.13 Mucocele of the Lower Lip. (From Callen JP, Paller AS, Greer KE, et al: *Color atlas of dermatology*, ed 2, Philadelphia, 2000, WB Saunders.)

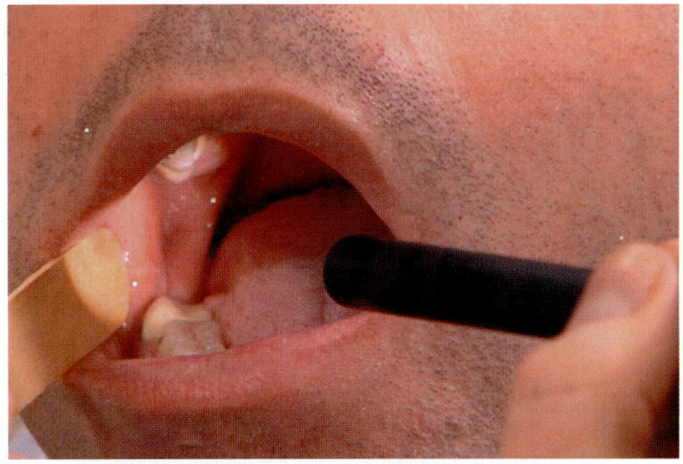

Fig. 12.14 Inspection of the Buccal Mucosa.

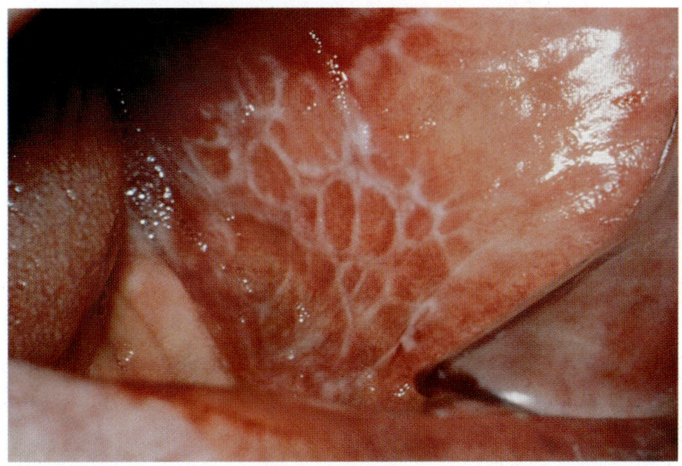

Fig. 12.15 Nonerosive Lichen Planus of the Buccal Mucosa.

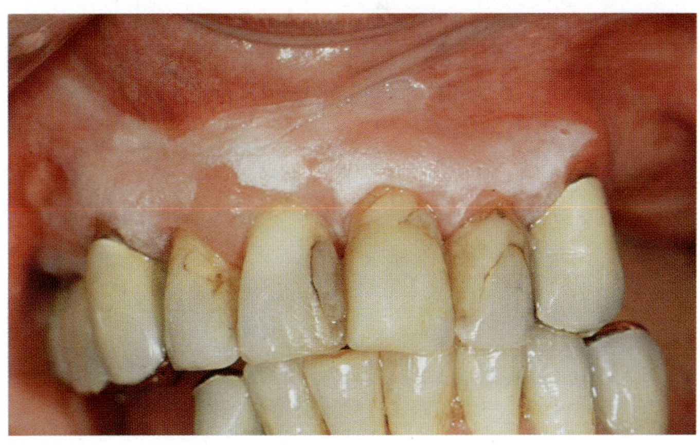

Fig. 12.16 Leukoplakia of the Gingiva.

asymmetry or areas of injection (dilated vessels, usually indicative of inflammation). The buccal mucosa, teeth, and gingivae are easily evaluated using a tongue depressor to retract the cheek away from the gums, as shown in Fig. 12.14. The examiner should inspect for discolorations, evidence of trauma, and the condition of the parotid duct orifice.

Are there any ulcerations of the buccal mucosa? Are there *white lesions* on the buccal mucosa? A common painless white lesion in the mouth is *lichen planus,* a reticulated, or lacelike, eruption bilaterally on the buccal mucosa. An erosive, painful variant is similar in appearance except for the presence of hemorrhagic and ulcerated lesions. Nonerosive lichen planus is shown in Fig. 12.15. Is *leukoplakia* present? In the mouth, leukoplakia can manifest as a painless, precancerous white plaque on the cheeks, gingivae, and tongue. Leukoplakia of the gingiva is pictured in Fig. 12.16. Over 15 years, this lesion developed into verrucous hyperplasia, verrucous carcinoma, and squamous cell carcinoma. As a result, a resection of the maxilla and palate was required. Fig. 12.17 depicts leukoplakia of the tongue in another patient. The thick, white, adherent patches are sharply demarcated and cannot be denuded from the tongue.

Small, pinhead-sized, yellow papules on the buccal mucous membrane are usually *Fordyce spots* or *granules.* Fordyce spots are normal, prominent, ectopic sebaceous glands commonly seen on the lips or buccal mucosa near the exit of the parotid duct. They are probably the most common lesions in the mouth. Fig. 12.18 depicts Fordyce spots on the buccal mucosa. Ectopic sebaceous glands can also be found on the shaft of the penis (see Fig. 18.11) and on the labia (see Fig. 19.13).

Fig. 12.19 shows angiokeratomas of the buccal mucosa, or *angiokeratoma corporis diffusum,* in a patient with *Fabry disease.* Fig. 18.18 depicts angiokeratomas on the scrotum of the same

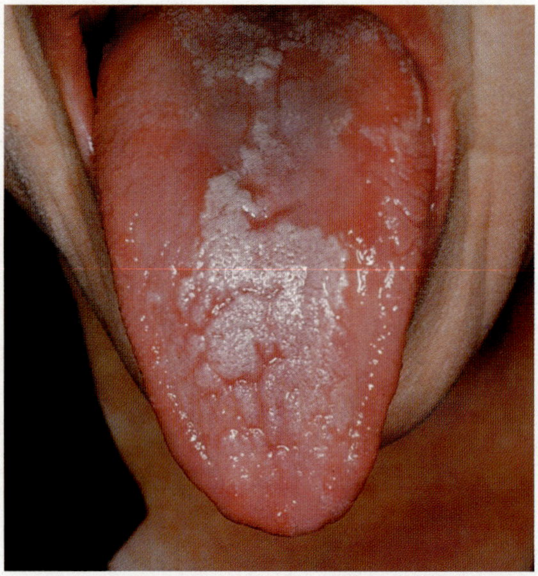

Fig. 12.17 Leukoplakia of the Tongue.

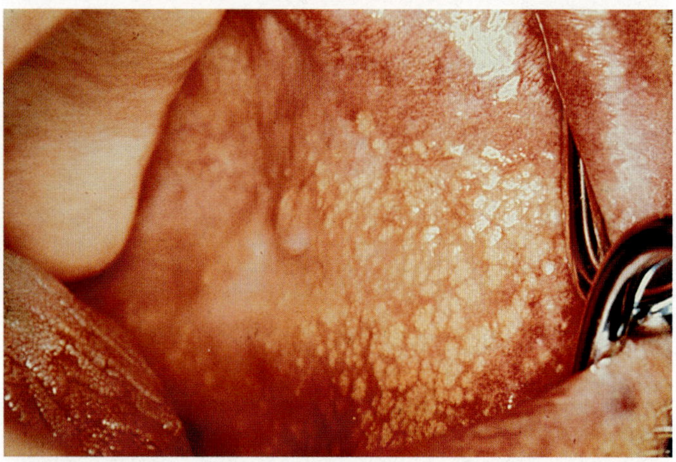

Fig. 12.18 Fordyce Spots (Granules) on the Buccal Mucosa. (From Eisen D, Lynch DP: *The mouth: diagnosis and treatment*, St. Louis, 1998, Mosby.)

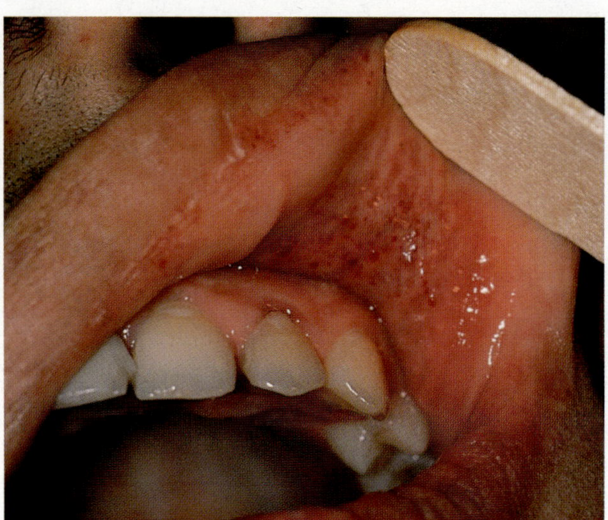

Fig. 12.19 Angiokeratomas of the Buccal Mucosa.

patient. Fabry disease is an inherited disorder resulting from the deposition of buildup of a type of fat, globotriaosylceramide, in the body's cells. It is a storage disorder more common in males and can affect many organs, including the heart, kidney, and skin.

Inspect the Gingivae

Normal gingivae are stippled, pink, and firm. Does the gingival tissue completely occupy the interdental space? Are the roots of the teeth visible, indicating recession of the periodontal tissue? Is there pus or blood along the gingival margin? Are the gingivae swollen? Is there evidence of bleeding? Is gingival inflammation present? Is abnormal coloration present? *Erythroplakia* is an area of mucous membrane on which there are granular, erythematous papules that bleed. Erythroplakia has a more significant potential for malignancy than leukoplakia. Fig. 12.20 shows a patient's mouth with erythroplakia of the gingiva (on the right) and inflammatory gingivitis (on the left).

There are many causes of *gingival hyperplasia,* including heredity, hormonal imbalances of puberty and pregnancy, medications, and leukemia. Gingival hyperplasia is common in patients taking phenytoin (Dilantin®), an antiepilepsy medication, and those taking nifedipine, a calcium channel blocker. It has been estimated that gingival hyperplasia develops in 30% to 50% of all patients taking phenytoin. The hyperplastic gingival changes of hormonal imbalances usually recede once the hormones have returned to their normal, lower levels. Fig. 12.21 depicts marked gingival hyperplasia in a patient taking phenytoin. Dense leukemic infiltration of the gingiva is commonly seen in acute monocytic and acute monomyelocytic leukemia. Fig. 12.22 shows gingival enlargement and bleeding caused by acute monomyelocytic leukemic infiltration.

Inspect the Teeth

There are 32 teeth in the total adult dentition. Is the dentition appropriate for the patient's age? The teeth should be inspected for caries and malocclusion. Are the teeth clean, especially around the gum line? Is there discoloration of the teeth? Is there tooth loss? Teeth inspection often provides insight into the patient's attitude toward general hygiene.

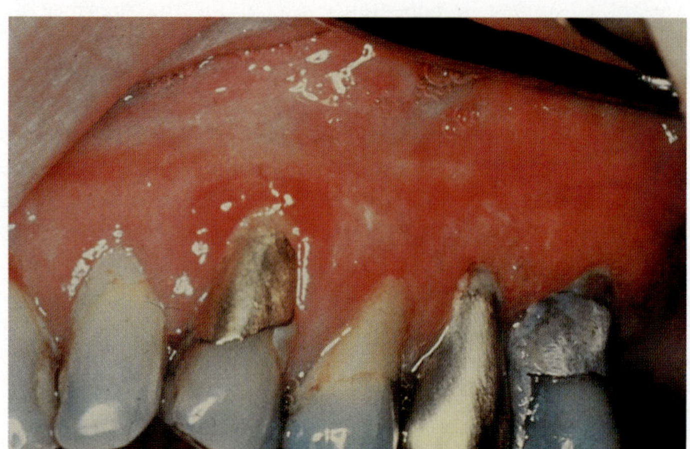

Fig. 12.20 Erythroplakia of the Gingiva *(right)*.

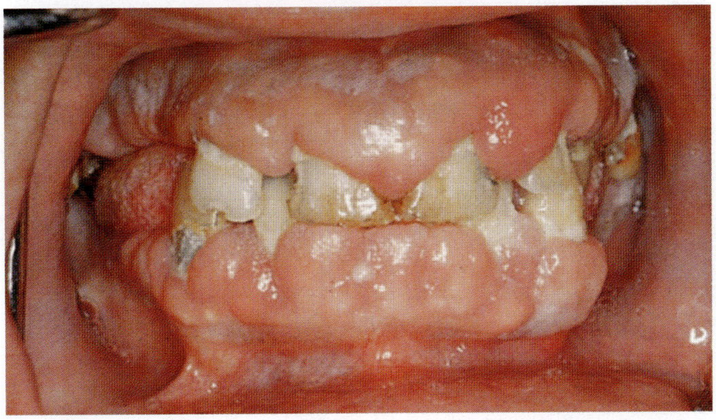

Fig. 12.21 Gingival Hypertrophy in a Patient Taking Phenytoin (Dilantin).

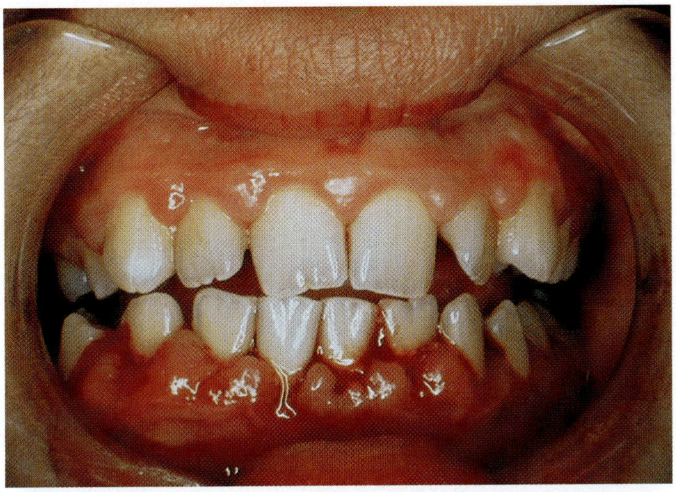

Fig. 12.22 Gingival Hypertrophy in a Patient With Acute Monomyelocytic Leukemia. Note the bleeding gingivae.

Are the teeth appropriately aligned? Ask the patient to bite normally while you retract the buccal mucosa with a tongue depressor. How many teeth bear force on mastication? Repeat this inspection on the other side. Do the maxillary teeth overlap the mandibular ones, and are they in contact with them? If so, the bite is probably normal.

If the patient is wearing dental appliances such as dentures or bridges, they should remove them for a complete evaluation.

Inspect the Tongue

Inspect the mucosa, and note any masses or ulceration. Is the tongue moist? Ask the patient to stick out the tongue. Neuromuscular weakness may be present if the tongue cannot protrude in the midline or move rapidly in all directions. Are there any mass lesions on the sides or undersurface of the tongue? Ask the patient to lift the tongue to the roof of the mouth so that the inferior aspect of the tongue can be inspected. In older individuals, the prominent veins on the ventral aspect of the tongue may be tortuous. These varicosities never bleed spontaneously and have no clinical significance. Fig. 12.23 shows a patient with sublingual varices. Fig. 12.24 shows a patient with a benign lipoma of the tongue.

A *geographic tongue* is a benign condition in which the dorsum of the tongue has smooth, localized red areas denuded of filiform papillae, surrounded by well-defined, raised yellowish-white margins and normal filiform papillae. These areas together give the tongue a maplike appearance. The tongue's appearance gradually changes as the depapillated areas heal and new areas of depapillation occur. A *black hairy tongue* is another benign condition in which the filiform papillae on the dorsum of the tongue are greatly elongated; these enlarged, "hairy" papillae become pigmented with a brownish-black color caused by staining from food or tobacco or proliferating chromogenic microorganisms. More commonly seen in males, this condition may be a sequela to antibiotic therapy. A *scrotal,* or *fissured, tongue* is another normal variant; approximately 5% of the population has fissures in the tongue. The fissures first develop in late childhood and become deeper with age. The fissure pattern is quite variable. Food debris may collect in the fissures, causing inflammation, but the condition is otherwise benign. Halitosis may be a problem. Fig. 12.25 shows these three normal tongue variants.

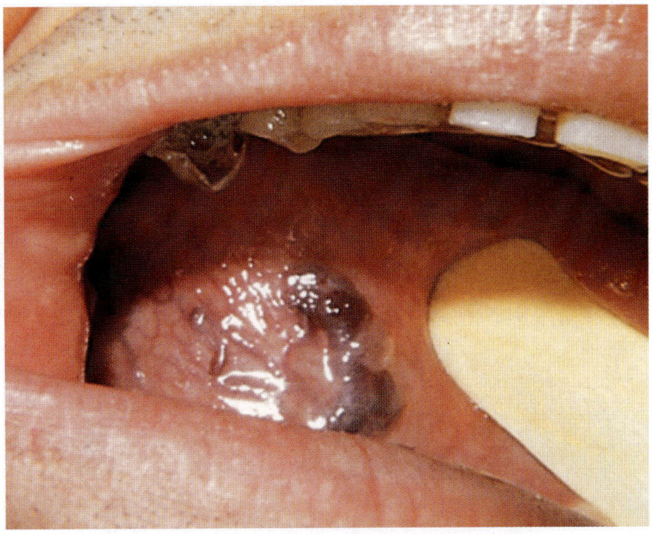

Fig. 12.23 Sublingual Varices of the Tongue.

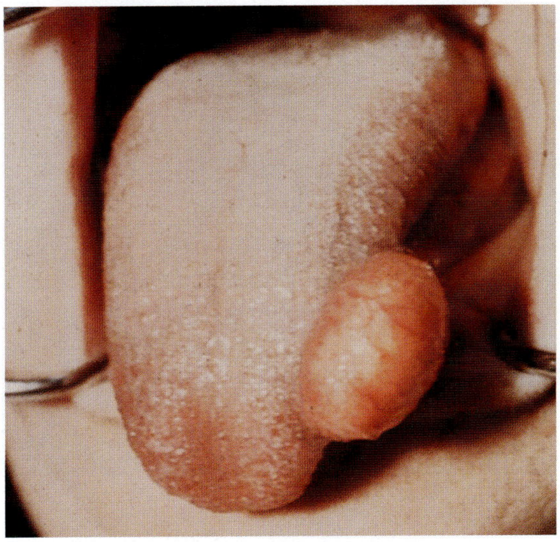

Fig. 12.24 Benign Lipoma of the Tongue.

Is *candidiasis* present? Candidiasis, also known as *moniliasis* or *thrush,* is an opportunistic mycotic infection. It frequently

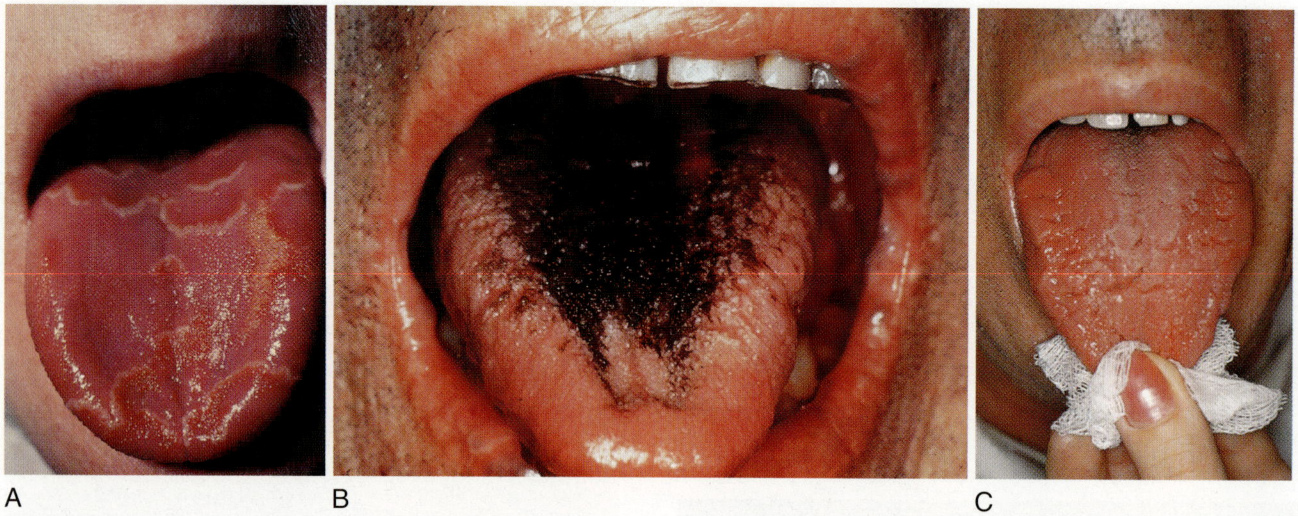

Fig. 12.25 Three Normal Tongue Variants. (A) Geographic tongue. (B) Black hairy tongue. (C) Scrotal, or fissured, tongue. (From Callen JP, Greer KE, Hood AF, et al: *Color atlas of dermatology*, Philadelphia, 1993, WB Saunders.)

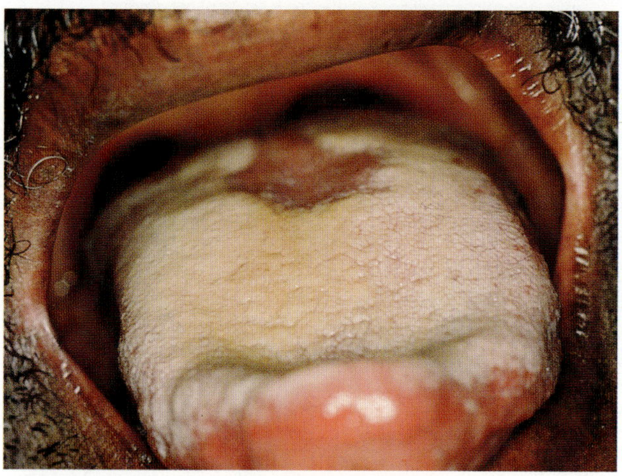

Fig. 12.26 Oral Candidiasis.

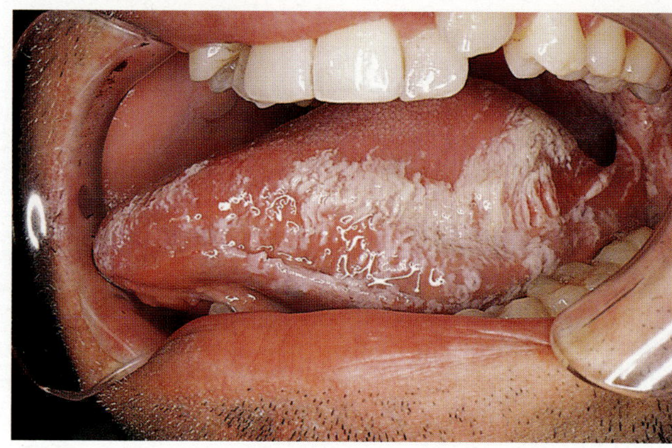

Fig. 12.27 Oral Hairy Leukoplakia. (From Silverman S: *Color atlas of oral manifestations of AIDS*, ed 2, St. Louis, 1996, Mosby-Year Book.)

involves the oral cavity, gastrointestinal tract, perineum, or vagina. The lesions appear as white, loosely adherent membranes beneath the fiery red mucosa. Oral candidiasis is the most common cause of white lesions in the mouth. It is uncommon in healthy individuals without broad-spectrum antibiotic or steroid-based therapies. The presence of thrush in such a patient may be an initial manifestation of acquired immune deficiency syndrome (AIDS). Candidiasis is the most common oral infection in patients with AIDS. The tongue of a patient with AIDS and oral candidiasis is pictured in Fig. 12.26.

Is leukoplakia present? One form of leukoplakia, *oral hairy leukoplakia,* is associated with the Epstein-Barr virus (EBV) and people infected with HIV. These raised white lesions appear corrugated, or "hairy," and range in size from a few millimeters to 2 to 3 cm. They are most commonly found on the lateral margins of the tongue but may also be seen on the buccal mucosa. In the absence of other causes of immunosuppression, oral hairy leukoplakia is diagnostic of HIV infection. It is seen in more than 40% of patients with HIV infection. The tongue of a patient with AIDS with oral hairy leukoplakia is pictured in Fig. 12.27.

Look for indurated ulcers or masses in the tongue's central and lateral aspect. This is the most common site for intraoral squamous cell carcinoma. Fig. 12.28 depicts squamous cell carcinoma of the tongue in the classic location.

Palpate the Tongue

See Video 12.2.

After a thorough inspection of the tongue, the examination proceeds with palpation. First, the patient sticks out the tongue onto a piece of gauze. The tongue is then held by the examiner's left hand as the sides of the tongue are inspected and palpated with the right hand. This is illustrated in Fig. 12.29. To examine the other side of the tongue, the examiner reverses hands.

The anterior two-thirds and the lateral margins of the tongue can be evaluated without stimulating the gag reflex. The examiner should palpate the lateral margins of the tongue because more than 85% of all lingual cancers arise in this area. All white lesions should be palpated. Is there evidence of induration (hardness)? Induration or ulceration is strongly suggestive of carcinoma. After the tongue is palpated, it is unwrapped, and the gauze is discarded. Any intraoral lesion, ulcer, or mass present for more than two weeks should be examined through biopsy and evaluated by an oral pathologist.

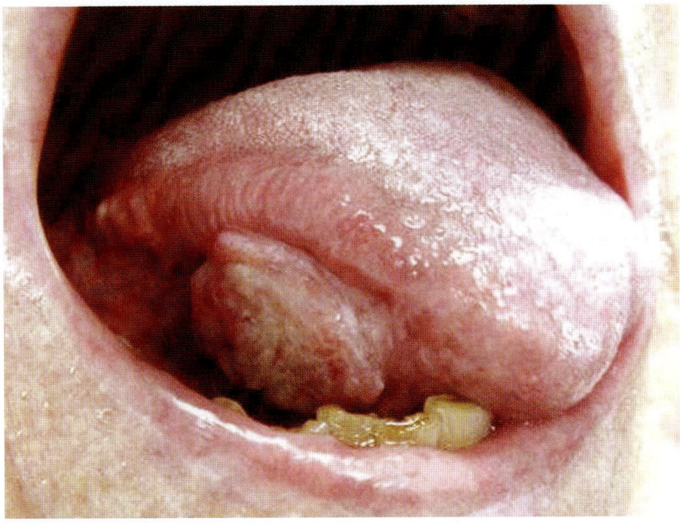

Fig. 12.28 Squamous Cell Carcinoma of the Tongue.

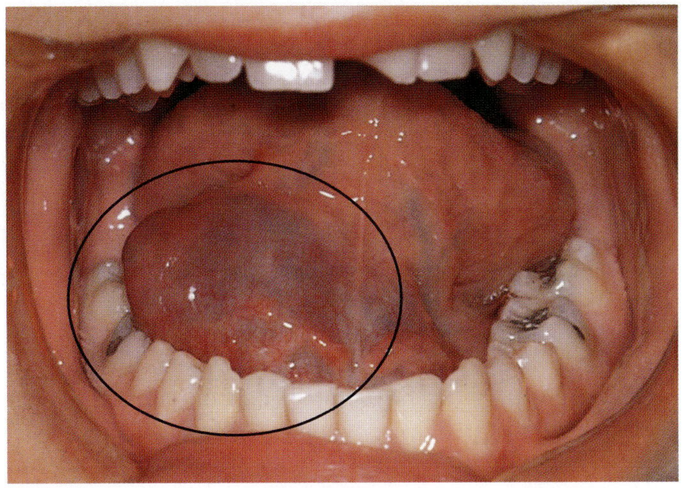

Fig. 12.30 Ranula.

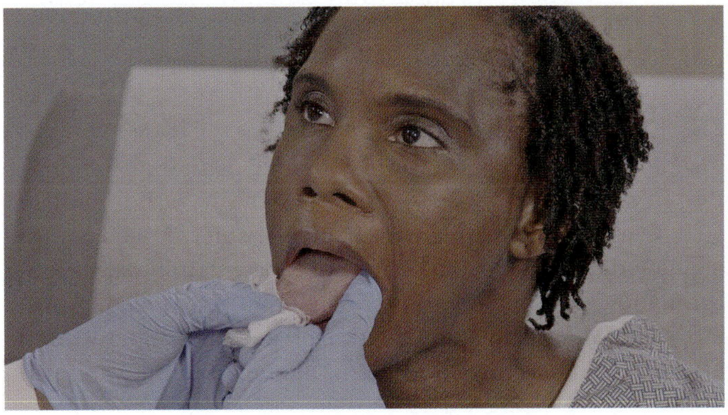

Fig. 12.29 Palpation of the Tongue.

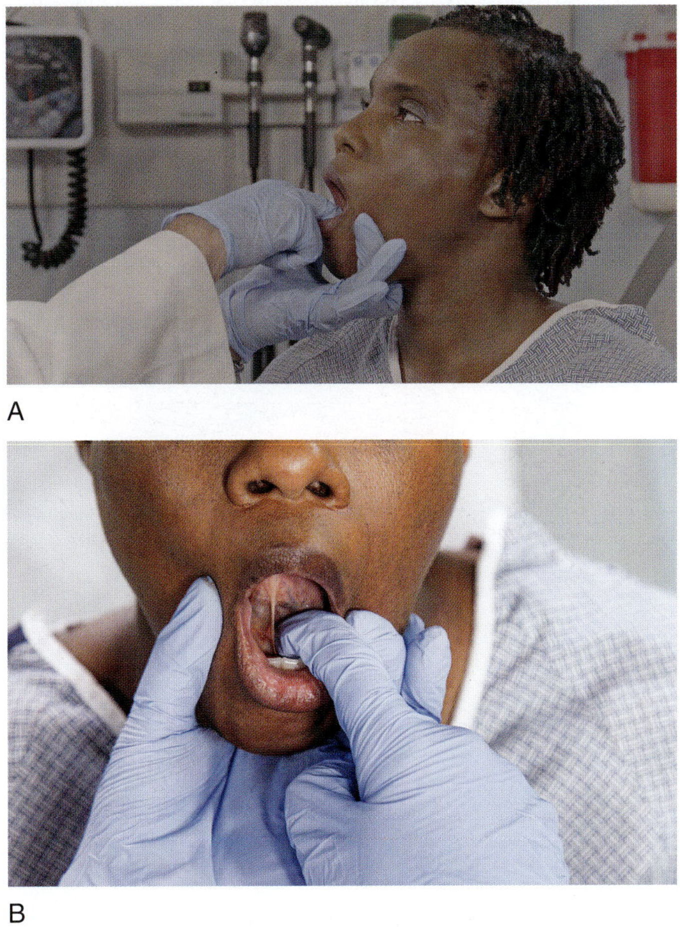

Fig. 12.31 (A) and (B) Technique for palpating the floor of the mouth.

Inspect the Floor of the Mouth

The patient is asked to lift the tongue to the roof of the mouth, and the examiner inspects the floor of the mouth. Is there edema on the floor of the mouth? The opening of the submandibular gland, the Wharton duct, should be observed. The examiner should look for leukoplakia, erythroplakia, or a mass.

A *ranula* is a large mucous retention cyst on the floor of the mouth in association with submandibular and sublingual glands. The lesion is unilateral, painless, and bluish. It is lateral to the frenulum and is typically larger than a mucocele. As a ranula increases in size, there may be a reduction in tongue movement and difficulty in speech and swallowing. An example of a ranula is pictured in Fig. 12.30.

Palpate the Floor of the Mouth

See Video 12.3.

The floor of the mouth should be examined by bimanual palpation. This is performed by placing one finger under the tongue and another under the chin to assess any thickening or masses. The examiner should hold the patient's cheeks whenever palpating a patient's mouth, as shown in Fig. 12.31. This is done as a precaution in case the patient suddenly tries to speak or bite down on the examiner's finger. The examiner's right index finger is placed under the tongue; the left thumb and third finger push the patient's cheeks inward to prevent biting; and the left index finger palpates under the patient's chin.

Inspect the Hard and Soft Palates

Inspect the rugae and vault shape of the palates. Also, inspect the palates for ulceration and masses. Masses are usually minor salivary gland tumors, primarily malignant. Are any white plaques present? Is the soft palate edematous? Is the uvula in the midline?

Is the palate intact? Fig. 12.32 shows a severe cleft palate. Clefts of the palate and lips are distinct entities but are closely related embryologically, functionally, and genetically. The incidence of an isolated cleft palate is 1 per 1000 births. Clefts of the palate vary widely in size and shape. They can extend from the soft palate to the hard palate and the incisive foramen. Recurrent otitis media, hearing loss, and speech defects are frequent complications.

In patients with impaired immunity or in those whose microbial flora has been altered by antibiotics, *Candida albicans,* a normal commensal organism of the gastrointestinal tract, can become highly invasive, as seen in Fig. 12.33. A patient who has AIDS has *pseudomembranous candidiasis* of the palate and uvula.

Are *petechiae* present? Petechiae are commonly associated with infective endocarditis, leukemia, oral sex, and viral infections such as infectious mononucleosis. Fellatio can result in palatal petechiae, characteristically at the junction of the hard and soft palates, as pictured in Fig. 12.34.

A common finding is a *torus palatinus,* a discrete, hard, lobulated swelling in the midline of the posterior portion of the hard palate. This benign lesion is an overgrowth of the palatine bone. It is painless and asymptomatic and occurs twice as often in females as males. It may remain undetected until it interferes with the fit of a denture. More than 20% of the population have at least a small torus palatinus. Fig. 12.35 shows tori palatini in two patients. Not uncommonly, individuals may have multiple tori palatini; Fig. 12.36 shows a patient with three tori palatini. A *torus mandibularis* is a hard, bony, often bilateral swelling that protrudes from the lingual surface of the mandible at the level of the premolar teeth. It is much less common than a torus palatinus. Approximately 5% to 10% of the population have a torus mandibularis; however, one-fifth of mandibular tori are unilateral. Fig. 12.37 shows bilateral mandibular tori in two patients.

Fig. 12.38 shows a patient with early invasive *erythroplakia* (red plaque) of the palate.

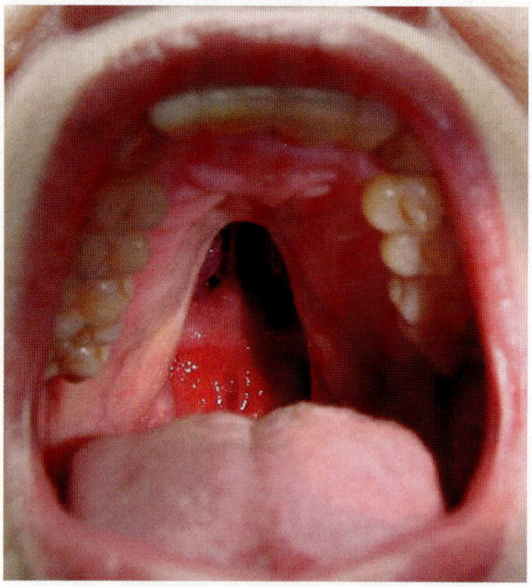

Fig. 12.32 Cleft Palate.

Inspect the Salivary Glands

The ductal orifices of the parotid gland and the submandibular gland should be visualized. The condition of the papillae should be inspected. Is there a flow of saliva? This is best evaluated by drying the papilla with a cotton applicator and observing the saliva flow produced by exerting external pressure on the gland.

The salivary glands are usually not visible. Careful observation of the face determines any asymmetry due to unilateral salivary gland enlargement. Obstruction to flow or infiltration of the gland results in glandular enlargement. Fig. 12.39 illustrates a patient with left parotid enlargement due to obstruction to flow by a stone.

Palpate the parotid and submandibular glands. Determine the consistency of each gland. Is tenderness present?

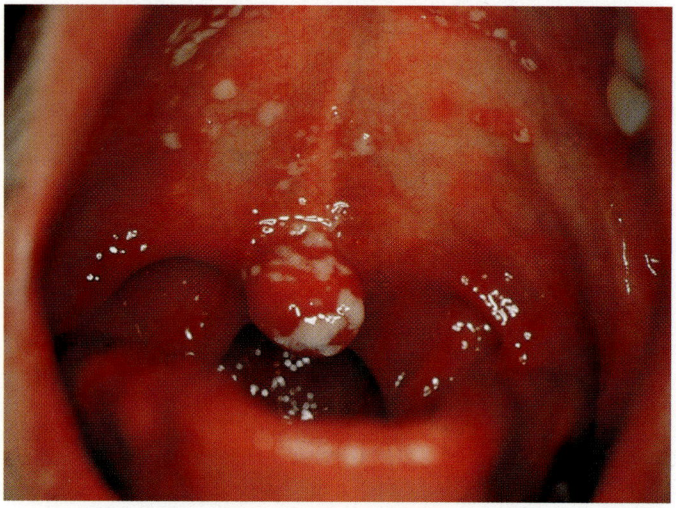

Fig. 12.33 Pseudomembranous Candidiasis.

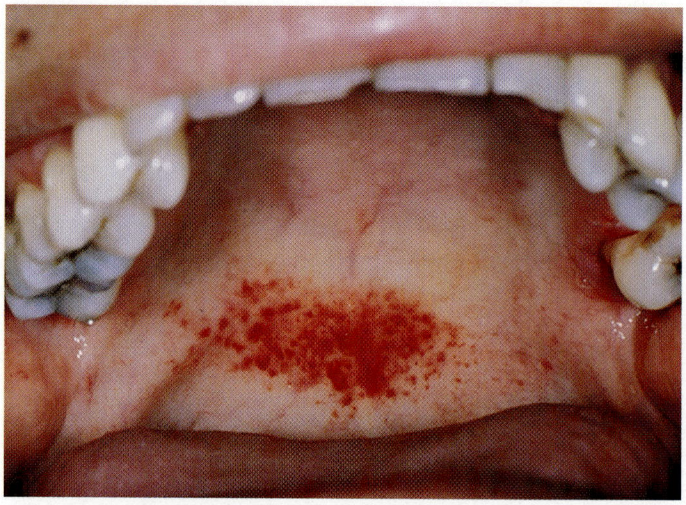

Fig. 12.34 Palatal Petechiae. (From Eisen D, Lynch DP: *The mouth: diagnosis and treatment*, St. Louis, 1998, Mosby.)

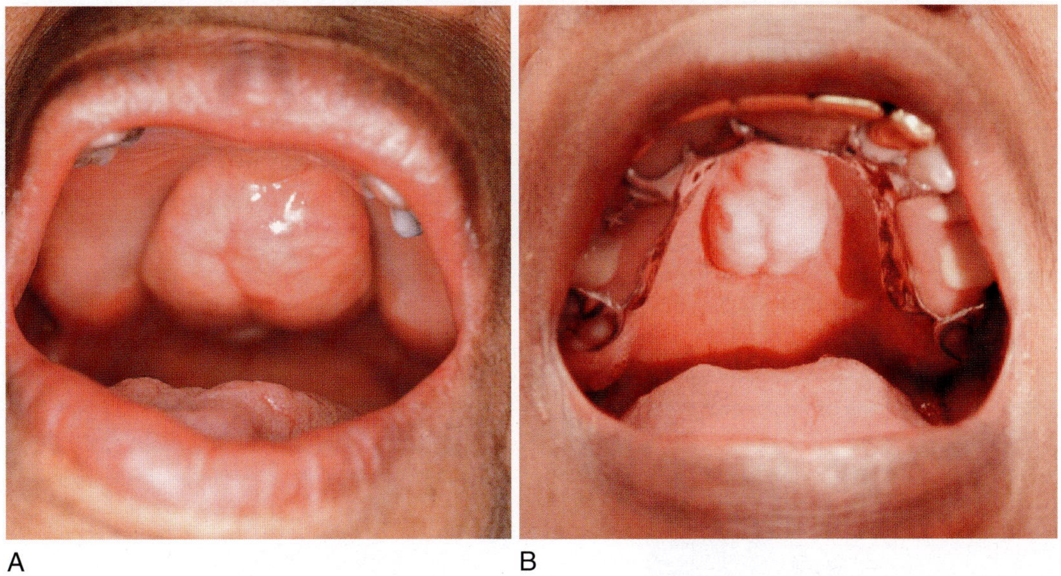

Fig. 12.35 (A) and (B) Torus palatinus.

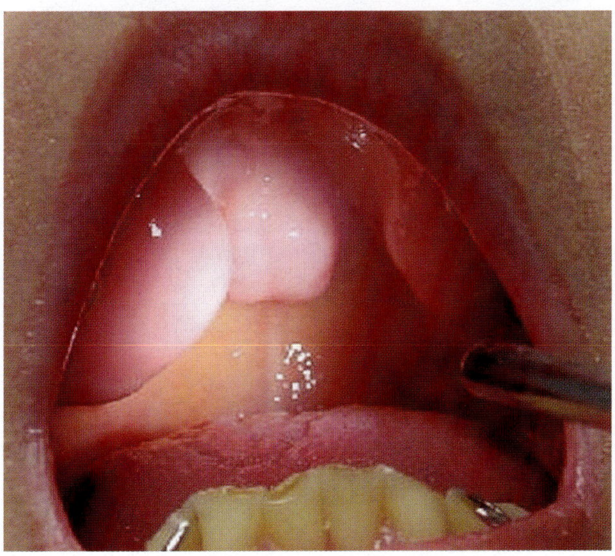

Fig. 12.36 Multiple Tori Palatini.

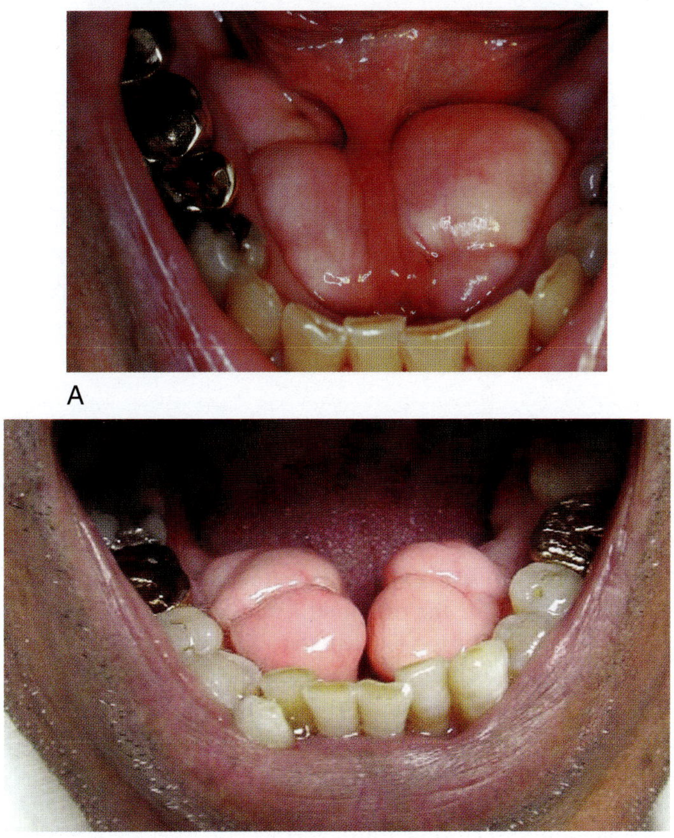

Fig. 12.37 (A) and (B) Bilateral mandibular tori. (A, From Eisen D, Lynch DP: *The mouth: diagnosis and treatment*, St. Louis, 1998, Mosby.)

Inspect the Twelfth Cranial Nerve

See Video 21.7.

Ask the patient to stick out the tongue. Does the tongue deviate to one side? A *hypoglossal,* or twelfth cranial, nerve palsy does not allow the lingual muscles on the affected side to contract normally. Consequently, the contralateral side "pushes" the tongue to the side of the lesion.

The Pharynx

Inspect the Pharynx

See Video 21.5.

Examination of the pharynx is limited to inspection. The examiner must use a tongue depressor to visualize the palate and oropharynx adequately. The patient is asked to open the mouth widely and breathe slowly through the mouth. On occasion, leaving the tongue on the floor of the mouth provides better visibility. The examiner should hold the tongue depressor in the right hand and a light source in the left. The tongue blade should be placed on the middle third of the tongue. The tongue is depressed and scooped forward *behind* the front teeth. The examiner should be careful not to press the patient's lower lip or tongue against the teeth with the tongue depressor. If the

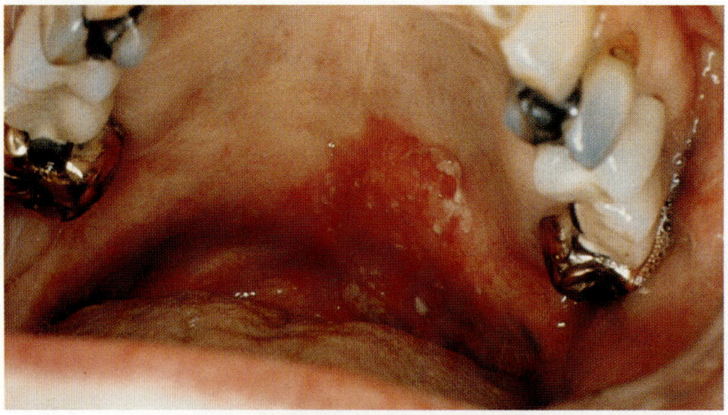

Fig. 12.38 Erythroplakia of the Palate.

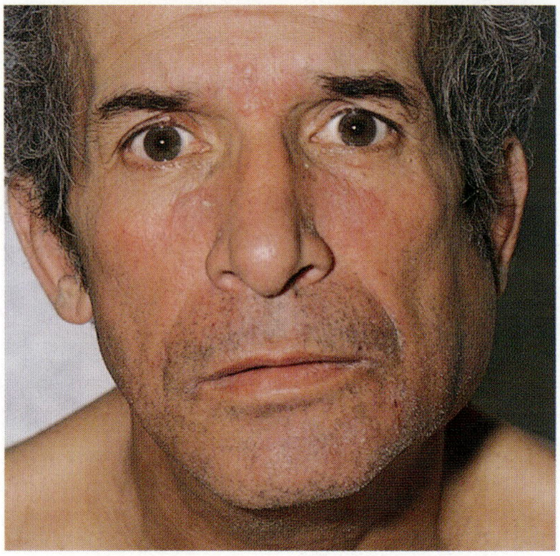

Fig. 12.39 Left Parotid Enlargement.

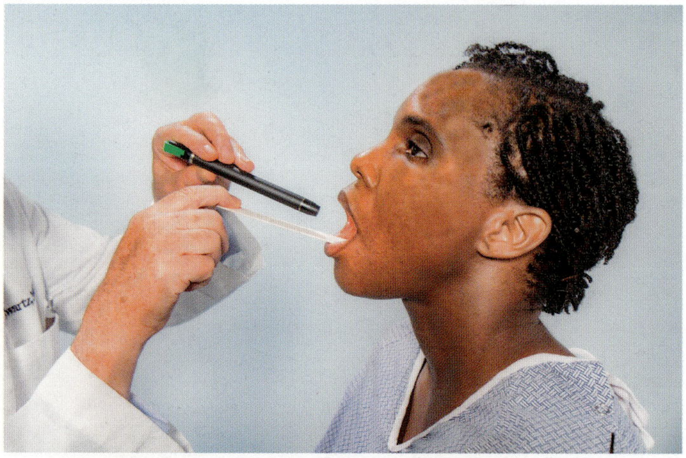

Fig. 12.40 Use of the tongue depressor to inspect the pharynx.

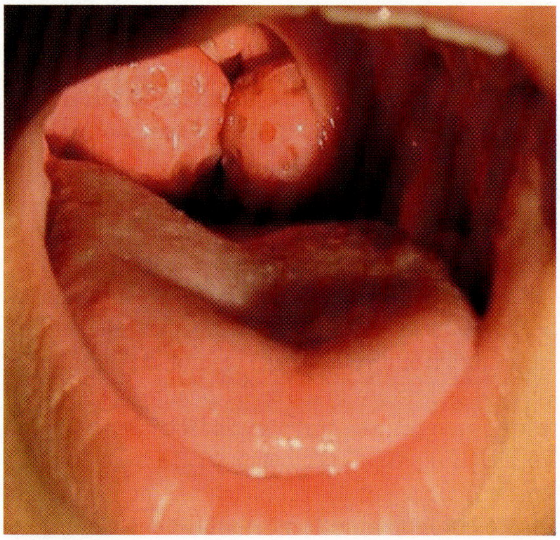

Fig. 12.41 "Kissing Tonsils." Notice the tonsillar crypts.

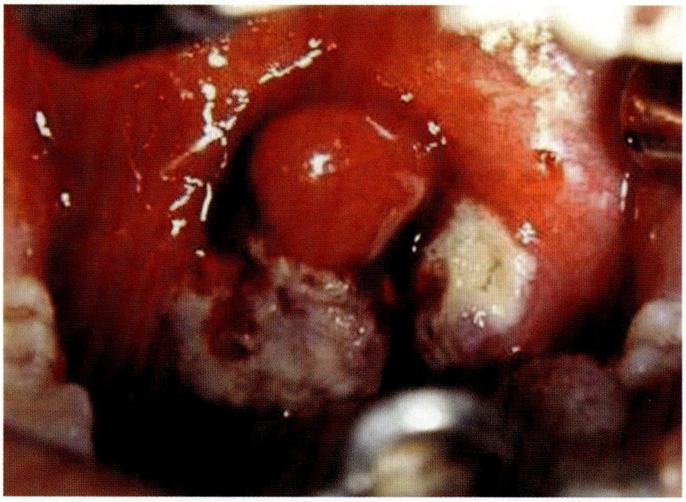

Fig. 12.42 Infectious Mononucleosis. Note the massive tonsillar enlargement and the cheeselike substance in the crypts.

tongue depressor is placed too anteriorly, the posterior portion of the tongue will mound up, making an inspection of the pharynx difficult; if placed too posteriorly, the gag reflex may be stimulated.

Is infection present? Is candidiasis present?

An accessory for the oto-ophthalmoscope handle is a light source that holds the tongue depressor and makes the examination easier. Both techniques of holding the tongue depressor are demonstrated in Fig. 12.40.

Inspect the Tonsils

Evaluate tonsillar size. Tonsillar enlargement results from infection or tumor. In chronic tonsillar infection, the deep tonsillar crypts may contain cheeselike debris. Fig. 12.41 shows enormous tonsillar growth, known as "kissing tonsils." Fig. 12.42 depicts massive tonsillar enlargement in a patient with infectious mononucleosis; the cheeselike deposit in the tonsillar crypts is visible.

Is a *pseudomembranous patch* or *membrane* present over the tonsils? A membrane is associated with acute tonsillitis, infectious mononucleosis, and diphtheria. Fig. 12.43 shows the oral cavity, characterized by erythema and a gray, membranous exudate, in a patient with diphtheria.

Inspect the Posterior Pharyngeal Wall

Is there a discharge, mass, ulceration, or infection present? Ask the patient to say, "Aahhh," as you observe for soft palate elevation.

Inspect the Gag Reflex

At the end of the inspection, tell the patient that you will test the gag reflex. The tip of the tongue depressor should gently touch the posterior surface of the tongue or the posterior pharyngeal wall. The gag reflex should follow rapidly.

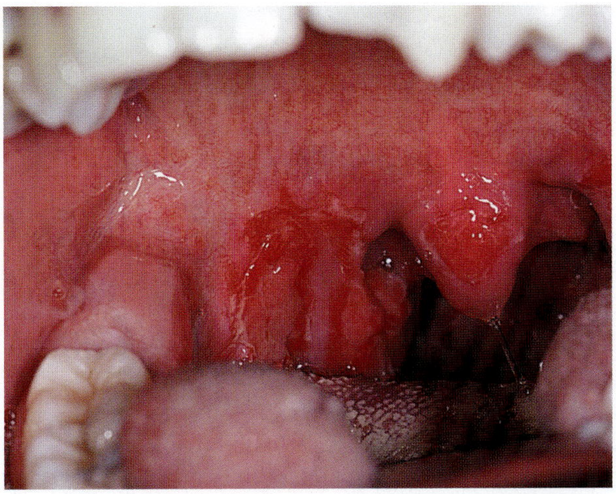

Fig. 12.43 Pseudomembrane Secondary to Diphtheria. (From Eisen D, Lynch DP: *The mouth: diagnosis and treatment*, St. Louis, 1998, Mosby.)

The Larynx

Using the Laryngeal Mirror

The tongue is held while a small, slightly warmed mirror is introduced into the mouth. The mirror should not be excessively warm and should avoid contact with the tongue. The patient is asked to breathe normally through the mouth. The mirror should be pushed upward against the uvula and positioned in the oropharynx. A light beam can then be reflected off the mirror onto the internal laryngeal structures. This technique is demonstrated in Fig. 12.44.

Although the examination of the larynx is essential, ear, nose, and throat (ENT) specialists usually perform indirect laryngoscopy. Any patient exhibiting symptoms of laryngeal disease should certainly be evaluated further.

CLINICOPATHOLOGIC CORRELATIONS

Lesions of the oral cavity are common. The most common acute oral ulcer is traumatic; the *aphthous or canker sore* is the next most common. Traumatic and aphthous lesions vary widely in size, although the latter is usually less than 1 cm in diameter. Both are relatively superficial with raised borders. Aphthous ulcers are typically located on the loose buccal or labial mucosa, whereas traumatic ulcers can occur anywhere. Despite the small

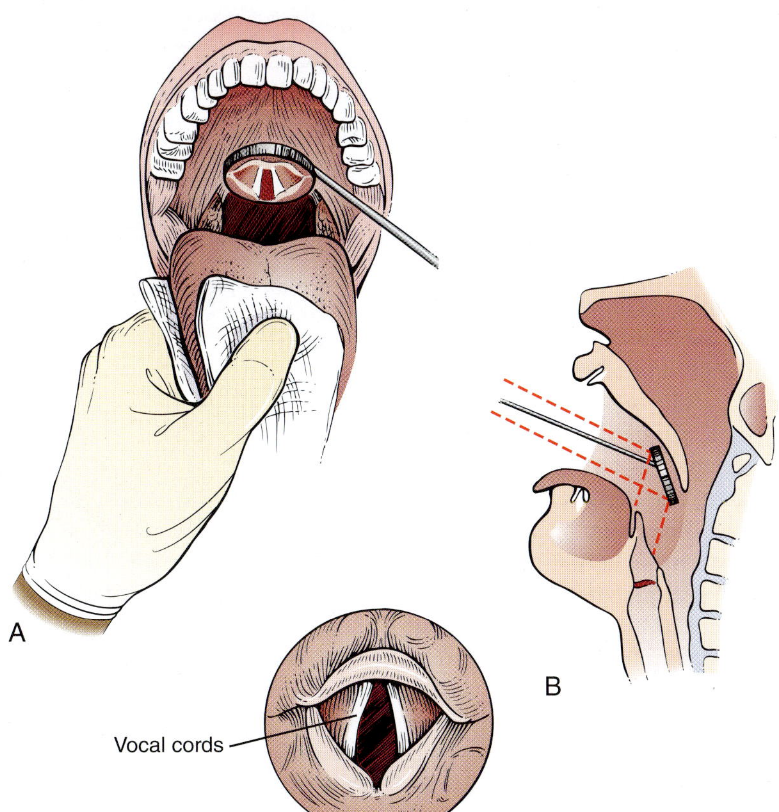

Fig. 12.44 Mirror Laryngoscopy. (A) Proper technique for holding the tongue and placement of the mirror. (B) Cross-sectional view through the pharynx, illustrating placement of the mirror. (C) Mirror reflection of the vocal cords.

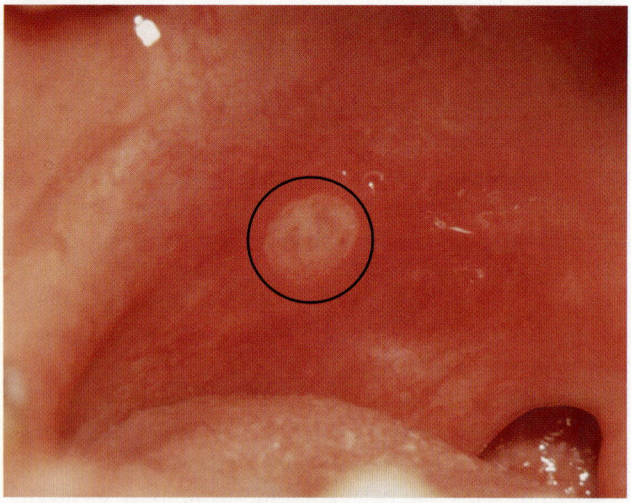

Fig. 12.45 Solitary Aphthous Ulcer.

size of many of these ulcers, they can be extremely painful. In addition, aphthous ulcers may recur in many patients. Both types of ulcers usually heal within 2 to 3 weeks without scarring. A *solitary,* or *giant,* aphthous ulcer of the palate is shown in Fig. 12.45. The patient has *periadenitis mucosa necrotica recurrens,* a major aphthous ulcer. These lesions are more significant than multiple aphthous ulcers and start as submucosal lesions that break down to form ulcers that may persist for many weeks before healing by secondary intention. Any oropharynx part may be affected, but the tonsils and soft palate are the most common sites.

Acute multiple ulcers preceded by or associated with vesicles may have infective or immunologic causes. Primary herpes simplex, herpes zoster, coxsackievirus, and HIV are causative infective agents. Allergic stomatitis, benign mucous membrane pemphigoid, pemphigus vulgaris, Behçet disease, and erythema multiforme are common immunologic causes. In addition, radiation therapy or chemotherapy may predispose an individual to develop multiple acute ulcers.

Benign mucous membrane pemphigoid, or *cicatricial pemphigoid,* is a chronic mucocutaneous bullous disease of older adults in which the lesions are commonly limited to the oral cavity and conjunctiva. Subepidermal bullae, up to 2 cm in size, and autoantibodies to the basement membrane are present; erosion may also be present. Skin involvement is rare and usually not severe. The Nikolsky sign[a] is generally positive, in which the bulla or external layer of mucous membrane or skin is easily separated from the underlying tissue by slight friction. Fig. 12.46 depicts benign mucous membrane pemphigoid. Note the denudation of the gingivae. Fig. 12.47 illustrates cicatricial pemphigoid. The most common oral finding is patchy, desquamative gingivitis, as seen in this figure.

Pemphigus vulgaris affects the oral cavity in 75% of cases. Autoantibodies to the epithelial intercellular substance are present. The Nikolsky sign is positive. The lesions are almost always

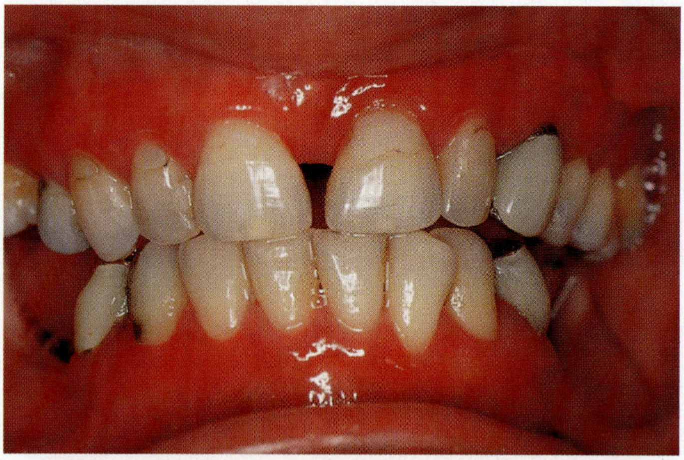

Fig. 12.46 Benign Mucous Membrane Pemphigoid.

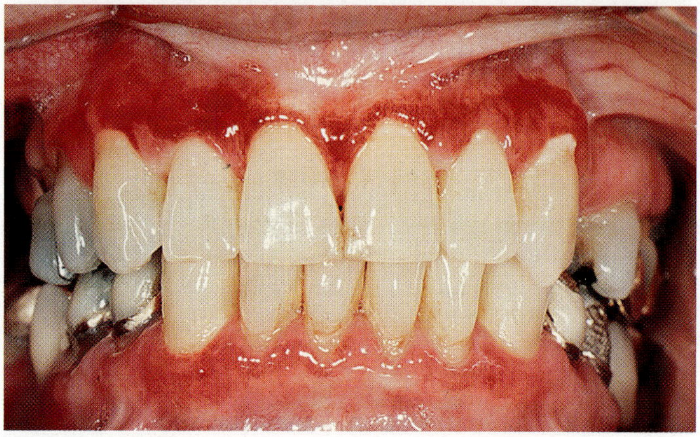

Fig. 12.47 Cicatricial Pemphigoid. (From Eisen D, Lynch DP: *The mouth: diagnosis and treatment*, St. Louis, 1998, Mosby.)

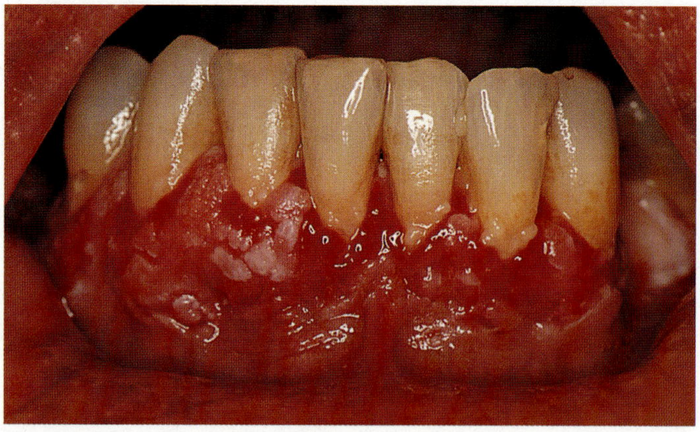

Fig. 12.48 Pemphigus Vulgaris. (From Eisen D, Lynch DP: *The mouth: diagnosis and treatment*, St. Louis, 1998, Mosby.)

painful. Fig. 12.48 depicts pemphigus vulgaris; the desquamative gingivitis is visible. Another case of pemphigus vulgaris is seen in Fig. 12.49. Note the large and confluent ulcerations, which were painful, on the soft palate.

Large chronic single ulcers may result from fungal infections such as aspergillosis or histoplasmosis. Infections by herpes

[a]Nikolsky sign is a dermatologic finding in which the top layers of the skin slip away from the lower layers when slightly rubbed. See Chapter 8, The Skin.

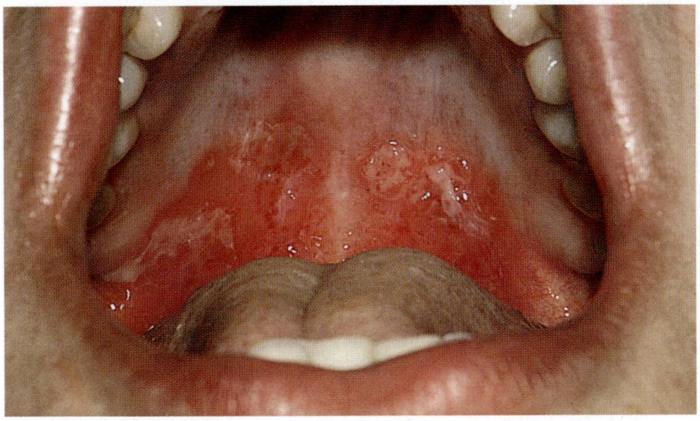

Fig. 12.49 Pemphigus Vulgaris. (From Eisen D, Lynch DP: *The mouth: diagnosis and treatment*, St. Louis, 1998, Mosby.)

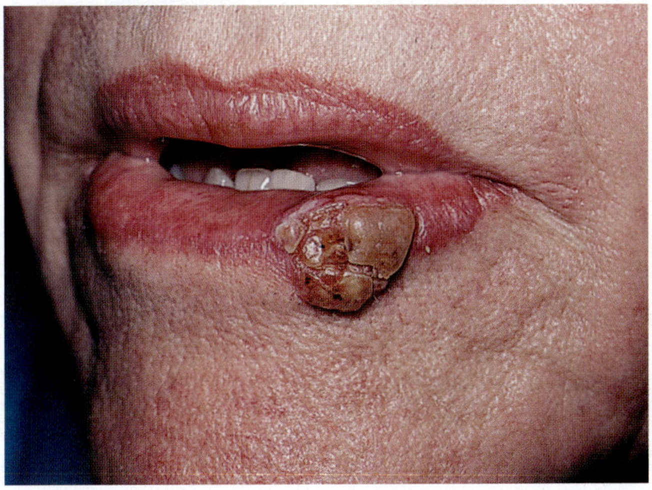

Fig. 12.50 Squamous Cell Carcinoma of the Lower Lip. (From Callen JP, Paller AS, Greer KE, et al: *Color atlas of dermatology*, ed 2, Philadelphia, 2000, WB Saunders.)

simplex virus, cytomegalovirus, *Mycobacterium* organisms (which cause tuberculosis), and *Treponema pallidum* (which causes syphilis) are also well-known causes of this type of ulcer. In addition, immunologic disorders such as pemphigus, systemic lupus erythematosus, bullous pemphigoid, and erosive lichen planus are often the cause of multiple chronic ulcers.

Cancer of the oral cavity is common. *Carcinoma of the lip* accounts for 30% of all cancers in this area and approximately 0.6% of all cancers. Most of these malignant tumors are squamous cell carcinomas. The lower lip is the site most frequently involved (95%). The patients are usually 50 to 70, with a strong male predominance (95%). Squamous cell carcinoma is characterized by a hard, infiltrative, usually painless ulcer. The risk factors that predispose to squamous cell carcinoma of the oral cavity are the same as for leukoplakia: smoking, spirits (alcohol), spices, syphilis, and spikes (ill-fitting dentures)—the "five Ss." Fig. 12.50 depicts a squamous cell carcinoma of the lower lip.

As mentioned earlier in this chapter, risk factors for oral cancers include tobacco use, alcohol consumption, and chewing *betel nuts*. Betel nuts are the seeds of the betel palm *(Areca catechu)*. Betel nut and leaf chewing are traditions that date back thousands of years. The nuts are chewed for their mildly euphoric stimulant effect, attributed to relatively high levels of psychoactive alkaloids. Chewing betel nuts can increase the capacity to work, create a warm sensation in the body, heighten alertness, and increase sweating. Although betel nut chewing is a part of many Asian and Pacific cultures and often takes place at ceremonies and gatherings, betel nuts are commonly sold at roadside booths in Taiwan decorated with multicolored neon lights for taxi and truck drivers to keep them awake while driving long distances or at night. Betel nut is so popular in Taiwan that it has been dubbed "Taiwanese chewing gum." It is Taiwan's No. 2 cash crop after rice. In India and Pakistan, betel nut preparation with or without the betel leaf is commonly called *paan*.

The International Agency for Research on Cancer regards the betel nut as a known human carcinogen. In Asian countries and communities, where betel nuts are consumed extensively, oral cancer accounts for up to 50% of all malignant cancers. Betel nut chewers in Taiwan were found to have a risk of acquiring oral cancer 28 times higher than that of nonusers, and people who chew betel nuts, smoke cigarettes, and drink alcohol are 123 times more likely to develop oral cancer. Of people with oral cancer in Taiwan, 9 out of 10 chew betel nuts. Fig. 12.51A shows the mouth of a patient from Taiwan with a long-standing habit of betel nut chewing; note the red stain on his teeth. Fig. 12.51B shows a betel nut wrapped in its leaf. In 2021, around 95,500 tons of betel nut had been produced in Taiwan. Fortunately, according to the country's health authorities, Taiwan has significantly reduced betel nut use in the past few years, thanks to a government-led promotion campaign to prevent oral cancer.[5] An effort has also been made to promote awareness of the detrimental effect of areca nut use on campuses and communities. The decrease is most significant among the 30 to 39 age group.

In addition to these risk factors, biologic factors include viruses and fungi, which have been found in association with oral cancers. For example, HPV has been implicated in some oral cancers.[6] HPV is a common sexually transmitted virus that infects approximately 40 million Americans. The virus can be passed from one person to another by skin-to-skin contact through sexual activity, including vaginal, anal, and oral sex. HPV can be spread even when an infected person has no visible signs or symptoms. HPVs are a large group of related viruses. Each virus in the group is given a number, which is called an HPV type. There are more than 80 types of HPV, most thought to be harmless.

HPV-16 and HPV-18 are high-risk strains known to significantly increase the risk of gynecologic cancer in females and penile cancer in males. However, 1% of persons infected have the HPV-16 strain, which is a causative agent in cervical cancer and is now linked to oral cancer as well (depending on where the infection is located).[6] Most HPV-related cancers are found in the back of the throat, including the base of the tongue and tonsils. These are the most common HPV-related cancers in males.

Condoms provide some protection against HPV, but they do not entirely prevent infection. An HPV vaccine can prevent

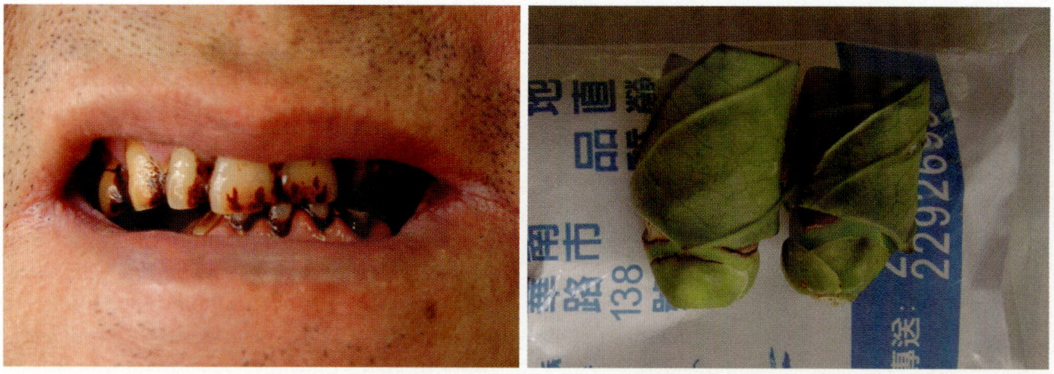

A B

Fig. 12.51 (A) Red teeth staining in a betel nut user. (B) Betel nut wrapped in its leaf.

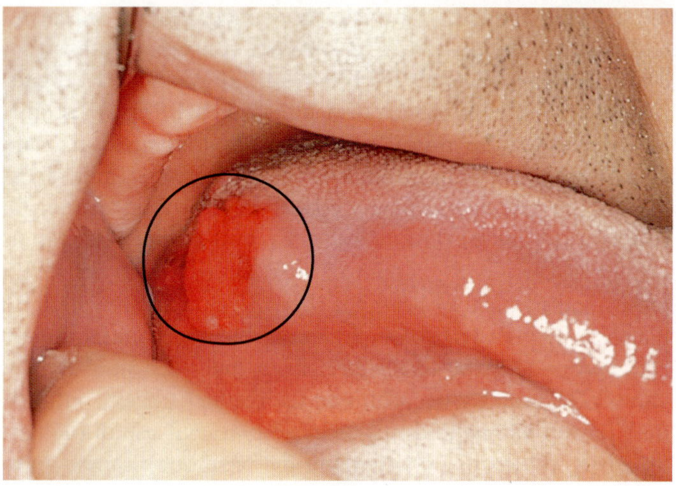

Fig. 12.52 Squamous Cell Carcinoma of the Tongue.

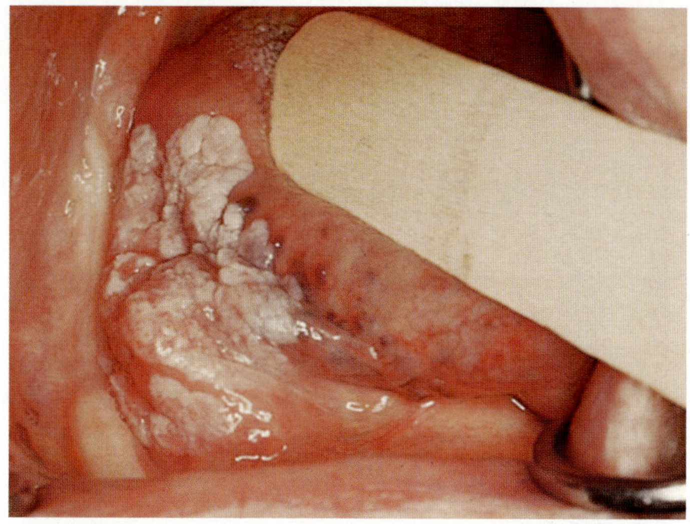

Fig. 12.53 Squamous Cell Carcinoma of the Tongue and Floor of the Mouth.

infection with certain types of HPV, including types linked to HPV-related cancers and types linked to anal and genital warts. It is approved for use in males and females and can *only* prevent HPV infection; the vaccine cannot be used to treat an existing infection. Gardasil 9® is the HPV vaccine approved by the U.S. Food and Drug Administration and is given in a series of shots. It should be given between the ages of 9 and 12. Teens and young adults ages 13 through 26 years who have not been vaccinated or received all their shots should get the vaccine as soon as possible. Vaccination of young adults will not prevent as many cancers as vaccination of younger children and teens. Studies have shown that Gardasil 9® gives long-lasting protection against HPV. See Chapter 19, Female Genitalia, for additional information on HPV and Gardasil 9®.

Another possible risk factor for oral cancer is lichen planus, an inflammatory disease of the oral soft tissues.

Lingual carcinoma is often easily missed because it is usually painless in its early stages. In 2018, there were 17,110 new cases of lingual cancer, with 2510 deaths from the disease. The percent surviving at five years was 65.8%. Lingual cancer generally occurs on the lateral aspects of the tongue or its undersurface; there is commonly extension onto the tongue from a lesion on the floor of the mouth. Fig. 12.52 depicts a carcinoma of the right lateral border of the tongue. Fig. 12.53 illustrates squamous cell carcinoma of the right lateral border of the tongue in another patient, with an extension on the floor of the mouth.

Carcinoma of the floor of the mouth accounts for 10% to 15% of all oral cancers and is the most common site of oral cancer in African Americans. It occurs primarily in males at an average age of 65 years. Approximately 20% of patients with carcinoma of the floor of the mouth have a second primary tumor. Cancer of the floor of the mouth has a strong association with alcohol consumption and tobacco smoking, particularly cigarettes; tobacco is implicated in more than 80% of cases of oral cancers. Smokers are up to 25 times more likely to develop head and neck cancer than their nonsmoking counterparts. Passive smoking, tobacco chewing, and cigar smoking are also risk factors for developing oral cancer. It is particularly important to examine the area behind the last molar tooth and the associated floor of the mouth and the base of the tongue. Fig. 12.54 shows a squamous cell carcinoma of the floor of the mouth.

Salivary gland neoplasms are not uncommon. They occur with an annual incidence of 6 per 100,000 individuals. More than 70% occur in the parotid gland. There are more

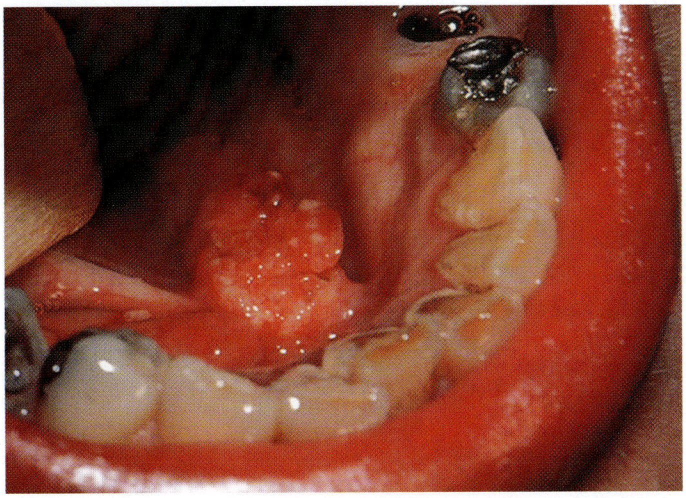

Fig. 12.54 Squamous Cell Carcinoma of the Floor of the Mouth.

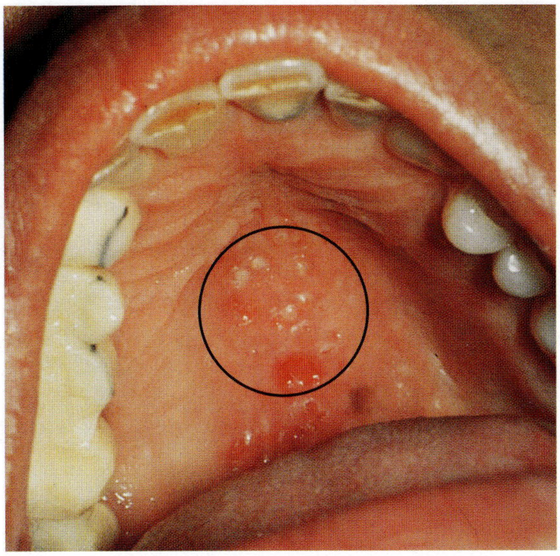

Fig. 12.56 Herpetic Lesions on the Palate.

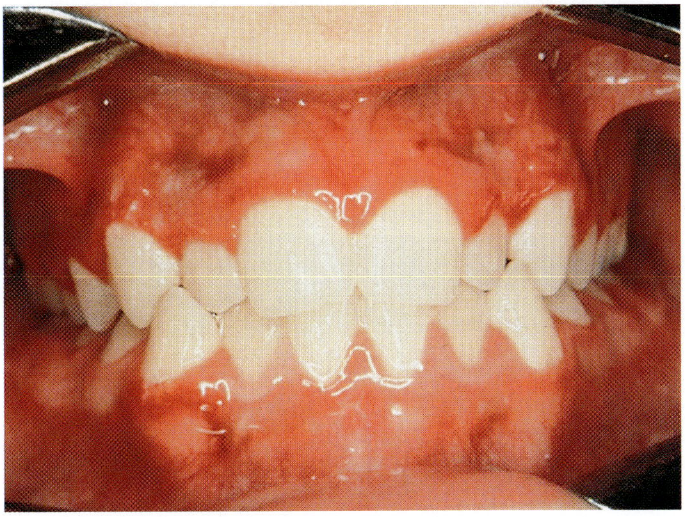

Fig. 12.55 Herpetic Gingivostomatitis.

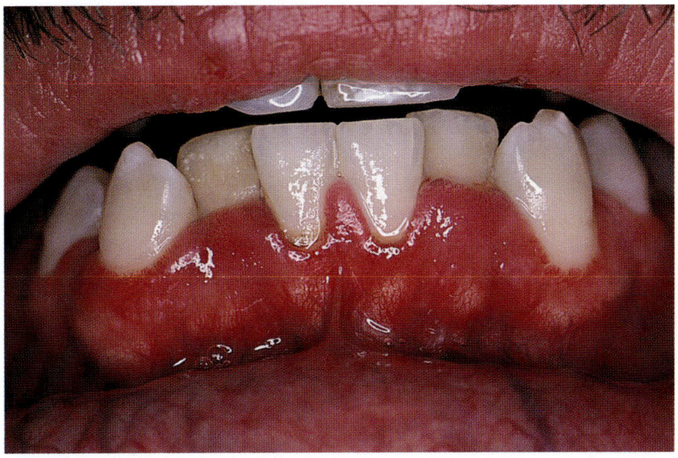

Fig. 12.57 Acute Necrotizing Gingivostomatitis. (From Eisen D, Lynch DP: *The mouth: diagnosis and treatment*, St. Louis, 1998, Mosby.)

than 50 types of salivary gland tumors. Salivary gland malignancies represent less than 5% of all head and neck cancers. They are a heterogeneous group of tumors with varied clinical behavior. About 60% of malignant salivary gland tumors arise in the parotid glands, about 30% occur in the submandibular glands, and 10% to 15% originate in the sublingual and minor salivary glands.[7]

Herpetic gingivostomatitis is an infection of the gums and oral mucosa by the herpes simplex virus. Small vesicles form on the oral mucous membrane and rapidly break down into painful ulcers on an intensely erythematous base. Fig. 12.55 depicts herpetic gingivostomatitis; the multiple erosions and marginal gingivitis are apparent. Fig. 12.56 shows herpetic lesions on the palate with ulceration.

Acute necrotizing gingivostomatitis (also known as *ulcerative gingivostomatitis* or *Vincent gingivitis*) is a severe, noncommunicable disease of young adults resulting from infection by *Fusobacterium nucleatum* or *Borrelia vincentii.* Most cases occur suddenly in the spring or autumn. The patients, commonly males with poor oral hygiene, present with gingival bleeding, alteration of taste, gingival pain, malaise, fever, and halitosis. As the disease progresses, a whitish pseudomembrane develops along the gingival margins, with ulceration and blunting of the interdental papillae. Acute necrotizing gingivitis, pictured in Fig. 12.57, may be an early feature of HIV infection.

On September 20, 2022, the Centers for Disease Control and Prevention (CDC) released a new report[8] on the incidence of HIV in the United States. Annual HIV infections and diagnoses were declining, which may be due to targeted HIV prevention efforts. There were 30,635 new HIV infections in 2022. Among all populations in the United States, the estimated number of annual infections declined by 8% from 2016 to 2019. By transmission categories, 7% were among people using injectable drugs; 22% were among heterosexual contacts; and 70% were

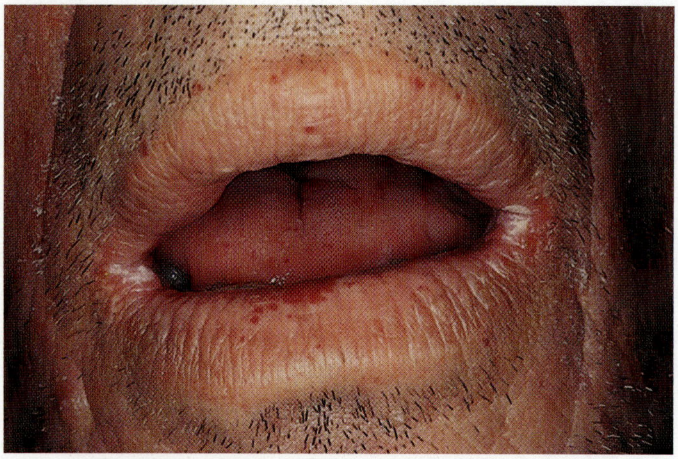

Fig. 12.58 Angular Cheilitis. (From Silverman S: *Color atlas of oral manifestations of AIDS*, ed 2, St. Louis, 1996, Mosby-Year Book.)

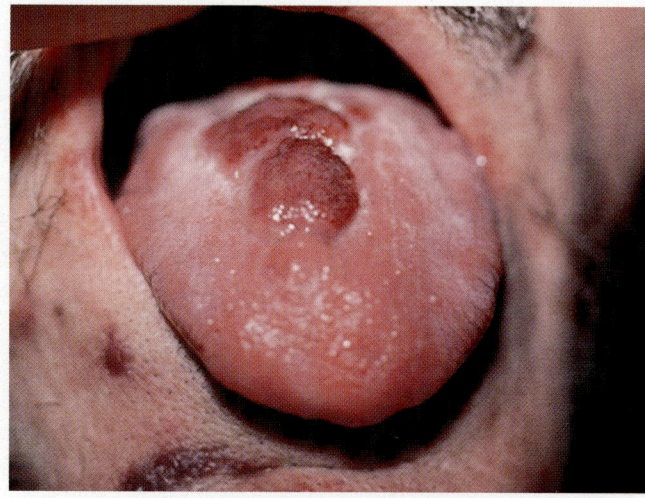

Fig. 12.59 Kaposi Sarcoma of the Tongue.

among gay, bisexual, and other males who reported male-to-male contact. Black/African American people account for a higher proportion of new HIV diagnoses and people with HIV than other races and ethnicities.[9] Racism, HIV stigma, homophobia, poverty, and barriers to healthcare continue to drive these disparities.

It has been estimated that more than 90% of patients infected with HIV will have at least one oral manifestation of their disease. As further immunologic impairment develops, the risk of oral lesions increases. It has also been shown that the oral manifestations can be used as a marker of immune compromise, independent of the $CD4^+$ T-lymphocyte count. If left untreated, the oral lesions may interfere with chewing, swallowing, and talking. Many patients have such severe pain that they reduce their oral intake, which results in additional weight loss, malnutrition, and further wasting.

A common oral manifestation of HIV infection is *angular cheilitis,* also known as *perlèche*. This painful condition is characterized by macerated, fissured, eroded, encrusted, and whitish (occasionally erythematous) lesions in the corners of the mouth. Accumulations of saliva gather in the skin folds and are subsequently colonized by yeast organisms such as *C. albicans*. Angular cheilitis may be associated with intraoral candidiasis. Angular cheilitis may also develop in patients with normal immunity who wear ill-fitting dentures or wear dentures during the night. An example of angular cheilitis is pictured in Fig. 12.58.

Figs. 12.26 and 12.33 show patients with *oral candidiasis,* another extremely common condition associated with HIV infection. Oral candidiasis is characterized by chronic severe pain in the throat that worsens on swallowing or eating. The curdlike white plaques are soft and friable and can easily be wiped off, leaving an area of intensely erythematous mucosa.

Fig. 12.27 shows a patient with *oral hairy leukoplakia.* As mentioned previously, this lesion is seen most frequently either unilaterally or bilaterally on the lateral margins of the tongue. The lesion is white, does not rub off, and occasionally occurs elsewhere in the mouth and oropharynx. Although not correlated with the stage of HIV infection, oral hairy leukoplakia may be the first sign of infection. It is seen most commonly in gay and bisexual males infected with HIV. It has been suggested that the Epstein-Barr virus may be a cofactor in developing oral hairy leukoplakia. The finding of oral hairy leukoplakia mandates HIV testing.

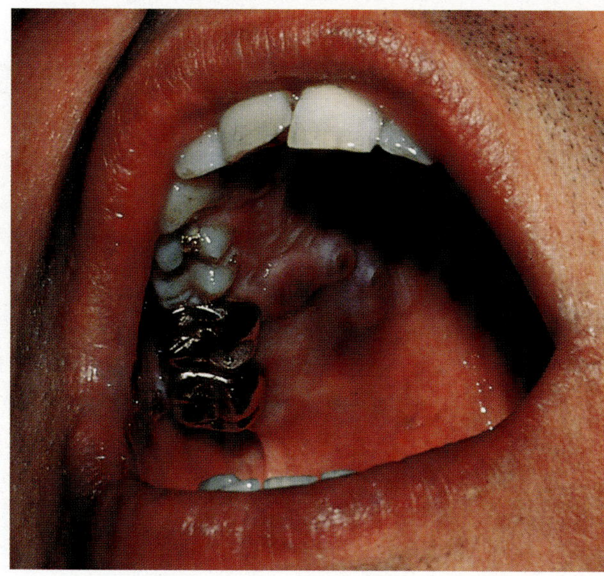

Fig. 12.60 Kaposi Sarcoma of the Hard Palate.

As discussed in Chapter 8, The Skin, the oral lesions of Kaposi sarcoma are common. Fig. 8.100 shows some of the typical oral lesions. Lesions of Kaposi sarcoma of the tongue (Fig. 12.59) and the hard palate (Fig. 12.60) are frequently found in patients with AIDS.

Table 12.1 summarizes the important signs and symptoms of some of the more common oral lesions. Table 12.2 reviews the most common oral lesions seen during the stages of HIV infection. Fig. 24.33 shows the chronology of primary teeth eruption.

TABLE 12.1 **Symptoms and Signs of Oral Lesions**

Lesion	Symptoms	Signs	Other Information
Aphthous ulcer (canker sore; see Fig. 12.45)	Painful, recurrent white sore with red border on lips, inner side of cheeks, tip and sides of tongue, or palate	Single lesion 0.5–2 cm in diameter that is first maculopapular but then ulcerates and has an area of erythema at its border; lesions usually on movable mucosal areas	Sixty percent of population have periodic canker sores lasting up to 2 weeks; cause is unknown
Herpetic ulcer (cold sore; fever blister; see Figs. 12.10, 12.55, and 12.56)	Painful, recurrent sores on the lips	Multiple vesicles, papules, or ulcers on the mucocutaneous junction, hard palate, or gingivae; as the bullae break, crusting occurs	*Primary* herpetic infection in children: multiple lesions in clusters on fixed mucous membranes; small, discrete, whitish vesicles before ulceration; ulcers approximately 1 mm in diameter, which may coalesce; tender lymphadenopathy, fever, and malaise present *Recurrent* form, common in adults: lip lesions *Both* forms: self-limited illness, 1–2 weeks
Chancre	Painless sore on lips or tongue lasting 2 weeks to 3 months	Single ulcerated lesion with indurated border; lesion without central necrotic material; tender lymphadenitis may be present	Examiner should look for genital lesions (see Figs. 18.13 and 19.33)
Squamous cell carcinoma (see Figs. 12.28, 12.50, and 12.52–12.54)	Ulcerated sore of the lips, floor of mouth, or tongue (especially lateral borders); erythroplakia of floor of mouth, soft palate	Single indurated lesion with indurated and raised border; often in an area of leukoplakia or erythroplakia; absence of necrotic material in crater; base often erythematous; speech alterations may result if lesion is large; painless lymphadenopathy may be present	Frequently in alcoholic patients or smokers
Erythema multiforme	Sudden onset of multiple painful ulcers in mouth or lips	Hemorrhagic areas of ulceration with erythematous bases, often with pseudomembrane; lesions start as bullae; skin involvement common (target lesions)	Many precipitating factors include drug reactions, herpesvirus infections, endocrine changes, and an underlying malignancy; most common in winter and spring in young adults; frequently recurring
Denture hyperplasia	Painless excess tissue at border of denture	Spongy, redundant, often erythematous tissue with impression of edge of denture; frequently seen on anterior maxillary mucosa	
Candidiasis (moniliasis; thrush; see Figs. 12.26 and 12.33)	Burning sensation in areas of tongue, inside of cheek, or throat	Whitish pseudomembrane, resembling milk curd, that can be peeled off, leaving a raw, erythematous area that may bleed; erythematous variant is secondary to broad-spectrum antibiotics	Often seen in individuals who are chronically debilitated, patients who are immunosuppressed, or patients receiving long-term antibiotic therapy; commonly seen in persons with AIDS
Erythroplakia (see Figs. 12.20 and 12.38)	Painless red area on inside of cheek, tongue, or floor of mouth	Granular, erythematous papules that bleed	High potential for malignancy
Leukoplakia (see Figs. 12.16, 12.17, and 12.27)	Painless white area on inside of cheek, tongue, lower lip, or floor of mouth	Hyperkeratinized, whitish lesion that cannot be scraped off; looks similar to flaking white paint; often speckled with reddish areas; associated adenopathy may indicate malignant changes of lesion	Patients are usually males over 40 years of age; linked to smoking, AIDS, alcoholism, and chewing tobacco high potential for malignancy
Lipoma (see Fig. 12.24)	Slow-growing, painless mass on inner surface of cheek or tongue	Yellowish, nontender, soft mass; freely mobile	
Lichen planus (see Fig. 12.15)	Usually no symptoms; erosive form causes painful, burning sores of inner side of cheek or tongue	White lesions on buccal mucosa bilaterally in the form of reticulated papules in lacelike pattern; erosive form appears as hemorrhagic ulcerated lesion with possible white areas or bullae; pseudomembrane may be present over lesion	Nonerosive form is a common cause of white lesions in the mouth; skin involvement in 10%–35% of affected patients and more frequently seen in patients with emotional stress
Traumatic ulcer	Pain in an area of a sore; short duration (1–2 weeks)	Single lesion with raised erythema at its border; center often with necrotic debris; occasionally purulent; mild lymphadenitis may be present	Patient frequently knows the cause (e.g., biting cheek while eating)
Mucocele (see Fig. 12.13)	Intermittent, painless swelling of the lower lip or inside of cheek; slightly bluish; occasionally ruptures	Dome-shaped, 1–2 cm in diameter, freely mobile cystic lesion	Related to trauma to ductal system of minor labial salivary glands

Continued

TABLE 12.1 Symptoms and Signs of Oral Lesions—cont'd

Lesion	Symptoms	Signs	Other Information
Black hairy tongue (see Fig. 12.25B)	Gagging sensation associated with "hairy" sensation of tongue; large brown or blackish painless lesion on top of tongue	Elongation of filiform papillae on the dorsum of tongue with a change in their color to almost black or brown	History of excessive antibiotic use, excessive use of mouthwash, poor oral hygiene, smoking, or alcohol use is common
Fordyce spots (see Fig. 12.18)	None	Clusters of small, yellowish, raised lesions best seen on the buccal mucosa opposite the molar teeth	Common in older individuals; they are normal, hyperplastic (ectopic) sebaceous glands

AIDS, Acquired immune deficiency syndrome.

TABLE 12.2 Occurrence of Oral Lesions During the Stages of HIV Infection

Oral Lesion	Occurrence During Primary HIV Infection	Occurrence During Early HIV Disease[a]	Occurrence During Advanced HIV Disease[b]
Candidiasis (see Figs. 12.26 and 12.33)	Common	Occasional	Very common
Oral hairy leukoplakia (see Fig. 12.27)	No	Occasional	Very common
Kaposi sarcoma (see Fig. 8.100, Figs. 12.59, and 12.60)	No	Rare	Very common
Linear gingival erythema	No	Common	Very common
Acute necrotizing gingivitis (see Fig. 12.57)	No	Rare	Common
Necrotizing stomatitis	No	No	Common
Herpes simplex–related (see Figs. 12.10, 12.55, and 12.56)	No	Occasional	Common
Aphthous ulcers (see Fig. 12.45)	Common	Occasional	Very common

[a]$CD4^+$ count >500 cells/mm^3.
[b]$CD4^+$ count <200 cells/mm^3.
HIV, Human immunodeficiency virus.
(Adapted from Weinert M, Grimes RM, Lynch DP: Oral manifestations of HIV infection, *Ann Intern Med* 125:485, 1996.)

USEFUL VOCABULARY

Listed here are the specific roots that are important in understanding the terminology related to diseases of the mouth and pharynx.

Root	Pertaining to	Example	Definition
arytenoid-	pitcher-shaped structure	***arytenoid***itis	Inflammation of the arytenoid cartilage
bucco-	cheek	***bucco***pharyngeal	Pertaining to the cheek and pharynx
cheil(o)-	lip	***cheil***itis	Inflammation of the lip
dent-	tooth	***dent***al	Pertaining to the teeth
gingiv-	gingiva(e)	***gingiv***ectomy	Surgical excision of diseased gingiva(e)
gloss(o)-	tongue	***glosso***plegia	Paralysis of the tongue
-labi-	lips	naso***labi***al	Pertaining to the nose and lip
leuko-	white	***leuko***plakia	White patch on mucous membrane; often premalignant
linguo-	tongue	***linguo***papillitis	Painful ulcers around the papillae of the tongue
-plakia	patch	erythro***plakia***	Red patch on mucous membrane; often premalignant
ptyal-	saliva	***ptyal***ism	Excessive salivation
stoma-	mouth; opening	***stoma***titis	Inflammation of the mouth

WRITING UP THE PHYSICAL EXAMINATION

Listed here are examples of the write-up for the examinations of the oral cavity and pharynx.

- The lips appear normal. The mucosa of the oral cavity is red and without masses, leukoplakia, or other lesions. There is good dentition and good dental hygiene. The tongue is midline and does not deviate to either side. The tonsils are absent. The pharynx appears normal. The palate is normal, without ulcers or masses.
- There is a 1- to 2-cm painful vesicular lesion at the mucocutaneous junction on the right side of the mouth. There is tonsillar hypertrophy with a purulent discharge in the crypts of both tonsils. There is bilateral anterior triangle lymphadenopathy, greater on the right. The remainder of the examination of the oral cavity is unremarkable.
- There is a whitish pseudomembrane over the hard and soft palates, and over the tongue. When it is lifted, its erythematous base is friable and bleeds. The rest of the mouth and throat appears normal.
- The lateral border of the tongue has an ulcerated, indurated lesion, 2 × 1 cm.
- The palate has a dome-shaped, 3-cm mass to the right of midline. Biopsy is recommended.

FULL VIDEO

- Video 12.4 Full Video: Examination of the oral cavity

REVIEW QUESTIONS

1. **In the examination of the mouth, which of the following symptoms is abnormal and needs further evaluation?**
   - **A.** Black hairy tongue
   - **B.** Sublingual varices
   - **C.** Buccal mucosa leukoplakia
   - **D.** Geographic tongue
   - **E.** Fissured tongue
2. **The small, pinhead-sized, yellow papules on the buccal mucosa shown below are:**

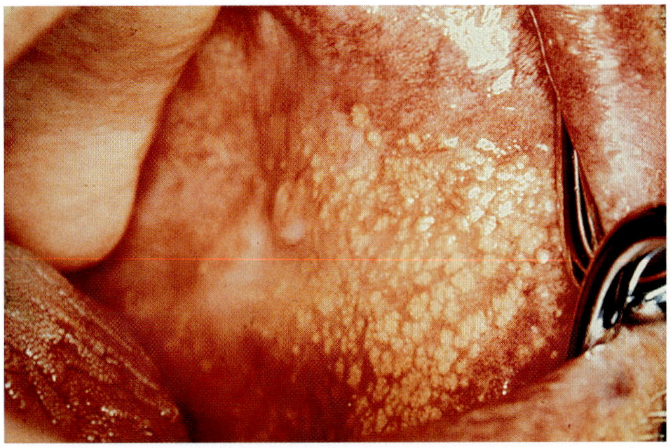

   - **A.** Premalignant
   - **B.** Sexually transmitted and similar to herpetic infection
   - **C.** Probably the most common lesions in the mouth
   - **D.** Ectopic apocrine glands
   - **E.** Related to HIV infection
3. **Which of the following statements is true?**
   - **A.** Carcinoma of the floor of the mouth accounts for 20% to 25% of all oral cancers.
   - **B.** Carcinoma of the tongue generally occurs on the lateral borders of the tongue.
   - **C.** Chewing betel nuts is the most common cause of oropharyngeal cancer in the United States.
   - **D.** Most of the strains of HPV (human papillomavirus) have been implicated in oral cancers.
   - **E.** Leukoplakia has a great potential for malignancy than erythroplakia.
4. **Regarding the occurrence of oral lesions during the stages of HIV infection, which of the following statements is true?**
   - **A.** Candidiasis is common during primary HIV infection.
   - **B.** Oral hairy leukoplakia is common during primary HIV infection.
   - **C.** Kaposi sarcoma is common during early HIV disease.
   - **D.** Acute necrotizing gingivitis is not common during advanced HIV disease.
   - **E.** Aphthous ulcers are not common during advanced HIV disease.
5. **Regarding carcinoma of the floor of the mouth, which of the following statements is *incorrect*?**
   - **A.** It is the most common site of oral cancers in African Americans.
   - **B.** About one-fifth of patients with carcinoma of the floor of the mouth have a second primary tumor.
   - **C.** Carcinoma of the floor of the mouth has a strong association with alcohol consumption and tobacco smoking.
   - **D.** Smokers are up to 25 times more likely to develop head and neck cancers than nonsmokers.
   - **E.** Passive smoking exposure is not a risk factor for developing oropharyngeal cancers.
6. **Regarding carcinoma of the lip, which of the following statements is correct?**
   - **A.** Most are squamous cell carcinomas.
   - **B.** The upper lip is the most common site.
   - **C.** There is a strong female predominance.
   - **D.** It is characterized by a painful ulcer.
   - **E.** Ill-fitting dentures are not a risk factor for carcinoma of the lip.
7. **Acute multiple oral ulcers that are preceded by or associated with vesicles may have infective causes such as:**
   - **A.** Herpes simplex
   - **B.** Herpes zoster
   - **C.** Coxsackie virus
   - **D.** HIV
   - **E.** All of the above
8. **The following figure shows a common oral finding. Which of the following statements is correct?**

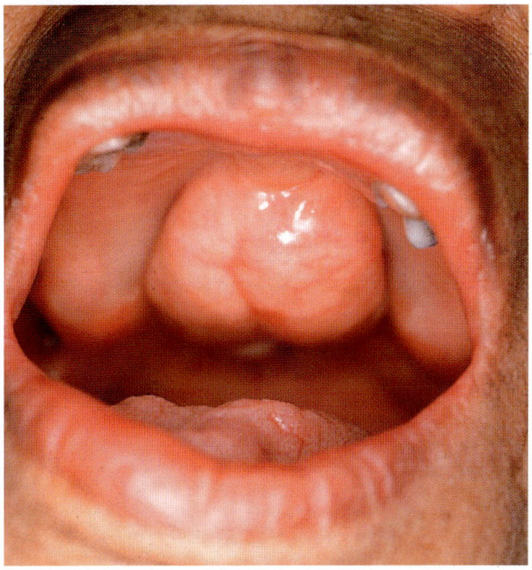

   - **A.** It is a discrete, soft swelling in the midline of the hard palate.
   - **B.** It is often premalignant.
   - **C.** It is painful.

D. It occurs twice as often in females as in males.
E. More than 50% of the population has this finding.

9. **The following figure shows oral hairy leukoplakia (OHL). Which of the following statements is *incorrect*?**

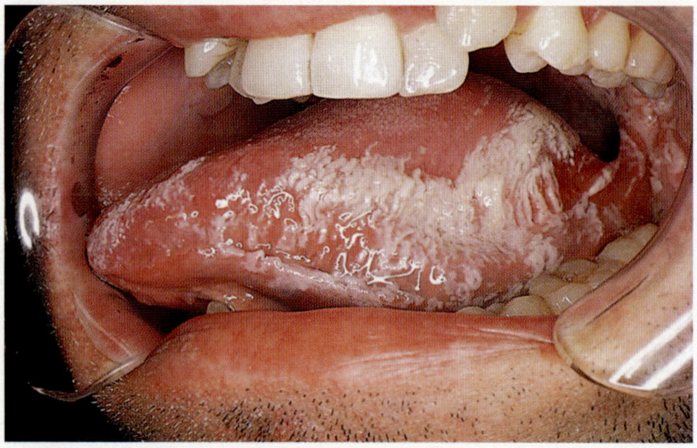

A. It is associated with the subsequent development of AIDS.
B. The lesions are raised white lesions appearing corrugated.
C. The lesions range in size from a few millimeters to 2 to 3 cm.
D. They are most commonly found on the lateral borders of the tongue.
E. OHL is not diagnostic of an HIV infection.

10. **Snoring is a common concern associated with obstructive sleep apnea. It is associated with which of the following symptoms?**
A. Morning headaches
B. Hypertension
C. Arrhythmias
D. Increased risk of heart attacks and strokes
E. All of the above

REFERENCES

Available online.

BIBLIOGRAPHY

Available online.

13

The Chest

Mark H. Swartz

In the beginning the malady [tuberculosis] is easier to cure but difficult to detect, but later it becomes easy to detect but difficult to cure.

Niccolò Machiavelli (1469–1527)

VIDEOS

Video 13.1	Assessing respiratory rate and pattern
Video 13.2	Palpating the posterior chest for tenderness
Video 13.3	Evaluating excursion of the posterior chest
Video 13.4	Evaluating tactile fremitus of the posterior chest
Video 13.5	Percussing the posterior chest
Video 13.6	Auscultating the posterior chest
Video 13.7	Evaluating the position of the trachea
Video 13.8	Evaluating tactile fremitus of the anterior chest
Video 13.9	Percussing the anterior chest
Video 13.10	Auscultating the anterior chest
Video 13.11	Full video: Examination of the posterior chest
Video 13.12	Full video: Examination of the heart and lungs (lying)

GENERAL CONSIDERATIONS

Oxygen enables the breath of life; without adequate lung function, lives cannot be sustained. Patients with pulmonary disease must work harder for adequate oxygenation. These patients are concerned with "air hunger" or "too little air." Anyone who has traveled to areas of high altitude, where the oxygen concentration is reduced, has experienced shortness of breath.

The magnitude of pulmonary disease is enormous. Five respiratory diseases are the most common causes of illness and death worldwide: chronic obstructive pulmonary disease (COPD), asthma, acute respiratory tract infection or pneumonia, tuberculosis (TB), and lung cancer.[1] Whereas the top two causes of death, heart disease and cancer, have seen a drop in their mortality rates, lung diseases such as COPD have seen the most significant rise of any leading cause of death. COPD is now the third leading cause of death worldwide. An estimated 200 million people have COPD, of which about 3.2 million die each year. Major risk factors include tobacco exposure, occupational and environmental exposures, respiratory infections, and genetics. The prevalence is highest in rural areas (8.4%) compared with large metropolitan areas (4.7%).

The symptoms of COPD include breathlessness, chronic coughing (with or without mucus), wheezing, chest tightness, and frequent throat clearing. Here are the facts:

- The National Heart, Lung, and Blood Institute estimates that 15.7 million American adults have COPD, and another 12 million are undiagnosed or developing COPD.
- More than 50% of adults with low pulmonary function were unaware of their COPD, so the actual number may be higher.[2]
- COPD kills more females than males each year. Moreover, the rate of females dying from the disease has been steadily climbing over the decades, reflecting the expansion of smoking among females in the mid-20th century.
- A person with COPD dies every 4 minutes in the United States.
- In 15 years, COPD is expected to become the leading cause of death.[3]
- COPD is relatively easy to diagnose using spirometry, which involves a machine in which the patient exhales as much as possible into a tube.
- Spirometry is noninvasive, takes less than 5 minutes, and yet is vastly underused. Only one-third or fewer of people with COPD ever undergo this test.

COPD is a preventable and treatable condition. Almost 90% of COPD is due to smoking, and smoking cessation at any age and stage is beneficial.

Cancer of the lung and bronchus is the first and most common cause of death from cancer in the United States. Lung and bronchus cancer represents 12.2% of all new cancer cases in the U.S.

In 2023, the American Cancer Society reported that there were 238,340 new cases of lung cancer, with 127,070 deaths. In 2023, there were 120,790 new cases in females with 59,910 deaths and 117,550 new cases in males with 67,160 deaths. Smoking is widely recognized as the leading cause of lung cancer. The rate of new lung and bronchus cancer cases was 50.0 per 100,000 males and females per year based on 2016–2020 cases, age-adjusted. The death rate was 35.0 per

100,000 males and females per year based on 2016–2020 deaths, age-adjusted.

Lung cancer death rates among females are falling more slowly than those among males because females began smoking in large numbers and subsequently quit later than males. As a result, lung cancer death rates have been declining since 1990 in males but have just begun to decline in females. Since 1987, more females have died yearly from lung cancer (59,910 in 2023) than from breast cancer (43,700 in 2023). Gender differences in lung cancer mortality patterns reflect historical differences in the uptake and reduction of cigarette smoking between males and females during the past 50 years.

In 2022, there were more than 8300 cases of TB reported with a rate of 2.5 cases per 100,000 persons.[4] TB is caused by infection with *Mycobacterium tuberculosis*. More than 13 million people in the United States live with latent TB infection. Latent TB infection occurs when the TB bacteria live in one's body without causing illness. Individuals with latent TB are asymptomatic, feel well, cannot spread the disease to others, usually have a positive TB skin test, and may develop TB if not treated for their latent infection. Fortunately, since 1992, the cases of TB and the incidence rates have steadily decreased. The timely diagnosis and treatment of active and latent TB infection are critical to eliminating TB worldwide.

TB can spread throughout the body, infecting almost every organ. The term disseminated TB, also known as miliary TB, includes pulmonary and extrapulmonary sites. It is estimated that extrapulmonary tuberculosis (EPTB) accounts for 15% to 25% of all cases of TB. HIV patients, especially those with low CD4 counts, have higher rates of EPTB. Children are more likely to have skeletal TB than adults. Pott disease is TB of the spine, secondary to the hematogenous spread from a primary site of infection, the lungs.[5] The lower thoracic and upper lumbar vertebrae areas of the spine are most commonly affected. If only one vertebra is affected, the disc is normal; however, if two vertebrae are involved, the disc between them collapses, as it is avascular and cannot receive nutrients. Caseation occurs, with vertebral narrowing and eventually vertebral collapse and spinal damage.

The COVID-19 pandemic may have subsided, but its impact highlights a global lung health crisis that has not gone away.

In 24 hours, the lungs oxygenate more than 5700 L of blood with more than 11,400 L of air. The surface area of the lungs' alveoli is larger than a tennis court.

STRUCTURE AND PHYSIOLOGY

The chest forms the bony case that houses and protects the lungs, the heart, and the esophagus as it passes into the stomach. The chest skeleton comprises 12 thoracic vertebrae, 12 pairs of ribs, the clavicle, and the sternum. The bony structure is illustrated in Fig. 13.1.

The lungs continuously provide oxygen and remove carbon dioxide from the circulatory system. The power required for breathing comes from the intercostal muscles and the diaphragm. These muscles act as bellows to suck air into the lungs. Expiration is passive. Elasticity helps during inspiration as well as alveolar compliance. The control of breathing is complex and is controlled by the *breathing center* in the brain's medulla.

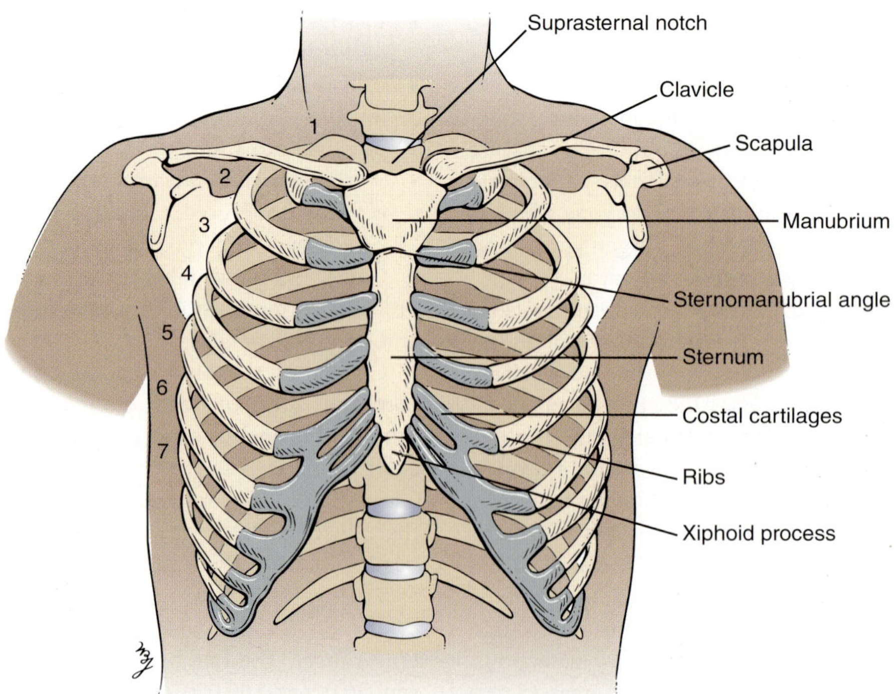

Fig. 13.1 Bony Chest Skeleton.

Inspired air is warmed, filtered, and humidified by the upper respiratory passages. After passing through the cricoid cartilage of the larynx, air travels through a system of flexible tubes, the *trachea.* The trachea bifurcates into the left and right bronchi at the fourth or fifth thoracic vertebra level. The right bronchus is shorter, wider, and straighter than the left bronchus. The bronchi continue subdividing into smaller bronchi and then into *bronchioles* within the lungs. Each respiratory bronchiole terminates in an *alveolar duct,* from which many *alveolar sacs* branch off. It is estimated that more than 500 million alveoli are in the lungs. Each alveolar wall contains elastin fibers that allow the sac to expand with inspiration and to contract with expiration by *elastic recoil.* This system of air-conducting passages is illustrated in Fig. 13.2.

The lungs are subdivided into lobes: the *upper, middle,* and *lower* on the right and the *upper* and *lower* on the left. The lungs are enveloped in a thin sac, the *pleura.* The *visceral* pleura overlies the lung parenchyma, whereas the *parietal* pleura lines the chest wall. The two pleural surfaces glide over each other during inspiration and expiration. The space between the pleura is the pleural cavity.

To describe physical signs in the chest accurately, the examiner must understand the topographic landmarks of the chest wall. The landmarks of clinical importance are as follows:

- Sternum
- Clavicle
- Suprasternal notch
- Sternomanubrial angle
- Midsternal line
- Midclavicular lines
- Anterior axillary lines
- Midaxillary lines
- Posterior axillary lines
- Scapular lines
- Midspinal line

Fig. 13.3 illustrates the anterior and lateral views of the thorax, and Fig. 13.4 illustrates the posterior thorax.

The *suprasternal notch* is located at the top of the sternum and can be felt as a depression at the base of the neck. The *sternomanubrial angle* is often referred to as the *angle of Louis.* This bony ridge lies approximately 5 cm below the suprasternal notch. When you move your fingers off the ridge laterally, the adjacent rib you feel is the second rib. The interspace below the second rib is the *second intercostal space.* Using this as a reference point, you should be able to identify the ribs and interspaces anteriorly. Try it on yourself.

To identify areas, several imaginary lines can be visualized on the anterior and posterior chest in Figs. 13.3 and 13.4. The *midsternal line* is drawn through the middle of the sternum. The *midclavicular lines* are drawn through the middle points of the clavicles and parallel to the midsternal line. The *anterior axillary lines* are vertical lines drawn along the anterior axillary folds parallel to the midsternal line. The *midaxillary lines* are drawn from each vertex of the axilla parallel to the midsternal

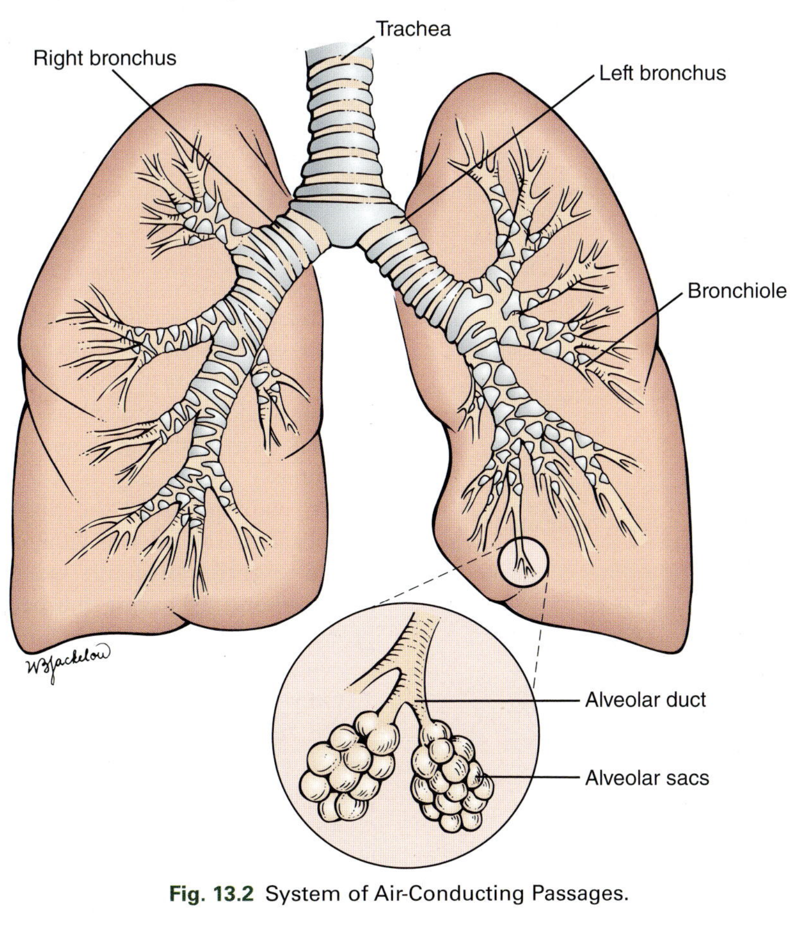

Fig. 13.2 System of Air-Conducting Passages.

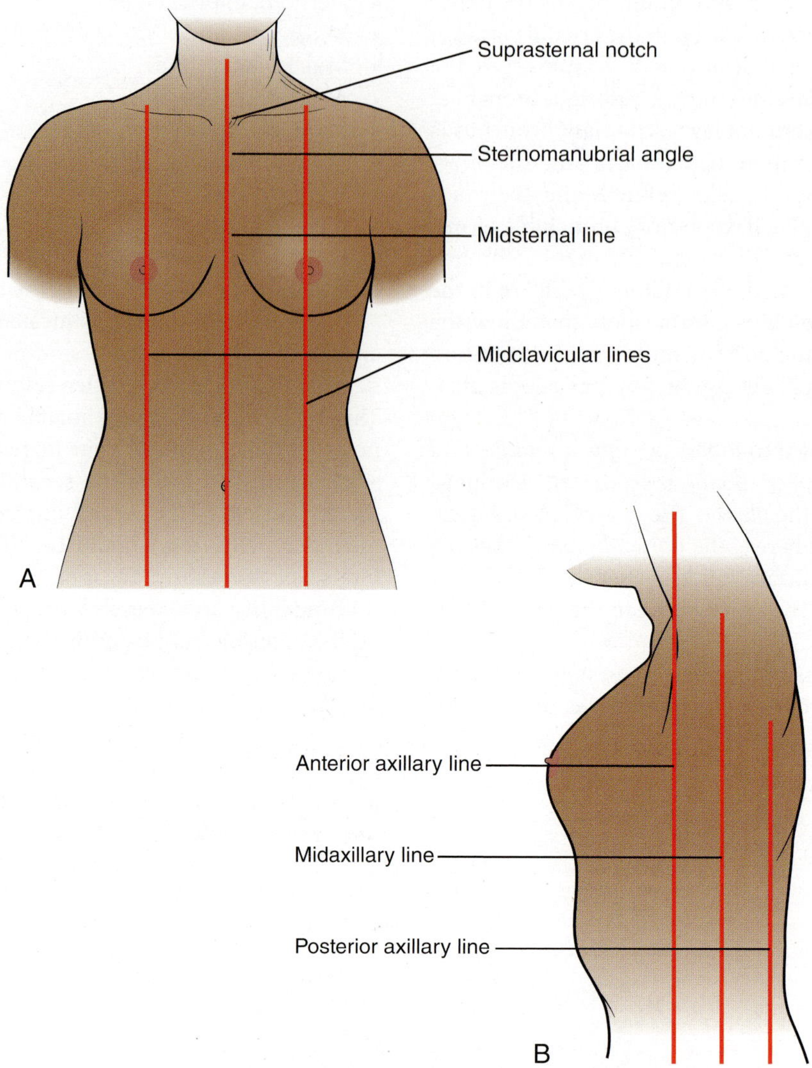

Fig. 13.3 Thoracic Cage Landmarks. (A) Topographic landmarks of the anterior thorax. (B) Landmarks on the lateral view.

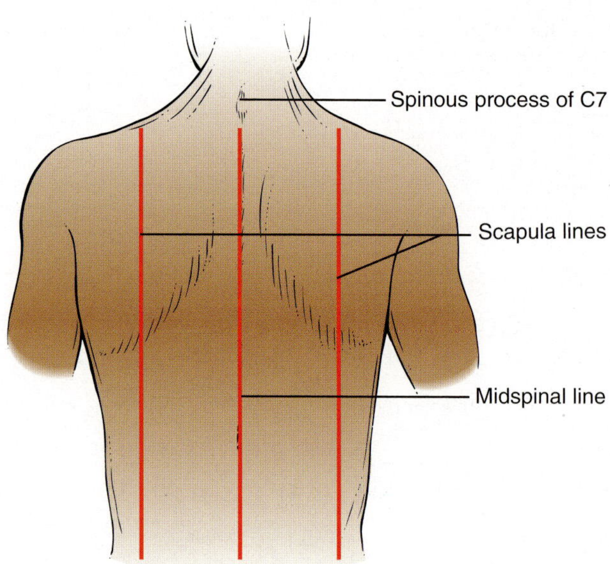

Fig. 13.4 Topographic Landmarks of the Posterior Thorax.

line. The *posterior axillary lines* parallel the midsternal line and extend vertically along the posterior axillary folds. The *scapular lines* are parallel to the midspinal line and pass through the inferior angles of the scapulae. The *midspinal line* is a vertical line that passes through the posterior spinous processes of the vertebrae.

Rib counting from the posterior chest is slightly more complicated. The inferior wing of the *scapula* lies at the level of the seventh rib or interspace. Another helpful landmark can be found by having the patient flex the neck; the most prominent cervical spinous process, the *vertebra prominens,* protrudes from the seventh cervical vertebra.

Only the first seven ribs articulate with the sternum. The eighth, ninth, and tenth ribs articulate with the cartilage above. The eleventh and twelfth ribs are floating ribs with free anterior portions.

The *interlobar fissures,* illustrated in Fig. 13.5, are situated between the lobes of the lungs. Both the right and the left lungs have an *oblique fissure,* which begins on the anterior chest at the

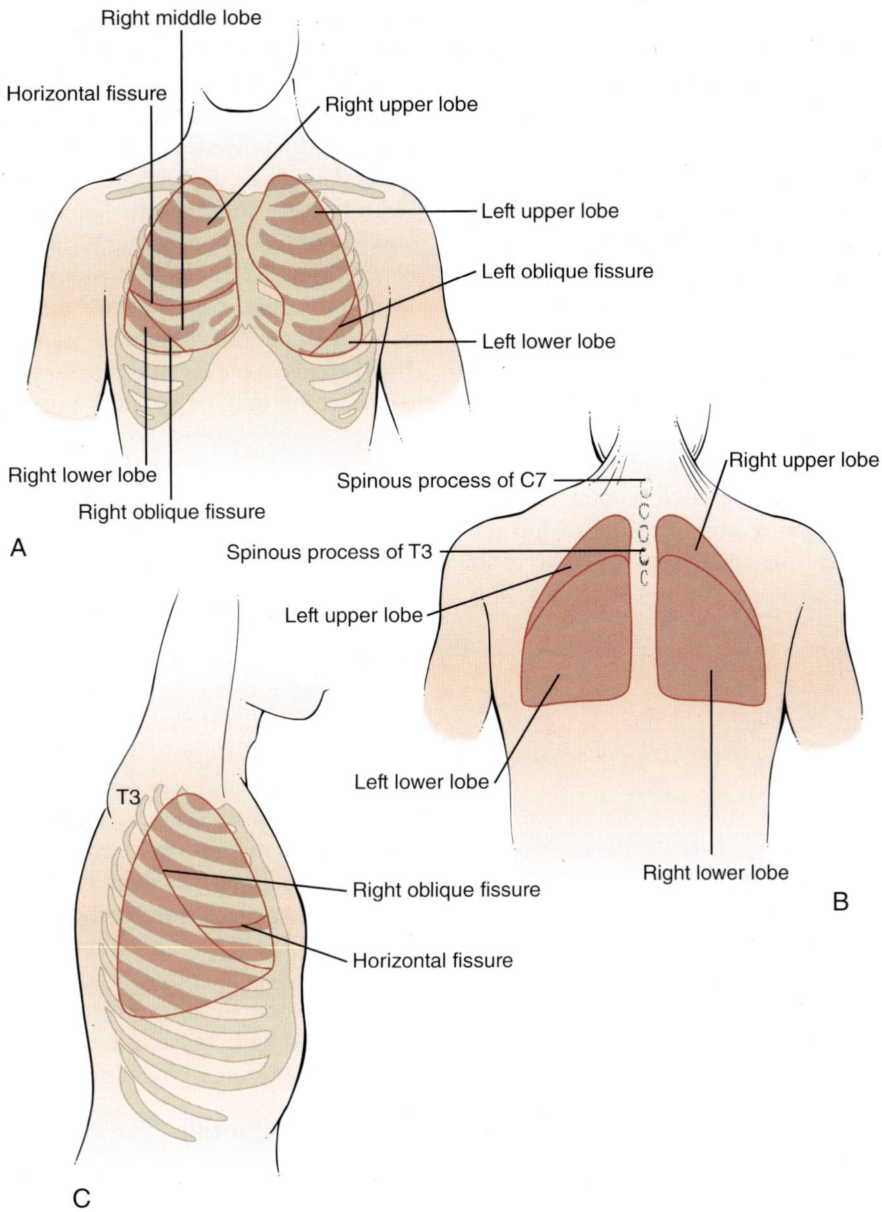

Fig. 13.5 Surface Topography and the Underlying Interlobar Fissures. (A) Anterior view. (B) Posterior view. (C) Lateral view.

level of the sixth rib at the midclavicular line and extends laterally upward to the fifth rib in the midaxillary line, ending at the posterior chest at the spinous process of T3. The right lower lobe is below the right oblique fissure; the right upper and middle lobes are superior to the right oblique fissure. The left lower lobe is below the left oblique fissure; the left upper lobe is superior to the left oblique fissure. The *horizontal fissure* is present only on the right and divides the right upper lobe from the right middle lobe. It extends from the fourth rib at the sternal border to the fifth rib at the midaxillary line.

The lungs extend superiorly approximately 3 to 4 cm above the medial end of the clavicles. The inferior margins of the lungs extend to the sixth rib at the midclavicular line, to the eighth rib at the midaxillary line, and between T9 and T12 posteriorly. This variation is related to respiration. The bifurcation of the trachea, the *carina,* is located behind the angle of Louis at approximately the level of T4 on the posterior chest. At the end of expiration, the right hemidiaphragm is situated at the level of the fifth rib anteriorly and T9 posteriorly. The presence of the liver on the right side makes the right hemidiaphragm slightly higher than the left.

During quiet breathing, muscle contraction occurs only during inspiration. Expiration is passive, resulting from the elastic recoil of the lungs and chest.

REVIEW OF SPECIFIC SYMPTOMS

The main symptoms of pulmonary disease are the following:

- Cough
- Sputum production
- Hemoptysis (coughing up blood)
- Dyspnea (shortness of breath)

- Wheezing
- Cyanosis (bluish discoloration of the skin)
- Chest pain
- Snoring
- Other symptoms

Cough

The most common symptom of lung disease is the *cough.* Coughing is so common that it is frequently regarded as a trivial concern. The cough reflex is a normal defense mechanism of the lungs that protects them from foreign bodies and excessive secretions. Infections of the upper respiratory tract are associated with coughing that usually improves in 2 to 3 weeks. However, a persistent cough necessitates further investigation.

Coughing is a coordinated, forced expiration interrupted by repeated glottis closure. The expiratory muscles contract against the partially closed glottis, creating high pressure within the lungs. When the glottis suddenly opens, an explosive rush of air clears the air passages. When a patient is concerned with coughing, ask these questions:

"Can you describe your cough?"
"How long have you had a cough?"
"Was there a sudden onset of coughing?"
"Do you smoke?" If so, *"What do you smoke? How much, and for how long?"*
"Does your cough produce sputum?" If so, *"Can you estimate the amount of your expectorations? What is the color of the sputum? Does the sputum have a foul odor?"*
"Does the cough occur for prolonged periods?"
"Does the cough occur after eating?"
"Is the coughing worse in any position?"
"What relieves the cough?"
"Are there any other symptoms associated with the cough? Fever? Headaches? Night sweats? Chest pain? Runny nose? Shortness of breath? Weight loss? Hoarseness? Loss of consciousness?"
"Do you have any birds as pets? Do you feed pigeons?"
"Have you ever been exposed to anyone with tuberculosis?"
"Have you been tested for tuberculosis?" If so, *"When and what were the results?"*
"Are you aware of any exposure, now or in the past, to hazardous materials, such as asbestos, dust, or other toxic agents?"

A complete occupational and environmental history is essential for any patient with chronic cough. Malignant *mesothelioma* is a cancer of the mesothelium that lines the lung, chest wall, and abdomen.[6] The primary risk factor for mesothelioma is asbestos exposure. Asbestos is a carcinogenic mineral of flexible fibers resistant to heat, electricity, and corrosion. These qualities make the mineral useful in many products. In the past, construction materials contained asbestos because it was an effective insulator. Asbestos in cloth, paper, cement, plastic, and other materials strengthens them.

Mesothelioma is almost always caused by exposure to asbestos. Inhaling or ingesting asbestos causes fibers to become trapped in the body. The trapped asbestos fibers can cause inflammation, scarring, and cancer. It usually takes many years for them to cause any apparent problems, with mesothelioma typically developing more than 20 years after asbestos exposure. The use of asbestos was banned entirely in the United States in 1999, so the risk of exposure is much lower nowadays. However, materials containing asbestos are still found in many older buildings. Individuals today involved with the demolition of older buildings are the most susceptible. Mesothelioma affects males more often than females. It is rare in people under age 45; 75% of people with mesothelioma are 65 and older. Mesothelioma is more common among Whites and Hispanics than among Blacks or Asians. The mesothelioma survival rate is typically 4 to 18 months after diagnosis, but there have been patients diagnosed with mesothelioma who have lived longer than 10 years. The current 5-year survival rate for the disease is just 10%.

Coughing may be voluntary or involuntary, productive or nonproductive. In *productive* cough, mucus or other materials are expelled. A *dry* cough does not produce any secretions.

Smoking is the most common cause of chronic cough. A *smoker's cough* results from inhalation of irritants in tobacco and is most marked in the morning. Coughing is usually decreased during sleep. When the smoker awakens, productive coughing increases attempting to clear the respiratory passages. Smoker's cough tends to sound different than regular coughing. It can involve wheezing and crackling noises associated with phlegm in the throat due to mucus and phlegm. Sometimes, the mucus is blood-tinged. In patients who stop smoking, the cough decreases and may disappear.

Coughing may also be *psychogenic.* This nonproductive cough occurs in individuals with emotional stress. When attention is drawn to it, the cough occurs more often. During sleep or when the patient is distracted, the coughing stops. Psychogenic coughing is a *diagnosis of exclusion:* Only after all other causes have been eliminated can this diagnosis be made.

Patients and healthcare professionals use many terms to describe a cough. Table 13.1 lists some of the more common descriptors and their possible causes.

Sputum Production

Sputum is the substance expelled by coughing. Approximately 75 to 100 mL of sputum is secreted daily by the bronchi. Ciliary action brings it up to the throat and then swallowed

TABLE 13.1 Descriptors of Coughing

Description	Possible Causes
Dry, hacking	Viral infections, interstitial lung disease, tumor, allergies, anxiety
Chronic, productive	Bronchiectasis, chronic bronchitis, abscess, bacterial pneumonia, tuberculosis
Wheezing	Bronchospasm, asthma, allergies, congestive heart failure
Barking	Epiglottal disease (e.g., croup)
Stridor	Tracheal obstruction
Morning	Smoking
Nocturnal	Postnasal drip, congestive heart failure
Associated with eating or drinking	Neuromuscular disease of the upper esophagus
Inadequate	Debility, weakness

unconsciously with the saliva. An increase in the quantity of sputum production is the earliest manifestation of bronchitis. Sputum may contain cellular debris, mucus, blood, pus, or microorganisms.

Sputum should be described according to color, consistency, quantity, the number of times it is brought up during the day and night, and the presence or absence of blood. An adequate description may indicate a cause of the disease process. Uninfected sputum is odorless, transparent, and whitish-gray, resembling mucus; it is termed *mucoid*. Infected sputum contains pus and is termed *purulent*; the sputum may be yellow, greenish, or red. Table 13.2 lists the appearances of sputum and its possible causes.

Hemoptysis

Hemoptysis is the coughing up of blood. Few symptoms produce as much alarm in patients as in hemoptysis. A detailed description of the hemoptysis is crucial because what is produced can include clots of blood, as well as blood-tinged sputum. The implications of each are very different. Coughing up blood clots is a symptom of extreme importance because it often heralds a severe illness. Blood clots usually indicate a cavitary lung lesion, a lung tumor, certain cardiac diseases, or pulmonary embolism. Blood-tinged sputum is generally associated with smoking, as previously mentioned, or minor infections but can also be seen with tumors and more severe conditions. When a patient is concerned with coughing up blood, the examiner should ask the following questions:

"Do you smoke?" If yes, *"What do you smoke? How much, and for how long?"*
"Did the coughing up of blood occur suddenly?"
"Have there been recurrent episodes of coughing up blood?"
"Is the sputum blood-tinged, or are there actual clots of blood?"
"How long have you noticed the blood?"
"What seems to bring on the coughing up of blood? Vomiting? Coughing? Nausea?"
"Have you ever had tuberculosis?"
"Have you ever been exposed to anyone with tuberculosis?"
"Have you been tested for tuberculosis?" If so, *"When and what were the results?"*
"Is there a family history of coughing up blood?"
"Have you had recent surgery?"
"Do you take any 'blood thinners'?"
"Are you aware of any bleeding tendency?"
"Have you had any recent travel on airplanes?"
"Have you had night sweats? Shortness of breath? Palpitations? Irregular heartbeats? Hoarseness? Weight loss? Swelling or pain in your legs?"
"Have you felt any unusual sensation in your chest after coughing up blood?" If so, *"Where?"*
(For a female with hemoptysis) *"Do you use oral contraceptives?"*

Any suppurative (associated with the production of pus) process of the airways or lungs can produce hemoptysis. Bronchitis is the most common cause of hemoptysis. Bronchiectasis and bronchogenic carcinoma are also major causes. Hemoptysis results from mucosal invasion, tumor necrosis, and pneumonia distal to bronchial obstruction by the tumor. Pneumococcal pneumonia characteristically produces rust-colored sputum. Pink and frothy sputum can result from pulmonary edema.

Occasionally, patients have a warm sensation in the chest at the location from which the hemoptysis originated. Therefore, it is helpful to ask patients with recent hemoptysis whether they experienced such a sensation. This information may lead to a more careful review of the physical examination and x-ray films of that area.

Patients who have undergone recent surgery or have traveled for long periods on airplanes are at risk for deep vein thrombophlebitis with pulmonary embolism. Females taking oral contraceptives are likewise at risk for pulmonary embolic disease. Hemoptysis occurs when pulmonary emboli result in infarction, with necrosis of the pulmonary parenchyma.

Recurrent episodes of hemoptysis may result from bronchiectasis, TB, or mitral stenosis. Atrial fibrillation is a common cause of "irregular heartbeats" and embolic phenomena.

Sometimes it is difficult to ascertain whether the patient coughed up or vomited blood. However, most patients can provide a sufficiently clear history. Table 13.3 lists characteristics

TABLE 13.2 Appearances of Sputum

Appearance	Possible Causes
Mucoid	Asthma, tumors, tuberculosis, emphysema, pneumonia
Mucopurulent	Asthma, tumors, tuberculosis, emphysema, pneumonia
Yellow-green, purulent	Bronchiectasis, chronic bronchitis
Rust-colored, purulent	Pneumococcal pneumonia
Red currant jelly	*Klebsiella pneumoniae* infection
Foul odor	Lung abscess
Pink, blood-tinged	Streptococcal or staphylococcal pneumonia
Gravel	Broncholithiasis
Pink, frothy	Pulmonary edema
Profuse, colorless (also known as *bronchorrhea*)	Alveolar cell carcinoma
Bloody	Pulmonary emboli, bronchiectasis, abscess, tuberculosis, tumor, cardiac causes, bleeding disorders

TABLE 13.3 Characteristics Distinguishing Hemoptysis From Hematemesis

Features	Hemoptysis	Hematemesis
Prodrome	Coughing	Nausea and vomiting
Past history	Possible history of cardiopulmonary disease	Possible history of gastrointestinal disease
Appearance	Frothy	Not frothy
Color	Bright red	Dark red, brown, or "coffee grounds"
Manifestation	Mixed with pus	Mixed with food
Associated symptoms	Dyspnea	Nausea

that help distinguish hemoptysis from hematemesis (vomiting blood).

Dyspnea

The *subjective* sensation of "shortness of breath" is *dyspnea.* Dyspnea is an important manifestation of cardiopulmonary disease, although found in other states such as neurologic, metabolic, and psychologic conditions. It is crucial to differentiate dyspnea from the *objective* finding of *tachypnea,* or rapid breathing. A patient may be observed breathing rapidly while stating they are not short of breath. The converse is also true: a patient may breathe slowly but have dyspnea. Never assume that a patient with a rapid respiratory rate is dyspneic.

The examiner needs to inquire when dyspnea occurs and in which position. *Paroxysmal nocturnal dyspnea* is the sudden onset of shortness of breath occurring at night during sleep. Patients are suddenly seized with an intense strangling sensation. They frantically sit up and, classically, run to the window for "air." As soon as they assume an upright position, the dyspnea usually improves. *Orthopnea* is difficulty breathing while lying flat. Patients require two or more pillows to breathe comfortably. *Platypnea* is a rare symptom of difficulty breathing while sitting up and is relieved by a recumbent position. *Trepopnea* is when patients are more comfortable breathing while lying on one side. (Some of the more common causes of positional dyspnea are listed in Table 13.4.) For any patient concerned with dyspnea, ask the following questions:

"How long have you had shortness of breath?"
"Did the shortness of breath occur suddenly?"
"Is the shortness of breath constant?"
"Does the shortness of breath occur with exertion? At rest? Lying flat? Sitting up?"
"What makes the shortness of breath worse? What relieves it?"
"How many level blocks can you walk without shortness of breath?"
"How many level blocks could you walk 6 months ago?"
"Is the shortness of breath accompanied by wheezing? Fever? Cough? Coughing up blood? Chest pain? Palpitations? Hoarseness?"
"Do you smoke?" If so, *"How much? For how long?"*
"Have you had any asbestos exposure? Sandblasting? Pigeon breeding?"

TABLE 13.4 Positional Dyspnea

Type	Possible Causes
Orthopnea	Congestive heart failure
	Mitral valvular disease
	Severe asthma (rarely)
	Emphysema (rarely)
	Chronic bronchitis (rarely)
	Neurologic diseases (rarely)
Trepopnea	Congestive heart failure
Platypnea	Postpneumonectomy status
	Neurologic diseases
	Cirrhosis (intrapulmonary shunts)
	Hypovolemia

"Have you had any exposure to individuals with tuberculosis?"
"Have you ever lived near the San Joaquin Valley? Midwestern or southeastern United States?"

It is essential to try to quantify the dyspnea. Questions such as "How many level blocks can you walk?" provide a framework for *exercise tolerance.* For example, if the patient answers, "two blocks," the patient is said to have *two-block dyspnea on exertion.* The interviewer can then ask, "How many level blocks were you able to walk 6 months ago?" and thus assess approximately the progression of the disease or the efficacy of therapy.

Careful questioning regarding *industrial exposure* is paramount for any patient with unexplained dyspnea. Examples of further questions regarding occupational and environmental history are discussed in Chapter 1, The Interviewer's Questions. Exposure to pigeons may result in psittacosis. In addition, psittacosis in humans is most commonly associated with pet birds, like parrots and cockatiels, and poultry, like turkeys and ducks. It is a bacterial infection caused by *Chlamydia psittaci.* Therefore, people who work in bird-related occupations (e.g., bird owners, aviary and pet shop employees, poultry workers, and veterinarians) are at increased risk. Psittacosis produces a mild illness; the most common symptoms include fever, chills, headache, muscle aches, and a dry cough.

Outbreaks of coccidioidomycosis[a] have occurred in individuals living in the southwestern United States. Living in the midwestern and southeastern United States has been linked to histoplasmosis[b] outbreaks.

Wheezing

Wheezing is an abnormally high-pitched noise resulting from a partially obstructed airway. It is usually present during expiration when slight bronchoconstriction occurs. Bronchospasm, mucosal edema, loss of elastic support, and tortuosity of the airways are the usual causes. Asthma causes bronchospasm,

[a]Coccidioidomycosis, also known as Valley Fever, is a disease caused by a fungus, *Coccidioides,* that grows in the soil and dirt in some areas of California and the southwestern United States. People and animals can get sick when they breathe in dust that contains the fungus. Most people who are exposed to the fungus never have symptoms. Other people may have symptoms, such as fatigue, cough, fever, shortness of breath, headache, sweats, rash, and muscle aches, that go away after weeks to months. Approximately 5% to 10% of people who get Valley Fever will develop serious or long-term problems in their lungs.

[b]Histoplasmosis is an infection caused by breathing in spores of a fungus, *Histoplasma capsulatum,* often found in bird and bat droppings. People usually get it from breathing in these spores when they become airborne during demolition or cleanup projects. People more likely to be exposed include farmers, pest control workers, poultry keepers, construction workers, roofers, landscapers, cave explorers, and demolition workers. In the United States, histoplasmosis commonly occurs in the Mississippi and Ohio River valleys. Most people with histoplasmosis never develop symptoms and aren't aware that they are infected. The most severe variety of histoplasmosis occurs mainly in infants and in people with weakened immune systems. Called disseminated histoplasmosis, it can affect nearly any part of your body, including the mouth, liver, central nervous system, skin, and adrenal glands. If untreated, disseminated histoplasmosis is usually fatal.

which results in the wheezing associated with this condition. Obstruction by intraluminal material, such as aspirated foreign bodies or secretions, is another important cause of wheezing. A well-localized wheeze, unchanged by coughing, may indicate that a foreign body or tumor partially obstructs a bronchus. When a patient is concerned with wheezing, the examiner must determine the following:

"At what age did the wheezing begin?"
"How often does it occur?"
"Are there any precipitating factors, such as foods, odors, emotions, animals, and so forth?"
"What usually stops the attack?"
"Have the symptoms worsened over the years?"
"Are there any associated symptoms?"
"Is there a history of nasal polyps?"
"Do you smoke?" If so, *"What do you smoke? How much, and for how long?"*
"Is there a history of heart disease?"

An important axiom to remember is that **asthma is associated with wheezing, but not all wheezing is asthma**.

Do not equate wheezing *only* with asthma. For example, although congestive heart failure is usually associated with abnormal breath sounds called *crackles* (discussed later in this chapter), sometimes there is such severe bronchospasm in heart failure that the primary physical finding is a wheeze rather than a crackle.

A decrease in wheezing may result from either an airway opening or a progressive closing of the air passage. A "silent" chest in a patient with an acute asthmatic attack is usually an ominous sign: It indicates the worsening of the obstruction.

Cyanosis

A family member or friend commonly detects cyanosis. However, the subtle bluish discoloration may go completely unnoticed by the patient. *Central* cyanosis occurs with inadequate gas exchange in the lungs, significantly reducing arterial oxygenation. Primary pulmonary problems or diseases that cause mixed venous blood to bypass the lungs (e.g., intracardiac shunt) are frequently the causative factors. The bluish discoloration is best seen in the mucous membranes of the mouth (e.g., the frenulum) and lips. *Peripheral* cyanosis results from an excessive extraction of oxygen at the periphery. It is limited to the extremities (e.g., the fingers, toes, nose). Ask the following questions:

"Where is the cyanosis present?"
"How long has the cyanosis been present?"
"Are you aware of any lung problems? Heart problem? Blood problem?"
"What makes the cyanosis worse?"
"Is there associated shortness of breath? Cough? Bleeding?"
"What types of work have you performed?"
"Is there anyone else in your family who has cyanosis?"

Cyanosis from birth is associated with congenital heart lesions. The acute development of cyanosis can occur in severe respiratory disease, especially acute airway obstruction. Peripheral cyanosis results from increased oxygen extraction in states of low cardiac output and is seen in cooler areas of the body, such as the nail beds and the outer surfaces of the lips. Peripheral cyanosis disappears as the area is warmed. Cyanosis of the nails and warmth in the hands suggest that the cyanosis is central. Central cyanosis occurs only after the oxygen saturation has fallen to less than 80%. Central cyanosis diffusely involves the skin and mucous membranes and does not disappear with the area's warming. At least 2 to 3 g of unsaturated hemoglobin per 100 mL of blood must be present for the patient to manifest central cyanosis. Exercise worsens central cyanosis because the muscles require increased oxygen extraction from the blood. Cyanosis may not be seen in patients with severe anemia, in whom hemoglobin levels are markedly decreased. Clubbing of the nails is seen in association with central cyanosis and significant cardiopulmonary disorders. See Fig. 8.12.

Some industrial workers, such as arc welders, inhale toxic levels of nitrous gases that can produce cyanosis by acquired *methemoglobinemia*. Methemoglobinemia is a condition with life-threatening potential in which there is a decrease in the oxygen-carrying capacity of hemoglobin.[7] Methemoglobin is a form of hemoglobin that has been oxidized, changing its heme iron configuration from the ferrous (Fe^{2+}) to the ferric (Fe^{3+}) state. Unlike normal hemoglobin, the affinity for oxygen of ferric iron is impaired, and, as a result, hemoglobin cannot deliver oxygen to the tissues. Increased levels of methemoglobin result in functional anemia. Other causes of acquired methemoglobinemia include various antibiotics, local anesthetics, nitrates, and aniline dyes. Instead of being red in color, the arterial blood of patients with methemoglobinemia is brownish; this results in the skin of white patients gaining a bluish hue.

Methemoglobinemia may also be congenital. Congenital methemoglobinemia is a primary hemoglobin abnormality causing congenital cyanosis. The signs and symptoms of methemoglobinemia include cyanosis, shortness of breath, mental status changes, headache, fatigue, dizziness, and loss of consciousness.

Chest Pain

Chest pain related to pulmonary disease usually results from the involvement of the chest wall or parietal pleura. Nerve fibers are abundant in this area. *Pleuritic pain* is a common symptom of inflammation of the parietal pleura. It is described as a sharp, stabbing pain usually felt during inspiration. It may be localized to one side, and the patient may *splint*[c] to avoid the pain. Chapter 14, The Heart, summarizes the critical questions for a patient concerned with chest pain.

Acute dilatation of the main pulmonary artery may also produce a sensation of dull pressure, often indistinguishable from angina pectoris. This results from nerve endings responding to the stretch on the main pulmonary artery.

Although chest pain occurs in pulmonary disease, chest pain is the cardinal symptom of cardiac disease and is discussed more thoroughly in Chapter 14, The Heart.

[c]*Splinting* means making the chest muscles rigid to avoid motion of that part of the chest.

Snoring

Snoring is a common concern. A significant problem often associated with heavy snoring is *obstructive sleep apnea.* Many affected patients are overweight and have a history of excessive daytime sleepiness. A bed partner may describe the patient as sleeping quietly at first; then, a transition occurs to louder snoring, followed by a cessation of snoring, during which time the patient becomes restless, has gasping motions, and appears to be struggling for breath. A loud snort terminates this period, and the sequence may begin again. It is common for patients with sleep apnea to have many of these episodes each night. Refer to Chapter 12, The Oral Cavity and Pharynx, for more information on snoring, sleep apnea, and sleep-disordered breathing.

Other Symptoms

In addition to the main pulmonary disease symptoms, there are other, less common symptoms. These include the following:

- Stridor (noisy, harsh breathing)
- Voice changes
- Swelling of the ankles (dependent edema)

Stridor is an abnormal, high-pitched respiratory sound that can be assessed during breathing.[8] It is typically produced by the irregular flow of air in the airways and is most prominently heard during inspiration. An obstruction in the extrathoracic region causes inspiratory stridor. During inspiration, the intratracheal pressure falls below the atmospheric pressure, causing airway collapse. However, stridor can also be present during both inspiration and expiration. Stridor can be due to congenital malformations and anomalies and in the acute phase from life-threatening obstruction or infection, especially in children. Generally, stridor is more common in pediatric patients than in adult patients. Acute stridor may be caused by foreign body aspiration (e.g., peanuts or unchewed food),[d] airway burns, bacterial tracheitis, epiglottitis, anaphylaxis, and croup.[e] In infants and young children, a small amount of inflammation can result in significant and rapid airway obstruction. **Stridor is considered a medical emergency. Urgent care may be required.**

The timing and the sound of stridor can provide clues to the type of airway disorder: *Inspiratory stridor* occurs when the individual breathes in; it generally indicates a collapse of tissue at the level of the supraglottis or glottis. Inspiratory stridor often occurs in children with croup. It may indicate serious airway obstruction from severe conditions such as epiglottitis, a foreign body lodged in the airway, or a laryngeal tumor. *Expiratory stridor* occurs when the individual exhales; it generally indicates a problem in the subglottic area, lower trachea, or bronchus. *Biphasic stridor* occurs when the individual breathes in and out; it typically indicates an obstruction at the subglottic area or upper trachea.

Given that the etiology of stridor is so varied, effective diagnosis and management of stridor relies on the clinical suspicion of the healthcare professional and appropriate imaging modalities.

Voice changes can occur with inflammation of the vocal cords or interference with the recurrent laryngeal nerve. *Swelling of the ankles* is a manifestation of dependent edema associated with right-sided heart failure, renal disease, liver disease, and obstruction of venous flow. As the condition worsens, abnormal fluid accumulations produce generalized edema of the entire body, known as *anasarca.*

Effect of Lung Disease on the Patient

The effect of lung disease on the patient varies greatly with the nature of the ailment, as does the subjective sensation of air hunger. Some patients with lung disease are hardly aware of the dyspnea. The decrease in exercise tolerance is so insidious that these patients may not be aware of any problem. Only when asked to try to quantify the dyspnea do these patients realize their deficiency. In other patients, dyspnea is so rapidly progressive that they experience severe depression. They recognize that little can be done to improve their lung conditions and thus markedly alter their lifestyle. Many become incapacitated and are forced to retire from work. They can no longer experience the slightest exertion without becoming dyspneic.

Often, chronic lung disease develops as a result of occupational hazards. Affected patients may become embittered and hostile. There has been much publicity about occupational exposure, but some industries still provide little employee protection.

COPD can be divided into two types: *emphysema* and *chronic bronchitis.* Both are characterized by a slowly progressive course, airflow obstruction, and lung parenchyma destruction. Classically, patients with emphysema are the "pink puffers." They are thin and weak from severe dyspnea associated with slight cough or sputum production. The classic "blue bloaters" suffer primarily from bronchitis. They are cyanotic and have a productive cough but are less troubled by dyspnea; they are usually short and stocky. These classic descriptions are interesting, but most patients with COPD have characteristics of both types.

Since ancient times, healthcare professionals have recognized that emotional factors play a role in the onset and maintenance of symptoms in bronchial asthma. Asthma attacks can be provoked by various emotions: fear, anger, anxiety, depression, guilt, frustration, and joy. The patient attempts to suppress the emotion, rather than the emotion itself, that precipitates the asthmatic attack.

A patient with an asthmatic attack becomes anxious and fearful, perpetuating the attack. Hyperventilation may contribute to the breathlessness of the frightened patient. Despite being given adequate medical therapy, these patients remain dyspneic. In such patients, the anxiety and its causes require attention. They need continuing medical *and* psychological support after an acute attack. As early as the 12th century, Maimonides

[d]Foreign body aspiration accounts for more than 17,000 emergency department visits per year in the United States, with most cases occurring before the age of 3 years.

[e]With croup, the peak incidence is between 6 months to 36 months, where there are about 5 to 6 cases per 100 toddlers. There is also a slight male predominance of 1.4:1.

is an abnormal increase. *Apnea* is the temporary cessation of breathing. *Hyperpnea* is an increased depth of breathing, usually associated with metabolic acidosis.

There are many types of abnormal breathing patterns. Neurological disease may affect breathing cycles and rhythms. Several classic central periodic breathing patterns have been described. *Biot's breathing*, or ataxic breathing, is a pattern in patients with acute neurological disease. Biot's breathing is an abnormal pattern characterized by groups of quick, shallow inspirations followed by regular or irregular periods of apnea. It has been associated with damage to the pons or medulla, often due to strokes or uncal herniation. It can also be caused by opioid use. *Cheyne-Stokes breathing*, also known as periodic respiration, is an abnormal pattern of breathing characterized by progressively deeper and sometimes faster breathing followed by a gradual decrease resulting in apnea. The pattern repeats, with each cycle lasting 30 seconds to 2 minutes. It has a crescendo-decrescendo pattern with a period of apnea between the cycles. It is associated with stroke, brainstem compression, bilateral cerebral dysfunction, severe congestive cardiac failure, renal failure, and narcotic poisoning. Cheyne-Stokes breathing may also be seen in those dying as the body attempts to deal with changing carbon dioxide levels. *Kussmaul's breathing* is characterized by deep, rapid breathing. However, Kussmaul's breathing does not feature the shallow breaths, apnea, or alternations in breathing patterns seen in Cheyne-Stokes or Biot's breathing respiration. Instead, respirations remain deep and rapid throughout the cycle. Kussmaul's respiration is seen in individuals with diabetic ketoacidosis or kidney failure. It is respiratory compensation for metabolic acidosis, most commonly occurring in people with diabetes with diabetic ketoacidosis. Fig. 13.10 illustrates and lists the more common types of abnormal breathing.

Inspect the Hands

Is *clubbing* of the fingernails present? The technique for evaluating clubbing is described in Chapter 8, The Skin. The earliest finding of clubbing is the loss of the angle between the nail and the terminal phalanx. For example, look at Fig. 8.12, in which a normal index fingernail is compared with a severely clubbed index fingernail of a patient with bronchogenic carcinoma.

Clubbing has been associated with several clinical disorders, such as the following:

- Intrathoracic tumors
- Mixed venous-to-arterial shunts
- Chronic pulmonary disease
- Chronic hepatic fibrosis

The pathogenesis of clubbing is unclear. In many conditions, however, arterial desaturation occurs. This may be the underlying problem. In some individuals, clubbing may be inherited without any pathologic process.

The Posterior Chest

Move behind the patient to examine the posterior chest.

Palpation

Palpation is used to assess the following:

- Areas of tenderness
- Symmetry of chest excursion
- Tactile fremitus

Palpate for tenderness. See Video 13.2.

With your fingers, firmly palpate chest areas where the patient experiences tenderness. A concern with "chest pain" may be related only to local musculoskeletal disease and not to disease of the heart or lungs. Be meticulous in assessing for areas of tenderness.

Evaluate posterior chest excursion. See Video 13.3.

The examiner can determine the degree of symmetry of chest excursion by placing their hands flat against the patient's back with the thumbs parallel to the midline at approximately the level of the tenth ribs and pulling the underlying skin slightly toward the midline. The patient is asked to inhale deeply, and the movement of the examiner's hands is noted. The hand movement should be symmetric. Localized pulmonary disease may cause one side of the chest to move less than the opposite. The placement of the examiner's hands is shown in Fig. 13.11.

Evaluate tactile fremitus. See Video 13.4.

Speech creates vibrations that can be heard when the examiner listens to the chest and lungs. These vibrations are termed *vocal fremitus*. When the examiner palpates the patient's chest wall while the patient is speaking, these vibrations can be felt and are termed *tactile fremitus*. Sound is conducted from the larynx through the bronchial tree to the lung parenchyma and the chest wall. Tactile fremitus provides valuable information about the underlying lung tissue and chest cavity density. Conditions that increase the density of the lung and make it more solid, such as consolidation, increase the transmission of tactile fremitus. Clinical states that decrease the transmission of these sound waves result in reduced tactile fremitus. If there is excess fat tissue on the chest, air or fluid in the chest cavity, or lung overexpansion, tactile fremitus is diminished.

Tactile fremitus can be evaluated in two ways. In the first technique, the examiner places the ulnar side of their right

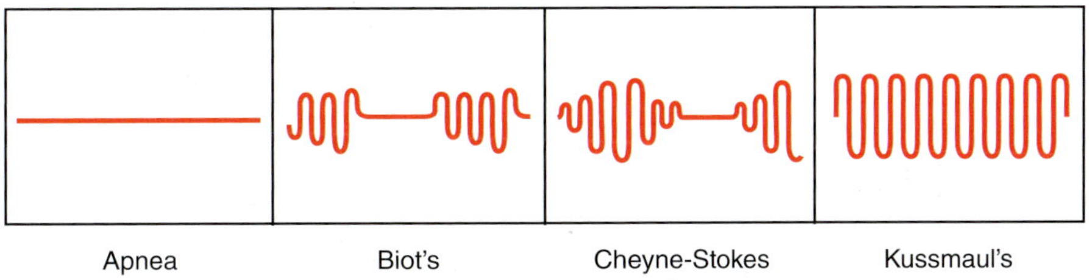

Fig. 13.10 Patterns of Abnormal Breathing.

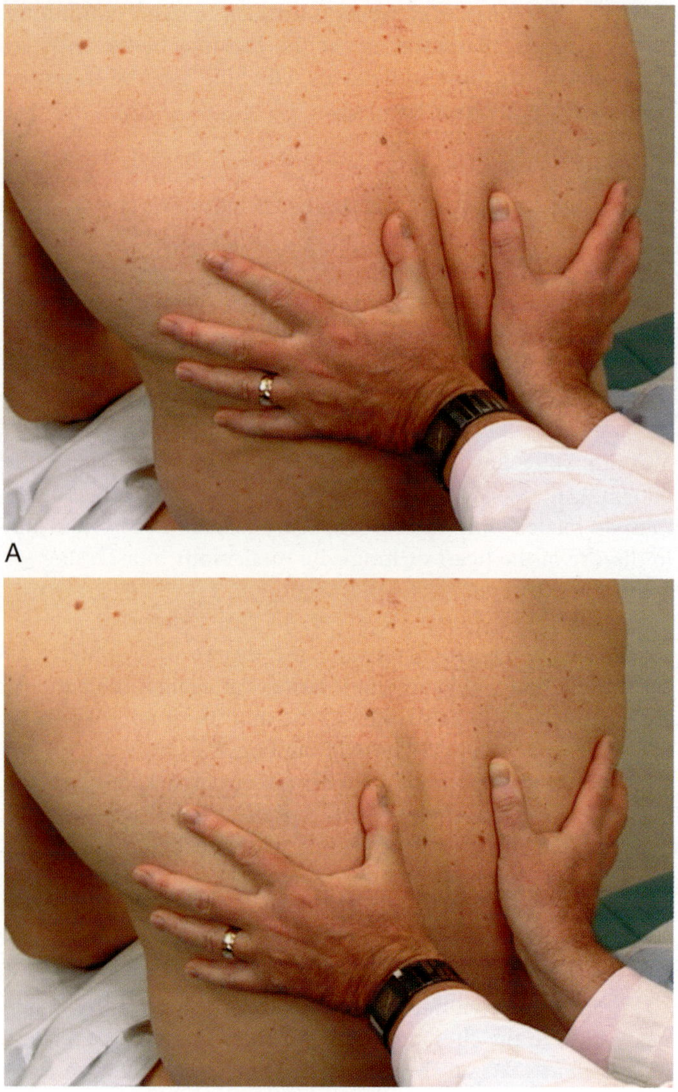

A

B

Fig. 13.11 Technique for Evaluating Posterior Chest Excursion. (A) Placement of the examiner's hands during normal expiration. (B) Placement of the examiner's hands after normal inspiration.

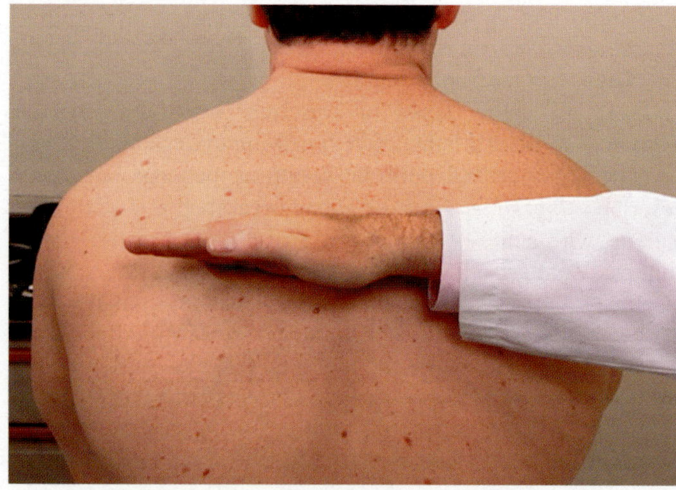

Fig. 13.12 Technique for Evaluating Tactile Fremitus.

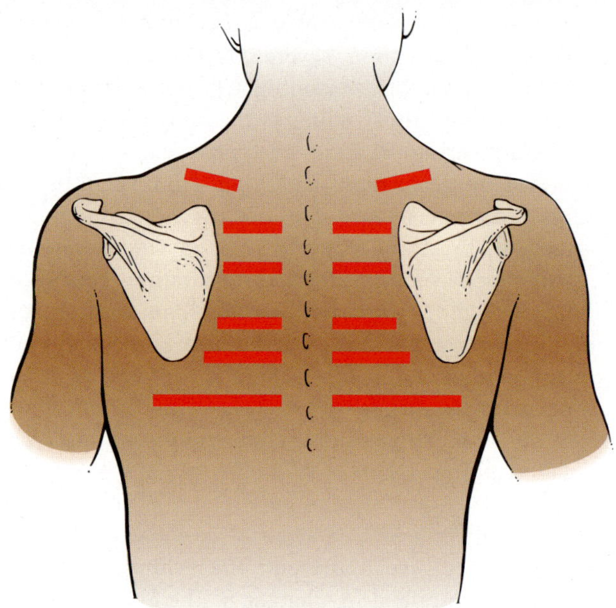

Fig. 13.13 Locations on the Posterior Chest for Evaluating Tactile Fremitus.

hand against the chest wall, as demonstrated in Fig. 13.12, and asks the patient to say, "Ninety-nine." Tactile fremitus is evaluated, and the examiner's hand is moved to the corresponding position on the other side. Tactile fremitus on the opposite side is then assessed and compared. By moving the hand from side to side and from top to bottom, the examiner can detect differences in the transmission of the sound to the chest wall. "Ninety-nine"[f] is one of the phrases used in English because it causes good vibratory tones. Alternatively, the patient could be asked to say, "One, two, three," or "Eee." The tactile sensation is enhanced if the patient speaks either louder or deeper. Tactile fremitus should be evaluated in the six locations illustrated in Fig. 13.13.

The other method of evaluating tactile fremitus is to use the fingertips instead of the ulnar side of the hand. The same side-to-side and top-to-bottom positions illustrated in Fig. 13.13 are used. The evaluation of tactile fremitus should be performed with only one of these techniques. The examiner should try both methods initially to determine which one is preferable.

Table 13.5 lists some of the important pathologic causes of changes in tactile fremitus.

Percussion

Percussion refers to tapping on a surface to determine the underlying structure. It is similar to a radar or echo detection system. Tapping on the chest wall creates vibrations transmitted to the underlying tissue, reflected, and picked up by the examiner's tactile and auditory senses. The sound heard and the

[f]Saying "ninety-nine" is derived from the German *neun und neunzig* meaning "99." These German words are very nasal and create a very vibratory sensation. Other languages may use different words or sounds to evaluate tactile fremitus.

TABLE 13.5 Causes of Changes in Tactile Fremitus

Increased Tactile Fremitus
Pneumonia
Decreased Tactile Fremitus
Unilateral
• Pneumothorax
• Pleural effusion
• Bronchial obstruction
• Atelectasis (incomplete expansion of lung tissue)
Bilateral
• Chronic obstructive lung disease
• Chest wall thickening (muscle, fat)

tactile sensation felt depend on the air-tissue ratio. The vibrations initiated by the percussion of the chest enable the examiner to evaluate the lung tissue to a depth of only 5 to 6 cm. Still, percussion is valuable because many changes in the air-tissue ratio are readily apparent.

Percussion over a solid organ, such as the liver, produces a *dull,* low-amplitude, short-duration note without resonance. Percussion over a structure containing air within a tissue, such as a lung, has a *resonant,* higher amplitude, lower pitched note. Percussion over a hollow air-containing structure, such as the stomach or bowel, produces a *tympanic,* high-pitched, hollow-quality note. Finally, percussion over a large muscle mass, such as the thigh, has a *flat,* high-pitched note.

Usually, dullness over the heart and resonance over the lung fields are heard and felt in the chest. As the lungs fill with fluid and become denser, as in pneumonia, resonance is replaced by dullness. The term *hyperresonance* has been applied to the percussion note obtained from a lung with decreased density, such as that found in emphysema. Hyperresonance is a low-pitched, hollow-quality, sustained resonant note bordering on tympany.

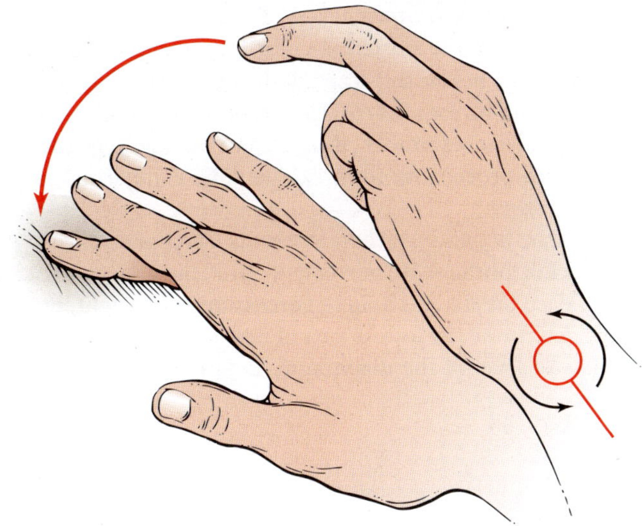

Fig. 13.14 Technique of Percussion.

In percussion of the chest, the examiner places the middle finger of one hand firmly against the patient's chest wall, parallel to the ribs in an interspace, with the palm and other fingers held off the chest. The tip of the right middle finger of the other hand strikes a quick, sharp blow to the terminal phalanx of the left finger on the chest wall. The motion of the striking finger should come from the wrist and not from the elbow. Paddleball players use this motion naturally, whereas tennis players must learn to concentrate on using this wrist motion. The percussion technique is diagrammed in Fig. 13.14 and demonstrated in Fig. 13.15.

Try percussion on yourself. Percuss over your right lung (resonant), stomach (tympanic), liver (dull), and thigh (flat).

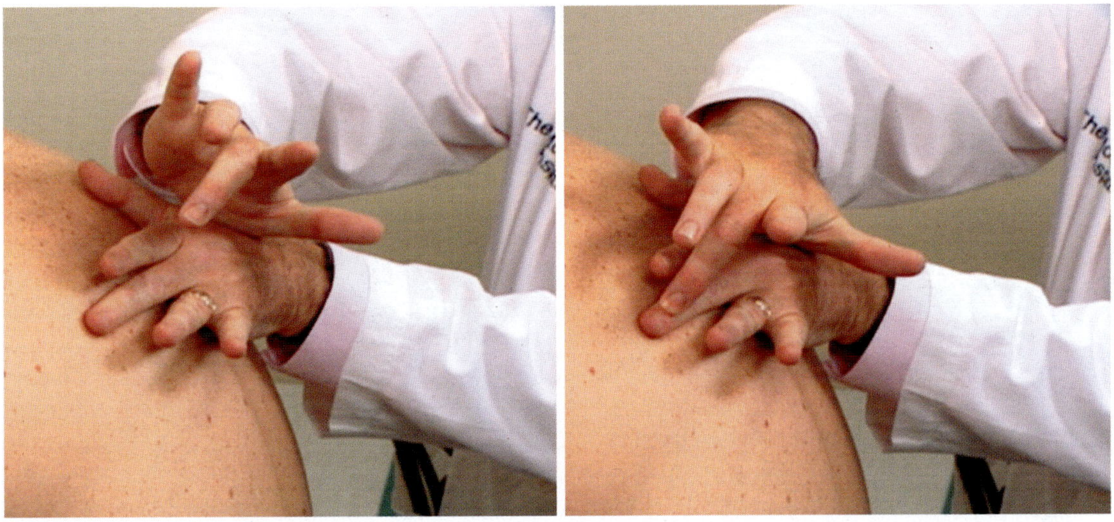

A B

Fig. 13.15 Percussion. (A) Position of the right hand ready to percuss. (B) Location of the fingers after striking. Notice that the motion is from the wrist.

Percuss the posterior chest. See Video 13.5.

The sites on the posterior chest for percussion are above, between, and below the scapulae in the intercostal spaces, as diagrammed in Fig. 13.16. The scapulae themselves are not percussed. The examiner should start at the top and work downward, proceeding from side to side, comparing one side with the other.

Evaluate diaphragmatic movement. Percussion is also used to detect diaphragmatic movement. First, the patient is asked to take a deep breath and hold it. Percussion at the right lung base helps determine the lowest area of resonance, which represents the lowest level of the diaphragm. Below this level is dullness from the liver. The patient is then instructed to exhale as much as possible, and the percussion is repeated. With expiration, the lung contracts, the liver moves up, and the same area becomes dull—the dullness level moves upward. The difference between the inspiration and expiration levels represents diaphragmatic motion, usually 4 to 5 cm. In patients with emphysema, the motion is reduced. In patients with phrenic nerve palsy, diaphragmatic motion is absent. This test is illustrated in Fig. 13.17.

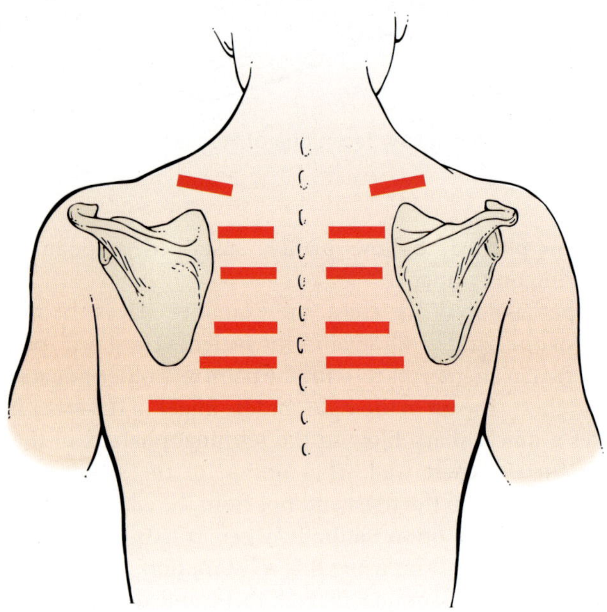

Fig. 13.16 Locations on the Posterior Chest for Percussion and Auscultation.

Auscultation

Auscultation is the technique of listening to sounds produced in the body. Auscultation of the chest is used to identify lung sounds. The stethoscope usually has two heads: the bell and the diaphragm. The bell detects low-pitched sounds, and the diaphragm is better at detecting higher-pitched sounds. The bell must be applied loosely to the skin; if pressed too tightly, the skin acts as a diaphragm, and the lower-pitched sounds are filtered out.

In contrast, the diaphragm is applied firmly to the skin. The bell may be more useful in very cachectic individuals because the protruding ribs in these patients make diaphragm placement difficult. The correct placements of the heads of the stethoscope are demonstrated in Fig. 13.18.

It is *never* acceptable to listen through clothing. The stethoscope's bell or diaphragm must *always* be in contact with the skin.

Types of breath sounds. Breath sounds are heard over most of the lung fields. They consist of an inspiratory phase followed by an expiratory phase. There are four types of normal breath sounds:

- Tracheal
- Bronchial
- Bronchovesicular
- Vesicular

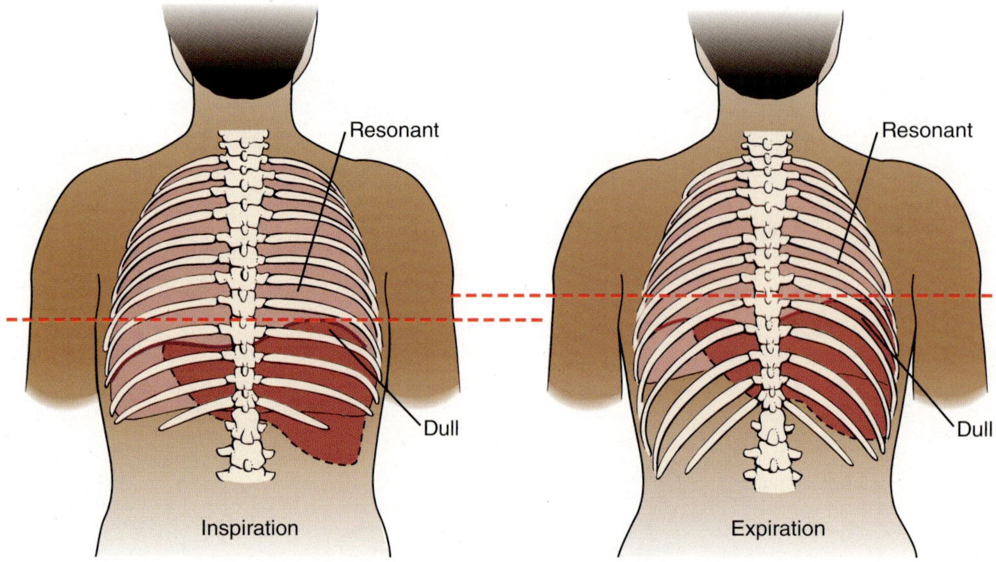

Fig. 13.17 Technique for Evaluating Diaphragmatic Motion. During inspiration *(left)*, percussion in the right seventh posterior interspace at the midscapular line would be resonant due to the presence of the underlying lung. During expiration *(right)*, the liver and diaphragm move up. Percussion in the same area would now be dull, owing to the presence of the underlying liver.

Tracheal breath sounds are harsh, loud, high-pitched sounds heard over the extrathoracic portion of the trachea. The inspiratory and expiratory components are approximately equal in length. Although these sounds are always heard when the examiner listens over the trachea, they are rarely evaluated because they do not represent any clinical lung problems.

Bronchial breath sounds are loud and high-pitched, like air rushing through a tube. The expiratory component is louder and longer than the inspiratory component. These sounds are usually heard when the examiner listens over the manubrium. A definite pause is heard between the two phases.

Bronchovesicular breath sounds are a mixture of bronchial and vesicular sounds. The inspiratory and expiratory components are equal in length. They are normally heard only in the first and second interspaces anteriorly and between the scapulae posteriorly. This is the area overlying the carina and mainstem bronchi.

Vesicular breath sounds are the soft, low-pitched sounds heard over most lung fields. The inspiratory component is much longer than the expiratory component, which is much softer and frequently inaudible.

The four types of breath sounds are illustrated and summarized in Fig. 13.19.

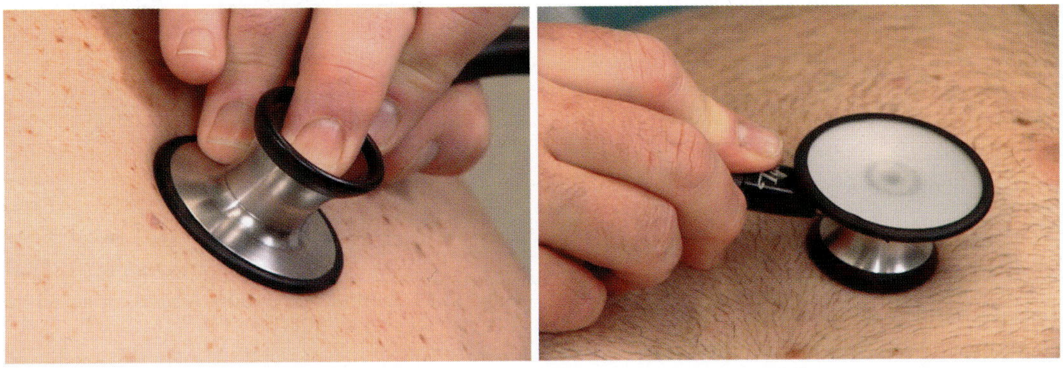

A B

Fig. 13.18 Placement of Stethoscope Heads. (A) Correct placement of the diaphragm. Notice that the head is applied tightly to the skin. (B) Placement of the bell. Notice that the bell is applied lightly to the skin.

Characteristic	Tracheal	Bronchial	Bronchovesicular	Vesicular
Intensity	Very loud	Loud	Moderate	Soft
Pitch	Very high	High	Moderate	Low
I:E ratio[a]	1:1	1:3	1:1	3:1
Description	Harsh	Tubular	Rustling but tubular	Gentle rustling
Normal locations	Extrathoracic trachea	Manubrium	Over mainstem bronchi	Most of peripheral lung

[a]Ratio of duration of inspiration to that of expiration.

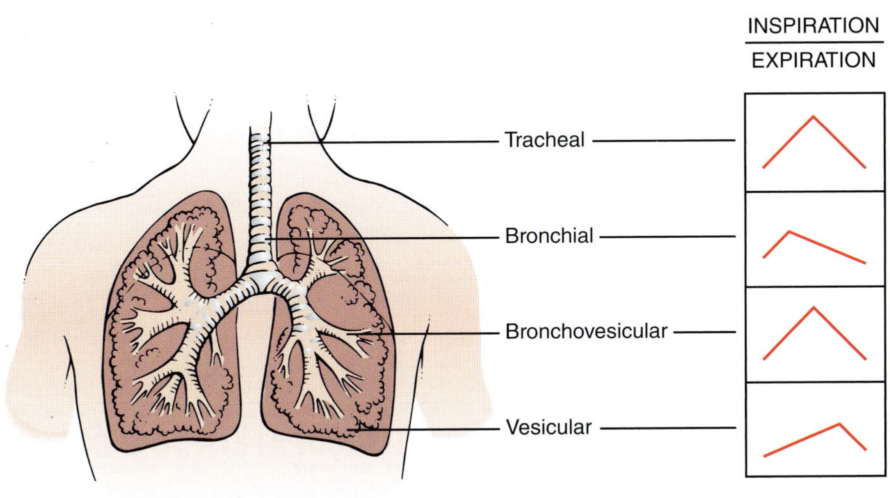

Fig. 13.19 Characteristics of Breath Sounds.

Auscultate the posterior chest. See Video 13.6.

Auscultation should be performed in a quiet environment. The patient is asked to breathe in and out through the mouth. The examiner should concentrate first on the length of inspiration and then on expiration. Very soft breath sounds are referred to as *distant.* Distant breath sounds are commonly found in patients with hyperinflated lungs, as in emphysema.

The examination should proceed from side to side and from top to bottom, comparing one side with the other. The positions are illustrated in Fig. 13.16. Because most breath sounds are high-pitched, the diaphragm is used to evaluate lung sounds.

The Anterior Chest

The examiner should now move in front of the patient. The first part of the examination of the anterior chest is performed with the patient seated, after which the patient is asked to lie down.

Evaluate the Position of the Trachea

See Video 13.7.

The examiner can determine the position of the trachea by placing their right index finger in the patient's suprasternal notch and moving slightly lateral to feel the location of the trachea. The examiner repeats this technique, moving the finger from the suprasternal notch to the other side. The space between the trachea and the clavicle should be equal. A shift of the mediastinum can displace the trachea to one side. This technique is demonstrated in Fig. 13.20.

Look at the patient pictured in Fig. 13.21. Notice that the trachea is markedly displaced to the right in this very cachectic female. The diagnosis of a mass in the left chest pushing the trachea or a mass in the right chest pulling the trachea is strongly suggested.

Now ask the patient to lie on their back for the rest of the examination of the anterior chest. The patient's arms are at the sides. If the patient is a female, either have her elevate her breasts or displace them as necessary during palpation, percussion, and auscultation. These examinations should not be performed over the breast tissue.

Evaluate Tactile Fremitus

See Video 13.8.

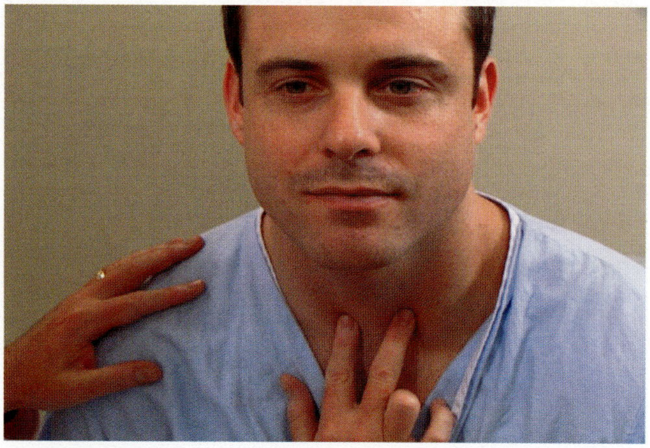

Fig. 13.20 Technique for Determining the Position of the Trachea.

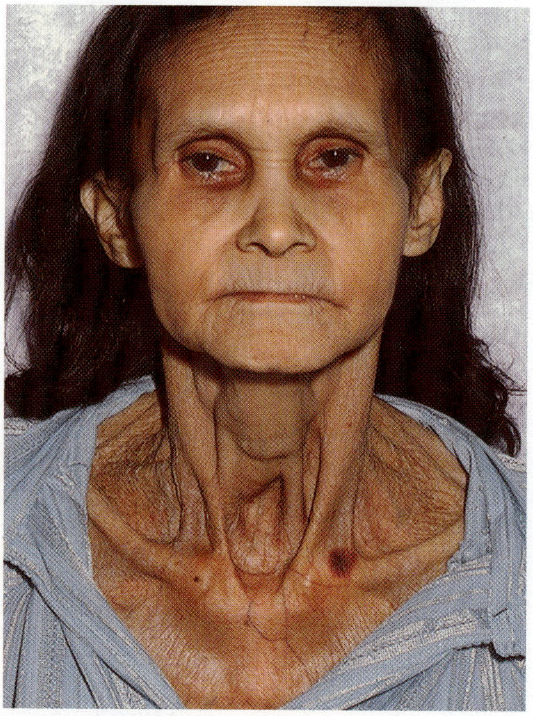

Fig. 13.21 Tracheal Deviation. Note the marked tracheal deviation to the patient's right.

Tactile fremitus is assessed in the supraclavicular fossae and alternate anterior interspaces, beginning at the clavicle. The techniques for evaluating tactile fremitus have already been discussed. Proceed from the supraclavicular fossae downward, comparing one side with the other.

Percuss the Anterior Chest

See Video 13.9.

Percussion of the anterior chest includes the supraclavicular fossae, the axillae, and the anterior interspaces, as illustrated in Fig. 13.22. The percussion note on one side is always compared with that elicited in the corresponding position on the other side. Dullness may be noted in the third to fifth intercostal spaces to the left of the sternum, which is related to the presence of the heart. Percuss high in the axilla because the upper lobes are best evaluated at these positions. Axillary percussion is sometimes easier to perform while the patient is sitting.

Auscultate the Anterior Chest

See Video 13.10.

Auscultation of the anterior chest is performed in the supraclavicular fossae, the axillae, and the anterior chest interspaces, as illustrated in Fig. 13.22. The techniques of auscultation have already been discussed. The breath sounds of one side are compared with the breath sounds heard in the corresponding position on the other side.

CLINICOPATHOLOGIC CORRELATIONS

In addition to the normal breath sounds discussed, other lung sounds may be produced in abnormal clinical states. These

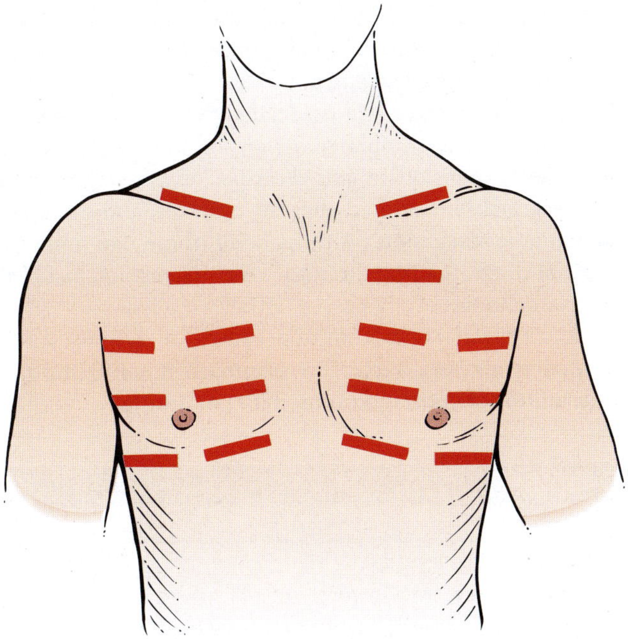

Fig. 13.22 Locations on the Anterior Chest for Percussion and Auscultation.

abnormal sounds heard during auscultation are called *adventitious* sounds. Adventitious sounds include the following:

- Crackles
- Wheezes
- Rhonchi
- Pleural rubs

Crackles are short, discontinuous, nonmusical sounds mainly heard during inspiration. Also known as *rales* or *crepitation,* the opening of collapsed distal airways and alveoli causes crackles—a sudden equalization of pressure results in a crackle. Coarser crackles are related to larger airways. Crackles are likened to the sound of rubbing hair next to the ear or when Velcro patches are pulled apart. They may be described as early or late, depending on when they are heard during inspiration. The timing of common inspiratory crackles is summarized in Table 13.6. The most common causes of crackles are pulmonary edema, congestive heart failure, and pulmonary fibrosis.

Wheezes are continuous, musical, high-pitched sounds mainly heard during expiration. They are produced by airflow through narrowed bronchi. Swelling, secretions, spasms, tumors, or foreign bodies may cause this narrowing. Wheezes are commonly associated with the bronchospasm of asthma.

TABLE 13.6 Timing of Common Inspiratory Crackles

Disease	Early Crackle	Late Crackle
Congestive heart failure	Very common	Common
Obstructive lung disease	Present	Absent
Interstitial fibrosis	Absent	Present
Pneumonia	Absent	Present

Rhonchi are lower-pitched, more sonorous lung sounds. They are believed to be more common with temporary mucous plugging and poor movement of airway secretions.

A *pleural rub* is a grating sound produced by the motion of the pleura, which is impeded by frictional resistance. It is best heard at the end of inspiration and the beginning of expiration. The sound of a pleural rub is like the sound of creaking leather. Pleural rubs are heard when pleural surfaces are roughened or thickened by inflammatory or neoplastic cells or fibrin deposits.

All the adventitious sounds should be described by location, timing, and intensity.

There is much confusion regarding the terminology of adventitious sounds. Table 13.7 summarizes the adventitious sounds.

On occasion, breath sounds are transmitted abnormally. This may result in auscultatory changes known by the following terms:

- Egophony
- Whispered pectoriloquy
- Bronchophony

Egophony (or *egobronchophony*) is said to be present when the spoken word heard through the lungs increases in intensity and takes on a nasal or bleating quality. For example, the patient is asked to say "eeee" while the examiner listens to an area where consolidation is suspected. If egophony is present, the "eeee" will be heard as "aaaah." This "e-to-a" change is seen in consolidation of lung tissue. For example, the area of a compressed lung above a pleural effusion often produces egophony.

Whispered pectoriloquy is the term for intensifying the whispered word heard in the presence of lung consolidation. The patient is instructed to whisper "one-two-three" while the examiner listens to the area suspected of having consolidation.

TABLE 13.7 Adventitious Sounds

Recommended Term	Older Term	Mechanism	Causes
Crackle	Rale Crepitation	Excess airway secretions	Bronchitis, respiratory infections, pulmonary edema, atelectasis, fibrosis, congestive heart failure
Wheeze	Sibilant rale Musical rale Sonorous rale Low-pitched wheeze	Rapid airflow through obstructed airway	Asthma, pulmonary edema, bronchitis, congestive heart failure
Rhonchus		Transient airway plugging	Bronchitis
Pleural rub		Inflammation of the pleura	Pneumonia, pulmonary infarction

Typically, whispering produces high-pitched sounds that tend to be filtered out by the lungs. When the examiner listens to a normal chest, little or nothing may be heard. However, if consolidation is present, the transmission of the spoken words is increased, and the words are heard.

Bronchophony is the increased transmission of spoken words heard in the presence of consolidation of the lungs. For example, the patient is asked to say "ninety-nine" while the examiner listens to the chest. If bronchophony is present, the words are transmitted more loudly than usual.

One of the most important principles concerning the chest examination is correlating the percussion, palpation, and auscultation findings. Dullness, crackles, increased breath sounds, and increased tactile fremitus suggest consolidation. Conversely, dullness, decreased breath sounds, and decreased tactile fremitus suggest a pleural effusion.

Many physical signs are associated with obstructive lung disease. These include impaired breath sounds, barrel chest, decreased chest expansion, impaired cardiac dullness, use of accessory muscles, absent cardiac impulse, cyanosis, and diminished diaphragmatic excursion. Although all these are important physical findings, the first three have the greatest intrinsic value as diagnostic tools.

Table 13.8 lists some common causes of dyspnea and its associated symptoms. Table 13.9 summarizes some important manifestations of common pulmonary conditions.

TABLE 13.8 Common Conditions Associated With Dyspnea

Condition	Dyspnea	Other Symptoms
Asthma	Episodic; symptom-free between attacks	Wheezing, chest pain, productive cough
Pulmonary edema	Abrupt	Tachypnea, cough, orthopnea, and paroxysmal nocturnal dyspnea with chronic state
Pulmonary fibrosis	Progressive	Tachypnea, dry cough
Pneumonia	Exertional, insidious onset	Productive cough, pleuritic pain
Pneumothorax	Sudden, moderate to severe	Sudden pleuritic pain
Emphysema	Insidious onset, severe	Cough as disease progresses
Chronic bronchitis	As disease progresses and with infection	Chronic, productive cough
Obesity	Exertional	

TABLE 13.9 Differentiation of Common Pulmonary Conditions

	FINDINGS				
Condition	**Vital Signs**	**Inspection**	**Palpation**	**Percussion**	**Auscultation**
Asthma[a]	Tachypnea; tachycardia	Dyspnea; use of accessory muscles; possible cyanosis; hyperinflation	Often normal; decreased fremitus	Often normal; hyperresonant; low diaphragm	Prolonged expiration; wheezes; decreased lung sounds
Emphysema	Stable	Increased anteroposterior diameter; use of muscles; thin individual	Decreased tactile fremitus	Increased resonance; decreased excursion of diaphragm	Decreased lung sounds; decreased vocal fremitus
Chronic bronchitis	Tachycardia	Possible cyanosis; patients tend to be short and stocky	Often normal	Often normal	Early crackles; rhonchi
Pneumonia	Tachycardia; fever; tachypnea	Possible cyanosis; possible splinting on affected side	Increased tactile fremitus	Dullness	Late crackles; bronchial breath sounds[b]
Pulmonary embolism	Tachycardia; fever; tachypnea	Often normal	Usually normal	Usually normal	Usually normal
Pulmonary edema	Tachycardia; tachypnea	Possible signs of elevated right-sided heart pressures[c]	Often normal	Often normal	Early crackles; wheezes
Pneumothorax	Tachypnea; tachycardia	Often normal; lag on affected side	Absent fremitus; trachea may be shifted to other side	Hyperresonant	Absent breath sounds
Pleural effusion	Tachypnea; tachycardia	Often normal; lag on affected side	Decreased fremitus; trachea shifted to other side	Dullness	Absent breath sounds
Atelectasis	Tachypnea	Often normal; lag on affected side	Decreased fremitus; trachea shifted to same side	Dullness	Absent breath sounds
Acute respiratory distress syndrome	Tachycardia; tachypnea	Use of accessory muscles; cyanosis	Usually normal	Often normal	Normal initially; crackles and decreased lung sounds, late

[a]The physical findings in asthma are often not reliable in predicting its severity.
[b]Bronchophony, whispered pectoriloquy, and egophony are also often present.
[c]Elevated jugular venous distention, pedal edema, and hepatomegaly.

USEFUL VOCABULARY

Listed here are the specific roots that are important for understanding the terminology related to diseases of the chest.

Root	Pertaining to	Example	Definition
bronch(o)-	bronchus	***bronch***itis	Inflammation of the bronchus
-capnia	carbon dioxide	hyper***capnia***	Excessive carbon dioxide in the blood
chondro-	cartilage	***chondr***oma	Hyperplastic growth of cartilage
costo-	ribs	***costo***chondritis	Inflammation of the rib cartilage
muc(o)-	mucus	***muco***lytic	Agent that dissolves mucus
phren(o)-	diaphragm	***phreno***hepatic	Pertaining to the diaphragm and liver
pleur(o)-	pleura	***pleu***ritic	Pertaining to inflammation of the pleura
-pne(o)-	breath	dys***pnea***	Difficulty in breathing; shortness of breath
pneumo-	lungs	***pneumo***nectomy	Surgical removal of lung tissue
spiro-	to breathe	***spiro***gram	A tracing of respiratory movements
-stern(o)-	sternum	costo***stern***al	Pertaining to the ribs and sternum

WRITING UP THE PHYSICAL EXAMINATION

Listed here are examples of the write-up for the examination of the chest.

- The trachea is midline. The chest is normal in appearance. Palpation is normal. The chest is clear to percussion and auscultation.
- The trachea is midline. A mild pectus excavatum is present. There is increased tactile fremitus at the left posterior chest, up one-third from the base. This area is also dull to percussion. Bronchial breath sounds and crackles are present in the area of dullness. Bronchophony and whispered pectoriloquy are also present in this area.
- The trachea is deviated to the left. The chest structure is within normal limits. There is decreased tactile fremitus on the right chest posteriorly, up three-fourths from the base. The percussion note is dull in the area of decreased fremitus. There are no breath sounds heard in this area. An area of egophony is present above the area of dullness.
- The trachea is midline. Tactile fremitus is normal, as is percussion. Auscultation reveals normal breath sounds with bilateral basilar crackles.

FULL VIDEOS

- Video 13.11 Full video: Examination of the posterior chest
- Video 13.12 Full video: Examination of the anterior chest (heart and lungs, lying)

REVIEW QUESTIONS

1. **Decreased tactile fremitus may be seen in all the following conditions except:**
   A. Pneumothorax
   B. Pleural effusion
   C. Pneumonia
   D. Bronchial obstruction
   E. Chronic obstructive lung disease
2. **Which physical findings support a diagnosis of a pleural effusion (fluid in the chest)?**
   A. **Palpation:** Increased tactile fremitus; **Percussion:** Dullness; **Auscultation:** Bronchial breath sounds
   B. **Palpation:** Normal; **Percussion:** Normal; **Auscultation:** Normal
   C. **Palpation:** Absent tactile fremitus; **Percussion:** Hyperresonant; **Auscultation:** Absent breath sounds
   D. **Palpation:** Decreased tactile fremitus; **Percussion:** Dullness; **Auscultation:** Absent breath sounds
3. **Which physical findings are supportive of a diagnosis of pneumonia (lung consolidation)?**
   A. **Palpation:** Increased tactile fremitus; **Percussion:** Dullness; **Auscultation:** Bronchial breath sounds
   B. **Palpation:** Normal; **Percussion:** Normal; **Auscultation:** Normal
   C. **Palpation:** Absent tactile fremitus; **Percussion:** Hyperresonant; **Auscultation:** Absent breath sounds
   D. **Palpation:** Decreased tactile fremitus; **Percussion:** Dullness; **Auscultation:** Absent breath sounds
4. **Hemoptysis may be seen in all the following diseases/conditions *except*:**
   A. Tuberculosis
   B. Lung cancer
   C. Pulmonary embolism
   D. Chronic smoking (especially e-cigarettes)
   E. Certain cardiac diseases
5. **Regarding positional dyspnea, which of the following statements is *false*?**
   A. Orthopnea can be seen commonly in congestive heart failure.
   B. Trepopnea can be seen commonly in congestive heart failure.
   C. Orthopnea can be seen commonly in neurologic disorders.
   D. Orthopnea can be seen in mitral valvular disease.
   E. Platypnea can be seen in hypovolemia.

6. **Regarding chest configuration, which of the following statements is false?**
   A. The anteroposterior chest diameter in a patient with chronic obstructive lung disease is increased.
   B. A flail chest is seen in a patient with multiple rib fractures.
   C. Although kyphoscoliosis results in abnormal anteroposterior diameter, the condition does not generally restrict pulmonary function.
   D. Patients with pectus excavatum commonly have abnormalities of the mitral valve.
   E. Pectus excavatum may be associated with abnormalities of the mitral valve.
7. **Regarding the descriptors of coughing, which of the following statements is false?**
   A. Dry, hacking cough may be associated with viral infections, tumors, allergies, or anxiety.
   B. Wheezing may be associated with bronchospasm, asthma, or congestive heart failure.
   C. Nocturnal cough may be associated with postnasal drip and congestive heart failure.
   D. Stridor may be associated with chronic smoking and debility.
   E. Neuromuscular disease of the upper esophagus may cause coughing associated with eating or drinking.
8. **Regarding the descriptors of sputum, which of the following statements is true?**
   A. Mucoid sputum is seen in pneumonia and tuberculosis.
   B. Mucopurulent sputum is seen in pulmonary edema.
   C. Pink, frothy sputum is seen in pulmonary embolism and *Klebsiella pneumoniae* infection.
   D. Foul-smelling sputum is seen in bronchiectasis.
   E. Bloody sputum is seen in broncholithiasis.
9. **Which of the following statements about stridor is correct?**
   A. Stridor is a medical emergency.
   B. Stridor is abnormal, low-pitched sound.
   C. Stridor is a specific pulmonary diagnosis.
   D. Stridor is seen in COVID-19.
   E. Inspiratory stridor generally indicates a collapse of tissue at the level of the supraglottis or glottis.
10. **Which statement about clubbing of the nails is correct?**
   A. It can be seen with intrathoracic tumors.
   B. It can be seen with mixed venous-to-arterial shunts.
   C. It can be seen in hepatic fibrosis.
   D. It can be seen in chronic pulmonary disease.
   E. It can be seen in all of these.

REFERENCES

Available online.

BIBLIOGRAPHY

Available online.

14

The Heart

Mark H. Swartz

For it is the heart by whose virtue and pulse the blood is moved, perfected, made apt to nourish and is preserved from corruption and coagulation. … It is indeed the fountain of life, the source of all action.

William Harvey (1578–1657)

VIDEOS

Video 14.1	Blood pressure cuff size selection
Video 14.2	Determining blood pressure by palpation
Video 14.3	Determining blood pressure by auscultation
Video 14.4	Evaluating for orthostatic hypotension
Video 14.5	Evaluating for supravalvular aortic stenosis
Video 14.6	Determining the cardiac rate
Video 14.7	Evaluating the carotid artery pulse
Video 14.8	Evaluating the jugular venous pulse
Video 14.9	Assessing the jugular venous wave form of tricuspid insufficiency. *Courtesy of Xiangya Hospital of Central South University, Changsha, China.*
Video 14.10	Palpating the cardiac point of maximum impulse (PMI)
Video 14.11	Palpating for generalized cardiac motion
Video 14.12	Palpating for cardiac thrills: Patient sitting
Video 14.13	Palpating for cardiac thrills: Patient lying
Video 14.14	Auscultating the heart
Video 14.15	Auscultating the heart: Using bell
Video 14.16	Full video: Examining the carotid artery and jugular venous pulses
Video 14.17	Full video: Examining the heart and lungs (sitting)
Video 14.18	Full video: Assessing blood pressure
Also see	
Video 13.12	Full video: Examination of the heart and lungs (lying)
Also see	
A.1	Aortic regurgitation
A.2	Aortic regurgitation and systolic flow murmur
A.3	Aortic stenosis
A.4	Early-systolic ejection sound
A.5	Mid-systolic click
A.6	Mitral regurgitation
A.7	Mitral stenosis and opening snap
A.8	Pericardial friction rub
A.9	S^3 gallop
A.10	S^4 gallop

GENERAL CONSIDERATIONS

The heart does not rest for more than a fraction of a second. During a lifetime, it contracts more than 4 billion times. To support this active state, the coronary arteries supply more than 10 million liters of blood to the myocardium and more than 200 million liters to the systemic circulation. Cardiac output can vary under physiologic conditions from 3 to 30 L/min, and regional blood flow can vary by 200%. This wide range occurs without any loss of efficiency in the normal state.

Diseases of the heart are common. The major disease categories are coronary heart disease (CHD), hypertension, rheumatic heart disease (RHD), bacterial endocarditis, and congenital heart disease. The clinical consequences of these conditions are usually severe.

During the past 50 years, significant advances have been made in preventing, diagnosing, and treating cardiovascular, lung, and blood diseases. Death rates from cardiovascular diseases (CVDs) have fortunately declined significantly, and Americans live longer healthier lives. Despite the tremendous progress that has been made, morbidity and mortality from cardiovascular, lung, and blood diseases continue to impose a significant burden on patients, their families, and the national healthcare system. The economic cost to the nation is substantial.

Nearly 83 million Americans have one or more forms of CVD. Although the death rates have declined, CVD is still the leading cause of death for males, females, and people of most racial and ethnic groups in the United States. Here are the facts about the medical and financial burden of heart disease in the United States:

- About 695,000 people died of heart disease in the United States in 2021: that's 1 in every 5 deaths.[1]
- Every 33 seconds, someone in the United States dies from CVD.[1]
- Every year, about 735,000 Americans have a heart attack. Of these, 525,000 are a first heart attack, and 210,000 occur in people who have already had a heart attack.
- Heart disease is the leading cause of death for both males and females. More than half the deaths resulting from heart disease are in males.
- In the United States, someone has a heart attack every 40 seconds.[2]
- One-half of the victims of sudden cardiac death are younger than 65.

- An estimated 90 million Americans have one or more types of heart disease.
- Approximately 9.3 million Americans have chest pain (angina).
- CHD costs the United States about $239.9 billion annually from 2018 to 2019. This includes the cost of healthcare services, medications, and lost productivity due to death.[2]

The key risk factors include high blood pressure (BP), high levels of low-density lipoprotein (LDL) cholesterol, and smoking. Approximately half of Americans (49%) have at least one of these risk factors. Several other medical conditions and lifestyle choices can also put people at a higher risk for heart disease, including:

- Diabetes
- Overweight and obesity
- Poor diet
- Physical inactivity
- Excessive alcohol use

CHD (43.8%) is the leading cause of death attributable to CVD in the United States, followed by stroke (16.8%), high BP (9.4%), heart failure (HF) (9.0%), and other CVDs (17.9%). By 2035, more than 130 million adults in the United States population (45.1%) are projected to have some form of CVD, and the total costs of CVD are expected to reach $1.1 trillion in 2035. Stroke prevalence in adults is 2.7% in the United States. The impact of hypertension management on stroke risk is evident, with a more significant risk reduction among those with more intense treatment.

The development of CHD appears to start early in life. Autopsy studies during the Korean War showed that 40% of all American soldiers killed in their early 20s already had atheromatous involvement in one or more of their coronary arteries.

CHD is also the leading cause of mortality in females in the United States. Here are the facts:

- Females account for about half of the total heart disease deaths in the United States each year, although many females continue to think of heart disease as a male's disease.
- CVD and stroke cause 1 in 3 deaths yearly, killing approximately one female every 80 seconds.
- Worldwide, 9.2 million females die from heart disease each year, accounting for one-third of all deaths in females.
- Of females with heart attacks, 42% die within 1 year, compared with 24% of males.
- Females' heart attacks experienced at younger than age 50 are twice as likely as males' to be fatal.
- An estimated 60 million females (44%) in the United States live with some form of heart disease.
- In the United States in 2021, 310,661 females died of heart disease.[1]
- In the United States, 267,000 females die each year from heart attacks: *six times more* than the number of females who die from breast cancer.
- Almost two-thirds (64%) of females who die suddenly of CHD have no previous symptoms.[3]

Unlike other forms of cardiac disease, CHD may be severe and life-threatening despite normal results on physical examination, electrocardiography, and chest radiography. The good news, however, is that from 1994 to 2004, the death rate from CHD declined by 33%, perhaps because of better control of hypertension, better cholesterol management, and cigarette smoking cessation.

Systemic arterial hypertension affects approximately 20% of the American population. It is a significant risk factor for coronary artery disease and a prime cause of congestive HF and strokes. It has been well established that there is a greater incidence of morbidity and mortality among patients with higher systolic or diastolic pressures.

Since the implementation of antibiotic therapy, the incidence of RHD has been decreasing in more affluent countries. RHD is the most commonly acquired heart disease in young people under 25. The global burden of disease caused by rheumatic fever and RHD currently falls disproportionately on children and young adults, often living in the poorest and most vulnerable countries, responsible for approximately 320,000 deaths annually. Some of the highest rates of acute renal failure (ARF) and RHD in the world are found in indigenous Australians (particularly across central and northern Australia), Maori, and Pacific Island populations.[4] The Pacific region, including Fiji, has the highest reported prevalence of RHD. The prevalence of RHD is also high in sub-Saharan Africa, Latin America, the Indian subcontinent, the Middle East, and Northern Africa. Indigenous people are up to eight times more likely than other groups to be hospitalized and nearly 20 times as likely to die from this disease. At least 33 million people are affected by RHD, with a significant number requiring repeated hospitalization and often unaffordable heart surgery in the following 5 to 20 years. Up to 1% of all schoolchildren in Africa, Asia, the Eastern Mediterranean region, and Latin America show signs of the disease.

Bacterial endocarditis remains a significant medical problem despite the wide use of antibiotics. The increasing number of cases is related to intravenous street drugs. Endocarditis is often not suspected in a patient until serious sequelae develop. In addition to causing valvular damage, persistent bacteremia can spread to the brain, myocardium, spleen, kidneys, and other sites in the body.

The incidence of congenital heart disease averages 5 per 1000 live births. If other commonly found congenital cardiovascular conditions, such as bicuspid aortic valve and mitral valve prolapse, are included, the incidence approaches 1 per 100 live births.

The *metabolic syndrome*, also known as *insulin resistance syndrome*, is a combination of medical risk factors that increases the risk of developing CVD, stroke, and type 2 diabetes (see Chapter 7, Assessment of Nutritional Status). According to the American Heart Association and the National Heart, Lung, and Blood Institute, five risk factors comprise metabolic syndrome. They are increased BP, a high blood sugar level, excess body fat around the waist (central obesity), and abnormal cholesterol and triglyceride levels. The metabolic syndrome is present if a patient has three or more of the following signs:

- BP equal to, or greater than, 130/85 mm Hg
- Fasting blood sugar equal to, or higher than, 100 mg/dL
- Large waist circumference (length around the waist):[a]
    - Males: 40 inches or more (102 cm or more)
    - Females: 35 inches or more (88 cm or more)

[a]For Asian Americans, the cutoff values are 35 inches (equal or greater than 90 cm) in males or 32 inches (equal or greater than 80 cm) in females.

- Low high-density lipoprotein cholesterol:
  - Males: less than 40 mg/dL
  - Females: less than 50 mg/dL
- Triglycerides equal to, or greater than, 150 mg/dL

According to the American Heart Association, 47 million Americans have metabolic syndrome. The syndrome runs in families and is more common among African Americans, Hispanics, Asians, and Native Americans. The risk of developing metabolic syndrome increases as one ages. There are more than 3 million cases in the United States annually; more than a third of all adults meet the definition and criteria for metabolic syndrome.

It is clear that the magnitude of cardiac disease is enormous, and the cost of morbidity and mortality is directly proportional.

STRUCTURE AND PHYSIOLOGY

The principal function of the cardiovascular system is to deliver nutrients to and remove metabolites from every cell in the body. A high-pressure delivery system, an area of exchange, and a low-pressure return system produce this metabolic exchange system. The high-pressure delivery system is on the *left* side of the heart and *arteries,* and the low-pressure return system includes the *veins* and the *right* side of the heart. The circulation of blood through the heart is illustrated in Fig. 14.1.

A thin pericardial sac envelops the heart. The bottom of this sac adheres to the diaphragm, and the top is loosely attached to the upper portion of the sternum. The *visceral* pericardium is the epicardial, or outermost, layer of heart cells. The *parietal* pericardium is the outer sac. Between these two surfaces, a small amount of pericardial fluid in the pericardial sac provides a lubricating interface for the constantly moving heart. The parietal pericardium is innervated by the phrenic nerve, which contains pain fibers. The visceral pericardium is insensitive to pain.

The synchronous contraction of the heart results from the conduction of impulses generated by the *sinoatrial (SA) node* and propagated through the *conduction system.* The SA node is located at the juncture of the superior vena cava and the right atrium. The SA impulse spreads from its point of origin concentrically. When the impulse reaches the *atrioventricular (AV) node* in the interatrial septum near the entrance of the coronary sinus, the impulse is slowed. It is then transmitted to the specialized conducting tissue known as the *right* and *left bundle branches,* which conduct the impulse to the specialized conducting pathways in the ventricles, *Purkinje fibers.* The impulse spreads from the endocardial to the epicardial surface of the heart. These conducting pathways are illustrated in Fig. 14.2.

The heart is innervated extensively by branches of the autonomic nervous system. Both sympathetic and parasympathetic fibers are present in the SA and AV nodes. Both types of fibers also innervate the atrial muscle. The ventricular musculature is innervated predominantly by the sympathetic nervous system.

The *parasympathetic fibers* travel along the vagus or tenth cranial nerve. The *sympathetic* fibers descend in the spinal cord to the level of T1 to T5, where they emerge through the ventral roots to form a synapse in the thoracic and cervical *sympathetic ganglia.* The postganglionic fibers travel through the cervical *cardiac nerves* to join the parasympathetic fibers in forming the *cardiac plexus,* located near the aortic arch and the tracheal bifurcation. These neural pathways are illustrated in Fig. 14.3.

Sympathetic stimulation by *norepinephrine* produces marked increases in heart rate and contractility. Parasympathetic

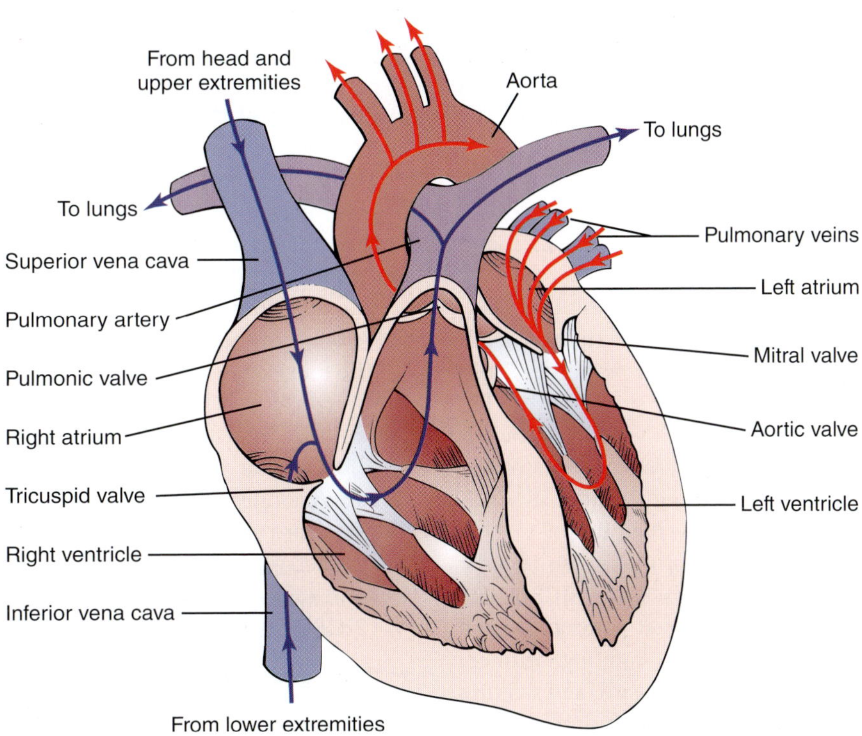

Fig. 14.1 Circulation of Blood Through the Heart.

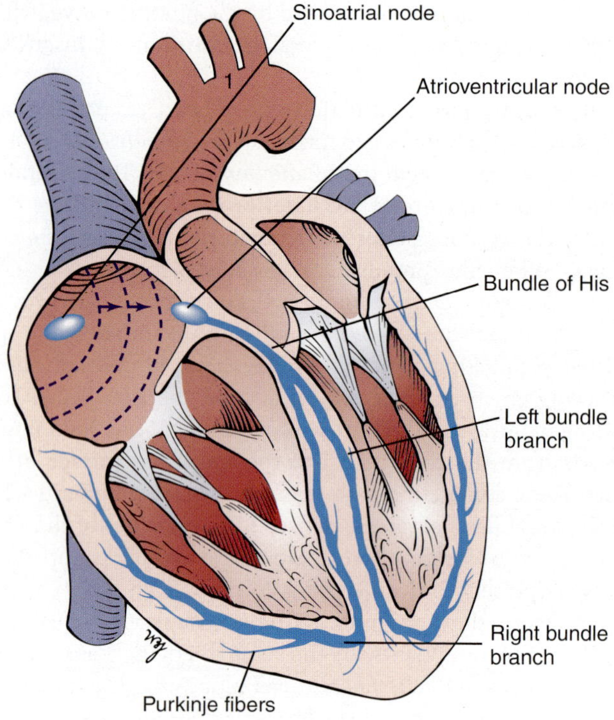

Fig. 14.2 Conducting Pathways of the Heart.

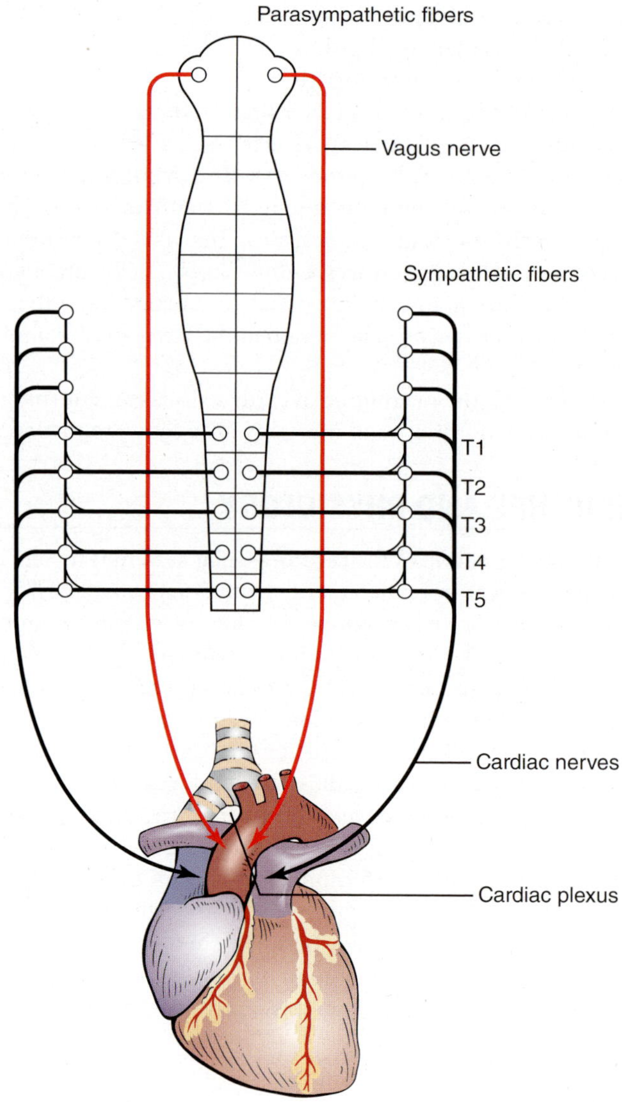

Fig. 14.3 Autonomic Neural Pathways of the Heart.

stimulation mediated by *acetylcholine* slows the heart rate and decreases contractility.

In addition, several receptor sites provide circulatory information to the *medullary cardiovascular center* in the brain. This center has cardioexcitatory and cardioinhibitory areas that regulate the neural output to the sympathetic and parasympathetic fibers. *Stretch receptors* in the aortic arch and the carotid sinus monitor BP. These *baroreceptors* respond to a decrease in BP by decreasing their impulses to the medullary center. The center senses this reduced activity, increases its sympathetic efferent activity, and decreases parasympathetic efferent activity. The net result is to increase the heart rate and contractility. An increase in BP causes an increase in afferent activity to the center, and the opposite changes occur.

To describe physical signs, the examiner must be able to identify the important chest surface topographic landmarks. Chapter 13, The Chest, describes these major areas (see Figs. 13.1, 13.3, and 13.4). These areas should be reviewed at this time.

The surface projection of the heart and great vessels is illustrated in Fig. 14.4. Most of the anterior cardiac surface is the right ventricle. The right atrium forms a narrow border from the third to the fifth ribs to the right of the sternum. The left ventricle lies to the left and behind the right ventricle. The left ventricular *apex* usually is in the *fifth intercostal space* at the *midclavicular line*. This location is commonly written as *5ICS-MCL* (fifth intercostal space at the midclavicular line).

The *apical impulse* is called the *point of maximum impulse* (PMI) or *apex beat* and is located generally at the 5ICS-MCL. This is where the cardiac impulse can be best palpated on the chest wall. The PMI results from the heart rotating counterclockwise (as viewed from below), moving forward, and striking against the chest wall during systole. Lateral and/or inferior displacement of the PMI usually indicates enlargement of the heart. The character of the apex beat may also provide information about cardiac function. For example, an overly forceful impulse may indicate a volume overload in the heart, and an uncoordinated, multiple tap PMI may indicate asynergy[b] of areas of the heart that can occur following a myocardial infarction.

The other heart chambers and vessels are usually not identifiable on examination.

The four classic *auscultatory areas* correspond to points over the precordium, where events originating at each valve are best heard. The areas are not necessarily related to the anatomic position of the valve, nor are all sounds heard in the area directly produced by the valve for which the area is named. The standard areas are as follows:

Aortic: Second intercostal space, right sternal border (2ICS-RSB)

Pulmonic: Second intercostal space, left sternal border (2ICS-LSB)

[b]Defective coordination of areas of the heart that normally act in unison as can result from a ventricular aneurysm.

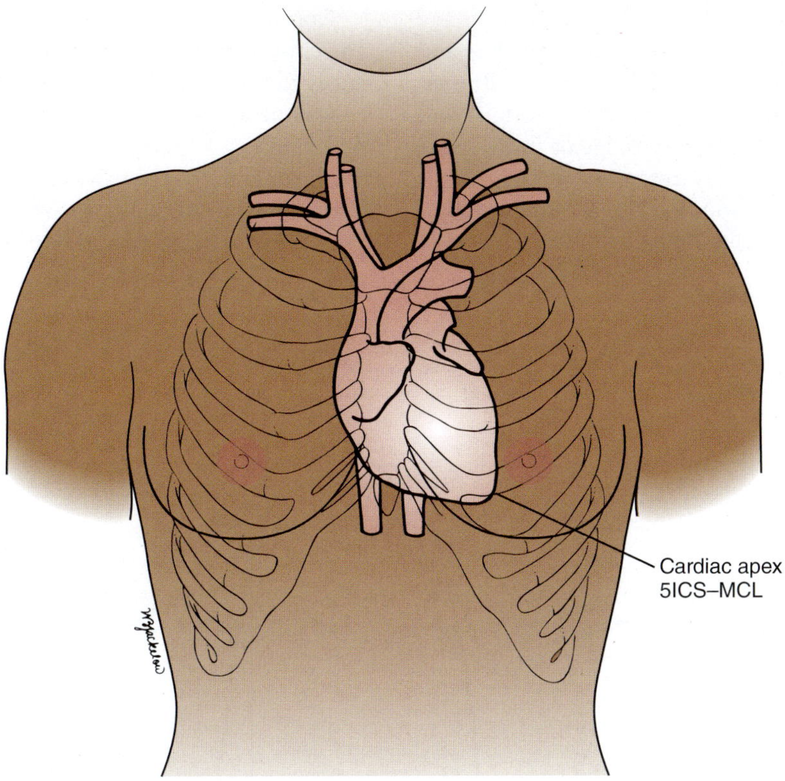

Fig. 14.4 Surface Topography of the Heart. *5ICS-MCL,* Fifth intercostal space at the midclavicular line.

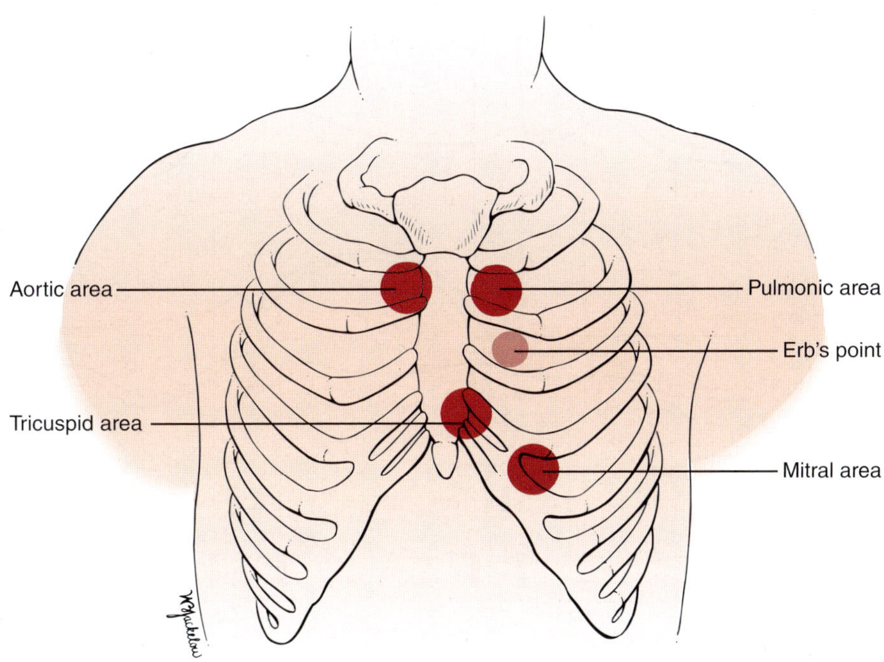

Fig. 14.5 Auscultatory Areas.

Tricuspid: Left lower sternal border (LLSB)
Mitral: Cardiac apex (5ICS-MCL)

In addition to these four areas, the third left intercostal space, known as *Erb's point,* is frequently where pulmonic or aortic sounds are best heard. The five areas are illustrated in Fig. 14.5. The second intercostal space to the right and left of the sternum is called the *base.*

Remember that the left atrium is the most posterior portion of the heart. When the left atrium enlarges, it extends posteriorly and to the right.

The Cardiac Cycle

To understand the cardiac cycle, the motion of the valves and the pressures within the chambers should be reviewed. The interrelationships of valve motion are critically important and must be understood. Only with the knowledge of these cycles can the healthcare professional fully comprehend the cardiac physical examination and heart sounds. The pressure tracings and valve motions are shown in Fig. 14.6.

Normally, only the closing of the heart valves can be heard. The closure of the *AV valves,* the tricuspid and the mitral, produces the *first heart sound* (S_1). The closure of the *semilunar valves,* the aortic and the pulmonic, produces the *second heart sound* (S_2).

The opening of the valves can be heard only if they are damaged. When an AV valve is narrowed or *stenotic,* the opening of the valve may be heard and is termed an *opening snap* (OS). If a

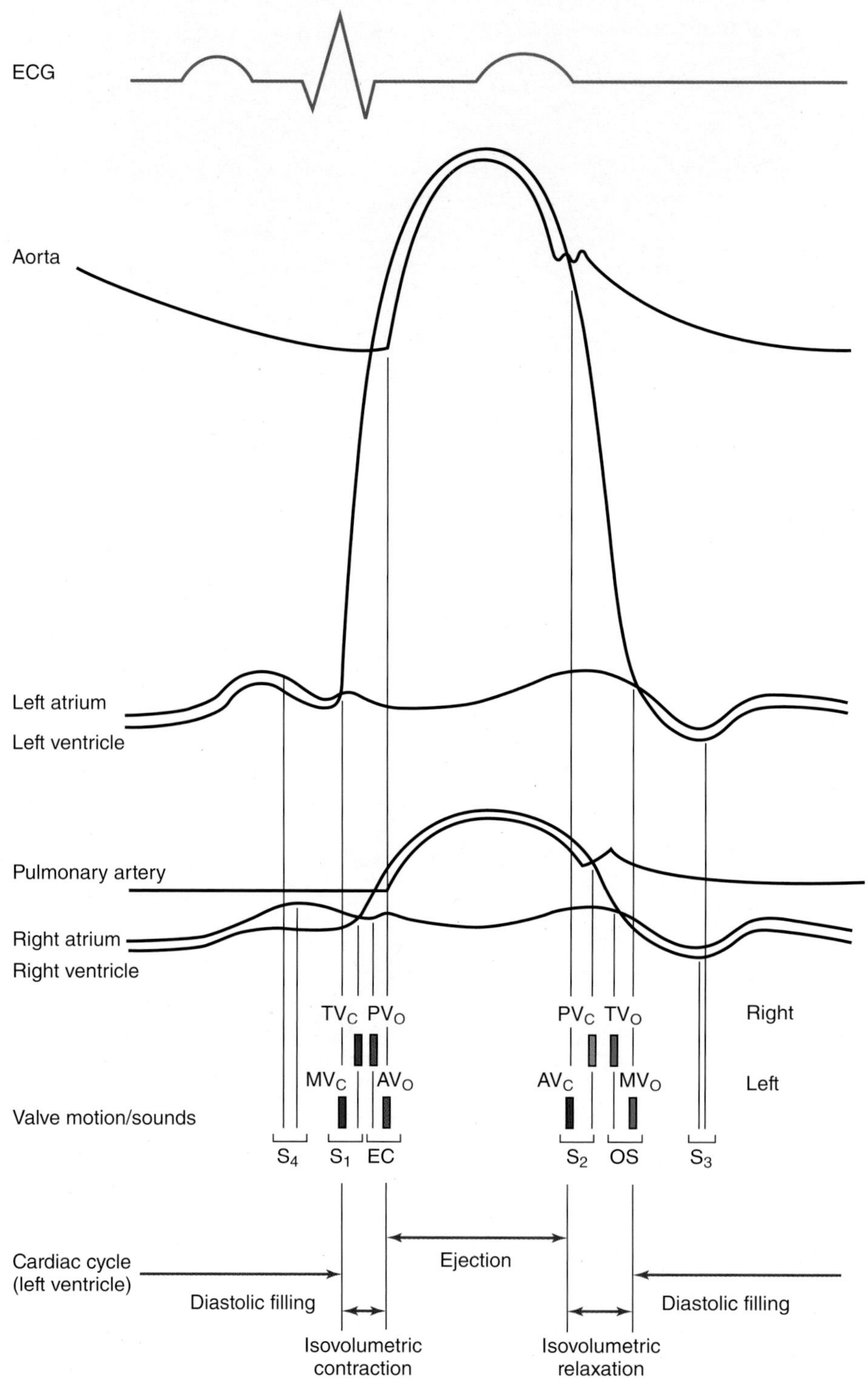

Fig. 14.6 The Cardiac Cycle. *AV_o,* Aortic valve opening; *EC,* ejection click; *ECG,* electrocardiogram; *MV_c,* mitral valve closing; *OS,* opening snap; *PV_o,* pulmonic valve opening; *S_1 to S_4,* first to fourth heart sounds; *TV_c,* tricuspid valve closing.

semilunar valve is stenotic, the opening may be heard and is called an *ejection click* (EC). It should be noted that in Fig. 14.6, the term *opening snap* refers to the opening of a pathologically damaged AV valve that occurs during *diastole,* and the term *ejection click* refers to the opening of a damaged semilunar valve that occurs during *systole.*

The sequence of the opening and closing of the four valves is as follows:

$$MV_c \quad TV_c \quad PV_o \quad AV_o \quad AV_c \quad PV_c \quad TV_o \quad MV_o$$

in which MV = mitral valve, TV = tricuspid valve, PV = pulmonic valve, AV = aortic valve, c = closing, and o = opening.

The mitral component of S_1 occurs as a result of the closure of the mitral valve when the left ventricular pressure rises to more than the left atrial pressure; it is written M_1. The tricuspid component of S_1 occurs due to closure of the tricuspid valve when right ventricular pressure rises to more than right atrial pressure; it is written T_1.

The period of isovolumetric contraction is the time between the AV valves' closure and the semilunar valves' opening. The pulmonic valve opens when the right ventricle's pressure exceeds the pulmonary artery's diastolic pressure. A pulmonic EC is heard at this time if the pulmonic valve is stenotic. When the pressure in the left ventricle exceeds the diastolic pressure in the aorta, the aortic valve opens. An aortic EC is heard at this time if the aortic valve is stenotic.

The systolic ejection period is between the semilunar valves' opening and closing. The point at which ejection is completed and the aortic and left ventricular curves separate is called the *incisura,* or *dicrotic notch,* and is simultaneous with the aortic component of S_2, or closure of the aortic valve; this is written A_2. The pulmonic valve closes at the point when the right ventricular pressure falls to less than the pulmonary diastolic pressure. This is the pulmonic component of S_2 and is commonly written P_2.

The time between the closure of the semilunar valves and the opening of the AV valves is called *isovolumetric relaxation.* The tricuspid valve opens when the pressure in the right atrium exceeds right ventricular pressure. A tricuspid OS may be heard if the tricuspid valve is stenotic. The mitral valve opens when the pressure in the left atrium exceeds left ventricular pressure. A mitral OS may occur at this time if the mitral valve is stenotic.

With the opening of the AV valves, the period of rapid filling of the ventricles occurs. Approximately 80% of ventricular filling occurs at this point. A third heart sound (S3) may be heard at the end of the rapid filling period. An S_3 occurs 120 to 170 ms after S_2. This period is approximately the same time it takes to say "Me too." The "me" is the S_2, and the "too" is the S_3. An S_3 is common in children and young adults. When present in individuals older than 30 years, it may signify a volume overload to the ventricle. Regurgitant valvular lesions and congestive heart failure (CHF) may be responsible.

At the end of diastole, *atrial contraction* and the additional 10% to 20% of ventricular filling occurs. A *fourth heart sound* (S_4) may be heard. The interval from the S_4 to the S_1 is approximately the time it takes to say "middle." The "mid-" is the S_4, and the "-dle" is the S_1. Note that the "mid" is much softer than the "dle," similar to the S_4 to S_1 cadence. An S_4 is commonly heard in children and young adults. When present in individuals older than 30 years, it generally indicates a *non-compliant* or "stiff" ventricle. Pressure overload on a ventricle causes concentric hypertrophy, which produces a noncompliant ventricle. In addition, CHD is a major cause of a stiff ventricle.

Two helpful mnemonics for remembering the cadence and pathophysiologic characteristics of the third and fourth heart sounds are as follows:

SLOSH' – ing – in	SLOSH' – ing – in	SLOSH' – ing – in
S_1 $\quad$ S_2 $\quad$ S_3	S_1 $\quad$ S_2 $\quad$ S_3	S_1 $\quad$ S_2 $\quad$ S_3
a – STIFF' – wall	a – STIFF' – wall	a – STIFF' – wall
S_4 $\quad$ S_1 $\quad$ S_2	S_4 $\quad$ S_1 $\quad$ S_2	S_4 $\quad$ S_1 $\quad$ S_2

The presence of an S_3 or an S_4 creates a cadence resembling the gallop of a horse. These sounds are therefore called *gallop* sounds or rhythms.

The first heart sound is loudest at the cardiac apex. *Splitting* of the first heart sound may be heard in the tricuspid area. The second heart sound is loudest at the base.

The terms A_2 and P_2 indicate the aortic and pulmonic components of S_2, respectively. A_2 normally precedes P_2, meaning the aortic valve closes before the pulmonic valve. With inspiration, the intrathoracic pressure lowers. This causes more blood to be drawn from the superior and inferior venae cavae into the right chambers of the heart. The right ventricle enlarges, and it takes longer for all the blood to be ejected into the pulmonary artery; thus, the pulmonic valve stays open longer. P_2 occurs later in inspiration, and the split between A_2 and P_2 is widened during inspiration compared to expiration. This is the cause of *physiologic splitting* of S_2, which is diagrammed in Fig. 14.7.

The blood in the right ventricle is then pumped into the large-capacitance bed of the lungs. Therefore, the blood return from the lungs to the left side of the heart decreases, and the left atrium and left ventricle become smaller. Atrial receptors trigger a reflex tachycardia that compensates for the decreased left ventricular volume. This increase in heart rate with inspiration is termed *sinus arrhythmia.* It is a misnomer because it is not an arrhythmia but a normal physiologic response to a decreased left ventricular volume during inspiration.

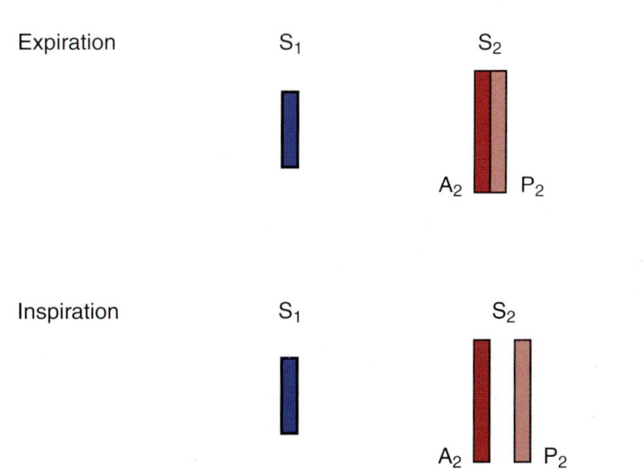

Fig. 14.7 Physiologic Splitting of the Second Heart Sound.

The Arterial Pulse

The arterial pulse is produced by the ejection of blood into the aorta. The normal configuration of the pulse consists of a smooth and rapid upstroke that begins approximately 80 ms after the first component of S_1. There is sometimes a slight notch in the arterial pulsation toward the end of the rapid ejection period. This is called the *anacrotic notch.* The peak of the pulse is smooth and dome-shaped and occurs approximately 100 ms after the onset of the pulse. The descent from the peak is less steep. There is a gradual descent to the dicrotic notch, representing the aortic valve's closure. The contour and volume of the arterial pulse are determined by several factors, including the left ventricular stroke volume, the ejection velocity, the relative compliance and capacity of the arteries, and the pressure waves that result from the antegrade flow of blood. Fig. 14.8 illustrates a characteristic arterial pulse.

As the arterial pulse travels to the periphery, there are several changes. The initial upstroke becomes steeper, the systolic peak is higher, and the anacrotic notch becomes less evident. In addition, the dicrotic notch occurs later in the peripheral pulse, approximately 300 ms after the onset of the pulse. The positive wave that follows the dicrotic notch is called the *dicrotic wave.*

Commonly, two waves may be present in the arterial pulse, which precedes the dicrotic notch. The *percussion wave* is the earlier wave and is associated with the rate of flow in the artery. The percussion wave occurs during the peak velocity of flow. The *tidal wave* is the second wave, is related to pressure in the vessel, and occurs during peak systolic pressure. The tidal wave is usually smaller than the percussion wave, but it may be increased in hypertensive or older patients.

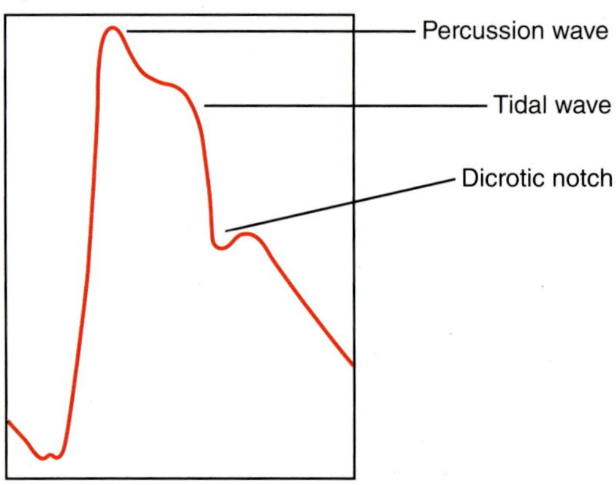

Fig. 14.8 The Arterial Pulse.

Blood Pressure

Arterial BP is the lateral pressure exerted by a column of blood against the arterial wall. It is the result of cardiac output and peripheral vascular resistance. BP depends on the volume of blood ejected, its velocity, the distensibility of the arterial wall, the viscosity of the blood, and the pressure within the vessel after the last ejection.

Systolic BP is the peak pressure in the arteries. The stroke volume and the compliance of the blood vessels regulate it. Diastolic BP is the lowest pressure in the arteries and depends on peripheral resistance. The difference in the systolic and diastolic pressures is the *pulse pressure.* Systolic BP in the legs is 15 to 20 mm Hg greater than in the arms, even while the individual is lying flat. This is in part related to Poiseuille's law, according to which the total resistance of vessels connected in parallel is greater than the resistance of a single large vessel. The BP in the aorta is less than the BP in the branched arteries of the lower extremities.

BP varies significantly according to the patient's excitement, degree of activity, smoking habits, pain, bladder distention, and dietary pattern. There is usually an inspiratory decline of up to 10 mm Hg in systolic BP during quiet respiration.

Jugular Venous Pulse

The jugular venous pulse provides direct information about the pressures in the right side of the heart because the jugular system is in direct continuity with the right atrium. During diastole, when the tricuspid valve is open, the jugular veins are continuous with the right ventricle as well. If there is no stenotic lesion at the pulmonic or mitral valves, the right ventricle indirectly monitors the pressures in the left atrium and left ventricle. The most common cause of *right*-sided CHF is *left*-sided CHF. Examination of the neck veins also provides information about the cardiac rhythm.

Understanding the normal physiologic characteristics is essential in considering jugular venous pulsation. Fig. 14.9 is an enlargement of the atrial and ventricular pressure curves in Fig. 14.6.

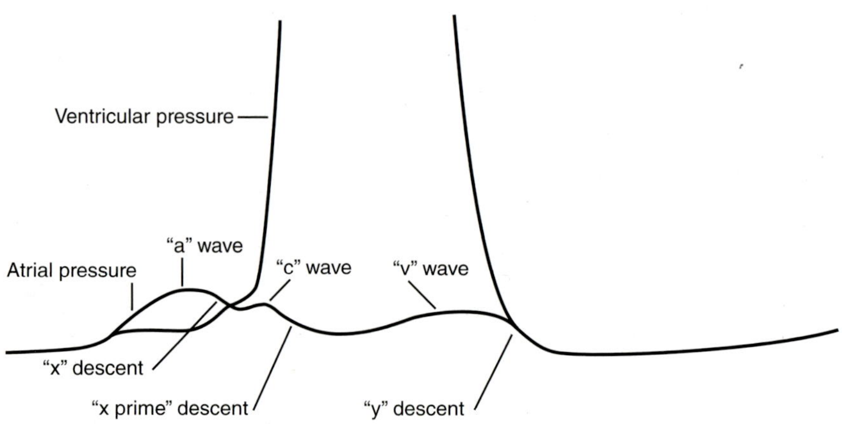

Fig. 14.9 The Atrial and Ventricular Pressure Curves Enlarged.

The *"a" wave* of the jugular venous pulse is produced by right atrial contraction. When the "a" wave is timed with the electrocardiogram, it is found to occur approximately 90 ms after the onset of the P wave. This time delay is related to the time from electrical stimulation of the atria to atrial contraction and to the resultant wave propagated in the neck. The *"x" descent* is caused by atrial relaxation, which occurs just before ventricular contraction. The "c" wave terminates this drop in right atrial pressure. The resulting increase in right atrial pressure is caused by tricuspid valve closure secondary to right ventricular contraction.

The descent of the AV valve rings, also known as the *descent of the base of the heart,* produces the next change in right atrial pressure, called the *"x prime" descent.* As the free wall of the right ventricle approaches the septum during contraction, the AV valve rings descend toward the apex as contraction progresses. This increases the size of the atrium, causing a fall in its pressure (hence the "x prime" descent). During ventricular systole, the right atrium fills with blood returning through the venae cavae. This increase in right atrial pressure due to its filling produces the ascending limb of the *"v" wave.* At the end of ventricular systole, right ventricular pressure falls rapidly. When it falls below the right atrial pressure, the tricuspid valve opens. This drop in right atrial pressure produces the *"y" descent.*

Usually, only the "a" and "v" waves are visible on examination. Because the "c" wave is frequently not observed, the "x" and "x prime" descents are summated into a single "x" descent. Occasionally, the later portion of the "c" wave may be enlarged by a carotid artery pulsation artifact.

Evaluation of the jugular venous pulse provides information about the venous pressure level and the type of venous wave pattern. These are described later in the section "The Jugular Venous Pulse."

REVIEW OF SPECIFIC SYMPTOMS

The important symptoms of cardiac disease are the following:

- Chest pain
- Palpitations
- Dyspnea
- Syncope
- Fatigue
- Dependent edema
- Hemoptysis
- Cyanosis

Chest Pain

Chest pain is the most important symptom of cardiac disease. It is not, however, pathognomonic for heart disease. It is well known that chest pain may result from pulmonary, intestinal, gallbladder, and musculoskeletal disorders. Ask the following questions of any patients complaining of chest pain:

"Where is the pain?"
"How long have you had the pain?"
"Do you have recurrent episodes of pain?"
"What is the duration of the pain?"
"How often do you get the pain?"
"What do you do to make it better?"
"What makes the pain worse? Breathing? Lying flat? Moving your arms or neck?"
"How would you describe the pain?[c] *Burning? Pressing? Crushing? Dull? Aching? Throbbing? Knifelike? Sharp? Constricting? Sticking?"*
"Does the pain occur at rest? With exertion? After eating? When moving your arms? With emotional strain? While sleeping? During sexual intercourse?"
"Is the pain associated with shortness of breath? Palpitations? Nausea or vomiting? Coughing? Fever? Coughing up blood? Leg pain?"

TABLE 14.1 Characteristics of Chest Pain

Feature	Angina	Not Angina
Location	Retrosternal, diffuse	Left inframammary, localized
Radiation	Left arm, jaw, back	Right arm
Description	"Aching," "dull," "pressing," "squeezing," "vise-like"	"Sharp," "shooting," "cutting"
Intensity	Mild to severe	Excruciating
Duration	Minutes	Seconds, hours, days
Precipitated by	Effort, emotion, eating, cold	Respiration, posture, motion
Relieved by	Rest, nitroglycerin	Nonspecific

Angina and other chest pain may manifest in a variety of ways. The characteristics listed here are the common manifestations. This list, however, is not exhaustive and should be used only as a guide.

Angina pectoris is the true symptom of coronary heart disease (CHD). Angina is commonly the consequence of hypoxia of the myocardium resulting from an imbalance of coronary supply and myocardial demand. Table 14.1 lists the characteristics that differentiate angina pectoris from the other types of chest pain.

Patients commonly describe angina by clenching their fist and placing it over the sternum. This is a pathognomonic sign of angina widely referred to as *Levine's sign.* Fig. 14.10 demonstrates this body language.

When chest pain is related to a cardiac cause, coronary atherosclerosis and aortic valvular disease are the most common. Table 14.2 lists some common causes of chest pain.

Sometimes patients may describe pain as "discomfort." Be aware of this situation.

Palpitations

Palpitations are the uncomfortable sensations in the chest associated with a range of arrhythmias. Patients may describe palpitations as "fluttering," "skipped beats," "pounding," "jumping," "stopping," or "irregularity." Determine whether the patient has had similar episodes and what was done to extinguish them. Palpitations are common and do not necessarily indicate serious heart disease. Any condition in which there is an increased stroke volume, as in aortic regurgitation, may be associated with

[c]In general, it is best to allow the patient to describe the character of the pain. These descriptions are provided for the interviewer to use only when the patient is unable to characterize the pain.

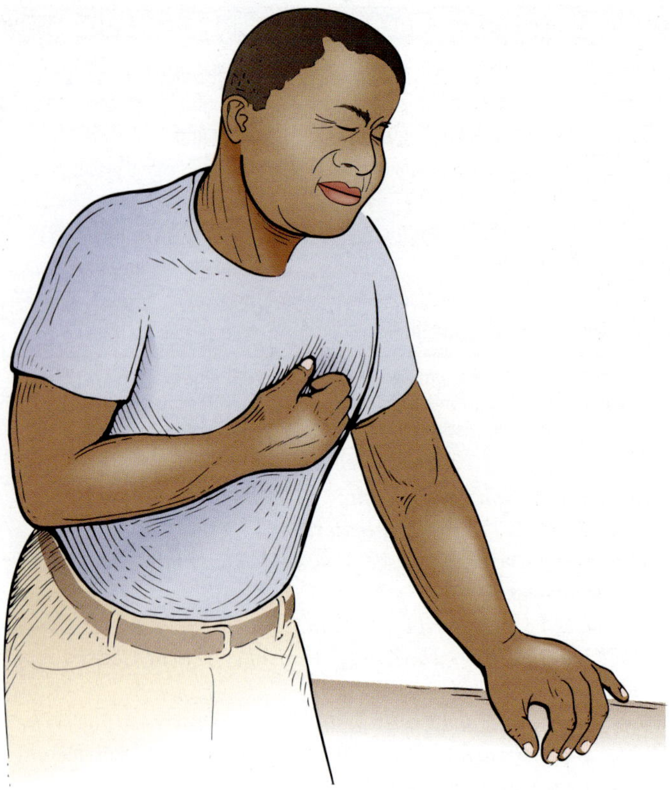

Fig. 14.10 Levine's Sign.

TABLE 14.2 Common Causes of Chest Pain

Organ System	Cause
Cardiac	Coronary artery disease Aortic valvular disease Pulmonary hypertension Mitral valve prolapse Pericarditis Idiopathic hypertrophic subaortic stenosis
Vascular	Dissection of the aorta
Pulmonary	Pulmonary embolism Pneumonia Pleuritis Pneumothorax
Musculoskeletal	Costochondritis[a] Arthritis Muscular spasm Bone tumor
Neural	Herpes zoster[b]
Gastrointestinal	Ulcer disease Bowel disease Hiatal hernia Pancreatitis Cholecystitis
Emotional	Anxiety Depression

[a]Tietze syndrome, which is an inflammation of the costal cartilages.
[b]Shingles, which is a viral invasion of the peripheral nerves in a dermatomal distribution.

a sensation of "forceful contraction." When a patient complains of palpitations, ask the following questions:

"How long have you had palpitations?"
"Do you have recurrent attacks?" If so, *"How frequently do they occur?"*
"When did the current attack begin?"
"How long did it last?"
"What did it feel like?"
"Did any maneuvers or positions stop it?"
"Did it stop abruptly?"
"Could you count your pulse during the attack?"
"Can you tap out on the table what the rhythm was like?"
"Have you noticed palpitations after strenuous exercise? On exertion? While lying on your left side? After a meal? When tired?"
"During the palpitations, have you ever fainted? Had chest pain?"
"Was there an associated flush, headache, or sweating associated with the palpitations?"[d]
"Have you noticed an intolerance to heat? Cold?"
"What kind of medications are you taking?"
"Do you take any medications for your lungs?"
"Are you taking any thyroid medications?"
"Have you ever been told that you had a problem with your thyroid?"
"How much tea, coffee, chocolate, or cola sodas do you consume daily?"
"Do you smoke?" If yes, *"What do you smoke?"*
"Do you drink alcoholic beverages?"
"Did you notice that you had to urinate after the palpitations?"[e]

In addition to primary cardiovascular causes, thyrotoxicosis, hypoglycemia, fever, anemia, pheochromocytoma, and anxiety states are commonly associated with palpitations. Hyperthyroidism is an important cause of rhythm disturbances outside the cardiovascular system. Caffeine, tobacco, and drugs are also important factors in arrhythmogenicity. Sympathomimetic amines used in the treatment of bronchoconstriction are potent stimuli for arrhythmia as well. In patients with panic disorders and other anxiety states, the sensation of palpitations may occur during periods of normal rate and rhythm.

Patients who have had previous attacks of palpitations should be asked the following:

"How was your previous attack terminated?"
"How often do you get the attacks?"
"Are you able to terminate them?" If so, *"How?"*
"Have you ever been told that you have Wolff-Parkinson-White syndrome or WPW?"[f]

Table 14.3 outlines the common causes of palpitations.

[d]Symptoms associated with a pheochromocytoma.

[e]After an attack of paroxysmal atrial tachycardia, patients often have an urge to urinate. The pathophysiologic process is not well understood, but the association is present.

[f]This technical term is appropriate because a patient with this form of preexcitation may have been told of this condition and may recognize the name. Wolff-Parkinson-White (WPW) syndrome is a congenital abnormality involving an abnormal conductive pathway between the atria and ventricles that bypasses the AV node, which can result in symptomatic and life-threatening arrhythmias.

TABLE 14.3 Common Causes of Palpitations

Extrasystoles	Bradyarrhythmias
Atrial premature beats[a]	Heart block
Nodal premature beats	Sinus arrest
Ventricular premature beats[b]	Drugs
Tachyarrhythmias	Bronchodilators
Paroxysmal supraventricular tachycardia	Digitalis
	Antidepressants
Atrial flutter	Smoking
Atrial fibrillation	Caffeine
Multifocal atrial tachycardia	Thyrotoxicosis
Ventricular tachycardia	

[a]Also known as atrial premature contractions or premature atrial contractions.
[b]Also known as ventricular premature contractions or premature ventricular contractions.

TABLE 14.4 Common Causes of Dyspnea

Organ System or Condition	Cause
Cardiac	Left ventricular failure Mitral stenosis
Pulmonary	Obstructive lung disease Asthma Restrictive lung disease Pulmonary embolism Pulmonary hypertension
Emotional	Anxiety
High-altitude exposure	Decreased oxygen pressure
Anemia	Decreased oxygen-carrying capacity

Dyspnea

The complaint of dyspnea is important. Patients report that they have "shortness of breath" or that they "can't get enough air." Dyspnea is commonly related to cardiac or pulmonary conditions. The questions about dyspnea are discussed in Chapter 13, The Chest. This section further delineates dyspnea as a *cardiac* symptom.

Paroxysmal nocturnal dyspnea (PND)[g] occurs at night or when the patient is supine. This position increases the intrathoracic blood volume, and a weakened heart may be unable to handle this increased load; congestive HF may result. The patient is awakened from sleep, is markedly dyspneic, is often coughing, and may seek relief by running to a window to "get more air." Episodes of PND are relatively specific for CHF.

The symptom of PND is often associated with *orthopnea,* the need for using more pillows to sleep. Ask all patients, "How many pillows do you need to sleep?" "Can you sleep flat without a pillow?" To help quantify the orthopnea, you can state, for example, "Three-pillow orthopnea for the past 4 months."

Dyspnea on exertion (DOE) is usually caused by chronic congestive HF or severe pulmonary disease. Quantify the severity of the dyspnea by asking, "How many level blocks can you walk now?" and "How many level blocks could you walk 6 months ago?" You can now attempt to quantify the dyspnea: for example, "The patient has had one-block DOE for the past 6 months. Before 6 months ago, the patient could walk four blocks without shortness of breath. In addition, during the last 3 months, the patient has noted four-pillow orthopnea."

Two uncommon types of breathlessness are trepopnea and platypnea. *Trepopnea* is a rare form of positional dyspnea in which dyspnea occurs in one lateral decubitus position instead of the other. It results from disease of one lung, one major bronchus, or chronic congestive HF. Patients with trepopnea from lung disease prefer to lie on the opposite side of the diseased lung. Patients with chronic congestive HF prefer to lie mainly on the right side.

Platypnea is breathlessness that occurs in the upright position and is relieved with recumbency. Platypnea was initially described in chronic obstructive pulmonary disease and was attributed to an increased wasted ventilation ratio in the upright position.

Table 14.4 lists the common causes of dyspnea.

[g]Be careful about the use of abbreviations. Although *PND* often abbreviates *paroxysmal nocturnal dyspnea,* the acronym can also indicate *postnasal drip* or *postnasal discharge.*

Syncope

Fainting, or syncope, is the transient loss of consciousness that results from inadequate cerebral perfusion. Ask patients what *they* mean by "fainting" or "dizziness." Syncope may have cardiac or noncardiac causes. When a patient describes fainting, ask the following questions:

"What were you doing just before you fainted?"
"Have you had recurrent fainting spells?" If so, *"How often do you have these attacks?"*
"Was the fainting sudden?"
"Did you lose consciousness?"
"In what position were you when you fainted?"
"Was the fainting preceded by any other symptom? Nausea? Chest pain? Palpitations? Confusion? Numbness? Hunger?"
"Did you have any warning that you were going to faint?"
"Did you have any black, tarry bowel movements after the faint?"

The activity that preceded the syncope is important because some cardiac causes are associated with syncope during exercise (e.g., valvular aortic stenosis, idiopathic hypertrophic subaortic stenosis, and primary pulmonary hypertension). If a patient describes palpitations before the syncope, an arrhythmogenic cause may be present. Arrhythmias or obstructive lesions may reduce cardiac output.

The patient's position just before fainting is important because this information may help determine the cause of the syncope. For example, if a patient faints after rising suddenly from bed in the middle of the night (e.g., to run to answer the telephone), *orthostatic hypotension* may be the cause. Orthostatic hypotension is a common form of postural syncope resulting from a peripheral autonomic limitation. There is a sudden fall in systemic BP resulting from a failure of adaptive reflexes to compensate for an erect posture. Symptoms of orthostatic hypotension include dizziness, blurring of vision, profound weakness, and syncope. Many drugs can cause orthostatic hypotension, leading to intravascular volume or tone changes. Older patients are most prone to orthostatic hypotension. *Micturition syncope* usually occurs in males during straining with nocturnal urination. It may occur after considerable alcohol consumption.

Vasovagal syncope is the most common fainting type and most challenging to manage. It has been estimated that 40% of all syncopal events are vasovagal. Vasovagal syncope occurs during sudden, stressful, or painful experiences, such as receiving bad news, surgical manipulation, trauma, losing blood, or even seeing blood. It is often preceded by pallor, nausea, weakness, blurred vision, lightheadedness, perspiring, yawning, diaphoresis, hyperventilation, epigastric discomfort, or a "sinking feeling." There is a sudden fall in systemic vascular resistance without a compensatory increase in cardiac output due to increased vagotonia. If the patient sits or lies down promptly, frank syncope can be aborted.

Carotid sinus syncope is associated with a hypersensitive carotid sinus and is most common in older adults. Whenever a patient with carotid sinus syncope wears a tight shirt collar or turns the neck in a certain way, there is increased carotid sinus stimulation. This causes a sudden fall in systemic pressure and syncope results. Two types of carotid sinus hypersensitivity exist: a cardioinhibitory (bradycardia) type and a vasodepressor (hypotension without bradycardia) type. *Posttussive syncope* usually occurs in patients with chronic obstructive lung disease. Several mechanisms have been postulated to explain its occurrence. It is generally accepted that coughing increases intrathoracic pressure, decreasing venous return and cardiac output. There may also be a rise in cerebrospinal fluid pressure, with decreased brain perfusion.

There are other suggested questions to ask a patient with syncope that direct attention to a neurologic cause. These are summarized in Chapter 21, The Nervous System. Table 14.5 lists the common causes of syncope.

TABLE 14.5 Common Causes of Syncope

Organic System or Condition	Cause
Cardiac	Decreased cerebral perfusion secondary to cardiac rhythm disturbance Left ventricular output obstruction
Metabolic	Hypoglycemia Hyperventilation Hypoxia
Psychiatric	Hysteria
Neurologic	Epilepsy Cerebrovascular disease
Orthostatic hypotension	Volume depletion Antidepressant medications Antihypertensive medications
Vasovagal	Vasodepression
Micturition	Visceral reflex (vasodepressor)
Cough	Chronic lung disease
Carotid sinus	Vasodepressor response to carotid sinus sensitivity

Fatigue

Fatigue is a common symptom of decreased cardiac output. Patients with CHF and mitral valvular disease frequently complain of fatigue. Fatigue, however, is not specific to cardiac problems. The most common causes of fatigue are anxiety and depression. Other conditions associated with fatigue include anemia and chronic diseases. You must attempt to differentiate organic from psychogenic fatigue. Ask the following questions:

"How long have you been tired?"
"Did the fatigue start suddenly?"
"Do you feel tired all day? In the morning? In the evening?"
"When do you feel least tired?"
"Do you feel more tired at home than at work?"
"Is the fatigue relieved by rest?"

Patients with psychogenic fatigue are tired "all the time." They are often more tired at home than at work but occasionally describe being more tired in the morning. They may feel their best at the *end* of the day when most patients with organic causes feel the worst.

Dependent Edema

Swelling of the legs, a form of *dependent edema,* is a frequent complaint of patients. Ask the following questions:

"When was the swelling first noted?"
"Are both legs swollen equally?"
"Did the swelling appear suddenly?"
"Is the swelling worse at any time of the day?"
"Does it disappear after a night's sleep?"
"Does elevation of your feet reduce the swelling?"
"What kind of medications are you taking?"
"Is there a history of kidney, heart, or liver disease?"
"Do you have shortness of breath?" If so, *"Which came first, the edema or the shortness of breath?"*
"Do you have pain in the legs?"
"Do you have any ulcers on your legs?"

If the patient is a female, ask the following questions:

"Are you taking oral contraceptives?"
"Is the edema associated with menstrual changes?"

The patient with CHF has symmetric edema of the lower extremities that worsens as the day progresses. It is least in the morning after sleeping with the legs elevated. If the patient also complains of dyspnea, it is helpful to determine which symptom came first. In patients with dyspnea and edema secondary to cardiac causes, the dyspnea usually precedes the edema. Bedridden patients may have dependent edema in the sacral area.

Hemoptysis

Hemoptysis is discussed in Chapter 13, The Chest. In addition to the pulmonary causes, mitral stenosis is an important cause of hemoptysis. The rupture of the bronchial veins, which are under high back pressure in mitral stenosis, produces hemoptysis.

Cyanosis

Cyanosis is also discussed in Chapter 13, The Chest. The critical questions regarding cyanosis are indicated in that chapter.

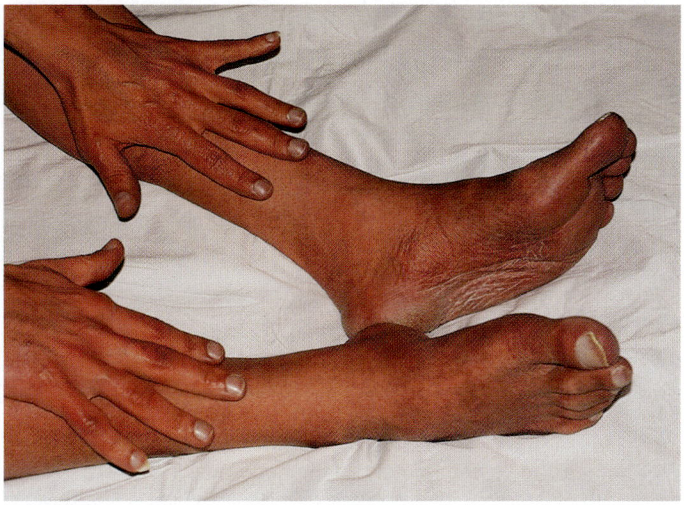

Fig. 14.11 Differential Cyanosis of the Extremities: Patent Ductus Arteriosus.

On occasion, cyanosis is noted only in the lower extremities. This is termed *differential cyanosis.* It is related to a right-to-left shunt through a patent ductus arteriosus (PDA). In a right-to-left shunt resulting from pulmonary hypertension, blood in the pulmonary artery crosses the PDA, which is located below the level of the carotid and left subclavian arteries; deoxygenated blood is pumped only to the lower extremity, producing cyanosis in only that location. Some blood does get to the lungs for oxygenation and is ultimately pumped out through the aorta to have normal skin color in the upper extremity.

The patient whose feet are shown in Fig. 14.11 is a 30-year-old immigrant who was evaluated in the United States for cyanosis. Until the age of 20 years, he had marked "bluish discoloration" of his lower extremities and relatively normal color in his upper extremities. Over the next 10 years, there was a gradual darkening of his upper extremities. Note the marked cyanosis of the extremities and nail beds of the fingers and toes. The patient had a PDA with marked pulmonary hypertension.

EFFECT OF CARDIAC DISEASE ON THE PATIENT

Patients with cardiac disease are intensely fearful. Once cardiac disease has been diagnosed, a series of reactions occur. Fear, depression, and anxiety are the outcomes. The patients, who were asymptomatic until their episode of "sudden death" resulting from coronary occlusion, are scared. They were resuscitated the first time; will an attack happen again? When? During recovery in the hospital, they are afraid to leave the intensive care unit because "no one will be watching." At the time of discharge from the hospital, they are filled with anxiety. Although they desperately want to go home, they ask themselves, "What will happen if I have chest pain at home? Who will provide medical assistance?" They go through a period of depression, recognizing what they have gone through. After convalescence, they fear daily situations that may provoke another attack. Can they go back to the daily "hassles" at work? Is it safe to have sexual intercourse? Despite appropriate reassurances from the healthcare professional, their anxiety level may remain high.

Many patients with cardiac disease who have witnessed a fatal cardiac arrest in another patient in their room refuse to admit how stressful this event was. The patients freely discuss the efficiency of the cardiac arrest team or complain that the noise kept them from sleeping. They refuse to identify with the deceased patient.

The patient with cardiac disease approaching surgery has the same fears as all surgical patients; these fears are discussed in Chapter 2, The Patient's Responses. However, surgical procedures for the patient with cardiac disease involve the "nucleus" of the body. The conscientious healthcare professional takes time to explain the nature of the problem and the surgical approach. Before the procedure, the healthcare professional should allow the patient, especially the family, to visit the intensive care unit where the patient will be for a few days after surgery. Patients should be reassured that everything possible will be done on their behalf. Their courage and determination and the healthcare professional's support are essential.

PHYSICAL EXAMINATION

The equipment for examining the heart is a stethoscope, a sphygmomanometer, a penlight, and an applicator stick.

The physical examination of the heart includes the following:

- Inspection of the patient
- Assessment of BP
- Assessment of the arterial pulse
- Assessment of the jugular venous pulse
- Percussion of the heart
- Palpation of the heart
- Auscultation of the heart
- Examination for dependent edema

The patient should be supine, and the examiner should stand on the right side of the bed. The head of the bed may be elevated slightly if the patient is more comfortable in this position.

Inspection

Evaluate General Appearance

The general inspection of the patient offers clues to cardiac diagnosis. Is the patient in acute distress? What is the patient's breathing like? Is it labored? Are accessory muscles being used?

Inspect the Skin

The skin can reveal many changes associated with cardiac disease. Inspect the skin color. Is cyanosis present? If so, does it appear central or peripheral? Is pallor present?

The *temperature* of the skin may reflect cardiac disease. Severe anemia, beriberi, and thyrotoxicosis tend to make the skin warmer; intermittent claudication is associated with coolness of the lower extremity in comparison with the upper extremity.

Are *xanthomata* present? Tendon xanthomata are stony-hard, slightly yellowish masses commonly found on the extensor tendons of the fingers and are pathognomonic for familial hypercholesterolemia. The soles' Achilles tendon and plantar tendons are common locations for tendon xanthomata. Fig. 14.12 shows tendon xanthomata on the extensor surfaces of a patient's

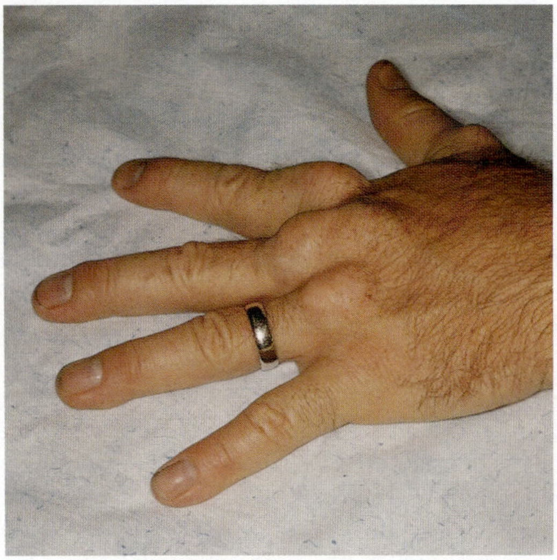

Fig. 14.12 Tendon Xanthomata.

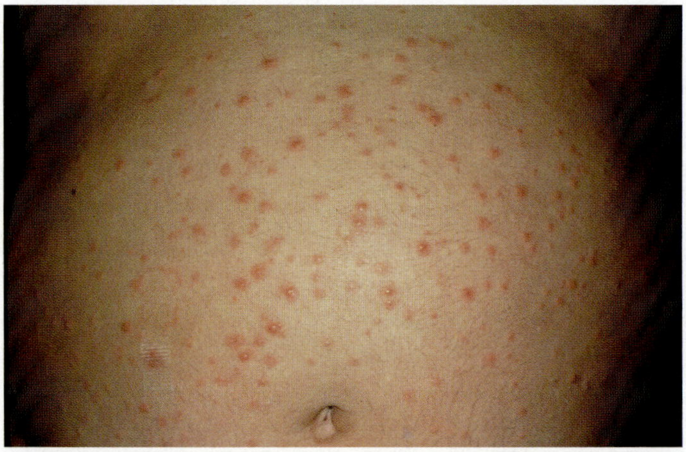

Fig. 14.14 Eruptive Xanthomata on the Abdomen. (From Lebwohl MG, editor: *Atlas of the skin and systemic disease*, New York, 1995, Churchill Livingstone.)

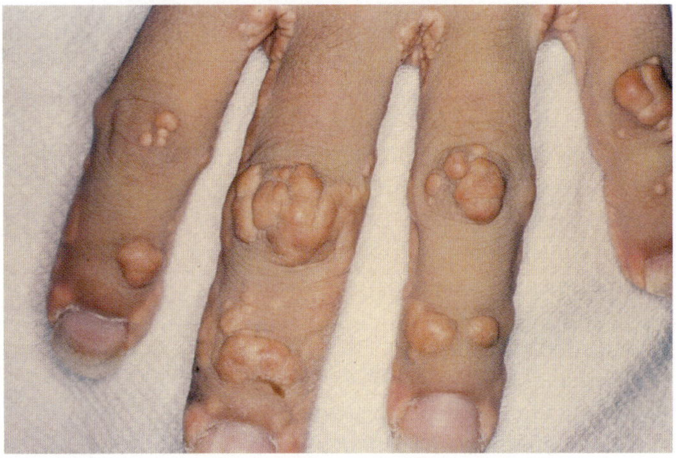

Fig. 14.13 Multiple Tuberous Xanthomata of the Hand. (From Callen JP, Greer KE, Hood AF, et al: *Color atlas of dermatology*, Philadelphia, 1993, WB Saunders.)

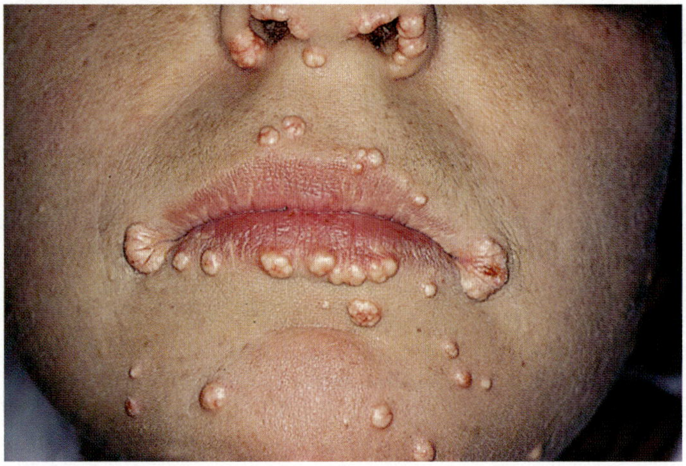

Fig. 14.15 Eruptive Xanthomata on the Face. (From Callen JP, Paller AS, Greer KE, et al: *Color atlas of dermatology*, ed 2, Philadelphia, 2000, WB Saunders.)

fingers with a total serum cholesterol concentration higher than 450 mg/dL.[h]

Fig. 14.13 shows multiple tuberous xanthomata of the hand of another patient. This patient had *primary biliary cirrhosis* and highly elevated cholesterol levels. Primary biliary cirrhosis is a rare, progressive, and often fatal liver disease occurring primarily in females. Pruritus is a common symptom. Xanthomata develop in approximately 15% to 20% of affected patients and are typically found on the palms, soles, knees, elbows, and hands. The serum cholesterol, usually LDL, is often as high as 1000 to 1500 mg/dL. Antimitochondrial antibody is present in nearly 90% of patients.

Eruptive xanthomata are seen in several familial disturbances of fat metabolism, specifically hyperlipidemia types I and IV. The chest, buttocks, abdomen, back, face, and arms are most commonly affected. Fig. 14.14 shows eruptive xanthomata on a patient's abdomen with uncontrolled diabetes mellitus and hypertriglyceridemia. Eruptive xanthomata on a patient's face are pictured in Fig. 14.15. Eruptive xanthomata result from elevated plasma triglyceride concentrations, often exceeding 1500 mg/dL.[i] These lesions developed in this patient after excessive alcohol consumption; his serum triglyceride concentrations exceeded 2000 mg/dL. The lesions, frequently found on the abdomen, buttocks, elbows, knees, and back, are yellowish papules on an erythematous base (1 to 3 mm in diameter). With a reduction in the level of triglycerides, the lesions may recede.

Is a rash present? The presence of *erythema marginatum* (erythema in which the reddened areas are disc-shaped with raised edges) in a febrile patient suggests acute rheumatic fever.

Are any painful lesions on the fingers or toes present? *Osler nodes* are painful lesions in the tufts of the fingers and toes in

[h]The desirable total cholesterol concentration for an adult is normally less than 200 mg/dL. For patients with coronary artery disease, the desirable level is less than 170 mg/dL.

[i]The desirable total triglyceride concentration for an adult is normally less than 150 mg/dL.

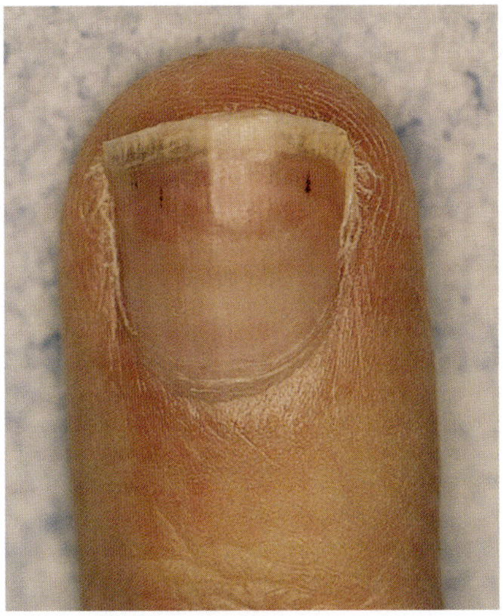

Fig. 14.16 Splinter Hemorrhages.

patients with infective endocarditis. They are evanescent but are said to occur in 10% to 25% of patients with infective endocarditis.

Inspect the Nails

Frequently, *splinter hemorrhages* are visible as small, reddish-brown lines in the nail bed. These hemorrhages run from the free margin proximally and are classically associated with infective endocarditis. However, the finding is nonspecific because it is seen in many other conditions, commonly local trauma to the nail. A nail with splinter hemorrhages in a patient with endocarditis is shown in Fig. 14.16.

Inspect the Facies

Abnormalities of the heart may also be associated with peculiarities of the face and head. Supravalvular aortic stenosis, a congenital problem, occurs associated with widely set eyes, strabismus, low-set ears, an upturned nose, and hypoplasia of the mandible. Moon facies and widely spaced eyes are suggestive of pulmonic stenosis. Expressionless facies with puffy eyelids and loss of the outer third of the eyebrow is seen in hypothyroidism. Affected individuals may have a cardiomyopathy. The *earlobe crease,* or Lichstein's sign, is an oblique crease, often bilateral, seen frequently in patients older than 50 with significant CHD. This sign is shown in Fig. 14.17. Although it is a helpful sign, many false-positive and false-negative findings exist.

Inspect the Eyes

Yellowish plaques on the eyelids, called *xanthelasma,* should raise the suspicion of underlying hyperlipoproteinemia, even though this lesion is less specific than the xanthoma. Xanthelasma in a patient with hypercholesterolemia is shown in Fig. 14.18.

Examination of the eyes may reveal an *arcus senilis.* An arcus (see Figs. 10.57 and 10.58) seen in a patient *younger than* 40 should raise the suspicion of *hypercholesterolemia.* Opacities in the cornea may be evidence for sarcoidosis, which may be

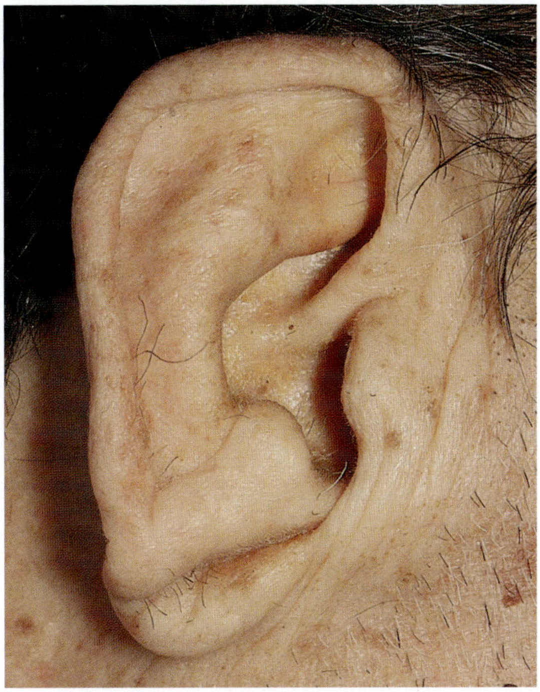

Fig. 14.17 Earlobe Creases.

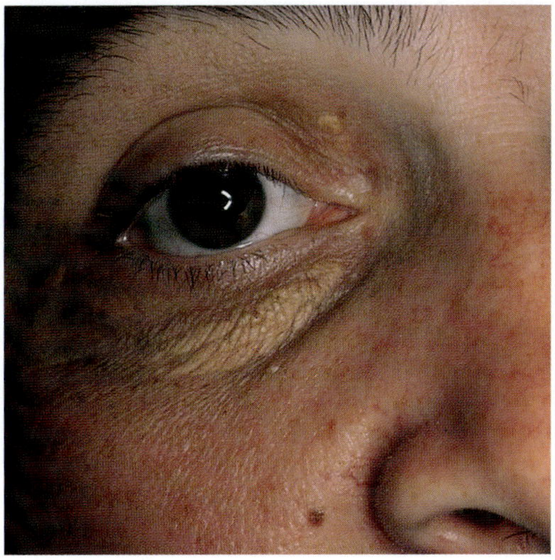

Fig. 14.18 Xanthelasma.

responsible for cor pulmonale or myocardial involvement. Displacement of the lens is frequently seen in patients with *Marfan syndrome,* an important cause of aortic regurgitation (see Fig. 10.74). Conjunctival hemorrhages are commonly seen in infective endocarditis. *Hypertelorism,* or widely set eyes, is often associated with congenital heart disease, especially pulmonic stenosis and supravalvular aortic stenosis. A retinal evaluation may furnish valuable information about diabetes (see Figs. 10.93 to 10.105), hypertension (see Figs. 10.84 and 10.106 to 10.110), and atherosclerosis. Roth's spots may develop in patients with infective endocarditis (see Fig. 10.114).

Inspect the Mouth

Have the patient open their mouth widely. Inspect the palate. Is the palate highly arched? A high-arched palate may be

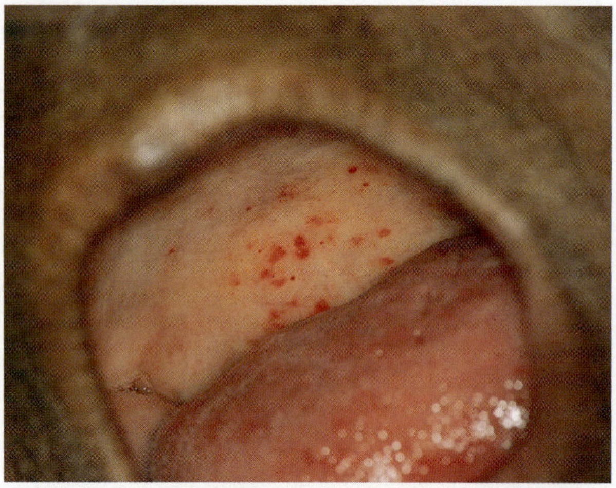

Fig. 14.19 Palatal Petechiae.

associated with congenital heart problems such as mitral valve prolapse.

Are there *petechiae* on the palate? Infective endocarditis may be associated with palatal petechiae, as seen in Fig. 14.19 (see also Fig. 12.34).

Inspect the Neck

Examination of the neck may reveal webbing. Webbing is seen in individuals with *Turner syndrome,*[j] who may have coarctation of the aorta, and in patients with *Noonan syndrome.*[k] Pulmonic stenosis is the associated cardiac abnormality in this condition.[5]

Inspect the Chest Configuration

Inspection of the chest often reveals information about the heart. Because the chest and the heart develop at about the same time during embryogenesis, it is not surprising that anything interfering with the development of the chest may interfere with the heart. A *pectus excavatum,* or caved-in chest, is seen in Marfan syndrome and mitral valve prolapse (see Fig. 13.7). *Pectus carinatum,* or pigeon breast, is also associated with Marfan syndrome (see Fig. 13.8) and Ehlers-Danlos Syndrome.

Assess the presence of visible cardiac motions.

Inspect the Extremities

Some congenital abnormalities of the heart are associated with abnormalities of the extremities. Patients with atrial septal defects (ASDs) may have an extra phalanx, an extra finger, or an extra toe. Long, slender fingers may suggest Marfan syndrome and aortic regurgitation. Short stature, cubitus valgus, and medial deviation of the extended forearm are typical of patients with Turner syndrome.

Blood Pressure Assessment

The Principles

BP can be measured directly with an intraarterial catheter or indirectly with a *sphygmomanometer.* The sphygmomanometer consists of an inflatable rubber bladder within a cloth cover, a rubber bulb to inflate the bladder, and a manometer to measure the pressure in the bladder. Indirect measurement of BP involves the auscultatory detection of the appearance and disappearance of the Korotkoff sounds over the compressed artery. *Korotkoff sounds* are low-pitched sounds originating in the vessel related to turbulence produced by partially occluding an artery with a BP cuff. Several phases occur in sequence as the occluding pressure drops. Phase 1 occurs when the occluding pressure falls to the systolic BP. The tapping sounds are clear and gradually increase in intensity as the occluding pressure falls. Phase 2 occurs at a pressure approximately 10 to 15 mm Hg lower than that in phase 1 and consists of tapping sounds followed by murmurs.[l]

Phase 3 occurs when the occluding pressure falls enough to allow a large volume to cross the partially occluded artery. The sounds are similar to the sounds of phase 2, except that only the tapping sounds are heard. Phase 4 is the abrupt muffling and decreased intensity of the sounds as the pressure approaches the diastolic BP. Phase 5 is the complete disappearance of the sounds. The occluding cuff no longer compresses the vessel. Turbulent flow is no longer present.

The normal BP for adults is less than 120 mm Hg systolic and less than 80 mm Hg diastolic (Fig. 14.20). Elevated (prehypertensive) BP is 120 to 129 systolic and less than 80 diastolic. When systolic and diastolic BPs fall into different categories, the higher category should be used to classify BP levels. The BP ranges in the table apply to most adults (aged 18 and older) who do not have serious short-term illnesses. For the diastolic BP reading, the Korotkoff sounds' disappearance is probably more accurate than the point of muffling. However, if the point of disappearance is more than 10 mm Hg lower than the point of muffling, the point of muffling is probably more accurate. Recording both the point of muffling and disappearance frequently helps in communication. A BP might be recorded as 125/75 to 65: the systolic BP is 125; the point of muffling is 75; the point of disappearance is 65 (the diastolic BP).

BP should be recorded only to the nearest 5 mm Hg because all sphygmomanometers have a ±3 mm Hg accuracy limit. In addition, normal BP changes occur from moment to moment, and measuring to less than 5 mm Hg provides a false sense of accuracy.

Two types of hypertension need to be recognized. *White coat hypertension* is a common phenomenon (approximately 15% to 20% of all stage 1 hypertensives) in which the patient's BP is higher in the doctor's office than measured at home or work.

[j]Short stature, retarded sexual development, and webbed neck in a female patient, associated with an abnormality of the sex chromosomes (45, XO).

[k]Noonan syndrome, also known as *male Turner syndrome*, is a genetically inherited disorder (46, XY) with heterogeneous phenotypic manifestations. The most consistent features are wide-set eyes, low-set ears, short stature, and pulmonic stenosis. The inheritance pattern is autosomal dominant. At least eight gene mutations are causing this syndrome, and the patient presentation ranges from mild to severe.

[l]A murmur is a blowing auscultatory sign produced by turbulence in blood flow. These vibrations can originate in the heart or in blood vessels as a result of hemodynamic changes.

Blood Pressure Category	SYSTOLIC mm Hg (Upper number)		DIASTOLIC mm Hg (lower number)
Normal	Less than 120	and	Less than 80
Elevated	120–129	and	Less than 80
High Blood Pressure (Hypertension) Stage 1	130–129	or	80–89
High Blood Pressure (Hypertension) Stage 2	140 or higher	or	90 or higher
Hypertensive Crisis (consult your doctor immediately)	Higher than 180	and/or	Higher than 120

Fig. 14.20 Blood Pressure Categories. (Reused from https://www.heart.org/en/health-topics/high-blood-pressure/understanding-blood-pressure-readings Reprinted with permission ©American Heart Association, Inc.)

These patients are at low cardiovascular risk. In contrast, *masked hypertension* is more serious because these individuals have normal BPs in the medical facility but have much higher BPs throughout the day, indicative of an increased risk of CVD. Masked hypertension has been estimated to occur in 10% of the general population.

See Video 14.1.

The size of the cuff is essential for accurately determining BP. It is recommended that the cuff be snugly applied around the arm, with its lowest edge 1 inch above the antecubital fossa. The cuff should be approximately 20% wider than the diameter of the extremity. The bladder should overlie the artery. Using a too narrow cuff for a large arm results in an erroneously high BP reading.

Another cause of falsely elevated BP readings is the lack of support of the patient's arm. To obtain an accurate measurement, the cuff must be at heart level. If the arm is not supported, the patient performs isometric exercise, raising the recorded pressure. In contrast, excessive pressure on the stethoscope's diaphragm produces a spuriously lower reading of the diastolic BP without any significant alteration of systolic pressure. If the arm is held correctly, no skin indentations should occur.

The *auscultatory gap* is the silence between the disappearance of the Korotkoff sounds after the initial appearance and their reappearance at a lower pressure. The auscultatory gap is present when there is a decreased blood flow to the extremities, as found in hypertension and aortic stenosis. Its clinical importance lies in that the systolic BP may be mistaken for the lower BP, the point of *reappearance*.

Determine Blood Pressure by Palpation

See Video 14.2.

BP assessment is performed by supporting the patient's right arm under the right arm/elbow of the examiner. The cuff bladder is centered over the right brachial artery. If the arm is obese, a large adult or thigh cuff should be used. The arm should be slightly flexed, and it should be supported at approximately the level of the heart. **To adequately determine the systolic BP and exclude an error resulting from an auscultatory gap, BP is first assessed by palpation.** In this procedure, the right brachial or radial artery is palpated while the cuff is inflated above the pressure required to obliterate the pulse. The adjustable screw is opened slowly for deflation. The reappearance of the brachial pulse identifies the systolic pressure. The adjustable screw is opened for rapid deflation when the pulse is felt. Holding of the arm and the BP assessment is demonstrated in Fig. 14.21.

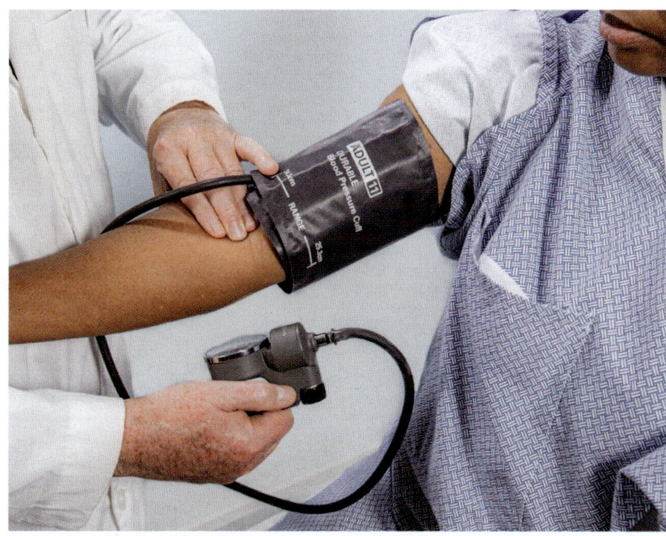

Fig. 14.21 Technique for Blood Pressure Assessment by Palpation.

Blood Pressure by Auscultation

See Video 14.3.

BP by auscultation is assessed in the right arm by inflating the cuff to approximately 20 mm Hg above the systolic pressure determined by palpation. The arm is supported as described previously. The stethoscope's diaphragm should be placed over the artery as close to the edge of the cuff as possible, preferably

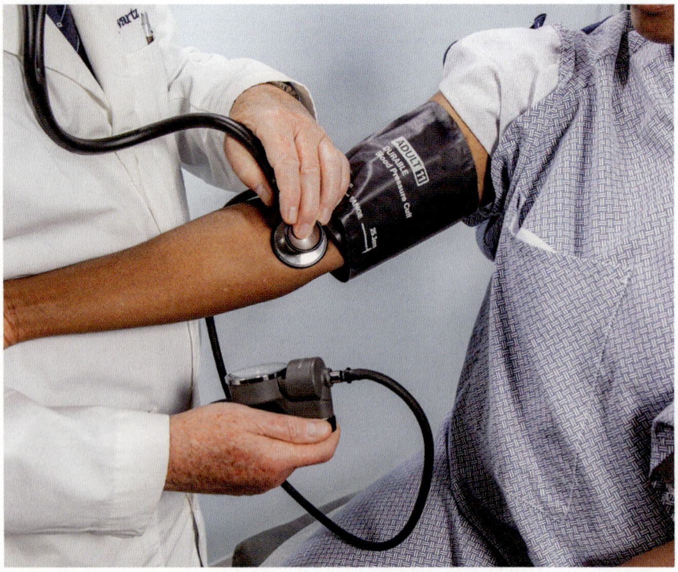

Fig. 14.22 Technique for Blood Pressure Assessment by Auscultation.

just under the edge. The cuff is deflated *slowly* while the Korotkoff sounds are evaluated. The systolic BP, the point of muffling, and the point of disappearance are determined. The systolic BP is the point at which the initial tapping sounds are heard. The technique for determining auscultatory BP is shown in Fig. 14.22. If the BP is high, measuring it again at the end of the examination is helpful when the patient may be more comfortable.

Rule Out Orthostatic Hypotension

See Video 14.4.

After the patient has been recumbent for at least 5 minutes, measure the baseline BP and pulse. Then have the patient stand and repeat the measurements immediately.

Orthostatic hypotension, or *postural hypotension*, is diagnosed when the systolic BP drops by ≥20 mm Hg or diastolic BP drops by ≥10 mm Hg within 3 minutes of standing compared to BP from the sitting or supine position. The development of symptoms such as dizziness may accompany the drop in BP. In most affected patients, there is also an increase in heart rate. Once orthostatic hypotension is diagnosed, a cause must be sought. The risk factors for orthostatic hypotension include older age, medications,[m] cardiac conditions, heat exposure, prolonged bed rest, pregnancy, and drinking alcohol.

Rule Out Supravalvular Aortic Stenosis

See Video 14.5.

If hypertension is detected in the right arm, perform the following test: Place the cuff on the patient's left arm and determine the auscultatory pressure. It is not necessary to remeasure the palpatory pressure or reevaluate for orthostatic changes. In supravalvular aortic stenosis, there is a difference in the BP in the arms; hypertension may be detected in the right arm, whereas hypotension may be present in the left arm.

Rule Out Coarctation of the Aorta

Coarctation of the aorta[6] is a relatively common defect that accounts for 5% to 8% of all congenital heart defects. Coarctation of the aorta may occur as an isolated defect or in association with various other lesions, most commonly bicuspid aortic valve and ventricular septal defect (VSD). The diagnosis of coarctation of the aorta may be missed in a child or adult unless an index of suspicion is maintained. It is a surgically correctable form of hypertension. Always check the BP in the lower extremity in any new patient with hypertension!

If the BP is elevated in the arms, determination of the BP in the lower extremities is essential for ruling out coarctation of the aorta. The patient is asked to lie on the abdomen while the thigh cuff, which is 6 cm wider than the arm cuff, is placed around the posterior aspect of the midthigh. The stethoscope is placed over the artery in the popliteal fossa. The Korotkoff sounds are determined as in the upper extremity. If a thigh cuff is unavailable, the regular cuff can be applied to the lower leg with the distal border just at the malleoli. The stethoscope is placed over either the posterior tibial or the dorsalis pedis artery, and the auscultatory BP is taken. *A leg systolic BP lower than that in the arm should raise suspicion of coarctation of the aorta, especially if the femoral pulse is delayed compared to the radial.* These two pulses typically peak at the same time.

Rule Out Cardiac Tamponade

In the presence of low arterial BP and a rapid and feeble pulse, it is necessary to rule out the existence of cardiac tamponade. *Cardiac tamponade*[7] results when fluid accumulates in the pericardial sac compressing the heart and interfering with normal diastolic filling, leading to decreased cardiac output and shock. The pericardial fluid that builds up slowly is better tolerated than a rapid accumulation.

A valuable clinical sign suggestive of cardiac tamponade is the presence of a marked *paradoxical pulse* (also known as a *pulsus paradoxus*), characterized by an exaggeration of the normal inspiratory fall in systolic pressure. There needs to be more clarity about the definition of a normal paradoxical pulse. A normal paradoxical pulse should be defined as the *normal* fall (approximately 5 mm Hg) in systolic arterial pressure during inspiration. The magnitude of the phenomenon should determine whether the pulsus paradoxus is normal or abnormal.

The technique for assessing the magnitude of a paradoxical pulse is as follows: Have the patient breathe as normally as possible. Inflate the BP cuff until no sounds are heard. Gradually deflate the cuff until sounds are heard in expiration only. Note this pressure. Continue to deflate the cuff slowly until sounds are heard during inspiration. Note this pressure. If the difference in these two pressures exceeds 10 mm Hg, a marked (abnormal) pulsus paradoxus is present; cardiac tamponade may be the cause.

[m]Medications used to treat BP, such as diuretics, alpha-blockers, beta-blockers, calcium channel blockers, angiotensin-converting enzyme (ACE) inhibitors, and nitrates, may be responsible for orthostatic hypotension. In addition, medications used to treat Parkinson disease, antidepressants, antipsychotics, muscle relaxants, narcotics, and medications to treat erectile dysfunction increase the risk of orthostatic hypotension.

A marked paradoxical pulse is not a specific phenomenon for tamponade because it is also seen in large pericardial effusions, constrictive pericarditis, and conditions associated with increased ventilatory effort, such as asthma and emphysema.

The Arterial Pulse

The following information is gained from palpation of the arterial pulse:

- The rate and rhythm of the heart
- The contour of the pulse
- The amplitude of the pulse

Determine the Cardiac Rate

See Video 14.6.

The radial pulse routinely assesses cardiac rate. The examiner should stand in front of the patient and grasp both radial arteries. The second, third, and fourth fingers should overlie the radial artery, as shown in Fig. 14.23. **Never palpate the radial pulse with your thumb,** as its pulse may be stronger than the patient's radial pulse. In doing so, you will record your heart rate! The examiner should count the pulse for 30 seconds and multiply the beats by two to obtain the beats per minute. This method is accurate for most *regular* rhythms. A *pulse deficit* may be present if the patient has an irregularly irregular rhythm, as is found in atrial fibrillation. In atrial fibrillation, many impulses bombard the AV node and ventricles. Due to the varying lengths of diastolic filling periods, some contractions may be very weak and unable to produce an adequate pulse wave despite ventricular contraction. A pulse deficit, which is the difference between the apical (precordial) and radial pulses, occurs. In such cases, only auscultation of the heart, not the radial pulse, accurately assesses the cardiac rate.

Determine the Cardiac Rhythm

When palpating the pulse, carefully evaluate the regularity of the rhythm. The slower the rate, the longer you should palpate. If the rhythm is irregular, is there a pattern to the irregularity?

Cardiac rhythm may be described as *regular, regularly irregular,* or *irregularly irregular.* A regularly irregular rhythm is a pulse with an irregularity that occurs in a definite pattern. An irregularly irregular pulse has no pattern.

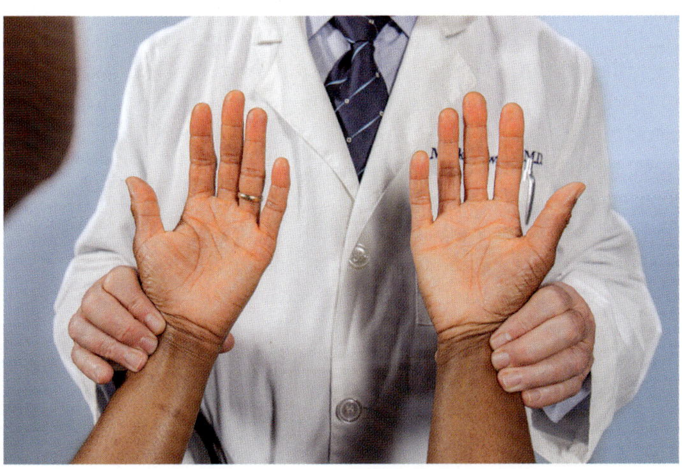

Fig. 14.23 Technique for Evaluating the Radial Artery Pulses.

Electrocardiography is the best medium for diagnosing the rhythm, but the physical examination may provide some clues. *Premature beats* may be recognized by isolated extra beats during a regular rhythm. *Bigeminy* is a coupled rhythm of beats in pairs. The first is the sinus beat, followed by a premature, usually ventricular, beat. If the premature beat is very early in the diastolic period, the pulse from this beat may be missed if the examiner evaluates the rhythm by palpation alone. A grossly irregular rhythm with no pattern is irregularly irregular and is the pulse felt in patients with *atrial fibrillation.*

Palpate the Carotid Artery

See Video 14.7.

Assess the carotid artery pulse by standing on the patient's right side, with the patient lying on the back. **Always auscultate the patient's carotid arteries for bruits *first*** (see Chapter 15, The Peripheral Vascular System). If a bruit is present, do not palpate the carotid artery. If a cholesterol plaque is present, palpation may produce an embolus to the brain.

To palpate the carotid artery, place your index and third fingers on the patient's thyroid cartilage and slip them laterally between the trachea and the sternocleidomastoid muscle. You should be able to feel the carotid pulsations just medial to the sternocleidomastoid muscle. Palpation should be performed low in the neck to avoid pressure on the carotid sinus, which would cause a reflex drop in BP and heart rate. Each carotid artery is evaluated separately. ***Never* press on both carotid arteries at the same time**. After the right carotid artery is evaluated, stand in the same position, place the same fingers back on the patient's trachea, and slip them laterally to the left to feel the left carotid artery. This technique is demonstrated in Fig. 14.24.

Evaluate the Characteristics of the Pulse

The carotid artery is used to assess the contour and amplitude of the pulse. *Contour* is the shape of the wave. It is frequently described as the speed of the upward slope, downward slope, and wave duration. Place a hand firmly against the carotid artery until a maximal force is felt. At this moment, the waveform should be discernible. The pulse may be *normal, diminished, increased,* or *double-peaked.* The normal carotid pulse wave is smooth, with the upward stroke steeper and more rapid than the downward stroke. A diminished pulse is a small, weak pulse. The palpating finger feels a gentle pressure rise with a distinct peak. An increased pulse is a large, strong, hyperkinetic pulse. The palpating finger feels an increased rate of rise of the ascending limb of the pulse and a quick tap at its peak. A double-peaked pulse has a prominent percussion and tidal wave with or without a dicrotic wave. Arterial pulse abnormalities are summarized in Fig. 14.25.

The Jugular Venous Pulse

The *external and internal jugular veins* provide information about the waveforms and right atrial pressure. The external jugular vein is easier to visualize than the internal jugular vein. The pulsations of the internal jugular vein are beneath the

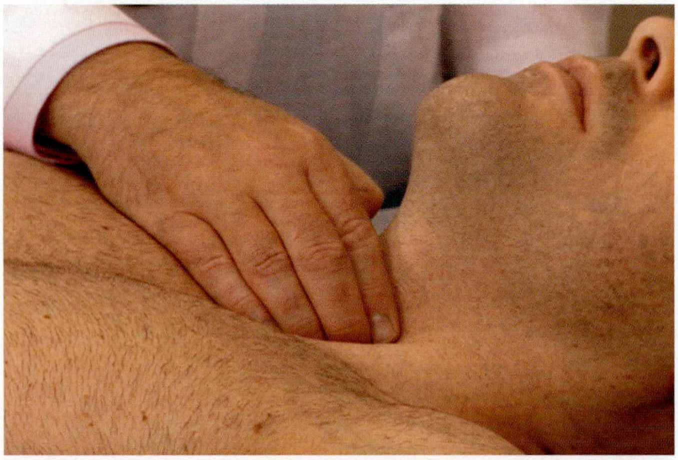

A

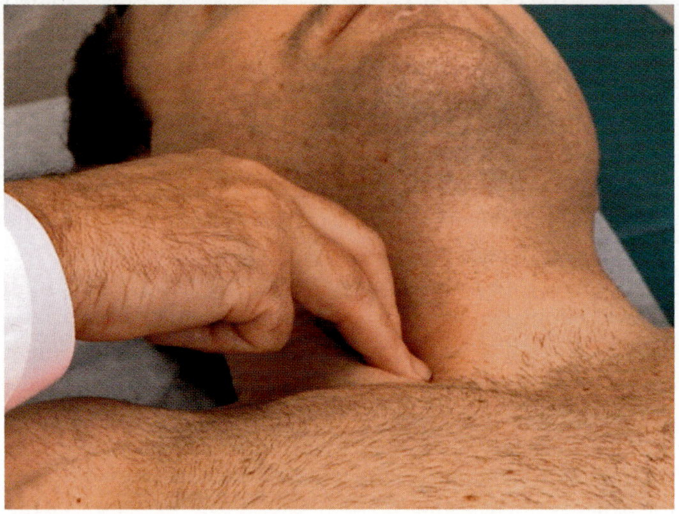

B

Fig. 14.24 (A) and (B) Technique for evaluating the carotid artery pulsations.

sternocleidomastoid muscle and are visible as they are transmitted through the surrounding tissue. The vein itself is not visible. Because the right internal jugular vein is straighter than the left, *only the right jugular vein is evaluated, usually.*

Determine the Jugular Wave Forms

See Video 14.8.

To visualize the *jugular waveforms,* the patient should lie flat without a pillow so that their neck is not flexed and does not interfere with the pulsations. The patient's trunk should be at approximately 25 degrees to the horizontal. The higher the venous pressure, the greater the elevation required; the lower the pressure, the lower the elevation needed. The patient's head should be turned to the right and slightly down to relax the right sternocleidomastoid muscle. Standing on the patient's right side, the examiner should place their right hand, holding a small pocket flashlight, on the patient's sternum and shine the light tangentially across the right side of the neck. Shadows of the "a," "c," and "v" waveforms and their descents will be cast on the sheet behind the patient. The light and shadows magnify the waveforms. This technique is demonstrated in Fig. 14.26. If no waveforms are seen, the angle of elevation of the head of the bed should be reduced.

To help identify the waveforms, the examiner can time the cardiac cycle by palpating the cardiac impulse beneath their right hand or by feeling the left carotid impulse with their left hand. The descents, rather than the waves themselves, tend to be more prominent. If the neck veins are visible at the jaw margin while the patient is seated, the examiner should watch for the waveforms at the angle of the jaw with the patient seated upright.

Variations of the jugular vein waveforms can provide valuable information about the patient's diagnosis. Some of the more common abnormal waveforms are:

- Increased "a" wave
  - Resistance to right atrial emptying that can occur at or beyond the tricuspid valve, as in:
  - Pulmonary hypertension
  - Tricuspid stenosis
  - Right atrial mass or thrombus, less common
- Cannon (Giant) "a" wave
  - Large positive venous pulse during "a" wave. It occurs when an atrium contracts against a closed tricuspid valve during AV dissociation, as in:
    - Premature atrial/junctional/ventricular contractions
    - Atrial flutter
    - Complete AV block
    - Ventricular tachycardia
- Absent "a" wave
  - No atrial contraction, as seen in atrial fibrillation
- Giant "cv" wave
  - Tricuspid regurgitation

Look at the patient shown in Video 14.9. This 48-year-old male presented with severe shortness of breath. Only 8 months earlier, he was diagnosed for the very first time with an atrial septal defect (ASD), a congenital defect. An ASD is characterized by a defect in the interatrial septum allowing pulmonary venous return from the higher-pressure left atrium to pass directly to the lower-pressure right atrium. With time, due to increased blood flow to the right atrium, right ventricle, and lungs, right-sided pressure increases above the left atrium and pulmonary hypertension develops, reversing blood flow from the right to the left atrium. Physical examination of this patient showed that he had now developed significant pulmonary hypertension resulting in significant hypoxemia and cyanosis due to the reversal of his shunt. This condition is known as *Eisenmenger syndrome.*[8] As a consequence of the increased pressure in the pulmonary circuit and increased volume in the right heart, the patient developed severe tricuspid regurgitation with a giant "cv" wave in his jugular pulse. Eisenmenger syndrome is a relatively rare disorder usually seen in persons with poor healthcare access in whom significant anatomical defects may go undetected for many years. Patients with Eisenmenger syndrome have reduced life expectancies, with high mortality in the third and fourth decades. Patients are at risk for paradoxical emboli, in which a blood clot from the veins in the lower extremity may pass through a septal defect from the right heart,

Type	Description	Cause
Anacrotic*	Small, slow rising, delayed pulse with a notch or shoulder on the ascending limb	Aortic stenosis
Waterhammer (Corrigan's)	Rapid and sudden systolic expansion	Aortic regurgitation
Bisferiens	Double-peaked pulse with a midsystolic dip	Aortic regurgitation
Alternans	Alternating amplitude of pulse pressure	Congestive heart failure
Paradoxical (marked)	Detected by blood pressure assessment. An exaggerated drop in systolic blood pressure during inspiration	Tamponade Constrictive pericarditis Chronic obstructive lung disease

*Also known as plateau pulse or pulsus parvus et tardus.

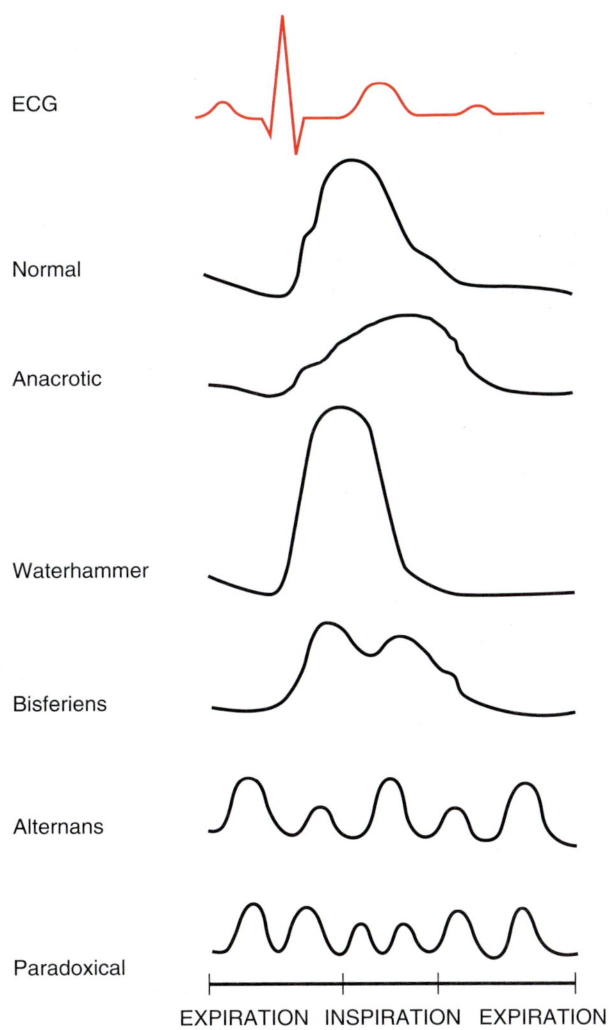

Fig. 14.25 Arterial Pulse Abnormalities. *ECG,* Electrocardiogram.

bypass the lungs, and instead enter the systemic circulation. This may result in devastating cerebrovascular accidents. Ventricular failure, hemoptysis, pregnancy complications, and strokes are common causes of death.[9]

The jugular pulse must be differentiated from the pulsation of the carotid artery. Table 14.6 lists the essential characteristic differences of these pulses.

Estimate the Jugular Venous Pressure

To assess the pressure on the right side of the heart, it is necessary to establish a reference level. The standard reference is the *manubriosternal angle.* At any degree of elevation, this position is used to measure the pressure in the jugular venous system and right heart. The patient should be positioned at whatever angle between the supine and upright positions best

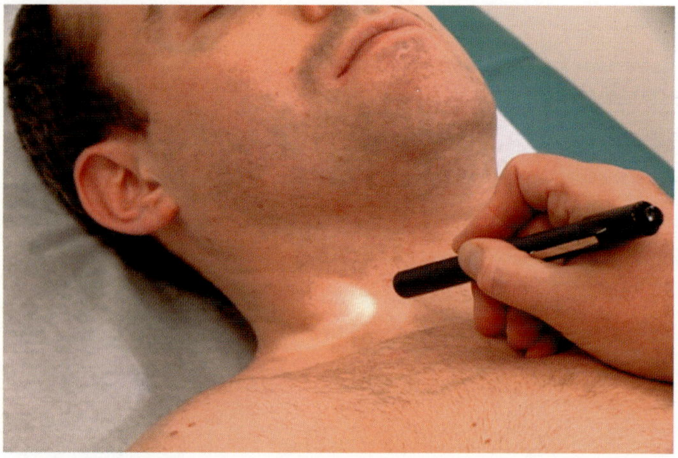

Fig. 14.26 Technique for Evaluating the Jugular Wave Forms.

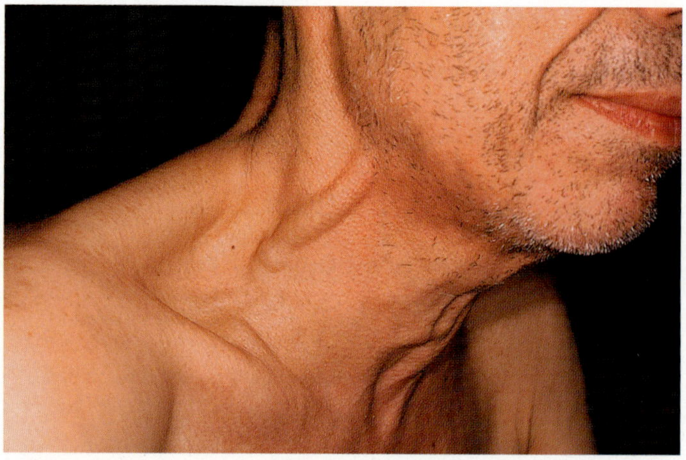

Fig. 14.27 Neck Vein Distention. (*My thanks to the patient and to Xiangya Hospital of Central South University in Changsha, China, for permission to show this patient in Video 14.9 during my bedside rounds.*)

TABLE 14.6 Differentiation of Jugular and Carotid Pulses

Feature	Jugular Pulse	Carotid Pulse
Palpation	Not palpable	Palpable
Wave forms	Multiform: two or three components	Single
Quality	Soft, undulating	Vigorous
Pressure[a]	Wave forms obliterated	No effect
Inspiration	Decreased height of wave forms	No effect
Sitting up	Decreased height of wave forms	No effect
Valsalva maneuver	Increased height of wave forms	No effect

[a]Light pressure on the vessel above the sternal end of clavicle.

demonstrates the top of the neck veins. An imaginary horizontal line is drawn from this height to above the sternal angle. The heart is approximately 5 cm below the sternal angle; thus, if the height of the column is 3 cm above the sternal angle, the estimated venous pressure is 3 + 5 cm or 8 cm water. If the top of the column is 3 cm above the sternal angle, central venous pressure is probably elevated. The specificity of this finding is estimated to be from 93% to 96%.[10] If there is neck vein distention up to the jaw margin while the patient is seated at 90 degrees, the right atrial pressure usually exceeds 15 mm Hg.[n] In the patient shown in Fig. 14.27, the neck veins are distended to the angle of the jaw while the patient is seated upright. The patient's right atrial pressure was 21 mm Hg.

Evaluate the Hepatojugular Reflux

A helpful test in assessing high jugular venous pressure is that of the *hepatojugular reflux*, also known as *abdominal compression*. The examiner can grossly assess right ventricular function by applying pressure over the liver. Patients with right ventricular failure have dilated sinusoids in the liver. Pressure on the liver pushes blood out of these sinusoids and into the inferior vena cava and right side of the heart, causing further distention of the neck veins. The procedure is performed with the patient lying in bed, mouth open, breathing normally; this prevents a Valsalva maneuver. The examiner places their right hand over the patient's liver in the right upper quadrant and applies a firm, progressive pressure. Compression is maintained for 10 seconds. The normal response is for the internal and external jugular veins to show a transient increase in distention during the first few cardiac cycles, followed by a fall to baseline levels during the latter part of the compression. In patients with right ventricular failure or elevated pulmonary artery wedge pressure, the neck veins remain distended during the entire period of compression; this distention diminishes rapidly (at least 4 cm) on sudden release of the compressing hand. If the examination is incorrectly performed with the patient's mouth closed, a Valsalva maneuver results and produces inaccurate results of the hepatojugular reflux test.

Like most other clinical maneuvers, the hepatojugular reflux test must be performed in a standardized manner. If performed correctly, this test can be of considerable value in the bedside assessment of the patient. The test result correlates best with the pulmonary artery wedge pressure and, as such, signifies increased central blood volume. The Ewy study[11] evaluated this test and showed that in the absence of right ventricular failure, a positive result suggests a pulmonary artery wedge pressure of 15 mm Hg or greater.

Percussion

Percuss the Heart's Borders

The technique of percussion is discussed in Chapter 13, The Chest. Percussion of the heart is performed at the third, fourth, and fifth intercostal spaces from the left anterior axillary line to the right anterior axillary line. Usually, there is a change in the percussion note from resonance to dullness approximately 6 cm lateral to the left of the sternum. This dullness is attributable to the presence of the heart.

A percussion dullness distance greater than 10.5 cm in the left fifth intercostal space has a sensitivity of 91.3% and a specificity of 30.3% for detecting increased left ventricular end-diastolic volume (LVEDV) or left ventricular mass. Percussion

[n]The normal end-expiratory right atrial pressure is approximately 3 to 7 mm Hg.

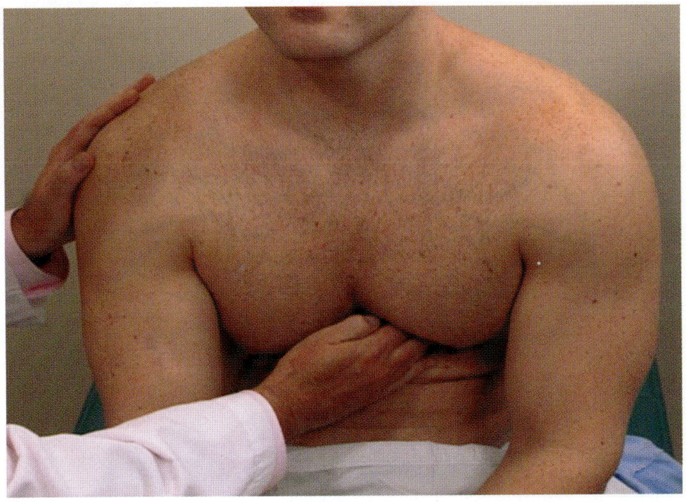

Fig. 14.28 Technique for Assessing Point of Maximum Impulse.

dullness of more than 10.5 cm in the fifth intercostal space has a sensitivity of 94.4% and a specificity of 67.2% in detecting cardiomegaly. In patients with a palpable apical impulse greater than 3 cm in the left decubitus position, the sensitivity of detecting increased LVEDV or left ventricular mass increases to 100%, and the specificity is 40%.

Palpation

Palpation is performed to evaluate the apical impulse, the right ventricle, the pulmonary artery, and the left ventricular motions. The presence or absence of *cardiac thrills*° is also determined by palpation. The PMI describes the outward motion of the cardiac apex as it rotates counterclockwise, as viewed from below, to strike the anterior chest wall during isovolumetric contraction.

Palpate the Point of Maximum Impulse

See Video 14.10.

The examiner should stand on the patient's right side, with the bed at a level comfortable for the examiner. Palpation for the PMI is most easily performed with the patient sitting. Only the examiner's fingertips should be applied to the patient's chest in the fifth intercostal space, midclavicular line because they are the most sensitive for assessing localized motion. The PMI should be noted. This technique is demonstrated in Fig. 14.28. If the apical impulse is not felt, the examiner should move their fingertips in the area of the cardiac apex. The PMI is usually within 10 cm of the midsternal line and is no larger than 2 to 3 cm in diameter. A PMI that is laterally displaced or is felt in two interspaces during the same phase of respiration is suggestive of cardiomegaly.

The PMI is felt in approximately 70% of normal individuals sitting or leaning forward. If it cannot be felt sitting, the patient should be reevaluated while supine and in the left lateral decubitus position. The position of the PMI in the left lateral decubitus position must be assessed with the understanding that the normal cardiac impulse is now shifted slightly to the left. If the patient is in the left lateral decubitus position and the PMI is not laterally displaced, the examiner can suspect that cardiomegaly is absent.

°Low-frequency cutaneous vibrations associated with loud heart murmurs.

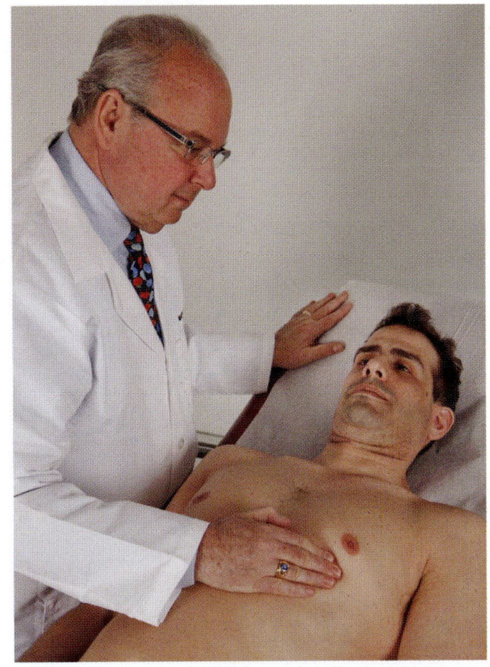

Fig. 14.29 Technique for Assessing Localized Cardiac Motion.

In a patient without conditions predisposing to left ventricular hypertrophy, a palpable apical impulse felt in the left lateral decubitus position that is greater than 3 cm is said to be a specific (91%) and sensitive (92%) indicator of left ventricular enlargement. An apical diameter greater than 3 cm is predictive (86%) of an increased LVEDV. In patients with an apical diameter of less than 3 cm and a normal LVEDV, the negative predictive value is 95%.

The PMI usually corresponds to the *left* ventricular apex. Still, in patients with an enlarged right ventricle, the heart is rotated clockwise, as viewed from below, and the right ventricle may actually produce the PMI. This rotation turns the left ventricle posteriorly and makes it difficult to palpate. The apical impulse by the right ventricle is diffuse, whereas the left ventricle tends to be more localized.

In patients with chronic obstructive lung disease, the overinflation of the lungs displaces the PMI downward and to the right. The PMI in such patients is felt in the *epigastric* area at the lower end of the sternum. In patients with chronic obstructive lung disease, a PMI in the normal location suggests cardiomegaly.

Palpate for Localized Motion

The patient should now lie down so that all four main cardiac areas can be palpated. The examiner uses their fingertips to assess any localized motion. This technique is demonstrated in Fig. 14.29.

A systolic impulse in the second intercostal space to the left of the sternum is suspect of pulmonary hypertension. This impulse is caused by the closure of the pulmonic valve under

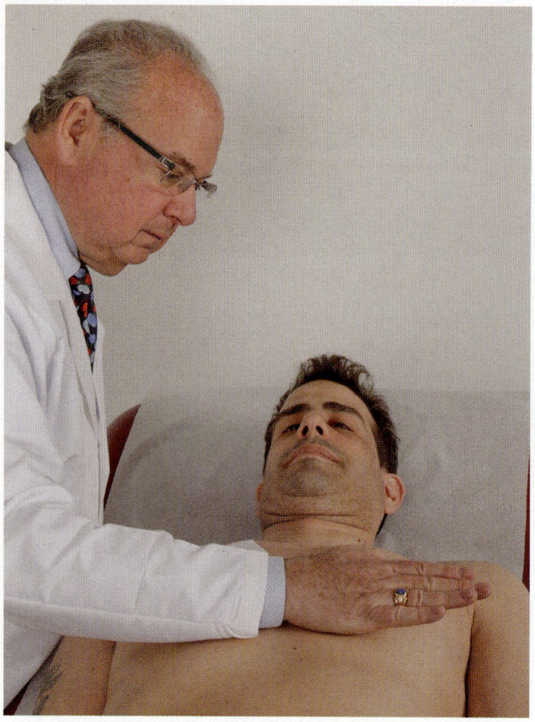

Fig. 14.30 Technique for Assessing Generalized Cardiac Motion.

increased pressure. This impulse suggests a dilated pulmonary artery, but it may also be felt in thin individuals without pulmonary hypertension.

Palpate for Generalized Motion

See Video 14.11.

After the chest has been palpated with the fingertips, the examiner uses the proximal portion of their hand to palpate for any large area of sustained outward motion, called a *heave* or *lift*. The examiner again palpates each of the four main cardiac areas. The technique for assessing heaves is demonstrated in Fig. 14.30. A *right ventricular rock,* a sustained left parasternal impulse associated with lateral retraction, suggests a large right ventricle.

Any condition that increases the ventricular filling rate during early diastole can produce a palpable impulse *after* the main left ventricular impulse. This second impulse in the area of the PMI is usually felt in association with an S_3. Frequently, an S_3 is more easily felt than heard.

Using a tongue blade or an applicator stick can be helpful to reinforce visually what has been palpated. The tip of the stick is placed directly over the area and held in place by the examiner's finger. This acts as a fulcrum, and the motions tend to be magnified by the stick's movement. The technique is demonstrated in Fig. 14.31.

Palpate for Thrills

See Video 14.12 and Video 14.13.

Thrills are the superficial vibratory sensations felt on the skin overlying an area of turbulence. The presence of a cardiac thrill indicates a loud murmur. Thrills are best felt using the heads of your metacarpal bones rather than the fingertips and applying

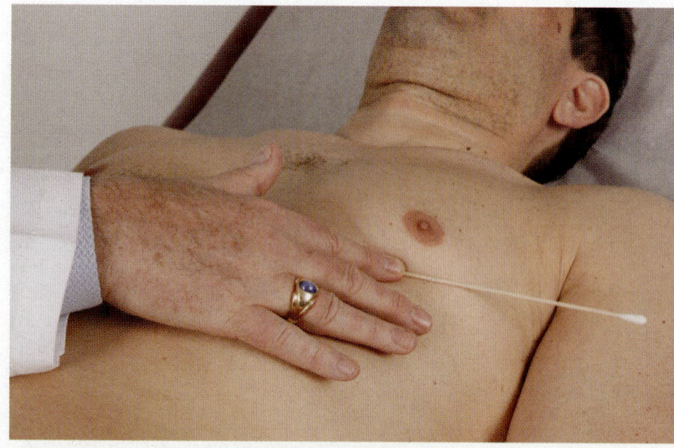

Fig. 14.31 Technique for Amplifying Detection of Cardiac Movement.

very gentle pressure on the skin. If too much pressure is applied, thrills are not felt. The palpation of thrills is generally of little importance because auscultation reveals the presence of the loud murmur that has produced the turbulence. Therefore, finding a thrill adds little to the diagnosis, but it is an interesting physical sign to alert the examiner as to what will be heard. The only importance of a thrill is that on an intensity grading scale from I to VI, with VI being the loudest murmur, the presence of a thrill makes a grade of IV or higher.

Auscultation

The Technique

Proper auscultation requires a quiet area. Every attempt should be made to eliminate extraneous noise from radios, televisions, etc. The earpieces of the stethoscope are directed anteriorly or parallel to the direction of the external auditory canal. If the earpieces are put in backward, the openings of the earpieces impinge on the wall of the external canal and lower the intensity of the sounds. The earpieces should fit properly to be comfortable but tight enough to exclude external noises.

It is often helpful to close your eyes when listening to the heart. Sounds that are more difficult to hear sound louder with your eyes closed because the brain is flooded with all types of sensory input when the eyes are open. The input from the eyes is the most important. The following important sensory input processed is auditory, followed by tactile input. If you eliminate the distraction of visual stimuli, the brain concentrates more on the auditory input, and the sounds become more evident.

As Chapter 13, The Chest, indicates, the stethoscope bell should be applied lightly to the skin, whereas the diaphragm should be pressed tightly against the skin. High-pitched sounds, such as valve closure, systolic events, and regurgitant murmurs, are better heard with the diaphragm. Low-pitched sounds, such as gallop rhythms or the murmur of AV stenosis, are better heard with the bell.

It is common in many countries to examine patients through their clothing or a hospital gown. In the United States, however, *never* listen through *any* clothing.

There are several other pitfalls in auscultation. Ensure the stethoscope is in good shape: Cracked tubing certainly interferes with good listening. Both the examiner and the patient must be comfortable for the best hearing. An examiner who is straining over the patient and is uncomfortable will want to finish the examination quickly without a proper assessment. Always inspect and palpate *before* auscultation. Accumulate as much information as possible before listening.

Auscultate the Cardiac Areas

The examiner should be on the patient's right side while the patient lies flat on the back. If not already at the proper height, the bed should be adjusted to make the examiner comfortable. The examiner should listen in the aortic, pulmonic, tricuspid, and mitral areas. However, the examiner should not limit auscultation to these areas alone. The examiner should start at any area and move the stethoscope gradually over the precordium from area to area. The areas have been established to provide some degree of standardization.

While listening at the apex and LLSB with the bell, the examiner should determine whether an S_3 or an S_4 is present.

Cardiac murmurs may radiate widely. The examiner should determine where the sounds are loudest or best heard. There are no acoustic walls in the chest. A murmur typically heard at the apex with radiation to the axilla may be heard in the neck if it is loud enough. The murmur in this example is most audible at the apex and axilla.

The Standard Auscultation Positions

See Video 14.14 and Video 15.15.

The four standard positions for auscultation are shown in Fig. 14.32. They are as follows:

- Supine
- Left lateral decubitus
- Upright
- Upright, leaning forward

All precordial areas are examined while the patient is supine. Using a systematic approach, the examiner starts at either the aortic area or the apex and carefully listens to the heart sounds. After examining all areas, the patient is instructed to turn onto the left side. The examiner should now listen at the apex for the low-pitched diastolic murmur of *mitral stenosis,* which is best heard with the stethoscope bell. Then the patient sits upright,

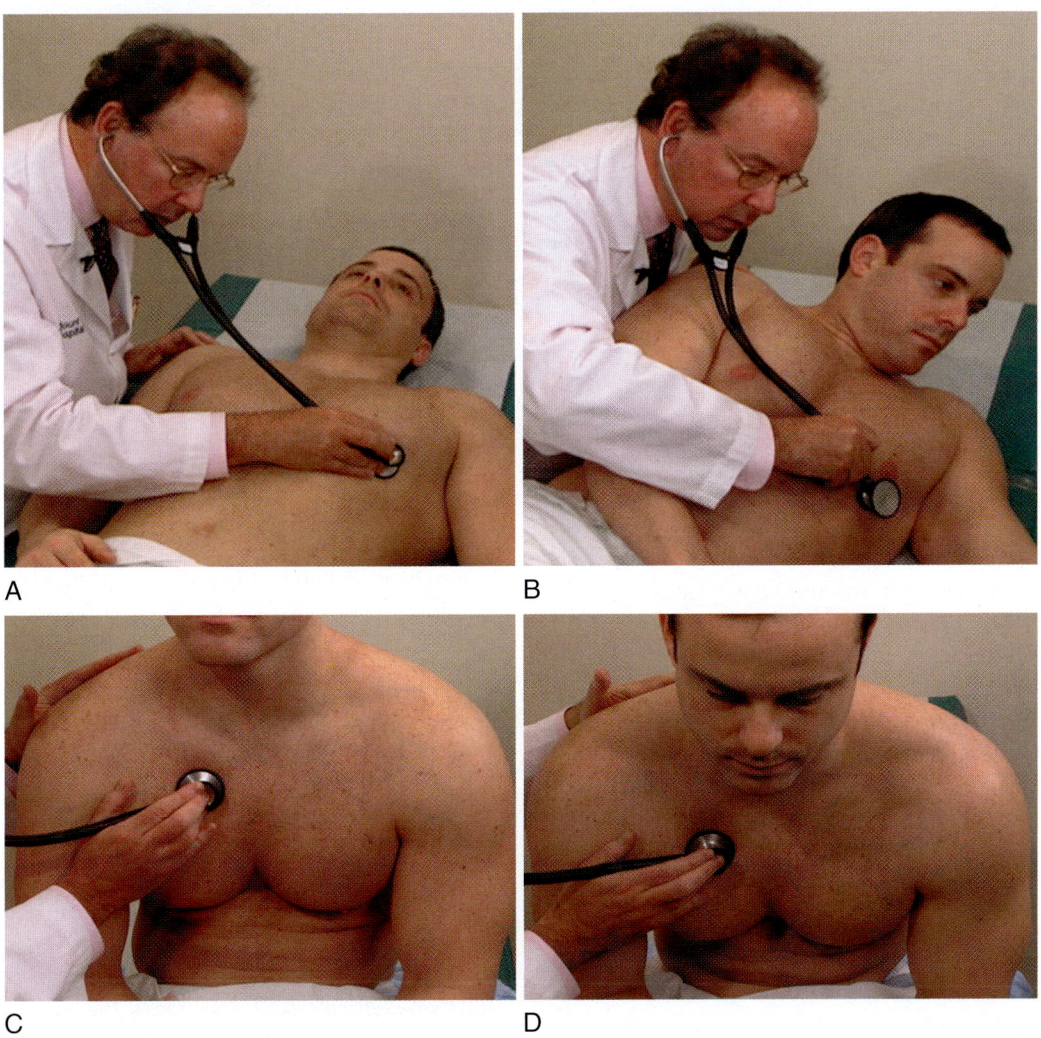

A B C D

Fig. 14.32 Positions for Auscultation. (A) The supine position used for listening to all areas. (B) The left lateral decubitus position used for listening with the bell in the mitral area. (C) The upright position used for listening to all areas. (D) The upright, leaning-forward position used for listening with the diaphragm at the base positions (i.e., aortic and pulmonic areas).

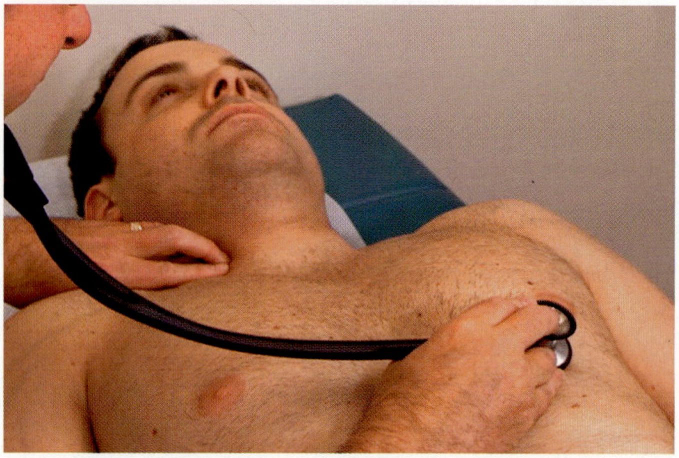

Fig. 14.33 Technique for Timing the Heart Sounds.

and all areas are examined with the stethoscope's diaphragm. Finally, the patient sits up and leans forward. The patient is asked to exhale and hold their breath. At the same time, the examiner, using the diaphragm, listens for the high-pitched diastolic murmur of *aortic regurgitation* at the right and left second and third intercostal spaces.

The influence of breathing. The examiner should pay special attention to the influence of breathing on the intensity of heart sounds. Most murmurs or sounds originating in the right heart are accentuated with inspiration. This is related to the increased return of blood that occurs with inspiration and increased right ventricular output. In addition, an S_3 or an S_4 originating on the right side of the heart is accentuated during inspiration.

Time the Cardiac Events

To interpret heart sounds accurately, the examiner must be able to time the cardiac cycle events. The most reliable way of identifying S_1 and S_2 is to time the sounds by palpating the carotid artery. While the examiner's right hand positions the stethoscope, the left hand is placed on the patient's carotid artery. This technique is demonstrated in Fig. 14.33. The sound that precedes the carotid pulse is the S_1. The S_2 follows the pulse. The carotid, *not* the radial pulse, must be used. The time delay from S_2 to the radial pulse is significant, and errors in timing will result.

Approach to Careful Auscultation

Until the examiner gains expertise in cardiac examination, heart sounds should be evaluated as suggested in Table 14.7. The examiner should take time in each area before continuing to the next area. The examiner should listen to several cardiac cycles at each position to be sure of the observations, including respiratory effects.

Describe Any Murmurs Present

If a murmur is present, attention should be directed to the following features:

- Timing in the cardiac cycle
- Location
- Radiation
- Duration
- Intensity
- Pitch
- Quality
- Relationship to respiration
- Relationship to body position

Timing of murmurs as to systole and diastole is paramount. Does the systolic murmur begin with, or after, S_1? Does it end before, with, or after S_2? Does the murmur occupy the entire systolic period? Murmurs occurring throughout systole are termed *holosystolic* or *pansystolic*. These murmurs begin with S_1 and end *after* S_2. A *systolic ejection* murmur begins after S_1 and ends *immediately before* S_2. Does the murmur occur only in early systole, midsystole, or late systole? Does the murmur persist throughout the entire diastolic period? Such murmurs are termed *holodiastolic*. In which area is the murmur best heard?

The *radiation* of the murmur can provide a clue as to its cause (Fig. 14.34). Does it radiate to the axilla? The neck? The back?

TABLE 14.7 Approach to Cardiac Auscultation

Position	Evaluate
Supine	S_1 in all areas S_2 in all areas Systolic murmurs or sounds in all areas
Left lateral decubitus	Diastolic events at apex with bell of stethoscope
Upright	S_1 in all areas S_2 in all areas Systolic murmurs or sounds in all areas Diastolic murmurs or sounds in all areas
Upright, leaning forward	Diastolic events at base with diaphragm of stethoscope

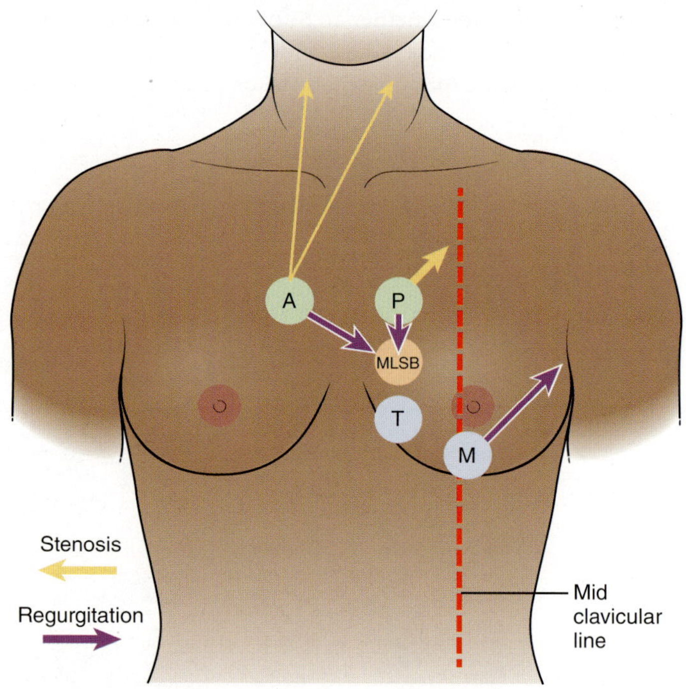

Fig. 14.34 Patterns of Radiation for Different Heart Murmurs.

The intensity of a murmur is graded from I to VI, based on increasing loudness. The following grading system, although antiquated, serves as a means of communicating the intensity of the murmur:

I: Lowest intensity, often not heard by inexperienced listeners
II: Low intensity, usually audible to inexperienced listeners
III: Medium intensity without a cardiac thrill
IV: Medium intensity with a cardiac thrill
V: Loudest murmur that is audible when the stethoscope is placed on the chest; associated with a cardiac thrill
VI: Loudest intensity: audible when the stethoscope is removed from the chest; associated with a cardiac thrill

Murmurs can be described, for example, as "grade II/VI," "grade IV/VI," or "grade II-III/VI." Any murmur associated with a thrill must be at least a grade IV/VI. A grade IV/VI murmur is louder than a grade II/VI murmur only because there is more turbulence; both or neither may have clinical significance. The "/VI" is used because there is another, less popular grading system involving only four categories. An important axiom to remember is the following:

In general, the intensity of a murmur tells nothing about the severity of the clinical state.

The quality of a murmur can be described as rumbling, blowing, harsh, musical, machinery, or scratchy.

Describe Any Pericardial Rubs

Friction rubs are extracardiac sounds of short duration with a unique quality resembling the sound of scratching on sandpaper. Rubs may result from irritation of the pleura (i.e., a pleural rub) or the pericardium (i.e., a pericardial rub). Pericardial rubs typically have three components: one systolic and two diastolic. The systolic component occurs during ejection; the two diastolic components occur during rapid filling and atrial contraction. Pericardial rubs are best heard with the patient sitting while holding their breath in expiration. Patients with pericardial rubs commonly have chest pain lessened by sitting forward. A rub that disappears while the patient holds the breath originates from the pleura.

The Goals of Auscultation

The goals at the end of auscultation are to be able to describe the following:

- The intensity of S_1 in all areas
- The intensity of S_2 in all areas
- The characterization of any systolic sounds
- The characterization of any diastolic sounds

With experience, the examiner can listen to all parts of the cardiac cycle in one area and compare the sounds and events with those of other areas. Normally, S_1 is loudest at the apex and S_2 at the base. The splitting of S_2 into A_2 and P_2 during inspiration is best heard in the pulmonic area with the patient lying on their back. This increases venous return and widens the A_2–P_2 split.

Examination for Edema

When peripheral venous pressure is high, as in congestive HF, pressure in the veins is distributed retrograde to the smaller vessels. Transudation of fluid occurs, and edema of dependent areas results. This increase in tissue fluid produces edema that "pits." Dependent edema occurs most commonly in patients with heart, kidney, or liver failure and those who have received excessive intravenous fluids.

Test for Edema

To test for pitting edema, the examiner presses their fingers into a dependent area, such as the patient's shin, for 2 to 3 seconds. If pitting edema is present, the fingers sink into the tissue, and the impression of the fingers remains when the fingers are removed. This technique is demonstrated in Fig. 14.35.

Pitting edema is usually quantified from 1+ to 4+, depending on the depth and how long the indentation persists. The grading for pitting edema is:

- 1+ roughly 2 mm in depth; disappears rapidly
- 2+ roughly 4 mm in depth; disappears in 10 to 15 seconds
- 3+ roughly 6 mm in depth; may last more than 1 minute; dependent extremity swollen
- 4+ 8 mm pit or deeper, may last 2 to 5 minutes; dependent extremity grossly distorted

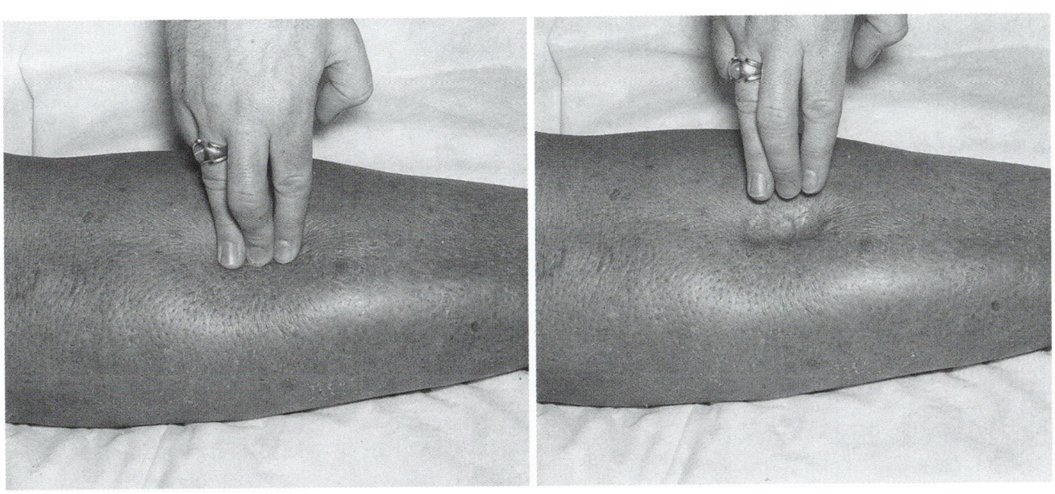

A B

Fig. 14.35 Technique for Testing for Pitting Edema. (A) The examiner presses into the patient's shin area. (B) When pitting edema is present, indentation occurs after the fingers are lifted.

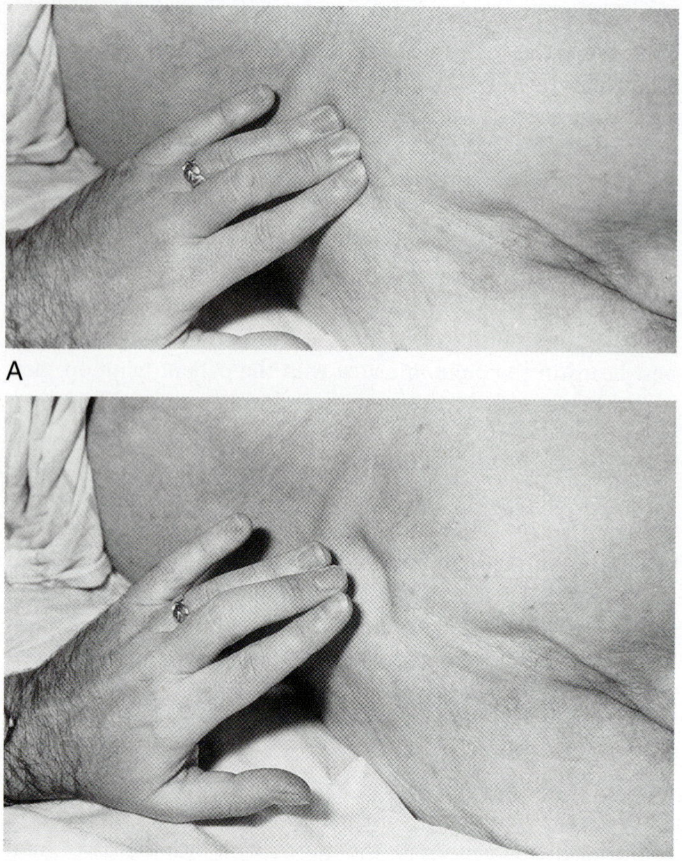

A

B

Fig. 14.36 Technique for Testing for Pitting Edema Over the Sacrum. (A) The examiner presses into the sacrum of a bedridden patient. (B) The pitting edema is evident.

In bedridden patients, the dependent area is usually the sacrum, not the shins. The examiner should evaluate for edema over the sacrum in these patients. Fig. 14.36 illustrates a 4+ sacral edema in a bedridden patient.

CLINICOPATHOLOGIC CORRELATIONS

The discussion now focuses on the pathologic changes that result in the following auscultatory events:

- Abnormalities of S_1
- Abnormalities of S_2
- Systolic clicks
- Diastolic opening snaps
- Murmurs

Abnormalities of the First Heart Sound

The factors that are responsible for the intensity of S_1 are as follows:

- The rate of rise of ventricular pressure
- The condition of the valve
- The position of the valve
- The distance of the heart from the chest wall

The faster the *rise* of left ventricular pressure, the louder the mitral component of S_1. Increased contractility increases the intensity of S_1. Decreased contractility softens S_1.

When the AV valve stiffens due to fibrosis or calcification, its closure is louder. The pathologically deformed valve of mitral stenosis produces an accentuated or louder S_1. After many years, as the valve becomes increasingly calcified, it becomes unable to move, causing S_1 to soften.

The *position of the valve* at the time of ventricular contraction affects the intensity of S_1. The *arc of coaptation* is the angle through which the valve closes. If the valve is in a midposition, it travels less than when it closes from a widely opened position. The more it is opened, the wider the arc of coaptation and the louder is S_1. This situation is directly related to the pressure in the left atrium when the left ventricular pressure exceeds it and closes the valve. This can occur in conditions with a shortened PR interval on the electrocardiogram. The mitral valve is opened normally during diastole for ventricular filling. The P wave of the electrocardiogram corresponds to atrial contraction, which elevates left atrial pressure (the "a" wave of the left atrial tracing), further opening the mitral valve in late diastole. If the PR interval is short, ventricular contraction occurs so quickly after atrial contraction that the atrial pressure is still high when the left ventricular pressure exceeds it. The mitral valve stays open longer and closes later than normal during the rapid rate of rise of pressure of the ventricle, which accentuates S_1.

In general, the longer the PR interval, the softer the S_1. Lengthening of the PR intervals, as is seen in the Wenckebach phenomenon,[p] produces an S_1 that softens until the dropped beat occurs.

Whenever the heart is *farther from the chest wall,* the S_1 is softer than normal. In patients who are very obese or have chronic obstructive lung disease, the intensity of the S_1 is softer than normal. In patients with a large pericardial effusion, the S_1 is likewise soft.

Abnormalities of the Second Heart Sound

Abnormalities of the Intensity of the Second Heart Sound

The conditions that change the intensity of S_2 are the following:

- Changes in systolic pressure
- Condition of the valve

Any condition that produces an increase in the systolic pressure increases the intensity of the S_2. Conversely, conditions that lower the systolic pressure soften the S_2. Hypertension raises aortic systolic pressure and produces a loud A_2 component of S_2.

[p]Wenckebach phenomenon, also known as Mobitz I block (type I second-degree AV block), is a progressive prolongation of the PR interval culminating in a non conducted P wave. The PR interval is the longest immediately before the dropped beat, and the PR interval is the shortest immediately after a dropped beat. Wenckebach is usually due to a reversible conduction block at the level of the AV node. It is usually a benign rhythm, causing minimal hemodynamic disturbance and a low risk of progression to third-degree heart block. It may be caused by drugs such as beta-blockers, calcium channel blockers, digoxin, and amiodarone. The prognosis for a patient with the Wenckebach phenomenon is excellent. It is usually asymptomatic and requires no intervention in asymptomatic patients.

Calcification or *fibrosis* of the semilunar valves produces a softening of their closure, S_2. Because the semilunar valves are a morphologically different type of valve, fibrosis does not cause an increased intensity, as in the closure of a fibrotic AV valve.

Abnormalities of Splitting of the Second Heart Sound

Normal physiologic splitting of S_2 was discussed in the section, "The Cardiac Cycle." This section deals with abnormalities of splitting.

Any condition that delays right ventricular systole, either electrically or mechanically, delays P_2 and produces a widened splitting of S_2. Right ventricular emptying is delayed by a right bundle branch block or pulmonic stenosis. The pulmonic component of S_2 is delayed during both inspiration and expiration, and *wide splitting* of S_2 occurs.

Any condition that shortens left ventricular systole allows A_2 to occur earlier than normal, and wide splitting likewise occurs. Conditions such as mitral regurgitation, VSD, and PDA shorten left ventricular systole, and the S_1 to A_2 interval is shorter than normal. In these conditions, there is a "double outlet" to the left ventricle, and systole is shorter. In a VSD, with a left-to-right shunt, not only is the left ventricular systole shorter, but also right ventricular systole is prolonged. Both factors are crucial in producing the wide splitting of S_2.

Any electrical or mechanical condition that delays left ventricular emptying produces *paradoxical splitting* of S_2. Left bundle branch block or aortic stenosis delays left ventricular emptying. These conditions delay the closure of the aortic valve after right ventricular systole and P_2 have occurred. The normal sequence of A_2 to P_2 is reversed. During inspiration, P_2 moves normally away from S_1 toward A_2. The split is said to be *narrowed.* With expiration, P_2 moves normally and approaches S_1; the P_2 to A_2 split widens. This widening during expiration is paradoxical. Other conditions, such as left ventricular failure and severe hypertension, delay left ventricular ejection and cause paradoxical splitting of S_2.

Fixed splitting of S_2 is the auscultatory hallmark of an atrial septal defect. In this situation, the split is wide and does not change with respiration. This is because inspiratory increases in venous return to the right atrium normally raise its pressure. During expiration, the right atrial pressure is lower, but the left-to-right atrial shunt keeps the volume in the right atrium constant during respiration; therefore, normal splitting does not occur.

Normal physiologic splitting of the second heart sound and abnormalities of splitting are illustrated in Fig. 14.37.

Systolic Clicks

Ejection clicks (ECs) are high-pitched sounds that occur early in systole at the onset of ejection and are produced by opening pathologically deformed semilunar valves. Pulmonic or aortic stenosis may produce ECs. The sounds are short and have the quality of a "click." Pulmonic ECs are best heard in the pulmonic area, and aortic ECs are heard in the aortic area. As calcification progresses, the mobility of the valve decreases, and the EC disappears.

Midsystolic clicks are not ECs. They occur in the middle of systole. They may be single or multiple, and they may change position during the cardiac cycle with various maneuvers that change ventricular geometry. The most common condition associated with a midsystolic click is prolapse of the mitral or tricuspid valve.

Diastolic Opening Snaps

An AV valve's opening is usually silent and occurs approximately 100 ms after S_2. This is about the time it takes to say "ma-ma" quickly. An *opening snap* (OS) is a diastolic event that

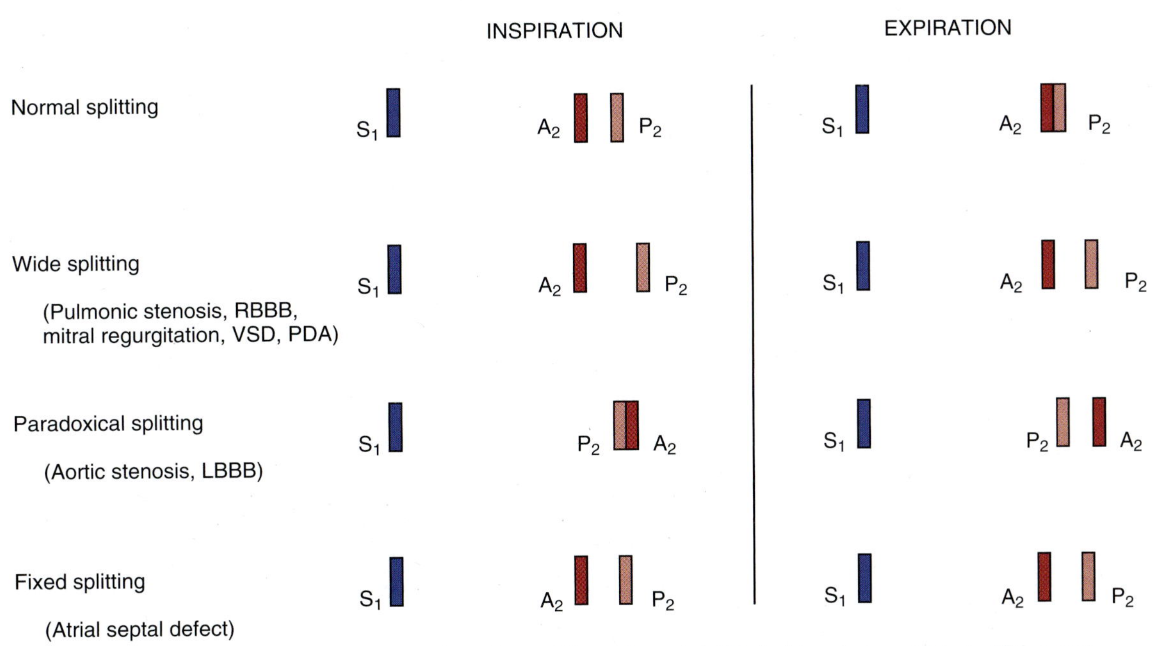

Fig. 14.37 Abnormalities of Splitting of the Second Heart Sound. *LBBB,* Left bundle branch block; *PDA,* patent ductus arteriosus; *RBBB,* right bundle branch block; *VSD,* ventricular septal defect.

is the sound of the opening of a pathologically deformed AV valve. The sound is sharp and high-pitched. The mitral OS of mitral stenosis occurs after A_2; the tricuspid OS of tricuspid stenosis occurs after P_2.

The interval between S_2 and the OS is termed the *S_2 to OS interval* and has specific significance as to the severity of the stenosis. As mitral stenosis worsens, the resistance and obstruction to flow increase. Pressure in the left atrium increases, and the gradient across the mitral valve increases. The mitral valve, therefore, opens earlier than normal when the left ventricular pressure falls below left atrial pressure. The S_2 to OS time shortens as the severity increases. Try saying "ma-da" as quickly as possible. This interval is about 50 to 60 msec and approximates a very short S_2 to OS interval, as heard in severe mitral stenosis.

Murmurs

Murmurs are produced when there is turbulent energy in the walls of the heart and blood vessels. Obstruction to flow or flow from a narrow vessel to a large-diameter vessel creates turbulence. Turbulence sets up eddies that strike the walls to produce vibrations that the examiner recognizes as a murmur. Murmurs can also be produced when there is a large volume of blood through a normal opening. The normal opening is relatively stenotic for the increased volume in this circumstance. "Blowing" murmurs are produced by large gradients with variable flow volumes. "Rumbling" murmurs result from areas of small gradients that depend on flow. "Harsh" murmurs result from large gradients and high flow.

An ejection murmur is produced by turbulence across a semilunar valve during systole, such as in aortic or pulmonic stenosis. Ejection murmurs appear diamond-shaped and are described as "crescendo-decrescendo." They begin slightly after S_1 and end before S_2. An EC from stenosis of the semilunar valve may precede the murmur. These murmurs are medium-pitched and are best heard with the diaphragm of the stethoscope. Because they are based on flow, the intensity of these murmurs does not indicate the degree of severity. Increased flow across a minimally narrowed aortic valve produces a loud murmur; decreased flow across a severely stenotic aortic valve may produce a barely audible murmur. Any increase in flow or volume may produce an ejection murmur, even in the presence of a normal valve. An ejection murmur as a sign of aortic stenosis is a high sensitivity but low specificity finding. Fig. 14.38 illustrates an ejection murmur.

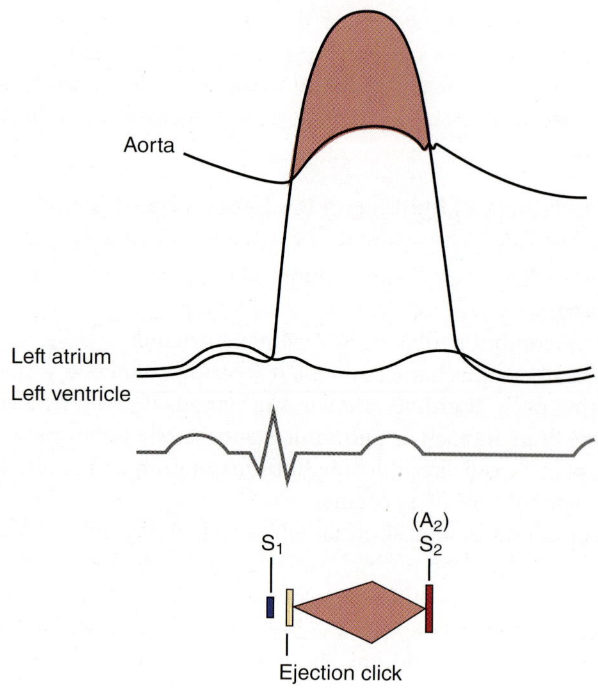

Fig. 14.38 A Systolic Ejection Murmur Such as That Occurs in Aortic Stenosis.

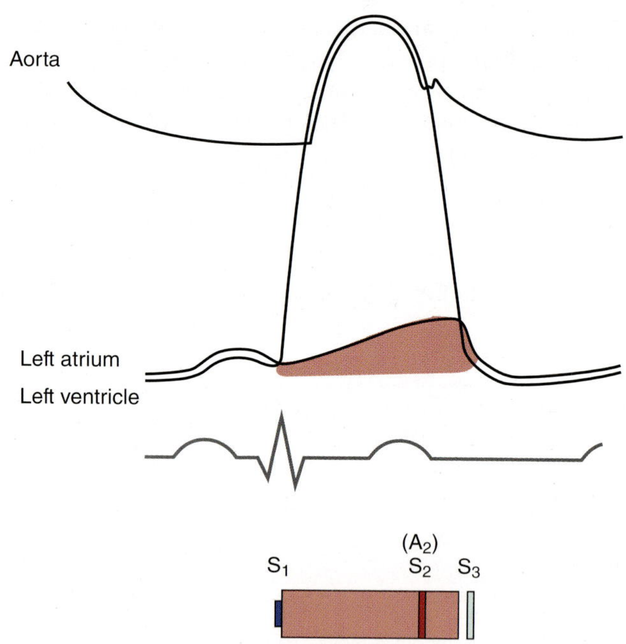

Fig. 14.39 A Systolic Regurgitant Murmur Such as That Occurs in Mitral Regurgitation.

Regurgitant systolic murmurs are produced by retrograde flow from a higher-pressure area to a lower one during systole, such as mitral or tricuspid regurgitation. These murmurs are holosystolic or pansystolic. They begin with S_1 and end after S_2. They extend past S_2 because ventricular pressure is higher than atrial pressure, even after the closure of the semilunar valve. An S_3 indicative of volume overload to the ventricle is often heard. These murmurs are high-pitched and best heard with the stethoscope's diaphragm. The terms *regurgitation, incompetence,* and *insufficiency* are often used synonymously for this type of murmur. The preferred term is *regurgitation* because it implies the retrograde direction of flow. The holosystolic murmur of AV valve regurgitation is a finding of high sensitivity. Fig. 14.39 illustrates a regurgitant murmur.

Diastolic AV murmurs begin after S_2 with the opening of the AV valve. Mitral stenosis and tricuspid stenosis are examples of this type of murmur. There is a pause between S_2 and the beginning of the murmur. Isovolumetric relaxation occurs during this period. The murmur is decrescendo in shape,

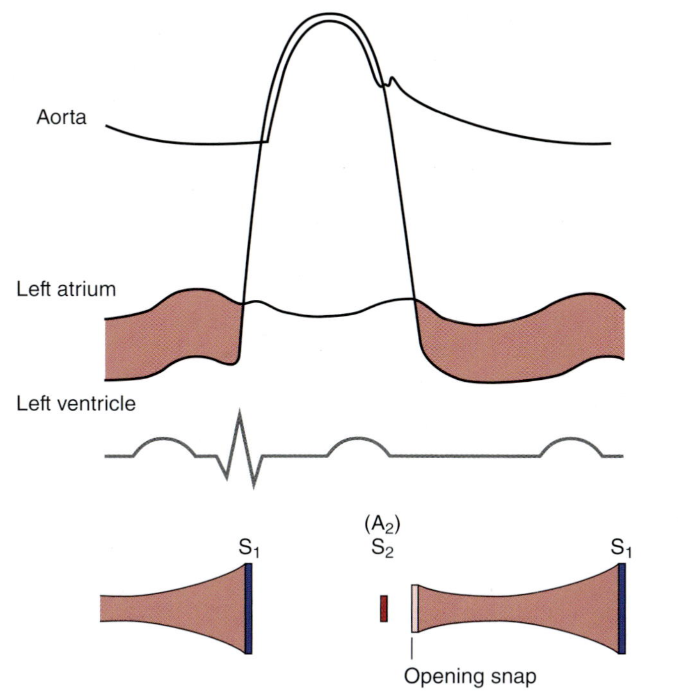

Fig. 14.40 A Diastolic Atrioventricular Murmur Such as That Occurring in Mitral Stenosis.

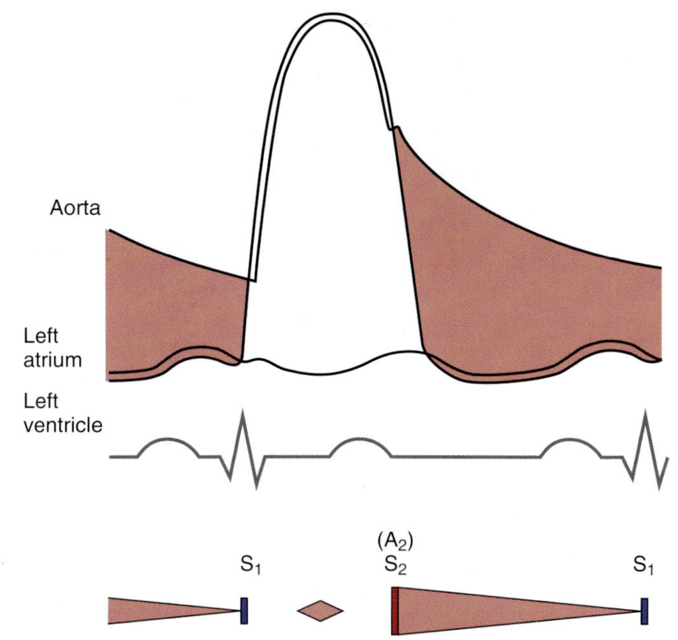

Fig. 14.41 **A Diastolic Semilunar Murmur Such as That Occurring in Aortic Regurgitation.** Note the systolic flow murmur related to the increased volume across the aortic semilunar valve.

beginning with an OS if the valve is mobile. These murmurs are low-pitched and are best heard with the bell of the stethoscope, with the patient lying in the left lateral decubitus position. Because the AV valve is stenotic, rapid filling does not occur, and a gradient persists throughout diastole. If the patient is in normal sinus rhythm, atrial contraction increases the gradient at the end of diastole or presystole, and there is an increase in the murmur then. This is known as *presystolic accentuation*. The diastolic AV murmur is a sensitive and specific sign of AV valve stenosis.

The first heart sound is the loudest. The cadence and emphasis of the sounds are best heard by saying the following mnemonic:

MIT′ – ral – vaaaalve MIT′ – ral – vaaaalve
S_1 S_2 OS DM S_1 S_2 OS DM

in which OS is the mitral OS, and DM is the diastolic murmur. The "aaaalve" is the presystolic accentuation heard when a patient with mitral stenosis is in normal sinus rhythm. Fig. 14.40 illustrates a diastolic AV murmur.

Diastolic semilunar murmurs begin immediately after S_2, as heard in aortic or pulmonic regurgitation. In contrast to the diastolic murmurs, there is no delay after S_2 to the beginning of the murmur. The high-pitched murmur is decrescendo in shape and is best heard with the stethoscope's diaphragm while the patient is sitting up and leaning forward. A diastolic semilunar murmur is a sign of low sensitivity but high specificity. Fig. 14.41 illustrates the pressure curves responsible for the generation of a diastolic semilunar murmur.

Table 14.8 lists important cardiac sounds according to the cardiac cycle. Fig. 14.42 lists and illustrates the characteristics of the systolic murmurs of aortic stenosis and mitral regurgitation. Table 14.9 summarizes the differentiation of some other systolic murmurs. Fig. 14.43 lists and illustrates the characteristics of the diastolic murmurs of mitral stenosis and aortic regurgitation.

TABLE 14.8 Cardiac Sounds

Cardiac Cycle	Sound
Early systolic	Ejection click Aortic prosthetic valve opening sound[a]
Midsystolic to late systolic	Midsystolic click Rub
Early diastolic	Opening snap S_3 Mitral prosthetic valve opening sound[b] Tumor plop[c]
Mid-diastolic	S_3 Summation gallop[d]
Late diastolic (sometimes called *presystolic*)	S_4 Pacemaker sound

[a]Opening and closure of the prosthetic aortic valve are heard with many prosthetic valves. The opening is comparable to an ejection click; the closing is a "prosthetic" S_2.
[b]Opening and closure of the prosthetic mitral valve are heard with many prosthetic valves. The opening is comparable to an opening snap; the closing is a "prosthetic" S_1.
[c]A left atrial myxoma that is pedunculated may "plop" in and out of the mitral annulus, simulating the auscultatory signs of mitral stenosis.
[d]At fast heart rates, the diastolic period shortens. If an S_3 and S_4 are present, the sounds may be summated into a single sound called a *summation gallop*.

Systolic Murmurs Differentiating Aortic Stenosis from Mitral Regurgitation

Feature	Aortic Stenosis	Mitral Regurgitation
Location	Aortic Area	Apex
Radiation	Neck	Axilla
Shape	Diamond	Holosystolic
Pitch	Medium	High
Quality	Harsh	Blowing
Associated signs	Decreased A_2 Ejection click S_4 Narrow pulse pressure Slow rising and delayed pulse	Decreased S_1 S_3 Laterally displaced diffuse PMI

PMI, Point of maximum impulse.

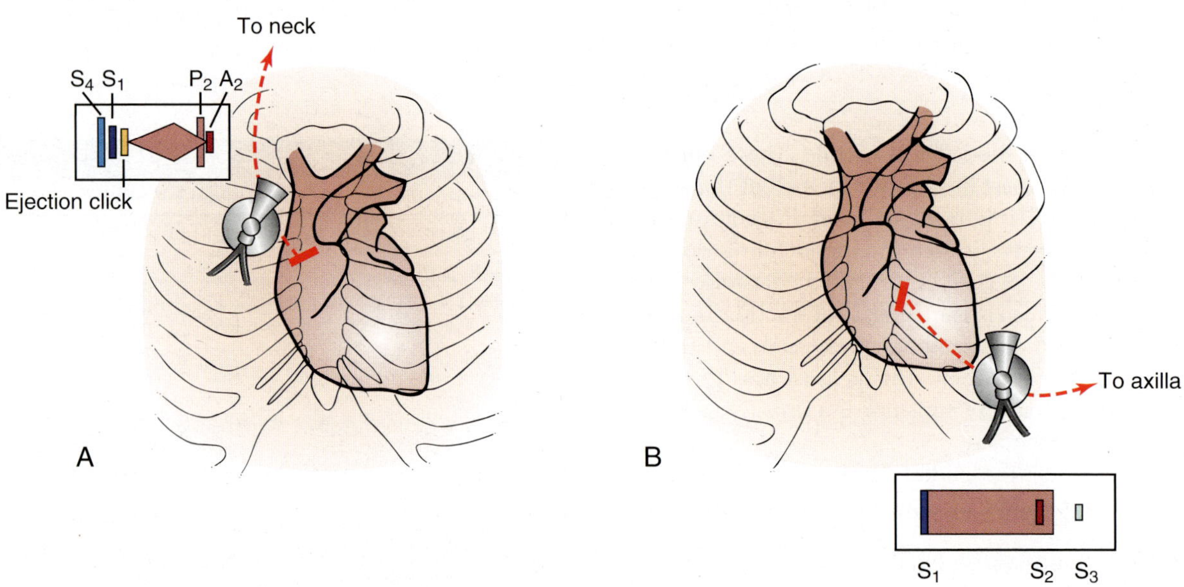

Fig. 14.42 Systolic Murmurs. (A) Pathophysiology of aortic stenosis. Note the paradoxical splitting of the second heart sound *(S_2)*, the *S_4*, and the ejection click. (B) Mitral regurgitation. Note that the murmur ends after *S_2* and note the presence of the *S_3*.

TABLE 14.9 Differentiation of Other Systolic Murmurs

Feature	Pulmonic Stenosis	Tricuspid Regurgitation	Ventricular Septal Defect	Venous Hum	Innocent Murmur
Location	Pulmonic area	Tricuspid area	Tricuspid area	Above clavicle	Widespread[a]
Radiation	Neck	Right of sternum	Right of sternum	Right neck	Minimal
Shape	Diamond	Holosystolic	Holosystolic	Continuous	Diamond
Pitch	Medium	High	High	High	Medium
Quality	Harsh	Blowing	Harsh	Roaring; humming	Twanging; vibratory

[a]Usually between the apex and the left lower sternal border.

Diastolic Murmurs Differentiating Mitral Stenosis from Aortic Regurgitation

Feature	Mitral Stenosis	Aortic Regurgitation
Location	Apex	Aortic Area
Radiation	No	No
Shape	Decrescendo	Decrescendo
Pitch	Low	High
Quality	Rumbling	Blowing
Associated signs	Increased S_1 Opening snap RV rock* Presystolic accentuation	S_3 Laterally displaced PMI Wide pulse pressure† Bounding pulses Austin Flint murmur‡ Systolic ejection murmur§

PMI, Point of maximum impulse; RV, right ventricular.

*Right ventricular impulse at lower left sternal border.

†The wide pulse pressure is the cause of the many physical signs of aortic regurgitations: Quincke's pulse, De Musset's sign, Duroziez's sign, Corrigan's pulse, and so forth.

‡An apical diastolic murmur head in association with aortic regurgitation, mimicking that of mitral stenosis.

§A flow murmur across a valve that is relatively narrow for the increased blood volume as a result of aortic regurgitation. It is relatively stenotic and need not be anatomically stenotic, as in true aortic stenosis.

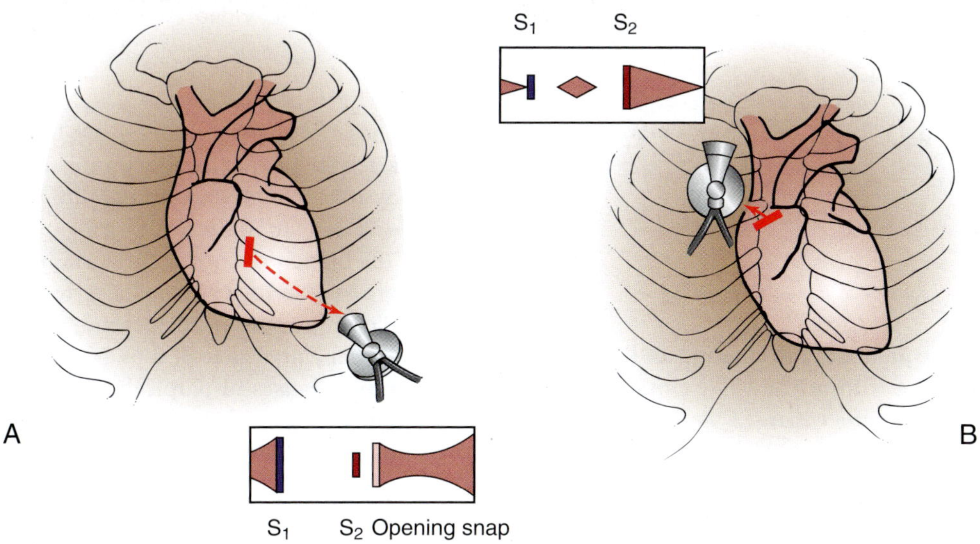

Fig. 14.43 Diastolic Murmurs. (A) Pathophysiology of mitral stenosis. Note the intensity of S_1 and the accentuation of the diastolic murmur in late diastole. (B) Aortic regurgitation. Note the mid-systolic flow murmur.

USEFUL VOCABULARY

Listed here are the specific roots that are important for understanding the terminology related to cardiac disease.

Root	Pertaining to	Example	Definition
brady-	slow	***brady***cardia	Slow heart rate
-cardio-	heart	***cardio***megaly	Enlargement of the heart
sphygmo-	pulse	***sphygmo***manometer	Instrument for measuring blood pressure
supra-	above	***supra***ventricular	Above the level of the ventricles
tachy-	fast	***tachy***cardia	Rapid heart rate

WRITING UP THE PHYSICAL EXAMINATION

Listed here are examples of the write-up for the examination of the heart.

- No abnormal jugular venous distention or abnormal jugular waveforms are present. The PMI is in the fifth intercostal space, midclavicular line. S_1 and S_2 are normal.[q]
- Physiologic splitting is present. No murmurs, gallops, or rubs are heard. There is no clubbing, cyanosis, or edema.
- The jugular venous pressure is elevated. There is a prominent "v" wave present in the neck. The jugular vein is distended 8 cm above the sternal angle at 45 degrees. The PMI is in the sixth intercostal space, anterior axillary line. S_1 is soft. S_2 is widely split on inspiration and expiration. A grade III/VI, high-pitched, holosystolic murmur is heard with radiation to the axilla at the apex. A palpable S_3 is present at the apex. There is 2+ pitting edema on the shins bilaterally. No cyanosis or clubbing is present.
- No abnormal jugular venous distention is seen. The PMI is in the fifth intercostal space, midclavicular line. S_1 is normal. S_2 is soft. An S_4 is present at the apex. A grade IV/VI, harsh, medium-pitched, crescendo-decrescendo murmur, beginning slightly after S_1 and ending before S_2, is present in the aortic area. This murmur radiates to both carotid arteries. No clubbing, cyanosis, or edema is present.
- The jugular venous pressure is significantly elevated. The jugular vein is distended to the jaw margin when the patient is seated at 90 degrees. The PMI is in the fifth intercostal space, midclavicular line. S_1 is accentuated. S_2 is normal. An RV rock is present at the left lower sternal border. There is a grade II/VI, low-pitched, diastolic rumble heard at the apex, best heard in the left lateral decubitus position. A grade III/VI, high-pitched, holosystolic murmur is heard at the left lower sternal border, which increases in intensity with inspiration. A right ventricular S_3 may be present at the left lower sternal border.[r]
- There is 4+ pitting sacral edema. No cyanosis or clubbing is present.

[q]The descriptors for S_1 and S_2 are *normal, increased, decreased, widely split, narrowly split, fixed split,* or *paradoxically split.* Never indicate that S_1 and S_2 are present.
[r]Notice that in this example the examiner stated that a finding may be present.
PMI, Point of maximum impulse; *RV,* right ventricular.

FULL VIDEOS

- Video 14.16 Full video: Examining the carotid artery and jugular venous pulses
- Video 14.17 Full video: Examining the heart and lungs (sitting)
- Video 14.18 Full video: Assessing blood pressure

REVIEW QUESTIONS

1. **Which of the following can put people at a higher risk of heart disease?**
   A. Diabetes
   B. Obesity
   C. Poor diet
   D. Alcohol misuse
   E. All of the above
2. **What is the correct sequence of the opening and closing of the four valves starting with mitral valve closure? *MV = mitral valve; PV = pulmonic valve; TV = tricuspid valve; AV = aortic valve; o = opening; c = closing***
   A. MVc-PVo-TVc-AVo-PVc-AVc-TVo-MVo
   B. MVc-TVc-PVo-AVo-AVc-PVc-TVo-MVo
   C. MVc-TVc-AVo-PVo-PVc-AVc-MVo-TVo
   D. MVc-AVo-TVc-PVc-PVo-AVc-TVo-MVo
   E. None of the above
3. **Which statement regarding chest pain is incorrect?**
   A. Chest pain is not pathognomonic for heart disease.
   B. Chest pain may result from pulmonary, intestinal, gallbladder and musculoskeletal disorders.
   C. Angina pectoris is the true symptom of coronary heart disease.
   D. Levine's sign is not a pathognomonic sign for angina pectoris.
   E. Occasionally patients with coronary heart disease may describe their pain as "discomfort" or "pressure."
4. **Which of the following statement about blood pressure is correct?**
   A. Blood pressure does not depend on the volume of blood ejected, its velocity, and the distensibility of the arterial wall.
   B. Diastolic blood pressure is not the lowest pressure in the arteries; it depends only on the peripheral resistance.
   C. Systolic blood pressure in the legs is 15-20 mm Hg greater than in the arms.
   D. The blood pressure in the aorta is greater than the blood pressure in the branched arteries of the lower extremity.
   E. Blood pressure is not dependent on a person's degree of excitement, degree of activity, pain, or bladder distension.
5. **Common causes of palpitations include all the following *except:***
   A. Bronchodilators
   B. Caffeine
   C. Smoking
   D. Antidepressants
   E. Medications for diarrhea
6. **According to the American Heart Association, a blood pressure of 135/85 is considered:**
   A. Normal
   B. Prehypertension (borderline)
   C. High blood pressure (stage 1)
   D. High blood pressure (stage 2)
   E. Hypertensive crisis
7. **An anacrotic pulse (also known as a plateau pulse or a *pulsus parvus et tardus*) is seen in which of the follow clinical conditions?**
   A. Aortic stenosis
   B. Aortic regurgitation
   C. Congestive heart failure
   D. Tamponade
   E. Constrictive pericarditis

8. **The factors that are responsible for the intensity of the first heart sound (S_1) are:**
   A. The rate of rise of ventricular pressure
   B. The condition of the valve
   C. The position of the valve
   D. The distance of the heart from the chest wall
   E. All of the above
9. **Which of the following conditions is *not* associated with wide splitting of the second heart sound (S_2)?**
   A. Pulmonic stenosis
   B. Right bundle branch block
   C. Mitral regurgitation
   D. Aortic stenosis
   E. Ventricular septal defect
10. **Comparing the systolic murmurs of aortic stenosis and mitral regurgitation, which of the following statement is false?**
   A. The murmur of aortic stenosis is best heard in the aortic area.
   B. The murmur of mitral regurgitation radiates to the axilla.
   C. The murmur of aortic stenosis is diamond shaped.
   D. The murmur of mitral regurgitation has a blowing quality.
   E. The murmur of aortic stenosis has a rumbling quality.
11. **Comparing the diastolic murmurs of mitral stenosis and aortic regurgitation, which of the following statement is true?**
   A. The murmur of mitral stenosis is best heard at the left sternal border.
   B. The murmur of aortic regurgitation does not radiate.
   C. The murmur of mitral stenosis is holodiastolic.
   D. The murmur of aortic regurgitation is low-pitched.
   E. The quality of the murmur of mitral stenosis is harsh.

REFERENCES

Available online.

BIBLIOGRAPHY

Available online.

15

The Peripheral Vascular System

Mark H. Swartz

"Veins which by the thickening of their tunicles in the old restrict the passage of blood, and by this lack of nourishment destroy their life without any fever, the old coming to fail little by little in slow death."

Leonardo da Vinci (1452–1519)

VIDEOS

Video 15.1	Palpating the radial artery pulse
Video 15.2	Palpating the brachial artery pulse
Video 15.3	Auscultating the carotid artery pulse
Video 15.4	Palpating the femoral artery pulse and evaluating for coarctation of the aorta
Video 15.5	Palpating the popliteal artery pulse
Video 15.6	Palpating the dorsalis pedis artery pulse
Video 15.7	Palpating the posterior tibial artery pulse
Video 15.8	Full video: Examining the peripheral vascular system
Also, see	
Video 14.16	Full video: Examining the carotid artery and jugular venous pulses

GENERAL CONSIDERATIONS

Diseases of the peripheral vascular system are common and may involve the arteries, veins, or lymphatic vessels. The arterial conditions include cerebrovascular, aortoiliac, femoropopliteal, renal, aortic occlusive, and aneurysmal diseases. The two most important diseases of the peripheral arteries are atherosclerosis of the larger arteries and microvascular disease. Peripheral vascular disease (PVD) is a nearly pandemic condition that can potentially cause the loss of a limb or even loss of life.

The most common cause of peripheral arterial occlusive disease is atherosclerosis that affects the medium-sized and large vessels of the extremities. Narrowing of the vessel causes a decreased blood supply, resulting in ischemia. PVD is a common disorder that usually affects males older than age 50. People are at higher risk if they have a history of:

- Abnormal cholesterol
- Diabetes
- Coronary artery disease
- Hypertension
- Kidney disease involving hemodialysis
- Smoking
- Strokes

Fig. 15.1 summarizes the risk factors for PVD according to the Framingham Heart Study.[a] This study established the traditional risk factors, such as high blood pressure, diabetes, and cigarette smoking for coronary heart disease and PVD. The study showed that cigarette smoking was associated with increased risk of heart disease. Increased cholesterol and blood pressure also increase the risk of heart and PVD. It has been more than 75 years since this small, middle-class community 23 miles west of Boston became the foundation in helping to solve the mysteries of heart and vascular disease.[1]

The classic symptoms of PVD are pain, heaviness, fatigue, burning, or discomfort in the muscles of your feet, calves, or thighs. These symptoms usually appear during walking or exercise and go away after several minutes of rest. At first, these symptoms may occur only when the patient walks uphill, walks faster, or walks for longer distances. Slowly, these symptoms come on more quickly and with less exercise. The legs or feet may feel numb while at rest. The legs also may feel cool to the touch, and the skin may look pale. When peripheral artery disease becomes severe, the patient may experience:

- Erectile dysfunction
- Pain and cramps at night
- Pain or tingling in the feet or toes, which can be so severe that even the weight of clothes or bedsheets is painful
- Pain that is worse when raising the leg and improves when dangling the legs over the side of the bed
- Skin that looks dark and blue
- Sores that do not heal

Atherosclerosis may become manifest by aneurysmal dilatation. The abdominal aorta is commonly affected. An abdominal aortic aneurysm (AAA) is a focal dilation 50% greater than the normal diameter of the aorta. The aneurysm is commonly below the renal arteries and may extend as far as the external iliac arteries. There are several well-defined risk factors associated with the development of AAA. They include advanced age, male sex, White race, a positive family history, smoking, other

[a]A project of the National Heart Institute (now known as the National Heart, Lung, and Blood Institute) and Boston University (1948).

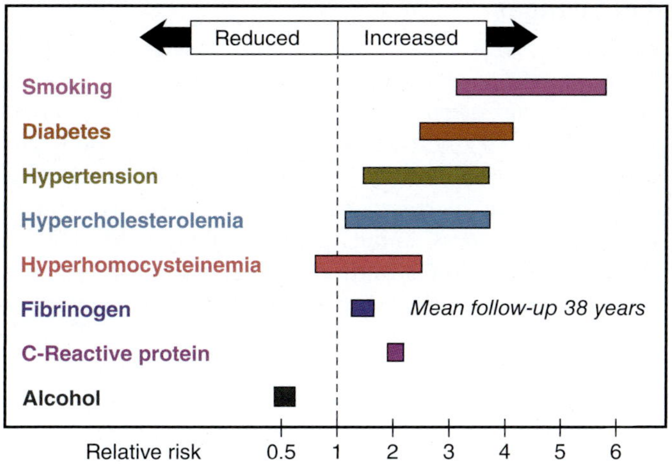

Fig. 15.1 Risk Factors for Peripheral Vascular Disease: Framingham Heart Study.

large vessel aneurysms, and atherosclerosis. AAA is 5 times more common in males than females and 3.5 times more common in White males than Black males.[2] Ruptured AAA is a vascular surgical emergency in which 50% of patients die before reaching the hospital and may carry an overall mortality rate of 80% to 90%.[3] The Centers for Disease Control ranks AAA as one of the top 15 causes of mortality in the United States in individuals between the ages of 85 to 89. In 2019, aortic aneurysms or aortic dissections were the cause of 9904 deaths.[4]

Often, AAA produces few, if any, symptoms. The examiner may discover a pulsatile mass as an incidental finding. Frequently, the first manifestation is the catastrophic rupture of the aneurysm. An AAA larger than 5 cm in diameter carries a 20% risk of rupturing within the first year of discovery and a 50% risk within five years.

Vesalius described the first AAA in the 16th century. Before the development of surgical intervention for the process, attempts at medical management failed. The initial surgical attempts at control entailed ligation of the aorta, with poor results. In 1923, Rudolph Matas performed the first successful aortic ligation on a patient. Attempts were made to induce thrombosis by inserting intraluminal wires. In 1948, C. E. Rea wrapped reactive cellophane around the aneurysm to induce fibrosis and limit expansion. This technique was used on Albert Einstein in 1949, and he survived 6 years before dying of rupture. However, not until 1951 was an abdominal aneurysm surgically treated by resection and grafting. That year, C. Dubost performed the first AAA repair with a homograft. Since then, great strides have been made in understanding the natural history of vascular disease and developing new technology to help diagnose and treat it.

Microvascular arterial disease occurs in patients with diabetes. Changes develop in the small arterioles that impair circulation to the skin or nerves, especially of the lower extremities, producing symptoms of ischemia. Peripheral neuropathy is a common sequela of microvascular disease. This neuropathy may manifest as a sensory, motor, or autonomic system defect. Microvascular disease affects more than 15 million individuals in the United States. In patients with diabetes, there is the tragic "Rule of 15," which states:

- Fifteen percent of all people with diabetes will develop a foot ulcer sometime in life.
- Fifteen percent of those foot ulcers will lead to osteomyelitis.
- Fifteen percent of foot ulcers lead to amputation.

Also, in patients with diabetes, the "Rule of 50" states that:

- Fifty percent of amputations are at the transfemoral/transtibial level.
- Fifty percent of patients have a second amputation in 5 years or less.
- Fifty percent of patients die in 5 years or less.

Peripheral venous disease often progresses to venous stasis and thrombotic disorders. One of the dreaded complications of thrombotic disease is pulmonary embolism (PE). More than 175,000 deaths annually are attributed to acute PE in the United States.

STRUCTURE AND PHYSIOLOGY

Diseases of the peripheral *arterial* system cause ischemia of the extremities. When the body is at rest, collateral blood vessels may be able to provide adequate circulation. During exercise, when oxygen demand increases, this circulation may not be sufficient for the actively contracting muscles, and ischemia may result. Remember that blood pressure in the lower extremity is higher than in the upper extremity. This forms the basis for the ankle-branchial index test, discussed later in this chapter.

The *venous system* consists of a series of low-pressure capacitance vessels. Nearly 70% of the blood volume is contained in this system. Although offering little resistance, the veins are controlled by various neural and humoral stimuli that enhance venous return to the right side of the heart. In addition, valves aid in the return of blood.

When an individual is upright, the venous pressure in the lower extremity is the highest. Over many years, the veins dilate due to the weakening of their walls. The veins cannot close adequately as the walls dilate, and blood reflux occurs. In addition, the venous pump becomes less efficient in returning blood to the heart. Both factors are responsible for the venous stasis in patients with chronic venous insufficiency. Complications from venous stasis include pigmentation, dermatitis, cellulitis, ulceration, and thrombus formation.

The *lymphatic system* is an extensive vascular network that returns tissue fluid (lymph) to the venous system. The extremities are richly supplied with lymphatic tissue. Lymph nodes, many located between major proximal joints, aid in filtering the lymphatic fluid before it enters the blood. The most important clinical symptoms of lymphatic obstruction are *lymphedema* and *lymphangitis.*

REVIEW OF SPECIFIC SYMPTOMS

Many patients with PVD are asymptomatic. When patients are symptomatic, vascular disease causes the following:

- Pain
- Changes in skin temperature and color
- Edema
- Ulceration

- Emboli
- Stroke
- Dizziness

Pain

Pain is the principal symptom of atherosclerosis. Whenever a patient complains of pain in the calf, arch of the foot, thighs, hips, or buttocks while walking, PVD of the arteries must be considered. The symptom of pain in the lower extremity during exercise and relieved by rest is called *intermittent claudication*. The site of the pain is always distal to the occlusive disease. **Supply does not equal demand.** As the disease progresses, pain at rest occurs. This is often severe and is aggravated by cool temperatures and elevation, especially during sleep in bed. Pain may also occur with deep vein thrombosis (DVT), a condition known as *venous claudication*. The combination of venous valvular incompetence, outflow obstruction, and calf muscle pump function derangement generates the hemodynamic setting most often associated with developing venous claudication. A unique feature of venous claudication is that motionless standing is often more difficult than walking. This is because the contraction of the muscles in our legs while walking pumps blood through the veins and back to the heart. *Neurogenic claudication* is a common symptom of lumbar spinal stenosis or inflammation of the nerves emanating from the spinal cord. The pain is often related to posture. The combination of the stenosis with specific back postures, such as arching, puts pressure on the lumbosacral nerve roots and the cauda equina. Table 15.1 describes the differences between intermittent claudication, venous claudication, and neurogenic claudication.

If a male patient complains of pain in the buttocks, hips, or thighs while walking, the examiner should inquire about erectile dysfunction. The patient may also experience leg numbness or weakness. *Leriche syndrome*[5] is commonly referred to as aortoiliac occlusive disease; the patient presents with intermittent claudication and erectile dysfunction. Leriche syndrome presents a triad of claudication, impotence, and absence of femoral pulses. In this condition, severe atherosclerosis at the aortic bifurcation involves the terminal aorta and iliac arteries. While impotence and sexual dysfunction may occur in most patients, the hallmark of Leriche syndrome is reduced or absent femoral pulses.[6]

Patients occasionally complain of bilateral leg pain or numbness while walking and resting. This is called *pseudoclaudication*, a symptom of musculoskeletal disease in the lumbar area.

Skin Changes

Skin color changes are common with vascular disease. In chronic *arterial insufficiency*, the affected extremity is cool and pale. In chronic *venous insufficiency*, the extremity is warmer than usual. The leg becomes erythematous, and erosions produced by excoriation result. With chronic insufficiency, stasis changes produce increased pigmentation, swelling, and an "aching" or "heaviness" in the legs. These changes characteristically occur in the lower third of the extremity and are more prominent medially. When venous insufficiency occurs, edema of dependent areas results.

Patients with acute DVT have secondary inflammation of the tissue surrounding the vein. This produces signs of inflammation: warmth, redness, and fever. Swelling is the most reliable symptom and sign associated with venous obstruction. This finding indicates severe deep vein obstruction because the superficial veins of the lower extremity carry only 20% of the total drainage and are not associated with swelling. The extremities should be compared, and a difference in circumference of 2 cm at the ankle or midcalf should be considered significant.

Edema

Lymphedema results from a primary abnormality in the lymphatic system's development or an acquired flow obstruction. Whether the congenital or the acquired form is involved, the net result is stasis of lymph fluid in the tissues, producing a *firm, nonpitting edema*. Over several years, the skin develops a rough consistency similar to a pigskin's. Because lymphedema is usually painless, the only symptom is "heaviness" of the extremity. Look at Fig. 16.8, which shows a patient with marked lymphedema secondary to inflammatory breast carcinoma. Her only complaint was the "heaviness" of her left arm!

Ulceration

Persistent ischemia of a limb is associated with ischemic ulceration and gangrene. Ulceration is almost inevitable once the skin has thickened and the circulation is compromised. Ulceration related to arterial insufficiency occurs due to trauma to the toes and heel. These painful ulcers have discrete edges that produce a "punched-out" appearance and are often covered with crust. When infected, the tissue is erythematous.

In contrast to arterial insufficiency ulceration, venous insufficiency leads to stasis ulceration, which is painless and occurs in the ankle area or lower leg just above the medial malleolus. The classic manifestation is a diffusely reddened, thickened area

TABLE 15.1 Differential Diagnosis of Intermittent Claudication

	Intermittent Claudication	Venous Claudication	Neurogenic Claudication
Quality of pain	Cramping	Aching, heaviness, tightness	"Pins and needles" sensation going down the leg, weakness
Onset	Gradual, consistent	Gradual; can, however, be immediate	Can be immediate
Relieved by	Stopping walking	Activity, elevation of leg	Sitting down, stooping, flexion at the waist
Location	Muscle groups (e.g., buttocks, thigh, calf)	Whole leg	Poorly localized, but can affect whole leg
Legs affected	Usually one	Usually one	Often both

over the medial malleolus. The skin has a cobblestone appearance resulting from fibrosis and venous stasis. Ulceration occurs with the slightest trauma. Rapidly developing ulcers are commonly caused by arterial insufficiency, whereas slowly developing ulceration is usually the result of venous insufficiency. Figs. 15.2 and 15.3 show stasis dermatitis and ulcerations over the medial malleoli. Patients with leg ulcers should be asked the following:

"What did the ulcer look like when it first appeared?"
"What do you think started the ulcer?"
"How quickly did it develop?"
"How painful is the ulcer?"
"What kind of medications have you been taking?"

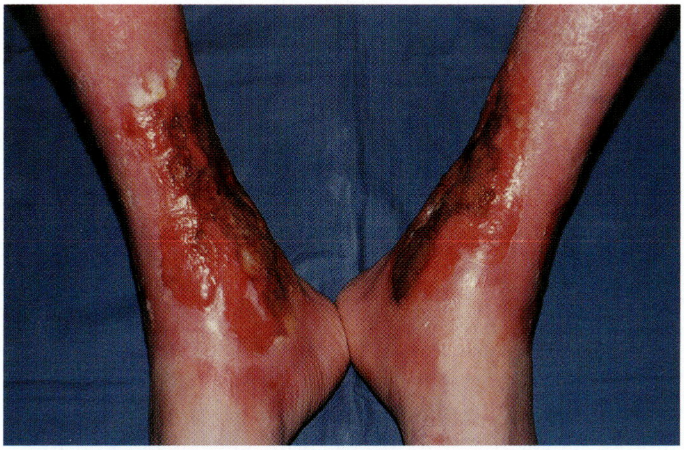

Fig. 15.2 Stasis Dermatitis and Bilateral Ulceration From Venous Insufficiency Over the Medial Malleoli.

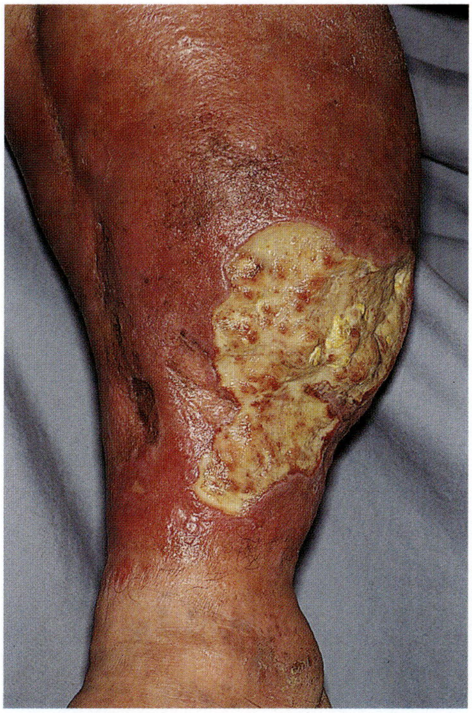

Fig. 15.3 Stasis Dermatitis and Ulceration From Venous Insufficiency Over the Medial Malleolus. (From Callen JP, Paller AS, Greer KE, et al: *Color atlas of dermatology*, ed 2, Philadelphia, 2000, WB Saunders.)

"Is there a history of any generalized diseases, such as anemia? Rheumatoid arthritis?"
"Is there a family history of leg ulcers?"

Emboli

Taking a history of emboli is essential. Thrombus formation results from stasis and hypercoagulability. It appears, however, that venous stasis is the most crucial cause of thrombus formation. Bed rest, congestive heart failure, obesity, pregnancy, recently extended airplane travel, and oral contraceptives have been linked to thrombus formation and emboli.

Symptoms secondary to emboli include shortness of breath from pulmonary emboli; abdominal pain from splenic, intestinal, or renal artery emboli; neurologic symptoms from carotid or vertebrobasilar artery emboli; and pain and paresthesias from peripheral artery emboli.

Neurologic Symptoms

Cerebrovascular occlusive disease causes many neurologic symptoms, including strokes,[b] dizziness, and changes in consciousness. Occlusion of the internal carotid artery (ICA) produces a syndrome of contralateral hemiplegia, blurred vision or vision loss, contralateral sensory deficits, and problems with thinking, reasoning, memory, and speech. Acute ICA occlusion is associated with large infarcts and poor clinical outcomes and contributes to morbidity and mortality worldwide. It has an incidence rate of approximately 6 per 100,000 individuals and may account for 15,000 to 20,000 ischemic events in the United States annually.[7]

Vertebrobasilar insufficiency (VBI)[8] represents inadequate blood flow through the posterior circulation of the brain, which is supplied by the two vertebral arteries that merge to form the basilar artery. The vertebrobasilar arteries supply the cerebellum, medulla, midbrain, and occipital cortex. Because the cerebellum is involved, survivors are often left with dysfunction of many organs, including ataxia, hemiplegia, gaze abnormalities, dysarthria,[c] dysphagia,[d] and cranial nerve palsies. About a quarter of strokes and TIAs occur in the vertebrobasilar distribution.

EFFECT OF VASCULAR DISEASE ON THE PATIENT

A patient with chronic arterial insufficiency has worsening pain while walking. As the condition progresses, ulceration of the toes, feet, and areas susceptible to trauma, such as the shins, develops. Pain may become excruciating. Gangrene of a toe may develop, and amputation of the toe is frequently followed

[b]A stroke is also known as a *cerebrovascular accident (CVA)*.
[c]Dysarthria is a motor speech disorder caused by muscle problems; it can make it hard to talk. This happens when brain or nerve damage changes the way muscles work. People may have trouble understanding what is being said.
[d]Dysphagia is a disorder of difficulty swallowing or moving food and liquids from the mouth to the stomach. Dysphagia can be painful. In some cases, swallowing may be impossible.

by amputation of the foot and leg. In addition, the patient becomes increasingly depressed due to the ongoing mutilation of the body.

PHYSICAL EXAMINATION

The equipment necessary to examine the peripheral vascular system consists of a stethoscope, a tourniquet, and a tape measure.

The physical examination of the peripheral vascular system consists of inspection, palpation, auscultation, and some additional tests if the disease is thought to be present.

General Inspection

The patient should be examined in the standing position and suitably undressed to preserve the modesty of the patient but also to permit complete examination of the entire lower extremity from the groin to the toes. The upper extremity should be exposed from the hands to the axilla. Both upper and lower limbs should be inspected carefully from the front and behind. Examine the four extremities for erythema, cyanosis, swelling, asymmetry, deformities, edema, hair loss, surgical scars, and skin color changes.

Inspect the Upper Extremities

The extremities should be compared for asymmetries in size, color, temperature, and venous patterns. Fig. 15.4 depicts massive lymphedema of the right upper extremity secondary to a right total mastectomy 18 years earlier.

Inspect the Lower Extremities

The lower extremities should be inspected for asymmetries in size, pigmentary abnormalities, ulcers, edema, and venous patterns. Is cyanosis present? Is edema present? If edema is present, does it pit? Bilateral color changes and swelling of the legs of the patient are pictured in Fig. 15.5. The patient had chronic venous insufficiency. She died of a massive pulmonary embolus 1 day after this photograph was taken.

Assess the Skin Temperature

Evaluate the temperature by using the back of your hand. Compare similar areas of each extremity. The coolness of an extremity is typical of arterial insufficiency.

Inspect for Varicosities

Inspect the lower extremities for varicosities. Look at the area of the proximal femoral ring and the distal portion of the legs. Varicose veins in these locations may not have been visible when the patient was lying down.

Varicosities of the *long saphenous vein* appear on the medial side of the leg, running anterior to the medial malleolus, up the medial aspect of the leg, before emptying into the femoral vein in the femoral triangle. The *short saphenous vein* runs on the posterior side of the leg, running posterior to the lateral malleolus, along the posterior aspect of the calf, before emptying into the popliteal vein between the two heads of the gastrocnemius muscle.

The patient in Fig. 15.6 was a 37-year-old female with severe right-sided heart failure. Notice the marked dilated and tortuous veins in the popliteal fossa. Also, notice the increased pigmentation of the skin over the lower legs. Fig. 15.7 shows another female, 65 years of age, with marked bilateral lower extremity varicosities extending from the groin down the entire legs. This most likely indicates insufficiency of the long saphenous vein. Despite the appearance, she suffered no other symptoms.

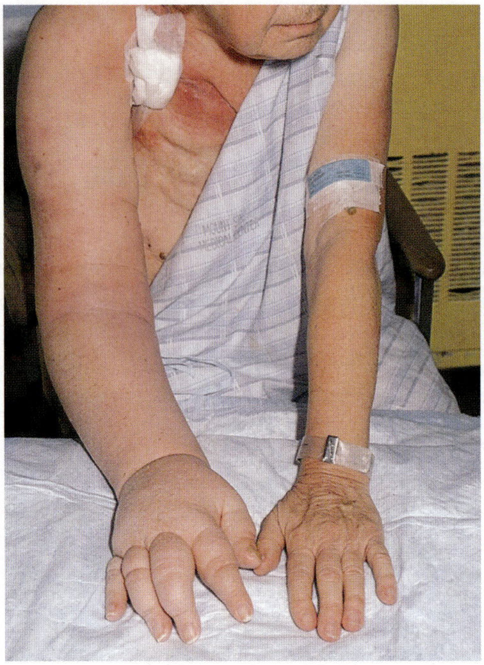

Fig. 15.4 Lymphedema.

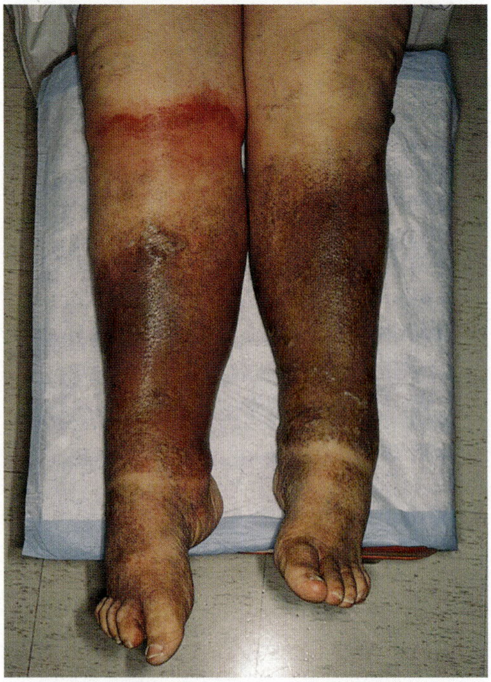

Fig. 15.5 Chronic Venous Insufficiency.

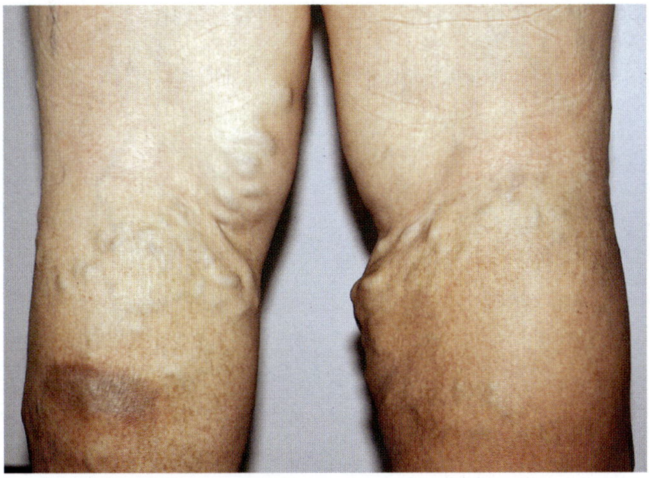

Fig. 15.6 Marked Varicosities of the Popliteal Fossa.

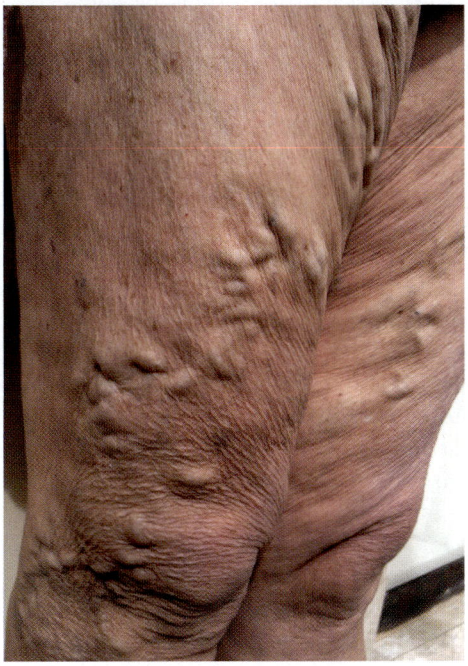

Fig. 15.7 Marked Bilateral Varicosities on the Lower Extremity.

Inspect for Ulceration

Arterial ulcerations are generally painful, found distally on the extremities, and have discrete borders. Venous ulcerations are usually painless, found above or over the medial malleolus, shallow, and have poorly defined borders (see Figs. 15.2 and 15.3). The entire leg will often become swollen with venous ulceration, and the skin will become firm and reddish-brown in color, known as *stasis dermatitis*.

Venous ulcers, also known as *stasis, insufficiency,* or *varicose ulcers*, result from malfunctioning venous valves causing pressure increase in the veins. This resulting venous hypertension causes blood pooling and stretching of the thin venous wall. This wall thinning allows fluid to seep into the surrounding subcutaneous tissue, causing edema. There is an eventual breakdown of tissue due to lack of oxygen; ulceration and necrosis result. Infection of the damaged tissue is a common complication.

In addition to chronic venous insufficiency, various other conditions and risk factors can affect blood flow in the legs and feet and lead to stasis dermatitis. These include being female, over 50 years of age, high blood pressure, obesity, having multiple pregnancies, heart or kidney failure, having low levels of physical activity, and a history of cellulitis.

Palpation

The patient should be supine for venous and arterial palpation of the lower extremities.

Venous Palpation

Palpate the saphenofemoral junction (SFJ) that is approximately 3 to 4 cm inferolateral to the pubic tubercle near the inguinal ligament. Ask the patient to cough while palpating this area and determine whether any impulse or thrill is felt. A palpable thrill results from turbulent retrograde flow at the SFJ. A *saphena varix* is a varicosity where the saphenous vein meets the femoral vein in the SFJ. It is often seen as a bluish swelling at the SFJ. It may be mistaken for a femoral hernia.

Saphenopopliteal reflux may be present in about 25% of patients with primary varicose veins. It is invariably associated with a palpable short saphenous vein in the popliteal fossa. Palpation of the short saphenous vein in the popliteal fossa has a sensitivity of 98% and a specificity of 75% in the diagnosis of saphenopopliteal incompetence.[9]

Arterial Palpation

When examining the peripheral arterial tree, a decreased or absent pulse is the most critical finding. When examining pulses, consistently record the amplitude, rate, and if any blood vessel tenderness, tortuosity, or nodularity exists. A warm environment is preferable, as a cool environment may cause peripheral vasoconstriction that can reduce the intensity of the peripheral pulse.

The patient's socks or stockings must be removed when the examiner assesses the peripheral pulses of the lower extremities. If there is confusion about whether you are feeling the patient's pulse or your pulse, you can palpate the patient's pulse with your right hand and use your left hand to palpate your right radial pulse. If the pulses are different, you are feeling the patient's pulse with your right hand. The thumb carries the greatest likelihood of confusion with the examiner's pulse, especially with a lower amplitude pulse like the radial pulse.

The radial, brachial, femoral, popliteal, dorsalis pedis, and posterior tibial pulses are routinely evaluated, although examination of the arterial pulses may miss up to 50% of PVD.

Grading of Amplitude of the Pulse

The description of the amplitude of the pulse is most important. The following pulse four-point scale is the most widely accepted grading system:

0 No palpable pulse; absent

1+ Faint, but detectable pulse; easily obliterated with pressure

2+ Normal, easily identified; not easily obliterated with pressure

3+ Increased pulse; obliterated with moderate pressure

4+ Strong, bounding pulse; cannot be obliterated with pressure

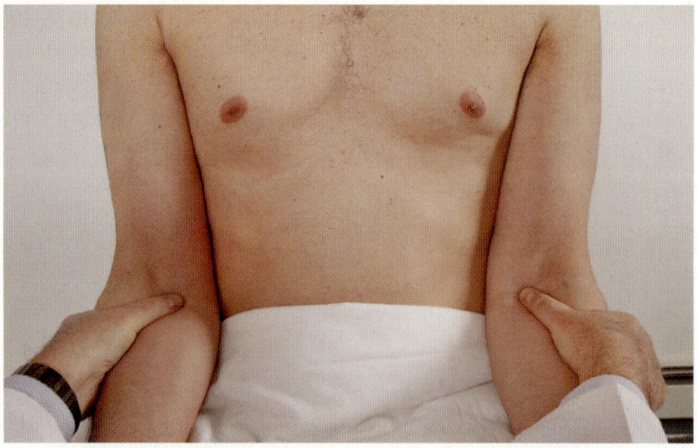

Fig. 15.8 Technique for Brachial Artery Palpation.

Palpate the Radial Pulse

See Video 15.1.

It would be best if you stood in front of the patient. The radial pulses are evaluated by grasping the patient's wrists and palpating the pulses with your index, middle, and fourth fingers. Hold the patient's right wrist with your left fingers and the patient's left wrist with your right fingers, as demonstrated in Fig. 14.23. The symmetry of the pulses is evaluated for timing and strength.

Palpate the Brachial Pulse

See Video 15.2.

Because the brachial pulse is stronger than the digital pulse, the examiner may use thumbs or other fingers to palpate the patient's brachial pulses. The brachial artery can be felt medially just under the belly or tendon of the biceps muscle. With the examiner standing before the patient, both brachial arteries can be palpated simultaneously. The examiner's left hand holds the patient's right arm, and the examiner's right hand holds the patient's left arm. Once the examiner's thumbs feel the brachial pulsation, the examiner should apply progressive pressure until the maximal systolic force is felt. Fig. 15.8 shows an alternate method of evaluating the brachial artery pulse bilaterally simultaneously.

Auscultate the Carotid Artery

See Video 15.3.

The patient should be supine. Auscultation for carotid bruits[e] is performed by placing the stethoscope's diaphragm over the patient's carotid artery while lying supine. This is demonstrated in Fig. 15.9. The patient's head should be slightly elevated on a pillow and turned slightly away from the carotid artery being evaluated. It is often helpful to ask the patient to hold their breath during the auscultation. Usually, either nothing or transmitted heart sounds are heard. After one carotid artery is evaluated, the other is examined. After auscultation of the carotid arteries, they are palpated (see Chapter 14, The Heart). As mentioned in Chapter 14, **always listen to the carotid artery before palpating it.**

[e]A bruit is a sound or murmur heard in a vessel as a result of increased turbulence.

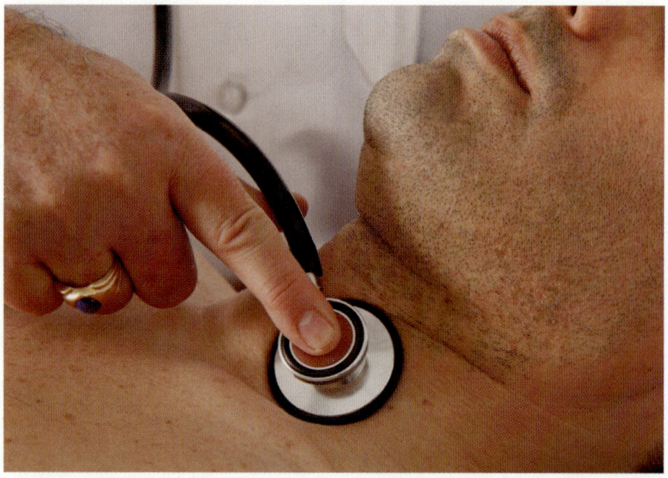

Fig. 15.9 Technique for Auscultation of the Carotid Artery.

The presence of a murmur should be noted. This may be a bruit resulting from local atherosclerotic disease of the carotid artery. Loud murmurs originating from the heart can occasionally be transmitted to the neck. With experience, the examiner can determine whether the disorder is local in the neck or distal in the heart.

Palpate the Abdominal Aorta

AAAs kill approximately 10,000 people in the United States each year. Many of these deaths could have been prevented if the patients were aware of the presence of this defect. Once the defect is recognized, the operative mortality rate for a nonruptured aneurysm is less than 5%, and after the operation, the survival rate equals that of the general population. An AAA that ruptures carries a mortality rate of nearly 90%. Even among patients who reach the operating room alive, the surgical mortality rate is 50%.

The patient should be supine. The examination is performed by palpating deeply, but gently, into the midabdomen. The presence of a mass with laterally expansive pulsation suggests an AAA. Aortic palpation's sensitivity to finding AAA is 60%, and the sensitivity of finding a pulsatile mass is only 50% of patients with diagnosed aortic ruptures. Some caution is urged in making this diagnosis in thin individuals, in whom the normal pulsatile aorta can be easily palpated. The high false-positive rate with this examination should be acceptable, however, because confirmation with abdominal ultrasonography is safe and inexpensive.

Other findings associated with an AAA include an abdominal bruit, a femoral bruit, and a femoral pulse deficit. A bruit may be present in at most 10% of patients with AAAs. Acute rupture of an AAA is suggested when a bruit is associated with severe pain in the abdomen or back and when the distal pulse is absent or diminished and later returns.

Table 15.2 summarizes the operating characteristics of the physical signs helpful in detecting an AAA.

Rule Out Abdominal Bruits

The patient should be supine. The examiner places the diaphragm of the stethoscope in the midline of the patient's abdomen about 2 inches (5 cm) above the umbilicus and listens

TABLE 15.2 Characteristics of Physical Signs for Detecting an Abdominal Aortic Aneurysm

Physical Sign	Sensitivity (%)	Specificity (%)
Definite pulsatile mass	28	97
Definite or suggestive pulsatile mass	50	91
Abdominal bruit	11	95
Femoral bruit	17	87
Femoral pulse deficit	22	91

Data from Lederle FA, Walker JM, Reinke DB: Selective screening for abdominal aortic aneurysms with physical examination and ultrasound, *Arch Intern Med* 148:1753, 1988.

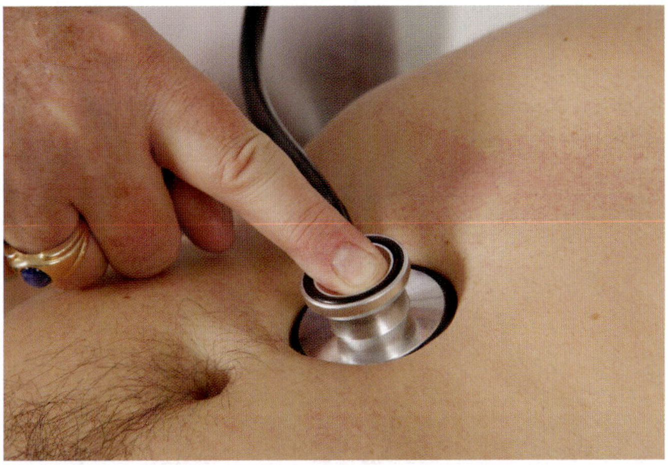

Fig. 15.10 Technique for Auscultation of the Abdominal Aorta.

carefully for the presence of an *aortic bruit.* This technique is demonstrated in Fig. 15.10. A definite or suggestive pulsatile mass carries a sensitivity of 50%, and a solid pulsatile mass carries a specificity of 97%.

A *renal bruit* may be the only clue to renal artery stenosis, a surgically correctable form of hypertension. Auscultation should be approximately 2 inches (5 cm) above the umbilicus and 1 to 2 inches (2.5 to 5 cm) laterally to the right and the left of midposition.

Abdominal bruits present only during systole are frequently of little clinical value because they are found in normal individuals and patients with essential hypertension. However, a systolic-diastolic abdominal bruit should raise the suspicion of renovascular hypertension. Nearly 60% of all patients with renovascular hypertension have such a bruit.

The presence of a combined systolic-diastolic abdominal bruit has a sensitivity of 39% and a specificity of 99% for detecting renovascular hypertension. The presence of this type of bruit has a positive likelihood ratio (LR+) of 39 and, if absent, a negative likelihood ratio (LR−) of 0.6. In a study that evaluated the presence of any epigastric or flank bruit and its association with renovascular hypertension, the sensitivity was 63%, but the specificity dropped to 90%. The presence of any abdominal bruit confers a much lower LR+ for renovascular hypertension (i.e., 6.4).

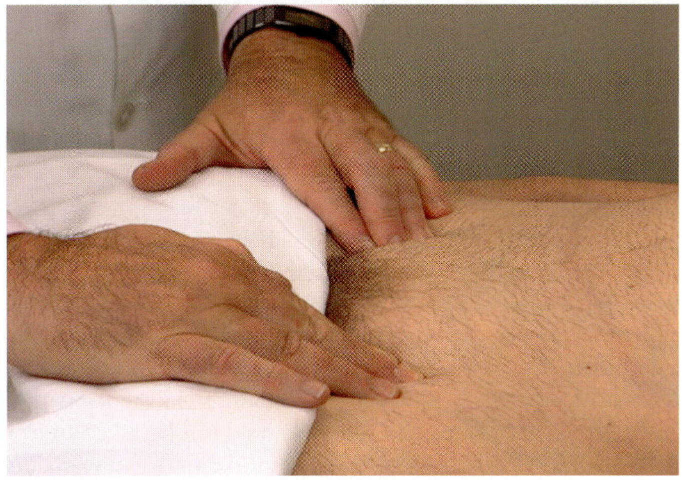

Fig. 15.11 Technique for Palpation of the Femoral Arteries.

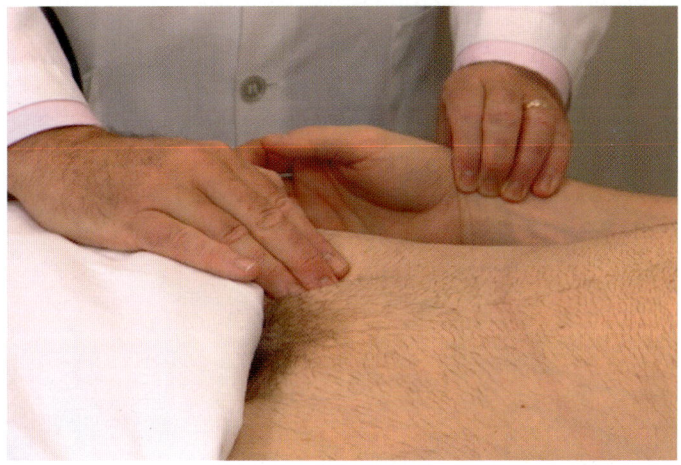

Fig. 15.12 Technique for Timing the Femoral and Radial Pulses.

Palpate the Femoral Pulse and Rule Out Coarctation of the Aorta

See Video 15.4.

The femoral pulse is evaluated with the patient lying supine and the examiner on the patient's right side. The lateral corners of the pubic hair triangle are observed and palpated. The femoral artery should run obliquely through the corner of the pubic hair triangle inferior to the inguinal ligament midway between the pubic tubercle and the anterior superior iliac spine. Both femoral pulses may be compared simultaneously. The technique is demonstrated in Fig. 15.11.

Auscultation for a bruit is necessary if one of the femoral pulses is diminished or absent. The diaphragm of the stethoscope is placed over the femoral artery. The presence of a bruit may indicate obstructive aortoiliofemoral disease.

The timing of the femoral and radial pulses is essential. Usually, these two pulses peak either simultaneously or with the femoral pulse preceding the radial pulse. By placing one hand on the patient's femoral artery and the other on the radial artery, the examiner can determine the peaking of these pulses. This technique needs to be performed on one side only and is demonstrated in Fig. 15.12. Any delay in the femoral pulse relative to the radial pulse should raise suspicion of coarctation of the aorta,[10] especially in an individual with hypertension. These individuals will be hypertensive in the upper extremity and hypotensive in the lower extremity.

Palpate the Popliteal Pulse

See Video 15.5.

The popliteal artery is often challenging to assess. Each artery is evaluated separately. While the patient is lying on the back, the examiner's thumbs are placed on the patella, and the remaining fingers of both hands are pressed in the popliteal fossa medial to the lateral biceps femoris tendon, as demonstrated in Fig. 15.13. The examiner should hold the leg with a mild degree of flexion. The patient should not be asked to elevate the leg because this tightens the musculoskeletal elements (i.e., muscles, tendons, ligaments) and makes it more challenging to feel the pulse. The examiner should squeeze both hands in the popliteal fossa. Firm pressure is usually necessary to feel the pulsation.

Palpate the Dorsalis Pedis Pulse

See Video 15.6.

The dorsalis pedis pulse is best palpated when the foot is dorsiflexed. The dorsalis pedis artery passes along a line from the extensor retinaculum of the ankle to a point just lateral to the extensor tendon of the great toe. It is usually easily palpated in the groove between the extensor digitorum longus and hallucis longus tendon. The dorsalis pedis pulses may be felt simultaneously, as demonstrated in Fig. 15.14.

Palpate the Posterior Tibial Pulse

See Video 15.7.

The posterior tibial artery can be palpated just posterior to the medial malleoli between the tibialis posterior tendon and the flexor digitorum longus tendon. Both arteries can be evaluated simultaneously. Fig. 15.15 demonstrates this procedure. Although posterior tibial pulses are absent in 15% of normal subjects, the most sensitive sign of occlusive peripheral arterial disease in patients older than 60 is the absence of the posterior tibial pulse. See Video 15.8 for a complete overview of the peripheral vascular system.

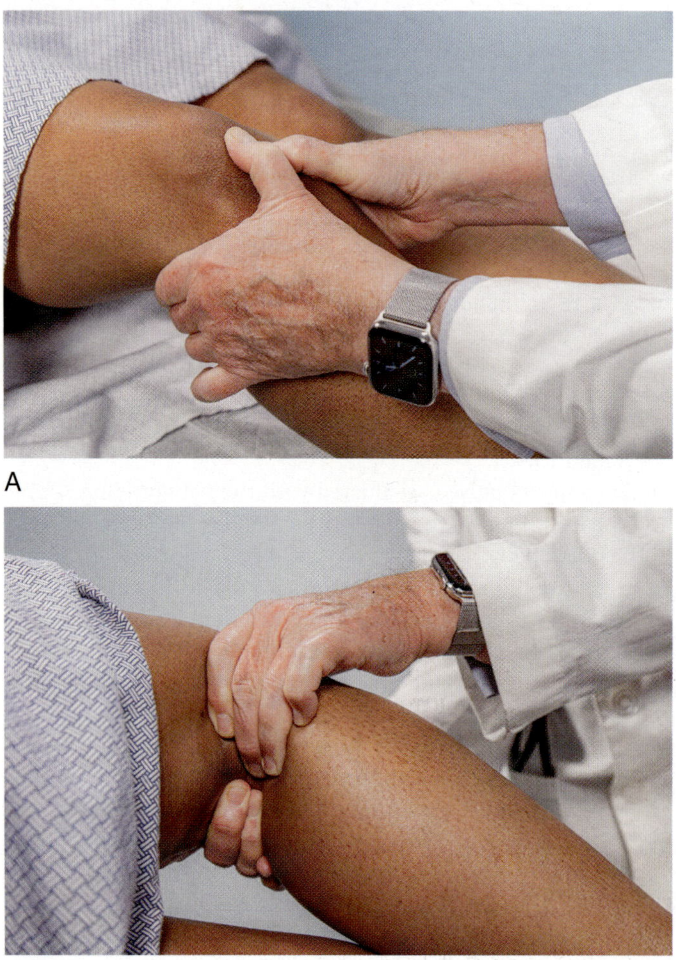

A

B

Fig. 15.13 Technique for Palpation of the Popliteal Artery. (A) Correct position of the hands from the front. (B) View from behind the popliteal fossa.

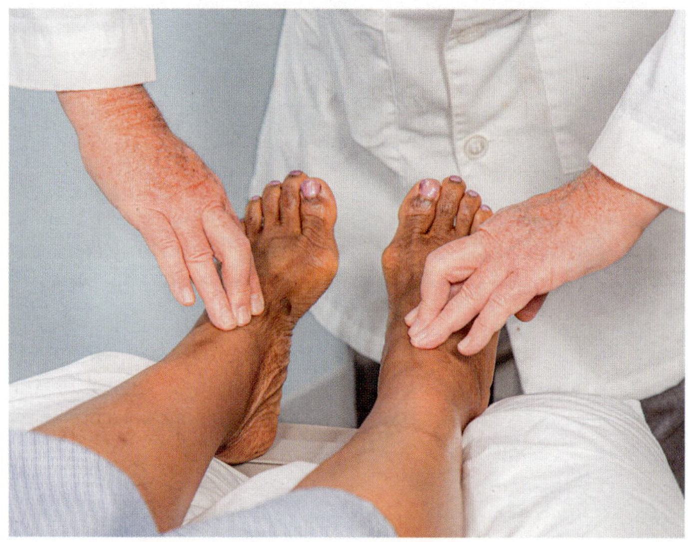

Fig. 15.14 Technique for Palpation of the Dorsalis Pedis Arteries.

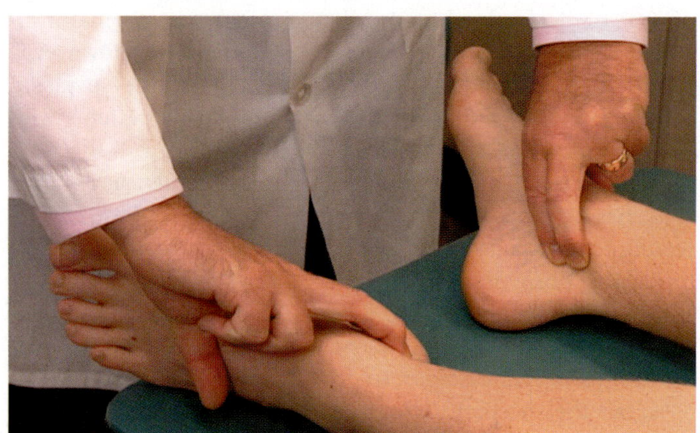

Fig. 15.15 Technique for Palpation of the Posterior Tibial Arteries.

Examination of the Lymphatic System

Physical signs of lymphatic system disease include the following:

- Palpable lymph nodes
- Lymphangitis
- Lymphedema

Lymph nodes should be described as *painless* or *tender*, *single* or *matted*, and *mobile* or *fixed*. Lymph nodes that are tender, matted, and fixed to surrounding overlying or underlying tissue strongly suggest a pathologic condition. Generalized lymphadenopathy and localized lymphadenopathy are suggestive of different diagnoses. *Generalized* lymphadenopathy is the presence of palpable lymph nodes in three or more lymph node chains. Lymphoma, leukemia, collagen vascular disorders, and systemic bacterial, viral, and protozoal infections may be responsible. *Localized* lymphadenopathy is usually the result of localized infection or neoplasm.

Lymphangitis is an inflammation of the lymphatic channels due to infection at a site distal to the lymphatic channel. When pathogens enter the lymphatic channels, invading directly through trauma to the skin, local inflammation and subsequent infection ensue manifesting as red streaks on the skin, the hallmark of lymphangitis. The inflammation or infection then extends proximally toward regional lymph nodes. Bacteria can proliferate in the lymphatic system. Individuals with lymphangitis often have fever, chills, and malaise, and some may report a headache, loss of appetite, and muscle aches. Lymphangitis can progress rapidly to bacteremia and disseminated infection, mainly caused by group A β-hemolytic streptococci species, which are the most common causes of lymphangitis. Individuals with diabetes, immunodeficiency, varicella, chronic steroid use, or other systemic illnesses have an increased risk of developing severe or rapidly spreading lymphangitis.

Obstruction to lymphatic flow produces *lymphedema,* which is usually indistinguishable from other types of edema. Look at Fig. 16.8; this patient has marked lymphedema of her left arm secondary to inflammatory breast carcinoma and lymphatic obstruction in her axilla.

The examinations for lymphadenopathy of the head, neck, and supraclavicular areas are described in Chapter 9, The Head and Neck, and Chapter 13, The Chest. Chapter 16, The Breast, describes the examination for palpating axillary adenopathy. Chapter 18, Male Genitalia and Hernias, describes the technique for palpating inguinal lymph nodes. The epitrochlear nodes are the other important lymph node chain, discussed in the following section.

Palpate for Epitrochlear Nodes

To palpate epitrochlear nodes, have the patient flex the elbow approximately 90 degrees. Feel for the nodes in the fossa about 3 cm proximal to the medial epicondyle of the humerus, in the groove between the biceps and the triceps muscles, as shown in Fig. 15.16. Epitrochlear nodes are rarely palpable, but their size, consistency, and tenderness should be described if they are present. Acute infections of the ulnar aspect of the forearm and hand may be responsible for epitrochlear adenopathy. Epitrochlear nodes are also observed in non-Hodgkin lymphoma.

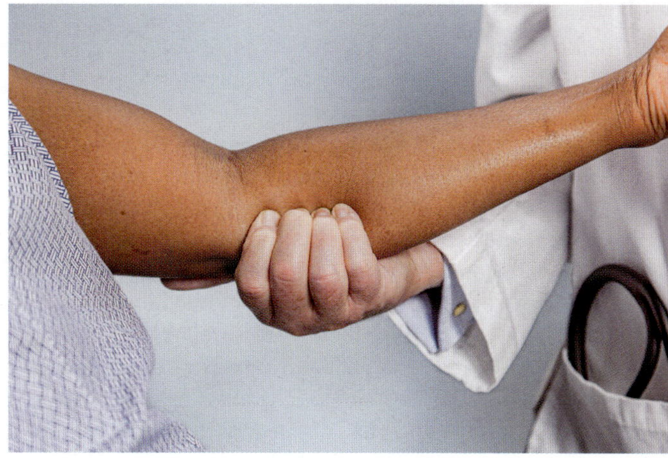

Fig. 15.16 Technique for Evaluating Epitrochlear Nodes.

Other Special Techniques

All the special tests described here are to be used in conjunction with other forms of testing. Each of these vascular techniques is associated with many false-positive and false-negative findings. The results, therefore, must be considered as part of the total evaluation.

Evaluate Arterial Supply in the Lower Extremity

The most critical sign of arterial insufficiency is a decreased pulse. Another test may be helpful in patients with suspected chronic arterial insufficiency of the lower extremity. The amount of pallor that develops after elevation and dependency on the ischemic extremity provide an approximate guide to the extent of decreased circulation. The *elevation test* is performed by having the patient lie on the back, and the examiner elevates the patient's legs at approximately 60 degrees above the bed. The patient is asked to move the ankles to help drain the blood from the venous system, making the color changes more apparent. After approximately 60 seconds, the feet are inspected for pallor. Typically, no pallor is present (grade 0). Definite pallor in 60 seconds is grade 1, in 30 to 60 seconds is grade 2, in less than 30 seconds is grade 3, and without elevation is grade 4. The patient is then asked to sit dangling the feet off the side of the bed, and the examiner assesses the time for color return *(rubor dependency test)*. It usually takes 10 to 15 seconds for color to return and 15 seconds for the superficial veins to fill. If it takes 15 to 30 seconds for color to return, moderate occlusive disease is present and indicates adequate collaterals; severe ischemia is present if it takes more than 40 seconds for color to return. A dusky or cyanotic color may also develop. This test is valid only if the valves of the superficial veins are competent. These tests are summarized in Table 15.3.

TABLE 15.3 Dependency Test for Arterial Insufficiency of the Lower Extremity

	Color Returns (s)
Normal	10–15
Moderate ischemia	15–30
Severe ischemia	>40

Ankle-Branchial Index

The *ankle-brachial index* (*ABI*[11]), or *ankle brachial pressure index (ABPI)*, is a quick, noninvasive test cornerstone of lower extremity vascular evaluation. It is the ratio of the blood pressure in the lower legs to the blood pressure in the arms measured by ultrasound. The ABI is calculated using three arteries: the brachial artery for the upper extremity and the dorsalis pedis and or posterior tibial artery at the ankle. Compared with the arm, lower blood pressure in the leg indicates PVD. The ABI/ABPI is calculated by dividing the systolic blood pressure at the ankle by the systolic blood pressure in the arm. The higher systolic reading of the left and right arm brachial artery is generally used in the assessment. The pressures in each foot's posterior tibial artery and dorsalis pedis artery are measured with the higher values used as the ABI for that leg.

$$ABPI_{leg} = P_{leg}/P_{arm}$$

where P_{leg} is the systolic blood pressure of dorsalis pedis or posterior tibial arteries, and P_{arm} is the highest of the left and right arm brachial systolic blood pressure.

Calculated ABPI values should be recorded to 2 decimal places. An ABPI between and including 0.90 and 1.30 is considered normal (i.e., free from significant PVD), while a lesser than 0.90 indicates some degree of PVD. An ABPI value of 1.30 or greater is also considered abnormal, suggestive of calcification of the walls of the arteries and noncompressible vessels. Table 15.4 indicates ABPI ratios that can be used to predict the severity of PVD.

The ABI test is a popular tool for the noninvasive assessment of PVD. Studies have shown the test's sensitivity to be 90% with a corresponding 98% specificity for detecting hemodynamically significant stenosis of more than 50% in major leg arteries as defined by angiography. A resting ABPI may be insensitive to mild peripheral arterial disease. Treadmill tests of 6 minutes are sometimes used to increase ABPI sensitivity.

Table 15.5 summarizes the most likely location of occlusive PVD based on the site of the patient's pain. Symptoms depend on which artery is blocked, how severe the blockage is, and whether the artery is gradually narrowed or suddenly blocked. Occlusive PVD most commonly develops in the arteries of the legs, including the iliac arteries and the femoral arteries, the popliteal arteries, and the tibial and peroneal arteries.

TABLE 15.4 Ankle-Brachial Pressure Index Ratios Can Be Used to Predict the Severity of Peripheral Vascular Disease

ABPI Ratio	Interpretation
Above 1.3	Abnormal—noncompressible calcified vessel
1.0–1.3	Normal range
0.90–0.99	Acceptable
0.80–0.89	Some PVD
0.50–0.79	Moderate PVD
Under 0.50	Severe PVD
Under 0.25	Severe limb-threatening PVD

ABPI, Ankle-brachial pressure index; *PVD,* peripheral vascular disease.

TABLE 15.5 Location of Occlusive Peripheral Vascular Disease

Location of Pain	Artery Involved
Buttocks and hip	Aortoiliac (Leriche syndrome)
Thigh	Common femoral (also pain in calf or both thigh and calf)
Calf	Upper ⅔ of calf—superficial femoral
	Lower ⅓ of calf—popliteal

Evaluate Capillary Refill Time

Pressure on the arteriolar capillaries under the nail blanches or whitens the nail bed so that when the skin is uncompressed, the blood can flow back into the vessels, and the nail bed returns to a normal color. Capillary refill time[12] is the amount of time it takes for the skin to return to normal, usually under 2 seconds.

The capillary refill time can be determined by compressing the nail bed until it blanches. Prolongation of the time it takes for normal coloration to return after release is synonymous with arterial vascular insufficiency. The capillary refill test is best performed in a room-temperature environment. A cool environment can cause peripheral vasoconstriction and alter the test results: dehydration, hypothermia, and most types of shock cause a prolonged capillary refill time without arterial insufficiency.

Evaluate Arterial Supply in the Upper Extremity

Chronic arterial insufficiency of the upper extremity is much less common than that of the lower extremity. The *Allen test,* which determines the patency of the radial and ulnar arteries, can be used to assess whether arterial insufficiency exists in the upper extremity. This test takes advantage of the radial-ulnar loop. Use one of your hands to occlude the radial artery and the other to occlude the ulnar artery. The patient is asked to clench the fist tightly. The patient is then asked to open the fist, and the color of the palm is observed. The palm should be pale at this point. Release the pressure on the radial artery while maintaining pressure on the ulnar artery. Observe the color of the palm. If normal, the color returns within seconds. If abnormal, the color will return slowly, suggesting radial artery insufficiency. The test is repeated with occlusion of the ulnar artery. Pallor of the palm during compression of one artery indicates occlusion of the other.

Test for Incompetent Saphenous Veins

It is easy to demonstrate incompetent saphenous vein valves on examination. The patient is asked to stand, and the dilated varicose vein becomes obvious. The examiner compresses the proximal end of the varicose vein with one hand while placing the other approximately 15 to 20 cm below it at the distal end of the vein. When saphenous valves in the portion of the vein examined are incompetent, an impulse is transmitted to the examiner's distal fingers.

Test for Retrograde Filling

The *Brodie-Trendelenburg maneuver* assesses venous valvular competency in the communicating veins and the saphenous system. The patient is positioned supine. Raise the affected leg 45 degrees for 15 to 20 seconds to drain venous blood. Place a tourniquet around the patient's proximal thigh with the leg still elevated to compress the superficial veins.

The patient is then instructed to stand while the examiner watches for the reappearance of the varicose veins. Rapid filling of the varicosities with the tourniquet still on suggests incompetent perforators *below* the level of the SFJ. If no filling is seen at this point, the tourniquet is released. Rapid filling of the varicosities at this stage suggests SFJ incompetence. The location of the incompetent perforator can then be determined by varying the position of the tourniquet. The Brodie-Trendelenburg maneuver is highly sensitive (91%) for identifying superficial reflux but poorly specific (15%).[13]

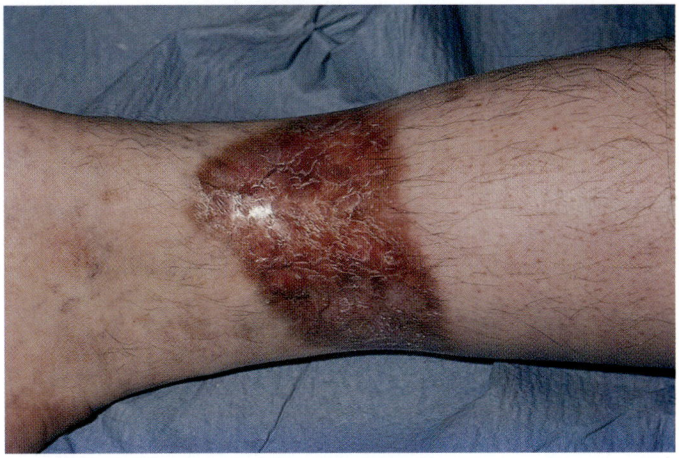

Fig. 15.18 Necrobiosis Lipoidica Diabeticorum. Note the shiny, waxy surface.

CLINICOPATHOLOGIC CORRELATIONS

The signs of an acute arterial occlusion are the *five Ps*: *p*ain, *p*allor, *p*aresthesia, *p*aralysis, and *p*ulselessness.

Chronic progressive small-vessel disease is characteristic of diabetes mellitus. It is commonly observed that arterial pulses are present despite gangrene in the extremity. Fig. 15.17 depicts dry gangrene of the toes in a patient with diabetes.

Diabetes has been associated with many skin disorders. The cutaneous hallmark of diabetes is a waxy, yellow, or reddish-brown, sharply demarcated, plaque-like lesion known as *necrobiosis lipoidica diabeticorum.* These lesions are classically found on the anterior surface of the lower legs. They are shiny and atrophic, with marked telangiectasia over their surface. The lesions tend to ulcerate, and the ulcers, once present, heal very slowly. Necrobiosis lipoidica diabeticorum often predates the development of frank diabetes. The severity of the cutaneous lesion is not related to the severity of diabetes. Fig. 15.18 shows necrobiosis lipoidica diabeticorum; Fig. 15.19 is a close-up photograph of the lesion in another patient with diabetes.

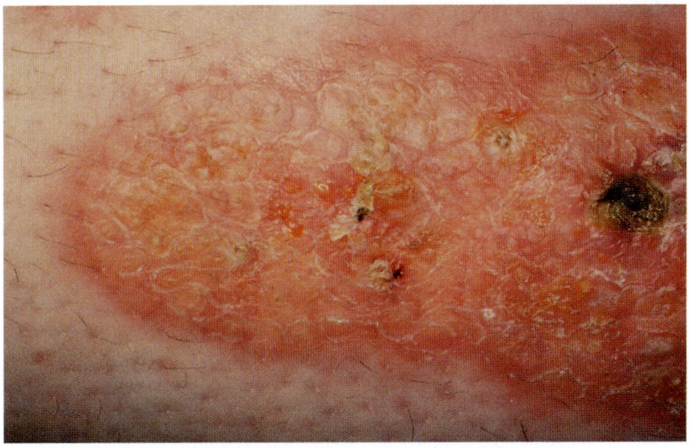

Fig. 15.19 Close-Up of a Necrobiosis Lipoidica Diabeticorum Lesion.

DVT of a lower extremity is diagnosed when there is marked unilateral swelling, venous distention, erythema, pain, increased warmth, and tenderness. There is often resistance to dorsiflexion of the ankle. Calf swelling is present in most patients with femoral or popliteal venous involvement, whereas thigh swelling occurs with iliofemoral thrombosis. Fig. 15.20

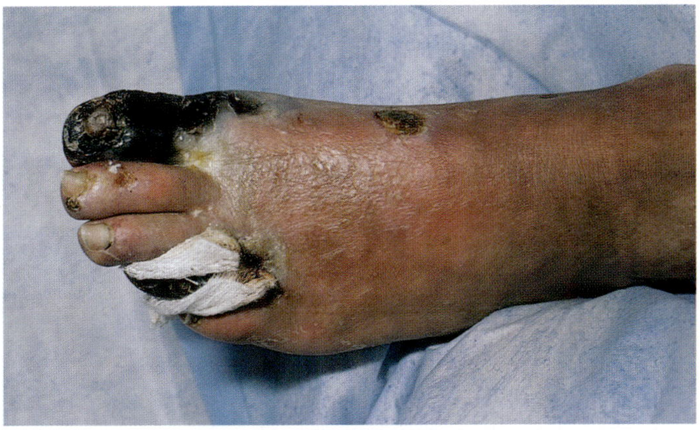

Fig. 15.17 Diabetic Gangrene.

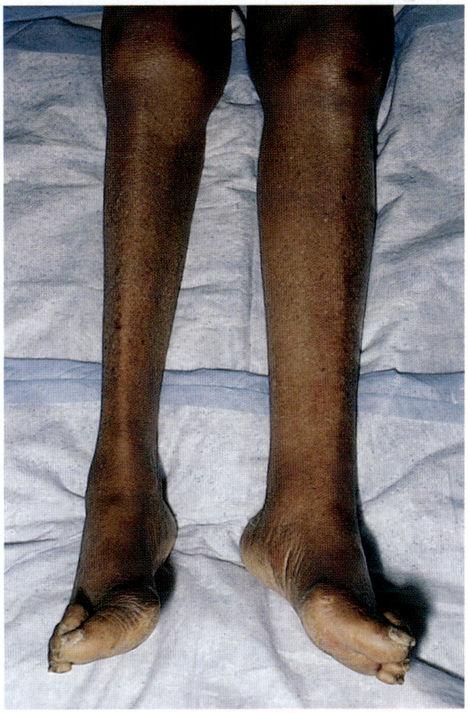

Fig. 15.20 Deep Vein Thrombosis, Left Leg.

shows deep femoral vein thrombosis secondary to cancer. Notice the marked swelling of the left leg.

The gentle squeezing of the affected calf or slow dorsiflexion of the ankle may produce calf pain in approximately 50% of patients with femoral vein thrombosis. Pain elicited by this technique is referred to as the *Homans sign,* or the *dorsiflexion sign.* Unfortunately, owing to the low sensitivity of the Homans sign, this finding should not be used as a single criterion for diagnosing DVT. A variety of unrelated conditions also may elicit a false-positive response. It can be of value if used in addition to more accurate diagnostic procedures like ultrasonography and venography.[14]

Many risk factors can increase the risk of DVT. These include, among others, prolonged bed rest, sitting for long periods, injury, surgery, birth control pills, pregnancy, a blood-clotting disorder, being overweight, smoking, congestive heart failure, cancer, inflammatory bowel disease, age, or family history of DVT or PE.

Secondary to venous thrombosis, inflammation around the vein may result. Erythema, warmth, and fever then occur, and *thrombophlebitis* is present. The examiner can often palpate this tender, indurated vein in the groin or medial thigh. This is commonly referred to as a *cord.*

DVT is associated with symptomatic PE in approximately 10% of patients. It usually happens when a part of a blood clot from a DVT breaks off from its original location in a vein and travels through the heart to the pulmonary arteries. If the embolus is large, main pulmonary artery obstruction may occur, which can result in death. It is estimated that an additional 45% of patients with DVT have asymptomatic, small pulmonary emboli. The Centers for Disease Control and Prevention estimate that DVT, PE, or both might affect up to 900,000 people in the United States annually.

Several factors important in precipitating thromboembolism are outlined in Table 15.6.

TABLE 15.6 Precipitating Factors in Thromboembolism

Factor	Cause
Stasis	Arrhythmia
	Heart failure
	Immobilization
	Obesity
	Varicose veins
	Dehydration
Blood vessel injury	Trauma
	Fracture
Increased coagulability	Neoplasm
	Oral contraceptives
	Pregnancy
	Polycythemia
	Previous thromboembolism

An important and common peripheral vascular condition is *Raynaud disease* or *phenomenon.* Classically, this condition is associated with three color changes of the distal fingers or toes: white *(pallor),* blue *(cyanosis),* and red *(rubor).* These color changes are related to artery spasm and decreased blood supply (pallor), increased peripheral extraction of oxygen (cyanosis), and return of blood supply (rubor). The patient may experience pain or numbness in the involved area due to the causes of pallor and cyanosis. During the hyperemic or rubor stage, the patient may complain of burning paresthesias. Between episodes, there may be no symptoms or signs of the condition.

TABLE 15.7 Differential Diagnosis of Raynaud Disease and Raynaud Phenomenon

Feature	Raynaud Disease	Raynaud Phenomenon
Sex	Female	Female
Bilaterality	Present (often symmetric)	± (asymmetric)
Precipitated by cold	Common	Increases symptoms
Ischemic changes	Rare	Common
Gangrene	Rare	More common
Disease association[a]	No	Yes

[a]Such as scleroderma, systemic lupus erythematosus, dermatomyositis, or rheumatoid arthritis.

Raynaud disease, which is *primary* or idiopathic, must be differentiated from the Raynaud phenomenon, which is *secondary.* Table 15.7 lists some of the different characteristics of these conditions.

Gangrene is necrosis of the deep tissues resulting from a decreased blood supply. Gangrene commonly affects the extremities, including the toes, fingers, and limbs. Any condition that affects blood flow increases the risk of gangrene, including diabetes, atherosclerosis, PVD, smoking, Raynaud disease, trauma, obesity, and a compromised immune system. Features of the primary vascular diseases causing gangrene of the lower extremities are summarized in Table 15.8.

TABLE 15.8 Differential Diagnosis of the Main Vascular Diseases Causing Gangrene

Feature	Diabetes	Atherosclerosis	Thromboangiitis Obliterans	Raynaud Disease	Arterial Embolism
Age	Any	Older than 60 years	Younger than 40 years	Younger than 40 years	Any
Sex	Either	Either	Male	Female	Either
Onset	Gradual	Gradual	Gradual	Gradual	Sudden
Pain	Moderate	Moderate	Severe	Moderate	Often severe
Distal pulses	May be absent	May be absent	May be absent	Present	Absent[a]

[a]Affected artery does not have pulsation.

USEFUL VOCABULARY

Listed here are the specific roots that are important for understanding the terminology related to vascular disease.

Root	Pertaining to	Example	Definition
angi(o)-	blood vessel	***angio***graphy	Radiographic visualization of blood vessels
embol(o)-	wedge; stopper	***embol***ism	Sudden blocking of a vessel by a clot
phleb(o)-	veins	***phlebo***tomy	Incision into a vein for blood removal
thrombo-	clot	***thrombo***embolism	Obstruction of a blood vessel by a clot that has broken loose from its site of formation
varico-	twisted; swollen	***varico***se	Unnaturally swollen and twisted

WRITING UP THE PHYSICAL EXAMINATION

Listed here are examples of the write-up for examining the vascular system.

- The extremities are normal in color, size, and temperature. All pulses in the upper and lower extremities are grade 2 and are equal. No bruits are present. No clubbing, cyanosis, or edema is present.
- There are yellow, waxy, sharply demarcated lesions on both anterior shins. Both legs appear slightly cool, the left greater than the right. There is a punched-out ulceration on the lateral aspect of the left ankle. The left big toe is blackened, with a sharp demarcation. The femoral pulses are grade 2 bilaterally. No distal pulses are felt. There is 1+ pretibial edema present bilaterally. No clubbing or cyanosis is present.
- The right lower extremity is 3 cm larger than the left, measured 4 cm below the inferior aspect of the patella. The right calf is tender, warm, and erythematous. A cord is palpated in the right groin. Both lower extremities are edematous and hyperpigmented. There is 3+ pretibial edema on the right and 2+ on the left. A small ulceration is present above the left medial malleolus. The arterial pulses are grade 2 at the femoral arteries and grade 1 at the popliteal arteries. No pulses are palpated distally to the popliteal arteries. No clubbing or cyanosis is present.

FULL VIDEOS

- Video 15.8 Full video: Examining the peripheral vascular system

REVIEW QUESTIONS

1. **People who are at a higher risk of peripheral vascular disease are all of the following *except:***
   A. People with diabetes
   B. People with abnormally high cholesterol
   C. People with hypertension
   D. People with multiple sclerosis
   E. People who are smokers
2. **When peripheral vascular disease becomes severe, the patient may experience all the following *except:***
   A. Sores that do not heal
   B. Skin that looks lighter than normal
   C. Pain or tingling in the lower extremity
   D. Night cramps
   E. Erectile dysfunction
3. **According to the Framingham Heart Study, of all the risk factors for peripheral vascular disease, the one factor which has a reduced relative risk is:**
   A. Smoking
   B. Hypercholesterolemia
   C. Alcohol
   D. Fibrinogen
   E. C-reactive protein
4. **According to the "Rule of 15," all the following statements are true *except:***
   A. 15% of all diabetic patients will develop a foot ulcer sometime in life
   B. 15% of diabetic foot ulcers will lead to osteomyelitis
   C. 15% of foot ulcers lead to amputation
   D. 15% of diabetic amputations are at the transfemoral/transtibial level
   E. 50% of patients die in 5 years or less
5. **Which of the following statements regarding the Leriche syndrome is correct?**
   A. Pain is experienced in the calf.
   B. Females and males can experience the pain.
   C. Atherosclerosis in the mid-aorta is the cause of the syndrome.
   D. The pain is often at rest.
   E. The patient may experience leg numbness or weakness.
6. **The physical sign for detecting an abdominal aortic aneurysm with the highest specificity is:**
   A. Abdominal bruit
   B. Femoral bruit
   C. Definity pulsatile mass
   D. Femoral pulse deficit
   E. Umbilical area darkening
7. **Patients with lymphangitis often experience all of the following symptoms *except:***
   A. Fever
   B. Chills
   C. Malaise
   D. Loss of appetite
   E. Vomiting

8. **Regarding the ankle branchial index (ABI), or the ankle branchial pressure index (ABPI), which of the following statements is true?**
   - **A.** It is the ratio of the blood pressure in the upper extremity to the lower extremity.
   - **B.** Compared with the upper extremity, lower blood pressure in the lower extremity indicates peripheral vascular disease.
   - **C.** The ABI/ABPI is calculated by dividing the systolic blood pressure in the arms by the systolic blood pressure at the ankle.
   - **D.** An ABPI between and including 0.80 and 1.30 is considered normal.
   - **E.** Studies have shown that the test's sensitivity is about 76%.

9. **Many factors can increase the risk of deep vein thrombosis (DVT). They include all the following *except:***
   - **A.** Long airplane rides
   - **B.** Smoking
   - **C.** Birth control pills
   - **D.** Inflammatory bowel disease
   - **E.** Multiple sclerosis

10. **Which of the following causes is *not* a precipitating factor in thromboembolism?**
    - **A.** Heart failure
    - **B.** Obesity
    - **C.** Alcohol
    - **D.** Malignancy
    - **E.** Polycythemia

REFERENCES

Available online.

BIBLIOGRAPHY

Available online.

16

The Breast

Mark H. Swartz and Farida G. Nentin

"Your breast is the only organ in your body that you are not born with. You come into the world with a nipple and lots of potential: some cells behind the nipple that, given the right hormonal stimulation, will grow and become a breast."

Susan Love, M.D. (1948–)

VIDEOS

Video 16.1	Inspecting the breasts
Video 16.2	Performing an axillary examination
Video 16.3	Palpating the breast
Video 16.4	Examining the nipple
Video 16.5	Full video: Examination of the female breast

GENERAL CONSIDERATIONS

The National Cancer Institute estimates that one of every eight females (approximately 13%) will develop breast cancer during their lifetime. Among the malignant diseases in females, breast cancer is the most common to develop and is the second most common cancer cause of death, after cancer of the lung and bronchus. In the United States in 2023, approximately 297,790 females and 2800 males were newly diagnosed with breast cancer. It is estimated that there were 48,470 deaths from breast cancer: 43,170 in females, 5300 in males. Breast carcinoma in situ, a very early form of the disease, will be diagnosed in another 55,720 females.[1]

The incidence of cancer of the breast is higher in the United States than in European or Asian countries. It has been well established that females in underdeveloped nations have lower rates of breast cancer than females from more affluent societies. Among racial and ethnic groups, White and Black females have the highest incidence rates of breast cancer (136.3 and 128.3 per 100,000 population, respectively). Asian/Pacific Islander females, Native American/Alaskan Native females, and Hispanic females have a lower risk (106.4, 107.4, and 98.5 per 100,000 population, respectively). The incidence rate for female breast cancer began to decline in 2000 after increasing for the previous two decades. The dramatic decline of almost 7% from 2002 to 2003 alone has been attributed to reductions in the use of hormone replacement therapy following the publication of results from the Woman's Health Initiative in 2002[2] indicating that combined estrogen and progesterone therapy was associated with an increased risk of breast cancer and coronary artery disease. Since 2003, breast cancer incidence rates have been stable.

There are several risk factors for breast cancer: age, genetics, family history of breast cancer, personal history of breast cancer, early menarche, late menopause, excessive alcohol consumption, obesity, nulliparity,[a] use of hormone replacement therapy, and a history of chest radiation.

If there is a family history of breast cancer, the risk of developing breast cancer increases significantly. The risk doubles if a first-degree relative, such as a parent, sibling, or child, has been affected, and triples if there are two affected first-degree relatives. If the relative was diagnosed before menopause, the risk increases threefold. In patients with a personal history of invasive breast cancer, the incidence of contralateral breast cancer is increased by 4%. This risk is doubled in patients with a family history of breast cancer and is even higher if the relative was diagnosed before menopause.

The age when a female begins menstruation and their reproductive cycle may contribute to the likelihood of developing breast cancer. Research suggests that females who start menstruating before the age of 12 have a higher incidence of breast cancer. Additionally, females who give birth for the first time at the age of 30 or older have a threefold higher risk of developing breast cancer than those who have their first child at a younger age.

Most breast cancers are detected as painless masses, noticed by either the patient or the examiner during a routine physical examination. The earlier the diagnosis is made, the better the prognosis is. Screening for breast cancer is best accomplished by a thorough clinical breast examination, breast self-examination (BSE), and mammography. Mammography is a sensitive method for detecting breast cancer and has been demonstrated to reduce the breast cancer mortality rate. The sensitivity of digital mammography is 72.4% and its specificity is 46.4%.[3]

[a]The status of a female who has never borne a child.

STRUCTURE AND PHYSIOLOGY

The *mammary glands* are the distinguishing feature of all mammals. Human breasts are conical in form and are often unequal in size. The breast extends from the level of the second or third rib to the level of the sixth or seventh rib, from the sternal edge to the anterior axillary line. The "tail" of the breast extends into the axilla and tends to be thicker than the other breast areas. This upper outer quadrant contains the greatest bulk of mammary tissue and is frequently the site of neoplasia. Fig. 16.1 illustrates the normal breast.

The normal breast consists of glandular tissue, ducts, supporting muscular tissue, fat, blood vessels, nerves, and lymphatic vessels. The glandular tissue consists of 15 to 25 lobes, each of which drains into a separate excretory duct that terminates in the nipple. Each duct dilates as it enters the base of the nipple to form a *milk sinus*. This serves as a reservoir for milk during lactation. Each lobe is subdivided into 50 to 75 lobules, which drain into a duct that empties into the excretory duct of the lobe.

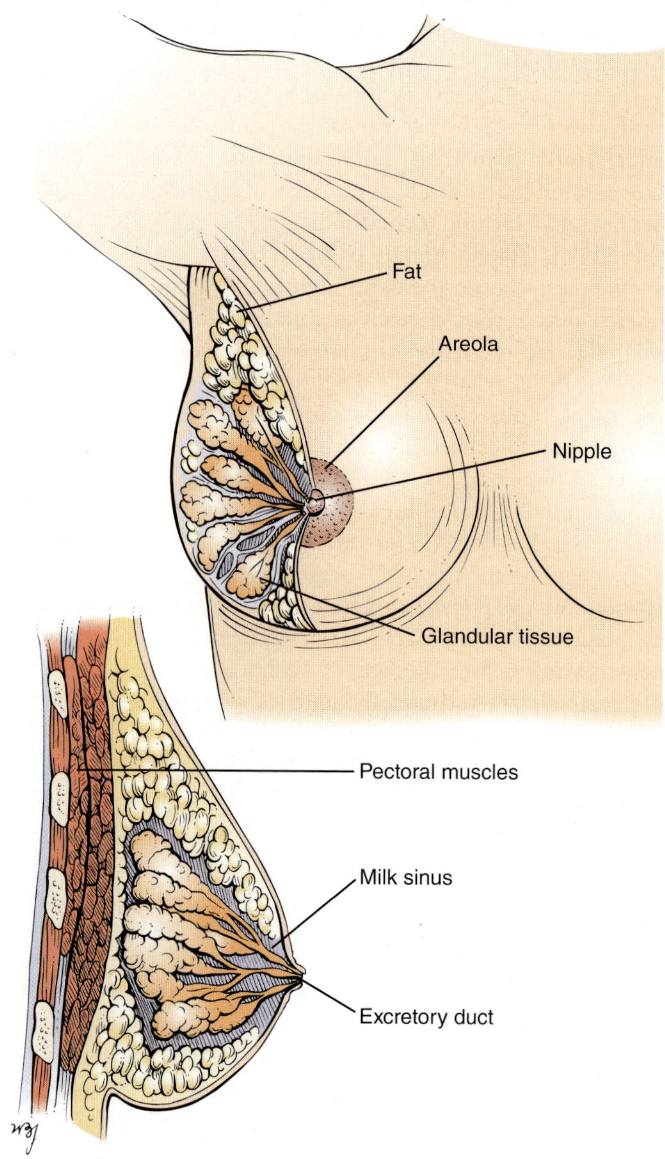

Fig. 16.1 Anatomy of a Normal Breast.

Both the nipple and areola contain smooth muscle that serves to contract the areola and compress the nipple. Contraction of the smooth muscle makes the nipple erect and firm, thereby facilitating the emptying of the milk sinuses.

The skin surrounding the nipple is hairless and has a dark pigment. It contains numerous sebaceous glands that are clustered near the milk sinuses. The skin of the areola, which also has a dark pigment, may have occasional hair follicles and small nodules called *Montgomery tubercles*, which are actually sebaceous glands.

Cooper ligaments are projections of the breast tissue that fuse with the outer layers of the superficial fascia and serve as suspensory structures.

The internal mammary artery carries the blood supply to the breast. The breast has an extensive network of venous and lymphatic drainage. Most of the lymphatic drainage empties into the nodes in the axilla. Other nodes lie beneath the lateral margin of the pectoralis major muscle, along the medial side of the axilla, and in the subclavicular region. The main lymph node chains and lymphatic drainage of the breast are illustrated in Fig. 16.2.

Several physiologic changes occur in the breast. These changes are a result of the following factors:

- Puberty and aging/menopause
- The menstrual cycle
- Pregnancy

At birth, the breasts contain a branching system of ducts emptying into a developed nipple. There is elevation of only the nipple at this stage. Shortly after birth, there is a slight secretion of milky material. After 5 to 7 days, this secretory activity stops. Before puberty, there is elevation of the breast and nipple, called the *breast bud stage*. The areola has increased in size. At the onset of puberty, the areola enlarges further and darkens. A distinct mass of glandular tissue begins to develop beneath the areola. By the onset of menstruation, the breasts are well developed, and there is a forward projection of the areola and nipple at the apex of the breast. When the breast has reached maturity 1 to 2 years later, only the nipple projects forward; the areola has receded to the general contour of the breast. The stages of breast development from birth to adulthood are illustrated in Fig. 16.3. Fig. 24.45 further illustrates and describes the Tanner stages of breast and pubic hair development.

The size, density, and shape of an adult's breasts can be influenced by various factors, with the presence of excess adipose tissue being one of the most significant. This is because the mammary gland is predominantly made up of adipose tissue, which can result in larger breasts for overweight females. The characteristics of the breasts can also change due to pregnancy and breastfeeding, often resulting in softer and less nodular breasts for those who have breastfed. However, the size of the breast is not necessarily related to nursing, as the glandular tissue is similar in all females. As females age and reach menopause, their breasts may decrease in size and become less dense due to a decrease in elastic tissue.

A significant physiological change that occurs during the menstrual cycle is engorgement, which takes place 3 to 5 days

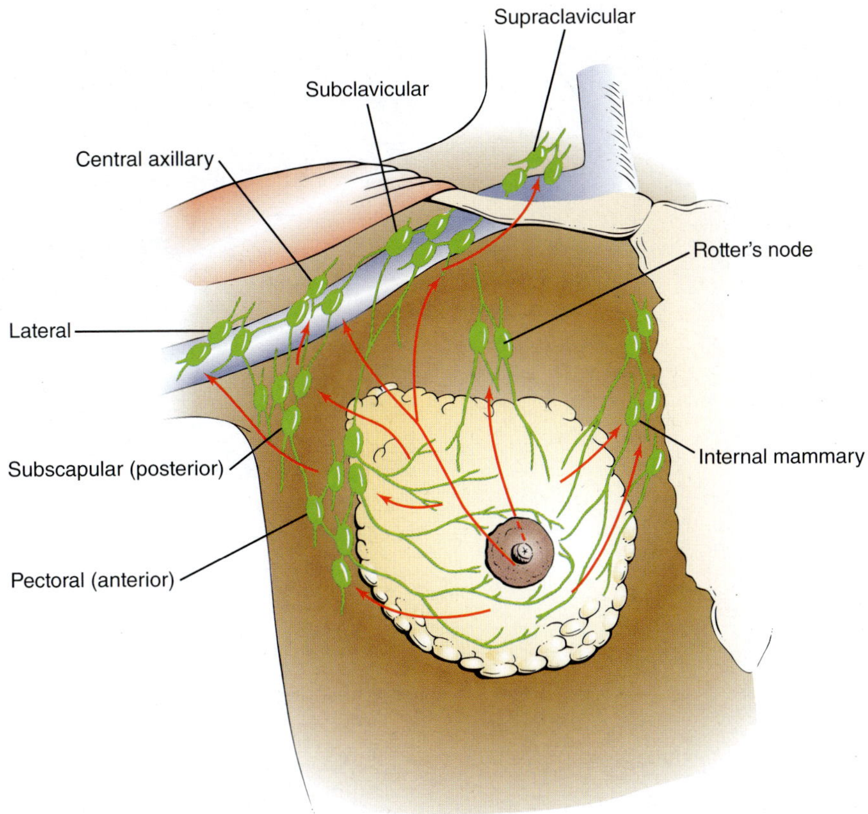

Fig. 16.2 **Lymphatic Drainage of the Breast.** Rotter's nodes are small interpectoral lymph nodes between the major and minor pectoral muscles. They are a frequent site for metastatic breast cancer.

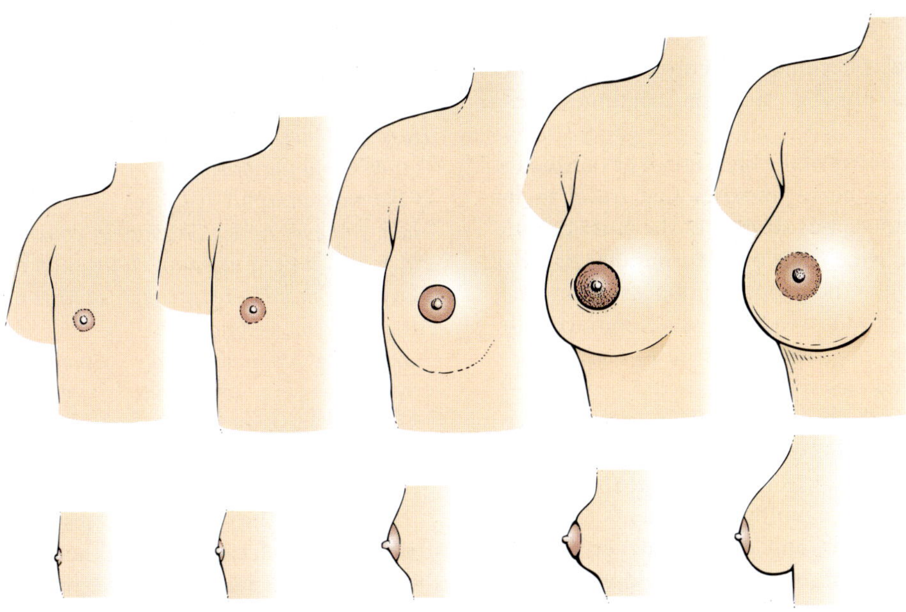

Fig. 16.3 Stages of Breast Development.

before menstruation. This results in the breasts becoming larger, denser, and more nodular, and heightened sensitivity. As a result of the increased nodularity, it is not advisable for an examiner to diagnose a breast mass during this time. It is recommended that the patient be reevaluated during the mid-period of the next cycle.

With pregnancy, the breasts become fuller and firmer. The areolae darken, and the nipples become erect as they enlarge. As the female approaches the third trimester, a thin, yellowish secretion called *colostrum* may be noted. After the birth of the child, if the birthing parent begins nursing within 24 hours, the secretion of colostrum stops, and the secretion of milk begins.

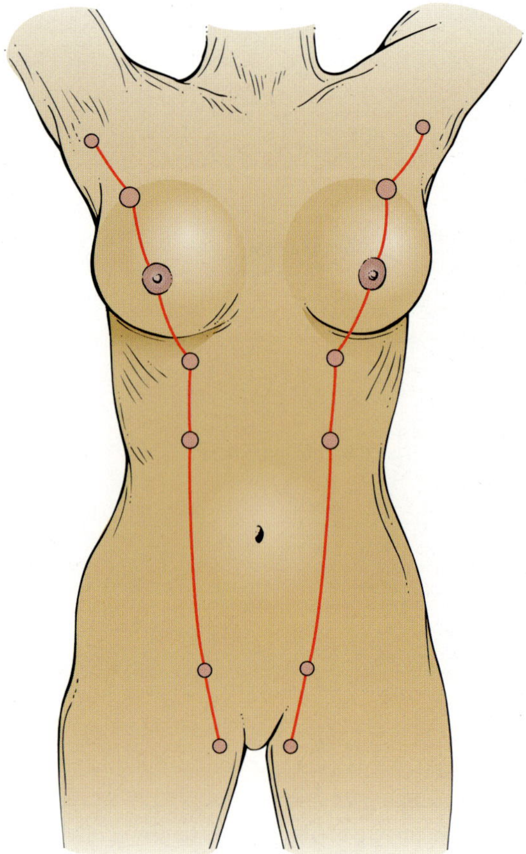

Fig. 16.4 The Milk Line.

During nursing, the breasts become markedly engorged. After the female has stopped nursing, lactation continues for a short time.

The neuroendocrine control of the breasts can be outlined as follows. Suckling produces nerve impulses that travel to the hypothalamus. The hypothalamus stimulates the anterior pituitary to secrete *prolactin,* which acts on the glandular tissue of the breast to produce milk. The hypothalamus also stimulates the posterior pituitary to produce *oxytocin,* which stimulates the muscle cells surrounding the glandular tissue to contract and force the milk into the ductular system.

Many abnormalities of the breast are related to its embryologic characteristics. An epithelial ridge called the *milk line* forms along each side of the body from the axilla to the inguinal region. Along this milk line are multiple rudiments for future breast development. In humans, only one rudimentary pair in the pectoral region persists and eventually develops into normal breasts. Accessory breasts or nipples are present in as many as 2% of White females. Accessory breasts may exist as glandular tissue, nipple, or only the areola. The axilla is the most common site for these anomalous structures, followed by a site just below the normal breast. In more than 50% of all patients with accessory breast tissue, the anomalies are bilateral. In general, accessory breast tissue is of little clinical significance. It usually has no physiologic function and is rarely associated with disease. Fig. 16.4 illustrates the milk line. Fig. 16.5 shows an accessory nipple.

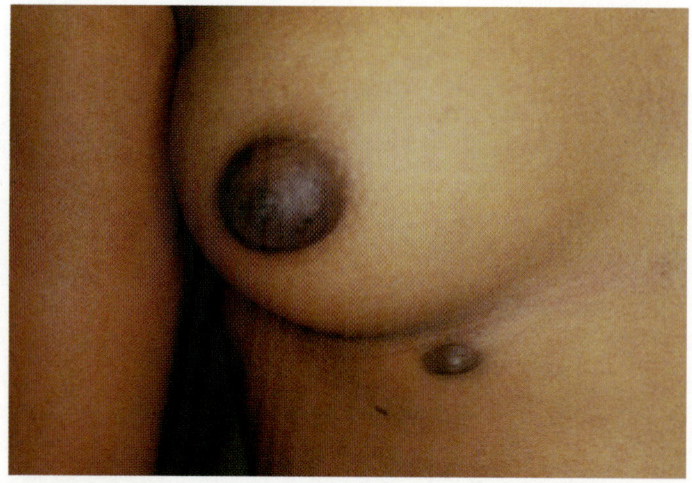

Fig. 16.5 Accessory Nipple. (From Callen JP, Greer KE, Hood AF, et al: *Color atlas of dermatology,* Philadelphia, 1993, WB Saunders.)

REVIEW OF SPECIFIC SYMPTOMS

The most important symptoms of breast disease are the following:

- Mass or swelling
- Pain
- Nipple discharge
- Change in skin over breast

Mass or Swelling

During self-examination, a patient may discover a breast mass. Ask the following questions:

"When did you first notice the lump?"
"Has the mass changed since you first noticed it?"
"Have you noticed that the mass changes in size during your menstrual periods?"
"Is the mass painful?"
"Have you ever noticed a mass in your breast before?"
"Have you noticed any skin changes on the breast?"
"Have you had any recent injury to the breast?"
"Are you breastfeeding?"
"Is there any nipple discharge? Nipple retraction?"
"Do you have breast implants?" If yes, *"What are they made of?"*
"Do you know of any family history of breast masses or cancer?"
"Have you ever had a mammogram or breast ultrasound in the past?"

If a lump in the breast increases in size during the premenstrual and menstrual phases of the menstrual cycle, it is probable that the female is only detecting natural nodularity or fibrocystic changes in her breast. However, if there is nipple discharge, nipple inversion, or changes in the skin overlying the lump, it is advisable to seek further investigation through imaging and possibly a biopsy to exclude the possibility of cancer. Refer to Fig. 16.6 for an example of a significant breast mass identified through self-examination.

Pain

Breast pain or tenderness is a common symptom. Most often, these symptoms are attributable to the normal physiologic

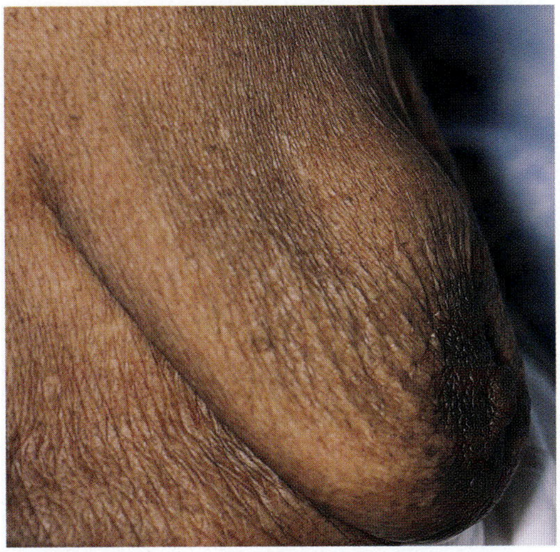

Fig. 16.6 Large Breast Mass Found on Self-Examination.

cycle. Ask the following questions of any patient with breast pain:

"Can you describe the pain?"

"When did you first experience the pain?"

"Is the pain constant throughout the month? Or does it increase and decrease at different times of the month? Do you notice these changes around your menstrual cycle?"

"Do you have pain in both breasts?"

"Have you had any injury to the breast?"

"Is the pain associated with a mass in the breast? Nipple discharge? Nipple retraction?"

"Has there been a change in your bra size?"

"Do you have any shoulder, neck, or back pain associated with it?"

If the patient experiences cyclic pain, it is likely due to changes in hormone levels throughout the menstrual cycle, and no further evaluation is needed. While having fibrocystic changes of the breast is usually painless, rapidly enlarging cysts may be painful. Although breast pain is a relatively uncommon manifestation of breast cancer, its presence does not exclude the diagnosis. **Never delay the evaluation of a painful breast mass.** If the evaluation of breast pain does not show any abnormalities, the patient should be counseled to wear tight-fitting bras, apply warm or cold compresses, and use nonsteroidal anti-inflammatory drugs (NSAIDs)[b] to relieve the discomfort. Consultation with a breast specialist can be obtained if conservative measures do not alleviate the pain.

Nipple Discharge

Nipple discharge is not a common symptom, but it should always raise suspicion of breast disease, especially if the discharge occurs spontaneously. Any patient who describes a nipple discharge should be asked the following questions:

"How long have you been having nipple discharge?"

"What color is the discharge? (typically clear, yellow, white, green, or red)

"Do you have a discharge from both breasts?"

"Does the discharge come spontaneously (on its own) or only when expressed from nipple?" "Is the discharge related to your menstrual cycle?"

"When was your last menstrual cycle?"

"Is the discharge associated with nipple retraction? A breast mass? Breast pain?"

"Do you have headaches or visual changes?"

"Are you taking any medications?"

"Are you using oral contraceptives?"

If the patient has recently delivered a child, ask:

"Were there any problems during the delivery of your last child?"

The two most common types of discharge are serous and bloody. *Serous discharge* is characterized by its thin, watery consistency and can appear as a yellowish stain on clothing. This type of discharge often results from an intraductal papilloma in one of the large subareolar ducts. Females taking oral contraceptives may experience bilateral serous discharge, while those with breast carcinoma may also have this type of discharge.

A *bloody* discharge is associated with an intraductal papilloma, which is common among pregnant and menstruating females. It may, however, be associated with a malignant intraductal papillary carcinoma. The presence of any nipple discharge is more important than its character because both types of discharge are associated with benign or malignant disease.

A *milky* discharge is usually milk. The secretion of milk while not nursing is known as *galactorrhea*. It is common for females to continue to secrete milk for a few months after they stop breastfeeding. In rare instances, the secretion may continue for a year. Abnormal lactation may also result from a pituitary tumor that interferes with the normal hypothalamic-pituitary feedback loop or from the use of certain psychiatric tranquilizing medications. Mechanical stimulation or suckling may produce physiologic stimulation.

Change in Skin Over Breast

A change in the color or texture of the skin of the breast or areola is an important symptom of breast carcinoma. The presence of dimpling, puckering, or scaliness warrants further investigation. The presence of unusually prominent pores, indicative of edema of the skin, is an important sign of malignancy. This clinical sign is called *peau d'orange* which is a French term meaning "orange peel" or "orange skin." It is used to describe a symptom in which the skin becomes thick and pitted, with a texture and appearance similar to that of orange peel. During the early stages of breast carcinoma, the lymphatic vessels of the breast are dilated and contain occasional emboli of carcinoma cells. Limited peau d'orange over the lower half of the areola is present. As the disease progresses, more lymphatic vessels become filled with carcinoma cells that block them, creating more generalized edema. The classic appearance of peau d'orange is pictured in Fig. 16.7.

General Suggestions

The interviewer should pay special attention to the family history of any female presenting with symptoms of breast disease.

[b]The five most common NSAIDs are aspirin, celecoxib (Celebrex®), ibuprofen (Advil®, Motrin®), naproxen (Aleve®, Naprosyn®), and indomethacin (Indocin®).

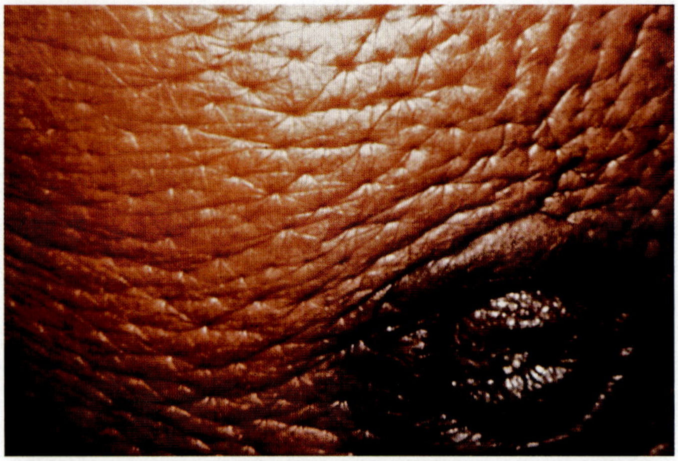

Fig. 16.7 Peau d'Orange.

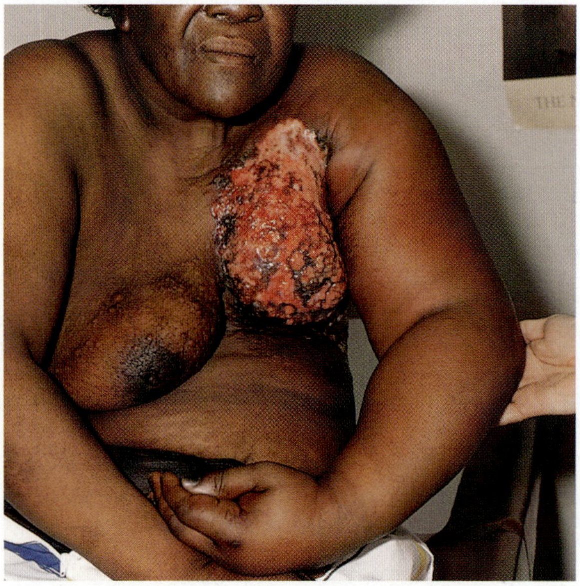

Fig. 16.8 Inflammatory Breast Carcinoma.

As indicated earlier, breast cancer may be a familial disorder. The occurrence of breast disease in a close relative and the age at which it developed are relevant to the patient's disease. Ask the patient the following questions:

"Have you had a mammogram?" If yes, *"When and what was the result?"*

"Have you had any breast biopsies or surgeries in the past?"

"Have you had breast cancer?" If yes, *"How was the cancer treated? Lumpectomy? Mastectomy? Chemotherapy? Radiation?"*

"Have you ever had radiation treatment to your chest for other cancers? If yes, *"Premenopausal or postmenopausal? At what age was the diagnosis made?"*

"Do you have any family members with a history of breast cancer?" If yes, *"Premenopausal or postmenopausal?" "At what age was their diagnosis made?"*[c]

"Do you use birth control pills?"

"Do you take estrogen replacement therapy?"

IMPACT OF BREAST DISEASE ON THE PATIENT

The psychosocial impact resulting from breast cancer is far-reaching. The diagnosis of breast cancer raises a whole mix of emotions, from the stress of treatment options to anxiety about the future and fear of recurrence. Patients may suffer a loss of self-identity with the change in appearance after a mastectomy, breast reconstructive surgery, or hair loss due to chemotherapy. Patients may also experience anxiety about their sexuality and fertility after undergoing treatment for breast cancer. Chemotherapy and chemoprophylaxis can alter hormone levels, alter a female's sexual arousal/response, and cause early menopause. This in turn would affect their ability to expand their family.

A new diagnosis of cancer is a great source of stress for patients. Each phase in the fight against cancer may induce psychological instability and can potentially contribute to the onset of depression or other mood-related conditions. The rates of anxiety and depression in those patients with breast cancer are estimated to be 10 to 30%.[4] Regardless of a patient's response to receiving this diagnosis, as a healthcare professional, it is imperative to treat the patient holistically. Open communication and emotional support among the patient, partner/spouse, family, healthcare professional, and healthcare team are important factors in the physical and psychological care of the patient.

The patient pictured in Fig. 16.8 had inflammatory carcinoma of their left breast, with massive lymphedema of the left arm. The patient had noticed that their arm had been swelling for the past few months, and she now needed support to raise it. She presented to the clinic complaining only about the heaviness of their arm. When examination revealed the breast lesion, she stated that she had noticed the breast changes "only a few days ago." This is an example of denial of illness (see also the patient shown in Fig. 2.1).

Over the last three decades, medical advancements in surgery and radiation therapy have led to alternative treatments for mastectomy. Breast conservation and breast reconstruction following mastectomy are now established options for many patients. For small, early cancers, lumpectomy with radiation provides comparable survival rates to mastectomy. Deciding on the right treatment for breast cancer is a complex and individual process. It's important for the patient and their healthcare professional to thoroughly explore all options with respect and understanding, as making an uninformed decision may lead to future regret.

PHYSICAL EXAMINATION

No special equipment is necessary for the examination of the breast. The examination of the breast consists of the following:

- Inspection
- Axillary examination
- Palpation

Breast examination is a two-part process. The first part is done while the patient is sitting up. This involves inspecting the breasts and palpating the lymph nodes. The second part is done

[c]It is important to include male family members because this family history should prompt a consultation with a genetic counselor.

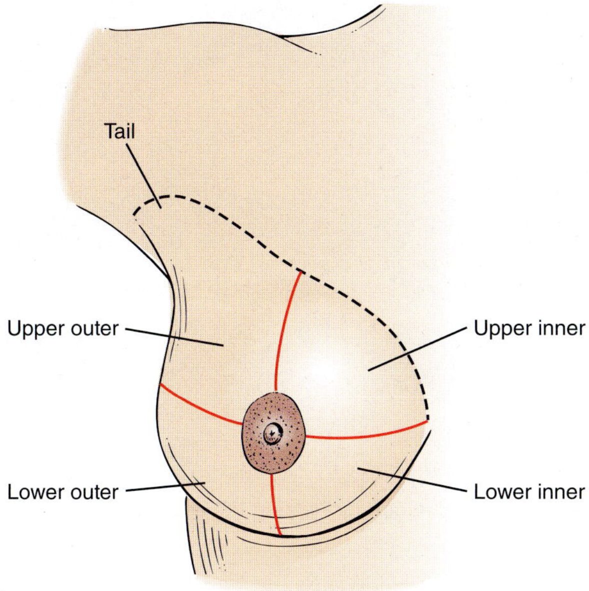

Fig. 16.9 The Four Breast Quadrants.

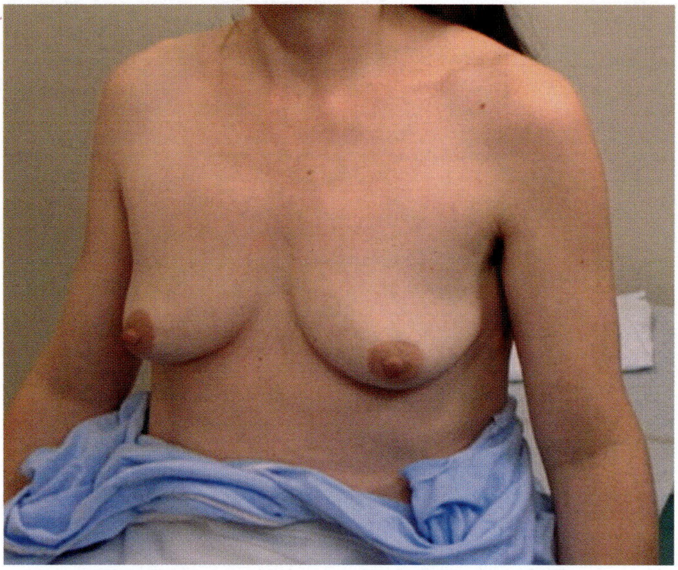

Fig. 16.10 Position of Patient for Inspection of the Breasts.

while the patient is lying supine. The examiner will palpate the entire breast systematically using the pulp of their fingers, instead of their fingertips, with firm and gentle pressure.

To facilitate communication, the breast is pictorially divided into four quadrants. Two imaginary lines run through the nipple at right angles to each other. By visualizing the breast as a face of a clock, one line is the "12 o'clock–6 o'clock" line, and the other is the "3 o'clock–9 o'clock" line. The resulting four quadrants are the upper outer, upper inner, lower outer, and lower inner. The "tail" is an extension of the upper outer quadrant. These regions are illustrated in Fig. 16.9.

Inspection

The patient should be seated on the edge of the examination table, facing the examiner. The examiner should ask the patient to remove the gown to their waist.

Inspect the Breasts

See Video 16.1.

Inspection is first accomplished with the patient's arms at their sides, as shown in Fig. 16.10. Tell the patient, "I am inspecting the breasts for any changes in the skin, contour, or symmetry." The breasts are inspected for size, shape, symmetry, contour, color, and edema. The nipples are inspected for size, shape, inversion, eversion, or discharge. The nipples should be symmetric. Is any abnormal bulging present?

The skin of the breast is observed for edema. Edema of the skin of the breast that overlies a malignancy may manifest as peau d'orange.

Is erythema present? Erythema is associated with infection and with inflammatory carcinoma of the breast. Fig. 16.11 shows marked erythema of the breast secondary to inflammatory breast carcinoma. The scar above the areola is from a previous biopsy of a benign breast mass.

Is dimpling present? The examiner must inspect the breasts for the presence of *retraction phenomena.* Dimpling is a sign of retraction phenomena that are caused by an underlying neoplasm and its fibrotic response. Skin retraction is commonly associated with malignancy that causes abnormal traction on Cooper ligaments. The shortening of the larger mammary ducts by cancer produces flattening or inversion of the nipple. A change in the position of the nipple is important because many females have a congenitally inverted nipple on one or both sides. The dimpling of the breast in Fig. 16.12 is associated with a bloody nipple discharge; both are secondary to carcinoma.

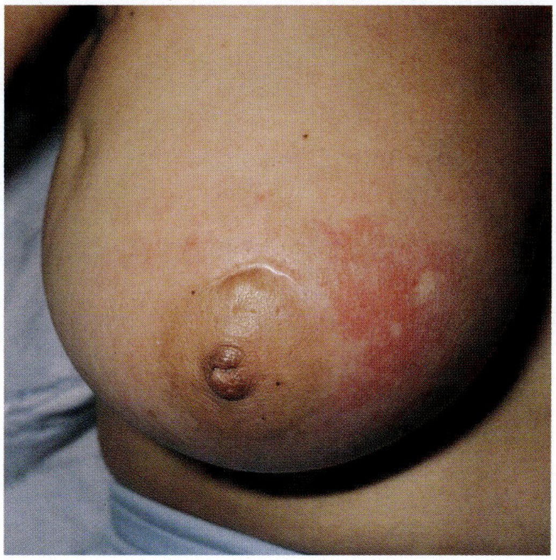

Fig. 16.11 Erythema of the Breast.

Is there a red, scaling, crusting plaque around one nipple, areola, or surrounding skin? *Paget disease* of the breast is a surface manifestation invariably associated with an underlying invasive or intraductal carcinoma. The lesion appears eczematous, but unlike eczema, it is unilateral. The skin may also weep and be eroded. A much less common form is extramammary Paget disease, which is seen around the anus or genitalia and is usually associated with malignant disease of the adnexa, bowel,

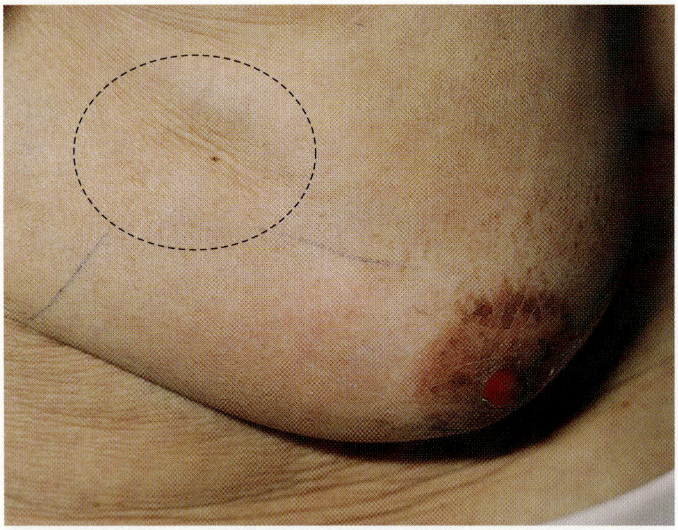

Fig. 16.12 **Breast Carcinoma.** Note dimpling of the breast and bloody nipple discharge.

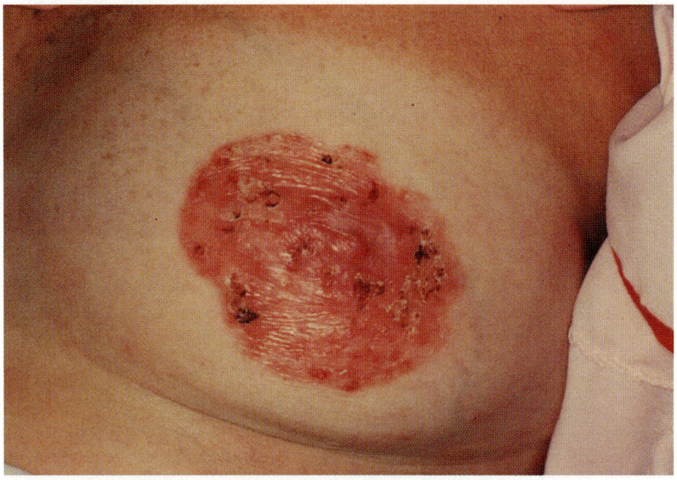

Fig. 16.13 **Paget Disease of the Breast.** (From Callen JP, Greer KE, Hood AF, et al: *Color atlas of dermatology*, Philadelphia, 1993, WB Saunders.)

or genitourinary tract. Fig. 16.13 shows Paget disease of the breast; an underlying ductal adenocarcinoma was present.

Inspect the Breasts in Various Postures

Inspection is next performed while the patient assumes several postures that may bring out signs of retraction that were less evident previously. Ask the patient to press their arms against their hips. This maneuver tenses the pectoralis muscles, which may bring out dimpling caused by the fixation of the breast to the underlying muscles. This technique is shown in Fig. 16.14. If a malignancy is present, the abnormal attachment of the tumor to the fascia and pectoralis muscle pulls on the skin and may produce skin dimpling. Any bulging may also indicate an underlying mass.

Another maneuver, which is useful for a patient with pendulous breasts, involves bending at the waist and allowing the breasts to hang free from the chest wall. This technique is illustrated in Fig. 16.15. A carcinoma causing

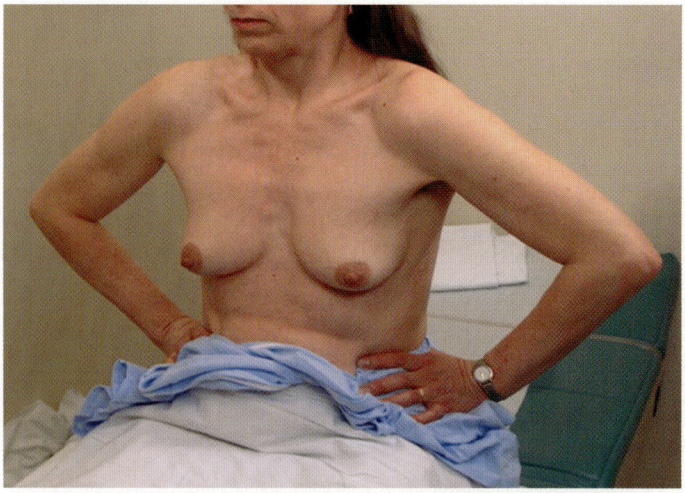

Fig. 16.14 Technique for Tensing the Pectoralis Muscles.

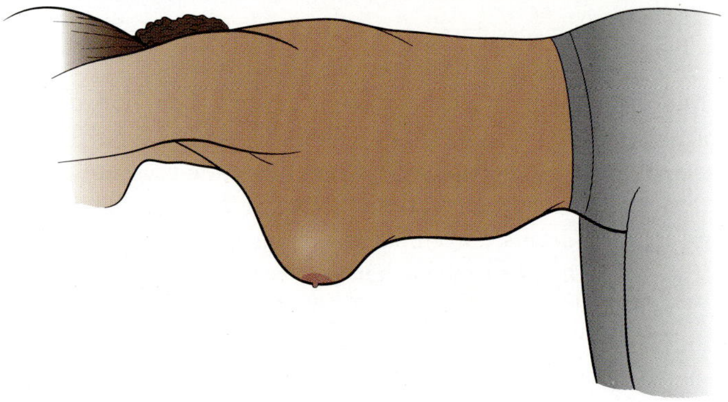

Fig. 16.15 Position of Patient for Inspecting the Breasts.

fibrosis in one breast produces a change in the contour of that breast.

Axillary Examination

See Video 16.2.

The axillary examination is performed with the patient seated facing the examiner. Examination of the axilla is best accomplished by relaxing the pectoral muscles. To examine the right axilla, the patient's right forearm is supported by the examiner's right hand. The tips of the fingers of the examiner's left hand start low in the axilla, and as the patient's right arm is drawn medially, the examiner advances the left hand higher into the axilla. This technique is demonstrated in Fig. 16.16. The supraclavicular, subclavian, and axillary regions are palpated.

To detect adenopathy, a technique involving small circular motions of the fingers over the ribs is used. Nodes that are freely mobile and measure between 3 to 5 mm in diameter are commonly found, and are typically indicative of lymphadenitis caused by minor hand and arm trauma. After examining one axilla, the examiner then evaluates the other using their opposite hand.

Palpation

The patient is asked to lie down and is told that the breast will next be palpated. The examiner stands at the right side of

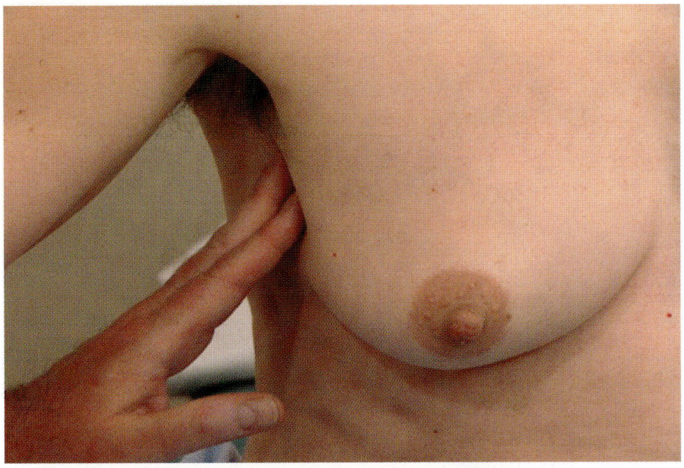

A

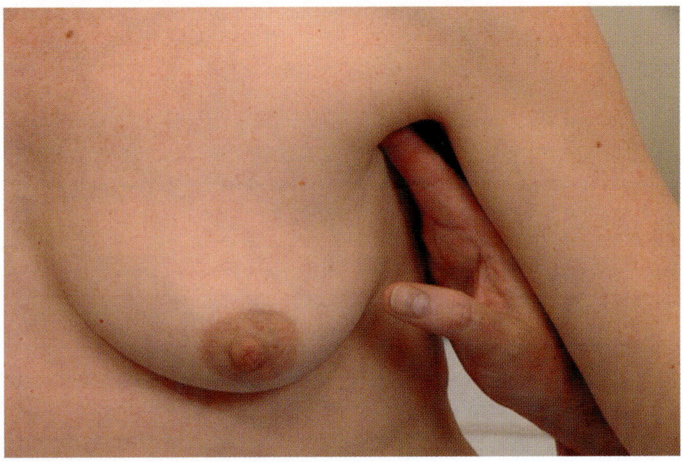

B

Fig. 16.16 Technique for Axillary Examination. (A) Low axilla *(right side)*. (B) High axilla *(left side)*.

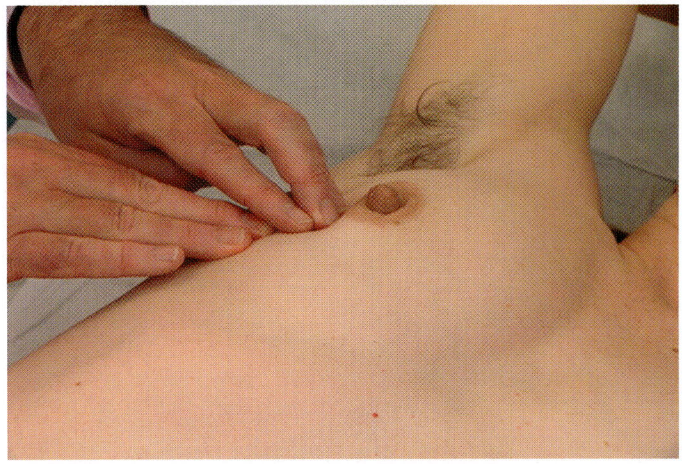

A

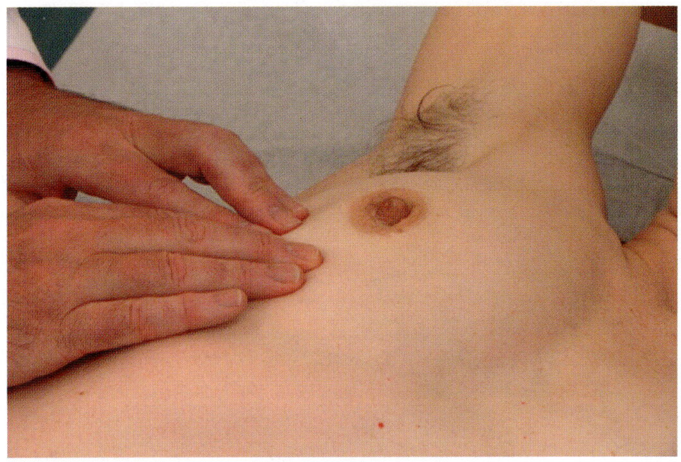

B

Fig. 16.17 Technique for Breast Palpation. (A) "Spokes of a wheel." (B) Concentric circles.

the patient's bed. Although the examiner can usually palpate each breast from the patient's right side, it is often better with large-breasted females to examine the left breast from the left side.

To properly examine the breast, it should be positioned evenly on the chest wall. Small-breasted individuals may keep their arms at their sides while larger-breasted individuals are advised to place their hands behind their head. Placing a pillow under the shoulder of the side being examined can help make the examination easier.

Palpate the Breast

See Video 16.3.

In palpation of the breast, the examiner should use both the flat of the hand and the fingertips, as demonstrated in Fig. 16.17. Palpation should be performed by the "spokes of a wheel," the concentric circle, or the vertical strip method. The "spokes of a wheel" method starts at the nipple (see Fig. 16.17A). The examiner should start the palpation by moving outward from the nipple to the 12 o'clock position. The examiner then should return to the nipple and move along the 1 o'clock position and continue the palpation around the breasts. The concentric circles approach (see Fig. 16.17B) also starts at the nipple, but the examiner moves from the nipple in a continuous circular manner around the breast. Any lesion found by either technique is described as being a certain distance from the nipple in clock time: for example, "3 cm from the nipple along the 1 o'clock line." These techniques are illustrated in Fig. 16.18.

Another method is the vertical strip, or grid, technique. The breast is divided into eight or nine vertical strips, each approximately one finger's width. The examiner's three middle fingers are held together and slightly bowed to ensure contact with the skin. The pads, not the tips, of the fingers must be used for palpation. Using dime-sized circles, the examiner evaluates the breast at each of three different levels of pressure: light, medium, and deep. Each strip consists of 9 or 10 areas of palpation, slightly overlapping the previous area, and each vertical strip is evaluated with the three pressures. Although this method has been shown to be superior to the other traditional types of breast palpation, it is more time-consuming and may be best used by females for BSE.

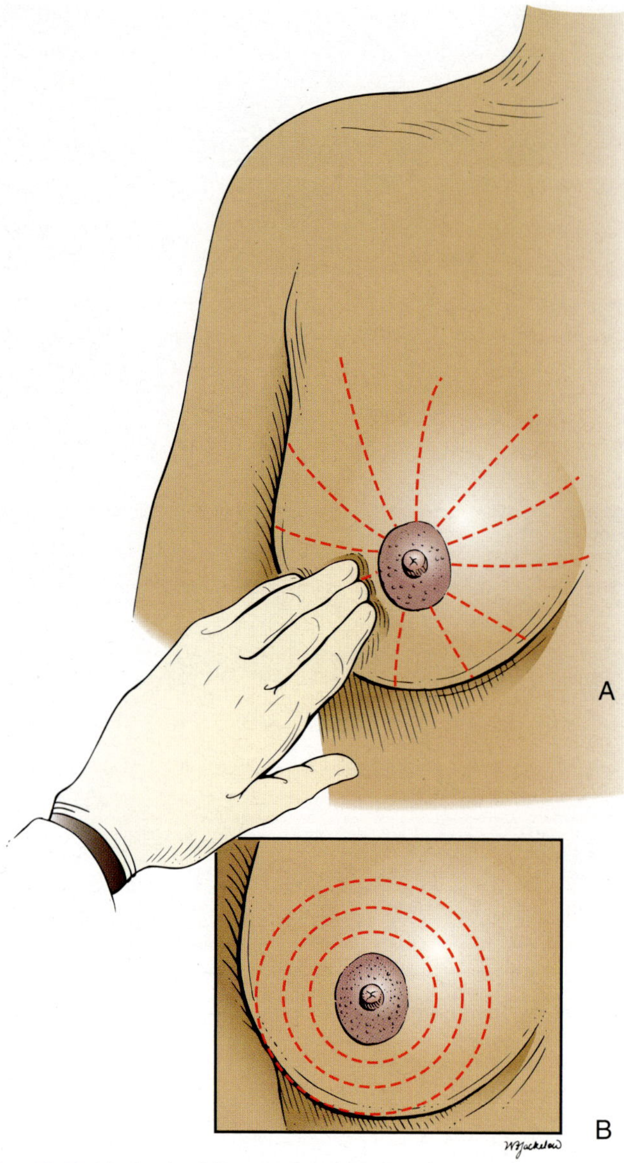

Fig. 16.18 Method of Breast Palpation. (A) "Spokes of a wheel." (B) Concentric circles.

The examiner should be careful when evaluating the *inframammary fold.* This fold is commonly observed in older females and is the area where the mammary tissue is bound tightly to the chest wall. Often, this ridge is mistaken for a breast disorder.

Describe the Findings

If a mass is palpated, the following characteristics should be described:

1. The *size* of the mass in centimeters and its position
2. The *shape* of the mass
3. The *delineation*, referring to the borders of the mass: Is it well delineated, as with a cyst? Are the edges diffuse, as with a carcinoma?
4. The *consistency*, describing the "hardness" of the mass: a carcinoma is often stony hard. A cyst has some elastic qualities.

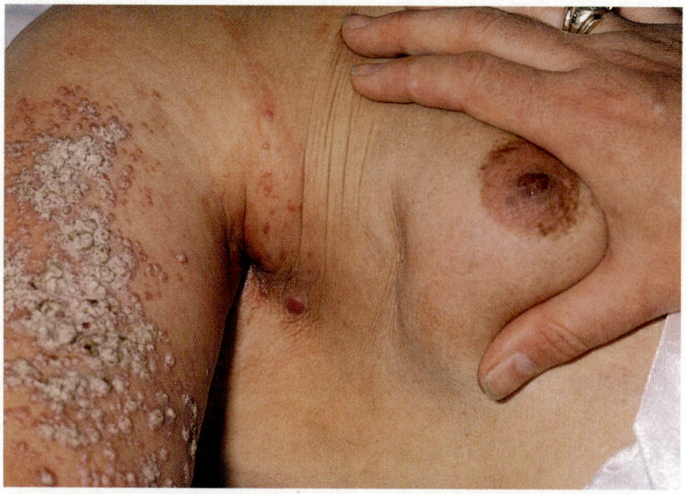

Fig. 16.19 Breast Dimpling. Note the satellite skin lesions of metastatic breast cancer on the upper arm.

5. The *mobility* of the lesion: Is the lesion movable in the tissue that surrounds it? Benign tumors and cysts are freely mobile. Carcinomas are usually fixed to the skin, underlying muscle, or chest wall.

Evaluate for Retraction Phenomenon

If a mass is detected, *molding* of the skin may be useful to determine whether the retraction phenomenon is present. The examiner should elevate the breast around the mass. Dimpling may occur if carcinoma is present. Fig. 16.19 demonstrates the technique of molding and its result in a patient with carcinoma of the breast. Notice the marked dimpling of the breast. This patient also had metastatic lesions of breast carcinoma on her arm, together with lymphedema. She presented to the clinic stating that she had discovered the swollen arm the day before.

Palpate the Subareolar Area

The subareolar area, the area directly under the areola, should be palpated while the patient is lying supine. In the subareolar area, the breast tissue is less dense. An abscess of Montgomery glands in the areola may cause a tender mass in this area.

Examine the Nipple

See Video 16.4.

Examination of the nipple concludes the examination of the breast. Inspect for nipple retraction, fissures, and scaling. To examine for discharge, place each hand on either side of the nipple and gently compress the nipple, noting the character of any discharge. This technique is demonstrated in Fig. 16.20. Ask the patient whether they would prefer to perform this part of the examination themselves.

Examination of the Male Breast

Examination of the breast should be performed on all males. The nipples should be inspected for swelling, discharge, and ulceration. The areola and the subareolar tissue should be palpated for any masses. The axillary examination is as indicated for females.

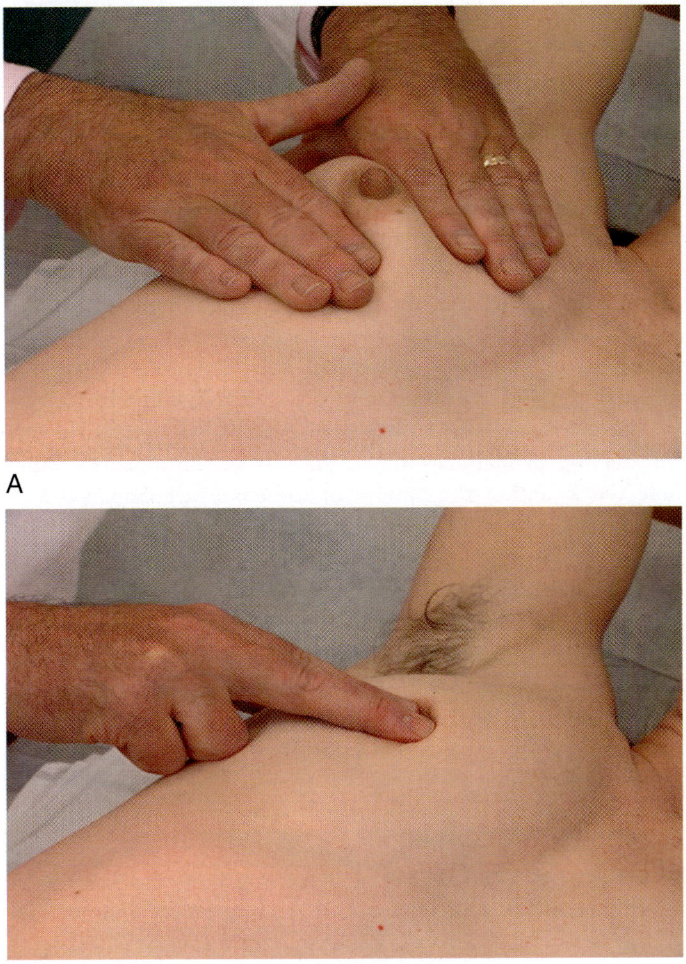

A

B

Fig. 16.20 Technique for Nipple Examination. (A) Examination for discharge. (B) Examination for masses below the nipple.

Breast Self-Examination[d]

Although monthly BSE was recommended for many years, it has been recognized that BSE has limited value in detecting early cancer. Organizations such as the American Cancer Society, American College of Obstetrics and Gynecology, and the U.S. Preventative Service Task Force have found insufficient evidence to recommend BSE. The emphasis on monthly BSE has been replaced by the concept of "breast self-awareness" whereby females older than 20 years become knowledgeable about the normal appearance and feel of their breasts but without a specific schedule or examination technique. A healthcare professional should help educate the patient so that they can have the awareness to report any skin changes, dimpling, nipple discharge or presence of new lumps or bumps. Although medical attention should be sought for any of these findings, they can be reassured that most findings are not cancer.

Many females will want to know how best to examine their breasts. The techniques of BSE are included here for the purpose of patient education:

1. Stand with your arms at your sides in front of a mirror. Inspect both breasts for anything unusual, such as dimpling, redness, puckering, discharge from the nipples, or scaling of the skin.
2. Raise your arms and clasp your hands behind your head. Press your hands forward. Look in the mirror for any changes in the breast tissue.
3. Put your hands down and place them on your hips. Bend slightly toward the mirror as you pull your shoulders and elbows forward.
4. Raise your right arm; using the pads of your left fingers, press into your right breast firmly, carefully, and thoroughly. Start at the upper outer edge and move in small circles, moving the circles slowly around the breast. Pay special attention to the breast tissue between the breast and the underarm. Use a massaging motion.
5. Gently squeeze your nipple and look for any discharge.
6. Repeat steps 4 and 5 while lying down with a small pillow under your right shoulder. Place your right arm over your head.
7. Repeat the examination on your left breast.
8. Examine each underarm while sitting or standing with your arm only slightly raised so that you can more easily feel in this area. Lifting the arm straight up will tighten the skin and make the examination more difficult.

THE MALE BREAST

Gynecomastia is the enlargement of one or both breasts in a male. It often occurs at puberty, occurs with aging, or is drug related. Fig. 16.21 shows a 90-year-old male who was treated with diethylstilbestrol for carcinoma of the prostate and developed gynecomastia.

It is estimated that in 2023, there were around 2800 new cases of invasive carcinoma in the male breast and roughly 530 deaths as a result of metastatic disease. The typical age of diagnosis is 59 years. The primary symptom, present in 75% of cases, is a solid and painless lump located either under the areola or in the upper outer quadrant of the breast.

Breast cancer in males and females is most prevalent in North America and the British Isles, while it is least common in Japan and Finland. Like in females, male breast cancer often spreads to various parts of the body, such as the bone, lung, liver, pleura, lymph nodes, skin, and other visceral sites.

[d]The importance of BSE has been recognized for more than 60 years. However, to date, the efficacy of this examination is not definitive. A large, randomized, controlled trial was conducted in 1997 by Thomas and associates in Shanghai and included more than 267,040 females, half of whom were given intensive training in BSE; the other half were asked to attend training sessions on the prevention of low back pain. All females were observed for 5 years for the development of breast diseases. The study showed neither a significant difference in mortality rate in the two groups nor an earlier identification of breast disease in the group trained in BSE. The authors' conclusion was that "there was insufficient evidence to recommend for or against the teaching of BSE." Based upon this important Chinese study, in 2009, the U.S Preventive Services Task Force recommended against doctors teaching females about BSE. The American Cancer Society no longer recommends BSEs.

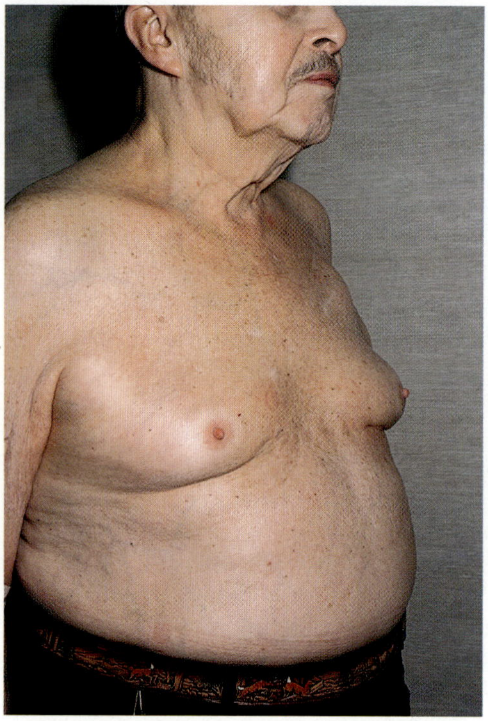

Fig. 16.21 Gynecomastia.

CLINICOPATHOLOGIC CORRELATIONS

Cancer of the Breast

There is mounting evidence that defects in DNA repair may be significant factors for the development of breast cancer. Two genes, *BRCA1* and *BRCA2,* have been identified as *tumor suppressor genes* or *breast cancer susceptibility genes* and appear to be involved with gene repair.[5] Tumor suppressor genes keep cellular growth in control but can cause cancer when their function is blocked. More than 2000 mutations have been described for these tumor suppressor genes. When mutations or deletions occur in these suppressor genes, the incidence of neoplastic transformation is much greater. *BRCA1* and *BRCA2* are associated with proteins, such as p53 and RAD51, which are involved with DNA repair and transcriptional activation. Carriers of germline mutations in *BRCA1,* located on chromosome 17, or *BRCA2,* located on chromosome 13, have an increased incidence of early-onset, familial breast, or ovarian cancer. Mutant *BRCA1* and *BRCA2* genes account for 50% of hereditable breast cancers.

Mutations in these tumor suppressor genes have been found in only 5% to 10% of females with early-onset breast cancers. If a mutation in the *BRCA1* gene is present, however, it is estimated that the lifetime risk for the development of breast cancer is approximately 60% to 80%, and the development of ovarian cancer is approximately 33%. A male with a mutant allele of the gene has an increased incidence of prostate cancer. *BRCA2* is associated with an increased incidence of breast cancer in males and females. Some population groups, such as individuals of Ashkenazi Jewish descent, have an increased prevalence of *BRCA1* and *BRCA2* mutation carriers. Researchers have discovered that 2.5% of these females may carry the mutation—an occurrence that is approximately five times greater than that of the general population. Although these mutations account for less than 10% of all breast cancer cases, they are very rare in the general population (less than 1%), so *widespread genetic testing is not recommended.*

The finding of a breast mass on palpation, even in the presence of a normal mammogram, necessitates a biopsy. However, breast palpation has a much lower true-positive rate (sensitivity) than mammography. There are many false-negative findings in breast palpation. This error is related to the difficulty in palpating a small mass in large breasts, the inherent properties of breast tissue, and poor technique. The limitations of physical examination and mammography are shown in Table 16.1.

The physical examination is of great importance in determining the probability that a mass is cancerous. Any lump detected by either the patient or the examiner carries a 20% risk of cancer. As indicated in Table 16.2, benign lesions usually are freely mobile, have well-delineated borders, and feel soft or cystic. However, of all breast cancers, 60% are freely mobile, 40% have well-delineated borders, and 50% feel soft or cystic. A fixed lesion has a 50% chance of being malignant. If this lesion has irregular borders, the likelihood of being malignant rises to 60%. The sensitivity and specificity of certain physical findings in evaluating a breast mass for malignancy are shown in Table 16.3.

Screening Guidelines for Early Detection of Cancer of the Breast

1. The National Cancer Institute recommends that females begin receiving screening mammograms every 1 to 2 years starting at 40 years of age and every year once they reach

TABLE 16.1 Limitations of Physical Examination and Mammography

Operating Characteristic	Physical Examination	Mammography
Sensitivity (%)	24	62
Specificity (%)	95	90

Data from Bond WH: The treatment of carcinoma of the breast. In Jarrett AS, editor: *Proceedings of a symposium on the treatment of carcinoma of the breast,* Amsterdam, 1968, Excerpta Medica.

TABLE 16.2 Differentiation of Breast Masses

Characteristic	Cystic Disease	Benign Adenoma	Malignant Tumor
Patient age	25–60 years	10–55 years	25–85 years
Number	One or more	One	One
Shape	Round	Round	Irregular
Consistency	Elastic, soft to hard	Firm	Stony hard
Delimitation	Well delimited	Well delimited	Poorly delimited
Mobility	Mobile	Mobile	Fixed
Tenderness	Present	Absent	Absent
Skin retraction	Absent	Absent	Present

TABLE 16.3 Characteristics of Breast Masses Suspect for Cancer

Characteristic	Sensitivity (%)	Specificity[a] (%)
Fixed mass	40	90
Poorly delimited mass	60	90
Hard mass	62	90

[a]Based on the assumption that nonmalignant breast masses have benign characteristics.
Data from Venet L, Strax P, Venet W, et al: Adequacies and inadequacies of breast examination by physicians in mass screening, *Cancer* 28(6):1546–1551, 1971.

50 years of age, continuing for as long as a female is in good health.[6] (The American College of Obstetrics and Gynecology recommends annual mammograms beginning at age 40.)[7] Screening mammography involves taking low-dose radiographs from two views of each breast, typically from above (craniocaudal view) and from an oblique or angled position (mediolateral-oblique view). Mammography can detect approximately 85% of breast cancers. If the mammogram indicates an abnormality, further breast imaging (i.e., with spot-view mammography, ultrasonography, or other imaging tests) is recommended. If further imaging confirms or reveals an abnormality, the patient may be referred for a biopsy to determine whether she has breast cancer. Screening mammography can miss 10% to 15% of breast cancers. These tumors can be missed (1) if the tumor is very small, (2) if the tumor is in an area not easily imaged (e.g., in the axilla), or (3) if other shadows obscure the tumor.

2. A clinical breast examination should be part of a periodic health examination, approximately every 3 years for females in their 20s and 30s and every year for females 40 years of age and older.
3. Females should know how their breasts normally feel. They should report any changes immediately to their healthcare professional. BSE should be taught to females in their 20s.
4. Females at increased risk (e.g., family history, genetic tendency, past history of breast cancer) should speak to their healthcare professional about the benefits and limitations of starting mammography screening earlier, having additional tests (e.g., breast ultrasonography, magnetic resonance imaging), or having more frequent examinations.

USEFUL VOCABULARY

Listed here are the specific roots that are important for understanding the terminology related to breast disease.

Root	Pertaining to	Example	Definition
gyne(co)-	female	***gyneco***mastia	Excessive development of the male breast
lact(o)-	milk	***lact***ation	Secretion of milk
mammo-	breast	***mammo***graphy	Radiographic visualization of the breast
mast(o)-	breast	***mast***itis	Inflammation of the breast

WRITING UP THE PHYSICAL EXAMINATION

Listed here are examples of the write-up for the examination of the breast.

- The breasts are symmetric, with both nipples everted. The overlying skin is normal. No dimpling is present. There are no masses or discharge. Axillary examination reveals no lymphadenopathy.
- The left breast is slightly larger than the right. There is a serosanguineous discharge from the left nipple. When the patient presses her arms against her hips, a dimple is seen 4 cm from the nipple at the 2 o'clock position of the left breast. Palpation reveals a 2 × 3 cm stony mass under the area of dimpling. The mass appears fixed to the underlying muscle and overlying skin. Examination of the left axilla reveals numerous hard, fixed lymph nodes.
- The right breast is larger than the left. The skin is erythematous and warm to the touch, especially around the areola. The right nipple is inverted. No masses are felt. Dimpling cannot be appreciated. No axillary adenopathy is present.
- The breasts are pendulous and symmetric. Both nipples are everted. There are multiple round, freely mobile masses in both breasts, more on the right. The masses are 2 to 3 cm in diameter, elastic in consistency, and somewhat tender. Skin retraction is absent. No discharge is present. No axillary adenopathy is present.

FULL VIDEO

- Video 16.5 Full video: Examination of the female breast

REVIEW QUESTIONS

1. Which of the following is NOT a risk factor for breast cancer?
  A. Frequent exercise
  B. Early menarche
  C. Excessive alcohol consumption
  D. Late menopause
  E. Family history of breast cancer

2. What is the function of the smooth muscle in the nipple and areola?
  A. It aids in milk production.
  B. It regulates hormonal changes.
  C. It controls the size of the breast.
  D. It provides structural support to the breast.
  E. It contracts to make the nipple erect.

3. **Which factor primarily determines the size of the adult breast?**
   A. Presence of excess adipose tissue
   B. Hormonal changes during menstruation
   C. Number of milk ducts
   D. Age at the onset of puberty
   E. Genetics
4. **When is cyclic breast pain most likely to occur?**
   A. During pregnancy
   B. After menopause
   C. Throughout the menstrual cycle
   D. During breastfeeding
   E. During the premenstrual and menstrual stages of the cycle
5. **What is the most likely cause of spontaneous nipple discharge?**
   A. Fibrocystic changes
   B. Hormonal fluctuations
   C. Intraductal papilloma
   D. Peau d'orange
   E. Galactorrhea
6. **Which breast symptom is associated with "peau d'orange"?**
   A. Mass or swelling
   B. Pain
   C. Nipple discharge
   D. Change in skin color or texture
   E. Nipple retraction
7. **During breast examination, which technique is recommended for detecting adenopathy in the axillary region?**
   A. Linear palpation
   B. Circular palpation
   C. Small, circular motions over the ribs
   D. Vertical strip, or grid, technique
   E. Molding of the skin around the mass
8. **Which technique is used to examine the nipple for discharge during a breast examination?**
   A. Firm pressure on the nipple
   B. Gently compress the nipple between the fingers
   C. Squeeze the nipple with both hands
   D. Pinch the nipple with thumb and forefinger
   E. Rotate the nipple in a circular motion
9. **What concept has replaced monthly breast self-examination (BSE)?**
   A. Breast self-examination (BSE) remains the gold standard for early breast cancer detection.
   B. Females are advised to perform BSE on a monthly basis.
   C. The concept of "breast self-awareness" without a specific schedule or technique is recommended.
   D. BSE should only be performed under the guidance of a healthcare professional.
   E. BSE is no longer recommended, and patients should rely solely on clinical examinations.
10. **According to the screening guidelines for early detection of breast cancer, what is the recommended frequency for clinical breast examinations for females in their 20s and 30s?**
    A. Every 1 to 2 years
    B. Every year
    C. Approximately every 3 years
    D. Only when a lump is detected
    E. It is not recommended for females in their 20s and 30s

REFERENCES

Available online.

BIBLIOGRAPHY

Available online.

17

The Abdomen

Mark H. Swartz

The way to a man's heart is through his stomach.

Fanny Fern (1811–1872)

VIDEOS

Video 17.1	Inspecting the contour of the abdomen and evaluating for abdominal hernias
Video 17.2	Evaluating bowel sounds
Video 17.3	Evaluating for abdominal bruits
Video 17.4	Evaluating for shifting dullness
Video 17.5	Evaluating the abdomen by light palpation
Video 17.6	Evaluating the abdomen by deep palpation
Video 17.7	Palpating the liver
Video 17.8	Palpating the spleen
Video 17.9	Performing the rectal examination
Video 17.10	Full video: Examination of the abdomen

GENERAL CONSIDERATIONS

Abdominal diseases are prevalent, with about 10% of adults in the United States experiencing peptic ulcer disease (PUD). This condition occurs when there are defects in the gastrointestinal mucosa, which extend through the muscularis mucosae. Peptic ulcer disease is responsible for causing a significant amount of morbidity and healthcare expenses, affecting over six million people in the United States annually. It is characterized by a discontinuation in the inner lining of the gastrointestinal tract due to gastric acid secretion or pepsin, extending into the muscularis propria layer of the gastric epithelium. Typically, it occurs in the stomach and proximal duodenum, but it can also involve the lower esophagus, distal duodenum, or jejunum.

PUD has multiple causes, but the majority of cases are attributed to *Helicobacter pylori*–associated PUD and NSAID-associated PUD.[1] Some medications such as NSAIDs, corticosteroids, bisphosphonates, potassium chloride, and fluorouracil have been linked to the development of PUD. *H. pylori* is a type of bacteria that is commonly found in the gastric epithelial cells and is responsible for causing 90% of duodenal ulcers and 70% to 90% of gastric ulcers. Approximately 30% to 40% of people in the United States are infected with *H. pylori*, which can lead to inflammation and PUD by breaking down the stomach's inner protective coating. Although *H. pylori* infection typically does not cause any noticeable symptoms, the lifetime prevalence of the infection is around 20% among those infected. The proportion of people with the infection increases with age, with only about 10% of young people having *H. pylori* infection.

It's been noted that 5% of people over the age of 40 are affected by *diverticular disease*. This condition leads to the formation of small bulging pouches in the colon walls, which is commonly referred to as diverticula. These pouches are most commonly found in the sigmoid colon. Although sometimes asymptomatic, diverticular disease can commonly cause symptoms like abdominal pain, rectal bleeding, and fever. There are two types of diverticular disease: diverticulosis and diverticulitis. Diverticulosis is the presence of diverticula and may lead to cramps, bloating, constipation, and bleeding. On the other hand, diverticulitis is an infection of the diverticula and can cause symptoms like pain, fever, chills, cramping, and constipation.

Colorectal cancer is the fourth most common type of cancer that affects both males and females in America, after excluding skin cancers. It is the second most common cause of cancer deaths in all patients. In 2023, there were 153,020 new cases of colorectal cancer diagnosed, and there were 52,550 deaths.[2] Colorectal death rates declined 52% from 1970 to 2015 among all patients because of increased screening and improvements in therapy. There was a significant decline, however, in 2020 cancer incidence counts, which may in part be due to the impact of the COVID-19 pandemic on health services and subsequential delays and reductions in cancer screening, diagnosis, and reporting to some central cancer registries. The average lifetime risk of developing colorectal cancer is 1 in 23 males and 1 in 25 females. The risk for this type of cancer differs widely among individuals. Ashkenazi (Eastern European) Jewish people have the highest risk of developing colorectal cancer of any ethnic group in the world. The second highest incidence is in African Americans, who have a rate of 50.4 cases per 100,000 population. The reason is not fully understood. The lowest incidence is in the Native American population, at 16.4 per 100,000. In 2020, the incidence rates were highest in Europe, Australia, and New Zealand, and the mortality rates were highest in Eastern Europe.

Some patients, such as those with congenital polyposis or ulcerative colitis, have a higher likelihood of developing colon cancer, often at a younger age. The risk for colonic cancer in patients with ulcerative colitis increases by 20% with each decade of life. Diet is also a factor in the incidence of colonic cancer, with individuals who consume a low-fiber, high-fat diet being at a higher risk. Consuming a diet high in red meats like beef, pork, lamb, or liver, and processed meats like hot dogs and some luncheon meats, can also increase the risk of colorectal cancer. Timely physical diagnosis has been proven to reduce mortality rates for colorectal cancer.

Every year, about 25,000 males and 11,000 females are diagnosed with *liver cancer*, and about 19,000 males and 9000 females die of the disease.[3] Liver cancer cases are mostly hepatocellular carcinoma, originating from hepatocytes, with more than 80% of cases falling under this category. Since 1992, liver cancer incidence has been increasing by 3.4% and 3% per year in males and females, respectively. Unlike other common cancer sites, incidence rates are highest among Asian Americans, Pacific Islanders, and Hispanics. In Western countries, liver cancer cases are mostly attributed to alcohol-related cirrhosis and nonalcoholic fatty liver disease associated with obesity. Chronic infections with hepatitis B virus (HBV) and hepatitis C virus (HCV) are associated with less than half of liver cancer cases in the United States, although they are the major risk factors for the disease worldwide. Liver cancer has several other risk factors, especially in developing countries. These include parasitic infections like schistosomiasis and liver flukes, as well as consumption of food that's contaminated with aflatoxin. Aflatoxin is a toxin that's produced by mold during the storage of agricultural products in warm and humid environments.

Gallbladder cancer is a rare malignancy but represents almost 50% of all biliary tract cancer. Biliary cancers are highly fatal malignancies with a 5-year survival rate of 17.6% (2007–2013).[4] Gallbladder cancer has a poor prognosis due to its aggressive tumor biology, complicated anatomic position, late presentation, and advanced stage at diagnosis. The incidence of gallbladder cancer is high in certain populations outside of the United States, including South America, India, Pakistan, Japan, and Korea. This is because these areas have a high prevalence of gallstones and chronic gallbladder infections. According to the American Cancer Society, there are an estimated 11,740 new cases of gallbladder cancer and 3830 deaths in the United States, with a higher incidence in females. While the overall incidence of gallbladder cancer decreases in patients over 50 years old, it increases in younger populations. Gallbladder cancer is more common in Whites, southwestern Native Americans, and Mexican Americans but less common in African Americans.

In 2023, there were 64,050 adults (33,130 males and 30,920 females) in the United States diagnosed with *pancreatic cancer*.[5] The disease accounts for approximately 3% of all cancers. Pancreatic cancer ranks as the eighth most prevalent cancer among females and the tenth most prevalent among males. The incidence of pancreatic cancer has been steadily increasing by approximately 1% per year for both genders since the late 1990s. Globally, approximately 495,773 individuals were diagnosed with pancreatic cancer in 2020. Smoking tobacco and using smokeless tobacco products are major risk factors for pancreatic cancer, with incidence rates being nearly two times higher for smokers than for nonsmokers.

Esophageal cancer is a deadly malignancy with very low survival, even with treatment.[6] Esophageal cancer is the fifth most frequently occurring gastrointestinal cancer in the United States, with an estimated 16,940 cases annually, and the sixth most common type of cancer globally. In the United States, almost 90% of esophageal squamous cell carcinoma cases are attributed to factors such as a history of smoking, alcohol consumption, and a diet that lacks fruits and vegetables. Symptoms of esophageal cancer include weight loss and pain or difficulty when swallowing.

STRUCTURE AND PHYSIOLOGY

To provide clear descriptions, the abdominal cavity is typically visually divided into four quadrants. These quadrants are divided by two imaginary perpendicular lines that intersect at the umbilicus. This results in the abdomen being divided into the right upper, right lower, left upper, and left lower quadrants. One of these lines extends from the sternum to the pubic bone, passing through the umbilicus. At the level of the umbilicus, there is a second line that intersects with the first at a right angle. This creates four quadrants, as shown in Fig. 17.1, each containing different abdominal organs.

Another way to divide the abdomen is into nine areas: *epigastric, umbilical, suprapubic, right and left hypochondrium, right and left lumbar, and right and left inguinal.* To do this, two imaginary lines are drawn by extending the midclavicular lines to the middle of the inguinal ligaments. These lines form the lateral extent of the rectus abdominis muscles. Then, two parallel lines are drawn at right angles to these lines: one at the costal margins and the other at the anterosuperior iliac spines. You can see this nine-area system in Fig. 17.2.

It is important for the examiner to be able to identify the abdominal structures in each quadrant. Refer to Table 17.1 for a list of the organs present in each of the four quadrants.

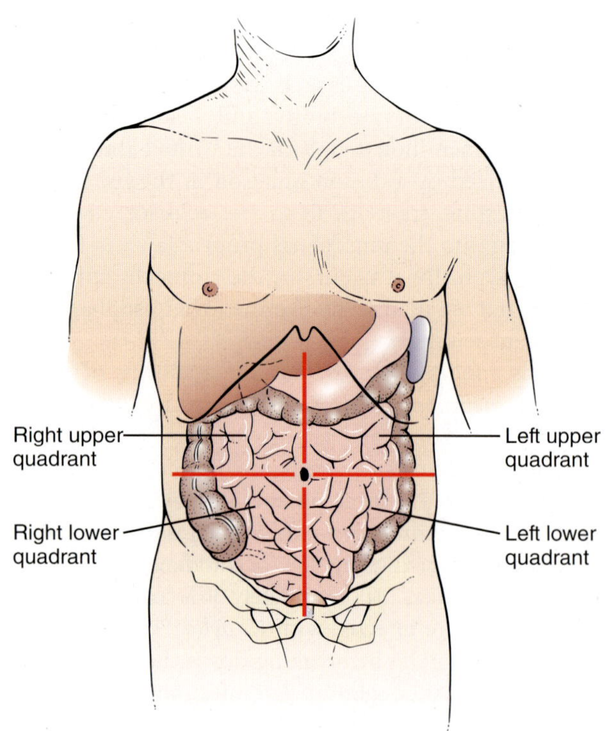

Fig. 17.1 The Four Abdominal Quadrants.

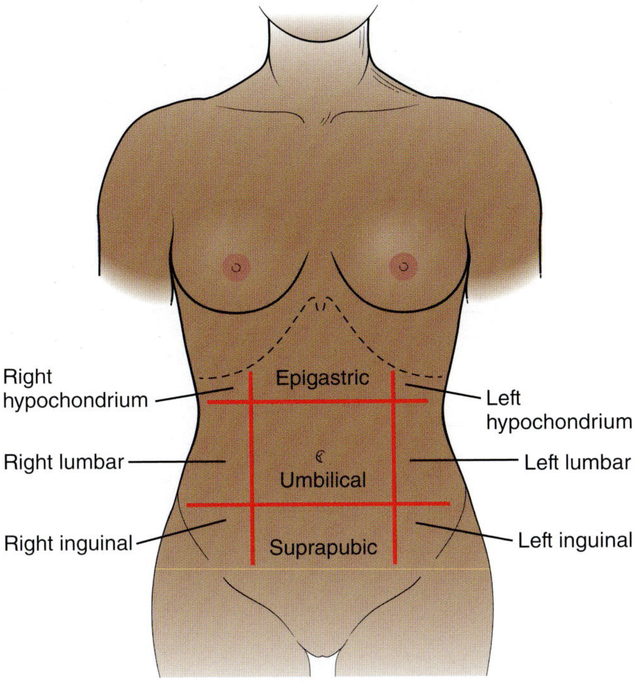

Fig. 17.2 The Nine Abdominal Areas.

TABLE 17.1 Abdominal Structures by Quadrants

Right	Left
Upper Quadrant	
Liver	Liver, left lobe
Gallbladder	Spleen
Pylorus	Stomach
Duodenum	Pancreas: body
Pancreas: head	Left adrenal gland
Right adrenal gland	Left kidney: upper pole
Right kidney: upper pole	Splenic flexure
Hepatic flexure	Transverse colon: portion
Ascending colon: portion	Descending colon: portion
Transverse colon: portion	
Lower Quadrant	
Right kidney: lower pole	Left kidney: lower pole
Cecum	Sigmoid colon
Appendix	Descending colon: portion
Ascending colon: portion	Left ovary
Right ovary	Left fallopian tube
Right fallopian tube	Left ureter
Right ureter	Left spermatic cord
Right spermatic cord	Uterus (if enlarged)
Uterus (if enlarged)	Bladder (if distended)
Bladder (if distended)	

In adults, it is unlikely that abnormalities in posterior (retroperitoneal) organs such as the kidneys, duodenum, and pancreas can be detected through palpation. However, in very young children with less developed abdominal muscles and little obesity, renal masses, particularly on the right side, can sometimes be felt.

This text does not provide a comprehensive breakdown of the pathophysiologic features of the gastrointestinal system. Nonetheless, a brief overview of the fundamental physiological features can help link the indications and indications of abdominal illnesses.

When we swallow food, it travels through the esophagus. However, if there is a blockage, it can cause difficulty swallowing, also known as *dysphagia.* In addition, gastroesophageal reflux can cause heartburn. Once the food reaches the stomach, it should relax to digest the food properly. If the stomach fails to relax, it can cause early satiety or pain. The stomach holds food and produces gastric juice to aid digestion. The stomach lining produces around 2 to 3 L of gastric juice daily, which is essential for protein digestion. The creamy substance formed after gastric digestion of food is called chyme. If someone has a gastric ulcer, secretion of gastric juice can cause pain. The pyloric sphincter helps to empty the stomach. Normally, the stomach empties within 6 hours after eating. However, any obstruction to gastric emptying can cause vomiting.

When chyme moves from the stomach to the duodenum, it triggers the release of pancreatic enzymes and the contraction of the gallbladder. The pancreas produces the highest amount of juice about 2 hours after eating, and the daily output ranges from 1 to 2 L. Chyme contains three enzymes—lipase, amylase, and trypsin—that break down fats, starches, and proteins, respectively. When there is a lack of pancreatic enzymes, the stool appears pale and bulky and has an unpleasant odor. These enzymes help neutralize the acidity of the duodenal contents, which can alleviate the pain from peptic duodenal ulcers. However, the pain from an inflamed gallbladder or pancreatitis may worsen during this phase of the digestive cycle.

The digested food continues its course through the small intestine, in which further digestion and absorption occur. Failure of bile production or its release from the gallbladder results in decreased digestion and absorption of fats, leading to diarrhea. Gallstones may form as a result of diet or hereditary predisposition.

The liver plays several important roles in the body, including producing bile, detoxifying byproducts from food digestion, and metabolizing proteins, lipids, and carbohydrates. On a daily basis, the liver produces around 1 L of bile. If the liver isn't functioning properly, it can lead to jaundice, ascites, and even coma.

The jejunum and ileum are responsible for the final stages of nutrient digestion and absorption. Specifically, bile acids and vitamin B_{12} are absorbed in the ileum. The color of stool is affected by stercobilin, a metabolite of bilirubin that is secreted in the bile. Without bile flowing into the small intestine, stools can become pale brown or gray and are referred to as *acholic*, meaning they lack bile.

The colon has a crucial function in eliminating water and electrolytes from the chyme. Typically, the colon receives about 600 mL of fluid per day, yet only 200 mL of water is expelled in the stool each day. If the colon is not functioning properly, it can result in either diarrhea or constipation. In the presence of diverticula, bleeding and pain can occur. Additionally, colonic obstruction can lead to intense pain. Tumors within the colon can cause obstruction or bleeding.

REVIEW OF SPECIFIC SYMPTOMS

The most common symptoms of abdominal disease are as follows:

- Pain
- Nausea and vomiting
- Change in bowel movements
- Rectal bleeding
- Jaundice
- Abdominal distention
- Mass
- Pruritus (itching)
- Loss of appetite

Pain

Abdominal pain is a crucial symptom of abdominal disease. While abdominal neoplasia may not cause pain, most abdominal diseases cause some degree of pain. Pain can be caused by mucosal irritation, smooth muscle spasms, peritoneal irritation, capsular swelling, or direct nerve stimulation. Rapid diagnosis and treatment are essential for abdominal pain.

Abdominal pain can generally be categorized into three types: visceral, parietal, and referred. *Visceral pain* occurs when the hollow organs of the abdomen, such as the stomach, intestines, or gallbladder, contract forcefully or their walls are stretched. Pain may also be felt if the capsule of the liver or spleen is stretched. This type of pain can be difficult to pinpoint and may be described as gnawing, burning, or aching. Severe pain may be accompanied by nausea, vomiting, and sweating.

Parietal pain is caused by inflammation of the peritoneum and is often experienced as extremely severe pain. Patients are typically able to pinpoint the pain to a specific organ and may lie very still, as movement can worsen the pain.

Referred pain refers to the experience of pain that originates in the internal organs but is felt by the patient in other areas of the body, such as the chest wall, abdomen, shoulder, or jaw. It seems that the pain originates in areas that are supplied by the same nerves as those responsible for sensation in the affected organ. The pain is usually specific to a particular area, such as the right shoulder or scapula in cases of acute cholecystitis, or the testicles in cases of renal colic or appendicitis. Fig. 17.3 illustrates common sites for referred pain, while Table 17.2 summarizes locations of pain associated with abdominal disease.

When a patient complains of abdominal pain, ask the following questions:

"Where is the pain?"
"Has the pain changed its location since it started?"
"Do you feel the pain in any other part of your body?"
"How long have you had the pain?"
"Have you had recurrent episodes of abdominal pain?"
"Did the pain start suddenly?"
"Can you describe the pain? Is it sharp? Dull? Burning? Cramping?"
"Is the pain continuous? Does it come in waves?"

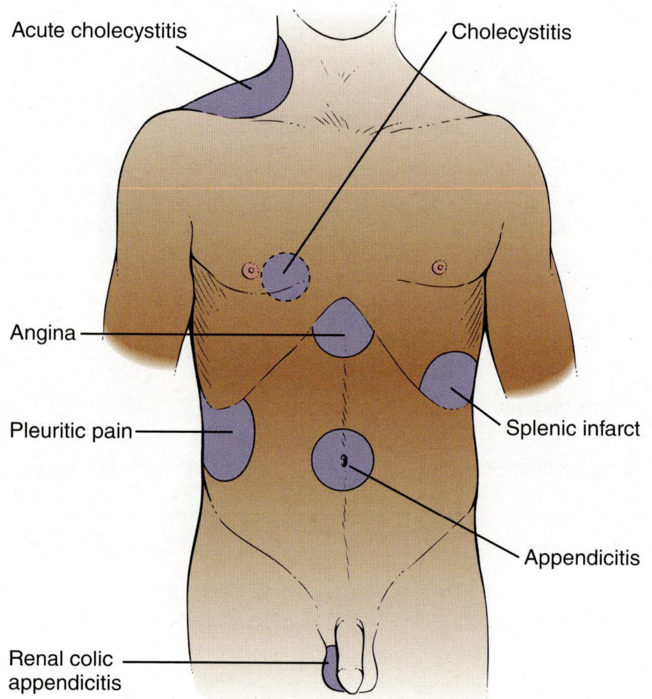

Fig. 17.3 Common Areas of Referred Pain. The *dotted area* is on the posterior chest.

TABLE 17.2 Location of Pain in Abdominal Disease

Area of Pain	Affected Organ	Clinical Example
Substernal	Esophagus	Esophagitis
Shoulder	Diaphragm	Subphrenic abscess
Epigastric	Stomach	Peptic gastric ulcer
	Duodenum	Peptic duodenal ulcer
	Gallbladder	Cholecystitis
	Liver	Hepatitis
	Bile ducts	Cholangitis
	Pancreas	Pancreatitis
	Small intestine	Obstruction
Right scapula	Biliary tract	Biliary colic
Midback	Aorta	Aortic dissection
	Pancreas	Pancreatitis
Periumbilical	Small intestine	Obstruction
Hypogastrium	Colon	Ulcerative colitis
		Diverticulitis
Sacrum	Rectum	Proctitis
		Perirectal abscess

"Has there been any change in the severity or nature of the pain since it began?"
"What makes it worse?"
"What makes it better?"
"Is the pain associated with nausea? Vomiting? Sweating? Constipation? Diarrhea? Bloody stools? Abdominal distention? Fever? Chills? Eating? Menstrual cycle?"
"Have you ever had gallstones? Kidney stones?"

"When you have the pain in your abdomen, do you feel the pain in any other part of your body at the same time?"

If the patient is female, ask this question:

"When was your last period?"

If the female patient is of child-bearing age and is sexually active, ask the question:

"Is there a possibility that you might be pregnant?"

It is important to take note of the *exact time* when the pain started and what the patient was doing at that time. A thorough assessment of the pain's timeline should also be obtained. If a patient is awakened from sleep by sudden, severe pain, it could be a sign of acute perforation, inflammation, or torsion of an abdominal organ. Intense pain can also be caused by a stone in the biliary or renal tract. The acuteness of the pain should also be noted, as conditions such as acute rupture of a fallopian tube due to an ectopic pregnancy, perforation of a gastric ulcer, peritonitis, and acute pancreatitis can cause such severe pain that it may lead to fainting.

It is crucial to determine the *location* of the pain at its onset, its *localization,* its *character,* and its *radiation.* Commonly, when an abdominal organ ruptures, pain is felt "all over the belly," without localization to a specific area. Pain arising from the small intestine is commonly felt in the umbilical or epigastric regions; for example, pain from acute appendicitis often begins at the umbilicus.

As time passes, the pain may start to affect other parts of the body. If someone experiences acute appendicitis, the pain initially occurs around the umbilicus but can then move to the lower right side of the abdomen within 1 to 3 hours. If someone has chest pain followed by abdominal pain, it's important to consider the possibility of a dissecting aortic aneurysm.

When identifying the source of pain, it's important to pay attention to its characteristics. Pain resulting from a perforated gastric ulcer is typically described as "burning," while a dissecting aneurysm may cause a "tearing" sensation. Intestinal obstruction often results in a "gripping" feeling, and pyelonephritis may cause "dull" or "aching" pain. Biliary or renal colic, on the other hand, can cause a "crampy" or "constricting" sensation.

It's important to pay attention to when symptoms occur and what makes them better or worse (e.g., meals or bowel movements). If a patient experiences periodic pain in the upper abdomen within an hour after eating, it could be a sign of a gastric peptic ulcer. However, if the patient has a duodenal peptic ulcer, they may experience pain 2 to 3 hours after eating or before the next meal. Eating food may help alleviate the pain, especially in duodenal ulcers. If a duodenal ulcer perforates to the pancreas, the patient may experience back pain that resembles an orthopedic issue. People with duodenal PUD may also experience nocturnal pain. It's important to note that pain after eating could also be a sign of vascular disease in the abdominal area. Older patients with this condition experience postprandial pain, anorexia, and weight loss. This trio of symptoms is characteristic of abdominal angina caused by obstructive vascular disease in the celiac axis or superior mesenteric artery. Refer to Table 17.3 for a summary of effective techniques to alleviate abdominal pain.

TABLE 17.3 Maneuvers for Ameliorating Abdominal Pain

Maneuver	Affected Organ	Clinical Example
Belching	Stomach	Gastric distention
Eating	Stomach, duodenum	Peptic ulcer
Vomiting	Stomach, duodenum	Pyloric obstruction
Leaning forward	Retroperitoneal structures	Pancreatic cancer Pancreatitis
Flexion of knees	Peritoneum	Peritonitis
Flexion of right thigh	Right psoas muscle	Appendicitis
Flexion of left thigh	Left psoas muscle	Diverticulitis

If the patient experiences pain in the lower abdomen, it could be due to urinary bladder conditions like a bladder infection or cystitis. The pain is often described as a dull pressure, which can be accompanied by burning sensations during urination, incontinence, frequent urination, flank pain, fever, nausea, or vomiting.

Experiencing abdominal pain from a ureter or renal pelvis, known as *renal colic,* can be excruciating and accompanied by intense spasms. Finding a comfortable position can be challenging for the patient. Kidney stones, also known as renal calculi or *urolithiasis,* are a common disorder affecting 10% of the population. The discomfort is due to rapid swelling of the ureter and renal pelvis, often caused by the acute obstruction. Always ask if there are any additional symptoms, such as fever, chills, or blood in the urine. *Nephrolithiasis* refers to kidney stones, or renal calculi, and, in conjunction with ureteral calculi, are the primary cause of acute renal colic. Nephrolithiasis has a lifetime prevalence of 5% to 15% and an incidence of 0.5% in North America and Europe.[7]

In Chapter 18, Male Genitalia and Hernias, there are more questions regarding abdominal pain in males, and Chapter 19, Female Genitalia, includes more details and queries about abdominal pain in females.

Nausea and Vomiting

When the body needs to expel harmful substances from the stomach or react to an irritant in the intestine, vomiting is a natural response. *Gastroenteritis,* which is an infection of the gastrointestinal tract, is a frequent cause of vomiting in adults. This type of infection is typically caused by bacteria or a virus, such as *norovirus.* Norovirus[8] is a very contagious virus that causes vomiting and diarrhea. It is an RNA virus of the family *Caliciviridae,* and causes substantial morbidity across both healthcare and community settings.[9]

Norovirus is sometimes called the "stomach flu" or "stomach bug." However, norovirus illness is not related to the flu. Noroviruses are the most common cause of gastroenteritis in the United States. Each year, norovirus causes 19–21 million cases of vomiting and diarrhea illness, approximately 109,000 hospitalizations, nearly 2.3 million outpatient visits, and 900 deaths, mostly among adults aged 65 years and older.[10]

Vomiting can be caused by other serious factors, including severe irritation of the peritoneum due to the perforation of an abdominal organ; obstruction of the bile duct, ureter, or intestine; or toxins.

Generally, vomiting caused by perforation is not extensive. On the other hand, obstruction of the bile duct or other tube can lead to the stretching of the muscular wall, which results in episodic vomiting at the peak of pain. Intestinal obstruction prevents the intestinal contents from passing distally; consequently, vomiting may result in the expulsion of intestinal contents. *Toxins* generally cause persistent vomiting. Not all abdominal emergencies cause vomiting. Intraperitoneal bleeding may occur in the absence of vomiting. Vomiting is frequently also caused by inflammation of intra-abdominal structures, as well as by extra-abdominal conditions, including drug toxicity, central nervous system disorders, myocardial infarction, and pregnancy. Ask the following questions if a patient complains of nausea, vomiting, or both:

"How long have you had nausea or vomiting?"
"What is the color of the vomit?"
"Is there any unusually foul odor to the vomitus?"
"How often do you vomit?"
"Is vomiting related to eating?" If yes, *"How soon after eating do you vomit? Do you vomit only after eating certain foods?"*
"Do you have nausea without vomiting?"
"Is the nausea or vomiting associated with abdominal pain? Constipation? Diarrhea? A loss of appetite? A change in the color of your stools? A change in the color of your urine? Fever? Chest pain?"
"Have you noticed a change in your hearing ability?"
"Have you noticed ringing in your ears?"

If the patient is a female, ask this question:

"When was your last period?"

If the patient is of child-bearing age and sexually active, ask the question:

"Is there a possibility that you might be pregnant?"

Determining the relationship between pain and vomiting is crucial in making a diagnosis. Typically, in cases of acute appendicitis, pain occurs before vomiting, usually a few hours earlier. The nature of the vomit can help determine the underlying cause. For instance, patients with acute gastritis tend to vomit stomach contents, while those with biliary colic produce greenish-yellow vomit. Intestinal obstruction may cause bilious vomit followed by feculent-smelling fluid. *Feculent vomit* is generally linked to intestinal obstruction.

Patients with hepatocellular disease, metastatic disease, and pregnancy often experience nausea, even in the absence of vomiting. Patients with Ménière disease may also experience nausea, along with vertigo, fluctuating sensorineural hearing loss, and tinnitus.

For further information on nausea and vomiting in the female patient, Chapter 19, Female Genitalia, provides more details.

Change in Bowel Movements

Take a careful history of bowel habits. A change in bowel movements necessitates further elaboration. Ask these questions of the patient with *acute* onset of diarrhea:

"How long have you had the diarrhea?"
"How many bowel movements do you have a day?"
"Did the diarrhea start suddenly?"
"Did the diarrhea begin after a meal?" If yes, *"What did you eat?"*
"Have you traveled recently?" If so, *"To where?"*
"Are the stools watery? Bloody? Malodorous?"
"Is the diarrhea associated with abdominal pain? Loss of appetite? Nausea? Vomiting?"

If a patient suddenly experiences diarrhea after eating, it may indicate an infection or exposure to toxins. Watery stools can be a sign of inflammation in the small intestine or colon. Bloody diarrhea may be a symptom of colon diseases like shigellosis[11] or amebiasis.[12]

The patient with *chronic* diarrhea should be asked the following:

"How long have you had diarrhea?"
"Do you have periods of diarrhea alternating with constipation?"
"Are the stools watery? Loose? Floating? Malodorous?"
"Have you noticed blood in the stools? Mucus? Undigested food?"
"What is the color of the stools?"
"How many bowel movements do you have a day?"
"Does the diarrhea occur after eating?"
"What happens when you fast? Do you still have diarrhea?"
"Is the diarrhea associated with abdominal pain? Abdominal distention? Nausea? Vomiting?"
"Have you noticed that the diarrhea is worse at certain times of the day?"
"How is your appetite?"
"Has there been any change in your weight?"
"Have you had any recent travel?" If so, *"To where?"*

Patients with colon cancer, diverticulitis, and inflammatory bowel disease often experience alternating bouts of diarrhea and constipation. Loose bowel movements are common in left colon diseases, while watery movements are seen in severe cases of inflammatory bowel disease and protein-losing enteropathies. Malabsorption syndromes can cause floating stools. Patients with ulcerative colitis often have stools mixed with blood and mucus. Inflammatory processes in the small bowel or colon can result in blood mixed with stool or undigested food. Irritable bowel syndrome usually leads to severe morning diarrhea.

Patients complaining of constipation should be asked these questions:

"How long have you been constipated?"
"How often do you have a bowel movement?"
"What is the size of your stools?"
"What is the color of your stools?"
"Is the stool ever mixed with blood? Mucus?"
"Have you noticed periods of constipation alternating with periods of diarrhea?"
"Have you noticed a change in the caliber of the stool?"
"Do you have much gas?"
"How's your appetite?"
"Has there been any change in your weight?"

It's important to take note of any changes in stool caliber and color. If stools become pencil-thin, it could be a sign of anal or distal rectal carcinoma. Pale brown or gray stools could indicate a lack of bile due to gallbladder obstruction or decreased bile production. If a patient experiences constipation, changes in weight may also be significant. An increase in weight could be a symptom of hypothyroidism, while weight loss may be associated with colon cancer or other hypermetabolic conditions.

Black or *tarry stools* may be due to bleeding in the upper part of the gastrointestinal tract, such as the esophagus, stomach, or the first part of the small intestine. In this case, the stool is black and tar-like in consistency because it gets digested on its way through the gastrointestinal tract. See the next section for further information on rectal bleeding.

It is possible for *black-colored (non-tarry) stools* to be caused by certain medications such as bismuth subsalicylate found in Pepto-Bismol® and Kaopectate®, as well as iron supplements in one's diet. Consumption of black licorice or blueberries can also lead to this symptom. Bismuth subsalicylate is commonly used to alleviate indigestion, heartburn, nausea, and diarrhea.

Rectal Bleeding

Rectal bleeding may be manifested by bright red blood, blood mixed with stool, or black, tarry stools. Bright red blood per rectum,[a] also known as *hematochezia,* can occur from colonic tumors, diverticular disease, or ulcerative colitis. Blood mixed with stool can be the result of ulcerative colitis, diverticular disease, tumors, or hemorrhoids. Ask the patient who describes rectal bleeding the following questions:

"How long have you noticed bright red blood in your stools?"
"Is the blood mixed with the stool?"
"Are there streaks of blood on the surface of the stool?"
"Have you noticed a change in your bowel habits?"
"Have you noticed a persistent sensation in your rectum that you have to move your bowels, but you cannot?"

Tenesmus refers to the painful and prolonged straining during bowel movements that does not result in relief. This condition is often caused by inflammation, obstruction in the rectum or anus, or a space-occupying lesion such as a tumor. Hemorrhoids are a frequent cause of rectal bleeding and the appearance of blood in stool.

Melena is a type of stool that appears black and sticky, resembling tar. It occurs due to bleeding in the stomach or the first part of the duodenum, resulting in partial digestion of hemoglobin. **Melena is the most common symptom of major gastrointestinal bleeding.** Usually, 90% of significant bleeding episodes occur from sites above the ligament of Treitz. It takes at least 50 mL of blood in the stomach to cause a black stool. Therefore, a melanotic stool indicates recent hemorrhage, but it doesn't reflect the presence or speed of bleeding at the moment of passage. Rapid bleeding may not allow enough time for hemoglobin to be digested, leading to hematochezia, not melena!

It's important to ask the patient if they have experienced melena. One helpful technique is to show them the black tubing on a stethoscope and ask if their bowel movements have ever been this color. Asking directly if they have ever had black stools may lead the patient to incorrectly associate dark (normal) stools with black stools. Ask these questions of a patient who describes melena:

"Have you passed more than one black, tarry stool?" If yes, *"When?"*
"How long have you been having black, tarry stools?"
"Have you noticed feeling lightheaded?"
"Have you had any nausea associated with these stools? Any vomiting? Diarrhea? Abdominal pain? Sweating?"

The answers to these questions can provide some information regarding the acuteness and the amount of the hemorrhage. Lightheadedness, nausea, and diaphoresis are seen with rapid gastrointestinal bleeding and hypotension.

Finding *silver-colored stools,* known as Thomas sign,[13] is uncommon, but it can be a strong indication of a serious condition. This condition is known as acholic stools with melena, which is often associated with cancer in the ampulla of Vater in the duodenum. The cancer can cause biliary obstruction, leading to acholic stools, while the sloughing of cancerous fronds can result in bleeding, leading to melanotic stools. These two symptoms together can produce feces with a tarnished-silver or aluminum paint-like appearance.

Jaundice

Jaundice, or hyperbilirubinemia,[14] is a condition where excess bilirubin accumulates in the body tissue, causing a yellow discoloration. This can occur due to increased production or impaired excretion of bilirubin. The normal serum levels of bilirubin are less than 1 mg/dL, but jaundice becomes noticeable with peripheral yellowing of the eye sclera, or *scleral icterus,* when serum bilirubin levels exceed 3 mg/dL (see Fig. 17.5). As bilirubin levels continue to rise, the skin may turn yellow or green, especially with long-term cases, due to the presence of biliverdin.

If jaundice (icterus) is present, it should signal to the examiner that there may be either liver parenchymal disease or blockage of bile flow. The cause of jaundice, or icterus, is due to a decrease in the excretion of conjugated bilirubin into bile. This can be caused by intrahepatic biliary obstruction, also known as medical jaundice, or extrahepatic biliary obstruction, also known as surgical jaundice. In any patient with icterus, the examiner should search for clues by asking the following questions:

"How long have you noticed the jaundice?"
"Did the jaundice develop rapidly?"
"Is the jaundice associated with abdominal pain? Loss of appetite? Nausea? Vomiting? Distaste for cigarettes?"
"Is the jaundice associated with chills? Fever? Itching? Weight loss?"
"Have you ever had a blood transfusion? Tattooing? Inoculations?"
"Have you ever been injured with a needle from a syringe or a scalpel blade?"
"Do you use any recreational drugs?" If yes, *"Do you use any drugs intravenously?"*
"Do you eat raw shellfish? Oysters?"
"Have you traveled abroad in the past year?" If yes, *"Where? Were you aware that you may have consumed unclean water?"*
"Have you been jaundiced before?"
"Has your urine changed color since you noticed that you were jaundiced?"
"What is the color of your stools?"
"Do you have any friends or relations who are also jaundiced?"
"What type of work do you do? What other types of work have you done?"
"What are your hobbies?"

[a]Often abbreviated as *BRBPR.*

Viral hepatitis[15] is an infection that causes liver inflammation and damage. Several different viruses cause hepatitis, including hepatitis A, B, C, D, and E. The hepatitis A and E viruses typically cause only acute infections. The hepatitis B, C, and D viruses can cause acute and chronic infections.

If someone contracts *hepatitis A*, they may experience symptoms like nausea, vomiting, loss of appetite, and aversion to smoking. Hepatitis A is mainly spread through exposure to fecal matter and has an incubation period of 2 to 6 weeks. Consuming raw shellfish can also cause it. In 2020, there were approximately 19,900 registered infections. Taking the hepatitis A vaccine can provide protection against the disease.

Hepatitis B, also known as HBV, is a disease that is transmitted through blood and has an incubation period of 1 to 6 months. Healthcare professionals are at a higher risk of contracting the disease, and being in close contact with someone who has it can also increase the chances of getting infected. In 2020, there were approximately 14,000 reported cases of HBV, and over 880,000 adults were diagnosed with chronic hepatitis B. Shockingly, 2 out of 3 people who have HBV are unaware of their condition. Furthermore, in 2020, the rate of new cases was 12 times higher among Asian Pacific Islanders than non-Hispanic White individuals. Fortunately, getting vaccinated against hepatitis B can help protect against the disease.

Hepatitis C, also known as HCV, is the most prevalent chronic blood-borne infection in the United States. The year 2020 witnessed around 66,700 new infections, and approximately 2.2 million adults suffered from hepatitis C. Shockingly, almost 40% of individuals who contracted the virus were not even aware of their infection. The fatality rates linked to hepatitis C in 2020 were at their peak among Native American and non-Hispanic Black communities. Individuals born between 1945 and 1965, commonly referred to as baby boomers, are 5 times more likely to be infected with HCV than other age groups. It is estimated that 1 in every 30 baby boomers is affected with HCV. According to the Centers for Disease Control and Prevention (CDC), many baby boomers acquired the virus in the 1970s and 1980s when infection control standards were not as strict as they are today. HCV was only discovered in 1989, and donated blood was not screened for the virus until 1992. The symptoms of HCV can take years or even decades to appear, which means that baby boomers may only be experiencing them now.

The CDC has estimated that there are as many as 200,000 new HCV infections annually in the United States. It is estimated that as many as 3.9 million Americans have the antibody to HCV and are currently asymptomatic. They are, however, at risk for chronic liver disease, the tenth leading cause of death in the United States. Approximately 40% of chronic liver disease is HCV-related and results in 8000 to 10,000 deaths a year. End-stage liver disease secondary to HCV infection is the most common indication for liver transplantation. Once identified, a patient with chronic HCV infection is often curable with oral medications taken every day for 2 to 6 months. Several well-tolerated oral regimens are now approved to treat patients with various HCV genotypes, stages of liver disease, and comorbidities.[16] It is recommended that all adults between the ages of 18 and 79 undergo screening for hepatitis C. It is important to note that there is currently no vaccine available for this disease.

Hepatitis D virus (HDV) is a unique virus that only affects individuals who have already been infected with hepatitis B. This type of infection is known as a coinfection, which happens when someone contracts both hepatitis B and hepatitis D at the same time. HDV can be spread through contact with bodily fluids, blood, sharing contaminated needles and syringes, and during sexual intercourse. HDV is a virus that relies on HBV for replication, and it affects almost 5% of people worldwide who have a chronic HBV infection. However, HDV infection can be prevented by getting vaccinated against HBV.

Hepatitis E is a short-term infection that typically clears up on its own within a few weeks, without necessitating any medical intervention. The virus responsible for hepatitis E, known as HEV, causes inflammation of the liver. Approximately 20 million HEV infections occur globally each year, resulting in an estimated 3.3 million cases of symptomatic hepatitis E. HEV is present in the feces of infected individuals and can be transmitted when the virus is ingested, even in minute quantities, by someone unaware of its presence. In developing nations, hepatitis E is commonly contracted through the consumption of water contaminated with feces from individuals who have the virus. While hepatitis E is not prevalent in the United States and other developed nations, individuals have contracted the disease from consuming raw or undercooked pork, venison, wild boar, or shellfish. Most individuals recover from hepatitis E without complications, unless they have a weakened immune system, in which case they may develop chronic hepatitis E. Unfortunately, a vaccine for hepatitis E is not yet available in the United States.

Slowly developing jaundice that is accompanied by pale stools and cola-colored urine is *obstructive jaundice*, either intrahepatic or extrahepatic. Jaundice accompanied by fever and chills is considered *cholangitis* until proven otherwise. Cholangitis may result from stasis of bile in the bile duct that results from a gallstone or from cancer of the head of the pancreas. Determine whether chemicals are used in a patient's occupation or hobbies because they may be related to the cause of jaundice. Many industrial chemicals and drugs have been associated with liver disease. These agents may be responsible for a viral hepatitis-like illness, cholestasis, or for granulomas or hepatic tumors. Occupational exposure to carbon tetrachloride and vinyl chloride is well known to cause liver disease. Ask questions related to alcohol abuse. These are described in Chapter 1, The Interviewer's Questions.

Abdominal Distention

Abdominal distention can occur due to excess gas in the gastrointestinal tract or the presence of ascites. The excess gas can be caused by malabsorption, irritable colon, or air swallowing *(aerophagia)*. Ascites may have various underlying reasons, including cirrhosis, congestive heart failure, portal hypertension, peritonitis, or neoplasia. To identify the cause of abdominal distention, ask the following questions:

"How long have you noticed your abdomen to be distended?"
"Is the distention intermittent?"
"Is the distention related to eating?"

"Is the distention lessened by belching or by passing gas from below?"

"Is the distention associated with vomiting? Loss of appetite? Weight loss? Change in your bowel habits? Shortness of breath?"

Sometimes after eating, a person may experience bloating caused by gas that can be relieved by passing gas or burping. If a person has ascites, their abdomen may gradually expand, causing their belt size to increase. People with cirrhosis, malignancy, or end-stage congestive heart failure may experience a loss of appetite. Congestive heart failure can cause both shortness of breath and ascites, and shortness of breath may also be caused by a decrease in lung capacity due to ascites from another cause. Chapter 1, The Interviewer's Questions, contains inquiries that are particularly relevant to alcohol abuse.

Mass

An abdominal mass may be a neoplasm or a hernia. An abdominal *hernia* is a protrusion from the peritoneal cavity into which peritoneal contents are extruded. The contents may be omentum, intestine, or bladder wall. An abdominal hernia may be inguinal, femoral, umbilical, or internal, depending on its location. The most common complaint is swelling, which may or may not be painful. An inguinal hernia may manifest as a mass in the groin or scrotum. The major complications of a hernia are intestinal obstruction and intestinal strangulation from the interference of blood supply. A hernia is termed *reducible* when it can be emptied of its contents by pressure or a change in posture.

If an examiner notices a pulsatile abdominal mass, they should consider the possibility of an aortic aneurysm. This could be an important sign or symptom to pay attention to.

Pruritus

Pruritus, or itching, is a common symptom. Generalized itching may be a symptom of a diffuse skin disorder[b] or a manifestation of chronic renal or hepatic disease. It is worth noting that generalized pruritus, or itching all over the body, can be caused by systemic diseases in around 50% of individuals. Lymphoma or Hodgkin disease, as well as malignancies of the gastrointestinal tract, can cause intense itching. Thyroid dysfunction is also known to be a cause of generalized pruritus. In addition, certain medications such as opiates, hydroxychloroquine, aspirin, nonsteroidal anti-inflammatory drugs, and those that are metabolized by the liver can also lead to generalized itching.

In older individuals, pruritus may also be caused by dry skin alone. *Pruritus ani* is localized itching of the anal skin. It has many causes, including fistulas, fissures, psoriasis, intestinal parasites, frequent liquid stools, anal perspiration, human immunodeficiency virus (HIV) infection, and diabetes. Pruritus ani may be caused by eating certain foods, smoking, and drinking alcoholic beverages, especially beer and wine. Some of the food items that have been associated with pruritus ani include coffee, tea, carbonated beverages, milk products, tomatoes and tomato products such as ketchup, cheeses, nuts, and chocolate. Cleanliness is almost never a factor.

Loss of Appetite

It is crucial to determine if there is a loss of appetite or intolerance to certain or all foods. Individuals with hepatitis often experience a decrease in their appetite and lose interest in smoking if they were smokers before. They may also feel an unpleasant taste or fullness in their stomach after consuming even a small meal.

IMPACT OF INFLAMMATORY BOWEL DISEASE ON THE PATIENT

There is a group of diseases called inflammatory bowel disease that have an unknown cause. The symptoms vary depending on the location, extent, and acuteness of the inflammatory lesions. Common symptoms include fever, loss of appetite, weight loss, abdominal discomfort, diarrhea, rectal urgency, and rectal bleeding. This illness is chronic and can be potentially disabling, often resulting in the need for multiple surgeries, fistula repair, and cancer.

Inflammatory bowel disease can cause extended periods away from school or work, disturbance to family life, issues with malabsorption and malnutrition, and frequent hospital stays. Those affected may experience between 10 to 30 bowel movements per day, which can be watery or bloody. As a result, individuals with inflammatory bowel disease may suffer from various psychological challenges, especially during their young adult years. Patients with inflammatory bowel disease may experience malabsorption, which can lead to osteopenia in 40% to 50% of cases and osteoporosis in 5% to 30% of cases. This can result in hip, spine, and distal radius fractures. Research has shown that individuals with inflammatory bowel disease have a 40% higher risk of fractures compared to the general population.

Malnutrition can delay sexual and social development. Patients who need frequent access to a bathroom may struggle to develop typical dating patterns and can experience social delays. Many of these patients exhibit signs of social immaturity and introversion, which can limit their ability to leave home. Their daily routines are often dictated by their bowel habits.

It is commonly observed that physical disease severity is often linked to emotional disturbance. Patients with inflammatory bowel disease have reported having a strong dependency on others. Additionally, they tend to repress feelings of anger, suppress emotions, and experience anxiety frequently. Many patients also express a constant desire to move past events in their lives. Patients with this condition may exhibit symptoms such as diarrhea, as well as obsessive-compulsive behavior. This obsessive behavior may become more pronounced when the patient is ill. It is common for these patients to constantly worry about the state of their bowels. Additionally, many of these patients are intelligent and well-read, having extensively researched their disease, including medical literature.

Typically, denial is not a significant indicator. Instead, these patients tend to obsessively focus on the specifics of their bowel habits.

Sexual problems are common. Interest and participation in sexual activity tend to be at a low level. Many of these individuals prefer to be fondled like a child and largely reject any genital

[b]For example, *dermatitis herpetiformis* (a blistering disease predominantly on the buttocks, shoulders, elbows, and knees) or *lichen planus*.

contact. Patients are prone to regard sexual activity in anal terms, such as "dirty," "unclean," or "soiling." They are squeamish about body contact, odors, and secretions. The loss of libido and decreased sexual drive may be related to their fear of bowel action during intercourse, of perineal pain, or that sexual intercourse may in some way further damage the bowel.

The frequent hospitalizations cause anxiety and depression, which exacerbate the disease. The fear of cancer may be the basis of depression, which is a common response to the disease. It is well established that emotional factors are important in maintaining and prolonging an existing attack. Schoolwork deteriorates as young patients are forced to miss more and more school, further increasing their anxiety.

A significant but often overlooked complication of inflammatory bowel disease is substance abuse. Due to ongoing pain, up to 5% of patients with this condition become physically addicted to oral narcotics. Additionally, many others develop a psychological dependence on their pain medication.

Many patients with ulcerative colitis require an ileostomy. The fear of disfigurement, the loss of self-confidence, the potential lack of cleanliness, and the dread of unexpected spillage are common.

Time for listening and an interest in a patient's problem are important in gaining the patient's confidence. Listening may reveal and help unravel the emotional problems that may be the source of the exacerbation of the bowel disease. Talking with the patient may be more efficacious than prescribing antiinflammatory agents or tranquilizers. Careful and thoughtful discussion of the illness strengthens the healthcare professional–patient relationship and produces immeasurable therapeutic benefits.

PHYSICAL EXAMINATION

To examine the abdomen and rectum, you will need a stethoscope, gloves, lubricant, tissues, and an occult blood testing card with a Hemoccult developer.

The patient should lie supine in bed, and the abdomen should be exposed from the lower sternum to the upper thighs, with the genitalia covered. The arms should be at the sides and the legs flat. Frequently, patients tend to place their arms behind their heads, which tightens the abdominal muscles and makes the examination more difficult. Placing a pillow beneath the knees or just bending the knees often aids in the relaxation of the abdominal muscles. The examiner should be standing on the patient's right side. A gown covering the chest is appropriate.

It's advisable to evaluate the area of discomfort last when a patient complains of abdominal pain. Commencing the examination by touching the area that causes the most pain can result in the contraction of abdominal muscles, thereby making the entire abdominal examination more difficult.

The physical examination of the abdomen includes the following:

- Inspection
- Auscultation
- Percussion
- Palpation
- Rectal examination
- Special techniques

Inspection

Evaluate General Appearance

When evaluating a patient's condition, their physical appearance can provide valuable insight. Patients experiencing renal or biliary colic often writhe in bed, unable to find a comfortable position, while those with peritonitis remain still due to intense pain with movement. Peritonitis patients may have their knees drawn up to ease abdominal muscle tension. Pale, sweating patients may be experiencing *shock* from pancreatitis or a perforated gastric ulcer.

The presence of any of the following signs could be an indication of certain disorders. Distension of the abdomen could be present due to small bowel obstruction, masses, tumors, cancer, hepatomegaly, splenomegaly, constipation, abdominal aortic aneurysm, and pregnancy. Any abnormal masses may indicate umbilical hernia, ventral wall hernia, femoral hernia, or inguinal hernia, depending on the location. The patient may be asked to cough, which results in raised intra-abdominal pressure, causing the hernia to become more prominent.

Determine Respiratory Rate

The respiratory rate increases in patients with generalized peritonitis, intra-abdominal hemorrhage, or intestinal obstruction.

Inspect the Skin

Check the skin and sclera for signs of yellowing, which could indicate jaundice. It's best to examine the patient in natural light, as artificial light can sometimes make jaundice harder to detect. Jaundice becomes apparent when the serum bilirubin level exceeds 2.5 mg/dL in adults or 6 mg/dL in neonates. Fig. 17.4 shows a patient with jaundice. Notice the scleral icterus and the yellow discoloration of the skin. Hyperbilirubinemia can also result in intense generalized pruritus.

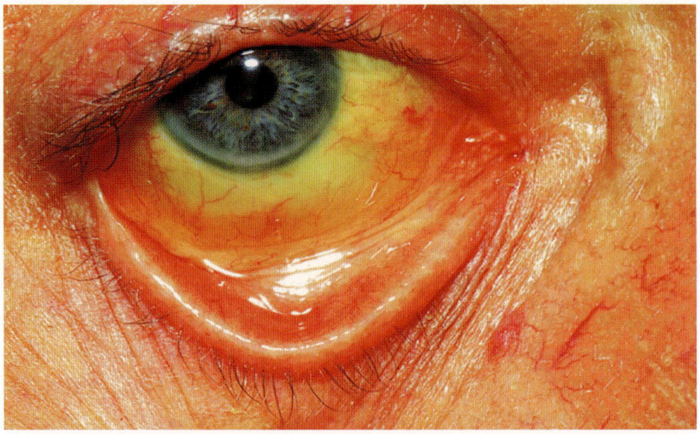

Fig. 17.4 Jaundice. (From Dover AR: *Macleod's clinical examination*, ed 15, London, 2024, Elsevier Ltd.)

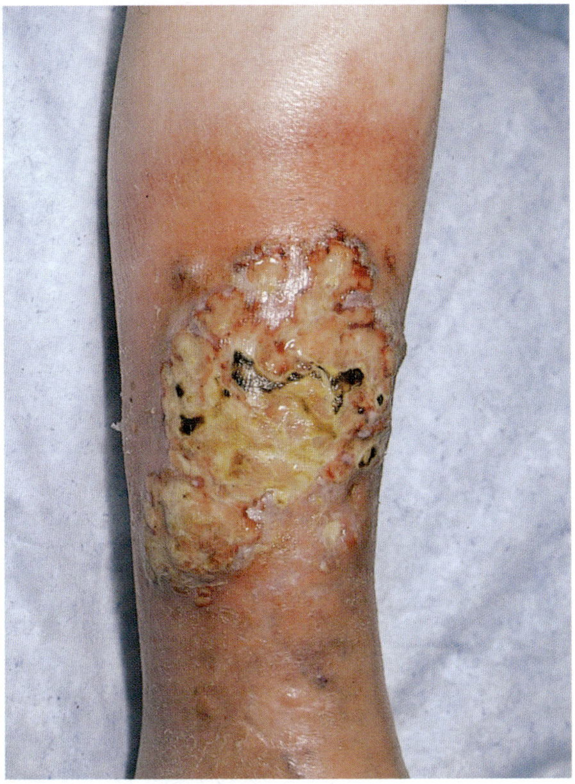

Fig. 17.5 Pyoderma Gangrenosum.

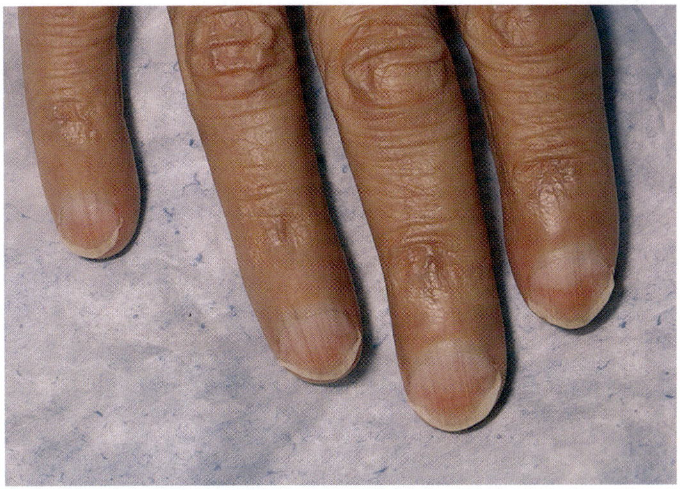

Fig. 17.6 Lindsay's Nails.

Inspect for *spider angiomas.* Spider angiomas have a high degree of sensitivity in patients with alcoholic cirrhosis but are nonspecific because they also occur in pregnancy and collagen vascular disorders (see Fig. 8.81).

Fig. 17.5 shows the leg of a patient with *pyoderma gangrenosum.* Notice the necrotic, undermined ulceration with pus. These tender ulcerations, commonly on the lower extremities, are associated with inflammatory bowel disease, especially ulcerative colitis. The clinical course of pyoderma gangrenosum generally follows the course of the bowel disease. This condition is also seen in patients with rheumatoid arthritis, myeloid metaplasia, and chronic myelogenous leukemia. See also Fig. 8.94.

Inspect the Hands

Is there muscle loss in the small muscles of the hands? This is associated with wasting.

The nails are examined for changes in the nail bed, especially an increase in the size of the lunula. The fingers of a patient with cirrhosis showing "half-and-half" nails are shown in Fig. 17.6. See also Fig. 8.8.

Inspect the Facies

Are the eyes sunken? Is temporal wasting present? These signs indicate wasting and poor nutrition.

The skin around the mouth and oral mucosa may provide evidence of gastrointestinal disorders. Melanin deposition around and in the oral cavity, especially the buccal mucosa, suggests *Peutz-Jeghers syndrome.*[17] Fig. 12.12 shows a patient's lips with the classic brown pigmentary changes of Peutz-Jeghers syndrome. This is an autosomal-dominant disorder characterized by generalized gastrointestinal, hamartomatous polyposis, and mucocutaneous pigmentation. The benign polyps are most common in the jejunum and colon. There is a greatly increased risk of developing certain types of other cancers. The polyps, however, may bleed, and cause intussusception[c] and obstruction. Telangiectasias of the lips and tongue are suggestive of *Osler-Weber-Rendu syndrome*[18] (see Fig. 12.11), in which multiple telangiectasias are present throughout the gastrointestinal tract. This autosomal dominant disorder is characterized by the presence of multiple mucocutaneous telangiectasias. These are small arteriovenous malformations that can often bleed, leading to significant discomfort for the patient. Common symptoms include nosebleeds, gastrointestinal bleeding, and anemia caused by iron deficiency. The classic oral lesions on the tongue and lower lip of a patient with Osler-Weber-Rendu syndrome are shown in Fig. 17.7.

Cushing syndrome, also known as hypercortisolism, presents with various clinical symptoms. The most prevalent signs include obesity, facial redness and swelling, excess hair growth, and high blood pressure. Nearly 90% of patients with hypercortisolism are obese. A common physical characteristic is a round and puffy face with a reddish hue, also known as moon facies. Patients may also have noticeable fat deposits in the areas above the collarbone and behind the neck, commonly referred to as buffalo hump. Fig. 17.8 shows a patient with Cushing syndrome and the typical moon facies.

[c]Intussusception is a grave medical condition that occurs when a section of the intestine slides into an adjacent section, causing a blockage that hinders the passage of food or fluid. This process also results in the interruption of blood flow to the affected area of the intestine, which can lead to infection, tissue death, or perforation.

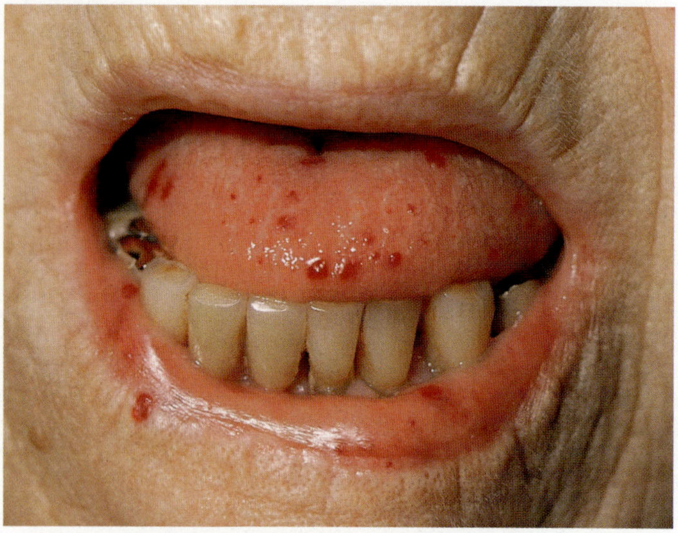

Fig. 17.7 Osler-Weber-Rendu Syndrome.

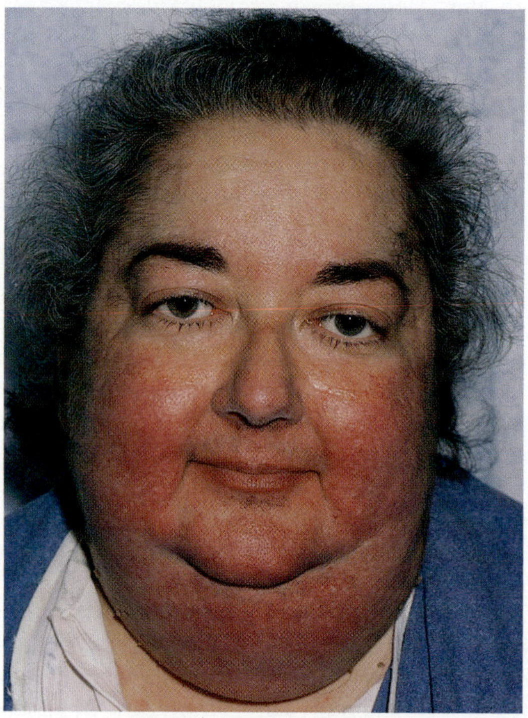

Fig. 17.8 Cushing Syndrome.

Evaluate the Mouth

If the patient has inflammatory lesions around the corner of the mouth, they could be experiencing *angular cheilitis*[19] (see Fig. 12.58), which might be an indication of iron or vitamin deficiency caused by malabsorption. It's important to get a thorough examination of the oral cavity to check for oral ulcers, which could be a sign of Crohn disease or celiac disease. If the tongue is pale, smooth, and shiny, it may mean an iron deficiency. On the other hand, if the tongue is beefy and red, it could be a sign of vitamin B_{12} and/or folate deficiency.

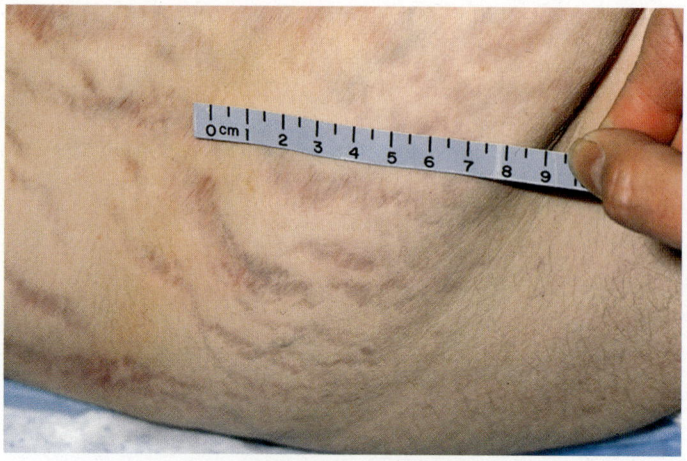

Fig. 17.9 Abdominal Striae.

Additionally, the smell of the patient's breath can indicate different disorders, such as *fetor hepaticus*, which is a strong musty smell associated with liver disorder. Fetor hepaticus is the characteristic breath of patients with severe parenchymal liver disease, which has been said to resemble the odor of a mixture of rotten eggs and garlic. In addition, a fruity breath could suggest *ketonemia*,[20] which is the presence of high concentration of ketones in the blood. Normally, when blood glucose decreases for more than a couple of hours, ketonemia develops in response to decreased insulin, and the will use ketones as an alternative endogenous fuel.

Inspect the Skin of the Abdomen

To properly assess the abdomen, the examiner should pay attention to the skin and any asymmetry, distention, masses, or visible peristaltic waves. This can be done by observing the abdomen from both a frontal and overhead view. Additionally, looking for striae and scars on the abdomen can provide useful information. Stretch marks, known as silver striae, can indicate weight loss, while pinkish-purple striae are a common sign of adrenocortical excess. An example of this can be seen in Fig. 17.9, which displays characteristic purplish striae in a patient with Cushing syndrome.

Is the umbilicus everted? An everted umbilicus is often a sign of increased abdominal pressure, usually from ascites or a large mass. An umbilical hernia may also cause an umbilicus to become everted.

During an inspection, a patch of ecchymosis on the abdomen can be a sign of internal bleeding. The *Grey Turner sign*, which is ecchymosis on the flank and groin, is commonly associated with hemorrhagic pancreatitis. Another sign is the *Cullen sign*, which is a periumbilical ecchymosis that can indicate retroperitoneal or intra-abdominal hemorrhage.

It can be important to identify traditional surgical scars. Fig. 17.10 displays the positions of several typical surgical scars.

Inspect the Superficial Veins

There are some physical indicators that could suggest portal hypertension or vena cava obstruction. One of these indicators

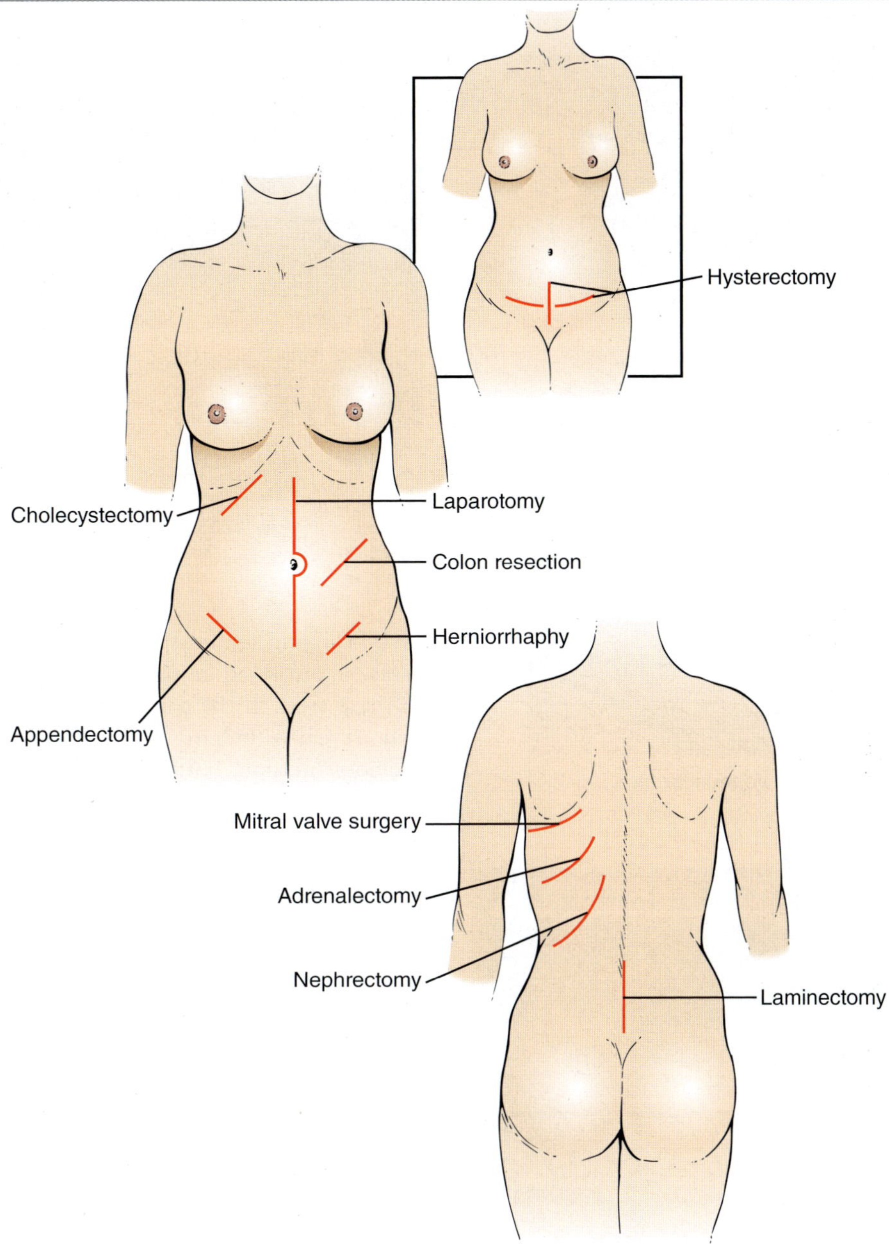

Fig. 17.10 Locations of Common Surgical Scars.

is superficial venous dilatation. The venous pattern of the abdomen is usually barely perceptible. If it is visible in the normal individual, the drainage of the lower two-thirds of the abdomen is downward. In vena caval obstruction, superficial veins may dilate, and the veins drain cephalad (toward the head). In patients with portal hypertension, the dilated veins appear to radiate from the umbilicus. This is caused by backflow through the collateral veins within the falciform ligament, and this pattern is called *caput medusae.* This condition has a 90% chance of indicating hepatic cirrhosis and portal hypertension.

If the superficial veins are distended, evaluate the direction of drainage by the following technique: Place the tips of your index fingers on a vein that is oriented cephalad-caudad, not transverse, and compress it. Using continuous pressure, slide your index fingers apart for approximately 3 to 4 inches (7.5 to 10 cm). Remove one finger and observe the refilling in the direction of flow. Repeat this procedure, but this time remove your other finger and observe the flow direction. Fig. 17.11 shows the abdomen of a patient with intrahepatic portal hypertension. Notice the engorged paraumbilical veins; the flow was away from the umbilicus toward the caval system.

Sinuses and fistulae can occur if there is a deep infection or an infection of a surgical tract. Crohn disease is often associated with the development of fistulas. If you identify a stoma, it's important to note various features to identify the type of stoma. These include the size and appearance of the stoma as well as the contents of the stoma bag.

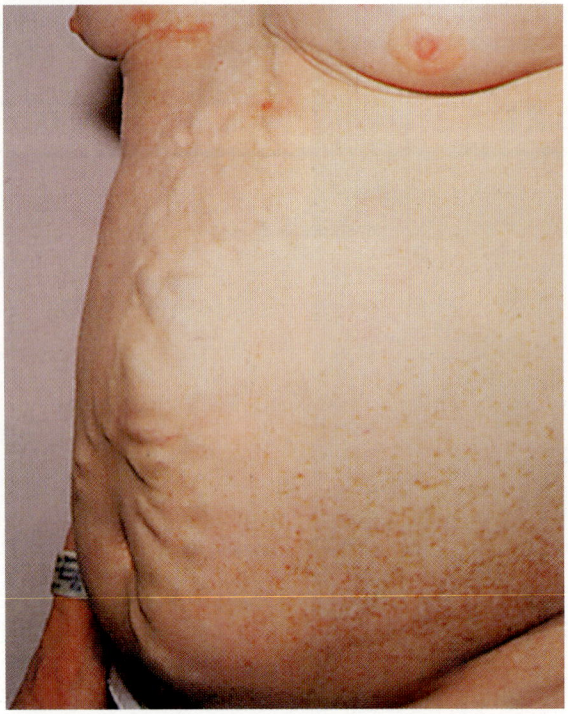

Fig. 17.11 Abdominal Venous Pattern.

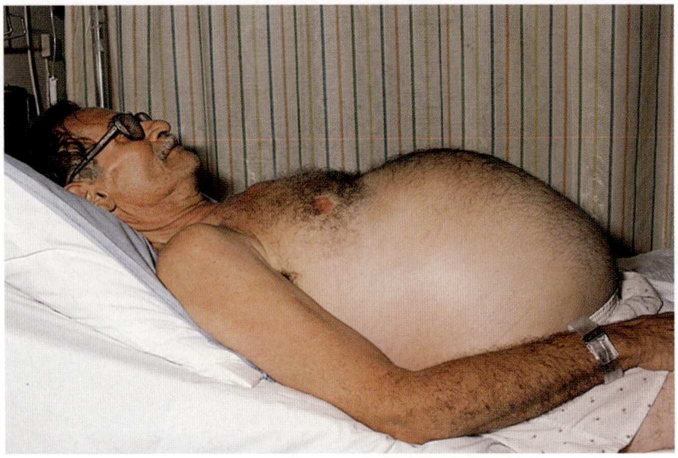

Fig. 17.12 Ascites.

Inspect the Contour of the Abdomen and Inspect for Hernias

See Video 17.1.

When assessing the abdomen, it's important to observe its contour. A sunken or concave appearance could be a sign of cachexia, while a protruding abdomen may indicate gaseous distention of the intestines, ascites, massive splenomegaly, or obesity. In patients with ascites, their fluid will sink into their lower abdomen when standing and bulge in their flanks when lying down. When lying on their side, the fluid will flow to the dependent lower side. A patient with a protuberant abdomen due to carcinomatous ascites is shown in Fig. 17.12.

To check for a hernia, it's important to have the patient lying in bed and ask them to cough while examining the inguinal, umbilical, and femoral areas. This maneuver can cause an increase in intra-abdominal pressure, leading to a sudden bulging in these areas. If the patient has had surgery before, coughing may reveal a bulging along the abdominal scar from the previous incision. Furthermore, coughing may also cause pain in a specific area. By using this technique, the examiner can pinpoint the area of greatest sensitivity and perform a thorough abdominal examination with minimal discomfort to the patient. Fig. 17.13 displays ascites caused by metastatic breast cancer and an umbilical hernia.

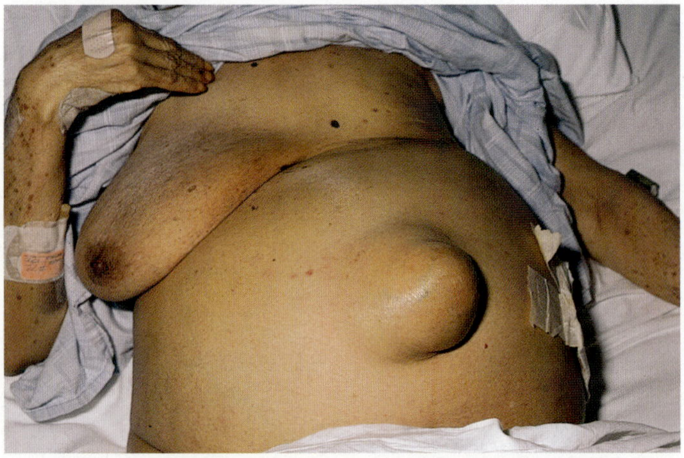

Fig. 17.13 Ascites With Umbilical Hernia.

Auscultation

Auscultation of bowel sounds can provide information about the motion of air and liquid in the gastrointestinal tract. **Always perform auscultation of the abdomen before percussion or palpation,** in contrast to the usual order. It is believed that percussion or palpation may change intestinal motility; therefore, auscultation should be performed first to ascertain whether bowel sounds are present or absent. The absence of bowel signs is a highly specific sign of peritonitis. Palpation may artificially stimulate the bowel, and one can lose this critical sign of peritonitis.

Evaluate Bowel Sounds

See Video 17.2.

The patient is placed in a supine position. To perform auscultation of the abdomen, the examiner places the diaphragm of the stethoscope over the midabdomen and listens for bowel sounds. This technique is illustrated in Fig. 17.14.

Normal bowel sounds occur approximately every 5 to 10 seconds and are low-pitched and gurgling. If after 2 minutes no bowel sounds are heard, "absent bowel sounds" may be noted. The absence of bowel sounds suggests a paralytic ileus that results from diffuse peritoneal irritation, *peritonitis.*

There may be rushes of low-pitched rumbling sounds, termed *borborygmi,*[21] which are associated with hyperperistalsis. These sounds resemble the sound of the word "borborygmi" itself. Stomach rumbling, or borborygmi, is usually a normal bodily occurrence. However, it can also be a symptom of an

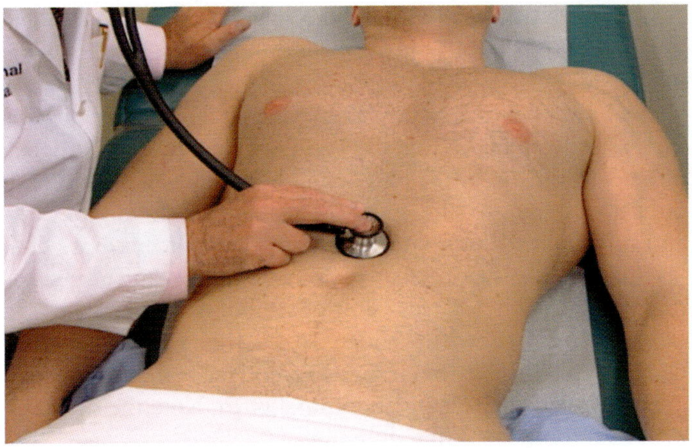

Fig. 17.14 Technique for Evaluating Bowel Sounds.

underlying issue. If the rumbling is accompanied by other symptoms, it may be caused by conditions such as Crohn disease, food intolerances, diarrhea, gastrointestinal bleeding, infectious enteritis, ulcerative colitis, or bowel obstruction. In some cases, loud stomach growling can simply be a sign of hunger after a long period without food.

Rule Out Obstructed Viscus

A *succussion splash* may be detected in a distended abdomen due to the presence of gas and fluid in an obstructed organ. The examiner applies the stethoscope over the patient's abdomen while shaking the patient's abdomen from side to side. The presence of a sloshing sound usually indicates distention of the stomach or colon. This technique is illustrated in Fig. 17.15.

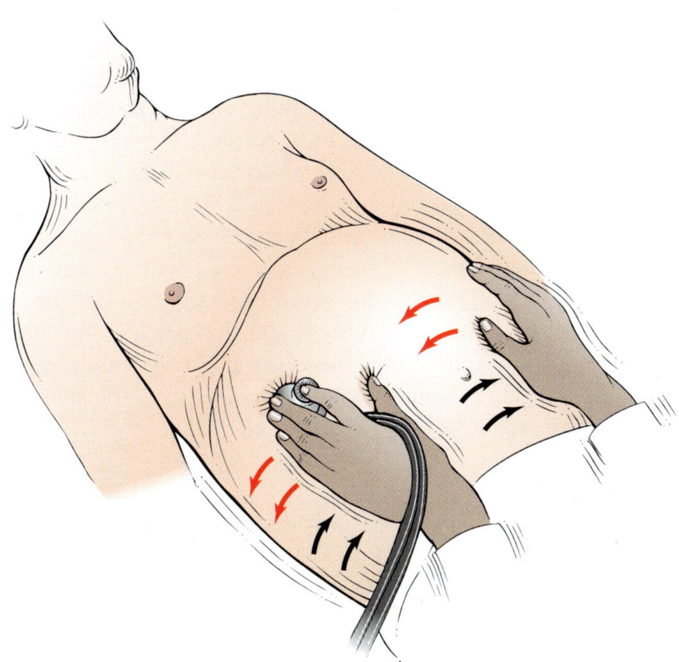

Fig. 17.15 "Succussion Splash" Technique for Assessing Distention of Abdominal Viscera.

Rule Out Abdominal Bruits

See Video 17.3.

Auscultation is important in identifying the presence of bruits. Assess each quadrant for their presence. Bruits may occur due to the narrowing of the renal artery or the abdominal aorta. (See the discussion of abdominal bruits in Chapter 15, The Peripheral Vascular System.)

Rule Out Peritoneal Rubs

A *peritoneal friction rub* is a rough, grating sound that occurs when the two layers of the peritoneum rub against each other, indicating inflammation in the peritoneum. Similar to pleural or pericardial rubs, this sound can be heard in the right or left upper quadrants during respiratory motion if there is inflammation of the liver or spleen, respectively.

Percussion

To obtain accurate information about abdominal pathology, it is essential to use the correct percussion technique. When performing percussion, it is crucial to recognize the sound of tympany over air-filled structures like the stomach, and dullness to percussion, which may indicate the presence of an underlying mass or an organ enlargement such as hepatomegaly or splenomegaly. In the normal examination, usually, only the size and location of the liver and spleen can be determined.

Some examiners prefer to palpate before percussion, especially if the patient complains of abdominal pain; either approach is correct. The technique of percussion is discussed in Chapter 13, The Chest.

Percuss the Abdomen

The patient lies supine. All four quadrants of the abdomen are evaluated by percussion. As mentioned, tympany is the most common percussion note in the abdomen. It is caused by gas in the stomach, small bowel, and colon. The suprapubic area, when percussed, may sound dull if the urinary bladder is distended or, in a female, if the uterus is enlarged.

Percuss the Upper Border of the Liver

The upper border of the liver is percussed in the right midclavicular line, starting in the midchest. As the chest is percussed downward, the resonant note of the chest becomes dull as the liver is reached. As percussion continues, this dull note becomes tympanic because the percussion is now over the colon. The upper and lower borders of the liver should be no more than 4 inches (10 cm) apart. The technique is illustrated in Fig. 17.16.

Predicting liver size by percussion can be challenging due to several issues. When ascites is present, it becomes difficult for the examiner to accurately determine the liver's actual size. A common reason for mistakenly measuring the liver as larger than it actually is (a false-positive measurement) is due to chronic obstructive lung disease. This condition can make it challenging to accurately percuss the upper border of the liver. When a patient is obese, it can be difficult to perform percussion and palpation. If the colon is distended, it can make it hard

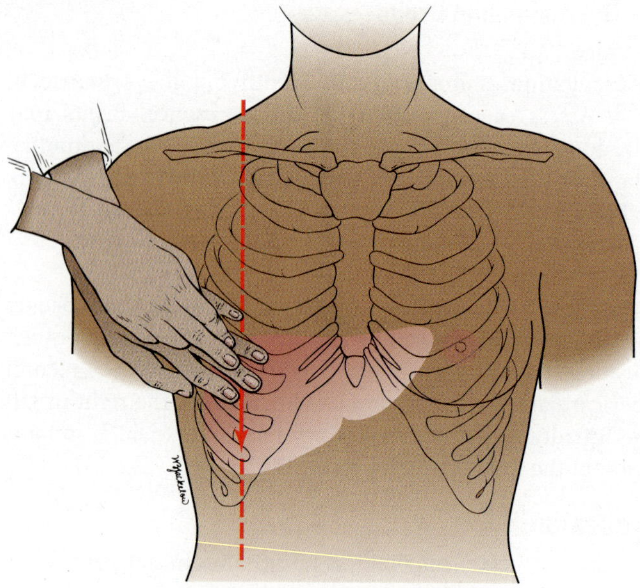

Fig. 17.16 Technique for Liver Percussion.

to detect the lower liver dullness. This can lead to underestimating the liver size, which is a false-negative measurement.

Percuss the Spleen

Although the size of the spleen is often challenging to determine, evaluation of the spleen should begin with percussion of splenic size. In normal individuals, the spleen lies within the rib cage against the posterolateral wall of the abdominal cavity in *Traube's space.* Traube space is defined by the sixth rib superiorly, the left anterior axillary line laterally, and the costal margin inferiorly. As the spleen enlarges, it remains close to the abdominal wall, and the tip moves downward and toward the midline. Because the early enlargement is in an anteroposterior direction, considerable enlargement may occur without becoming palpable below the costal margin.

Have the patient lie in the supine position. To check for splenomegaly, percussion is performed on the left anterior axillary line in the most inferior interspace while the patient takes a deep breath. If the percussion note changes from tympanitic to dull, it suggests the presence of splenomegaly with a sensitivity of 82% and specificity of 83%. Splenomegaly can occur due to various reasons such as trauma with hematoma formation, portal hypertension, hematologic malignancies, infections such as HIV and Epstein-Barr virus, and splenic infarction.

Rule Out Ascites

A special percussion test for shifting dullness may be performed on patients to check if they have ascites,[22] which is an accumulation of fluid in the abdomen. To conduct this test, the abdomen is percussed and checked if a dull area changes to a tympanic when the patient is turned from lying on their back to lying on their side. This test can identify ascites if the amount of fluid buildup in the abdomen is more than 500 mL.

While the patient is lying on their back, the examiner determines the borders of tympany and dullness. The area of tympany is present above the area of dullness and is caused by gas in the bowel floating on top of the ascitic fluid. The patient is then asked to turn on one side, and the examiner again determines the borders of the percussion notes. If ascites is present, dullness "shifts" to the more dependent position; the area around the umbilicus that was initially tympanic becomes dull. Shifting dullness has a sensitivity of 64% to 90% and a specificity of 72%. The test for shifting dullness is illustrated in Fig. 17.17 and shown in Video 17.4.[d] This 42-year-old male had a 15-year history of cirrhosis secondary to hepatitis C and presented with increasing abdominal girth. Note the dramatic demonstration of shifting dullness.

Another test for ascites is for the presence of a fluid wave. To do this, an examiner or the patient places their hand in the middle of the abdomen and presses down to stop the impulse transmission from subcutaneous adipose tissue. The examiner then taps one side of the abdomen while palpating the other. If a fluid wave is detected, it may indicate the presence of ascites. This technique is demonstrated in Fig. 17.18. A prominent fluid wave is considered the most specific physical diagnostic test for ascites, with a specificity of 84%–96% according to various studies. However, false-positive results may occur in obese individuals, and false-negative results may occur in cases of small to moderate ascites.

A third physical signs of ascites is the appearance of bulging flanks. This occurs when the weight of the abdominal fluid pushes outwards, causing the flanks to protrude. It has a sensitivity of 81% and specificity of 59% in detecting ascites.

To detect ascites, healthcare professionals rely on the presence of shifting dullness and a prominent fluid wave. However, the accuracy of these signs depends on the prevalence of the disease in a particular patient. Various studies have examined the effectiveness of physical examination tests for ascites, and the results are summarized in Table 17.4. The presence of a prominent fluid wave is the strongest indicator of ascites, while the absence of bulging flanks, flank dullness, or shifting dullness decreases the likelihood. Healthcare providers must consider these factors and use their clinical judgment to make an accurate diagnosis.

Among the more common historical items perceived by patients, an increase in abdominal girth or recent weight gain has the highest chance of being associated with ascites. An increase in abdominal circumference has a positive likelihood ratio (LR+) of 4.16; recent weight gain has an LR+ of 3.20. Conversely, the absence of the subjective increase in abdominal girth has a negative likelihood ratio (LR−) of 0.17; the absence of subjective ankle swelling carries an LR− of 0.10.

Palpation

Abdominal palpation is commonly divided into the following:

- Light palpation
- Deep palpation

[d]My thanks to the patient and Xiangya Hospital of Central South University in Changsha, China, for permission to make this video during my bedside rounds there.

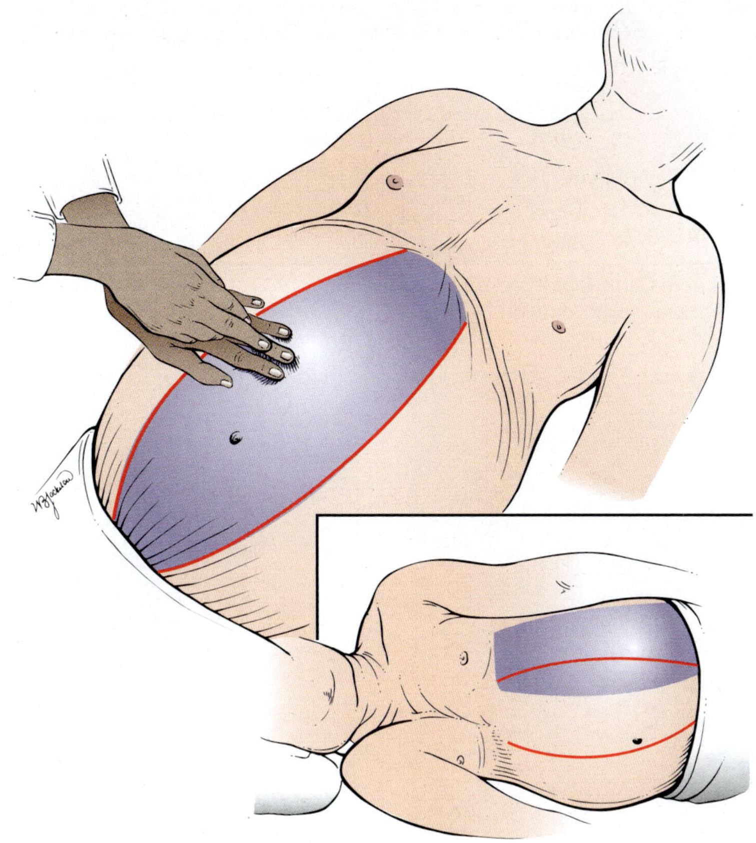

Fig. 17.17 Technique for Testing for Shifting Dullness. The *shaded areas* represent the areas of tympany.

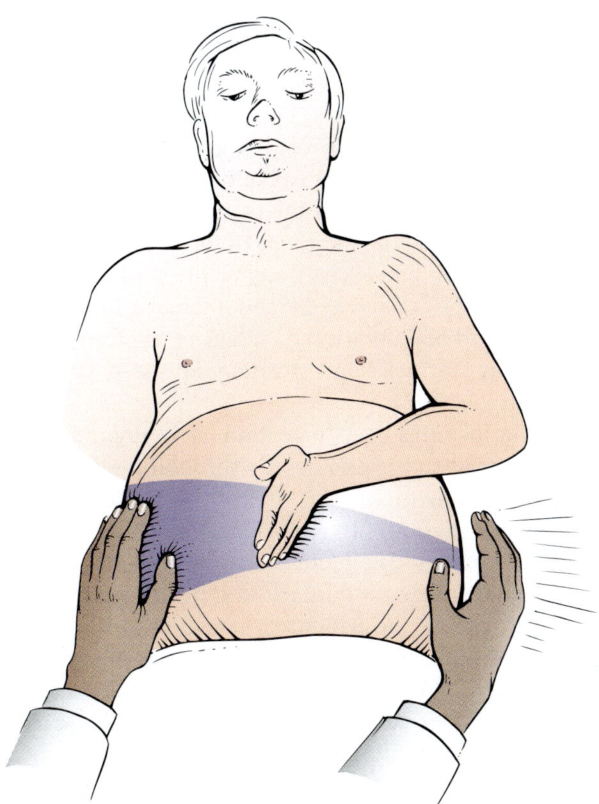

Fig. 17.18 Technique for Testing a Fluid Wave.

- Liver palpation, lower border
- Spleen palpation
- Kidney palpation

When performing palpation on the patient, they should be lying on their back. It's important to start palpation in a part of the abdomen that is furthest away from where the pain is being felt.

Light Palpation

See Video 17.5.

Light palpation is used to check for tenderness and muscle spasms. The examiner should use the flat part of their right hand or the pads of their fingers, keeping their fingers together and avoiding sudden jabs. Instead of sliding over the abdomen, they should lift their hand from one area to the next. Fig. 17.19 depicts how to perform light palpation. During the process, it's important to **observe the patient's face for any signs of discomfort or pain,** such as a wince, which is an involuntary facial contraction often triggered by pain.

When dealing with patients who are ticklish, it may prove helpful to place their hand between the examiner's hands, as shown in Fig. 17.20.

During exhalation, the rectus muscles typically loosen and become less stiff. However, if there is minimal change, it may indicate the presence of rigidity. This refers to involuntary contractions in the abdominal muscles, which can be a sign of peritoneal irritation. Rigidity can occur throughout the

TABLE 17.4 Characteristics of Physical Signs (Pooled Data) for Detection of Ascites[a]

	SENSITIVITY		SPECIFICITY			
Physical Sign	**%**	**Range**	**%**	**Range**	**LR+**	**LR−**
Bulging flanks	81	69–93	59	50–68	2.0	0.3
Flank dullness	84	80–94	59	47–71	2.0	0.3
Shifting dullness	86	64–90	72	63–81	2.7	0.3
Prominent fluid wave	62	47–77	90	84–96	6.0	0.4

[a]95% confidence interval; data pooled from Cummings et al. (1985), Simel et al. (1988), Cattau et al. (1982), and Williams and Simel (1992).
LR+, Positive likelihood ratio; *LR−*, negative likelihood ratio.

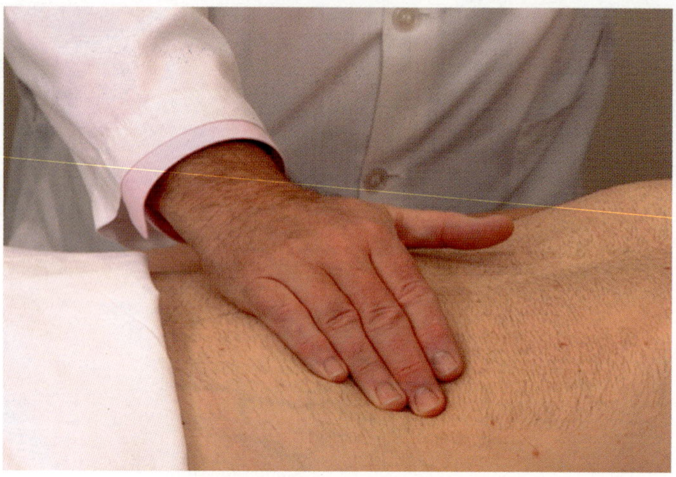

Fig. 17.19 Technique for Light Palpation.

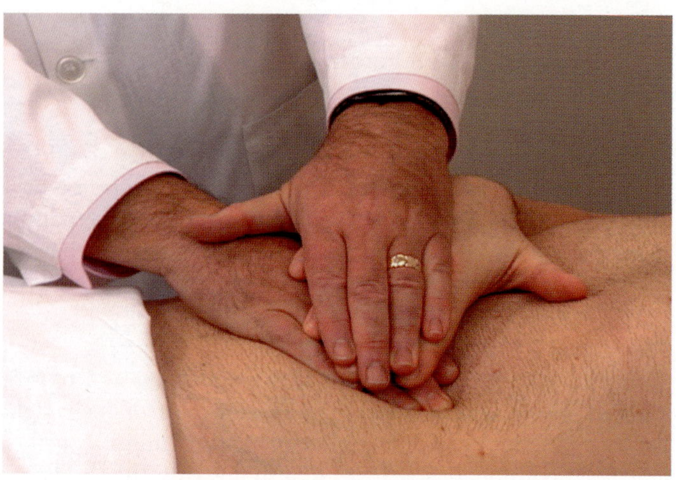

Fig. 17.20 Technique Used for Ticklish Patients. The patient's hand is sandwiched between the examiner's hands.

abdomen, as in the case of diffuse peritonitis, or in a specific area, such as over an inflamed appendix or gallbladder. When a patient has generalized peritonitis, the abdomen may be described as "board-like."

When patients report abdominal pain, it's important to perform gentle palpation. Using a pin to lightly stroke the abdomen can help identify areas of heightened sensitivity caused by inflammation of the visceral or parietal peritoneum. This condition is known as hyperesthesia. The patient is asked to compare the sharpness of the pin's sensation on one side of the abdomen to the corresponding area on the other side. While this technique can be helpful, it's important to consider all other findings and not rely solely on this observation.

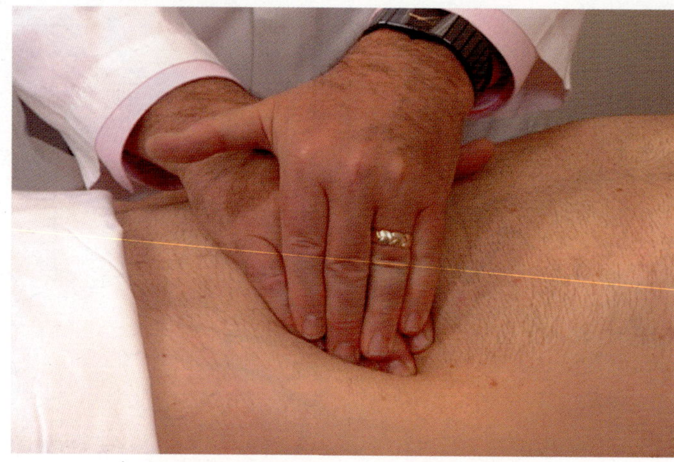

Fig. 17.21 Technique for Deep Palpation.

Deep Palpation

See Video 17.6.

To determine the size of organs and detect any unusual masses in the abdomen, deep palpation is used. The examiner places their right hand flat on the patient's abdomen and their left hand on top of it. The fingertips of the left hand apply pressure while the right hand senses any tactile stimulation. Gentle pressure should be applied to the abdomen in a steady manner. It is important to observe the patient's facial expressions during palpation. The correct hand position for deep palpation is illustrated in Fig. 17.21.

When performing deep palpation, it is important to instruct the patient to breathe quietly through their mouth and keep their arms at their sides. It may be helpful to ask the patient to open their mouth while breathing to promote relaxation of the muscles. The hands used for palpation should be warm to avoid causing voluntary muscular spasm known as guarding. Engaging the patient in conversation can also aid in relaxing their abdominal muscles. Patients with well-developed rectus muscles should be advised to flex their knees to help relax their abdominal muscles. Any tender areas should be identified.

Rule out rebound tenderness. If a patient experiences abdominal pain, it is important to check for rebound tenderness. This is a sign of peritoneal irritation that can be detected

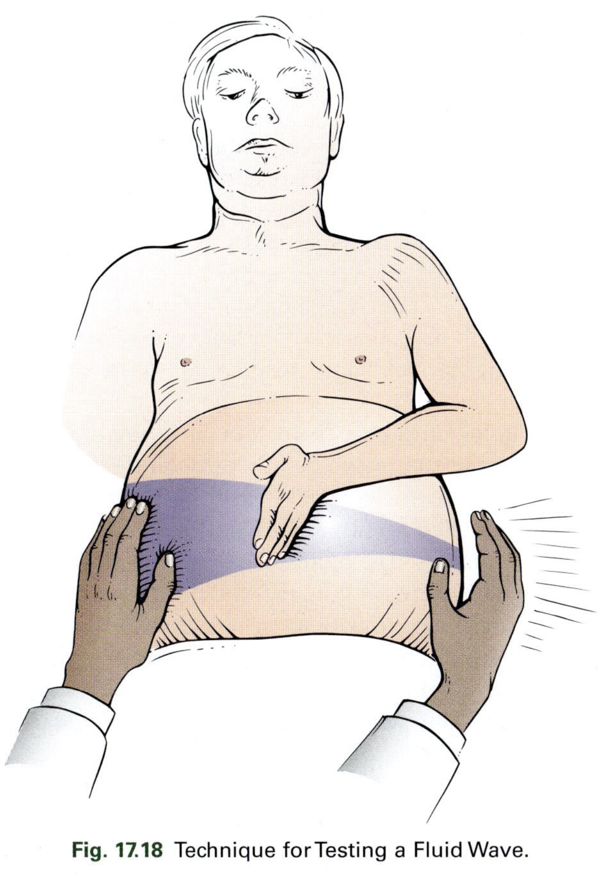

by pressing deeply and slowly on an area of the abdomen that is not suspected to be inflamed, and then quickly removing the hand. The pain felt on the side of the inflammation when pressure is released is known as rebound tenderness. If a patient has generalized peritonitis, they will feel pain in the palpation area. To determine which area hurts more, the patient should be asked if the pain is worse during press or release. This test is helpful but should be performed toward the end of the abdominal examination due to the possibility of eliciting generalized pain in patients with peritonitis.

Liver Palpation, Lower Border

See Video 17.7.

To perform palpation of the liver, place your left hand posteriorly between the patient's right twelfth rib and the iliac crest, lateral to the paraspinal muscles. Place your right hand in the patient's right upper quadrant parallel and lateral to the rectus muscles and below the area of liver dullness. The patient is instructed to take a deep breath as you press inward and upward with your right hand and pull upward with your left hand. You may feel the liver edge slipping over the fingertips of your right hand as the patient breathes. Start as low as the pelvic brim and gradually work upward. A markedly enlarged liver edge may be missed if the examination does not start low. The technique of liver palpation is demonstrated in Fig. 17.22.

A healthy liver edge is characterized by a firm, regular ridge with a smooth surface. If you are unable to detect the liver edge, simply repeat the maneuver by adjusting your right hand closer to the costal margin. Liver enlargement can occur due to factors such as vascular congestion, hepatitis, neoplasm, or cirrhosis.

Another helpful technique for palpating the liver is known as the "hooking" method. To perform this technique, the examiner stands close to the patient's head and places both hands together beneath the dullness area and right costal margin. While the patient takes a deep breath, the examiner presses upwards and inwards to "hook" around the edge of the liver. The technique for "hooking" the liver is shown in Fig. 17.23.

Sometimes, it can be challenging to determine the exact border of an enlarged liver. However, using the scratch test may help. To perform the test, the examiner holds the stethoscope's diaphragm with their left hand and places it below the patient's right costal margin over the liver. While listening through the stethoscope, the examiner uses their right index finger to scratch the abdominal wall at points in a semicircle equidistant from the stethoscope. As the finger scratches over the liver's edge, there may be a noticeable increase in the sound intensity. You can see an illustration of this technique in Fig. 17.24.

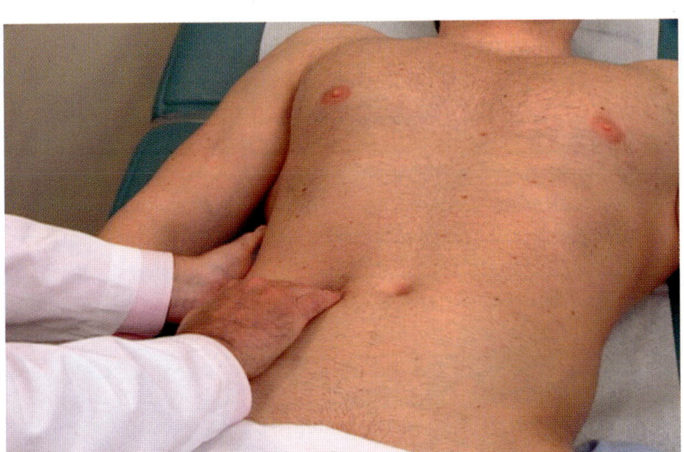

Fig. 17.22 Technique for Liver Palpation.

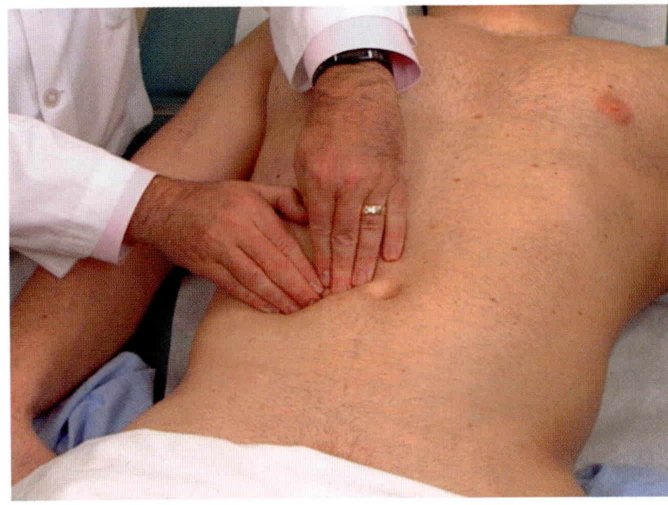

Fig. 17.23 Technique for "Hooking" the Liver.

A palpable liver is not necessarily enlarged or diseased; however, its being palpable does increase the possibility of hepatomegaly. Being nonpalpable does not rule out hepatomegaly, but it does reduce the likelihood that the liver is enlarged. The LR+ for hepatomegaly, if the liver is palpable, is 2.5; if the liver is not palpable or if the enlargement of the liver is detected by scintigraphic scanning, the LR− is 0.45.

Rule out hepatic tenderness. To check for tenderness in the liver, position your left hand over the patient's right upper quadrant, and use your right fist's ulnar surface to gently tap the area. Inflammatory conditions affecting the liver or gallbladder may cause tenderness when palpated. Refer to Fig. 17.25 for a demonstration of this procedure.

Sometimes, when the liver is being examined by palpation, the patient may experience sudden pain in the right upper quadrant during inspiration. This is known as *Murphy sign*[23] and can indicate acute cholecystitis. During inhalation, the lungs expand and push the liver, diaphragm, and inflamed gallbladder downwards against the examining hand causing severe pain and sudden inspiratory arrest. The sudden cessation of inspiration due to pain characterizes a positive Murphy sign.

Spleen Palpation

See Video 17.8.

Feeling for the spleen is more challenging than feeling for the liver. To perform this exam, the patient lies on their back while the examiner stands on their right side. The examiner places their left hand over the patient's lower left ribs and lifts the rib-cage. Then, the right hand is placed in the right lower quadrant and moved diagonally toward the left upper quadrant where the

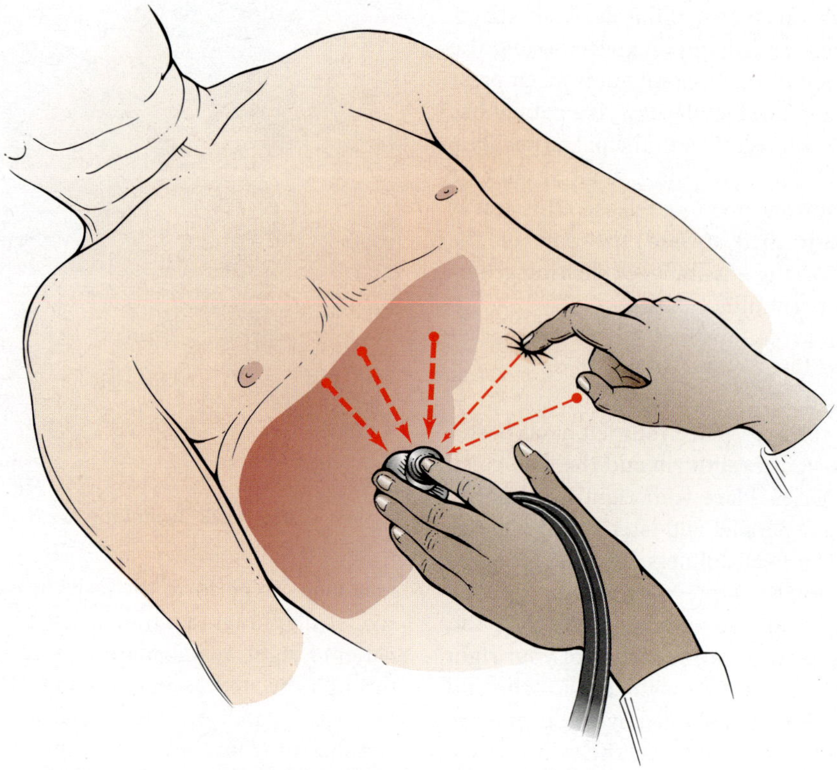

Fig. 17.24 The Scratch Test for Determining Liver Size.

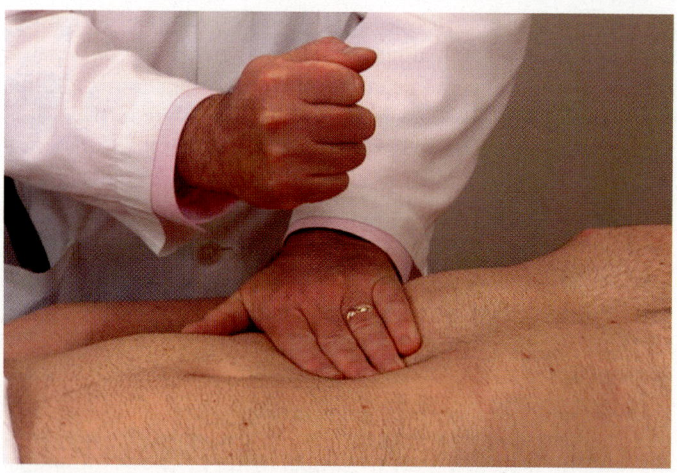

Fig. 17.25 Liver Tap Technique for Assessing Liver Tenderness.

splenic flexure is located. As the right hand approaches the left lower rib margin, the patient is asked to inhale and exhale deeply. The left hand applies pressure to push the spleen forward. The examiner should attempt to feel the tip of the patient's spleen as it descends during respiration. If the spleen is enlarged, it may be felt as a firm mass under the right hand with gentle pressure. There are various reasons why the spleen may be enlarged, and this should be considered in conjunction with the patient's medical history and other physical findings. Fig. 17.26 illustrates the positions of the hands for splenic palpation.

Another technique to palpate the spleen is to ask the patient to lie on their right side. This position helps to bring the spleen forward and downward with the assistance of gravity. The examiner will place their left hand on the patient's left costal margin while using their right hand to palpate the left upper quadrant. This technique in demonstrated in Fig. 17.27.

When examining a spleen, it's important to begin palpation near the umbilicus and gradually move toward the left upper quadrant. This is especially crucial in cases of massive enlargement, as starting too high could result in the examiner missing the splenic border.

Under normal conditions, the spleen cannot be felt by touch. However, to check for any abnormalities, both palpation techniques should be used. Splenic enlargement can occur due to various reasons such as hyperplasia, portal hypertension, infection, or tumor or myeloid infiltration. Fig. 17.28 shows a patient with massive splenomegaly secondary to chronic myelocytic leukemia.

Kidney Palpation

In adults, it is typically not possible to feel either kidney as they are retroperitoneal organs and can be obscured by fat and muscle. Although it can be challenging to assess them in this way, it is still a valuable skill to have, particularly when examining a newborn.

To check the right kidney, the examiner stands on the patient's right side and places their left hand behind the patient's right flank, between the costal margin and the iliac crest. With the right hand just below the patient's costal margin, the tips of the fingers should point to the left. This method of kidney palpation is shown in Fig. 17.29.

During deep palpation, it may be possible to feel the lower pole of the right kidney in the newborn or very young child as it descends while breathing in. The lower pole will feel like a smooth, rounded mass.

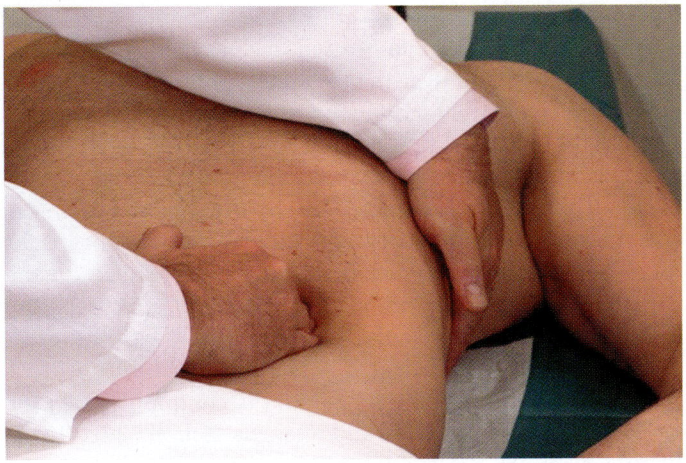

A

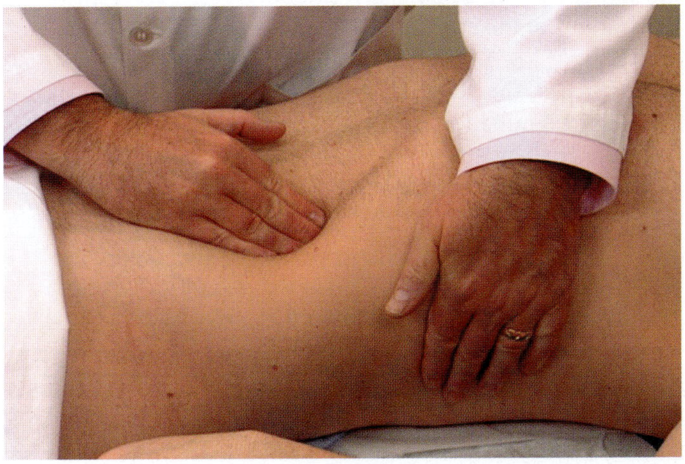

B

Fig. 17.26 (A) and (B) Technique for splenic palpation, with patient lying on the back.

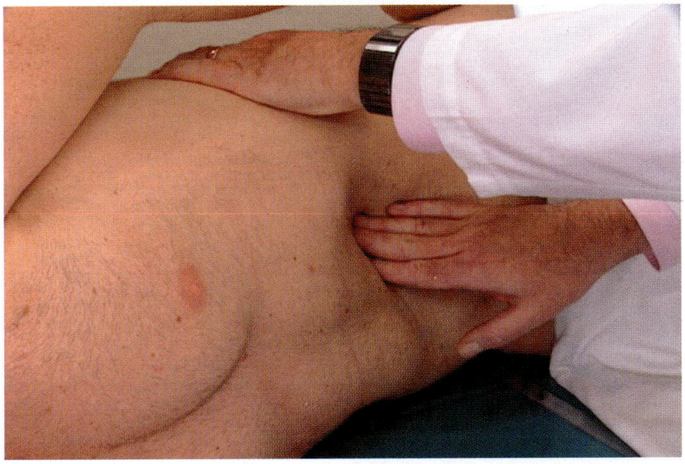

Fig. 17.27 Another Technique for Splenic Palpation, With Patient Lying on Right Side.

To examine the left kidney, the examiner stands on the patient's left side and follows the same procedure as for the right kidney. However, the left kidney is positioned higher than the right, so the lower pole of a healthy left kidney is usually not detectable even in a newborn or young child. Sometimes, the spleen may be wrongly identified as an

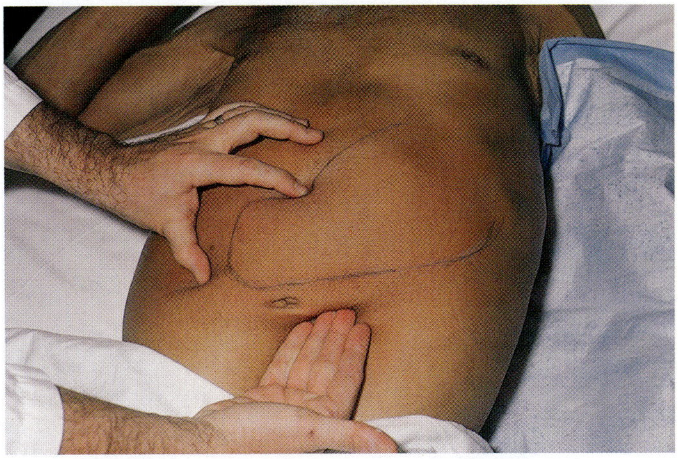

Fig. 17.28 Splenomegaly. Note the splenic notch.

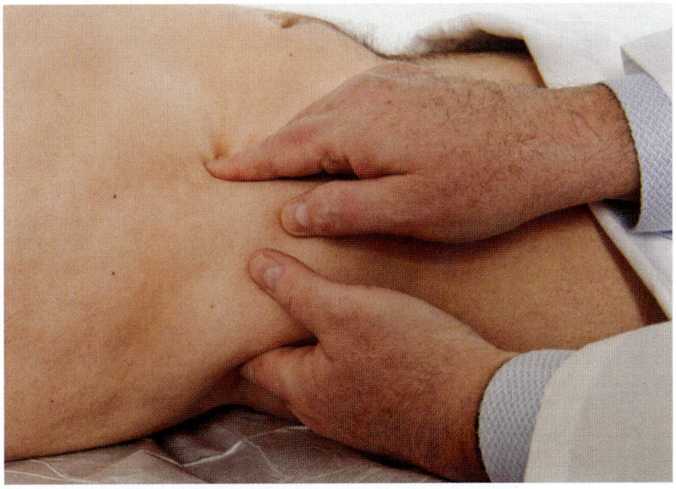

Fig. 17.29 Technique for Kidney Palpation.

enlarged left kidney. The medial notch of the spleen, however, can help distinguish it from the kidney.

Rule out renal tenderness. To rule out renal tenderness, the patient should be seated. The examiner, behind the patient, will make a fist and *lightly* tap the costovertebral angle on both sides, as shown in Fig. 17.30. If a patient has pyelonephritis, they will typically experience severe pain even with slight percussion in these regions. **Only digital pressure should be used if pyelonephritis is suspected.** As mentioned in Chapter 22, Putting the Examination Together, this part of the abdominal examination is often conducted during examination of the posterior chest.

Rectal Examination

See Video 17.9.

After conducting a routine abdominal examination, the healthcare professional may perform a digital rectal examination (DRE). If there is inflammation in the peritoneal surface of the anterior rectum, the DRE may reveal tenderness. Before the examination, it is advisable to instruct the patient to empty their bladder and bowels, if necessary.

This section is specifically about the rectal examination for male patients. The examination for female patients is discussed in Chapter 19, Female Genitalia.

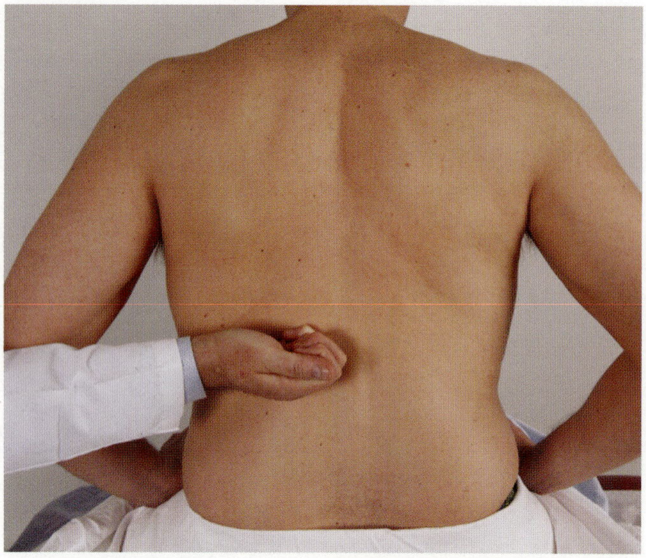

Fig. 17.30 Assessing Costovertebral Angle Tenderness.

Patient Positioning

The examination of the abdomen concludes with a DRE. It is essential to explain the procedure to the patient and ensure their privacy is maintained before proceeding. The rectal examination should be conducted using proper technique.

When examining the rectum of a male patient, there are different positions that can be used, such as lying on the back, left side, or bending over the examination table while standing. If the patient has difficulty standing, or if a detailed examination of the anus is not necessary, the modified lithotomy position is used. This involves the patient lying on their back with their knees bent. During the examination, the examiner passes their right hand under the patient's right thigh while using their left hand to apply pressure on the patient's abdomen. By using this bimanual approach, the examination can be conducted safely and with minimal disturbance to the ill patient.

The left lateral decubitus position, is commonly used for patients who are bedridden and weak (as seen in Video 17.9). In this position, the right upper leg should be bent while the left lower leg is partially extended. Fig. 17.31 provides illustrations of the modified lithotomy and left lateral decubitus position.

For males, the standing position is commonly used for a thorough examination of the anus and rectum. The patient is instructed to bend over while being supported by shoulders and elbows on a bed or examination table.

The Technique

The examiner should tell the patient that a cool-feeling lubricant will be used, and this will be followed by the sensation of having

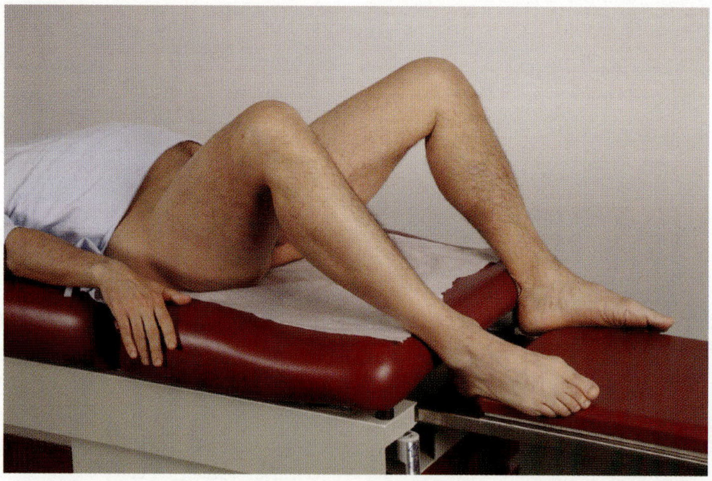

A

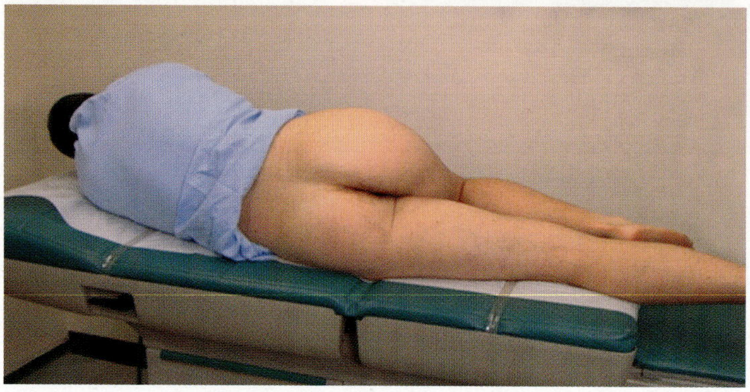

B

Fig. 17.31 Positions for the Rectal Examination for Bedridden Patients. (A) Modified lithotomy position. (B) Left lateral decubitus position.

to move the bowels; the patient should be assured that he will not do so since he has already emptied his bowels prior to the examination. Wearing gloves on both hands, the left hand carefully spreads the buttocks while the examiner uses their right hand to examine the anus and surrounding tissues. The anal skin is checked for any signs of abnormalities such as inflammation, excoriation, fissures, nodules, fistulas, scars, tumors, and hemorrhoids. Fig. 17.32 displays prolapsed internal hemorrhoids. Inspect the anus as shown in Fig. 17.33A. Any unusual areas are palpated, and patients are asked to strain while the examiner inspects the anus for hemorrhoids or fissures.

The examiner should place their lubricated, gloved right index finger against the patient's anal sphincter muscle to dilate the sphincter and slowly slide it into the rectum. To relax the sphincter, gently press the palmar surface of your finger. Fig. 17.34A shows this technique.

Instruct the patient to take a deep breath while you insert your right index finger into the anal canal as the sphincter relaxes (refer to Fig. 17.33B). The sphincter should completely close around your finger for proper assessment of sphincter tone. Fig. 17.34B illustrates this examination.

To properly examine the rectum, it is recommended to insert the finger as far as possible, although the maximum distance for digital exploration is likely around 4 inches or 10 centimeters. Once the finger is inserted, the examiner can move their left hand to the patient's left buttock while using their right index finger to examine the rectum.

Palpate the Rectal Walls

To examine the rectum, palpate its lateral, posterior, and anterior walls. You can do this by rotating your finger along the sides of the patient's rectum, as shown in Fig. 17.35. While doing so, you should be able to feel the ischial spines, coccyx, and lower sacrum. Look out for polyps as you palpate the walls; these may be sessile (attached by a base) or pedunculated (attached by a stalk). If you notice any irregularities or tenderness, take note of them. To fully examine the entire circumference of the rectal wall, you will need to turn your back to the patient and hyperpronate your hand. Otherwise, the portion of the rectal wall between the 12 o'clock and 3 o'clock positions may go undetected, and a small lesion in this quadrant may be missed.

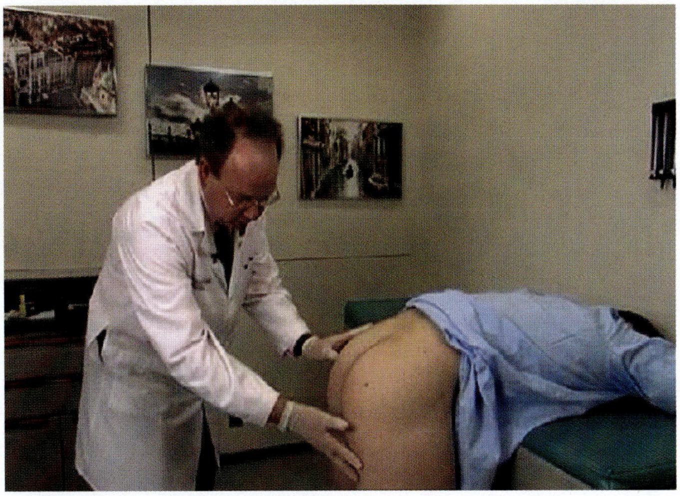

A

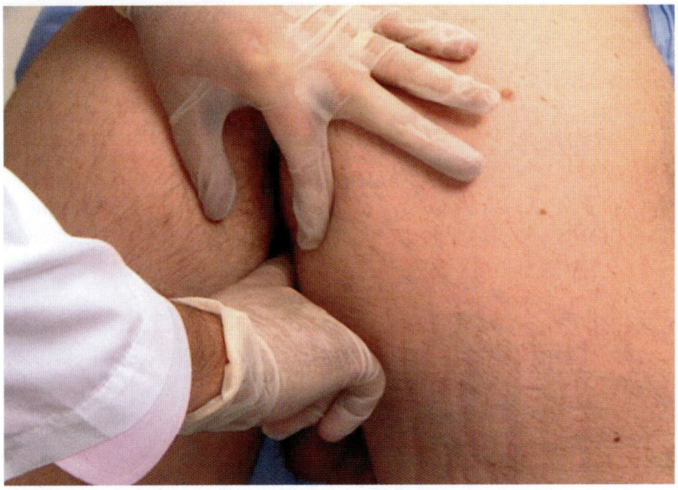

B

Fig. 17.33 Technique of the Rectal Examination. (A) Inspection. (B) Palpation. The examiner's finger is inserted with the palm of the hand facing downward.

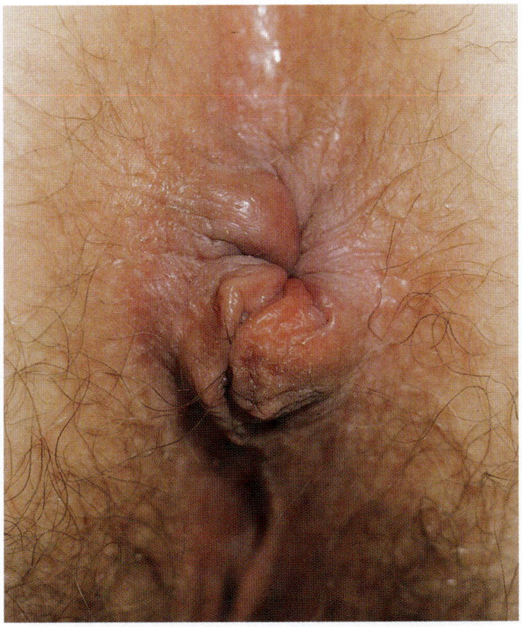

Fig. 17.32 Prolapsed Internal Hemorrhoids.

Intraperitoneal metastases may be palpated anterior to the rectum. These tumors are hard, and a shelf-like structure projects into the rectum due to infiltration of the Douglas pouch with neoplastic cells. This is *Blumer's shelf.*

Palpate the Prostate Gland

The prostate gland is located in front of the rectum wall and its size, surface, consistency, sensitivity, and shape should be evaluated. The prostate is a bilobed, heart-shaped structure approximately 1.5 inches (4 cm) in diameter. It is normally smooth and firm and has the consistency of a hard rubber ball. The apex of the heart shape points toward the anus. Identify the median sulcus and the lateral lobes. Note any masses, tenderness, and nodules. Only the lower apex portion of the gland is palpable.

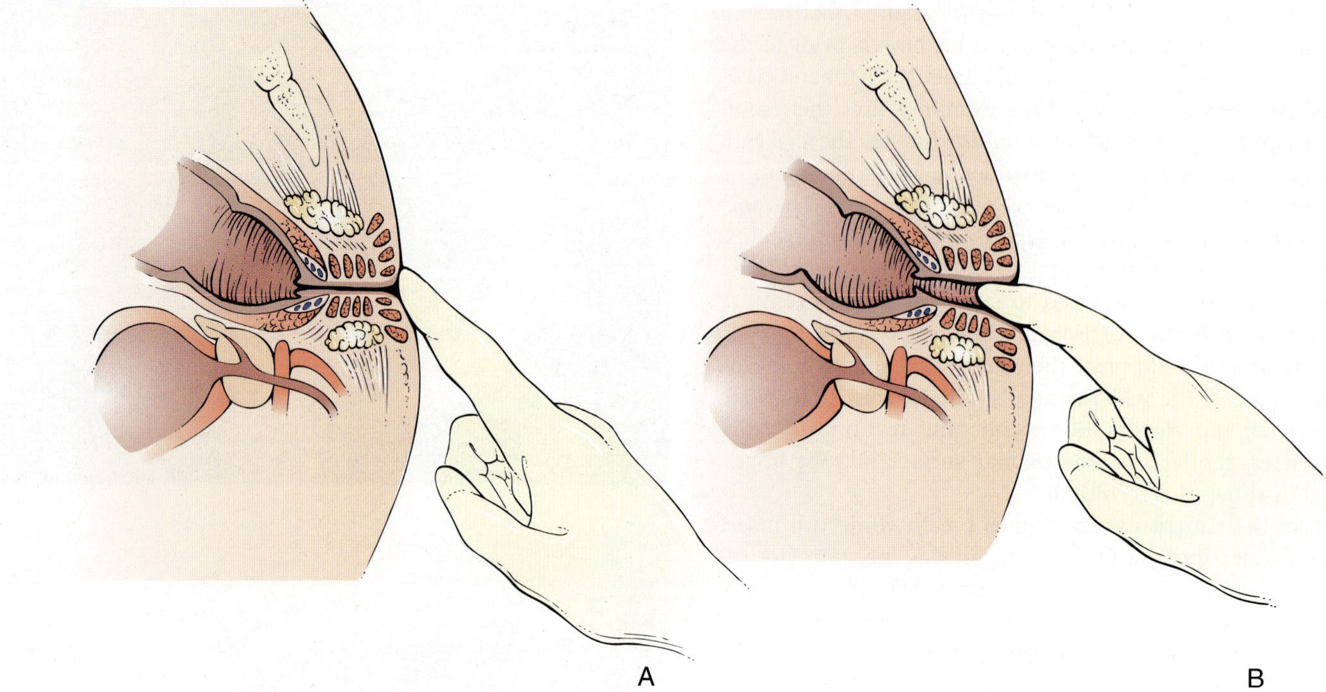

Fig. 17.34 Illustration of the Rectal Examination. (A) The sphincter is relaxed by gentle pressure with the palmar surface of the examiner's finger. (B) With the examiner's left hand spreading the patient's buttocks, examination is carried out with the examiner's right index finger.

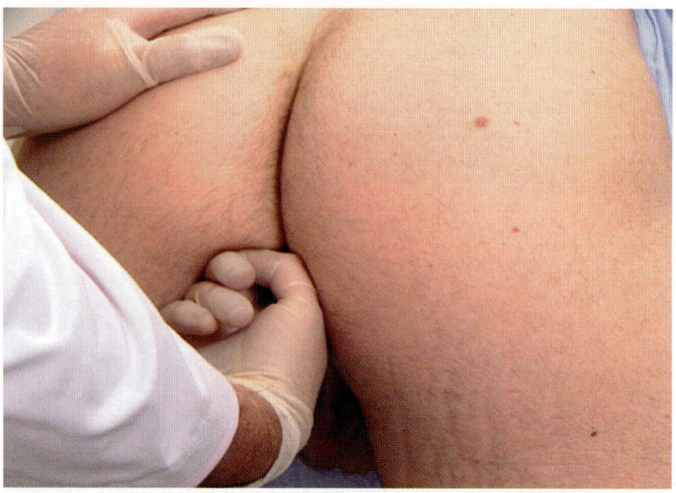

Fig. 17.35 Technique for Rectal Examination. Note position of the examiner's left hand.

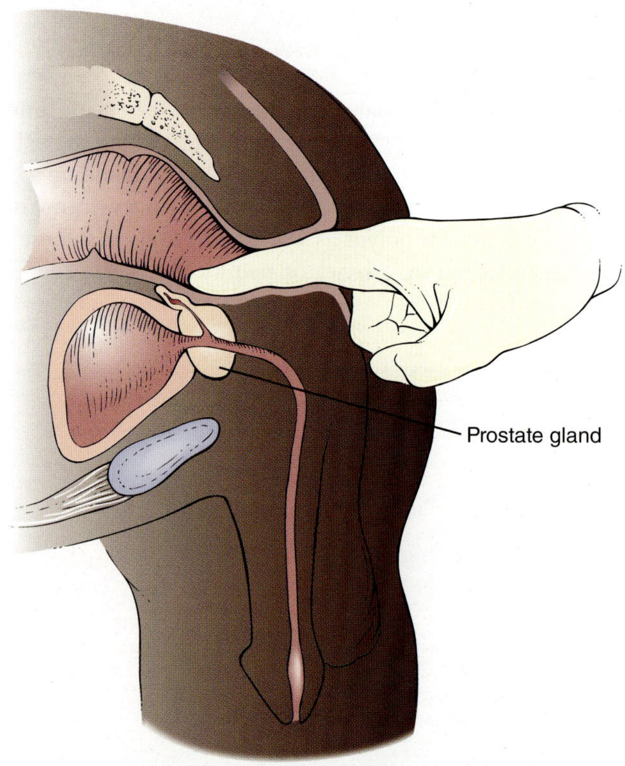

Fig. 17.36 Examination of the Prostate.

The superior margin is usually too high to reach. The examination of the prostate is illustrated in Fig. 17.36. The size of the prostate in relation to the examiner's finger is shown in Fig. 17.37.

If there is a hard, irregular nodule in the prostate gland, it may suggest the presence of cancer. Typically, prostate cancer[24] affects the posterior lobe, which can be easily identified during a DRE. Prostate cancer is the most commonly diagnosed malignancy worldwide and the fifth leading cause of cancer death in males. In 2020 worldwide, there were approximately 1,414,249 newly diagnosed cases and 375,000 deaths from this disease. However, most prostate cancers tend to grow slowly and are low-grade with relatively low risk and limited aggressiveness. Early detection is usually limited to detecting abnormalities during a DRE.

Benign prostatic hypertrophy (BPH)[25] is a very common condition that causes the prostate gland to become enlarged

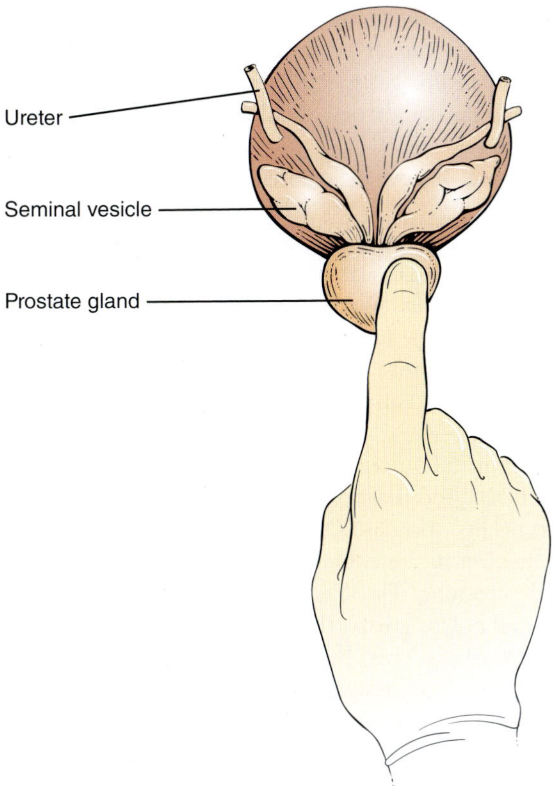

Fig. 17.37 Relationship of the Size of the Prostate Gland to the Examining Finger.

and soft, leading to protrusion into the rectal lumen. This condition is prevalent and occurs due to excessive growth of prostate tissue, which hinders the flow of urine by compressing the prostatic urethra. Another name for BPH is benign prostatic hyperplasia. It commonly affects males, with about 50% of those aged 60 and up to 90% of males over 85 experiencing it.

There are two distinct types of symptoms associated with BPH: obstructive symptoms and bladder-related symptoms. Obstructive symptoms include difficulty initiating urination, needing to strain, having a weak stream, and experiencing leaking or dribbling. Bladder-related symptoms, on the other hand, encompass frequent or urgent urination, an inability to completely empty the bladder, and waking up during the night to urinate (i.e., *nocturia*).

If a male has a swollen, painful, or tender prostate gland, it could be a sign of *acute prostatitis*. The seminal vesicles are located above the prostate gland and are not usually noticeable unless they become enlarged.

After completing the rectal examination, it is important to inform the patient that you will be withdrawing your finger. Carefully remove your examining finger and provide the patient with tissues to clean themselves.

Fecal Occult Blood Test

Inspect the examining digit and take note of the color of any fecal material. Place the fecal material on the fecal occult blood test (FOBT) card and examine it with the Hemoccult developer. The FOBT, also known as the guaiac or benzidine test, is a method used to detect hidden blood in the stool. If blood is present, it will cause a chemical reaction resulting in a blue coloration on the FOBT card. The intensity of the blue color indicates the amount of blood present, ranging from light blue (trace blood) to dark blue (4+ positive).

The FOBT is a screening test often used to detect colorectal cancer before symptoms appear. The presence of blood in the stool indicates bleeding in the digestive tract, which can be caused by various conditions such as polyps, hemorrhoids, diverticulosis, ulcers, colitis, and colorectal cancer.

Although the examination for inguinal hernias is part of the abdominal examination, it is discussed in Chapter 18, Male Genitalia and Hernias.

Special Techniques

If there is a suspicion of appendicitis, healthcare professionals may perform an *iliopsoas test.*[26] During this test, the patient lies on their unaffected left side and extends their right leg at the hip against the resistance of the examiner's hand placed above their right knee. If the patient experiences abdominal pain from the contraction of the psoas muscle, it may indicate a positive iliopsoas sign, which could be caused by an inflamed appendix resting on the psoas muscle. Fig. 17.38 shows how the test is performed, but it's important to note that the test is only positive if the inflamed appendix is positioned on the psoas muscle.

There is another helpful test to check for inflammation of the appendix called the *obturator test.* To perform this test, the patient's right thigh is flexed at the hip with the knee bent and rotated internally. If there is increased pain in the right lower quadrant, it could indicate inflammation of the internal obturator muscle due to appendicitis or an abscess. The obturator test is demonstrated in Fig. 17.39.

The Rovsing's sign test is a third test to help diagnose acute appendicitis. To perform the test, the patient must lie flat on their back. The healthcare professional will apply gentle pressure to the **left** lower quadrant of the abdomen and slowly release it. If the patient experiences sudden pain in the **right** lower quadrant, it is indicative of a positive Rovsing's sign, which suggests inflammation of the appendix.

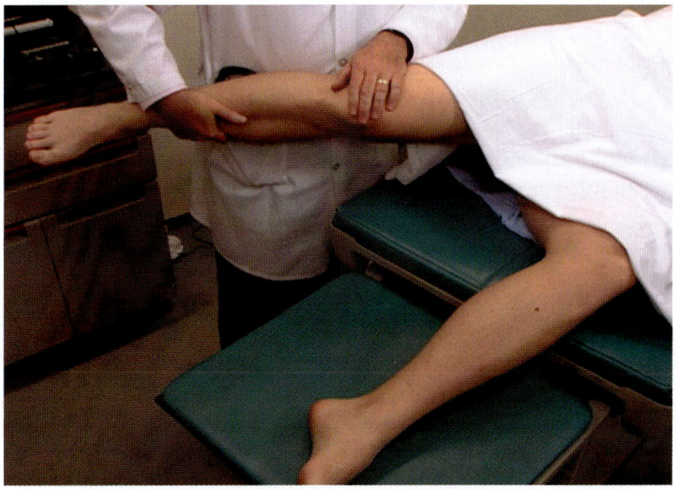

Fig. 17.38 The Iliopsoas Test.

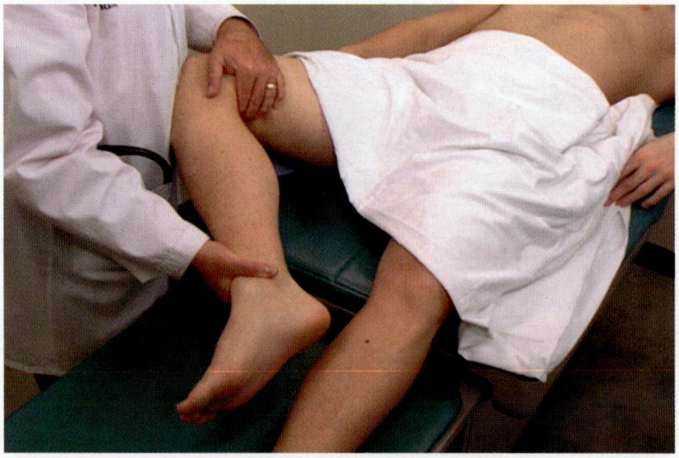

Fig. 17.39 The Obturator Test.

CLINICOPATHOLOGIC CORRELATIONS

There is evidence that detecting and removing polyps reduces the incidence of colorectal cancer and that detecting early cancers lowers the mortality rate from colorectal cancer. The COVID-19 pandemic led to the postponement of elective medical procedures, resulting in missed routine cancer screenings for many individuals. As a consequence, there may be an increase in the diagnosis of colorectal cancer in the coming years.

The American Cancer Society has suggested the following guidelines for the early detection of colorectal cancer in individuals without increased risk. Beginning at age 45 years, males and females should start regular colorectal cancer screening. People in good health and with a life expectancy of more than 10 years should continue routine screening through the **age of 75 years.** For people **aged 76 through 85,** the decision to be screened should be based on a person's preferences, life expectancy, overall health, and prior screening history. People **over 85** years should no longer get colorectal cancer screening.

Several test options for colorectal cancer screening are available.[27] The two main groups of evaluation are:

Visual (structural) exams (Tests that find polyps and cancer)

- Flexible sigmoidoscopy (FSIG) every 5 years,[e] *or*
- Colonoscopy every 10 years, *or*
- Computed tomography colonography (virtual colonoscopy) every 5 years[f]

Stool-based tests (Tests that primarily find cancer)

- Highly sensitive guaiac-based fecal occult blood test (gFOBT)[g] yearly, *or*
- Multitargeted stool DNA test (MT-sDNA) every 3 years, *or*
- Highly sensitive fecal immunochemical test (FIT) yearly[h]

People at increased risk of colorectal cancer might need to start colorectal cancer screening before age 45, be screened more often, and/or get specific tests. These individuals have:

- A strong family history of colorectal cancer or certain types of polyps
- A personal history of colorectal cancer or certain types of polyps
- A history of inflammatory bowel disease (i.e., ulcerative colitis or Crohn disease)[i]
- A known family history of a hereditary colorectal cancer syndrome[j] (e.g., familial adenomatous polyposis [FAP] or Lynch syndrome)
- A history of radiation to the abdomen or pelvic area to treat a prior cancer

The colorectal cancer mortality rate can be reduced by 15% to 33% by FOBT and diagnostic evaluation and treatment for positive test results. Annual FOBT screening leads to a more significant reduction in the colorectal cancer mortality rate than does biennial screening. Flexible sigmoidoscopy identifies nearly all cancers and polyps greater than 0.4 inches (1 cm) in diameter and 75% to 80% of small polyps in the portion of the bowel examined. Screening with flexible sigmoidoscopy has been shown to result in a 60% to 80% reduction in the risk of death from colorectal cancer in the part of the colon examined. Screening colonoscopy offers the potential both to identify and remove cancers and premalignant lesions throughout the colon and rectum.

A 2020 systematic review and meta-analysis in the *Journal of Cancer*[28] indicated that colonoscopy could significantly reduce the incidence and mortality of colorectal cancer. Usually, the recommended age by developed countries for regular colonoscopic screening is 50. Based on this study's results, the population aged 20 to 50 years old could also benefit from colonoscopic screening. Further research is ongoing.

Anal cancer[29] is increasing in both males and females worldwide. Most anal cancers are related to human papillomavirus (HPV) infection. Males who have sex with male patients, HIV-positive individuals, transplant recipients, and females with cervical neoplasia have a higher risk for anal cancer than the general population. Males who have sex with males have a 44% greater risk for anal cancer than the general population.[30] Anal cancer, like cervical cancer, is potentially preventable. Anal cytologic findings have been studied and found to be a useful screening test to detect anal cancer. It has been shown that a high proportion of males who have sex with male patients were infected with anal HPV (66%).

[e] If the test is positive, a colonoscopy should be performed.

[f] If the test is positive, a colonoscopy should be performed.

[g] The multiple stool take-home test should be used. One test done by a healthcare professional in the office in *not* adequate for testing. A colonoscopy should be done if the test is positive.

[h] The multiple stool take-home test should be used. One test done by a healthcare professional in the office in *not* adequate for testing. A colonoscopy should be done if the test is positive.

[i] For individuals diagnosed with inflammatory bowel disease, it is recommended that they undergo colonoscopies *(and not any other type of test)* at least 8 years after their diagnosis. Follow-up colonoscopies should be conducted every 1 to 3 years, depending on the person's risk factors for colorectal cancer as well as the findings of the previous colonoscopy.

[j] For some genetic syndromes, *colonoscopy is the only screening test*, as opposed to other tests. It may be recommended to start screening at a young age, including during teenage years, and the frequency of tests will vary based on the syndrome and other factors.

Table 17.2 lists the classic locations of pain referred from abdominal structures. Table 17.3 summarizes the maneuvers for ameliorating abdominal pain. Table 17.4 summarizes the sensitivities and specificities of the various maneuvers used to detect ascites. Table 17.5 is a comparison of the clinical manifestations of ulcerative colitis and Crohn disease. Table 17.6 lists the clinical features of cancer of the stomach, pancreas, and colon. Table 17.7 lists the variation of symptoms in right-sided and left-sided colon cancer and in rectal cancer. Table 17.8 compares the symptoms and signs of cirrhosis, which are numerous, as they relate to hepatocellular failure and portal hypertension.

Prostate cancer is the second leading cancer diagnosed among American males. In 2023, there were 288,300 new cases of prostate cancer in the United States and 34,700 deaths from prostate cancer. An estimated 1 in 8 males will be diagnosed with prostate cancer during their lifetime, but only 1 in 41 males will die of the disease. In the years from 2007 to 2014, there was a significant decrease in the number of prostate cancer diagnoses, likely due to a decrease in screening as a result of revised screening guidelines. However, since 2014, there has been a gradual increase of 3% annually in the overall incidence rate and a 5% increase per year in the incidence of advanced-stage prostate cancer.

The prostate cancer incidence rate among African American males (180.6 per 100,000) is more than seven times that among Koreans (24.2 per 100,000). Indeed, African Americans in the United States have the highest rates of this cancer in the world. Although the incidence among White persons is quite high, it is distinctly lower than that among African Americans. Asian and Native American males have the lowest rates.

Prostate cancer is often detected early, with 86% of cases diagnosed at a localized stage where the 5-year survival rate is 100%. Even for regional cancer, the 5-year survival rate is almost 100%. However, the incidence rates for prostate cancer are still rising partly due to increased screening tests. Regular DRE and measuring prostate-specific antigen (PSA) levels in blood samples can detect the cancer early. If any of these tests show abnormal results during yearly check-ups, it is likely that the cancer is caught at an early and more treatable stage.

During the early 1990s, the PSA test became available as a straightforward blood test to determine the possibility of having prostate cancer, marking the start of the current era for prostate cancer. PSA is a protein produced by both healthy and cancerous cells in the prostate gland. While most of it is found in semen, a small amount can also be detected in the blood. In general, the normal blood PSA level for males is under 4 ng/mL. However, this level can be affected by various factors, leading to many false positives for cancer. For example, it may increase due to noncancerous prostate enlargement (BPH) or prostatitis. Additionally, PSA levels typically increase gradually with age.

Prior to taking a PSA test, it is advisable for patients to refrain from ejaculation for at least 48 hours, as it may lead to a temporary spike in blood PSA levels. A false-positive test result can cause unnecessary anxiety for the patient and their family, and may lead to further medical procedures, such as a prostate

TABLE 17.5 Clinical Comparison of Ulcerative Colitis and Crohn Disease

Feature	Ulcerative Colitis	Crohn Disease
Diarrhea	Present	Present
Hematochezia	Common	Rare
Extraintestinal manifestations	Common	Common
Perirectal disease	Fissures	Fistulas Abscesses
Rectal disease	Present	Absent
Anal disease	Absent	Present

TABLE 17.6 Clinical Comparison of Cancer of the Stomach, Pancreas, and Colon

Cancer of Stomach	Cancer of Pancreas	Cancer of Colon
Major Symptoms		
Upper abdominal pain Occult bleeding Weight loss Vomiting Anorexia Dysphagia	Upper abdominal pain Back pain Weight loss Jaundice	Change in bowel habits Gastrointestinal bleeding Lower abdominal pain
Risk Factors		
Adenomatous polyps Pernicious anemia Family history Immigrants from Japan	Smoking Alcoholism (?)	Adenomatous polyps Ulcerative colitis Familial polyposis Gardner syndrome Villous adenomas

TABLE 17.7 Variation of Symptoms of Cancer of the Right Colon, Left Colon, and Rectum

Symptom	Cancer of Right Colon	Cancer of Left Colon	Cancer of Rectum
Pain	Ill defined	Colicky[a]	Steady, gnawing
Obstruction	Infrequent	Common	Infrequent
Bleeding	Brick-red	Red mixed with stool	Bright red coating stool
Weakness[b]	Common	Infrequent	Infrequent

[a]Worse with ingestion of foods.
[b]Secondary to anemia.

TABLE 17.8 Signs and Symptoms of Cirrhosis

Hepatocellular Failure
Spider angiomata (see Fig. 8.81)
Gynecomastia
Palmar erythema
Ascites (see Video 17.4)
Jaundice
Testicular atrophy
Erectile dysfunction
Bleeding problems
Changes in mental function
Portal Hypertension
Ascites (see Video 17.4)
Varices: esophageal
Hemorrhoids (see Fig. 17.32)
Caput medusae
Splenomegaly (see Fig. 17.28)

biopsy, that can potentially cause serious infections, pain, and bleeding. False negatives can also occur, which may give the patient, family, and healthcare professional false assurance that the patient does not have cancer, when in fact they may require treatment for cancer.

It's been proven that PSA screening can lower the mortality rate for prostate cancer. However, it's important to note that prostate cancer often develops very slowly and may not have any negative impact on a patient's life. For that reason, many males do not benefit from treatment for prostate cancer and may unnecessarily suffer from the treatment's side effects, such as incontinence, bowel dysfunction, and impotence. Overtreatment is the major potential harm of overdiagnosis.[31]

Until recently, many healthcare professionals and professional organizations encouraged yearly PSA screening for males beginning at age 50. Some organizations recommended that males who are at higher risk of prostate cancer, including African American males and males whose father or brother had prostate cancer, begin screening at age 40 or 45. However, as of 2013, as more has been learned about both the benefits and harms of prostate cancer screening,[k] there have been varying expert opinions on when and who should be screened for prostate cancer. However, all recommendations suggest using serum PSA testing as the primary method of initial screening. The expert recommendations aim to assist patients in making an informed decision about whether or not to undergo screening. They encourage patients to consider the benefits and potential risks, as well as their age, general health, comorbidities, and personal preferences.

[k]The Prostate, Lung, Colorectal, and Ovarian (PLCO) Cancer Screening Trial was a trial of 76,693 males, and the European Randomized Study of Screening for Prostate Cancer (ERSPC) trial consisted of 182,000 males. The results of these studies were conflicting. The PLCO trial showed no benefit from screening in reducing mortality. The ERSPC trial showed a 20% reduction in mortality in males ages 55 to 69 years of age but at a cost of overdiagnosis, with a 76% false-positive rate on biopsy.

The *"Ask-Tell-Ask"* approach derived from motivational interviewing is useful in counseling patients about the benefits and risks of screening. It is a back-and-forth, bidirectional cycle between the patient and the healthcare professional that addresses four essential components: the patient's perspective, information that needs to be delivered, response to the patient's emotions, and recommendations by the healthcare professional.

Related to PSA screening for prostate cancer, ***Ask* the patient** to describe his current understanding of the issue. You might say:

- *"What do you know about prostate cancer screening?"*
- *"Have you thought about whether you want to be screened for prostate cancer?"*

***Tell* the patient**. When communicating with the patient, use simple language to explain the screening, diagnostic, and treatment options for an elevated PSA level. Avoid giving lengthy lectures or overwhelming amounts of information. Keep the communication straightforward and clear.

Finally, ***Ask* the patient** if he understood what you just said or what are his feelings about cancer screening now after discussing the "pros and cons" of PSA screening.[l]

Researchers are now investigating ways to improve the PSA test to better distinguish cancerous from benign lesions and slow-growing cancers from fast-growing, potentially lethal cancers. Some of the methods being studied include:

- Free versus total PSA[m]
- PSA density of the transition zone[n]
- Age-specific PSA reference ranges[o]
- PSA velocity and PSA doubling time[p]
- Pro-PSA[q]

[l]The "***Ask-Tell-Ask***" (also called "Elicit-Provide-Elicit") approach is very useful also for speaking with female patients about mammography/breast sonography and breast cancer.

[m]The amount of PSA in the blood that is "free" (not bound to other proteins) divided by the total amount of PSA (free plus bound). Some evidence suggests that a lower proportion of free PSA may be associated with more aggressive cancer.

[n]The blood level of PSA is divided by the volume of the transition zone of the prostate. The transition zone is the interior part of the prostate that surrounds the urethra. Some evidence suggests that this measure may be more accurate at detecting prostate cancer than the standard PSA test.

[o]Because a male's PSA level tends to increase with age, it has been suggested that the use of age-specific PSA reference ranges may increase the accuracy of PSA tests. However, age-specific reference ranges have not been generally favored because their use may delay the detection of prostate cancer in many patients.

[p]PSA velocity is the rate of change in a patient's PSA level over time, expressed as ng/mL per year. PSA doubling time is the period over which a patient's PSA level doubles. Some evidence suggests that the rate of increase in a patient's PSA level may be helpful in predicting whether he has prostate cancer.

[q]Pro-PSA refers to several different inactive precursors of PSA. There is some evidence that pro-PSA is more strongly associated with prostate cancer than with BPH. One recently approved test combines measurement of a form of pro-PSA with measurements of PSA and free PSA. The resulting "prostate health index" can be used to help a patient with a PSA level of between 4 and 10 ng/mL decide whether they should have a biopsy.

USEFUL VOCABULARY

Listed here are the specific roots that are important for understanding the terminology related to abdominal disease.

Root	Pertaining to	Example	Definition
aer(o)-	air; gas	***aero***phagia	Air swallowing
celi(o)-	abdomen	***celi***ac	Pertaining to the abdomen
chol(e)-	bile	***chole***lith	Gallstone
cyst-	sac containing liquid	chole***cyst***itis	Inflammation of the gallbladder
enter(o)-	intestines	***enter***itis	Inflammation of the small intestines
gastr(o)-	stomach	***gastr***ectomy	Surgical removal of the stomach
lapar(o)-	loin; flank	***lapar***otomy	Surgical incision through the flank; generally, any abdominal incision
-phago-	eating	***phago***cyte	Any cell that ingests other cells or microorganisms
-tripsy	shock waves	litho***tripsy***	Noninvasive technique for breaking up stones via use of shock waves

WRITING UP THE PHYSICAL EXAMINATION

Listed here are examples of the write-up for the examination of the abdomen.

- The abdomen is scaphoid without scars. Bowel sounds are present. The liver is felt two fingerbreadths below the right costal margin for a total span of 10 cm (4 inches). Neither the spleen nor any masses are felt. The kidneys are not palpable. Rectal examination reveals normal sphincter tone. The prostate is soft, without any masses. The walls of the rectum are smooth, without masses. Results of testing of the stool for blood are negative. No CVAT is present.
- The abdomen has a scar in the right upper quadrant. Bowel sounds are absent. Marked tympany is present throughout the abdomen. Rigidity is present throughout. Marked tenderness is present in the abdomen, especially in the left lower quadrant. Examination of the rectum reveals tenderness in the same area. Stool guaiac test result is 4+. The liver, spleen, and kidneys are not felt. No CVAT is present.
- The abdomen is obese. Bowel sounds are present. Percussion notes are normal. There is an area of significant pain in the right lower quadrant, immediately above the right midposition of the inguinal ligament. Rectal examination discloses severe pain in the same area. The obturator and straight leg raising signs are positive on the right. Stool guaiac test result is negative. Right CVAT is present. No organomegaly is felt.
- The abdomen is protuberant, with a midline, well-healed scar. Bowel sounds are present. Shifting dullness and a fluid wave are present. A large mass 8 × 15 cm (3 × 6 inches) is felt in the right upper quadrant. Results of examination of the rectum are unremarkable except for a trace positive stool guaiac. There is no hepatosplenomegaly.
- The abdomen is scaphoid and soft, without guarding, rigidity, or tenderness. Bowel sounds are present. The liver measures 12 cm (4.7 inches) in span in the midclavicular line. The spleen tip is felt below the left costal margin. No masses are present. Rectal examination reveals a 2-cm (0.75-inch) hard nodule in the posterior lobe of the prostate, which is nontender. Stool guaiac test result is negative.

CVAT, Costovertebral angle tenderness.

FULL VIDEO

- Video 17.10 Full video: Examination of the abdomen

REVIEW QUESTIONS

1. **Related to the patient's description of pain, which of the following pairs is *incorrect*?**
   A. Perforated gastric ulcer – "burning"
   B. Dissecting aneurysm – "burning"
   C. Intestinal obstruction – "constricting"
   D. Pyelonephritis – "aching"
   E. Biliary colic – "crampy"
2. **Patients often describe maneuvers to ameliorate their pain. Which of the following pairs is *incorrect*?**
   A. Belching – stomach problem
   B. Eating – lower small bowel problem
   C. Vomiting – upper bowel problem
   D. Leaning forward – pancreatic problem
   E. Knee flexion – peritoneal problem
3. **Blood mixed with stool can be seen in all the following conditions *except*:**
   A. Crohn disease
   B. Ulcerative colitis
   C. Diverticular disease
   D. Colorectal cancer
   E. Hemorrhoids
4. **Which of the following statements is true?**
   A. Hematochezia may commonly result from gastric cancer.
   B. The acute onset of diarrhea after a meal suggests inflammatory bowel disease.
   C. Vomiting is frequently caused by inflammation of intra-abdominal structures and extra-abdominal conditions.
   D. Jaundice results from decreased excretion of unconjugated bilirubin into the bile.
   E. Loss of appetite is often seen in patients with Crohn disease.
5. **In examining the abdomen, inspecting the entire body for signs of abdominal disease is necessary. Which of the following statement is *false?***
   A. Patients with renal colic writhe in pain and are constantly moving.
   B. Spider angiomas have a high degree of sensitivity in patients with alcoholic cirrhosis.

C. "Half and half" nails (aka Lindsay's nails) are associated with chronic renal disease and azotemia.
D. The respiratory rate is increased in patients with generalized peritonitis.
E. A bluish discoloration of the umbilicus (known as the Cullen sign) is seen in hemorrhagic pancreatitis.

6. **Which of the following statements about abdominal palpation is *false?***
A. The patient must be supine during palpation.
B. Light palpation is used to detect tenderness and areas of muscular spasm or rigidity.
C. Palpation of the abdomen must always precede auscultation of the abdomen.
D. Always look at the patient's face during palpation.
E. A palpable liver is not necessarily enlarged or diseased.

7. **Regarding the digital rectal examination (DRE) in the male, which of the following statements is *incorrect?***
A. First ask the patient to relax.
B. The patient is instructed to empty their bladder and bowels prior to the examination.
C. The DRE may be performed with the patient standing and bent over the examination table, lying on their left side, or lying on their back.
D. The left lateral decubitus position is used most commonly in patients who are weak and bedridden.
E. The examining finger is inserted as far as possible into the rectum, although 4 inches is the probable limit of digital exploration.

8. **People at increased risk of colorectal cancer might need to start colorectal cancer screening before age 45. These people include:**
A. A strong family history of colorectal cancer
B. A history of colorectal cancer or certain types of polyps
C. A history of inflammatory bowel disease
D. A history of radiation to the abdomen or pelvic area
E. All of the above

9. **Regarding the clinical symptoms of inflammatory bowel disease, which of the following pairs is *incorrect?***
A. Diarrhea – ulcerative colitis
B. Hematochezia – Crohn disease
C. Extraintestinal manifestations – both ulcerative colitis and Crohn disease
D. Perirectal disease – both ulcerative colitis and Crohn disease
E. Rectal disease – ulcerative colitis

10. **All of the following signs and symptoms are common in cirrhosis *except:***
A. Gynecomastia
B. Palmar erythema
C. Jaundice
D. Erectile dysfunction
E. Dyspnea

REFERENCES

Available online.

BIBLIOGRAPHY

Available online.

18

Male Genitalia and Hernias

Mark H. Swartz

If a man's urine is like the urine of an ass, like beer yeast, like wine yeast or varnish, that man is sick…and through a bronze tube in the penis pour oil and beer and licorice.

From the Sushruta Samhita (ca. 3000 BCE)

VIDEOS

Video 18.1	Inspecting the external genitalia
Video 18.2	Inspecting the penis
Video 18.3	Inspecting the external meatus of the penis
Video 18.4	Palpating the penis and urethra
Video 18.5	Inspecting the scrotum
Video 18.6	Palpating the testes
Video 18.7	Palpating the epididymis and vas deferens
Video 18.8	Palpating for inguinal hernias
Video 18.9	Full video: Examining the male genitalia

GENERAL CONSIDERATIONS

Throughout recorded history, people have held a particular fascination with the external genitalia and urologic system. Antiquity documents described urologic surgery and kidney stones in great detail. In fact, one of the earliest known cases of kidney stones was discovered in a young boy who lived around 7000 BCE.

Male circumcision is a surgical procedure that has been in practice for centuries, with its origins dating back to 3000 BCE. It has been predominantly associated with religious rites, being an initiatory rite in Judaism and a sign of spiritual purification among Muslims. Temple walls often depict circumcision, although its exact origin remains unknown. The Egyptian Book of the Dead contains a passage that describes the Sun God beginning to incise himself and blood falling from his phallus. During the Roman takeover of Egypt in 30 BCE, circumcision had become a ritual practice with significant religious meaning. Only circumcised priests were allowed to perform certain religious rites. In Hindu culture, the penis and testicles were seen as a symbol of the center of life. The prepuce was sacrificed as a special offering to the gods.

The Bible contains several references related to urology. For instance, in Genesis 17:7, Abraham establishes a covenant with God on behalf of the Jewish people. In Genesis 17:14, it is stated that anyone who is an uncircumcised male and has not undergone the procedure will be cut off from their community, as they have broken the covenant with God. The book of Leviticus 12:3 instructs Jews to circumcise the flesh of the foreskin on the eighth day of life. In addition, Leviticus 15:2-17 discusses discharges that can make a male unclean. Currently, approximately 1 in 6 males globally undergoes circumcision. More than 15 million post-infancy circumcisions are performed annually, making it one of the most frequently performed surgical procedures.

The disease now believed to be gonorrhea was described in the Bible, Hindu literature, and Egyptian papyri. The Mesopotamian tablets contain information on different remedies. For instance, one cure involves boiling beer and milk and applying it to the pubic area if a male experiences pain during sexual activity. For many centuries, Avicenna's *Canon of Medicine* (c. 1012 CE)[a] was regarded as the foremost medical text. It contained a curious remedy for penile discharge, which involved placing a louse in the penis.

Although Albert Neisser was the first to describe gonococcus in 1879, the history of gonorrhea can be traced back to the earliest records of human civilization.[1] The Romans, Jews, and Arabs all have documents referring to the disease, and each society had its own description of symptoms and treatment. In 130 CE, the Roman physician Galen described the disease as an "involuntary escape of semen." The word "gonorrhea" itself comes from the Greek, meaning "the flow of seed." Gonorrhea has been referred to by various names over time, with the most popular one being "clap" for the last four centuries. The name originated from a district in Paris popular for prostitution, known as Le Clapier.

[a]Avicenna, a Persian physician who lived from 980 to 1037 CE, is recognized as one of the most influential medical writers of the Middle Ages. His book, the *Canon of Medicine*, is considered a historical masterpiece. It is a well-organized summary of all the medical knowledge available at that time, which includes a comprehensive list of drugs. Avicenna's works were highly regarded in Western medical studies from the 13th to the 17th centuries and were considered an authoritative source. They had a significant impact on modern medicine, and some universities used his works for teaching up to the 19th century.

The origin of syphilis remains uncertain. There was a lot of confusion between syphilis and gonorrhea, with some people thinking that gonorrhea was just a precursor to syphilis. The cause of both diseases was also a mystery, with some theories suggesting that syphilis was caused by floods, consumption of disguised human flesh, or contaminated water. It was not until 1500, when syphilis was pandemic in Europe, that the venereal origins of both diseases were understood. It is now believed that syphilis was introduced on the European continent in 1492 by the returning sailors who had been traveling with Columbus. Following France's invasion of Italy and the siege of Naples in 1495, the prevalence of syphilis increased rapidly throughout Europe. Syphilis was often referred to as "King's pox" or "French pox."

As male patients age, they commonly develop a non-cancerous growth in their prostate called benign prostatic hyperplasia (BPH). This condition, which was mentioned in Chapter 17, The Abdomen, affects a significant portion of the male population. By the time a male reaches 80 years of age, 1 in 4 requires treatment to alleviate symptoms caused by BPH. Fortunately, there are several treatment options available, such as watchful waiting, behavioral therapy, medical solutions, and surgical treatment. Every year, over 300,000 prostate surgeries are performed in the United States to treat BPH, with the most common procedure being transurethral resection of the prostate (TURP).[2,b] Despite being the gold-standard surgery for BPH, TURP carries risks such as ejaculatory and erectile dysfunction after the procedure.[c] TURP is recommended for patients with prostate sizes of less than 100 g, and approximately 150,000 patients undergo this surgery annually. However, open prostatectomy surgery is the preferred intervention for prostate sizes greater than 100 g and is widely practiced.

Cancer affecting the genitourinary system is prevalent. As previously discussed in Chapter 17, The Abdomen, *prostate cancer* is the second most frequently diagnosed cancer among males in America. To learn more about prostate cancer, please refer to Chapter 17.

Bladder cancer (BC) is a type of tumor that arises in the urinary bladder. Urothelial carcinoma is the most common type of BC, accounting for about 90% of cases. BC is the seventh most prevalent form of cancer globally. In the United States, there were 81,400 new cases of BC in 2020, with 62,100 occurring in males and 19,300 in females. Additionally, 17,980 people died due to BC, with 13,050 males and 4930 females being affected. BC is a prevalent cancer in the United States, ranking fourth among males and sixth among females. Whites are twice as likely to develop BC compared to African Americans, and the risk increases with age. Due to the high likelihood of recurrence, close monitoring is necessary for patients with BC. As a result, BC is among the costliest cancers.

BC has several known risk factors. The most important ones are smoking, schistosomiasis infection, and exposure to harmful chemicals in the workplace. Smoking poses the highest risk for BC, with smokers being 2 to 6 times more likely to develop it than nonsmokers. Studies show that around 50% of male and 30% of female BC cases are linked to smoking. Occupational exposure to certain chemicals such as *arylamines* can also contribute to up to 25% of all urinary BCs. Workers in industries such as dyeing, rubber, leather, truck driving, painting, and aluminum may be at greater risk of BC due to exposure to arylamines.

BC has varying 5-year relative survival rates depending on its stage. For those with carcinoma in situ of the bladder (abnormal cells found in the bladder lining), the survival rate is 97%. If the cancer is localized solely in the bladder, the survival rate is 71%. However, if it has spread beyond the bladder to nearby lymph nodes or organs, the survival rate drops to 39%.

Although *testicular cancer* accounts for only 1% of all cancers in males, testicular cancer is the most commonly diagnosed cancer in males between the ages of 20 and 34.[3] In 2023, 9190 males in the United States were diagnosed with testicular cancer with 470 deaths due to the cancer. It is estimated that about 1 in every 250 males will receive a testicular cancer diagnosis at some point in their life. In 2020, there were 74,458 reported cases of this disease worldwide. The 5-year survival rate for testicular cancer in the United States is a promising 95%. Fortunately, this form of cancer is highly responsive to treatment, even if it has spread to other areas of the body, with a success rate of 95%. Early detection can increase the chances of a full recovery to 98%. Sadly, the incidence of testicular cancer has been rising in recent decades, with a doubling in cases over the past 40 years.

Testicular cancer is more frequently observed in White males, with an incidence rate of 7.1 per 100,000 persons, as compared to 5.4 in Hispanic males and 1.7 in African American males. About 90% of all testicular tumors present as an asymptomatic testicular mass. Before undergoing therapy, a significant number of patients suffer from oligospermia or sperm abnormalities. During chemotherapy that involves platinum-based agents, nearly all patients become oligospermic. However, many of them can regain their sperm production and father children without having to use cryopreserved semen. Early detection through regular physical examination and self-examination is the most crucial prognostic factor. It is important to educate all males on how to perform testicular self-examinations, which will be further discussed later in this chapter.

Renal cancer is a prevalent disease in the United States, with about 63,000 new cases and almost 14,000 deaths annually. Renal cell carcinoma (RCC), also known as renal cell cancer or renal cell adenocarcinoma, is the most frequent form of kidney cancer, accounting for approximately 90% of all cases.[4]

[b]During a TURP procedure, a resectoscope, a slender metal tube equipped with a light, camera, and wire loop, is used to remove sections of the prostate that are causing the prostate symptoms. The resectoscope is inserted through the penile, or anterior, urethra; there is no need for skin incisions. The wire loop is heated to burn away the affected prostate tissue. To clear away the removed tissue, a catheter is placed in the urethra to irrigate the bladder with fluid.

[c]TURP is generally considered a safe procedure with a very low risk of serious complications. However, many patients who undergo a TURP procedure may experience *retrograde ejaculation*, which is the loss of ability to ejaculate semen during sexual activity or masturbation. Despite this, they can still experience the physical pleasure of an orgasm.

Renal pelvis carcinoma (7%) and Wilms tumor (1%),[d,5] which is a childhood cancer that manifests before the age of 5 years, are other types of renal cancer. About two-thirds of people are diagnosed when the cancer is located only in the kidney. This group boasts a 5-year relative survival rate of 93%. However, if kidney cancer has spread to surrounding tissues or organs and/or the regional lymph nodes, the 5-year relative survival rate drops to 72%. Symptoms of renal cell cancer include blood in the urine and a lump in the abdomen. Tobacco use significantly increases the risk of renal cancer, particularly in heavy smokers, with the greatest risk for cancer of the renal pelvis.

Difficulty achieving or maintaining an erection for satisfactory sexual performance is a prevalent issue known as *erectile dysfunction* (ED) or impotence. According to a study called the Massachusetts Male Aging Study,[e] over half of males between the ages of 40 and 70 have some level of ED. Of those surveyed, 17% reported minimal dysfunction, 25% reported moderate dysfunction, and 10% reported complete dysfunction. The study also found that ED tends to worsen with age. At age 40, only 5% of American males have complete ED, but by age 70, that number rises to 15%. Additionally, two-thirds (67%) of 70-year-old males experience some degree of ED.[6]

As the population ages, healthcare professionals will likely treat more male patients for ED, affecting up to 30 million individuals. Research has demonstrated that ED not only impacts a male's physical and sexual satisfaction but also his overall quality of life. ED has been linked to issues with self-image and sexual relationships and may even lead to significant psychological harm, especially severe depression.

STRUCTURE AND PHYSIOLOGIC CHARACTERISTICS

Cross-sectional and frontal views of the male genitalia are shown in Fig. 18.1.

The *penis* is composed of three elongated, distensible structures: two paired *corpora cavernosa* and a single *corpus spongiosum.* The urethra runs through the corpus spongiosum. The penis has two surfaces, dorsal and ventral (urethral), and consists of the root, the shaft, and the head. The shaft is composed of erectile tissue that, when engorged with blood, produces a firm erection necessary for sexual intercourse. The corpora cavernosa also contains smooth muscle that contracts rhythmically during ejaculation.

On the dorsal aspect of the penis in the midline runs the dorsal vein, with an artery and a nerve on either side. The distal end of the corpus spongiosum expands to form the head, or *glans penis.* The glans penis covers the end of the corpora cavernosa. The glans has a prominent margin on its dorsal aspect, the *corona.* A slit-like opening on the tip of the glans is the *external meatus* of the urethra.

The skin of the penis is smooth, thin, and hairless. At the distal end of the penis, a free fold of skin called the *prepuce* (foreskin) covers the glans. Secreted mucus and sloughed epithelial cells called *smegma* collect between the prepuce and the glans, providing a lubricant during sexual intercourse. The prepuce can be retracted to expose the glans as far as the corona. During circumcision, the prepuce is removed.

The root of the penis lies deep to the scrotum, in the perineum. At the root, the corpora cavernosa diverge. Each corpus cavernosum is enveloped in a dense, fibroelastic covering called the *tunica albuginea,* and these tunicae fuse to form the median septum of the penis. A cross-section through the penis is shown in Fig. 18.2.

The blood supply to the penis is from the internal pudendal artery, from which the dorsal and deep arteries of the corpora cavernosa are derived. The veins drain into the dorsal vein of the penis. In the flaccid state, the venous channels and arteriovenous anastomoses are widely patent, whereas the arteries are partially constricted.

The process of achieving an erection involves complex hemodynamic and neurophysiologic events. When the penis is flaccid, the smooth muscles of the penile arteries and sinusoid spaces are contracted. However, the erectile state is initiated in the brain and requires the relaxation of the smooth muscles of the penis. Neural signals are sent from the brain center to the corpora cavernosa, where the neurotransmitter nitric oxide is synthesized and released. Nitric oxide is the primary mediator responsible for relaxing the endothelial and cavernous smooth muscle. Nitric oxide activates guanylate cyclase to produce cyclic guanosine monophosphate (GMP), which decreases intracellular calcium levels, allowing smooth muscle relaxation and an increase in arterial inflow and corporal veno-occlusion in the penis. When the blood-filled sinusoidal spaces expand, they press against the veins, which are against the inner layer of the rigid tunica albuginea. This reduces the outflow of blood from the veins. When the penis is erect, the arteriovenous anastomoses are closed, and the arteries are widely opened. Muscular pillars are present in the walls of the arteries, veins, and arteriovenous anastomoses, which aid in occluding the lumina. Phosphodiesterase, predominantly type V in penile tissue, catalyzes the conversion of cyclic GMP to GMP and results in detumescence. There are oral medications, such as sildenafil (Viagra®), that selectively inhibit phosphodiesterase V, allowing the corpus cavernosum smooth muscle to relax and potentiate erections during sexual stimulation. These agents enhance the effect of the nitric oxide–mediated increase in cyclic GMP levels and significantly improve erectile function and sexual function. The anatomy of erection is illustrated in Fig. 18.3.

The *urethra* extends from the internal urinary meatus of the bladder to the external meatus of the penis. The urethra can be divided into three portions: the prostatic (posterior) portion, the membranous portion, and the cavernous (anterior) portion.

[d]Wilms tumor, or nephroblastoma, is the most common pediatric renal or abdominal cancer and the fourth most common pediatric cancer overall. Wilms tumor is typically found in children younger than five years old. Most Wilms tumors are unilateral. This tumor is more common in Africans and African Americans, while it is least common in East Asians.

[e]The Massachusetts Male Aging Study was a community-based, random sample observational survey of noninstitutionalized males 40 to 70 years old conducted from 1987 to 1989 in areas near Boston, Massachusetts.

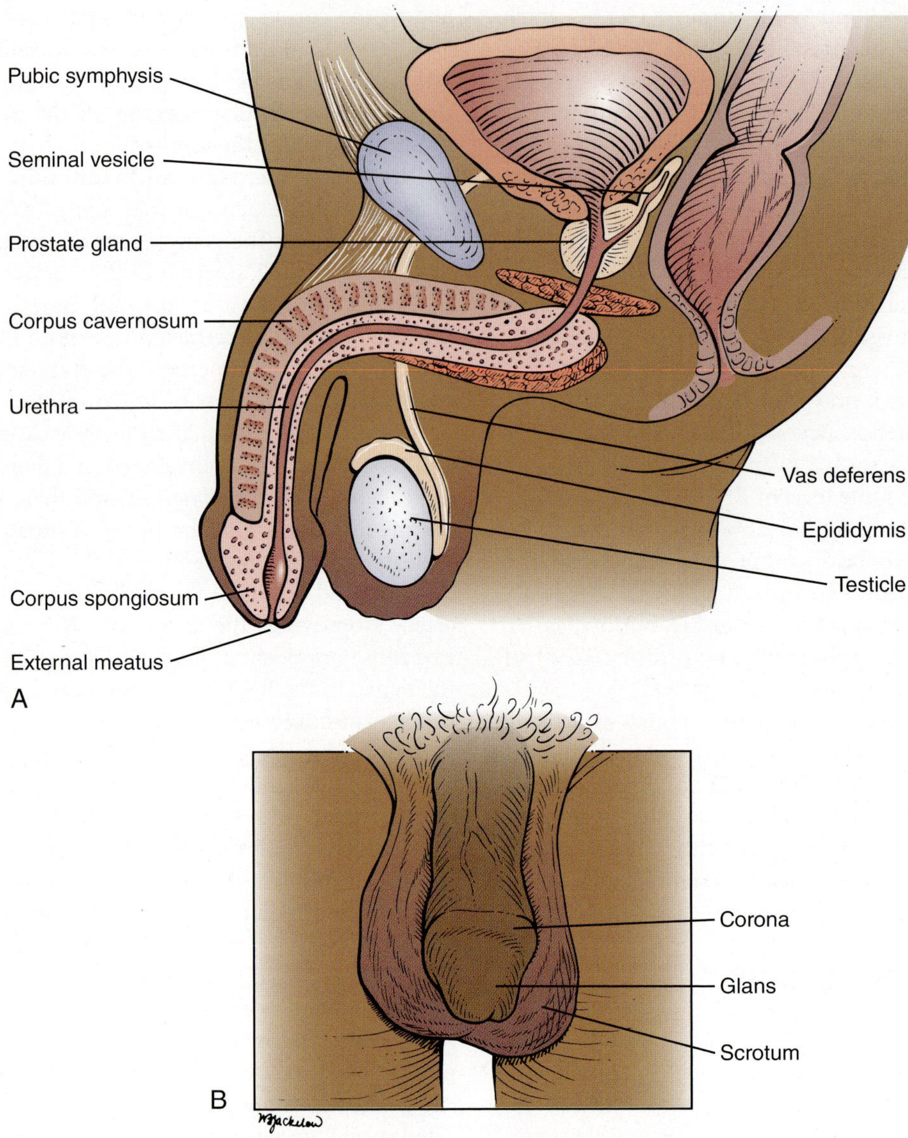

Fig. 18.1 Male Genitalia. (A) Diagram of cross-section. (B) Diagram of frontal view.

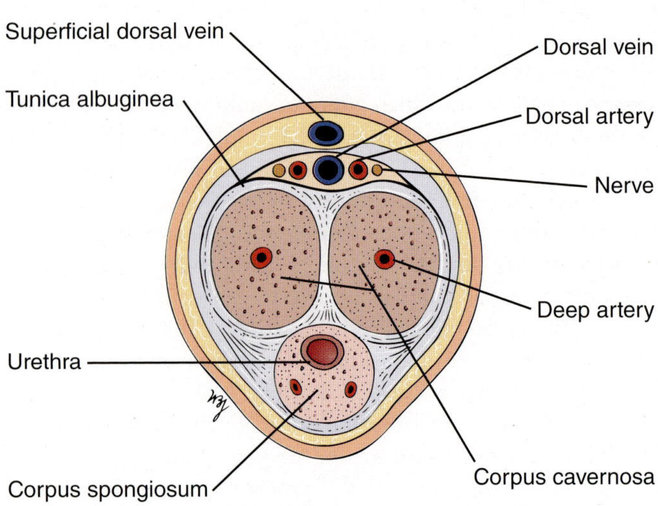

Fig. 18.2 Cross-Sectional View Through the Penis.

The short posterior portion passes through the prostate gland. The common ejaculatory duct and several prostatic ducts enter at the distal end of this portion. The external urethral sphincter surrounds the membranous urethra, and on either side lie Cowper bulbourethral glands. The anterior urethra is the longest portion and passes through the corpus spongiosum. The ducts of Cowper glands enter the anterior urethra near its proximal end.

The *scrotum* is the pouch containing the testes; it is suspended externally from the perineum. The scrotum is divided into halves by the intrascrotal septum, with one testis lying on each side. The wall of the scrotum contains involuntary smooth muscle and voluntary striated muscle. The scrotum plays a crucial role in regulating the temperature of the testes. It ensures that the testes are kept at a temperature that is about 2°C lower than the peritoneal cavity. This is important for spermatogenesis to occur. The size of the scrotum is variable according to the

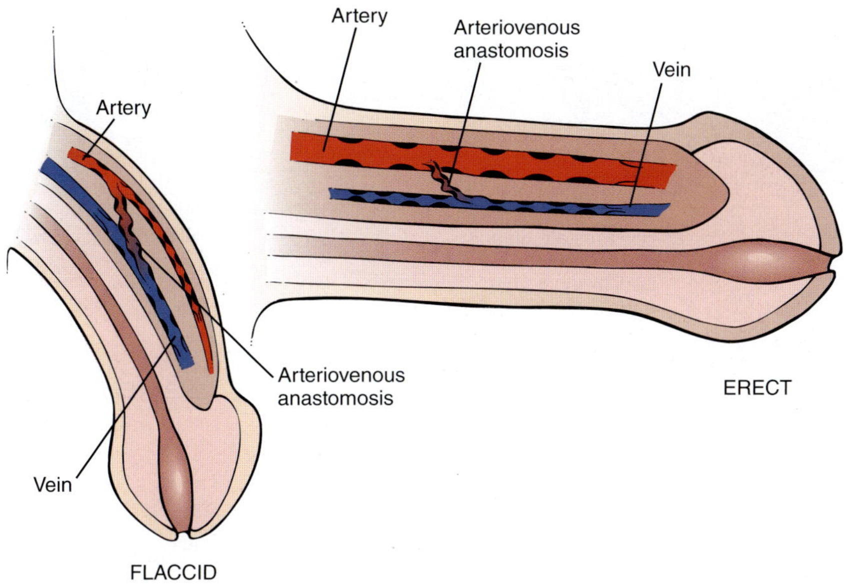

Fig. 18.3 Anatomy of Erection.

individual and his response to ambient temperature. During exposure to cold temperatures, the scrotum is contracted and very rugate. In a warm environment, the scrotum becomes pendulous and smoother.

The *testes,* or *testicles,* are ovoid, smooth, and approximately 1.5 to 2 inches (3.5 to 5 cm) in length. The left testicle commonly lies lower than the right. The testes are covered with a tough fibrous coat called the *tunica albuginea testis.* Each testicle has a long axis directed slightly anteriorly and upward and contains long, microscopic, convoluted seminiferous tubules that produce sperm. The tubules end in the *epididymis,* which is comma-shaped and located on the posterior border of the testis. It consists of a head that is swollen and overhangs the upper pole of the testicle. The inferior portion, or tail, of the epididymis continues into the *vas deferens.* The testicular artery enters the testicle in its posterior midportion. The veins draining the testicle form a dense network called the *pampiniform plexus,* which drains into the testicular vein. The right testicular vein drains directly into the inferior vena cava, whereas the left drains into the left renal vein. The lymphatic drainage of the testes is to the preaortic and precaval nodes, not to the inguinal nodes. This is important to recognize because the testes are embryologically intra-abdominal organs, and neoplasms and inflammations of the testis produce adenopathy of these nodal chains. In general, inguinal adenopathy is rare.

The relationship of the testicle and epididymis is illustrated in Fig. 18.4.

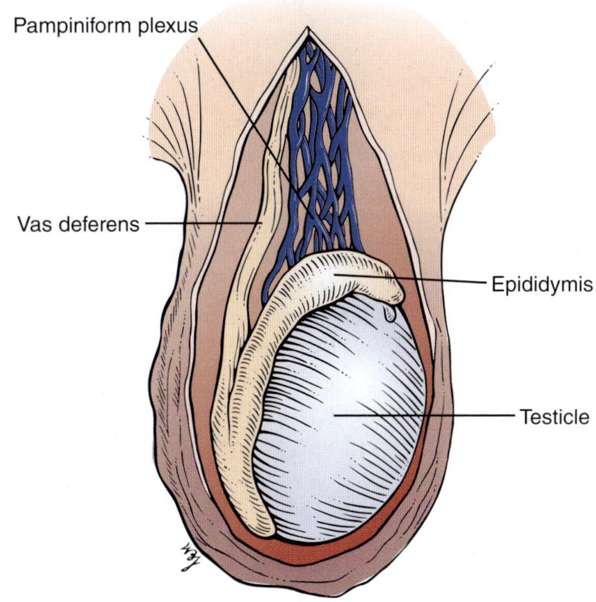

Fig. 18.4 Anatomy of the Testicle and Epididymis.

The vas deferens is a cord-like structure, easily felt in the scrotum. The vas deferens, testicular arteries, and veins form the *spermatic cord,* which enters the inguinal canal. The vas deferens passes through the internal ring and, after a convoluted course, reaches the fundus of the bladder. It passes between the rectum and the bladder and approaches the vas deferens on the opposite side near the seminal vesicles. Near the base of the prostate, the vas deferens joins with the duct of the corresponding seminal vesicle to form the *ejaculatory duct,* which passes through the prostate gland to enter the posterior urethra.

The *prostate gland* is approximately the size of two almonds, or approximately 1.5 inches (3.5 cm) long by 1.2 inches (3 cm) wide. Traversing the gland in the midline is the posterior urethra. On either side is an ejaculatory duct. The prostate gland is composed of five lobes, with the posterior lobe being of clinical importance due to its frequent involvement in prostate cancer. In cancer cases, the groove between the two lateral lobes may be eliminated. Meanwhile, the middle and lateral lobes, located above the ejaculatory ducts, are often affected by benign hypertrophy. The anterior lobe, however, is of limited clinical significance.

The sources and direction of seminal fluid flow in the male genitalia are illustrated in Fig. 18.5.

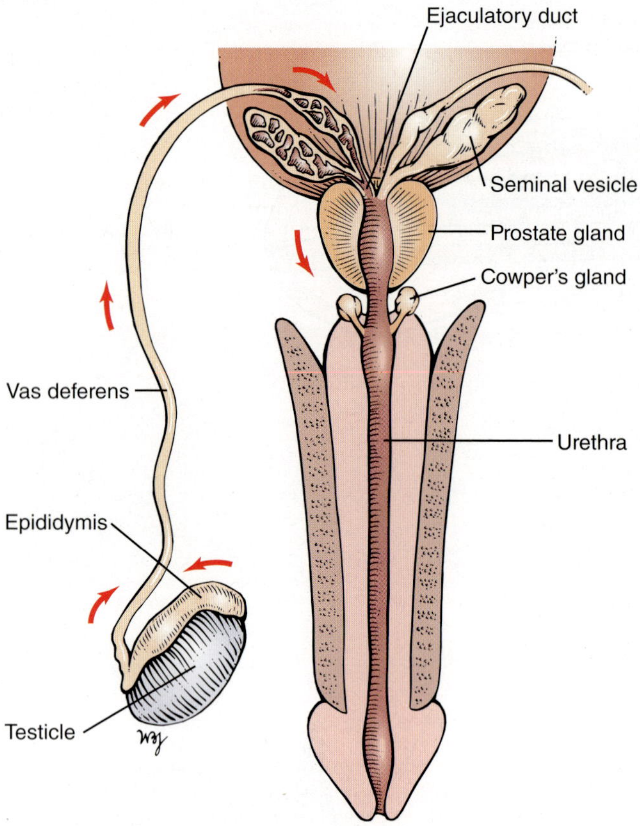

Fig. 18.5 Sources and Direction of Seminal Fluid Flow.

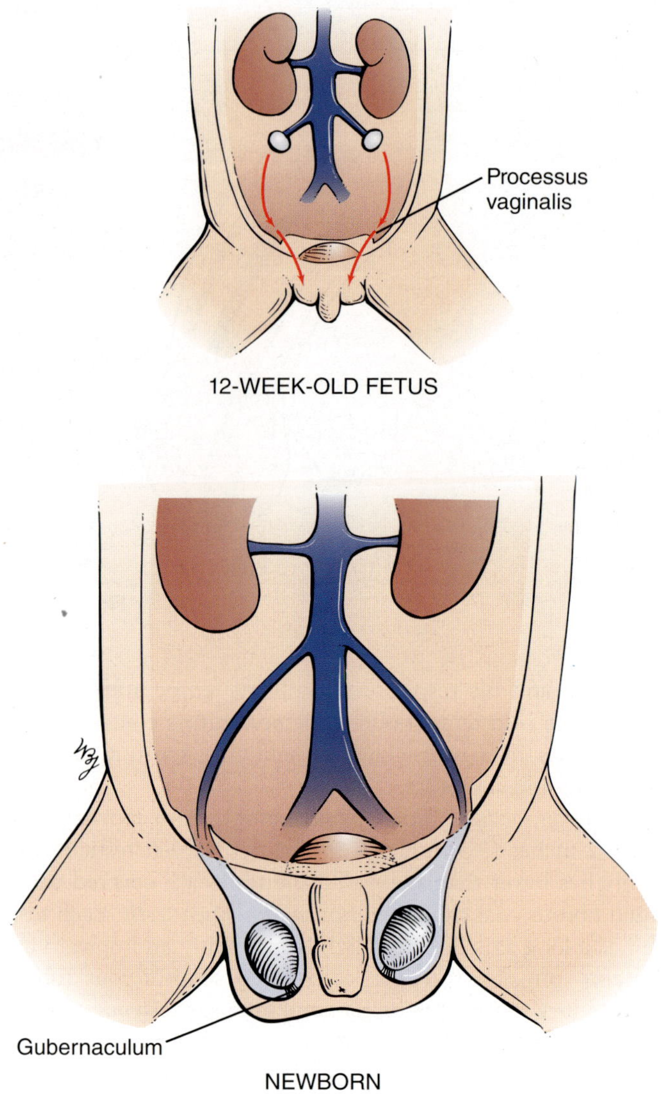

Fig. 18.6 Descent of the Testes.

It is important to review the descent of the testes. At birth, male newborns typically have both testes located in the scrotum. This descent occurs just before birth. During the 12th week of gestation, the gubernaculum begins to develop in the inguinal fold and grows through the body wall to reach the scrotum. This creates a tract that indicates the location of the inguinal canal. Additionally, a dimple called the processus vaginalis forms in the peritoneum and follows the path of the gubernaculum. During the seventh month of gestation, the processus vaginalis reaches the aponeurosis of the external oblique muscle, and the testes start to descend from the abdominal cavity through the internal ring to eventually reside in the abdominal wall. By the eighth month, the testes continue their descent through the inguinal canal, and at the time of birth, they are located in the scrotum. At birth, the gubernaculum is barely distinguishable, and the processus vaginalis becomes obliterated within the spermatic cord. In approximately 3% of full-term male infants, there is an incomplete descent of one or both testicles, also known as *cryptorchidism*.[f,7] An illustration of the descent of the testes is shown in Fig. 18.6.

[f]Cryptorchidism refers to the absence of at least one testicle in the scrotum and is the most commonly occurring birth defect related to male genitalia. It is noteworthy that around 80% of cryptorchid testes descend by the third month of life. In cases where testicles remain undescended, there is a greater likelihood of decreased fertility (in cases of bilateral cryptorchidism), testicular germ cell tumors (although the risk is under 1%), testicular torsion, inguinal hernias, and psychological issues.

The stages of genital development for male children are depicted in Fig. 24.48, which is further discussed in Chapter 24, The Pediatric Patient.

REVIEW OF SPECIFIC SYMPTOMS

The most common symptoms of male genitourinary disease are as follows:

- Pain
- Dysuria
- Changes in urine flow
- Red urine
- Penile discharge
- Penile lesions
- Genital rashes
- Scrotal enlargement
- Groin mass or swelling
- ED
- Infertility

Pain

Flank pain can be caused by a sudden distension of the ureter, renal pelvis, or bladder. It is important to ask the following questions to any patient experiencing flank pain:

"When did the pain begin?"
"Where did the pain begin? Can you point to the area?"
"Do you feel the pain in any other area of your body?"
"Did the pain start suddenly?"
"Have you ever had this type of pain before?"
"Is the pain constant?"
"What seems to make the pain worse? Less?"
"Has the color of your urine changed?"
"Is the pain associated with nausea? Vomiting? Abdominal distention? Fever? Chills? Burning sensation on urination?"

Gradual enlargement of any organ is usually painless. If a patient experiences a sharp pain in the costovertebral angle, it may result from the sudden swelling of the renal capsule caused by acute pyelonephritis or obstructive hydronephrosis. Additionally, spasmodic pain from upper ureteral dilation may result in referred pain in the testis on the same side while lower ureteral dilation may lead to pain in the scrotum. The pain caused by ureteral distention is intense and can cause discomfort regardless of the patient's position, leading to overall discomfort. Bladder distention can lead to feelings of fullness in the lower abdomen and pain in the suprapubic area, along with a strong urge to urinate. There are several potential causes of groin pain, including issues with the spermatic cord, testicles, or prostate gland, as well as lymphadenitis, hernias, herpes zoster, or a neurological disorder.

Testicular pain can result from nearly any disease of the testis or epididymis. Such diseases include epididymitis, orchitis, hydrocele, spermatic cord torsion, and tumor. Referred pain from the ipsilateral ureter must always be considered.

Priapism[8] is an involuntary, prolonged erection unrelated to sexual stimulation and unrelieved by ejaculation. The symptoms of priapism include a painful erection that lasts longer than 4 to 6 hours and is not relieved by orgasm, or a partial erection that lasts longer than several days, even if it is not painful. This condition is a true urologic emergency because the condition can result in impotence, sexual dysfunction, or penile infection.

Priapism is a condition that can affect males of any age, although it is more commonly seen in boys aged 5 to 10 years and males aged 20 to 50 years. The most common cause of priapism in young boys is sickle cell disease, while drug treatment for ED, specifically injection therapy, is a leading cause in adult males. Priapism can also be caused by blood-related diseases that cause sludging of blood in the penile veins, such as leukemia, macroglobulinemia, thalassemia, and multiple myeloma. In about one-third of cases, it is not possible to identify a specific cause.

A prolonged erection occurs when the veins in the corpora cavernosa become thrombosed. In individuals with sickle cell disease, sickled red blood cells can obstruct the blood vessels in the penis, leading to priapism in 35% of males. Additionally, certain psychotropic drugs like trazodone (Desyrel®) or chlorpromazine (Thorazine®) may also cause priapism.

Dysuria

Experiencing pain while urinating, known as *dysuria*, is often described as a "burning" sensation. Dysuria is a sign of inflammation in the lower urinary tract, which can cause discomfort in the penis or suprapubic area. It can also make urination difficult due to external meatal stenosis[g] or urethral stricture. Painful urination is typically accompanied by increased frequency and urgency to urinate. If the patient reports pain or difficulty during urination, inquire about the following:

"How long have you noticed a burning sensation on urination?"
"How often do you urinate each day?"
"How does your urination feel different?"
"Is your urine clear?"
"Does the urine smell bad?"
"Do you have a discharge from your penis?"
"Does the urine seem to have gas bubbles in it?"
"Have you noticed any solid particles in your urine?"
"Have you noticed pus in your urine?"
"Have you ever had urethral instrumentation, which is a catheter placed into your bladder through your penis?" If so, *"For how long?"*

Pneumaturia[9] is a condition in which there is air in the urine, causing the patient to notice "gas bubbles" in their urine. "*Bubbles in the pee*" may be the way to describe or characterize this condition. Generally, there should not be any gas present in the urinary tract. This symptom may indicate the introduction of air due to urinary tract instrumentation, fistula formation from the bowel (containing air) to the urinary system[h] (as often seen in cases of Crohn disease or diverticulitis), or a urinary tract infection caused by gas-producing bacteria like *Escherichia coli*, *Klebsiella pneumoniae*, or *Clostridia*.

Fecaluria is the presence of fecal material in the urine and is rare. The passage of feculent-smelling material results from either a verico-colic fistula or a urethrorectal fistula. Crohn disease is the most common cause of an ileovesical fistula. The diagnostic features of a fistula to the urinary system are pneumaturia, fecaluria, and recurrent or persistent urinary tract infections.

These fistulas result from ulceration from the bowel to the urinary tract. Diverticulitis and carcinoma are also frequent causes.

Enterovesical fistulae (EVF) are uncommon, accounting for about 1 out of every 3000 surgical admissions, according to a 2021 study.[10] The peak incidence is between the ages of 51 and 60, and according to a 2021 review,[11] males seem to be more affected than females by about 2:1 to 3:1. According to the study, the leading cause of EVF is diverticulitis, responsible for 60% to 70% of cases. The second most common causes are

---

[g]Meatal stenosis refers to the abnormal narrowing of the urethral opening, specifically the meatus located at the head of the penis. This condition can be present at birth or acquired later in life. When the narrowing becomes significant, it can impede the flow of urine from the bladder, leading to incomplete emptying of the bladder. If left untreated, this can increase the risk of urinary tract infections and subsequent kidney problems.

[h]Known as a vesico-colic fistula.

various types of cancer (including colorectal, bladder, and prostate) and Crohn disease. The same review cites Crohn disease as the cause of 27.5% of EVF cases, while cancers are responsible for 6.5% of cases.

Pyuria, also known as pus in the urine, is the body's response to inflammation of the urinary tract. The primary cause of inflammation leading to pyuria is typically bacteria; however, it can also be present in patients with neoplasms and kidney stones. Bowel bacteria are the most common cause of urinary tract infections, which typically occur in females due to their shorter and closer urethra proximity to the anus. Males have longer urethras, making it more difficult for bacteria to reach the bladder. Although males are less prone to urinary tract infections, it is crucial to take them seriously when they do occur. Infections in males can be caused by various factors, such as prostatitis, an enlarged prostate that causes incomplete bladder emptying, or bladder and kidney stones.

Changes in Urine Flow

Patients often encounter variations in their urine flow, including changes in frequency and incontinence.[i] Urinary frequency, which is passing urine more than usual, is the most common symptom of the genitourologic system. Nocturia is the term used to describe urinary frequency at night. There are various reasons why individuals experience frequency, such as bladder wall irritation, decreased bladder size, and increased urine volume. When the bladder is obstructed and cannot be emptied fully, it decreases its effective capacity. To define the problem, it's important to ask the following questions in addition to those related to dysuria.

"Do you find that you must wake up at night to urinate?"
"Can you estimate the amount of urine passed each time you urinate?"
"Do you have sudden urges to urinate?"
"Have you found that despite an urge to urinate, you cannot start the stream?"
"Has there been a change in the caliber of the stream?"
"Have you found that you must wait longer for the stream to start?"
"Do you have the sensation that after urination has stopped, you still have to urinate?"
"Do you have to strain at the end of urination?"
"Have you been drinking more fluids recently?"
"Do your drink coffee or tea before bedtime?"
"Do you involuntarily lose small amounts of urine?"
"Do you lose your urine constantly?"
"Do you lose your urine when lifting heavy objects? Laughing? Coughing? Bending over?"
"Do you have to press on your abdomen to urinate?"

Urinary incontinence is more than just a medical issue; it can have a significant impact on one's emotional, psychological, and social well-being. Those who experience urinary incontinence may feel anxious about engaging in regular daily activities and avoid venturing too far from a restroom. This condition can prevent individuals from fully enjoying life.

Prostatic hyperplasia is the most common cause of reduced usable bladder capacity in males. Symptoms include frequency of urination, nocturia, urgency, weak stream, intermittent stream, and a sensation of incomplete emptying. Long-standing prostatic hypertrophy can lead to an inability to urinate (a condition known as *urinary retention*[j])—necessitating urethral catheterization—or to urinary tract infections or bladder stones. Most bladder diseases, such as cystitis, cause frequency as a result of irritation of the bladder mucosa. *Polyuria,* or voiding large amounts of urine, is usually accompanied by excessive thirst, or *polydipsia.* Diabetes mellitus and diabetes insipidus are common causes of polydipsia.

Individuals with chronically distended bladders, such as those with prostatic hypertrophy, often retain a significant amount of urine. This causes the pressure within the bladder to remain elevated. Even a small increase in intra-abdominal pressure, such as when coughing, sneezing, laughing, or lifting heavy objects, can be enough to overcome the bladder neck resistance and result in urine leakage. Leakage may be steady or intermittent. This type of incontinence is *overflow* incontinence. *Stress* incontinence is leakage that occurs only when the patient strains. The primary defect is a loss of muscular support in the urethrovesicular region. Residual urine is insignificant. Any increase in intra-abdominal pressure causes leakage. This type of incontinence is more common in females and is discussed in Chapter 19, Female Genitalia.

Polyuria is the frequent or multiple episodes of urination in a 24-hour cycle, with a considerable amount of urine excreted each time. An individual with polyuria may excrete more than 3 L of urine daily. Typically, a person produces 1 to 2 L of urine daily. It is crucial to distinguish between diabetes mellitus, diabetes insipidus, and psychological diabetes insipidus. To help identify the condition, ask the following questions:

"How long have you been passing large amounts of urine?"
"Was the onset sudden?"
"How often do you have to urinate at night?"
"Is there any variability in the urine flow from day to day?"
"Do you have excessive thirst?"
"Do you prefer water or other fluids?"
"What happens if you don't drink? Will you still have to urinate?"
"How is your appetite?"
"Do you have any visual problems? Headaches?"
"Are you aware of any emotional problems?"

Patients with diabetes mellitus have a high osmotic load and, consequently, have polyuria. Increased appetite is also common. Diabetes insipidus is caused by a vasopressin deficiency related to a lesion in the hypothalamus or pituitary gland.

[i] *Urinary incontinence*, which is losing control of one's bladder, is a widespread issue that can be quite embarrassing. The severity of the problem ranges from occasional leakage when coughing or sneezing to a sudden and intense urge to urinate that may make it difficult to reach a toilet in time.

[j] Urinary retention is the condition where a person is unable to urinate voluntarily. Acute urinary retention is a sudden and often painful inability to urinate, even when the bladder is full. The primary reason for this condition is obstructive, with BPH accounting for 53% of cases. Other factors such as infection, inflammation, iatrogenic, and neurological reasons can also lead to urinary retention.

In these patients, the urine cannot become concentrated despite a rise in plasma osmolality. Patients with psychogenic diabetes insipidus, which is more common, have polyuria related to compulsive drinking of water. It is seen in patients with psychological problems. The onset of polyuria is abrupt in patients with psychogenic diabetes insipidus, and they have no preference for the type of fluid they drink. In contrast, patients with true diabetes insipidus prefer water. Since true diabetes insipidus is connected to intracranial lesions, it's common for those affected to experience headaches and visual disturbances, specifically issues with their visual field.

Red Urine

Red urine is usually a sign of *hematuria*, which means there is blood in the urine. Nevertheless, red urine can be caused by various factors, so it is not always an indication of bleeding. There are various reasons why urine can appear red, including the use of vegetable dyes, certain drugs like phenazopyridine (marketed as Pyridium®), or consuming excessive amounts of beets. However, if the red color is caused by the presence of blood, it is known as gross hematuria. This could be an indication of a serious urinary tract disease and should not be ignored. It is important to ask patients experiencing red urine the following questions:

"How long have you noticed red urine?"
"Have you had red urine previously?"
"Have you noticed that the urine starts red and then clears? Starts clear and then turns red? Is it red throughout?"
"Have you noticed clots of blood in the urine?"
"Have you done any severely strenuous physical activity recently, such as prolonged hiking, running, or marching?"
"Did you have an upper respiratory infection or a sore throat a few weeks ago?"
"Is the red urine associated with flank pain? Abdominal pain? Burning sensation on urination? Fever? Weight loss?"
"Are you aware of any bleeding problems?"
"Are you taking any medications?"
"Do you eat beets often?" If so, *"How much?"*

Individuals who participate in strenuous activities may traumatize blood cells as these cells travel through the small vessels in the feet. A condition called *march hemoglobinuria* may result, causing intravascular hemolysis and hemoglobinuria. The temporal relationship of blood in the urine is an important factor. Blood only at the beginning, or *initial* hematuria, usually has a source in the urethra. Blood only at the end of urination, or *terminal* hematuria, indicates a disorder at the bladder neck or the posterior urethra. Blood evenly distributed throughout urination is *total* hematuria and implies disease above the prostate gland (e.g., the kidney) or a massive hemorrhage at any level. Blood staining of undergarments without blood in the urine indicates pathologic processes in the external urethral meatus. Weight loss and hematuria are seen in RCC. Red urine that occurs 10 to 14 days after an upper respiratory infection may indicate acute glomerulonephritis.

Penile Discharge

Discharge from the penis is a continuous or intermittent flow of fluid from the urethra. Ask the patient whether he has ever had a discharge and, if he has, whether it was bloody or purulent. Bloody penile discharges are associated with ulcerations, neoplasms, or urethritis. Purulent discharges are thick and yellowish-green and may be associated with gonococcal urethritis or chronic prostatitis. Determine when the discharge was first noted. Fig. 18.7 shows a patient with a purulent penile discharge secondary to gonococcal urethritis. *Neisseria gonorrhoeae* causes gonorrhea. After exposure, approximately 25% of males and more than 50% of females contract the disease. In males, the acute symptoms of dysuria and a purulent urethral discharge begin 2 to 10 days after exposure. In female patients, a vaginal discharge and dysuria develop days to weeks after exposure; however, in up to 50% of females, the infection may be asymptomatic.

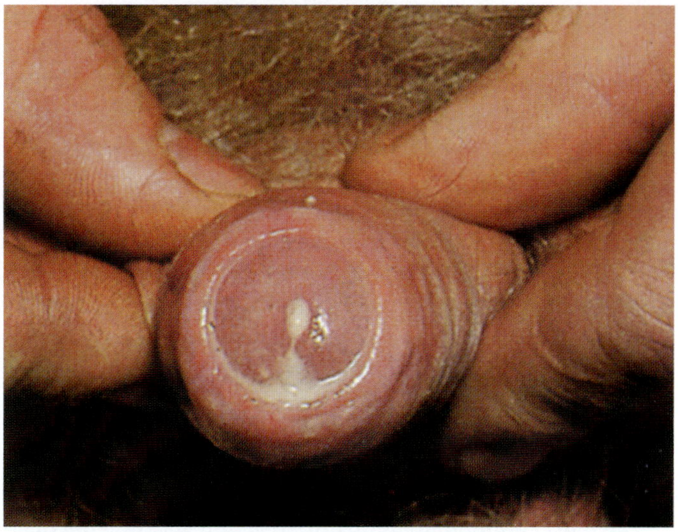

Fig. 18.7 Purulent Penile Discharge of Gonorrhea. (From Korting GW: *Practical dermatology of the genital region*, Philadelphia, 1980, WB Saunders.)

Tactful direct questioning about any history of or exposure to sexually transmitted diseases is essential. The interviewer should determine the patient's sexual orientation (see Chapter 5, Anti-Racist and Anti-Oppressive Clinical Skills) and the type of sexual exposure—oral, vaginal, or anal—because this information can help determine the types of bacteriologic cultures necessary. Asking direct questions about specific sexual practices (e.g., "Do you have anal intercourse?") is preferable to asking a more open-ended question (e.g., "In what type of sexual practices do you partake?"). It is appropriate to ask whether the patient has more than one sexual partner and whether the partner(s) have any known illnesses. **Make no assumption about the gender of the partner(s).** The interview questions regarding sexual history provided in Chapter 1, The Interviewer's Questions, and in Chapter 5, Anti-Racist and Anti-Oppressive Clinical Skills, should be reviewed.

Penile Lesions

If a person has a history of lesions on his penis, it may indicate the possibility of venereal disease. There are many possible causes for a genital rash, ranging from sexually transmitted infections,[k] allergies or autoimmune disorders,[l] fungal infections,[m] viral infections,[n] infecting parasites,[o] and balanitis.[p] To properly assess the genital rash, it's vital to gather a comprehensive medical history, focusing on recent sexual encounters, recent travels, hygiene routines, and whether the lesion is itchy or painful. Additionally, ask if the patient has had any sexually transmitted diseases in the past, such as gonorrhea, syphilis, herpes, trichomoniasis, or venereal warts.

Genital Rashes

Male genital rashes are very common. They may be confusing to identify and are often difficult to treat. Some rashes may occur exclusively on the genitalia; others, which are typically found on other parts of the body, have an atypical appearance when present on the genitalia. The skin over the genitalia is thin and moist, so typical dry scaliness may not be present.

The most common inflammatory reaction affecting the male genitalia is *psoriasis* (Fig. 8.57C). The patient develops bright red, well-defined, scaling plaques. Often the entire scrotum, inguinal folds, and penis are involved. The penis is a common location for psoriasis and, in some cases, is the sole area of involvement. Psoriatic lesions on the penis are typically red, scaly papules or raised plaques on the glans and shaft, with the exception of uncircumcised males who often experience no scaliness when lesions are located on the glans. Psoriatic patches on other body parts usually facilitate the diagnosis. Supportive findings include red scaly plaques on the elbows, knees (see Fig. 8.53), gluteal cleft (see Fig. 8.54), scalp (see Fig. 8.56), and periumbilicus, as well as pitting of the nail plates (see Fig. 8.14). Fig. 18.8 shows another patient with psoriasis of the penis.

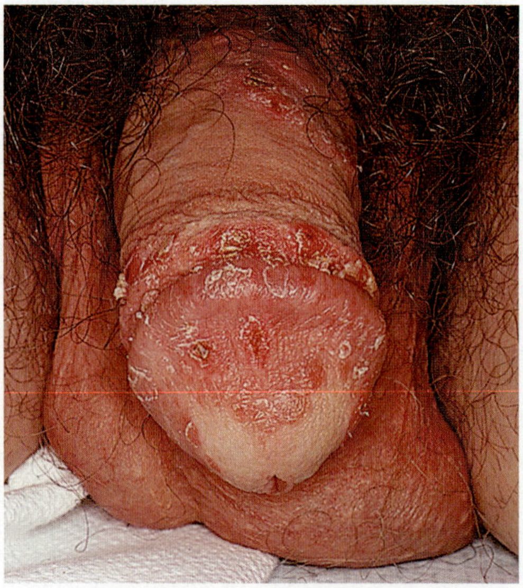

Fig. 18.8 Psoriasis. (From Callen JP, Paller AS, Greer KE, et al: *Color atlas of dermatology*, ed 2, Philadelphia, 2000, WB Saunders.)

Another form of genital rash is *contact dermatitis*. It may develop from soaps or disinfectants. Irritants used for facial actinic keratosis may inadvertently be transferred to the genitalia. Itching is a major symptom.

Fixed drug eruptions are unique reactions that occur in a specific part of the body every time a particular drug is given. These reactions present as multiple, well-defined, macular, eczematous, bullous patches that appear suddenly. When they occur on the genitalia, they can be very painful and usually appear on the distal penis and glans. The drugs responsible for these eruptions include nonsteroidal anti-inflammatory drugs, sulfonamides (especially co-trimoxazole), and laxatives containing phenolphthalein, tetracycline, and barbiturates. Fig. 18.9 displays an example of a fixed drug reaction on the penis that occurred after taking tetracycline. Over 500 medications have been associated with fixed drug reactions, so it is important for the examiner to obtain a detailed medication history.

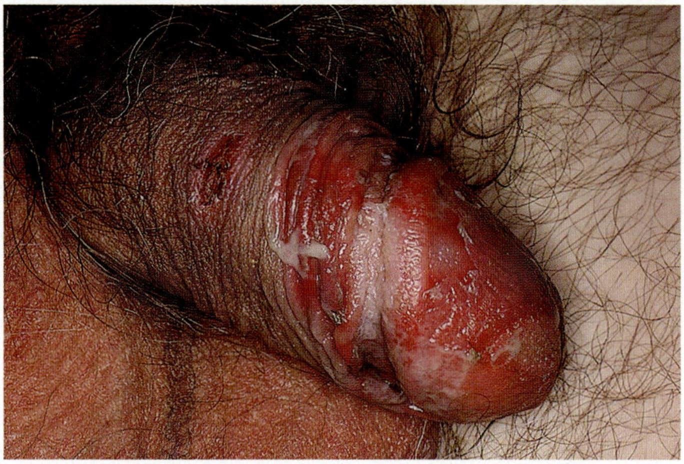

Fig. 18.9 Fixed Drug Reaction. (From Callen JP, Paller AS, Greer KE, et al: *Color atlas of dermatology*, ed 2, Philadelphia, 2000, WB Saunders.)

Lichen planus[12] is an inflammatory, common disorder of no known cause characterized on the skin by violaceous, flat, shiny papules ranging from 0.75 to 3 inches (2 to 8 mm) in diameter that are faintly erythematous to violet in color (Figs. 8.111A and B). Lichen planus inside the mouth appears as lacy patches of tiny white dots. These patches may occur on the inside of the cheeks or on the tongue (Fig. 12.15). Lichen planus of the genitals can cause bright red, painful areas (Fig. 18.10). The glans penis is frequently involved.

Scrotal Enlargement

It is not uncommon for a male to complain of enlargement of his scrotum, but it is often difficult for him to determine which

[k]Such as genital herpes (Figs. 18.34 and 18.35), genital warts (Fig. 18.40), and syphilis.

[l]Such as contact dermatitis, lichen planus (Fig. 8.111), and psoriasis (Fig. 8.57 and Fig. 18.8). A lubricant, cream, or lotion used for masturbation or sex can irritate the penile skin, causing a rash.

[m]Such as tinea cruris (i.e., jock itch, Fig. 8.62), tinea corporis (i.e., ringworm), and yeast infections caused by *Candida albicans*.

[n]Such as molluscum contagiosum (Figs. 18.36 and 18.37).

[o]Such as scabies (Fig, 18.16) and body lice.

[p]An inflammation of the foreskin or the head of the penis that's usually caused by bacterial or fungal growth and is more likely to occur in males who are uncircumcised. It leads to itchiness, redness, and a discharge (Fig. 18.17).

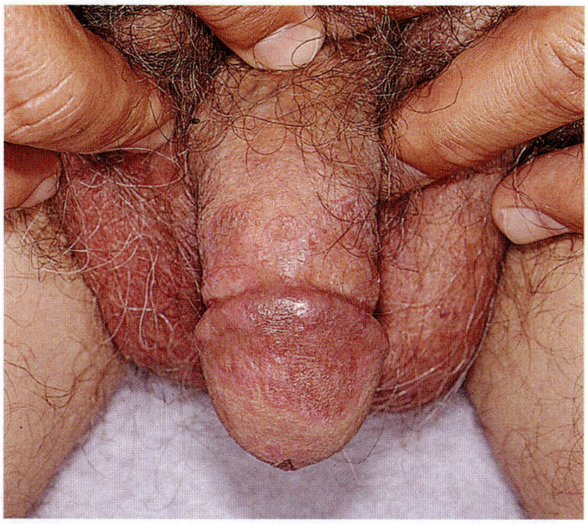

Fig. 18.10 Lichen Planus. (From Callen JP, Paller AS, Greer KE, et al: *Color atlas of dermatology*, ed 2, Philadelphia, 2000, WB Saunders.)

anatomic structures in the scrotum are enlarged. Ask these questions:

"When did you first notice the enlargement?"
"Is the enlargement painful?"
"Have you sustained any injury to your groin?"
"Does the enlargement change in size?"
"Have you ever had the enlargement before?"
"Have you ever had a hernia?"
"Have you had any problems with fertility?"

Scrotum swellings may be caused by enlargement of the testicles or epididymis, a hernia, varicocele,[13] spermatocele, or hydrocele.[14] Testicular enlargement can occur due to inflammation or a tumor, and it is usually one-sided. Painful swelling in the scrotum may be the result of acute inflammation in the epididymis or testis, torsion of the spermatic cord, or a strangulated hernia.

A *varicocele* is an abnormal dilation and enlargement of the scrotal venous pampiniform plexus which drains blood from each testicle. While usually painless, varicoceles are clinically significant because they are the most commonly identified cause of abnormal semen analysis, low sperm count, decreased sperm motility, and abnormal sperm morphology, thus contributing to male infertility.

Spermatoceles, also referred to as spermatic cysts, are noncancerous masses that are filled with fluid and grow near the testicles. They are typically painless and located near the upper and back part of the testicle but are not connected to it. The cysts can have a smooth texture and contain a cloudy, whitish fluid, often consisting of sperm.

A *hydrocele* is a buildup of fluid between the layers of tissue surrounding the testis and spermatic cord. This can happen when there is an imbalance between the amount of fluid produced and the amount that is resorbed. Normally, the testes move from the abdomen to the scrotum between 28 and 40 weeks of gestation with the process completed by the 33rd week. The process involves a fold of tissue called the processus vaginalis. If this fold doesn't close properly, it can create a pathway for fluid to accumulate resulting in a congenital hydrocele.

Groin Mass or Swelling

If a patient describes a mass in the groin, ask the following questions:

"When did you first notice the mass?"
"Is the mass painful?"
"Does the mass change in size with different positions?"
"Have you had any venereal diseases?"

The primary reason for swelling in the groin is often due to a hernia, which tends to decrease in size when the patient is lying down. Additionally, adenopathy caused by infections of the external genitalia can also result in inguinal swelling. However, enlargement of inguinal nodes occurs only if the scrotal skin is affected. It's important to note that when there is pathology in the testicles, it affects the paraaortic nodes rather than the inguinal nodes. This is because the testes initially develop in the retroperitoneum near the paraaortic nodes.

Erectile Dysfunction

Difficulty achieving or maintaining an erection during sexual activity is known as *erectile dysfunction* or impotence. A penile erection requires proper neurovascular function, but several neurologic and vascular conditions can contribute to ED. For instance, ED may be caused by vascular diseases such as atherosclerotic stenosis or occlusion of the cavernosal arteries, or vascular problems linked to smoking. Certain medications like antihypertensives, antidepressants, antiandrogens, histamine H2-receptor antagonists, tranquilizers, appetite suppressants, anti-seizure medications, and recreational drugs are also known to cause ED. Additionally, conditions such as type II diabetes, hypertension, hyperlipidemia, chronic kidney disease, multiple sclerosis, injury from prostate surgery, use of antiarrhythmics, muscle relaxants, and excessive alcohol consumption may increase the risk of ED.

A delicate approach must be taken. It is necessary to use tact and appropriate language that the patient will understand. Explaining that ED is a common problem often sets the tone. Deep-seated problems necessitate careful questioning. The interviewer may discover latent sexual identity problems; guilt and taboos experienced early in life may have left a lasting impression, affecting sexual performance. It is most important to classify the origin of the ED, because there are specific therapies for different causes.

Start by asking some of the following questions:

"If you were to spend the rest of your life with your sexual function just the way it is now, how would you feel about that?"
"Are you satisfied with your sexual function?" If not, *"What are the reasons?"*
"What is your relationship status?"
"Is your partner satisfied with your sexual function?" If not, *"What are the reasons?"*
"When was the last time you had a satisfactory erection?"
"Over the last 4 weeks, how would you rate your confidence that you could get and keep an erection?"
"When you had erections with sexual stimulation, how often were your erections hard enough for penetration (entering your partner)?"
"During sexual intercourse, how often were you able to maintain your erection after you had penetrated (entered) your partner?"

"During sexual intercourse, how difficult was it to maintain your erection to completion of intercourse?"

A careful history is the most essential component in the evaluation of ED. Key and direct questions are important:

"How much do or did you enjoy sexual intercourse?"

"When you have sexual stimulation or intercourse, how often do you ejaculate?"

"How easily can you reach an orgasm (climax)?"

"How strong is your sex drive?"

"How easily are you sexually aroused?"

"Are your orgasms satisfying?"

To determine the cause of ED, consider asking additional questions. If a male has a history of unusual anxiety, stress, sexual abuse, or ethnic, cultural, sexual, or religious inhibitions, psychogenic causes for ED should be suspected. Males younger than 40 years of age often experience psychogenic ED. To gather more information, ask the following questions:

"Do you have early morning erections or nighttime emissions?"

"Do any individuals other than your partner arouse you?"

"Are you able to masturbate to an erection or climax?"

If any of these questions receive a positive response, it is likely that the cause of the ED is psychological in nature. Allowing the patient to share their issues can give them a chance to express their concerns and alleviate some anxiety. However, it is crucial to ensure confidentiality to gain the patient's trust first.

During the interview related to your discussion about sexual behavior, it's important for the interviewer to address and overcome any personal sexual anxieties to conduct a clear and confident discussion. Creating an open dialogue about these anxieties can be helpful. It's crucial also for the interviewer to avoid imposing their own moral beliefs on the patient.

Infertility

Infertility is a prevalent problem, affecting about 15% of all couples in the United States and at least 180 million worldwide.[15] It is estimated that 1 in 6 couples who are trying to conceive struggle with this issue. In about 30% to 40% of all cases, male infertility plays a significant role. This implies that approximately 10% of all males in the United States who are attempting to conceive experience infertility.

Male infertility may result from low sperm production, abnormal sperm function, or blockages that impede sperm delivery. Various factors such as illnesses, injuries, chronic health issues, lifestyle choices, and others could contribute to male infertility.

Infertility refers to the inability to conceive or cause pregnancy. A couple is deemed infertile when pregnancy fails to occur after a year of regular intercourse without the use of contraceptives. Male patients with a history of infertility should be asked about mumps, testicular injuries, venereal disease, diabetes, varicoceles (see Fig. 18.27), radiation exposure, or urologic surgery. Diabetic males or those who have undergone TURP may experience infertility due to retrograde ejaculation, which is ejaculation into the urinary bladder. Sexual intercourse frequency and any difficulties in achieving or maintaining an erection should be determined. Patients' general work habits, medication use, alcohol consumption, and sleeping habits should be documented.

IMPACT OF ERECTILE DYSFUNCTION ON THE MALE

Difficulty achieving or maintaining an erection sufficient for sexual intercourse is known as ED. It can be either erectile or ejaculatory and may be partial or complete. Males may experience difficulty achieving or maintaining an erection or premature ejaculation. The incidence of ED ranges from 20% to 30%. Libido and potency naturally decline with age, but this generally does not occur before the age of 50. However, some males remain sexually active well into old age. If a male patient with ED occasionally has erections or can achieve orgasm during masturbation, it may be primarily an emotional issue. In nearly 90% of male patients complaining of ED, the cause is found to be emotional rather than anatomical factors.

Learning about a friend's sexual experiences, particularly if they are exaggerated, can lower a person's confidence, and make them feel inadequate. The cultural norms of the individual play a significant role in determining what is considered adequate. It is difficult to compare Western and Eastern cultural practices.

In 1948, Alfred Kinsey and his team collected accurate information on Anglo-American sexual behaviors.[q] The frequency of sexual activity ranged from one to four times per week. The period of maximum sexual activity was from 20 to 30 years of age. It was shown that there were marked variations among individuals as well as among socioeconomic groups. Kinsey stated that the lower the socioeconomic group, the more frequent the sexual encounters.

Boredom, anxiety, peer pressure, aging, deterioration of the stereotypical male role, and female "aggressiveness" are factors contributing to psychogenic ED. Guilt, anxiety, and hypochondriasis are common in males with psychogenic ED. Sexual indifference in a female may make the male feel more insecure in their own marital adjustment, worsening his ED. The male's self-image may be poor. It is common for a male with marginal difficulties to worry incessantly about their next attempt at coitus. Their fear of failure generates enormous anxiety, which reinforces their inadequacy, and a vicious circle begins. Each

[q]In 1948 and 1953, Kinsey published two reports titled *Sexual Behavior in the Human Male* and *Sexual Behavior in the Human Female*, respectively. According to Kinsey's data, Americans were participating in sexual activities more frequently and with greater variety than previously thought. These reports caused a stir of controversy during the 1940s and 1950s, and even today, more than 75 years after the first report was released, Kinsey's findings and methods are still hotly debated and remain controversial worldwide. Some individuals praised Kinsey, an American biologist, for transforming sexual norms, by encouraging open discussions about sex and challenging traditional beliefs about human desires and abilities; other individuals considered Kinsey an attention-seeker whose sole objective was to normalize and legitimize many sexual gratification practices.

failure worsens the next attempt. If the act of coitus is not satisfactory to the patient or their partner, embarrassment and guilt develop.

Some males may be able to maintain erections but have difficulty in ejaculation. They may become physically exhausted and have to stop intercourse before ejaculating. The ejaculatory ducts may become so inflamed or even ulcerated that if ejaculation does occur, blood is present in the semen. This produces further anxiety and emotional upset that aggravate the situation.

ED can have significant consequences regardless of its cause. Males may experience feelings of emasculation and develop an inferiority complex. It is common for them to also experience anger and depression. When a patient's ED is linked to an anatomic defect, it can lead to further impact on their self-image due to the physical illness. If sexual issues go unresolved, it could result in personality changes in the patient. The fear of losing a sexual partner can have a negative impact on one's work and ability to get proper sleep and rest. If sexual issues persist, it can lead to neurotic complaints. Without proper guidance, patients may experience complete ED and even develop suicidal tendencies.

Severe psychiatric disorders require treatment from a trained psychiatrist or sexual therapist. The success of the treatment largely depends on the healthcare professional and the patient's sexual partner being able to inspire confidence in the patient.

PHYSICAL EXAMINATION

The only equipment necessary for the examination of the male genitalia is disposable latex gloves.

Many students are concerned about the possibility that a patient will have an erection during the examination. Although this is possible, it is rare for a male to become sexually excited because the patient is usually somewhat uncomfortable under these circumstances. If the examination is performed in an objective manner, it should not be a source of stimulation to the patient. If the patient does develop an erection, do not proceed with the examination.

The examination of the male genitalia is conducted in two different positions, first lying down and then standing up. This is because certain conditions such as hernias or scrotal masses may not be visible when the patient is lying down. Therefore, postural changes are crucial for a comprehensive examination.

The examination of the male genitalia consists of the following:

- Inspection and palpation with the patient lying down
- Inspection and palpation with the patient standing
- Hernia examination

Inspection and Palpation With the Patient Lying Down

See Video 18.1.

Inspect the Skin and Hair

When the patient is in a supine position, it is important to examine the skin in the groin area for any signs of superficial fungal infections, rashes, or excoriations. The presence of excoriations may suggest a scabies infection.

Take a close look at the distribution of hair and check the pubic area for the presence of crab lice or nits, which are egg cases attached to the hair.

Inspect the Penis and Scrotum

In the examination of the penis and scrotum, note the following:

- Whether the patient is circumcised
- The size of the penis and scrotum
- Any lesions on the penis and penile edema

In Fig. 18.11, notice the *ectopic sebaceous glands* on the shaft of the penis. These glands are small, pinhead-sized, and have a whitish-yellow appearance. They are commonly seen in males on the corona, inner foreskin, and shaft of the penis. They are similar to the Fordyce spots of the oral mucosa (refer to Fig. 12.18). The papules become more visible during an erection when the skin of the penis is stretched. Females may also have ectopic sebaceous glands on their labia minora and labia majora (refer to Fig. 19.13).

Even though *pearly penile papules*[16] typically do not cause any symptoms, males who have them may confuse them with genital warts, leading to worries about having a sexually transmitted infection. Having pearly penile papules around the coronal sulcus is considered a normal anatomical variant with a prevalence ranging from 14% to 48% of males. These papules are seldom observed in children but are mainly seen in late adolescence and early adulthood. As patients age, the prevalence of these lesions tends to decline as they involute. These papules are skin-colored lesions that are asymptomatic, filiform in shape, and form rows where the glans penis and sulcus coronarius meet. They are more commonly found in uncircumcised males and should not be confused with condylomata acuminata. Fig. 18.12, which shows a patient with pearly penile papules.

Similar papules have never been described on the female genitalia.

Fig. 18.13 shows the penis of a patient with the chancre of *primary syphilis*. Although the typical syphilitic chancre is

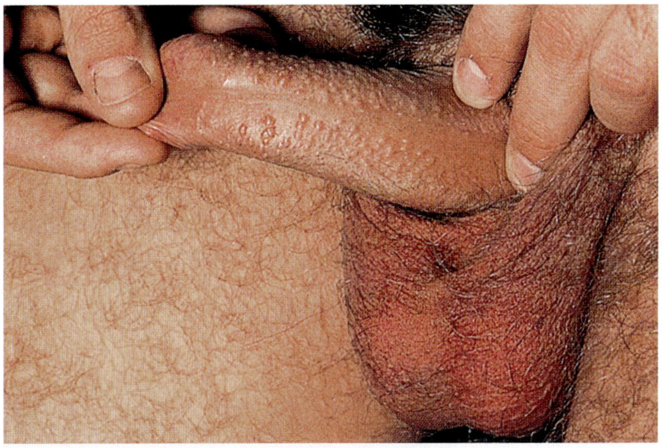

Fig. 18.11 Ectopic Sebaceous Glands on the Penis. (From Leibowitch M, Staughton R, Neill S, et al: An *atlas of vulval disease: a combined dermatological, gynecological and venereological approach*, ed 2, London, 1997, Mosby.)

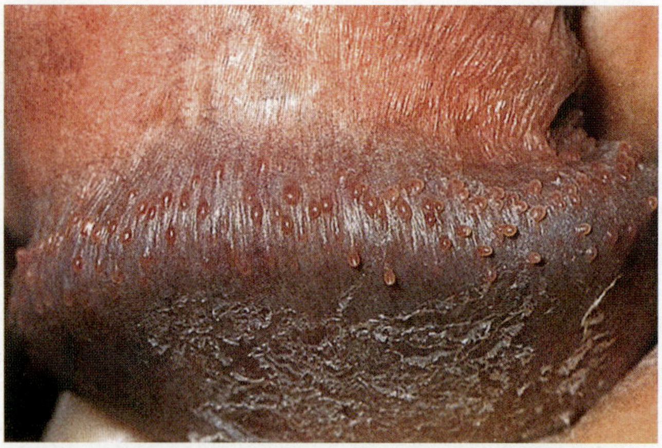

Fig. 18.12 Pearly Penile Papules. (From Leibowitch M, Staughton R, Neill S, et al: *An atlas of vulval disease: a combined dermatological, gynecological and venereological approach*, ed 2, London, 1997, Mosby.)

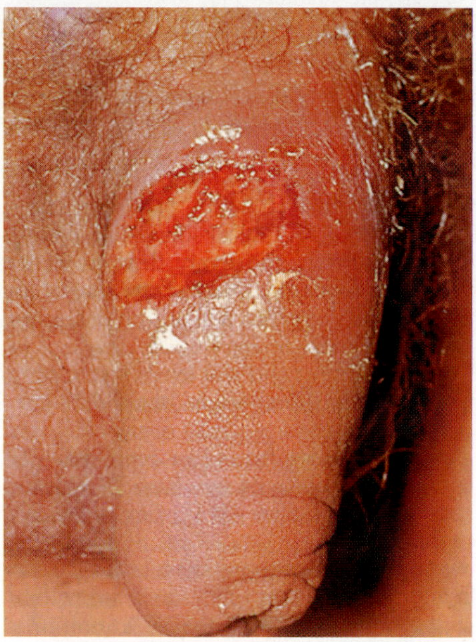

Fig. 18.13 Chancre of Primary Syphilis.

described as nontender, approximately 30% of patients with primary syphilis describe some tenderness. Usually only a single lesion is present. The edge of the chancre is usually indurated. Moderate nontender inguinal adenopathy was present in this patient.

Two patients with *chancroid* are depicted in Fig. 18.14. Unlike the relatively painless chancre of syphilis, the ulceration caused by chancroid is excruciatingly painful. The ulcer has a purulent, grayish surface that eventually becomes granulating. The base of the ulcer and the surrounding area are typically not infiltrated, making it easy to distinguish from other types of ulcers. Genital lesions are often accompanied by moderate tender adenopathy. It's important to note that chancroid ulceration differs from syphilis chancre also in that multiple lesions are frequently present in chancroid, as illustrated in Fig. 18.14A. A lesion similar to the one in Fig. 18.14B was found on the opposite side of this patient's penis.

Small, fleshy growths known as *venereal warts* or *condylomata acuminata* can appear in various areas around the genitals, including near the meatus, on the glans, in the perineum, at the anus, and on the shaft of the penis. These growths are a manifestation of human papillomavirus (HPV) infection and often have a bumpy, cauliflower-like appearance. They are highly contagious and can be transmitted in up to 60% of patients after just one instance of exposure. For reference, see Fig. 18.15, which shows a patient with condylomata acuminata on the shaft of his penis; Fig. 18.40 provides another example of these venereal warts.

It is crucial to examine the penis and scrotum for pruritic papules, as they may be a sign of *scabies* infection. This kind of rash typically manifests 4 to 6 weeks following exposure to the *Sarcoptes scabiei* var. *hominis* mite and is characterized by incessant itching, particularly at night. The symptoms of scabies result from the host's immune response to the mites and their byproducts as they burrow into the skin. Scabies is a contagious skin condition that can easily pass from one person to another through direct skin-to-skin contact. It only takes about 10 minutes of direct skin-to-skin contact for mites to spread

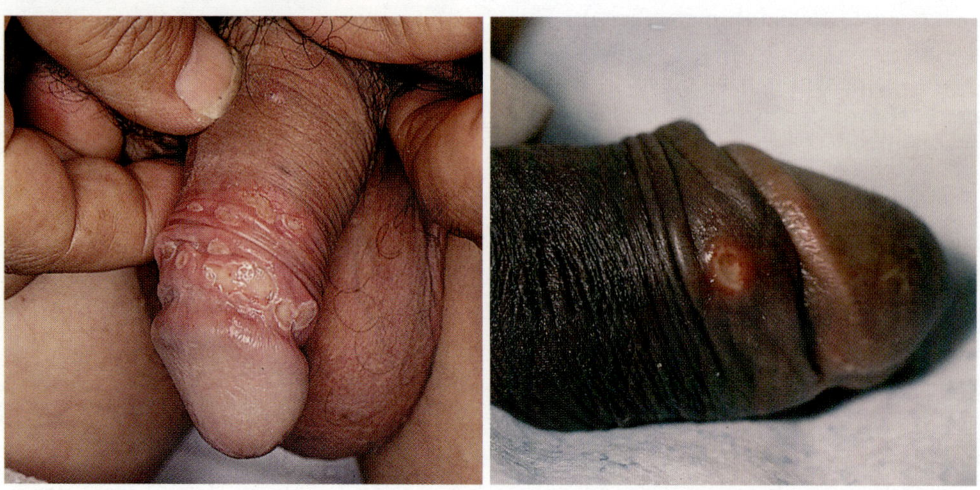

A B

Fig. 18.14 Chancroid. (A) Note the multiple lesions. (B) This patient had another lesion on the other side of his penis. (A, From Callen JP, Paller AS, Greer KE, et al: *Color atlas of dermatology*, ed 2, Philadelphia, 2000, WB Saunders.)

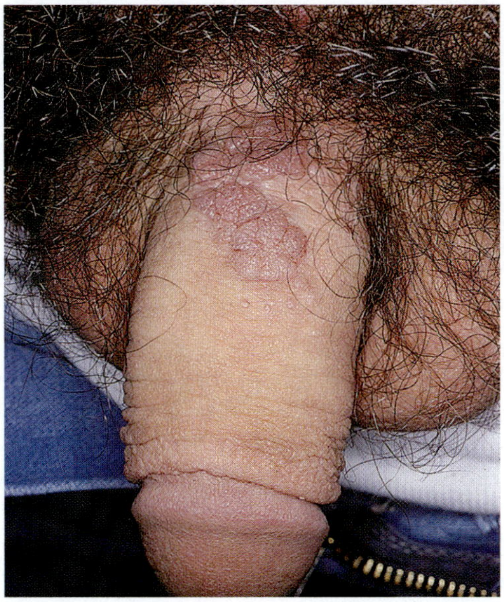

Fig. 18.15 Condylomata Acuminata of the Shaft of the Penis. (From Callen JP, Paller AS, Greer KE, et al: *Color atlas of dermatology*, ed 2, Philadelphia, 2000, WB Saunders.)

from one person to another. The disease can spread through fomite[r] transmission, which includes contamination through clothing or bed sheets. It's estimated that 300 million people worldwide are infected with scabies each year, making it a major health issue in many developing nations. In 2009, the World Health Organization classified it as a neglected skin disease. Fig. 18.16 shows the typical genital papular lesions in a scabies patient, with noticeable signs of scratching. Fig. 8.91 shows the hands of a patient with scabies.

Balanitis refers to the inflammation of the glans penis, which is more commonly found in uncircumcised males. *Candida* infection is the primary cause of this condition, usually facilitated by the warmth and moisture in the affected area that promotes the growth of the yeast organisms. At the onset of the infection, flat erythema appear on the inner side of the foreskin and glans, which eventually develop into pustules that break open and leave a moist, bright red, eroded surface. If the infection affects both the glans and foreskin, the term *balanoposthitis* is used. *Candida* balanitis can be identified by the erosions visible on the distal shaft and glans penis in Fig. 18.17, where the foreskin has been retracted.

Angiokeratomas are a type of benign skin condition. Fabry disease,[s] on the other hand, is a rare genetic disorder linked to the sex chromosomes, which affects the body's ability to metabolize glycosphingolipids. It is characterized by symptoms such as pain, fever, and the appearance of angiokeratomas in a "bathing suit" distribution, particularly around the umbilicus and scrotum. This is due to a deficiency in the enzyme responsible for removing lipids from the blood, leading to the accumulation of these substances in various organs and causing dysfunction. Because of this mechanism, Fabry disease is classified as a lysosomal storage disorder. The scrotum of a 15-year-old patient with Fabry disease and multiple angiokeratomas is shown in Fig. 18.18.

The patient in Fig. 18.19 has acquired immune deficiency syndrome (AIDS) and Kaposi sarcoma. Notice the marked penile and scrotal edema, as well as the lesions of Kaposi sarcoma on his thighs and scrotum.

Inspect the Perineum

The examiner raises the scrotum of the patient to thoroughly examine the perineum for signs of inflammation, ulcers, warts, abscesses, or any other abnormalities.

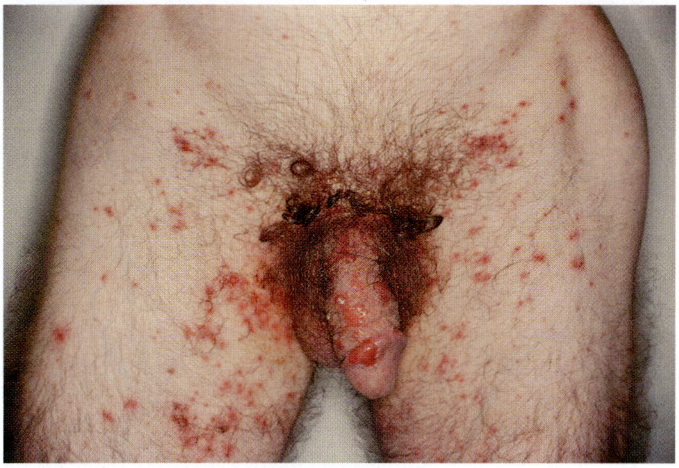

Fig. 18.16 Scabies in the Groin and on the Penis. (From Callen JP, Greer KE, Hood AF, et al: *Color atlas of dermatology*, Philadelphia, 1993, WB Saunders.)

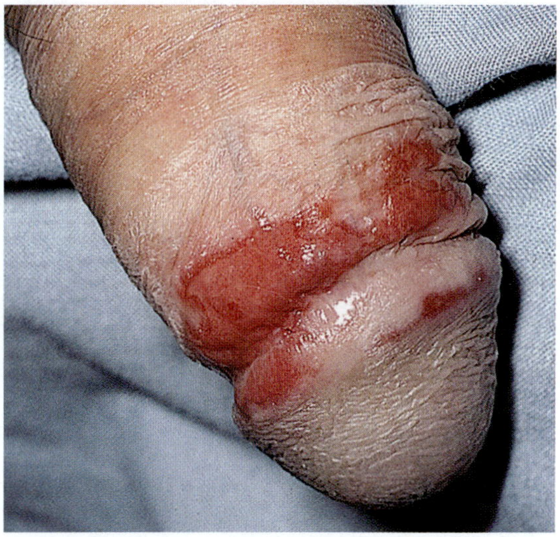

Fig. 18.17 *Candida* Balanitis. (From Callen JP, Paller AS, Greer KE, et al: *Color atlas of dermatology*, ed 2, Philadelphia, 2000, WB Saunders.)

[r]A fomite is any inanimate object that, when contaminated with or exposed to infectious agents (such as pathogenic bacteria, viruses, or fungi), can transfer disease to a new host.

[s]Fabry disease is an inherited disorder that results from the buildup of a type of fat, called globotriaosylceramide, in the body's cells. Beginning in childhood, this buildup causes signs and symptoms that affect many parts of the body. Characteristic features of Fabry disease include episodes of pain, particularly in the hands and feet (acroparesthesias); angiokeratomas; a decreased ability to sweat (hypohidrosis); corneal opacities; problems with the gastrointestinal system; tinnitus; and hearing loss.

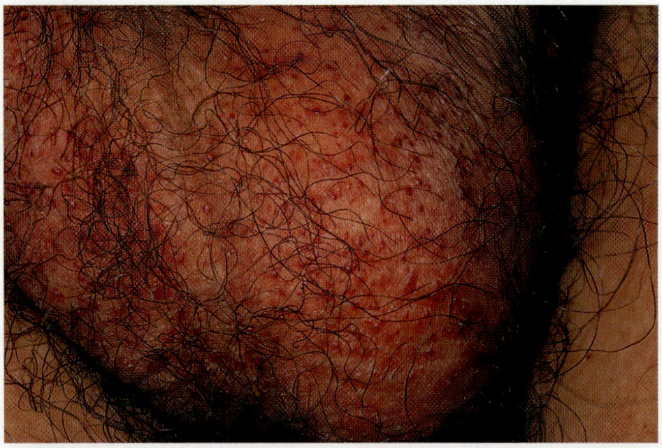

Fig. 18.18 Angiokeratomas in a Patient With Fabry Disease.

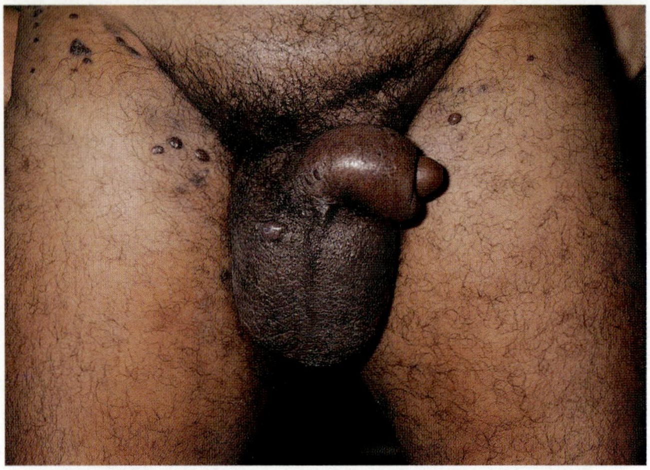

Fig. 18.19 Kaposi Sarcoma and Acquired Immune Deficiency Syndrome–Related Scrotal Edema.

To check for inguinal adenopathy, the examiner should roll their fingers along the inguinal ligament. In this area, small (0.2-inch [0.5-cm]), lymph nodes that can be moved easily, non-fixed, are typically present. This region is a common area for small lymph nodes as the lymphatic vessels from the perineum, legs, and feet drain into this area.

Inspect for Groin Masses

When examining the groin area, it may be helpful to ask the patient to cough or strain. This can help detect any sudden bulges, which could be a sign of an inguinal or femoral hernia.

Inspection and Palpation With the Patient Standing

Request the patient to stand while you position yourself in front of them.

Inspect the Penis

See Video 18.2.

If the patient is uncircumcised, it is necessary to retract the foreskin. Some examiners may ask the patient to do it themselves, while others may prefer to assess the tightness of the foreskin. The presence of cheesy, white material under the foreskin is known as smegma and is a natural occurrence.

Phimosis is a medical condition where the foreskin is tight and unable to retract back behind the head of the penis. This can cause smegma buildup, leading to inflammation of the glans and prepuce (*balanoposthitis*[t]). The chronic irritation from this condition may increase the risk of developing cancer of the penis.

The glans is inspected for ulcers, warts, nodules, scars, and signs of inflammation.

Inspect the External Meatus

See Video 18.3.

The examiner should note the position of the external urethral meatus. It should be central on the glans. To inspect the meatus, the examiner places their hands on either side of the glans penis and opens the meatus. The technique for examining the meatus is demonstrated in Fig. 18.20.

The meatus should be observed for any discharge, warts, and stenosis. Fig. 18.21 shows a patient with meatal condylomata acuminata.

Sometimes, a birth defect called *hypospadias* can cause the urethral meatus to open on the ventral surface of the penis, instead of at the tip of the glans penis. The meatus can occur anywhere along the urethral groove that runs from the tip of the penis along the ventral aspect of the shaft to where the penis joins with the scrotum or perineum. In nearly 50% of cases, the meatus location is subcoronal, 20% of cases have a middle location, and the rest are posterior (distal). Mild hypospadias is often an isolated birth defect that doesn't affect the rest of the reproductive or endocrine system, but in more severe cases, some infants may have additional structural anomalies of the genitourinary tract. Another, less common birth defect is *epispadias*, which causes the meatus to be located on the dorsal surface of the penis.

Palpate the Penis and Urethra

See Video 18.4.

Palpate the shaft from the glans to the base of the penis. The presence of scars, ulcers, nodules, induration, and signs of inflammation must be noted. To palpate the corpora cavernosa, hold the penis between the fingers of both your hands and use your index fingers to note any induration. Fig. 18.22 illustrates the method of palpation of the shaft of the penis.

If there are areas of hard tissue or induration under the skin of the penis shaft that do not hurt when touched, *Peyronie disease* may be present. This plaque, or scar tissue, may be felt as flat lumps or a band of hard tissue beneath the skin. The plaque builds up inside the penis, in the thick elastic membrane called the tunica albuginea. The tunica albuginea helps keep the penis stiff during an erection. As the condition develops, the plaque pulls on the surrounding tissues and causes the penis to curve or bend, usually during an erection. Curves in the penis can

[t]Acute balanoposthitis is a purulent, pyogenic infection of the prepuce. This condition leads to erythema and edema of the prepuce. Dysuria is common, and minor bleeding may occur. These episodes typically resolve with antibiotic treatment and require no further intervention unless recurrent episodes occur.

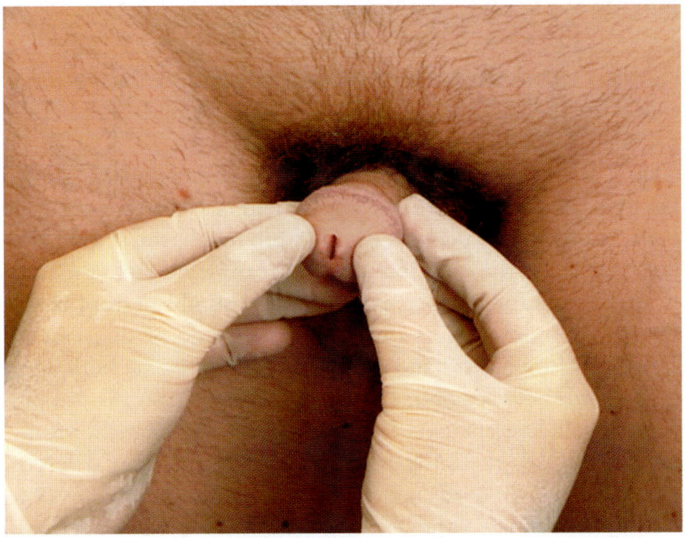

Fig. 18.20 Technique for Inspecting the External Urethral Meatus.

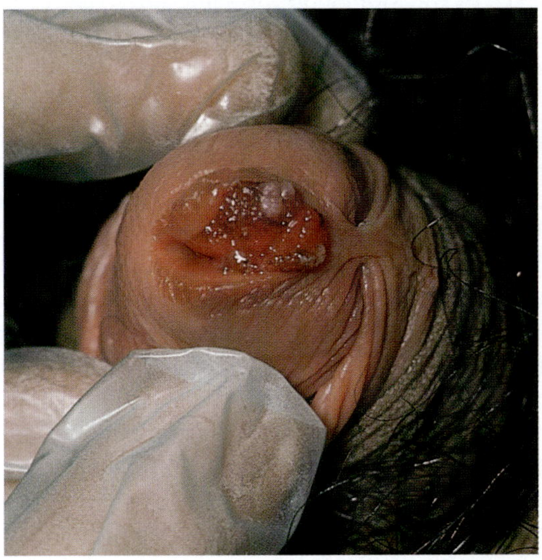

Fig. 18.21 Condylomata Acuminata of the Urethral Meatus.

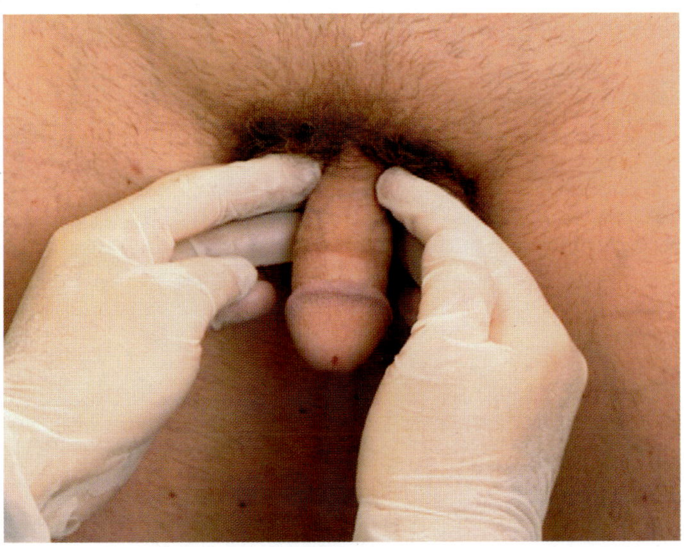

Fig. 18.22 Technique for Palpation of the Penis.

make erections painful and may make sexual intercourse painful, difficult, or even impossible.

Peyronie disease is an acquired condition that commonly affects the dorsum of the penis, particularly the middle or upper third. In Fig. 18.23, the erect penis of a patient with Peyronie disease is shown, with the tip of the penis pointing upward. This patient's wife complained of pain during sexual activity as the penis rubbed directly on her clitoris. The exact cause of Peyronie disease is unknown, but it is believed to result from repeated injury to the penis during sexual intercourse, sports, or accidental trauma. However, in most cases, there is no specific incident of trauma to the penis that can be recalled.

Approximately 1 in 100 males in the United States over the age of 18 have been diagnosed with Peyronie disease. However, based on studies of males who reported having symptoms of Peyronie disease, researchers estimate that the actual number of males who have Peyronie disease is more than 1 in 10.

The urethra should be palpated from the external meatus through the corpus spongiosum to its base. To palpate the base of the urethra, the examiner elevates the penis with the left hand while the right index finger invaginates the scrotum in the midline and palpates deep to the base of the corpus spongiosum. The pad of the examiner's right index finger should palpate the entire corpus spongiosum from the meatus to its base. This technique is demonstrated in Fig. 18.24. If a discharge is present, "milking the urethra" may allow a drop to be placed on a glass slide for microscopic evaluation.

The foreskin, if retracted, should be replaced. *Paraphimosis* is a condition in which the foreskin can be retracted but cannot be replaced and becomes caught behind the corona.

Inspect the Scrotum

See Video 18.5.

The scrotum is now reevaluated while the patient is standing. Observe the contour and contents of the scrotum. Two testicles should be present. Normally the left testicle is lower than the right. The presence of any fullness not seen while the patient was lying down should be noted.

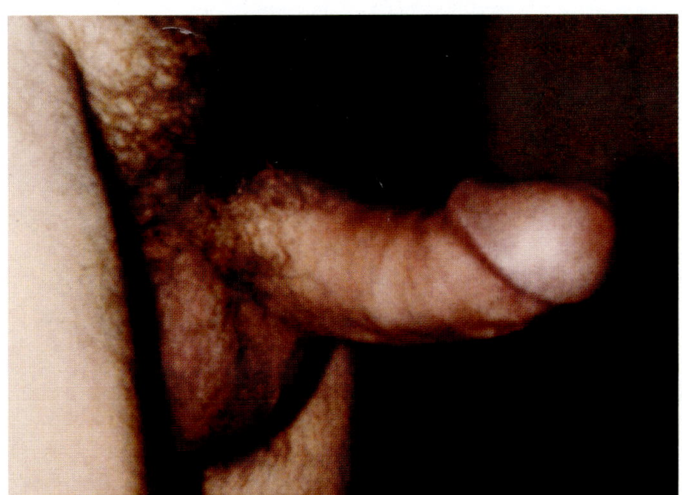

Fig. 18.23 Peyronie Disease.

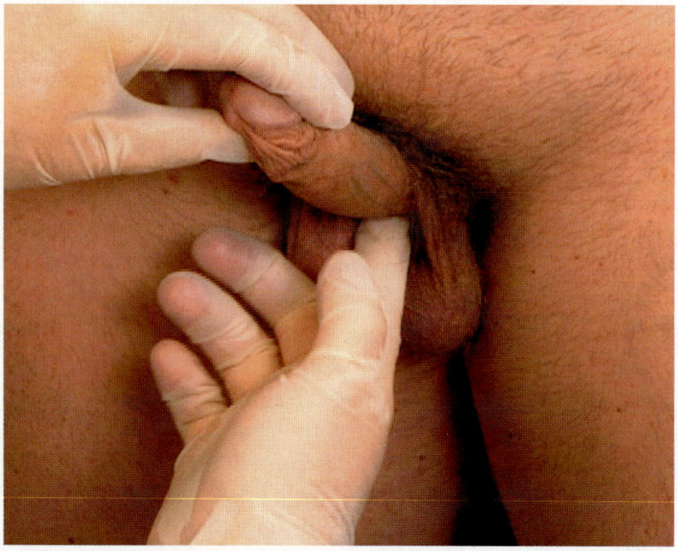

Fig. 18.24 Technique for Palpation of the Base of the Urethra.

Palpate the Testes

See Video 18.6.

Each testis is palpated separately. Use both hands to grasp the patient's testicle gently. While the left hand holds the superior and inferior poles of the testicle, the right hand palpates the anterior and posterior surfaces. The technique for palpation of the testicle is demonstrated in Fig. 18.25.

It's important to observe the size, shape, and texture of each testicle during a physical exam. There should be no signs of tenderness or lumps. Healthy testicles should feel firm and rubbery. It's also important to compare the size and texture of each testicle to the other. If one testicle feels heavier than the other or a mass is detected, the examining finger should be able to palpate above the mass within the scrotum. Because inguinal hernias arise from the abdominal cavity, the examining finger is unable to get above such a mass. In contrast, the examining finger can frequently get above a mass that arises from within the scrotum.

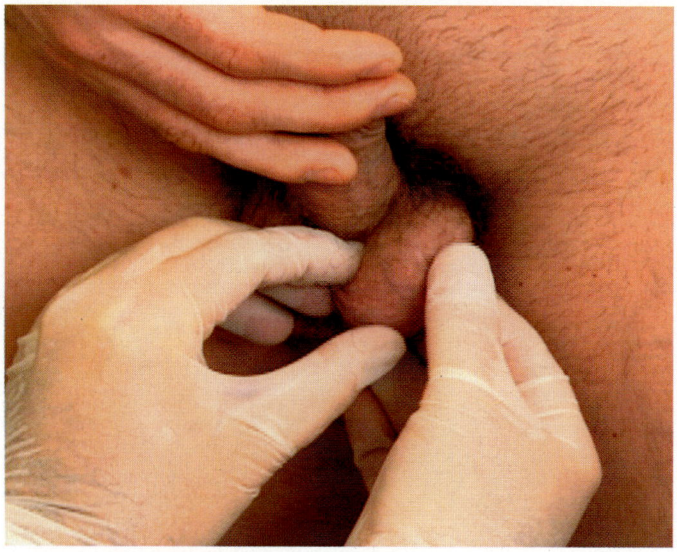

Fig. 18.25 Technique for Palpation of the Testicle.

Palpate the Epididymis and Vas Deferens

See Video 18.7.

Next, locate and palpate the epididymis on the posterior aspect of the testicle. The head and tail should be carefully palpated for tenderness, nodularity, and masses.

The spermatic cord is palpated from the epididymis up to the external abdominal ring. The patient is asked to elevate his penis gently. If the penis is elevated too much, the scrotal skin is reduced, and the examination is more difficult. Hold the scrotum in the midline by placing both your thumbs in front of and both your index fingers on the perineal side of the patient's scrotum. Using both hands, simultaneously palpate both spermatic cords between your thumbs and index fingers as you pull your fingers laterally over the scrotal surface. The most prominent structures in the spermatic cord are the vasa deferens. The vasa are firm cords approximately 0.08 to 0.15 inches (2 to 4 mm) in diameter and feel like "partially cooked spaghetti." The sizes are compared, and tenderness or beading is noted. The absence of the vas deferens on one side is often associated with the absence of the kidney on the same side. The technique of spermatic cord palpation is demonstrated in Fig. 18.26.

A common enlargement of the spermatic cord resulting from dilation of the pampiniform plexus is a *varicocele*. These varicosities are usually on the left side, and the impression on palpation has been likened to feeling a bag of worms. Because the varicocele is gravity dependent, it is usually visible only while the patient is standing or straining. Varicoceles occur in around 15% to 20% of all males but are found in about 40% of infertile males. The testicular veins originate in the testicle and form the pampiniform plexus. Venous blood then travels up through the inguinal canal as part of the spermatic cord, forms the internal spermatic vein, and terminates in the abdomen. As mentioned earlier, the right internal spermatic vein terminates directly into the low-pressure inferior vena cava while on the left side, it joins with the relatively high-pressure left renal vein. This anatomy explains why the majority of clinically detectable varicoceles are on the left side.

Varicoceles usually form during puberty and develop over time. They may cause some discomfort or pain, but they often

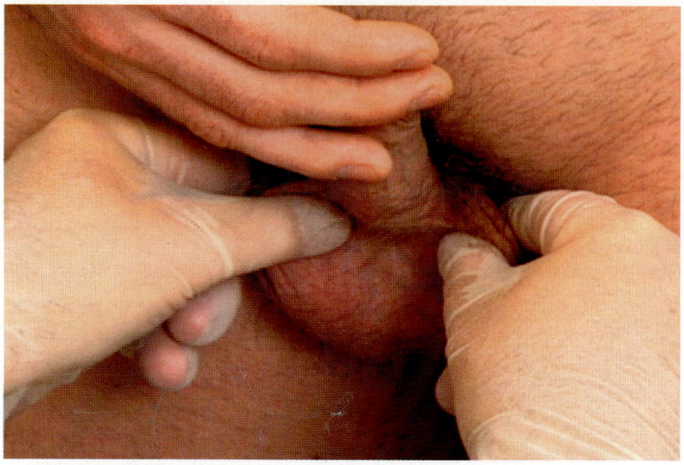

Fig. 18.26 Technique for Palpation of the Spermatic Cord.

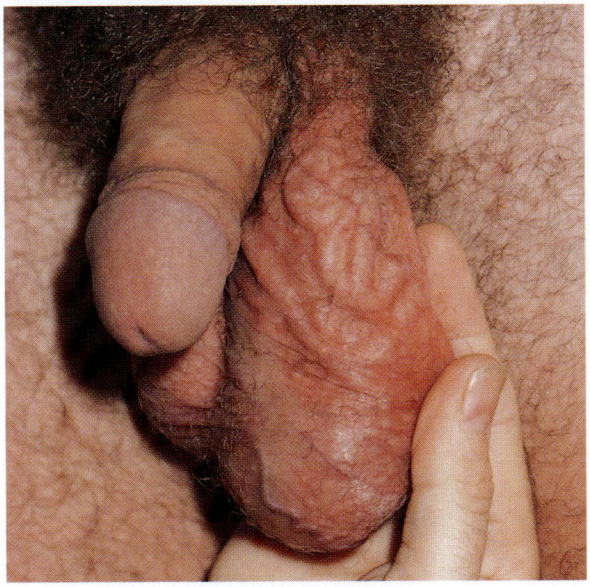

Fig. 18.27 Varicocele.

result in no symptoms or complications. While usually painless, varicoceles are clinically significant because they are the most commonly identified cause of abnormal semen analysis, low sperm count, decreased sperm motility, and abnormal sperm morphology that can lead to infertility.

The patient is asked to turn their head and cough while the spermatic cords are held between the examiner's fingers. A sudden pulsation, especially on the left side, suggests the diagnosis of a varicocele. Although the diagnosis is usually made from palpation, large varicoceles may be discovered on mere inspection, as can be seen in the patient in Fig. 18.27.

Transilluminate Scrotal Masses

When a lump is found in the scrotum, it is important to perform transillumination. To do this, a light is used to shine on the side of the scrotum in a dark room. Vascular structures, tumors, blood, hernias, and normal testicles will look solid when illuminated. However, if there is a fluid-filled cavity, such as a hydrocele or spermatocele, the light will pass through and create a red glow. The testis cannot be felt directly due to the cystic mass surrounding it. However, transillumination may allow visualization of the normal-sized testicle's position within the hydrocele. A hydrocele, seen only as massive scrotal enlargement, is shown in Fig. 18.28. Transillumination of a hydrocele in another patient is shown in Fig. 18.29. A cross-section illustration of a hydrocele is illustrated in Fig. 18.30.

Hernia Examination

Inspect Inguinal and Femoral Areas

Hernias typically refer to the protrusion of a viscus or a part of it through a normal or abnormal opening. However, 90% of all hernias occur in the inguinal area. Generally, the hernial impulse is more visible than palpable.

Ask the patient to stand and turn their head to the side, then cough or strain. Check for any sudden swelling in the inguinal and femoral areas, which could be a sign of a hernia. If you notice a sudden bulge, ask the patient to cough again and compare it to the other side. If the patient feels pain while coughing, find out where the pain is and check the area again.

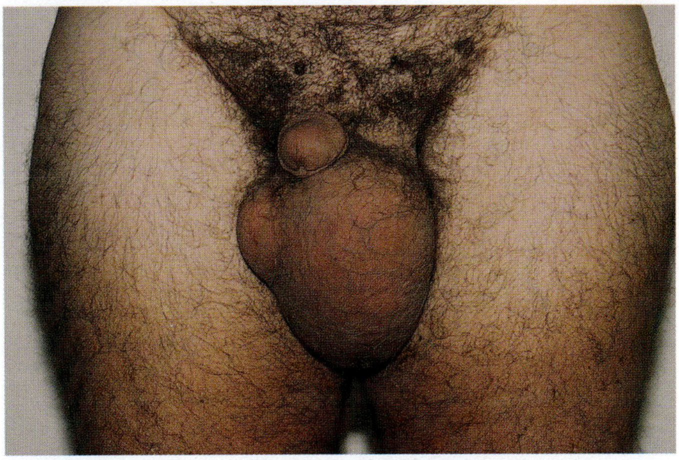

Fig. 18.28 Hydrocele.

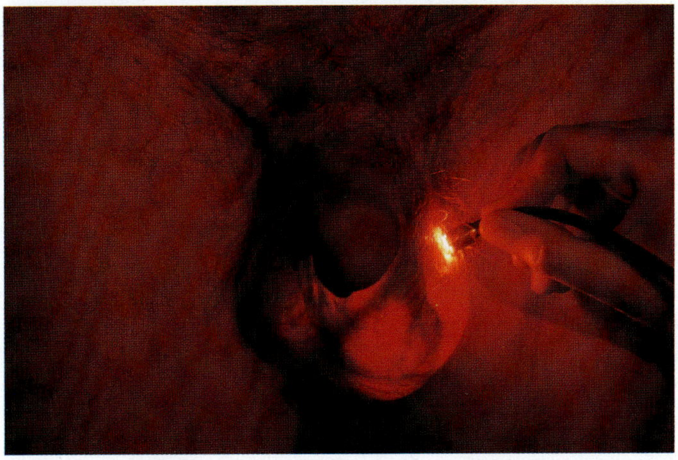

Fig. 18.29 Transilluminated Hydrocele.

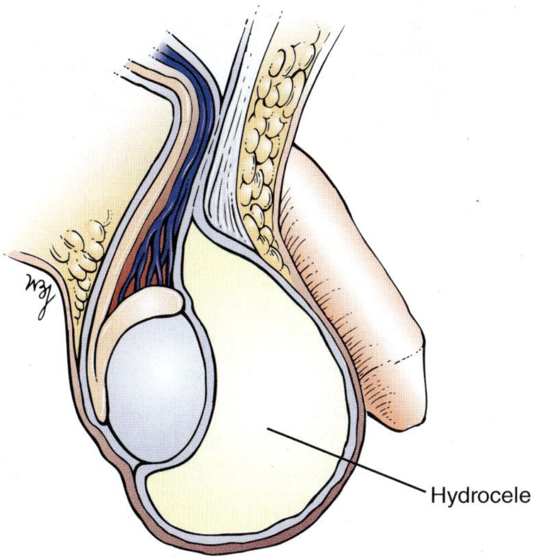

Fig. 18.30 Cross-section of a Hydrocele, Illustrating Its Anatomy.

Palpate for Inguinal Hernias

See Video 18.8.

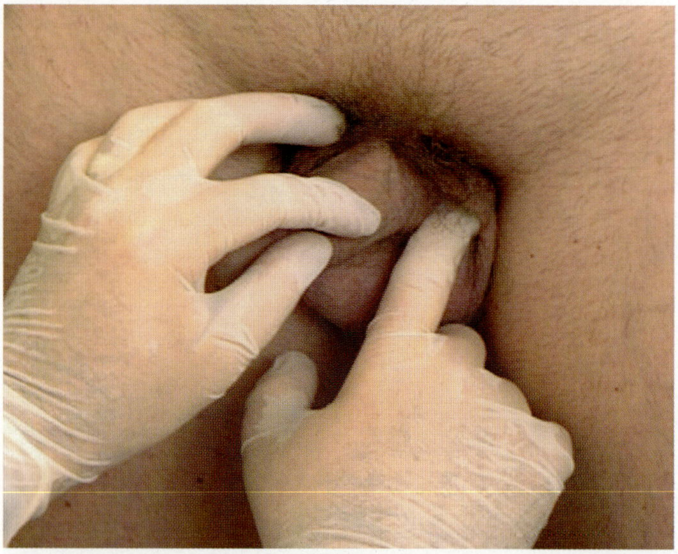

Fig. 18.31 Technique for Examination for Inguinal Hernias.

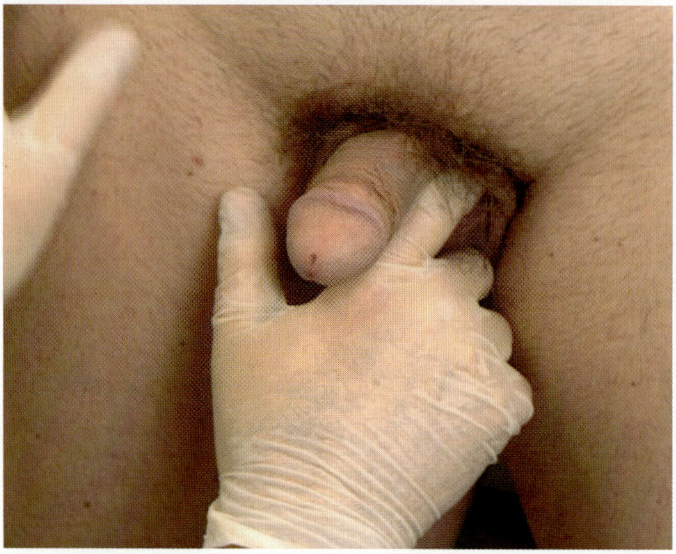

Fig. 18.32 Technique for Palpation of Inguinal Hernias.

To check for inguinal hernias, the examiner uses their right index finger in the patient's scrotum above the left testis. The examiner then pushes the scrotal skin inward to reach the external inguinal ring, making sure there is enough skin to do so. The finger is positioned with the nail facing outward and the pad of the finger inward, as shown in Fig. 18.31. The examiner may also place their left hand on the patient's right hip for additional support.

To properly examine, the healthcare professional should use their right index finger to trace the spermatic cord from the external inguinal ring, moving parallel to the inguinal ligament and up towards the internal inguinal ring. The internal inguinal ring can be found superior and to the side of the pubic tubercle. The external ring may be dilated and allow the finger to enter easily. The correct position of the right hand is shown in Fig. 18.32 and is illustrated in Fig. 18.33.

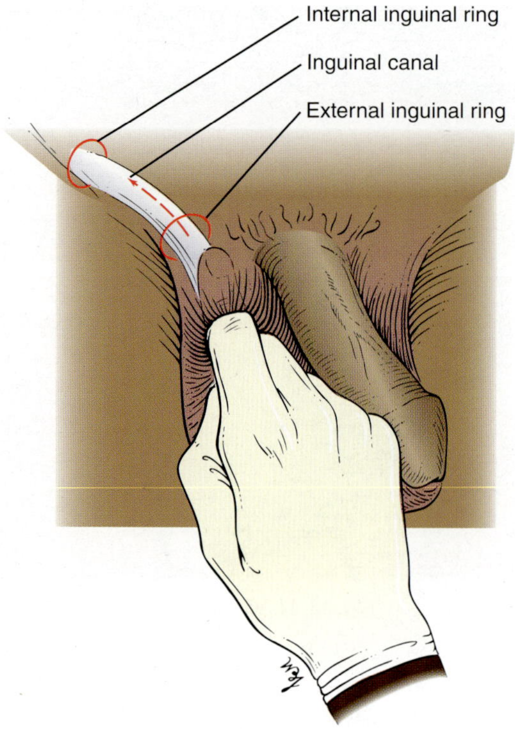

Fig. 18.33 Position of the Examining Finger in the Inguinal Canal.

To check for a hernia, place your index finger on the external ring or in the inguinal canal and ask the patient to turn their head to the side and cough or strain down. If there is a hernia, you will feel a sudden impulse against either the tip or the pad of your examining finger. When a hernia is discovered, instruct the patient to lie down and carefully apply constant pressure to the bulge to see if it can be reduced. When the hernia examination is conducted slowly and with sufficient scrotal skin, it is typically painless. In the following section, we will cover the characteristics of hernias.

Once you have finished evaluating the patient's left side, use your right index finger to examine their right side by repeating the procedure. Some examiners prefer to use the right index finger to examine the patient's right side and the left index finger for the patient's left side. Try both techniques to see which one is more comfortable for you.

If you notice a big lump in the patient's scrotum that doesn't let light pass through, it may indicate the presence of an indirect inguinal hernia. To confirm this, you can listen to the lump with your stethoscope and check if there are bowel sounds, which can be a helpful sign in diagnosing the hernia.

Chapter 17, The Abdomen, discusses the process of examining the prostate. If the rectal examination has not yet been conducted, this is the appropriate time to examine both the rectum and prostate.

CLINICOPATHOLOGIC CORRELATIONS

Gross hematuria that is usually painless is often the first indication of a urinary tract tumor, commonly located in the bladder. Table 18.1 lists the common causes of gross hematuria in different age groups and by sex.

TABLE 18.1 Causes of Hematuria by Age and Sex

Age (Years)	Male	Female
Younger than 20	Congenital urinary tract anomaly Acute glomerulonephritis Acute urinary tract infection	—
20–40	Acute urinary tract infection Kidney stone Bladder tumor	—
40–60	Bladder tumor Kidney stone Acute urinary tract infection	Acute urinary tract infection Kidney stone Bladder tumor
Older than 60	Prostatic disorder Bladder tumor Acute urinary tract infection	Bladder tumor Acute urinary tract infection

Scrotal disorders are quite prevalent. If a male experiences swelling in the scrotum, a detailed history and a comprehensive physical examination usually yield enough data to make an accurate diagnosis. Intrascrotal masses are frequently observed during a physical examination. While many masses are harmless, it is important to note that testicular cancer is the primary form of solid cancer found in males under the age of 35.

When considering a patient's medical history, there are several important factors to consider. These factors include the patient's age, when symptoms started (if there were any), any other problems experienced (such as fever, weight loss, or difficulty urinating), past medical history, and sexual history.

There are different types of intrascrotal masses, which can be classified based on their nature. They may be acute or non-acute, intratesticular or extratesticular, and neoplastic or non-neoplastic.

Acute, Non-Neoplastic Lesions

Among acute, non-neoplastic lesions, testicular torsion, epididymitis, and trauma are the most frequently observed pathologic disorders. *Testicular torsion* is a serious surgical emergency that occurs when a testicle rotates, twisting the spermatic cord that brings blood to the scrotum. The twisting of the testis results in venous obstruction, edema, and, ultimately, arterial obstruction causing sudden, severe pain and swelling. If torsion is recognized within 6 hours, healthcare professionals can usually save the testis in 70% to 90% of cases as testicular viability significantly decreases after that time period. Testicular torsion is a true urological emergency. This condition is commonly seen in adolescents aged 12 to 18 years, and patients typically experience sudden, one-sided testicular pain along with nausea and vomiting. During a physical exam, the testis is swollen, tender, and may be withdrawn, often resting in a horizontal position. Early identification of torsion is crucial to provide timely treatment.

Epididymitis is the most common cause of acute scrotal swelling. It accounts for more than 600,000 visits to healthcare professionals annually in the United States. Patients usually complain of recent onset of testicular pain that is associated with fever, dysuria, and scrotal swelling. Epididymitis is a frequently occurring condition that can be confused with testicular torsion. Medical management is used to treat epididymitis, whereas testicular torsion requires immediate surgery. Epididymitis is a condition that can affect males of all ages, but it is more common in those aged 20 to 39. This is usually associated with sexually transmitted diseases, with *Chlamydia trachomatis* and *Neisseria gonorrhea* accounting for around 50% of cases in males under 39. After the age of 39, the main cause of epididymitis is *Escherichia coli* and other coliform bacteria commonly found in the gastrointestinal tract. On physical examination, the epididymis is tender and indurated. The testis may also be enlarged and tender; this variant is called *epididymo-orchitis.*

Acute scrotal swelling can be caused by *trauma*, which may result in a hematoma in the scrotum or testicle. It's important to note that 10% to 15% of patients with testicular tumors may only seek medical attention after experiencing trauma.

Non-Acute, Non-Neoplastic Lesions

The most frequently occurring intrascrotal pathologic conditions are the non-acute, non-neoplastic lesions, which consist of hydrocele, spermatocele, and varicocele. Hydrocele, illustrated in Fig. 18.30, is a fluid buildup within the tunica vaginalis layers, causing painless swelling of the scrotum. Hydroceles can be congenital, acquired, or idiopathic. Acquired hydroceles may result from trauma, infection, renal transplantation, and neoplasm. Idiopathic hydroceles are the most common; patients may have no symptoms or may complain of a dull ache or scrotal heaviness. In general, hydroceles are anterior to the testis. They are smooth-walled and can be transilluminated. Fig. 18.29 depicts a transilluminated hydrocele.

Spermatoceles are painless, cystic collections of fluid in the epididymis. It is also known as a spermatic or epididymal cyst. They are frequently found on routine physical examination. A spermatocele feels like a smooth but separate, firm lump near the top of, or behind, the testicle. Because they are fluid-filled, they can often be transilluminated. In general, spermatoceles are not a cause of infertility. They may, however, reduce the quantity and quality of sperm produced, if the spermatocele is large.

A *varicocele* is a common intrascrotal mass resulting from abnormal dilation of the veins of the pampiniform plexus. Varicoceles are usually caused by faulty valves in the spermatic veins and pampiniform plexus. Normally, these veins have many valves that allow blood to flow in one direction. However, in patients with varicoceles, these valves are flawed, which causes blood to flow backwards and accumulate in the veins. Males with varicoceles usually don't experience any symptoms, but they may feel a sense of heaviness or pain in the testicle or scrotum or have trouble conceiving. Varicoceles are typically detected in patients between the ages of 15 and 30, and rarely occur after the age of 40. As mentioned earlier, varicoceles are mostly located on the left side. If a varicocele is found on the right side, it may indicate an obstruction of the inferior vena cava. On the other hand, if a left-sided varicocele appears relatively suddenly

TABLE 18.2 Differential Diagnosis of Common Scrotal Swellings

Diagnosis	Usual Age (Years)	Able to Be Transilluminated	Scrotal Erythema	Pain
Epididymitis	Any	No	Yes	Severe, increasing severity
Torsion of testes	<20	No	Yes	Severe, sudden
Testis tumor	15–35	No	No	Minimal or absent
Hydrocele (see Fig. 18.28)	Any	Yes (see Fig. 18.29)	No	None
Spermatocele	Any	Yes	No	None
Hernia (see Figs. 18.42 and 18.43)	Any	No	No	None to moderate[a]
Varicocele (see Fig. 18.27)	>15	No	No	None

[a]Unless the hernia is incarcerated, in which case pain may be severe.

after puberty, it could be a sign of a left renal tumor or hypernephroma. Fig. 18.27 shows a 23-year-old patient with a varicocele; his only symptom was a heaviness in his left scrotum. Notice the markedly dilated veins in the scrotum.

Neoplastic Lesions

Testicular cancer is among the most common malignancies in males aged 15 to 45. It is one of the most curable forms of cancer, with cure rates as high as 90% and a 5-year survival rate of more than 95%. It makes up 1% of male tumors and 5% of urological malignancies. The incidence of testicular cancer has been on the rise in recent years and is becoming increasingly significant due to the lasting impact it can have on patients and their treatment. In fact, the incidence of testicular cancer has doubled over the past 40 years. Although most testicular neoplasms are asymptomatic, some patients may experience acute pain due to trauma, hemorrhage, hydrocele, or epididymitis, and therefore seek medical attention. Some males might experience weight loss, fever, abdominal pain, edema in their lower extremities, or bone pain due to advanced metastatic disease. It's crucial to consider a history of cryptorchidism because there is a significant link between this condition and testicular malignancies. The physical examination usually reveals a painless swelling or nodule on one of the testicles. It's worth noting that only 1% to 3% of testicular tumors occur in both testicles. Extra-testicular tumors are uncommon and are usually benign. Pure seminomas constitute approximately 40% of all testicular cancer cases. Forty percent of testicular cancers have mixed histologic characteristics. The American Cancer Society recommends that males aged 15 to 35 perform a monthly testicular self-examination. It is suggested to perform this examination during or after a shower when the scrotal skin is warm and relaxed. It is best to do the test while standing.

For further information about testicular self-examination, visit: https://medlineplus.gov/ency/article/003909.htm.

1. Gently feel the scrotal sac to locate the testicle.
2. Hold the testicle with one hand while firmly but gently rolling the fingers of the other hand over the testicle to examine the entire surface.
3. Repeat the procedure with the other testicle.

Any change in the shape of the testicle, the presence of a painless lump, or swelling in the scrotum should be evaluated by a healthcare professional.

Table 18.2 provides a differential diagnosis of common scrotal swellings.

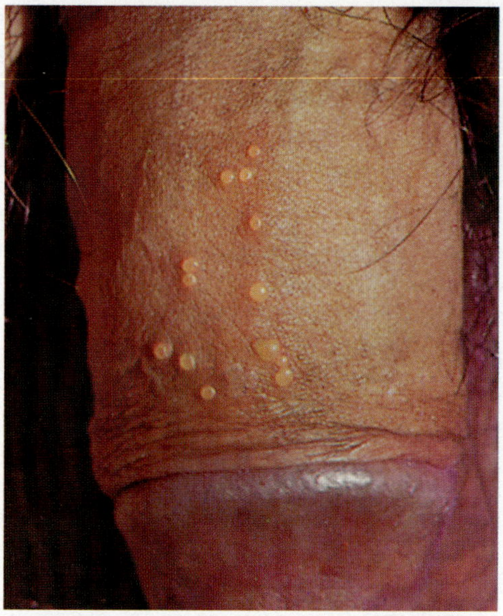

Fig. 18.34 Herpes Simplex Virus Type 2 Infection. (From Callen JP, Paller AS, Greer KE, et al: *Color atlas of dermatology*, ed 2, Philadelphia, 2000, WB Saunders.)

Sexually transmitted diseases are quite common. At a venereal disease clinic, out of every 100 outpatient visits by males, 25% have gonorrhea, 25% have nongonococcal urethritis, 4% have venereal warts, 3.5% have herpes, 1.7% have syphilis, and 0.1% have chancroid. Since the early 1980s, there has been a significant increase in the incidence of both gonococcal and nongonococcal urethritis. On university campuses, 85% of urethritis is nongonococcal.

There are two types of genital lesions associated with venereal diseases: ulcerative and nonulcerative. The frequency of these lesions has significantly shifted since the 1950s. In the past, chancroid was prevalent while herpes was uncommon. Nowadays, the opposite is true as herpes simplex virus type 2 (HSV-2) infection is widespread while chancroid is rare. Fig. 18.34 shows the vesicular stage of a herpetic infection. Another example of HSV-2 infection is shown in Fig. 18.35. Anal ulcerative lesions are becoming more common, particularly among males having sex with males.

Molluscum contagiosum is a common, usually self-limited, cutaneous eruption affecting the skin and mucous membranes. This condition is commonly observed in children and is caused by a large DNA poxvirus. Adults can contract the infection by engaging in sexual activity with infected individuals. The distinct sores

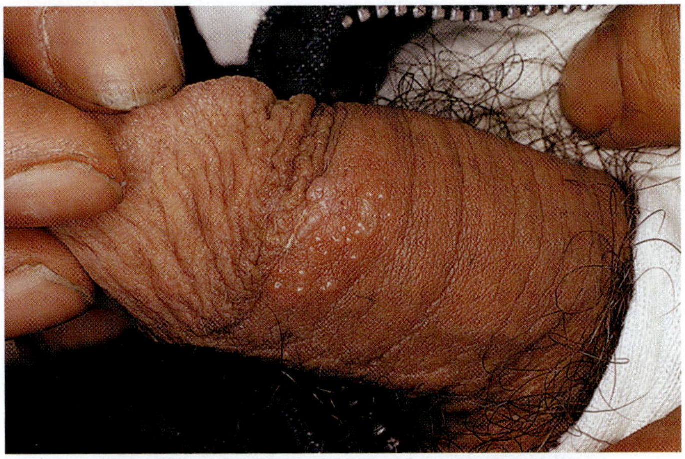

Fig. 18.35 Herpes Simplex Virus Type 2 Infection.

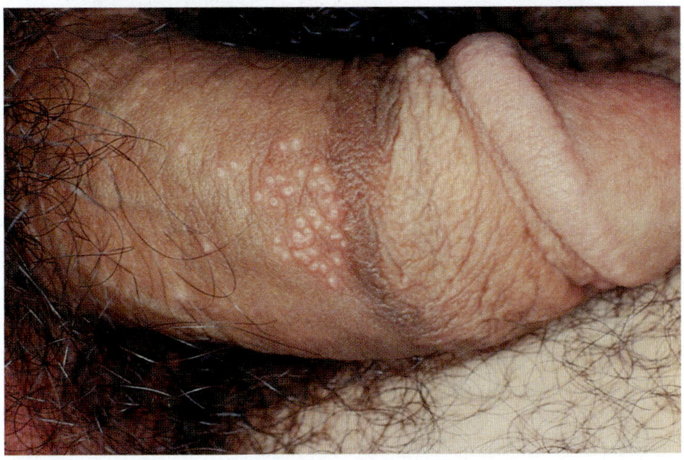

Fig. 18.36 Lesions of Molluscum Contagiosum of the Penis. (From Callen JP, Greer KE, Hood AF, et al: *Color atlas of dermatology*, Philadelphia, 1993, WB Saunders.)

appear as flesh-colored papules that vary in dimension from tiny dots to as large as 0.4 inches (1 cm) in diameter. The umbilication[u] is the most important diagnostic sign. Painful lesions can appear on any part of the body, including the face and trunk in children and around the genitals in adults. If an adult is diagnosed with this disease, it is important for them to get screened for other sexually transmitted diseases. Remember, the lesions are very contagious as the name suggests. As the lesions develop, there may be a surrounding patch of eczema. In patients with AIDS, the lesions become widespread, attaining sizes up to 0.8 inch (2 cm) in diameter. Fig. 18.36 shows lesions of molluscum contagiosum of the penis. Fig. 18.37 is a close-up photograph of the classic, umbilicated lesions of molluscum contagiosum. Table 18.3 lists a differential diagnosis of genital papular lesions.

The primary lesion of *syphilis* is the chancre (see Fig. 18.13), which occurs from 10 days to 3 weeks after infection at the site of the inoculation. The chancre is a painless ulcer with an indurated edge. It usually heals spontaneously within a month. If the patient is not treated for syphilis, the disease may evolve to the *secondary stage*. This occurs approximately 2 months after

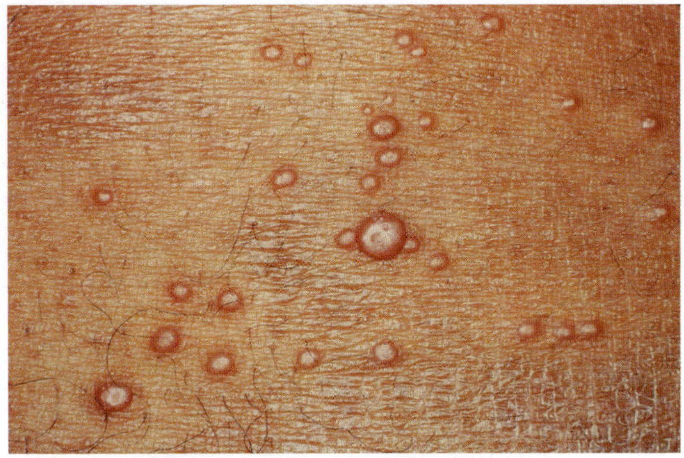

Fig. 18.37 Close-Up Photograph of the Umbilicated Lesions of Molluscum Contagiosum. (From Callen JP, Greer KE, Hood AF, et al: *Color atlas of dermatology*, Philadelphia, 1993, WB Saunders.)

the appearance of the chancre. The patient may present with a widespread, nonpruritic, maculopapular rash over the genitalia, trunk, palms, and soles. There is a tendency for cropping of the lesions. The healed chancre may still be evident. There is also generalized lymphadenopathy. In the genital and perianal areas, the papules may coalesce and erode. These large, moist, painful papules, which look as if they were "pasted" on the skin, are called *condylomata lata*. They are covered with exudate and teem with active spirochetes. If untreated, the patient may recover but may have a relapse of the eruption within 2 years. After this period, there is a long latent period during which the disease may progress to cardiovascular syphilis or neurosyphilis, a condition known as *tertiary syphilis*.

The skin lesions of syphilis are important to recognize. Fig. 18.38 shows the typical skin lesions of secondary syphilis on the feet. Fig. 18.39 shows condylomata lata in the perineum of the same patient. The healing chancre of primary syphilis is also seen on the penis of this patient.

HPV infection of the genital tract is one of the most common sexually transmitted diseases among young adults and is the cause of venereal warts and cancer. In the United States, it is estimated that 20 million people have genital HPV infections at any one time, with 5.5 million acquiring it annually. In the United States, 26,800 males and females develop HPV-related cancer annually. Risk factors associated with HPV infection include younger age, belonging to an ethnic minority, alcohol consumption, and a high frequency of anal or vaginal sexual encounters. About 80% of males and females will get an HPV infection at some point. Most people with HPV do not even know they are infected and never develop symptoms. The body most often clears the virus before it causes any health problems. For some, however, the infection persists and can lead to precancerous changes. The annual cost burden in the United States of genital HPV infection is $6 billion, which makes it the second most costly sexually transmitted disease after human immunodeficiency virus infection. Condylomata acuminata are typically caused by HPV 6 or HPV 11, which are considered low-risk HPV types because these strains are rarely found in association with genital dysplasias or invasive cancer. HPV 16 and HPV 18

[u]The term "umbilicated" comes from the Latin word "umbilicatus," which indicates a concave center, much like that of a navel.

TABLE 18.3 Differential Diagnosis of Genital Papules

Condition	Appearance	Pain	Lymphadenopathy
Herpes (see Figs. 18.34 and 18.35)	Multiple, ulcers, vesicles	Painful	Present
Condylomata lata (see Fig. 18.39)	Multiple, moist, flat, round	Painful	Present
Condylomata acuminata (see Figs. 18.15, 18.21, and 18.40)	Multiple, verrucous	Absent	Absent
Molluscum contagiosum (see Figs. 18.36 and 18.37)	0.04- to 0.2-inch (1- to 5-mm) umbilicated papules, often in clusters; caseous material expressible from center	Painful	Rarely

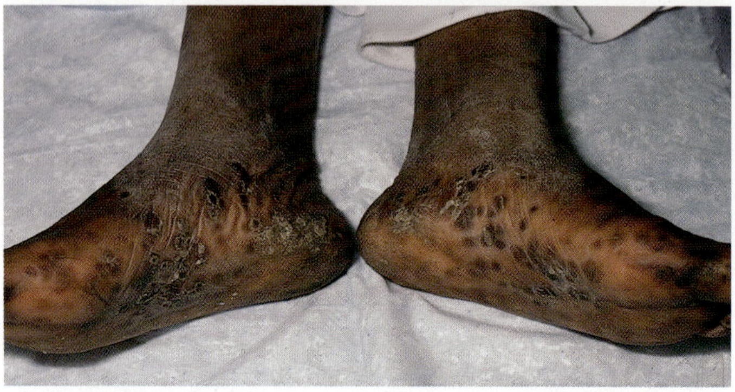

Fig. 18.38 Secondary Syphilis Lesions on the Feet.

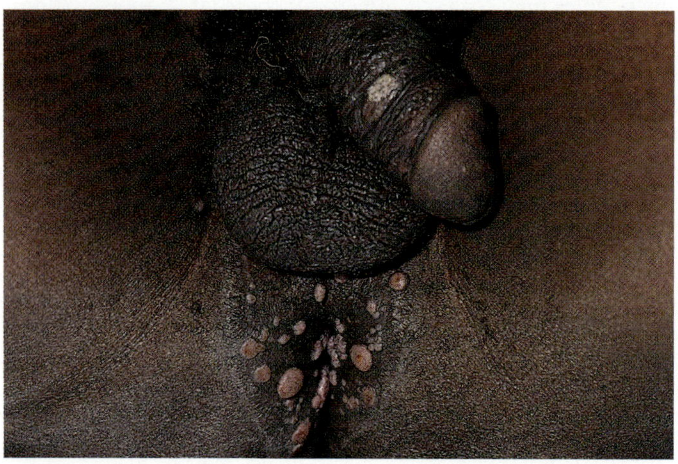

Fig. 18.39 Condylomata Lata. Note the healing primary chancre on the penis.

are the strains responsible for most HPV-related cancers. Patients with immunodeficiencies are at higher risk for persistent HPV infection and progressive disease. Fig. 18.40 shows the classic cauliflower lesions of condylomata acuminata on the penis of a renal transplant recipient (see also Figs. 18.15 and 18.21).

The HPV vaccine, *Gardasil 9®*,[17] is a safe and effective vaccination against HPV infection. All males and females ages 9 to 26 should get the vaccine. It is most effective when given at ages 11 or 12. The vaccine is given in two doses for males and females ages 9 to 14. Beginning at age 15 through 45, three doses are required for full immunity. Ninety percent of genital warts, 74% of all HPV cancers, and 81% of cervical cancers are prevented by the vaccine. The vaccine reduces the risk of most HPV-related cancers of the throat and the penis and also prevents HPV-related genital warts in both males and females.

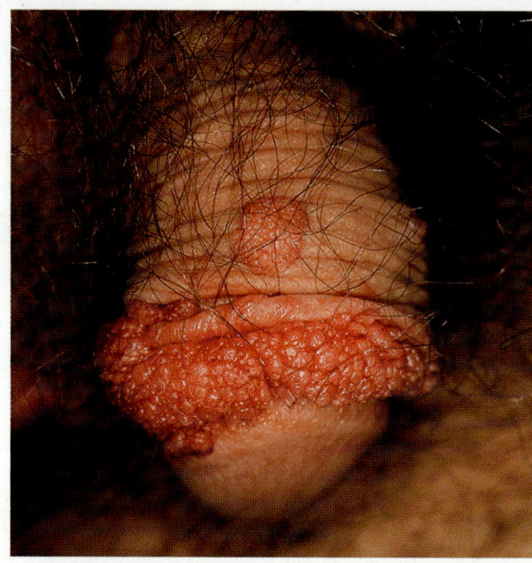

Fig. 18.40 Condylomata Acuminata of the Penis. (From Bolognia JK, Jorizzo JL, Rapini RP: *Dermatology*, London, 2003, Mosby.)

Reactive arthritis (ReA), previously known as *Reiter syndrome*,[V] is a relatively rare, inflammatory (aseptic) arthritis that manifests 1 to 6 weeks after a gastrointestinal or genitourinary infection. It is one of the most common causes of acute inflammatory arthritis in males. It is defined as the classic triad of nongonococcal urethritis, arthritis, and conjunctivitis. However, most patients do not present with the classic triad. it is believed that the disorder is due to an aberrant autoimmune response to a gastrointestinal or genitourinary infection caused by *salmonella*, *shigella*, *campylobacter*, or *chlamydia*. The incidence is about 2% to 4% after a urogenital infection, mainly with *Chlamydia trachomatis*, and varies from 0% to 15% after gastrointestinal infections with *Salmonella*, *Shigella*, *Campylobacter*, or *Yersinia*. ReA is more common in males in the second and third decades of their life, and over two-thirds of these patients are HLA-B27 positive. ReA is often associated with a psoriasis-like dermatitis on the palms and soles known as *keratoderma blennorrhagicum*,[W] This painless, papulosquamous, "barnacle-like" eruption is pictured in Fig. 18.41.

[V]The medical term "Reiter syndrome" has been discontinued due to the historical association with Hans Reiter, who was a member of the Nazi Party and the director of the Kaiser Wilhelm Institute of Experimental Therapy. It is alleged that war prisoners were subjected to inhumane experiments under his leadership.

[W]*Keratoderma blennorrhagicum* describes the appearance of skin lesions resembling psoriasis that appear first on the palms of the hands and soles of the feet but may eventually spread to the scalp, torso, and genitals.

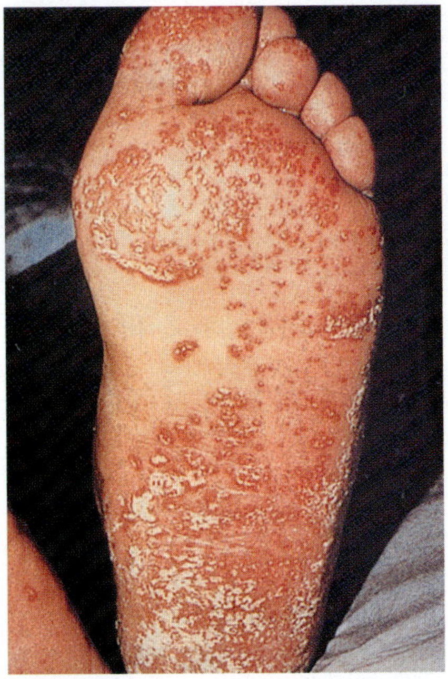

Fig. 18.41 Keratoderma Blennorrhagicum in a Patient With Reactive Arthritis. (From Leibowitch M, Staughton R, Neill S, et al: *An atlas of vulval disease: a combined dermatological, gynecological and venereological approach*, ed 2, London, 1997, Mosby.)

Inguinal and femoral hernias are prevalent conditions, with approximately 200,000 new cases reported annually in the United States. Most of these cases are self-diagnosed. In fact, more than 600,000 surgical repairs for inguinal hernias are carried out across the country every year, making it one of the most frequently performed general surgical procedures in the United States. The most common symptom of a hernia is a bulge or lump in the affected area. A hernia occurs when an organ, such as the intestines, pushes through an opening in a muscle or tissue that holds it in place. One common type of hernia, mainly affecting males, is an inguinal hernia. This occurs when the intestines protrude through a weakened area in the abdominal wall, particularly the internal ring and inguinal canal. In fact, inguinal hernias make up around 70% of all hernias. Such a hernia is caused by the intestines pushing through a weak spot or tear in the lower abdominal wall.

An *indirect inguinal hernia* is very common in males of all ages. It's important to keep in mind that the testicles move down through the inguinal canal, which may not completely close once they reach the scrotum. This can create a weakened area that is more susceptible to hernias when there is increased abdominal pressure or straining. As a result, the intestines may pass through the internal inguinal ring, into the inguinal canal, and eventually enter the scrotum.

A *direct inguinal hernia* is a tear in the transversalis fascia or a weakened muscular abdominal wall, allowing a portion of the intestine to push through the wall. This weakening can develop over time due to everyday activities and aging. The intestines do not enter the inguinal canal when a direct inguinal hernia is present. A direct inguinal hernia almost always develops in adulthood, usually later in life, unless the problem is the result of a specific injury.

A *femoral hernia* occurs when the intestines push through the wall of the femoral canal into the upper thigh. The femoral canal is situated below the inguinal ligament in the groin and contains the femoral arteries, veins, and nerves. Females are more susceptible to femoral hernias than males, and the condition is uncommon in general. Pregnant or overweight females are particularly vulnerable. Femoral hernias account for less than 3% of all hernia cases.

If a patient cannot push a hernia back in, the contents of the hernia may become trapped or incarcerated in the abdominal wall or inguinal canal. This can cause the hernia to become strangulated, which can lead to a compromised blood supply to the tissue that is stuck, creating the potential for necrosis. It is important to seek immediate medical attention for a strangulated hernia as it is a medical emergency if left untreated. It is less likely that a direct hernia will result in bowel strangulation.

The major types of external abdominal hernias are indirect and direct inguinal hernias and femoral hernias. Fig. 18.42 shows a patient with a left indirect inguinal hernia. Notice the lack of symmetry of the inguinal area due to the intestines that have pushed into the inguinal canal and scrotum. Fig. 18.43 shows a patient with a small right direct inguinal hernia. Notice the bulge that is medial to the internal inguinal ring and does not enter the scrotum. Fig. 18.44 illustrates and lists the major differences in the differential diagnosis of inguinal and femoral hernias.

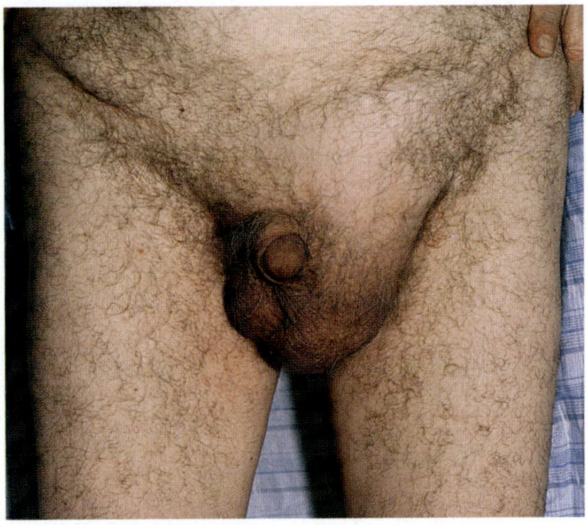

Fig. 18.42 Left Indirect Inguinal Hernia.

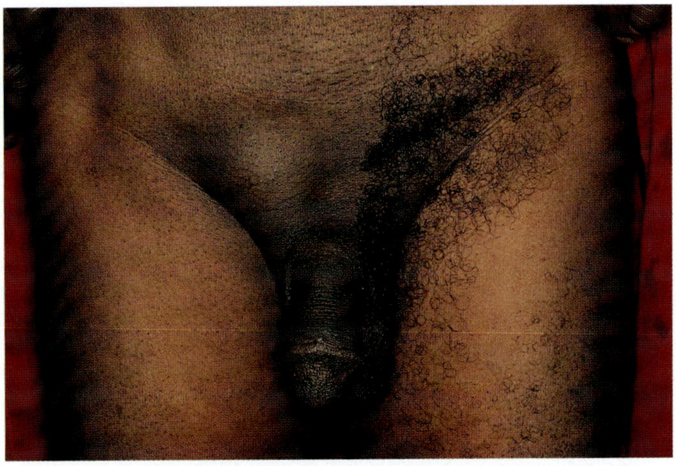

Fig. 18.43 Right Direct Inguinal Hernia.

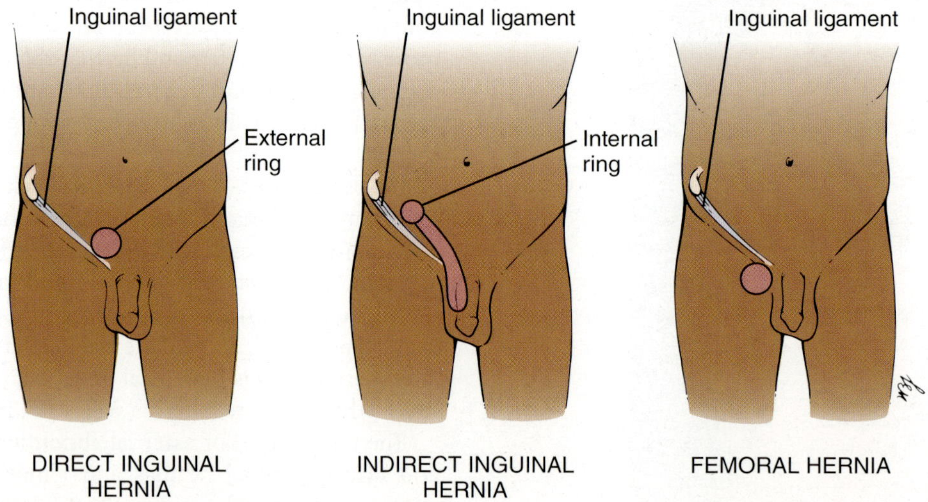

Feature	Direct Inguinal[a]	Indirect Inguinal[b]	Femoral
Occurrence	Middle-aged and elderly men	All ages	Least common: more frequently found in women
Bilaterality	55%	30%	Rarely
Origin of swelling	Above inguinal ligament; directly behind canal near external ring	Above inguinal ligament; hernial sac enters inguinal canal at internal ring and exits at external ring	Below inguinal ligament
Scrotal involvement	Rare	Common	None
Impulse location	At side of examining finger in inguinal canal	At tip of examining finger in inguinal canal	Not felt by examining finger in inguinal canal; mass below canal

[a]See Fig. 18.43.
[b]See Fig. 18.42.

Fig. 18.44 Differential Diagnosis of Inguinal and Femoral Hernias.

USEFUL VOCABULARY

Listed here are the specific roots that are important for understanding the terminology related to urologic disease.

Root	Pertaining to	Example	Definition
andr-	man	***andr***ogen	Substance possessing masculinizing properties
cyst(o)-	urinary bladder	***cysto***tomy	Incision of the urinary bladder
litho-	stone	***litho***tomy	Incision of an organ for the removal of a stone
nephro-	kidney	***nephro***pathy	Disease of the kidneys
orchi(o)-	testes	***orchi***tis	Inflammation of the testis
pyel(o)-	pelvis of kidney	***pyelo***gram	X-ray film of the kidney and ureter
ureter(o)-	ureter	***uretero***lith	A stone lodged or formed in the ureter
urethr(o)-	urethra	***urethro***plasty	Plastic surgery of the urethra
vas(o)-	vas deferens	***vas***ectomy	Excision of the vas deferens

WRITING UP THE PHYSICAL EXAMINATION

Listed here are examples of the write-up for the examination of the male genitalia.

- The penis is circumcised. Both testes are in the scrotum and are within normal limits. There are no abnormal scrotal masses. No inguinal hernias are present. No inguinal adenopathy is present.
- The penis is uncircumcised. The foreskin is easily retracted. The left hemiscrotum is markedly enlarged by a painless mass that can be transilluminated. The left testicle cannot be palpated. The right testicle is within normal limits. No inguinal hernias are present. A small, 2 × 2 cm (0.75 × 0.75 inch), soft, nonfixed, nontender lymph node is present in the right inguinal area.
- The penis is circumcised. There is a 1- to 2-cm (0.40- to 0.75-inch) verrucous mass at the external meatus. A thick, yellow, purulent urethral discharge, which can be milked from the urethra, is seen at the meatus. The scrotal contents are within normal limits. No inguinal hernias are present.
- The penis is uncircumcised. The foreskin is tight, although it can be retracted by the patient. A large amount of smegma is present behind the corona. There is a large mass of nontender, dilated veins present in the left hemiscrotum that can be seen and felt when the patient stands. An impulse is felt in the left spermatic cord upon coughing. No inguinal hernias are present.
- The penis is circumcised. The left testicle is soft and measures 2 × 3 cm (0.75 × 1.20 inch). The right testicle appears normal. The scrotal contents are within normal limits. The hernia examination on the left side reveals a prominent impulse when the patient coughs. This impulse is felt at the tip of the examiner's finger.
- The penis is circumcised. There is a 1-cm (0.4-inch) painless ulcer with a clean, nonpurulent base at the corona. The ulcer is indurated and has a smooth, regular, sharply defined border. Painless, firm, movable inguinal lymphadenopathy is present bilaterally. The testes are normal, as are the other scrotal contents. No inguinal hernias are present.

FULL VIDEO

- Video 18.9 Full video: Examining the male genitalia

REVIEW QUESTIONS

1. Regarding erection, which of the following statements is false?
   - **A.** Erection is a complex hemodynamic and neurophysiologic event.
   - **B.** The erectile state begins in the brain and requires contraction of the smooth muscles of the penis.
   - **C.** There is synthesis and release of nitric oxide in the corpora cavernosa.
   - **D.** Nitric oxide activates guanylate cyclase to produce cyclic guanosine monophosphate, which decreases intracellular calcium levels.
   - **E.** In the erect state, the arteriovenous channels are closed.
2. Testicular pain can commonly occur with all of the following *except:*
   - **A.** Epididymitis
   - **B.** Orchitis
   - **C.** Varicocele
   - **D.** Hydrocele
   - **E.** Spermatic cord torsion
3. Regarding priapism, which of the following statements is true?
   - **A.** Priapism is a medical emergency.
   - **B.** Priapism is seen exclusively in patients with sickle cell anemia.
   - **C.** Priapism is a nonpainful, persistent erection lasting more than 6 hours.
   - **D.** It is estimated that 50%–60% of males with sickle cell disease will have priapism at some point in their life.
   - **E.** Priapism can result from penile infections.
4. Which of the following statements about benign prostatic hypertrophy (BPH) is false?
   - **A.** BPH is the most common cause of reduced usable bladder capacity in males.
   - **B.** Symptoms of BPH include frequent urination, nocturia, and a sensation of incomplete bladder emptying.
   - **C.** Infrequently, BPH can lead to the complete inability to urinate.
   - **D.** BPH can lead to urinary tract infections.
   - **E.** BPH can be ameliorated by catheterization.
5. All of the following may cause red urine *except:*
   - **A.** Acute glomerulonephritis
   - **B.** Vegetable dyes
   - **C.** Strenuous exercise
   - **D.** Bladder neck disorder
   - **E.** Gonorrhea
6. Hematuria in a male between the ages of 20 to 40 may generally indicate any of the following *except:*
   - **A.** Acute urinary tract infection
   - **B.** Kidney stone
   - **C.** Bladder tumor
   - **D.** Prostatic disorder
   - **E.** All of the above
7. Which of the following associations is true?
   - **A.** Epididymitis – able to be transilluminated
   - **B.** Torsion of the testicle – no scrotal erythema
   - **C.** Testicular tumor – minimal or absent pain
   - **D.** Hydrocele – commonly seen in males younger than 15
   - **E.** Spermatocele – very painful
8. Which of the following genital lesions has the appearance of multiple lesions, ulcers, and vesicles?
   - **A.** Herpes simplex virus type 2 (HSV-2)
   - **B.** Condylomata lata
   - **C.** Condylomata acuminata
   - **D.** Molluscum contagiosum
   - **E.** Syphilis

9. In diagnosing inguinal and femoral hernias, which of the following statements is true?
   A. An indirect inguinal hernia is more common in middle-aged and elderly males.
   B. A femoral hernia is more commonly found in females.
   C. A direct inguinal hernia is rarely bilateral.
   D. An indirect inguinal hernia rarely is associated with scrotal involvement.
   E. A direct inguinal hernia is felt at the tip of the examining finger in the inguinal canal.

10. Which of the following statements about sexually transmitted diseases is incorrect?
    A. Genital lesions may be ulcerative or non-ulcerative.
    B. Today, herpes simplex virus type 2 (HSV-2) is more common than chancroid.
    C. Molluscum contagiosum is a common, self-limited eruption.
    D. The primary lesion of syphilis occurs from 3 to 6 weeks after infection.
    E. Risk factors associated with human papillomavirus (HPV) infection include younger age, alcohol consumption, and a high frequency of anal and vaginal encounters.

REFERENCES

Available online.

BIBLIOGRAPHY

Available online.

19

Female Genitalia

Mark H. Swartz and Farida G. Nentin

...The unique change of the small uterus into an enormous and powerful structure capable of containing a perfect child and sending it forth by tremendous efforts into the outer world; the changes in all the surrounding organs and tissues necessitated by the accomplishment of such a remarkable work in the short space of nine months; and the subjection of this great physical work to the law of individual freedom and perfection are facts which show the superior complication and importance of the female sexual organization.

Elizabeth Blackwell, M.D. (1821–1910)

VIDEOS

Video 19.1	Preparing for the pelvic examination
Video 19.2	Inspecting and palpating the female external genitalia
Video 19.3	Testing for pelvic organ prolapse
Video 19.4	Using the vaginal speculum
Video 19.5	Performing the traditional Pap smear
Video 19.6	Inspecting the vaginal walls
Video 19.7	Performing the bimanual palpation
Video 19.8	Palpating the rectovaginal septum
Video 19.9	Full video: Performing the speculum examination
Video 19.10	Full video: Performing the bimanual examination
Video 19.11	Full video: Performing the rectovaginal examination

GENERAL CONSIDERATIONS

The history of obstetrics and gynecology dates back to the time of Hippocrates in 400 BCE. He was one of the earliest physicians to describe midwifery, menstruation, sterility, symptoms of pregnancy, and puerperal (the period after labor) infections. Soranus, in the 2nd century CE, played a major role in the early gynecologic history. He wrote extensively on topics such as anatomy, menstruation, fertility, signs of pregnancy, labor, care of the infant, dysmenorrhea (painful menstruation), uterine hemorrhage, and the use of vaginal specula.

William Harvey, who developed the theory of blood circulation, also wrote a significant treatise on obstetrics. Published in 1651, this work included a detailed assessment of uterine changes throughout life.

During the 18th century, there was a growing understanding of pregnancy, labor, and fertility. However, it wasn't until the 19th century that diseases related to female genitalia were better comprehended. In 1872, Emil Noeggerath published his investigations on gonorrhea, which ultimately changed the medical world's opinion on the significance of this disorder. He was the first to suggest that "latent gonorrhea" was linked to sterility in females. Although the first cesarean section was described in 1596 by Scipione Mercurio, the current technique of Max Sänger was documented in 1882.

As of 2023, cancer of the uterine corpus, also known as *endometrial cancer,* accounted for approximately 3.4% of all new cancer cases and 2.1% of all cancer deaths in the United States. In 2023, there were 66,200 new cases and 13,030 deaths from cancer of the uterus. It is the fourth most common cancer in females, after breast cancer, lung cancer, and colorectal cancer. Obesity poses a significant risk for endometrial cancer due to the production of estrogen in adipose tissue. Around 40% of uterine cancer cases are linked to obesity. The exposure to increased estrogen levels is a prominent risk factor for endometrial cancer. Other factors that may increase estrogen exposure include menopausal estrogen therapy (without the use of progestin), early onset of menstruation, late menopause, low parity, and a history of polycystic ovary syndrome (PCOS) because of chronic anovulation. The lifetime risk of developing uterine cancer is 1 in 35. The 5-year relative survival rate for all cases of uterine cancer is 81%. Depending on the stage of diagnosis, the 5-year survival rate is 95%, 68%, or 16% if the cancer is diagnosed at a local, regional, or distant stage, respectively. Although the mortality rate has slightly decreased since the 1980s among White females, it has remained stable among other racial and ethnic groups. Black females are more likely to be diagnosed with later-stage disease, and Black and Hispanic females have been found to present with more aggressive disease.

Between the mid-1950s and 1992, deaths from invasive cancer of the cervix in the United States dropped by 74%. The decline in mortality from cervical cancer is largely attributed to early detection by physical examination. It has been estimated that noninvasive cervical cancer (carcinoma in situ) is approximately four times more common than invasive cervical cancer. In the United States, the widespread use of the

Papanicolaou (Pap)[a] *test* has decreased the incidence and mortality rate by 40% since the mid-1970s. Most invasive cervical carcinomas are found in females who have not had regular Pap tests. In 2023, there were 13,960 new cases of invasive cervical cancer diagnosed and 4310 deaths from this disease. The death rate continues to decline by approximately 2% per year. An American female has a 0.78% lifetime risk (1 per 128) for the development of cervical cancer and a 0.27% risk of dying from the disease. The 5-year relative survival rate for the earliest stage of invasive cervical cancer is 92%, and the overall (all cases considered together) 5-year survival rate is 65%.

Cervical cancer has been linked to several risk factors. Among these, the most commonly associated ones are young age at first sexual intercourse, having multiple sexual partners, being infected with human papillomavirus (HPV), herpes simplex virus or human immunodeficiency virus, having a history of cervical dysplasia, and smoking.

The most important risk factor for cervical cancer is infection with a high-risk strain of HPV. HPVs are a group of more than 100 types of viruses—some of which can cause warts—or papillomas, which are noncancerous (benign) tumors. Certain other types of HPV can cause cancer of the cervix. These are called *high-risk* or *oncogenic* types of HPV, and approximately 70% of all cervical cancers are caused by HPV types 16 and 18. It has been shown that younger patients, in their teens and early 20s, have the highest incidence of HPV infection, but are able to mount an immune response to clear the infection. The current guidelines indicate that females should be screened with cervical cytology, or Pap test, at the age of 21, regardless of when she initiated sexual activity. In females older than 30 years, an HPV test should be conducted at the same time as a Pap test.[1]

Vaccines have been developed that protect against infection with certain strains of HPV, which may reduce cervical cancer rates in the future. Gardasil9® is now the only approved vaccine in the United States, replacing the previously approved quadrivalent HPV recombinant vaccine (Gardasil®) and HPV bivalent vaccine (Cervarix®). Gardasil9® protects against types 6, 11, 16, 18, 31, 33, 45, 52, and 58. The Gardasil9® vaccine entails a series of three injections over a 6-month period. In October 2018, the FDA expanded the approved use of Gardasil9® for use in females and males 9 to 45 years of age (previously approved for use from age 9 to 26) to prevent all HPV-related lesions and cancers.[2] These vaccines cannot protect against established infections nor do they protect against all HPV types.

Although ovarian carcinoma accounts for only 3% of all cancers in females, it is the cause of 5% of all cancer deaths. It is the fifth leading cause of cancer death and the leading gynecologic malignancy in females in the United States. Cancer of the ovary accounts for nearly 50% of all deaths from gynecologic malignancies. This is due to the advanced stage of diagnosis in most patients. The most important risk factor is a strong family history of breast or ovarian cancer. In 2023, there were 19,710 new cases of ovarian cancer and 13,270 deaths from it. The lifetime risk for development of ovarian cancer is 1 per 59; the incidence is 1.4 per 100,000 females younger than 40 years, but it increases to 45 per 100,000 females older than 60 years. The incidence has been declining by 1% per year since 1992. The overall 5-year relative survival rate is 47%, with a 92% survival rate for the earliest stage of ovarian cancer and a 29% 5-year survival rate in late-stage disease. A carefully performed bimanual pelvic examination has been shown to be the cornerstone of diagnosis of ovarian cancer.

[a] The Pap test is named after George N. Papanicolaou, the healthcare professional who developed the screening technique. When performed correctly, this test can accurately diagnose cervical carcinoma in 98% of cases, making it a lifesaving screening tool for cervical cancer. It can detect abnormal cells in the cervix before they become cancerous. In addition to the Pap test, healthcare professionals often perform HPV tests to check for HPV, one of the leading causes of cervical cancer.

STRUCTURE AND PHYSIOLOGIC CHARACTERISTICS

The external female genitalia, known collectively as the vulva, are shown in Fig. 19.1. The *vulva* consists of the mons veneris, the labia majora, the labia minora, the clitoris, the vestibule and its glands, the urethral meatus, the fourchette, and the perineum. The *mons veneris* is a rounded prominence of fat tissue overlying the pubic symphysis. The *labia majora* are two large skinfolds that form the lateral boundaries of the vulva. They meet anteriorly at the mons veneris to form the anterior commissure. The labia majora and the mons veneris have hair follicles and sebaceous glands. The labia majora correspond to the scrotum in the man. The *labia minora* are two narrow, pigmented

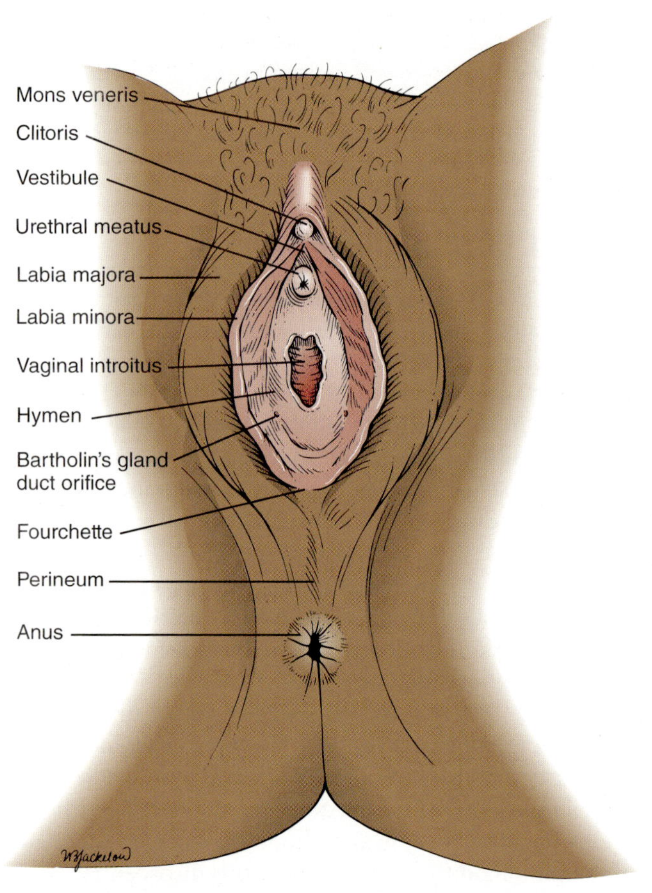

Fig. 19.1 The External Female Genitalia.

skinfolds that lie between the labia majora and enclose the *vestibule,* which is the area lying between the labia minora.

Anteriorly, the two labia minora join to form the prepuce of the *clitoris.* The clitoris, analogous to the penis, consists of erectile tissue and a rich supply of nerve endings. It has a glans, two corpora cavernosa (the body), and the crura. The crura are attached to the undersurface of the pubic ramus and are covered by the ischiocavernosus muscles. The external *urethral meatus* is located in the anterior portion of the vestibule below the clitoris. Paraurethral glands, or *Skene glands,* are small glands that open lateral to the urethra. Secretion of sebaceous glands in this area protects the vulnerable tissues against urine. The major vestibular glands are known as *Bartholin glands* or vulvovaginal glands. These pea-sized glands correspond to the male Cowper glands. Each Bartholin gland lies posterolaterally to the vaginal orifice. During sexual intercourse, a watery fluid is secreted that serves as a vaginal lubricant. Posteriorly, the labia minora unite at the posterior commissure to form the *fourchette.* The *perineum* is the area between the fourchette and the anus.

If the labia minora are reflected laterally, the vaginal introitus and hymenal ring are exposed. The *hymen* is a circular fold of tissue that partially occludes the *vaginal introitus.* There are marked variations in its size, as well as in the number of openings in it. The vaginal introitus is the border between the external and internal genitalia and is located in the lower portion of the vestibule.

The majority of the vulva is innervated by the pudendal nerve, with the exception of the area anterior to the urethral meatus, which is innervated by the ilioinguinal and genitofemoral nerves. The blood supply to the external genitalia and perineum is predominantly from the internal pudendal arteries. The lymphatic drainage is into the superficial and deep inguinal nodes.

The internal genitalia are shown in Fig. 19.2. The *vagina* is a muscularly walled, hollow canal that passes upward and slightly backward, at a right angle to the uterus. The vagina lies between the urinary bladder anteriorly and the rectum posteriorly. The vaginal walls are lined by transverse rugae, or folds. The lower portion of the cervix projects into the upper portion of the vagina and divides it into four fornices. The anterior fornix is shallow and is just posterior to the bladder. The posterior fornix is deep and is just anterior to the rectovaginal pouch, known as the *cul-de-sac (pouch) of Douglas*, and the pelvic viscera lie immediately above this pouch. The lateral fornices contain the broad ligaments. The fallopian tubes and ovaries may be palpated in the lateral fornices. The superficial cells of the vagina contain glycogen, which is acted on by the normal vaginal flora to produce lactic acid. This is in part responsible for the resistance of the vagina to infection.

The arterial supply to the vagina is derived from the internal iliac, uterine, and middle hemorrhoidal arteries. The lymphatic channels of the lower third of the vagina drain into the inguinal nodes. The lymphatic channels of the upper two-thirds enter the hypogastric and sacral nodes.

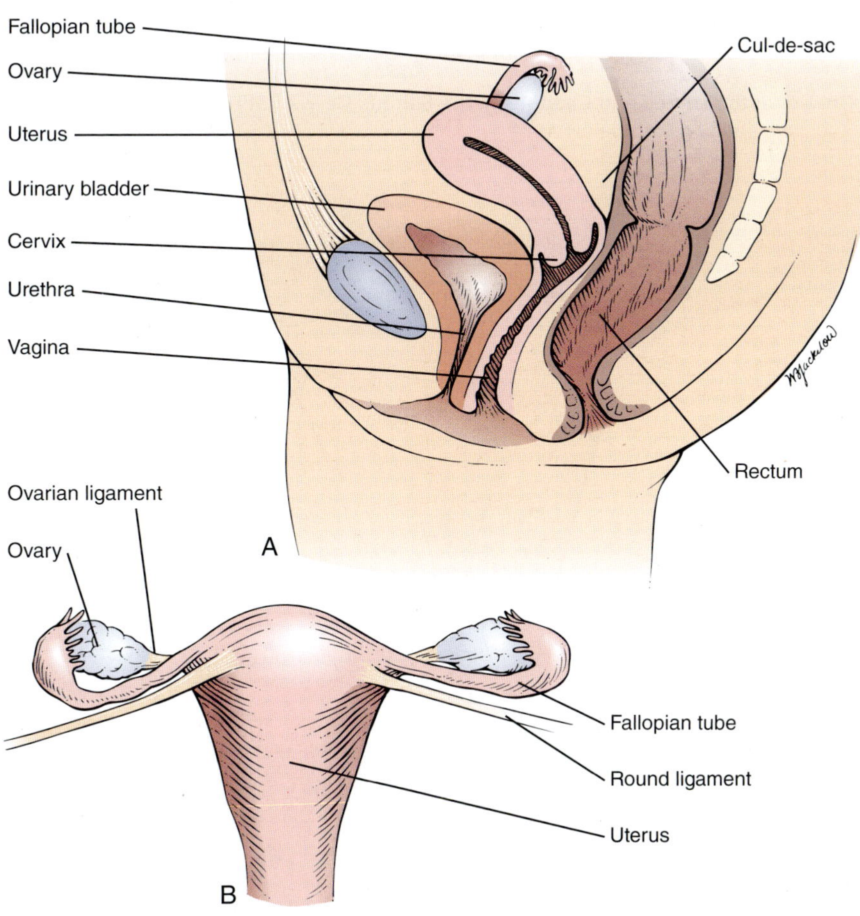

Fig. 19.2 (A) Cross-sectional view of the internal female genitalia. (B) Frontal view of the uterus, fallopian tubes, and ovaries.

The *uterus* is a hollow muscular organ with a small central cavity. The lower end is the *cervix,* and the upper portion is the *fundus.* The size of the uterus is different during various stages of life. At birth, the uterus is only 3 to 4 cm long. The adult uterus is 7 to 8 cm long and 3.5 cm wide, with an average wall thickness of 2 to 3 cm. The growth of the uterus and the relationship of the size of the fundus to the size of the cervix are shown in Fig. 19.3.

The triangular uterine cavity is 6 to 7 cm in length and is bounded by the *internal cervical os* inferiorly and the entrances of the fallopian tubes superiorly. The uterus can be anteverted, axial, or retroverted in position related to the axis extending from cervix to the uterine fundus. The uterine fundus may also be folded forward (anteflexed) or backward (retroflexed).

The uterus is freely mobile and is located centrally in the pelvic cavity. It is supported by the broad and uterosacral ligaments, as well as by the pelvic floor. The peritoneum covers the fundus anteriorly down to the level of the internal cervical os. Posteriorly, the peritoneum covers the uterus down to the pouch of Douglas. Fig. 19.4 is a detailed anatomic representation of the uterus.

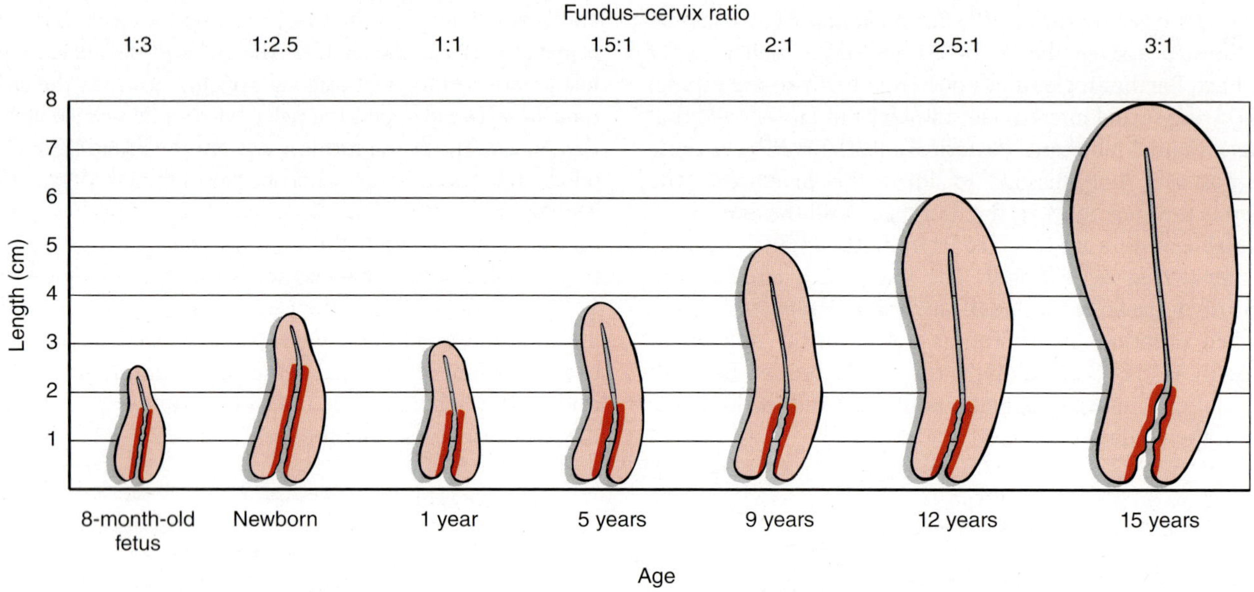

Fig. 19.3 Growth of the Uterus and Changes in the Fundus-Cervix Ratio With Development. The darker red area represents the length of the cervix.

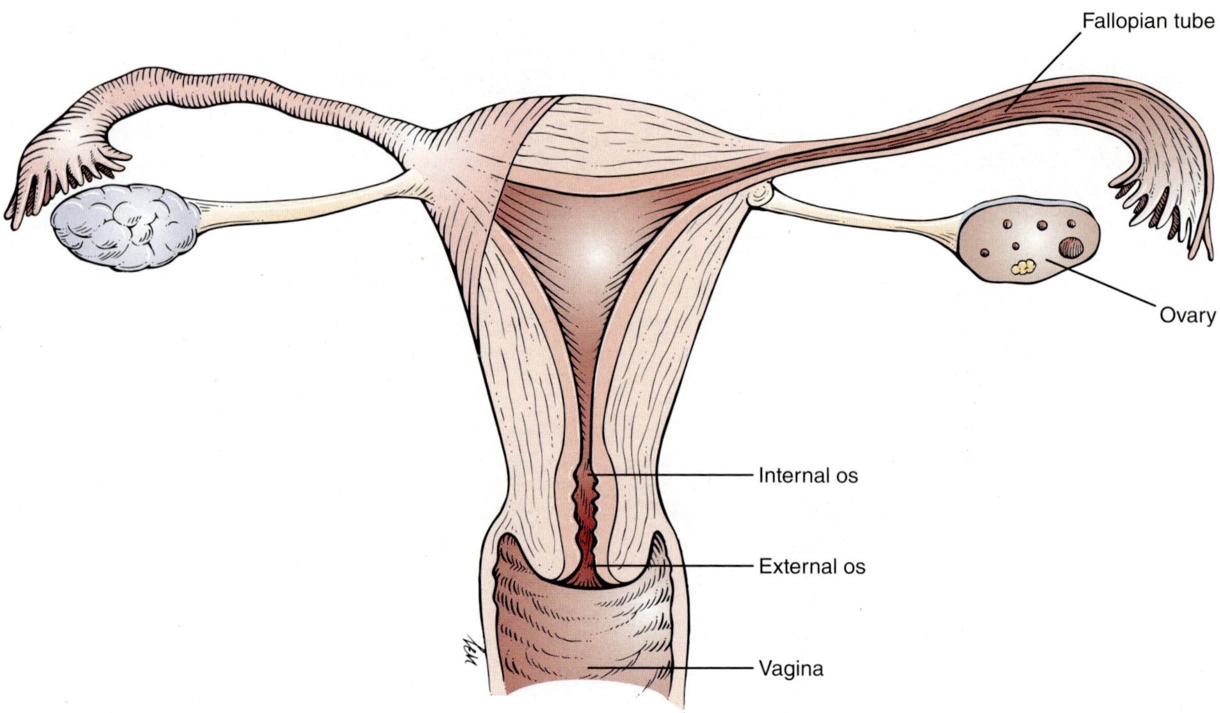

Fig. 19.4 Anatomy of the Uterus.

The cervix is the vaginal portion of the uterus. The greater portion of the cervix has no peritoneal covering. The cervical canal extends from the *external cervical os* to the internal cervical os, where it continues into the endometrial cavity up to the fundus of the uterus. The external cervical os in females who have not given birth vaginally is small and circular. In females who have had vaginal deliveries, the external cervical os is linear or oval.

With increasing levels of estrogens, the external cervical os begins to dilate, and cervical mucous secretion becomes clear and watery. With high levels of estrogens, cervical mucus, when placed between two glass slides that are then pulled apart, can be stretched 15 to 20 cm before breaking. This property of cervical mucus—the ability to be drawn into a fine thread—is termed *spinnbarkeit.* When cervical mucus is allowed to dry on a glass slide and is examined under low power by light microscopy, a *fern pattern* made up of salt crystals may be seen. Spinnbarkeit and *ferning* reach a maximum at the midpoint of the menstrual cycle. Sperm can more easily penetrate mucus with these characteristics.

The blood supply to the uterus comes from the uterine and ovarian arteries. The lymphatic vessels of the fundus enter into the lumbar nodes.

The *fallopian tubes,* or *oviducts,* enter the fundus at its superior aspect. They are small muscular tubes that extend outward into the broad ligament toward the pelvic wall. The other end of the oviduct opens into the peritoneal cavity near the ovary. These endings are surrounded by fringe-shaped projections called *fimbriae.* The primary function of the fallopian tube is to provide a conduit for the egg to convey it from the corresponding ovary to the uterus, a trip that takes several days. Sperm traverse the fallopian tube in the opposite direction, and it is usually in the fallopian tube that fertilization takes place.

The *ovaries* are almond-shaped structures about 3 to 4 cm long and are attached to the broad ligament. The blood supply to the ovaries arises from the ovarian arteries from the abdominal aorta; while the left ovarian vein drains into the left renal vein and the right ovarian vein drains directly into the inferior vena cava. The primary functions of the ovary are oogenesis and hormone production.

The ovaries, fallopian tubes, and supporting ligaments are termed the *adnexa.*

The female reproductive system is under the influence of the hypothalamus, whose releasing factors control the secretion of the anterior pituitary gonadotropic hormones: *follicle-stimulating hormone* and *luteinizing hormone.* In response to these hormones, the ovarian Graafian follicle secretes estrogens and discharges its ovum. After ovulation, the ovarian follicle is termed the *corpus luteum,* which secretes estrogens and progesterone. With the secretion of progesterone, the basal body temperature rises. This is a reliable sign of ovulation. Under the influence of the ovarian hormones, the uterus and breasts undergo the characteristic changes of the menstrual cycle.

If pregnancy does not occur, the corpus luteum regresses, and the level of ovarian hormones begins to fall. At this time, before menstruation, many females have symptoms of weakness, depression, and irritability. Breast tenderness is also common. These symptoms are termed *premenstrual syndrome.* Approximately 5 days after the fall in the level of hormones, the menstrual period begins. Menstrual fluid throughout the 5-day period measures 50 to 150 mL, only half of which is blood; the remainder is mucus. Because menstrual blood does not contain fibrin, it does not clot. When the menstrual flow is heavy, as it is on days 1 to 2, "clots" may be described. These clots are not fibrin clots but are combinations of red blood cells, glycoproteins, and mucoid substances that are believed to form in the vagina rather than in the uterine cavity.

Some of the hormone-dependent changes related to the menstrual cycle are shown in Fig. 19.5.

Approximately 1.5 years before puberty, gonadotropins are measurable in the urine. The ovaries enter a period of rapid growth at, on average, 8 to 9 years of age, which marks the onset of puberty. Secretion of estrogens begins to increase rapidly at approximately 11 years of age. Concomitant with estrogen production, the sexual organs begin to mature. During puberty, the secondary sex characteristics begin to develop. The breasts enlarge, hair develops on the pubis, the vulva enlarges, the labia minora become pigmented, and the body contour changes. Puberty lasts for 4 to 5 years. The first menstrual cycle, called *menarche,* occurs at the end of puberty at approximately 12.5 years of age. There is, however, a wide variation in the age at menarche. The cycles continue approximately every 28 days, with a flow lasting 3 to 5 days. The first day of the period is designated the first day of the cycle. It is rare for cycles to be absolutely regular, and cycles of 21 to 35 days are considered normal.

At the time of menarche, the menstrual cycle is usually anovulatory[b] and irregular. After 1 to 2 years, ovulation begins. After stabilization of the menses, ovulation occurs approximately midcycle in those with a regular cycle.

Menopause marks the ends of menstruation. *Menopause* is defined as the last uterine bleeding induced by ovarian function. It usually occurs between 45 and 55 years of age. Ovulation and corpus luteum formation no longer occur, and the ovaries decrease in size. The period after menopause is termed *postmenopausal.*

THE OBGYN HISTORY

Even in the absence of specific symptoms, all OBGYN patients, regardless of age, should be asked several important questions to provide a complete gynecologic, obstetric, and reproductive history. A comprehensive gynecologic history includes the following basic information: sex recorded at birth, menstrual history, obstetric history, sexual history, types of contraception (past and present), pap smear history, history of sexually transmitted infections (STIs), history of gynecology-related problems (such as PCOS, fibroids, and ovarian cysts), a gynecologic specific review of symptoms, and screening for intimate partner violence. It is always important to remember to use nonmedical terminology when taking a history.

[b]Not accompanied by the release of an ovum from the ovaries.

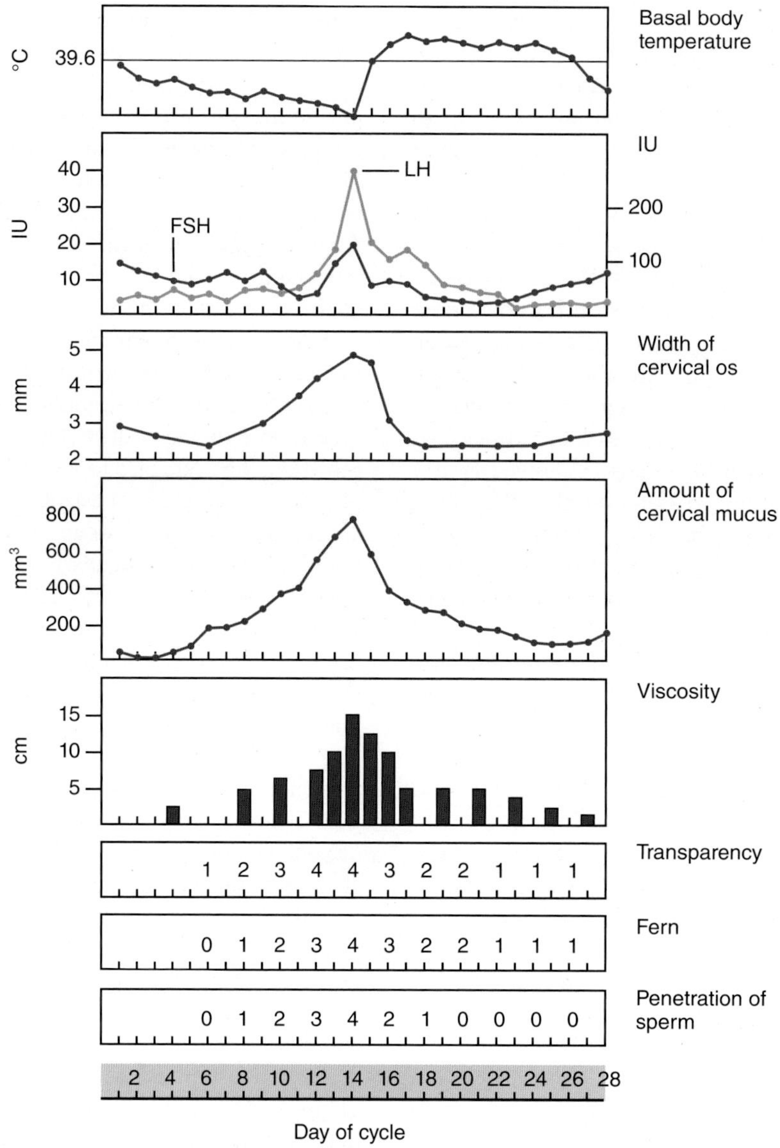

Fig. 19.5 Physiologic Changes Associated With the Menstrual Cycle. The numbers 0 to 4 indicate an increasing characteristic of cervical mucus. Notice that ferning, transparency, and penetration of sperm are maximal at midcycle. *FSH,* Follicle-stimulating hormone; *IU,* International units; *LH,* luteinizing hormone.

Sex Recorded at Birth

At birth, the sex (male or female) is recorded, most often based on the infant's anatomical and other biological characteristics. Sometimes referred to as birth sex, natal sex, gender assignment, biological sex, or sex; however, *sex recorded at birth* is the recommended term. This is what appears on the birth certificate.

Menstrual History

A menstrual history should begin by summarizing the age at menarche, the cycle length, and the duration of bleeding. If menarche was reached at age 12 years, periods are regular every 29 days lasting for 5 days, the menstrual history is written as "12 × 29 × 5." Examples of questions to use to elicit a menstrual history include:

"Are you having periods?"

"At what age did you start getting your period?"

"When was the first day of your last menstrual period (LMP)?"

"How often do your periods occur?"

"Are they regular?"

"How many days does the bleeding last?"

"How many pads or tampons do you use on the heaviest day of your period?"

"During your period, do you experience any menstrual cramps? Mood swings? Breast tenderness or breast pain? Bloating? Swelling? Headache?"

"Do you have any bleeding between periods?"

"Do you have any bleeding after intercourse?" (postcoital bleeding)

"Have you had any episodes of bleeding since stopping your periods?" (postmenopausal patients)

Obstetric History

The obstetric history includes the number of total pregnancies regardless of outcome, known as *gravidity,* and the number of

pregnancies reaching 20 weeks or beyond, known as *parity*. Parity is further broken down to:
t—term pregnancies (37 to 42 weeks)
p—preterm pregnancies (20 to <37 weeks)
a—spontaneous or induced abortions and ectopic pregnancies
l—live children.

Gravidity and parity are typically written as such: G# P *t-p-a-l*. For example: a female who has two children (one born at term, one born at 34 weeks), a history of an ectopic pregnancy and two miscarriages in the first trimester, and is currently pregnant would have a gravidity/parity representation of **G6 P1132**. A second example: a patient with a history of two prior full-term children and a 22-week miscarriage would have a gravidity/parity representation of **G3 P2102**.

When asking about abortions or miscarriages, it is advisable to keep in mind that in the United States, and in some other countries, the word "abortion" itself may be charged with many religious, political, and cultural feelings in different patients. Maintain sensitivity while asking the question, reminding the patient, if necessary, that the medical term "abortion" means loss of any pregnancy, including voluntary terminations, ectopic pregnancy, or spontaneous miscarriage.

Examples of questions for obtaining an obstetric history include:
"Have you ever been pregnant?"
"Do you have a history of any miscarriages, abortions, or ectopic pregnancies?" or *"What was the outcome of your pregnancies?"* (preferable)
"How were these pregnancies treated? Did you take medication or did you need surgery?"
"For each delivery, what was the date of delivery? How many weeks pregnant were you when you delivered?"
"Did you have any complications during your delivery?"
"Did you have any complications during your pregnancy, such has high blood pressure or diabetes?"
"Did any of your children have complications after delivery?"

Sexual History

Discussing sexual health with a patient can be very challenging for both the patient and the healthcare professional. A great majority of females with sexual concerns report that they are not asked about sexual health during medical visits, and if sexual health is discussed during their encounter, the conversation is initiated by the patient. Healthcare professionals should become comfortable asking open-ended questions about a patient's sexual habits at an initial visit, an annual visit, and when there is concern for an STI or sexual dysfunction disorder. Examples of questions for obtaining a sexual history include:
"Are you currently sexually active?" If yes, *"In the past 6 months, how many sexual partners have you had? In the past 12 months?"*
"When you are sexually active, are your partners male, female, or both?"
"What kind of sexual contact do you have? Genital? Anal? Oral?" (Ask for both male and female partners)
"Do you use any type of contraception?"
"Do you use any barrier protection to protect against STIs?" (Male/female condoms)
"Every time, most times, sometimes?"
If no to contraception and condoms, *"Are you trying to become pregnant?"*
If no contraception and not trying to conceive, *"Do you want to discuss contraception today?"*
"Do you (or any partners?) have a history of any STIs, such as herpes, HIV, gonorrhea, and chlamydia?" (Listing infections specifically can trigger patient's memory)
"When were you last tested for STIs?"
"Do you ever experience pain with intercourse? Pain on insertion, deep pelvic pain, etc."
"Do you have concerns about sexual function, like ability to achieve an orgasm? Changes in sexual desire or arousal? Or satisfaction during sex?"
"Do you feel safe in your sexual relationships?"

REVIEW OF SPECIFIC SYMPTOMS

The most common symptoms of female genitourinary disease are as follows:

- Abnormal (uterine/vaginal) bleeding
- Dysmenorrhea (painful menses)
- Masses or lesions
- Vaginal discharge
- Vaginal itching
- Abdominal or pelvic pain
- Dyspareunia (pain with intercourse)
- Changes in hair distribution
- Changes in urinary pattern
- Infertility

Abnormal (Uterine/Vaginal) Bleeding

Ask these questions in the setting of abnormal vaginal bleeding:
"How long have you noticed the vaginal bleeding?"
"Do you use contraceptives?" If yes, *"What types of contraceptives do you use?"*
"Are your periods regular or irregular?"
"How often are your periods?"
"How many days do your periods last?"
"How many tampons or pads do you use on the heaviest days of your period?"
"Are there any clots of blood?"
"What was the first day of your last period?"
"Have you noticed bleeding between your periods?"
"Do you have abdominal/pelvic pain during your periods?"
"Do you have hot flashes? Cold sweats?"
"Do you think you might be pregnant?"
"Have you ever been pregnant before?" If yes, *"Tell me about all of your pregnancies."*
"Are you under any unusual emotional stress?"
"Have you noticed that you were warm in a room and others were not? Have you noticed that you were cold in a room and others were not?"
"Have you noticed a change in your vision?"
"Have you had any headaches? Nausea? Change in hair pattern? Milk discharge from your nipples?"
"What is your diet like?"

Abnormal uterine bleeding (AUB) is classified by the bleeding pattern and its underlying cause. In 2011, a new classification system was introduced to characterize AUB.[3] AUB can be due to structural or nonstructural causes. Examples of structural causes of AUB include endometrial polyps, adenomyosis, leiomyomas, and endometrial hyperplasia and carcinoma. Nonstructural causes of AUB include coagulopathies, ovulatory dysfunction, or idiopathic causes.

The term *menorrhagia* has now been replaced with *heavy menstrual bleeding (AUB/HMB)* and is excessive bleeding at the time of the menstrual period. The flow may be increased, the duration may be increased, or both may occur. The number of pads or tampons a patient uses each day of the cycle helps quantify the flow. AUB/HMB in some cases may be associated with blood disorders such as leukemia, inherited clotting abnormalities, and decreased platelet states. Uterine fibroids are a leading cause of AUB/HMB. *Metrorrhagia* is now described as *intermenstrual bleeding (AUB/IMB)* and is uterine bleeding of normal amount at irregular, noncyclic intervals, particularly between normal menstrual cycles. Foreign bodies such as intrauterine devices, as well as uterine or cervical polyps, and ovarian and uterine tumors, can cause AUB/IMB. Often there is increased bleeding between cycles as well as heavier periods; this is described as *heavy and IMB,* previously known as *menometrorrhagia.*

Amenorrhea is the cessation or nonappearance of menstruation. Before puberty, amenorrhea is physiologic, as it is during pregnancy and after menopause. In primary amenorrhea, menstruation has never occurred; in secondary amenorrhea, menstruation has occurred but has ceased, as in pregnancy. Long-distance joggers, patients with anorexia or with abnormally low body fat may have secondary amenorrhea. Diseases of the hypothalamus, pituitary gland, ovary, uterus, and thyroid gland are associated with amenorrhea. *Galactorrhea,* or milk discharge from the nipples, occurs in many individuals with pituitary tumors. Chronic disease is also frequently associated with secondary amenorrhea.

Menopause is typically defined as having no menstrual cycle for 12 months. Bleeding that occurs after this 12-month time period is termed *postmenopausal bleeding.* Because many cancers of reproductive organs may present with bleeding, any postmenopausal bleeding must be investigated. Uterine fibroids or tumors of the cervix, uterus, or ovary may be responsible. Lower genital tract disease, such as vaginal atrophy, or even urinary tract problems may present with postmenopausal bleeding.

Dysmenorrhea

Dysmenorrhea, or painful menstruation, is a common symptom. It is often difficult to define as abnormal because many healthy females have some degree of menstrual discomfort. Typically, this pain should subside soon after the commencement of the menstrual flow. There are two types of dysmenorrhea: primary and secondary. Primary dysmenorrhea is far more common. It begins shortly after menarche, is associated with colicky uterine contractions, and occurs with every period. Childbirth frequently alleviates this state permanently. Secondary dysmenorrhea is caused by acquired disorders within the uterine cavity (e.g., intrauterine devices, polyps, or fibroids), obstruction to flow (e.g., cervical stenosis), or disorders of the pelvic peritoneum (e.g., endometriosis[c] or pelvic inflammatory disease [PID]). It usually occurs after several years of painless periods. Regardless of its cause, dysmenorrhea is described as intermittent, crampy pain accompanying the menstrual flow. The pain is felt in the lower abdomen and back, sometimes radiating down the legs. In severe cases, fainting, nausea, or vomiting may occur.

Masses or Lesions

Masses or lesions of the external genitalia are common. They may be related to STIs, cysts, skin changes, pre-malignancies, or cancerous lesions. Ask these questions in the setting of a lesion on the genitalia:

"When did you first notice the mass (lesion)?"
"Has it changed since you first noticed it?"
"Have you ever had it before?"
"Is it painful?" "Is it itchy?"
"Are you sexually active?" If yes, *"When was the last time you engaged in sexual activity?"*
"Have you been exposed to anyone with a known STI?"

Syphilis may result in a chancre on the labia (see Fig. 19.33). Often unnoticed, it is a small, painless ulcer with a sharply demarcated border. Small, acutely painful ulcers may be chancroid (see Fig. 19.34) or genital herpes (see Fig. 19.32). A patient with an abscess of Bartholin gland (see Fig. 19.17) may present with an extremely tender mass in the vulva. Benign lesions, such as genital warts (condylomata acuminate; see Figs. 19.14 and 19.15), and malignant conditions manifest as a mass on the external genitalia.

Some affected patients are concerned of a sensation of fullness or mass in the pelvis, incontinence, and sexual dysfunction as a result of pelvic organ prolapse. *Pelvic organ prolapse* refers to the descent or protrusion of the vaginal walls, cervix, or uterus into the vagina or through the vaginal introitus. This is caused by a weakening of the pelvic support ligaments. The anterior vaginal wall can descend, producing a *cystocele* that triggers urinary symptoms such as frequency and stress incontinence. The posterior vaginal wall can descend, producing a *rectocele,* which triggers bowel symptoms such as constipation, tenesmus, or incontinence. The uterus can also descend, which results in uterine prolapse. In the most severe state, the uterus may lie outside the vulva with complete vaginal inversion, a condition known as *procidentia.* The consequences of pelvic organ prolapse are discussed further in the section titled "Clinicopathologic Correlations" later in this chapter.

Vaginal Discharge

Vaginal discharge is a common concern. Is there an associated foul odor? Although a whitish discharge is often normally present, a malodorous discharge often indicates a pathologic problem. The most common pathologic odor, associated with bacterial vaginosis, is a foul, fishy odor related to the volatilization of amines that

[c]Endometriosis is the presence of endometrial tissue outside the uterus and is a common cause of chronic pelvic pain.

TABLE 19.1 Characteristics of Common Vaginal Discharges

Feature	Physiologic Discharge	Nonspecific Vaginitis	*Trichomonas*	*Candida*	Gonococcal
Color	White	Gray	Grayish-yellow	White	Greenish-yellow
Fishy odor	Absent	Present	Present	Absent	Absent
Consistency	Nonhomogeneous	Homogeneous	Purulent, often with bubbles	Cottage cheese–like	Mucopurulent
Location	Dependent	Adherent to walls	Often pooled in fornix	Adherent to walls	Adherent to walls
Discharge at introitus	Rare	Common	Common	Common	Common
Vulva	Normal	Normal	Usually normal	Erythematous	Erythematous
Vaginal mucosa	Normal	Normal	Usually normal	Erythematous	Normal
Cervix	Normal	Normal	May have red spots	Has patches of discharge	Has pus in os

are produced by anaerobic metabolism of a variety of bacteria. Is itching also present? Patients with candidiasis are concerned of intense pruritus and a white, dry discharge that looks like cottage cheese. Has the patient recently taken any medications, such as antibiotics? Antibiotics change the normal vaginal flora, and an overgrowth of *Candida* may result. Table 19.1 summarizes the important characteristics of vaginal discharge.

Vaginal Itching

Vaginal and vulvar itching is often associated with infections, glycosuria,[d] vulvar dermatitis, vulvar dystrophies, or vulvar neoplasia. Pruritus may also be a symptom of a systemic disease, such as Crohn disease.

An example of a vulvar dystrophy is *lichen sclerosus,* a relatively common condition in which the genital skin shows a uniform reddened, smooth, shiny, almost transparent appearance. It is a destructive inflammatory condition with a predilection for genital skin. It is much more common in females, although it can be seen in males with involvement of the glans penis and foreskin. Whitish atrophic patches of thin skin are typical, as is fine crinkling of the skin. Pruritus is a common symptom, and the fragile skin is susceptible to secondary infection. Although most common in White and Hispanic postmenopausal patients, lichen sclerosus may be seen in patients of all ages. It is rare in Black females. Lichen sclerosus should be thought of as a premalignant lesion because one complication is the development of squamous cell carcinoma. Fig. 19.6 shows an early stage of lichen sclerosus in a female patient. Notice the resorption of the labia minora; the clitoris is preserved. Fig. 19.7 shows a later stage in another patient. Notice the classic whitish crinkling of the skin and the resorption of the labia and clitoris. Fig. 19.8 shows vulvar squamous cell carcinoma with the background of lichen sclerosus in another patient.

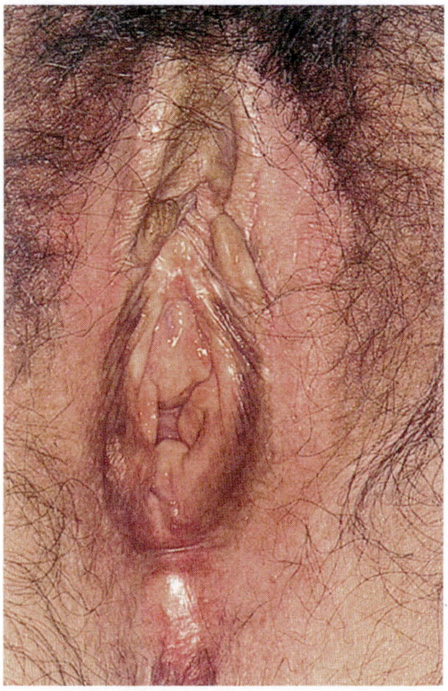

Fig. 19.6 **Lichen Sclerosus, Early Stage.** (From Leibowitch M, Staughton R, Neill S, et al: *An Atlas of Vulval Disease: A Combined Dermatological, Gynecological and Venereological Approach,* ed 2, London, 1997, Mosby.)

Pelvic Pain

Ask the following questions, in addition to those listed in Chapter 17, The Abdomen, in the setting of pelvic pain:

"How long have you been experiencing the pain?"
"What was the first day of your last menstrual period?"
"Are you using any contraceptives?" If no, *"Could you be pregnant?"*
"Do you notice the pain at any particular time of your menstrual cycle?"
"Are you sexually active?" If yes, *"When were you last sexually active?"*
"Is the pain related to intercourse?"
"Have you been sexually active with a partner with any known STIs?"
"Do you have abnormal vaginal discharge?"
"Do you experience a burning sensation when you urinate?"

Pelvic pain may be acute or chronic. Is the patient pregnant? Acute abdominal pain may be a complication of pregnancy. Spontaneous abortion, uterine perforation, and ectopic tubal pregnancy all are life-threatening situations. Acute inflammation, or PID, is caused by vaginal bacteria, such as gonorrhea, chlamydia, or bacterial vaginosis, moving from the vagina to the uterus, fallopian tubes, and ovaries. Acute lower pelvic pain localized to one side that occurs at the time of ovulation is termed *mittelschmerz.* This pain is related to a small amount of

[d]High levels of glucose in the urine, as in diabetes.

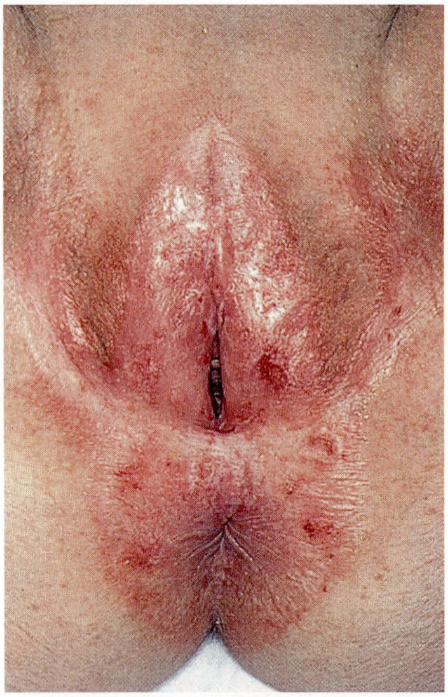

Fig. 19.7 **Lichen Sclerosus, Later Stage.** Note the classic whitish crinkling of the skin and resorption of the labia and clitoris. (From Leibowitch M, Staughton R, Neill S, et al: *An Atlas of Vulval Disease: A Combined Dermatological, Gynecological and Venereological Approach*, ed 2, London, 1997, Mosby.)

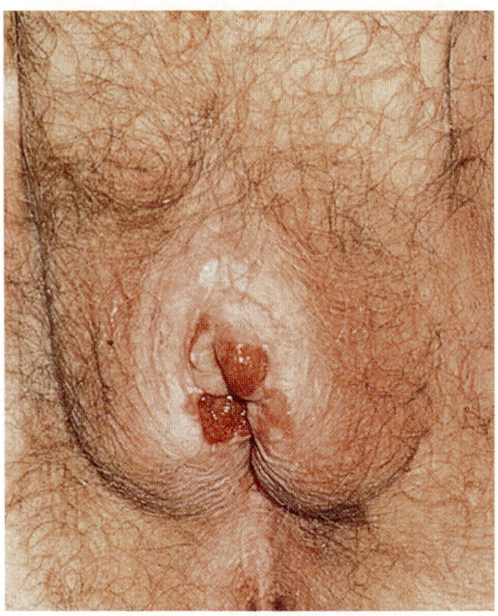

Fig. 19.8 **Squamous Cell Carcinoma With Background of Lichen Sclerosus.** (From Leibowitch M, Staughton R, Neill S, et al: *An Atlas of Vulval Disease: A Combined Dermatological, Gynecological and Venereological Approach*, ed 2, London, 1997, Mosby.)

intraperitoneal bleeding at the time of ovum release. Urinary tract infection may also cause acute suprapubic pain. Patients with urinary tract infections usually have associated urinary symptoms of burning sensation or frequency.

Chronic pelvic pain may result from ectopic endometrial tissue known as endometriosis, chronic PID, and fibroids, as well as from non-gynecologic causes such as interstitial cystitis, inflammatory bowel disease, musculoskeletal conditions, and psychological factors.

Dyspareunia

Dyspareunia is pain during or after sexual intercourse. To aid in the evaluation and diagnosis of dyspareunia, dyspareunia should be categorized as pain with insertion, vaginal pain, or deep pelvic pain during intercourse. Causes of pain with insertion may include vulvovaginal infections or dystrophies and vaginismus. *Vaginismus* is a condition of severe pelvic pain and involuntary spasm when there is any attempt at penetration. Patients with this condition may have a history of depression/anxiety, or trauma or abuse, and may require psychological therapy or couples therapy with desensitization to overcome this problem. Mid-vaginal pain is usually attributed to a lack of lubrication during intercourse. This can be alleviated with the use of lubricants during intercourse, or vaginal estrogen cream if there is vaginal atrophy present. Patients with sexual dysfunction, particularly arousal disorders, may also experience a lack of genital lubrication during intercourse. This is often treated symptomatically with lubricants and vaginal estrogen in the case of atrophy. Deep pelvic pain during intercourse is often due to endometriosis, PID, interstitial cystitis, irritable bowel syndrome, or a history of sexual abuse.

Changes in Hair Distribution

Hair loss or change in hair distribution may occur during certain states of hormonal imbalance. *Hirsutism* is an excessive growth of hair on the upper lip, face, earlobes, upper pubic triangle, trunk, or limbs. *Virilization* is extensive hirsutism associated with receding temporal hair, a deepening of the voice, and clitoral enlargement. Increased androgen production by the adrenal glands or ovaries may be responsible for these phenomena. Tumors of the ovary are commonly associated with amenorrhea, rapidly developing hirsutism and virilization. Polycystic ovarian disease is the most common ovarian cause of hirsutism, AUB, infertility, acne, and obesity. Fig. 19.9 shows the increased

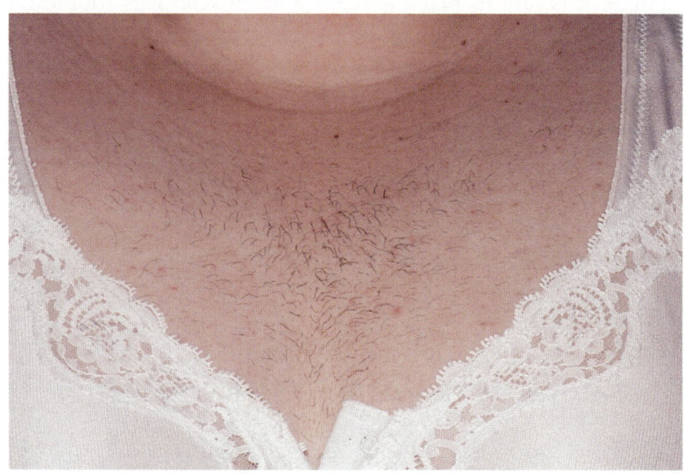

Fig. 19.9 **Increased Hair Growth in a Patient With Polycystic Ovary Syndrome.** (From Hordinsky MK, Sawaya ME, Scher RK: *Atlas of Hair and Nails*, Philadelphia, 2000, Churchill Livingstone.)

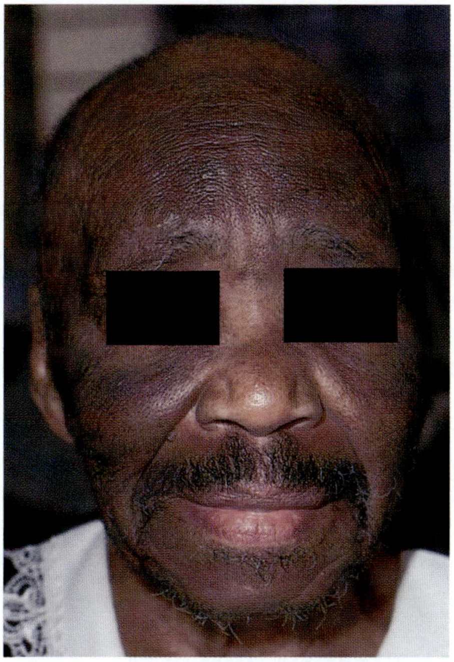

Fig. 19.10 Increased Hair Growth in a Patient With an Androgen-Secreting Ovarian Tumor. (From Hordinsky MK, Sawaya ME, Scher RK: *Atlas of Hair and Nails*, Philadelphia, 2000, Churchill Livingstone.)

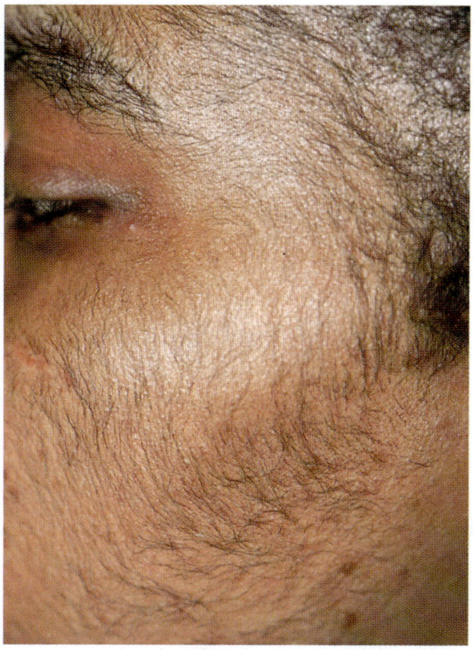

Fig. 19.11 Increased Hair Growth Caused by Minoxidil Antihypertensive Therapy. (From Hordinsky MK, Sawaya ME, Scher RK: *Atlas of Hair and Nails*, Philadelphia, 2000, Churchill Livingstone.)

hair growth on the chest of a 34-year-old female with PCOS. They also presented with amenorrhea and obesity. Fig. 19.10 shows the face of a 68-year-old female with an androgen-secreting ovarian tumor. Note the male-pattern baldness and the facial hair. This patient also had clitoral enlargement.

It is important to determine whether the patient is taking any medications. Several drugs such as cyclosporine, minoxidil, diazoxide, penicillamine, and glucocorticoids have the unexpected side effect of causing diffuse hair growth on the face. Fig. 19.11 shows such growth in a 42-year-old female who was taking minoxidil for hypertension. This drug is now used as a topical treatment for androgenic alopecia. The pathophysiologic process behind the increased hair growth is unknown.

Hair loss, or *alopecia,* is a distressing problem. Many drugs may have a profound effect on hair growth. The interviewer must inquire whether the patient has taken any chemotherapeutic agents or has been exposed to radiation. Different areas of the head seem to respond differently to androgens. The top and front of the scalp respond to increased androgen production by hair loss, whereas the face responds with increased hair growth. Has the patient been dieting? Because hair has a high metabolic rate, crash diets and infectious diseases reduce the nutrients available for hair growth, and secondary alopecia may result.

Changes in Urinary Pattern

Changes in the patterns of urination are common. Chapter 18, Male Genitalia and Hernias, reviews many of the symptoms associated with changes in the urinary pattern. These symptoms may occur in female patients as well.

Stress incontinence is urinary incontinence that occurs with straining or coughing. Stress incontinence is more common among females than among males. The female urinary bladder and urethra are maintained in position by several muscular and fascial supports. It has been postulated that estrogens may be responsible, at least in part, for a weakening of the pelvic support. With aging, the support of the bladder neck, the length of the urethra, and the competence of the pelvic floor are decreased. Repeated vaginal deliveries, strenuous exercise, and chronic coughing increase the chance for stress incontinence. Ask an affected patient these questions:

"Do you lose your urine on straining? Coughing? Lifting? Laughing?"
"Do you lose your urine constantly?"
"Do you lose small amounts of urine?"
"Are you aware of a full bladder?"
"Do you have to press on your abdomen to void?"
"Are you aware of any weakness in your limbs?"
"Have you ever had a loss of vision?"
"Do you have diabetes?"

Patients with pure stress incontinence describe urine loss without urgency that occurs during any activity that momentarily increases intra-abdominal pressure. Although stress incontinence is common among females, it is important to rule out other types of incontinence, such as neurologic, overflow, and psychogenic. *Neurologic incontinence* may result from cerebral dysfunction, spinal cord disease, and peripheral nerve lesions. Multiple sclerosis is a chronic relapsing neurologic disorder causing urinary incontinence. Most affected individuals suffer from an episode of temporary loss of vision as an early symptom. *Overflow incontinence* occurs when the pressure in the bladder exceeds the urethral pressure in the absence of bladder contraction. This may occur in patients with diabetes and an atonic bladder. In *psychogenic incontinence,* individuals have been known to urinate in bed at night to "warm" themselves or during the daytime in group settings to draw attention to themselves.

Infertility

Infertility is defined as the inability to become pregnant despite unprotected, properly timed intercourse for 12 months below the age of 35 years, or for 6 months over the age of 35 years. During this time, approximately 85% of females conceive. The average time it takes for a female to conceive is 4 to 5 months.

Infertility is not just a female health issue. About 40% of cases are attributed to female-factor infertility,[e] 30% of cases to male-factor infertility, and 30% of cases are of unknown etiology. Male-factor infertility can be caused by vas deferens obstruction, varicocele (see Fig. 18.27), chromosomal defects, testicular infection, autoimmune states, and decreased sperm count. Therefore, a semen analysis is one of the initial components of the infertility evaluation.

Female infertility can be caused by ovulatory dysfunction, diminished ovarian reserve, tubal disease, peritoneal factors (endometriosis, PID), or uterine/cervical abnormalities. The infertility evaluation in the female patient should include a relevant history, including duration of infertility; prior infertility evaluations; menstrual history; pregnancy history; frequency and timing of intercourse; surgical history; history of STI; symptoms pertaining to thyroid disorders; medication history; family history, particularly any known family members with birth defects or developmental delays; and history of toxic habits. A physical exam should include the body mass index (BMI), palpation of the thyroid, breast exam, and a pelvic exam. Care should be taken to look for signs of hyperandrogenism.

IMPACT OF INFERTILITY

The problem of infertility is not new. From ancient times, cultures have practiced fertility rites to ensure the continuation of their people. Many societies considered a female's worth in terms of her ability to have children. These trends continue today where, in some societies, the childless female is frequently stigmatized and marginalized.

According to estimates, around 1 in every 8 couples in the United States faces fertility problems. It is important to note that infertility is a problem that affects both sexes. Previously, it was believed that infertility had no demonstrable organ disorder in 30% to 50% of the cases. However, recent studies suggest that more than 90% of infertile couples have some kind of pathological cause. Nevertheless, only 50% of these couples are able to conceive. Factors contributing to infertility can be attributed to the female partner in one-third of cases, to the male partner in one-third of cases, and to a combination of both partners or unexplained in the remaining one-third of cases.

Infertility is one of several important developmental crises of adult life. Receiving the diagnosis of "infertility" can have profound impact on all aspects of a female's life: physical, emotional/mental, sexual, and financial. The patient may experience anxiety and depression, and if preexisting mental health conditions were present, undergoing evaluation and treatment for infertility may exacerbate these mental health conditions. Infertility can affect a patient's self-identity and self-esteem and riddle them with feelings of guilt, shame, and betrayal. Females may shy away from pregnant family members, friends, or colleagues due to feelings of jealousy or resentment, which can cause social isolation. Couples may experience strain and isolation, as well as a loss of spontaneity and a decrease in sexual desire while undergoing treatment for infertility. Couples may also experience stress and conflict over the financial burden of fertility treatment.

Regardless of the cause of infertility, the treatment must work to lessen the psychological side effects. Both partners must be encouraged to communicate. Education regarding the physical problem is important throughout the medical workup. Communication between the partners and the healthcare professional is paramount. The patient and partner need to be protected from their own insecurities and treated with empathy and compassion.

[e]In general, fallopian tubal patency or ovulation problems.

PHYSICAL EXAMINATION

The equipment necessary for the examination of the female genitalia and rectum consists of a vaginal speculum, lubricant, gloves, liquid media for cytology (which has replaced the traditional Pap smear), cervical scraper and brush, cotton-tipped applicators, glass slides, culture media (as appropriate), tissues, and a light source. A mirror is often handy so that the patient can participate in the examination.

General Considerations

Unlike most other parts of the physical examination, the pelvic examination is often viewed with apprehension by the patient. This is frequently related to a previous bad experience. An examination performed slowly and gently with adequate explanations goes a long way in developing a good doctor–patient relationship. Communication is the key to a successful pelvic examination. The examiner should talk to the patient and tell them exactly what is going to be done. Eye contact is also necessary to decrease the patient's anxiety. The patient's ability to relax enables a more accurate and less traumatic examination.

Regardless of the examiner's gender, the pelvic exam should always be performed in the presence of a female attendant. Although not required by law in all states, the presence of a female attendant is important for assistance, as well as for medicolegal considerations. At times, the patient may request that a family member be present. The examiner should grant such a request if no other attendant is available.

Throughout the world, various patient positions are preferred to facilitate the pelvic examination. These include the lying supine on an examining table, lying in bed on the left side, lying on supine in bed with the legs abducted, and sitting upright in a chair with the legs abducted. In the United States, the patient usually lies on their back on an examination table with their feet in heel rests, known as the dorsolithotomy position. Appropriate draping to ensure the patient's privacy can also ease the patient's apprehension during the pelvic exam.

PREPARATION FOR THE EXAMINATION

See Video 19.1.

The patient should be instructed to empty their bladder and bowels before the examination. The patient is assisted onto an examination table with the buttocks placed near its edge. The heel rests of the table are extended, and the patient is instructed to place their heels in them. If possible, some cloth should be placed over the rests. Alternatively, the patient can be given plastic foam booties to protect the feet from cold metal heel rests. Shortening the heel rest brackets helps the patient bend their knees to lower the position of the cervix. An older patient with osteoarthritis may need the heel rests to be longer because they may have limited hip and knee motion. Offer the patient a mirror that they can use to observe the examination.

The head of the examination table should be elevated so that eye contact between the healthcare professional and the patient can occur. A sheet is usually draped over the lower abdomen and knees of the patient. Some patients prefer not to have the sheet used. The patient should be asked their preference.

The knees are drawn up sufficiently to relax the abdominal muscles as the thighs are abducted. Ask the patient to let their legs fall to the sides or to drop their knees to each side. Never tell a patient to "spread their legs."

Gloves should be worn for the examination of the female genitalia. The examiner should be seated on a stool between the legs of the patient. Good lighting, including a light source directed into the vagina, is essential.

The examination of the female genitalia consists of the following:

- Inspection and palpation of external genitalia
- Examination with speculum
- Bimanual palpation
- Rectovaginal palpation

Inspection and Palpation of External Genitalia

See Video 19.2.

Inspect the External Genitalia and Hair

To make the patient more comfortable during inspection of the external genitalia, it is often useful to tell the patient that they will feel your touch on their leg. Start by placing the *back* of your hand on the patient's inner thigh so they can become more comfortable being touched for the exam.

The external genitalia should be inspected carefully. The mons veneris is inspected for lesions and swelling. The hair is inspected for its pattern and for pubic lice and nits. The skin of the vulva is inspected for redness, excoriation, masses, leukoplakia, and changes in pigmentation. Lesions should be palpated for tenderness.

Inspect the Labia

Tell the patient that you are now going to examine and separate the labia, as demonstrated in Fig. 19.12. Inspect the vaginal introitus.

The labia minora may show wide variation in size and shape; they may be asymmetrical. On occasion, yellowish-white, asymptomatic papules may be seen over the inner labia minora. These are called *Fordyce spots* and are normal; they represent ectopic sebaceous glands. Fig. 19.13 shows Fordyce spots. Ectopic sebaceous glands are also common in the mouth (see Fig. 12.18) and on the shaft of the penis (see Fig. 18.11).

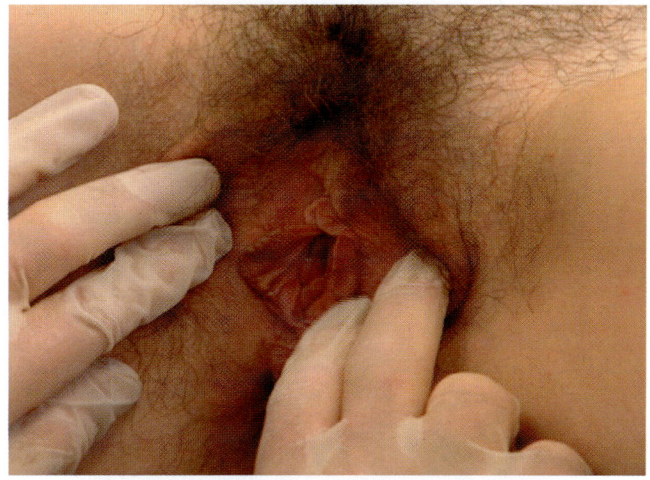

Fig. 19.12 Technique for Inspecting the Labia.

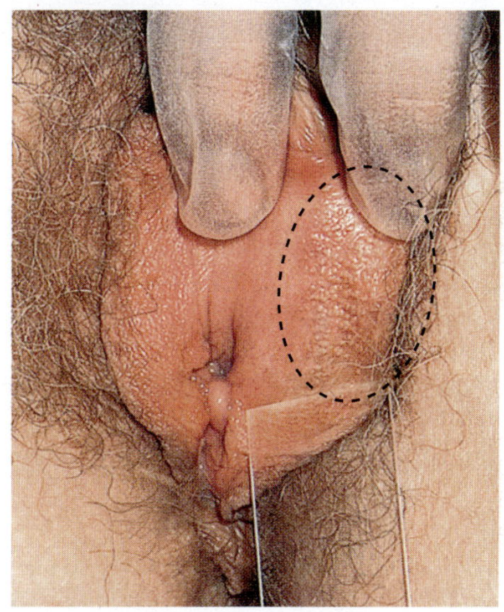

Fig. 19.13 Fordyce Spots of the Labia. (From Leibowitch M, Staughton R, Neill S, et al: *An Atlas of Vulval Disease: A Combined Dermatological, Gynecological and Venereological Approach*, ed 2, London, 1997, Mosby.)

Inflammatory lesions, ulceration, discharge, scarring, warts, trauma, swelling, atrophic changes, and masses are noted. Figs. 19.14 and 19.15 show condylomata acuminata of the labia.

Inspect the Clitoris

Inspect the clitoris for size and lesions. The clitoris is normally 3 to 4 mm in size.

Inspect the Urethral Meatus

Is pus or inflammation present? If pus is present, determine its source. Dip a cotton-tipped applicator into the discharge, send it to the laboratory for culture, and spread some of the sample on a microscope slide for later evaluation. Are any masses present?

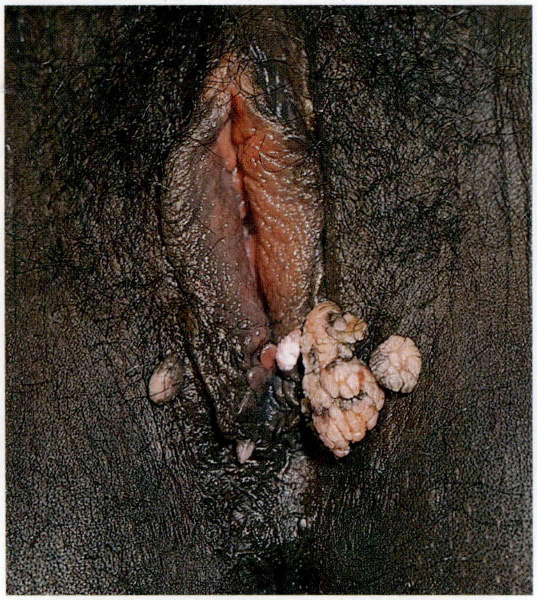

Fig. 19.14 Condylomata Acuminata.

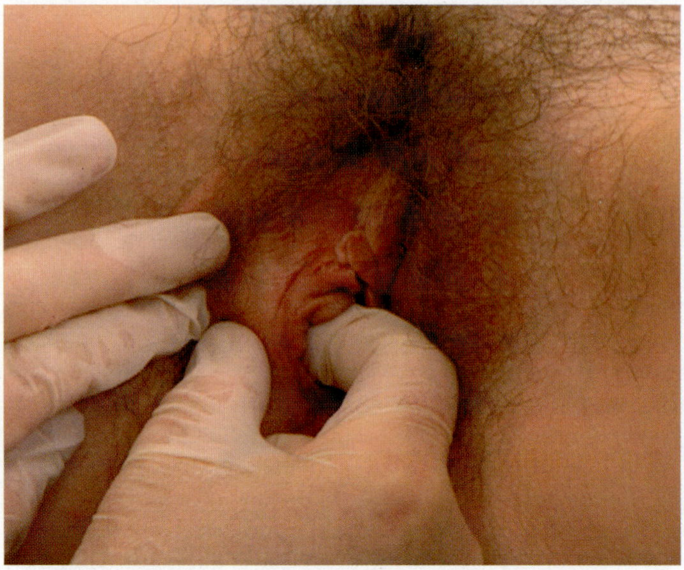

Fig. 19.16 Technique for Palpation of Bartholin Glands.

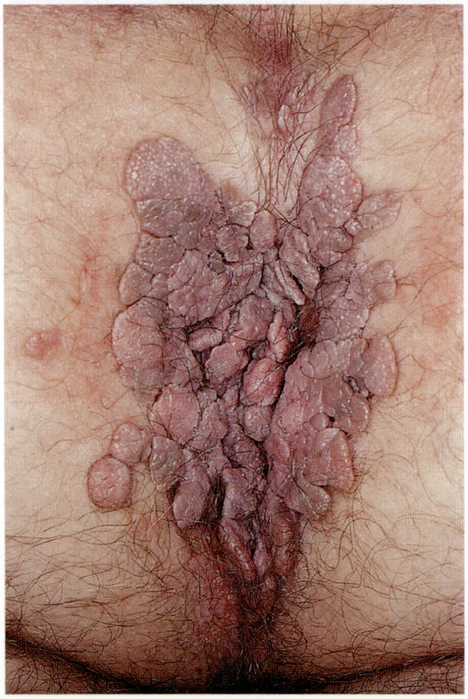

Fig. 19.15 Condylomata Acuminata. (From Callen JP, Paller AS, Greer KE, et al: *Color Atlas of Dermatology*, ed 2, Philadelphia, 2000, WB Saunders.)

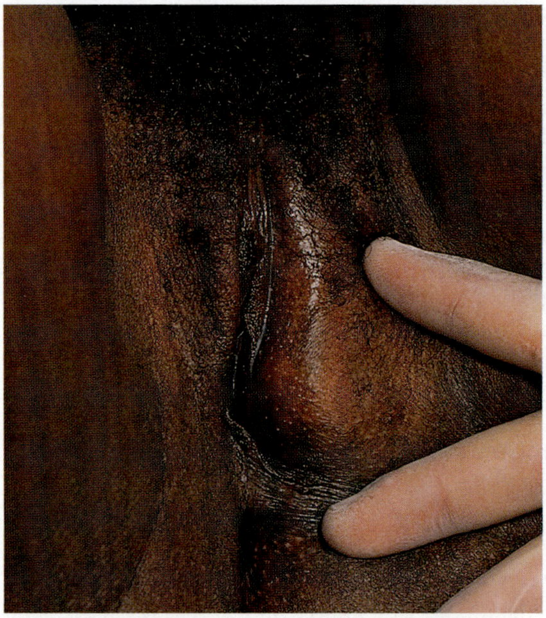

Fig. 19.17 Bartholin Gland Abscess.

A *urethral caruncle* is a small benign tumor at the urethral orifice and is relatively common in postmenopausal females. It appears as a bright red or flesh-colored mass extending through the urethral orifice. It may be asymptomatic or may cause pain or bleeding. Urethral caruncles must be differentiated from other tumors by biopsy.

Inspect the Area of Bartholin Glands

Tell the patient that you are going to examine the glands of the labia. With a lubricated glove, palpate the area of the right gland (at the 7 to 8 o'clock position) by grasping the posterior portion of the right labia between your right index finger in the vagina and your right thumb on the outside, as demonstrated in Fig. 19.16. Is any tenderness, swelling, or pus present? Normally, Bartholin glands can be neither seen nor felt. Use your left hand to examine the area of the left gland (at the 4 to 5 o'clock position).

Fig. 19.17 shows an abscess in the left Bartholin gland.

Inspect the Perineum

The perineum and anus are inspected for masses, scars, fissures, and fistulas. Is the perineal skin reddened? The anus should be inspected for hemorrhoids, condylomata, irritation, and fissures.

Test for Pelvic Organ Prolapse

See Video 19.3.

While you gently separate the labia and depress the perineum, ask the patient to bear down or cough. If prolapse is present, ballooning of the anterior or posterior walls may be seen. Bulging of the anterior wall is associated with a cystocele; bulging of the posterior wall is indicative of a rectocele. If stress incontinence is present, the coughing or bearing down may trigger a spurt of urine from the urethral orifice.

Examination With Speculum

Preparation

The speculum examination entails inspecting the vagina and cervix. There are several types of specula. The metal *Cusco,* or *bivalve,* speculum is the most popular. This speculum consists of two blades or bills that are introduced closed into the vagina and are then opened by squeezing the handle mechanism. The vaginal walls are held apart by the bills, and adequate visualization of the vagina and cervix is achieved. There are basically two types of bivalve specula: Graves and Pedersen. *Graves* speculum is more common and is used for most adult patients. The bills are wider and are curved on the sides. *Pedersen* speculum has narrower, flat bills and is used for patients with a small introitus. The plastic, disposable bivalve speculum is becoming more common. A disadvantage to its use is the loud click made as the lower bill is disengaged during removal from the vagina. If a plastic speculum is used, the patient should be informed that this sound will occur. Check the bills to make sure that there are no rough edges.

Before using the speculum in a patient, practice opening and closing it. If the patient has never had a speculum examination, show the speculum to them. You should warm the speculum with warm water and then touch it to the dorsum of your hand to ensure that the temperature is suitable. A small amount of jelly lubricant may be used, especially since liquid-based cervical cytologic examination has replaced the glass slide Pap test, and gonorrhea and chlamydia testing by polymerase chain reaction (PCR)[f] has replaced most bacterial and fungal cultures. Tell the patient that you are now going to perform the speculum part of the internal examination.

Technique

See Video 19.4.

While the examiner's left index and middle fingers separate the labia and firmly depress the perineum, the closed speculum, held in the examiner's right hand, is introduced *slowly* into the introitus at an oblique angle of 45 degrees from the vertical over the examiner's left fingers. This procedure is demonstrated in

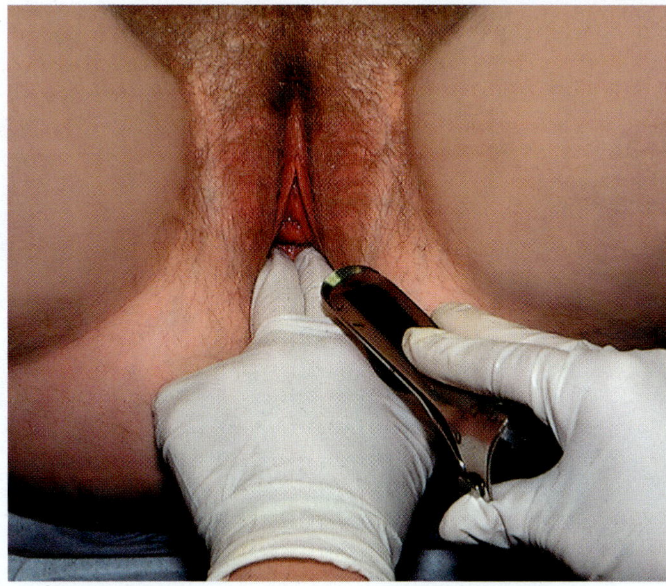

Fig. 19.18 Technique for Insertion of the Vaginal Speculum. Note the examiner's fingers pressing downward on the perineum. (Reused with permission from Wilson SF, Giddens J: *Health Assessment for Nursing Practice*, St. Louis, 2013, Elsevier.)

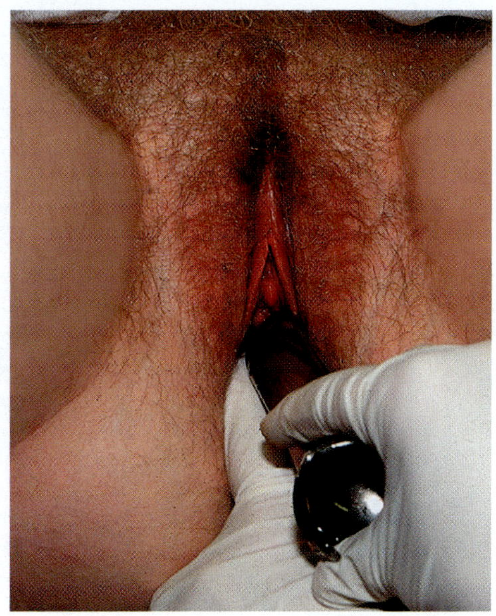

Fig. 19.19 Technique for Insertion of the Vaginal Speculum. Note that the speculum rides over the examiner's fingers, avoiding contact with the external urethral meatus and clitoris. (Reused with permission from Wilson SF, Giddens J: *Health Assessment for Nursing Practice*, St. Louis, 2013, Elsevier.)

Figs. 19.18 and 19.19 and is diagrammed in Fig. 19.20. *Do not introduce the speculum vertically*, because injury to the clitoris or urethral meatus may occur.

Inspect the Cervix

The speculum is introduced to full depth. When it is inserted completely, the speculum is rotated to the horizontal position, with the handle now pointing downward, and is opened *slowly.* With the bills open, the vaginal walls and cervix can be

[f]PCR is a method to analyze a short sequence of DNA or RNA even in samples containing only minute quantities of DNA or RNA. The test amplifies the genetic material to a level that can be detected. The technique is complex, consisting of many stages, and is expensive. PCR has many clinical uses. For example, it is used to diagnose genetic diseases, establish paternity or biological relationships, perform DNA fingerprinting and DNA forensics, and identify bacteria and viruses. The PCR test has been the gold standard test for diagnosing COVID-19 since authorized for use in February 2020.

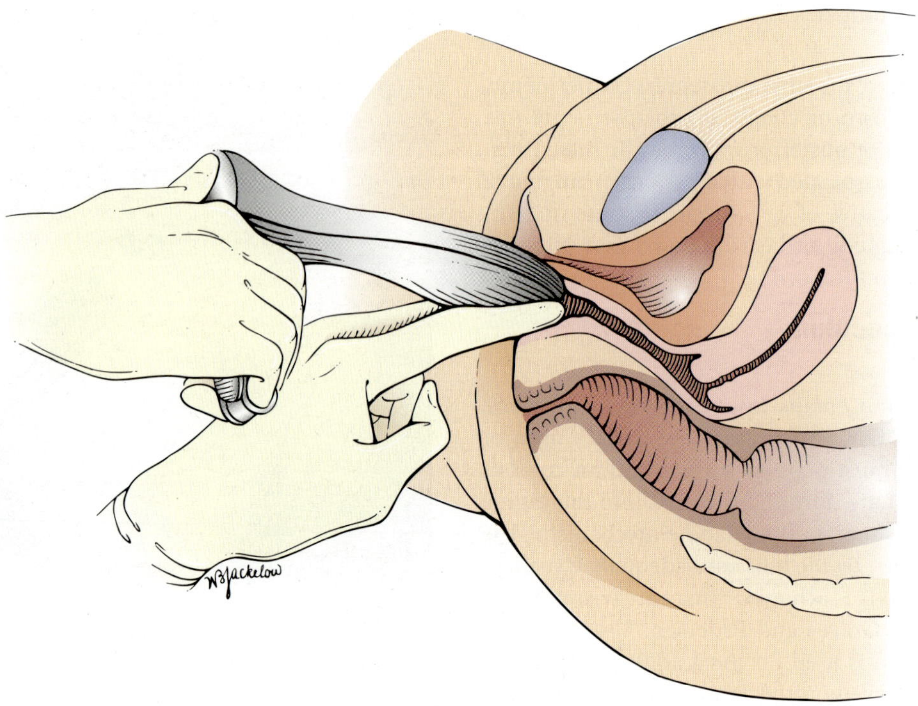

Fig. 19.20 Cross-Sectional View of the Speculum Examination.

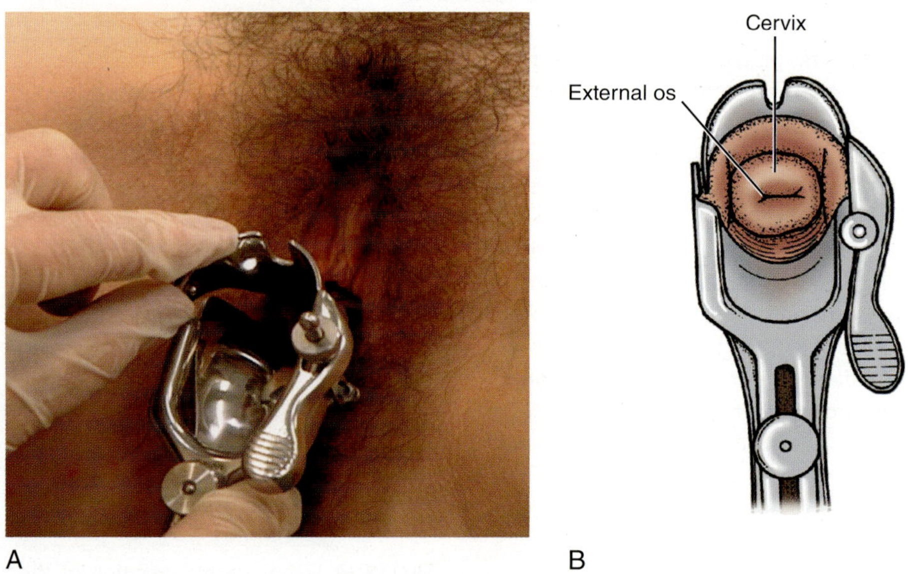

Fig. 19.21 **Technique for Inspecting the Cervix.** (A) Opening of the speculum bills after the speculum has been fully inserted and rotated to the transverse position. (B) Internal view of the cervix when the speculum is correctly inserted. (B reused with permission from Monahan FD, Drake DT, Neighbors M, editors: *Medical-Surgical Nursing: Foundations for Clinical Practice*, ed 2, Saunders.)

visualized. The cervix should rest within the bills of the speculum. This is demonstrated in Fig. 19.21 and diagrammed in Fig. 19.22. To keep the speculum open, the set screw can be tightened. If the cervix is not immediately seen, gently turn the bills in various directions to expose the cervix. The most common reason for not visualizing the cervix is failure to insert the speculum far enough before opening it.

If a discharge is obscuring any part of the vaginal walls or cervix, the discharge should be removed with a cotton-tipped applicator and spread onto a glass microscope slide. A culture may also be obtained.

Inspect the cervix for color, discharge, erythema, erosion, ulceration, leukoplakia, scars, and masses. What is the shape of the external cervical os? A bluish discoloration of the cervix may be an indication of pregnancy or a large tumor.

A normal cervix is seen in Fig. 19.23. Notice that the external cervical os is round, which is characteristic of the cervix of a female who has never had a vaginal delivery.

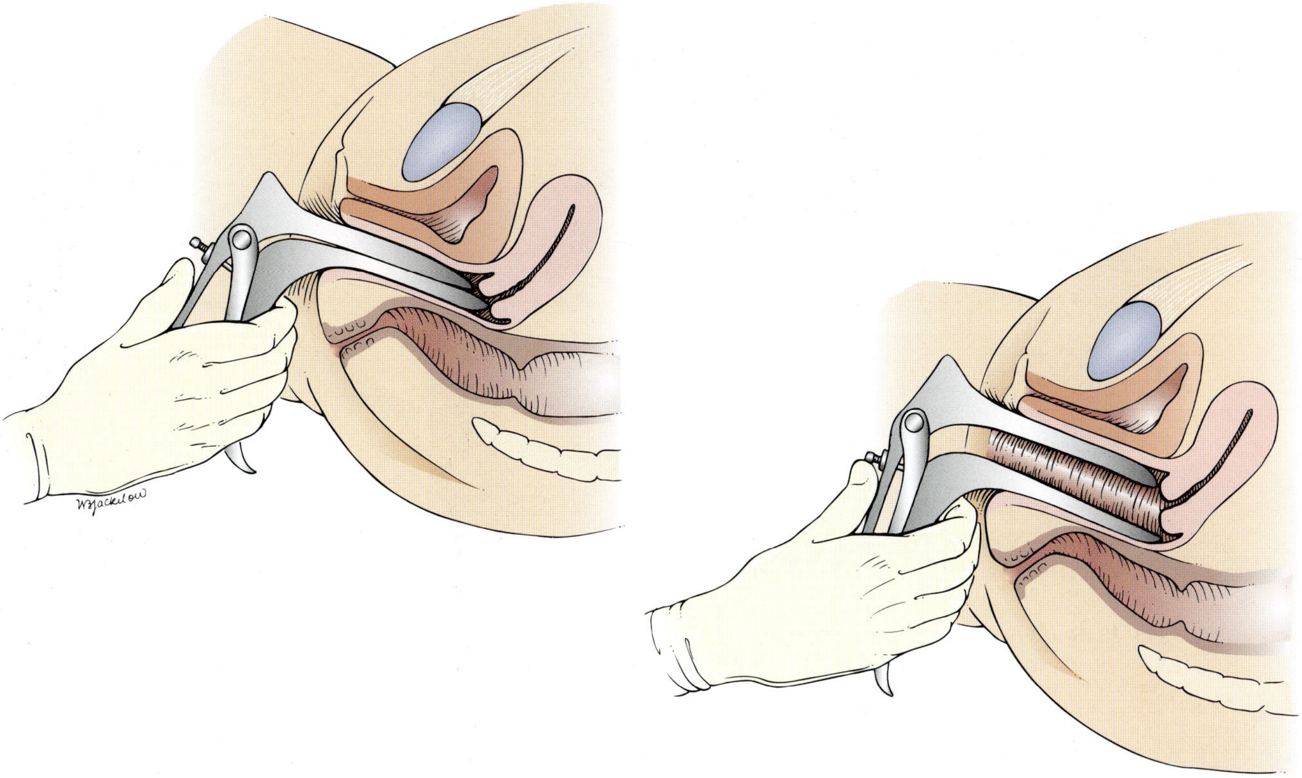

Fig. 19.22 Cross-Sectional View Illustrating the Position of the Speculum During Inspection of the Cervix.

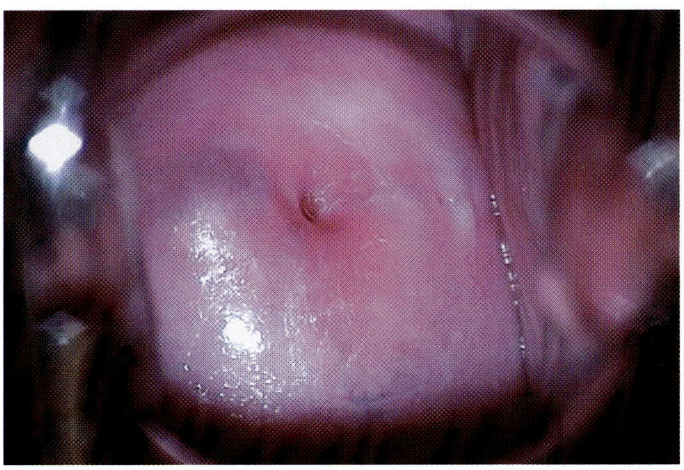

Fig. 19.23 A Normal Cervix. Note the round external cervical os in a nulliparous female.

Papanicolaou Smear

See Video 19.5.

Traditionally, the Pap smear was done by scraping cells from the cervix, applying it to a glass slide, then fixing the cells with a preservative spray and examining the smear under a microscope (Figs. 19.24 and 19.25). A newer method, the *liquid-based cytologic examination,* or *liquid-based Pap test,* can remove most of the blood, mucus, bacteria, yeast, and pus cells in a sample (which can mask the cervical cells) and can spread the cervical cells more evenly on the slide. The cervical or endocervical sample is collected by inserting a broom-type or Cytobrush and plastic spatula into the endocervix, then rotating 360 degrees while cells are scraped from the exo- and endocervix. Instead of being directly placed on a slide, the sample is placed into a vial with a special preservative solution. This new method, performed with the *ThinPrep®* or *SurePath™* system, also prevents cells from drying out and becoming distorted.

Studies have revealed that liquid-based testing can slightly improve detection of cancers, greatly improve detection of precancerous conditions, and reduce the number of tests that need to be repeated. The most significant advantage of the liquid-based test is the ability to co-test for HPV with the same specimen. In 2019, representatives from 19 organizations and consensus groups convened to develop and publish updated risk-based consensus guidelines for management of abnormal cervical cancer screening tests. All are based on Pap and HPV co-tests as done with the liquid-based methods.

Because the Pap smear may cause the cervix to bleed slightly, advise the patient that there may be mild spotting, which is normal. Any significant bleeding, however, should be evaluated. The results of the Pap smear are usually available in 2 to 3 weeks.

Inspect the Vaginal Walls

See Video 19.6.

The patient is told that the speculum will now be removed. The set screw is released with the examiner's right index finger, and the speculum is rotated back to the original oblique position. As the speculum is slowly withdrawn and closed, the vaginal walls are inspected for masses, lacerations, leukoplakia,

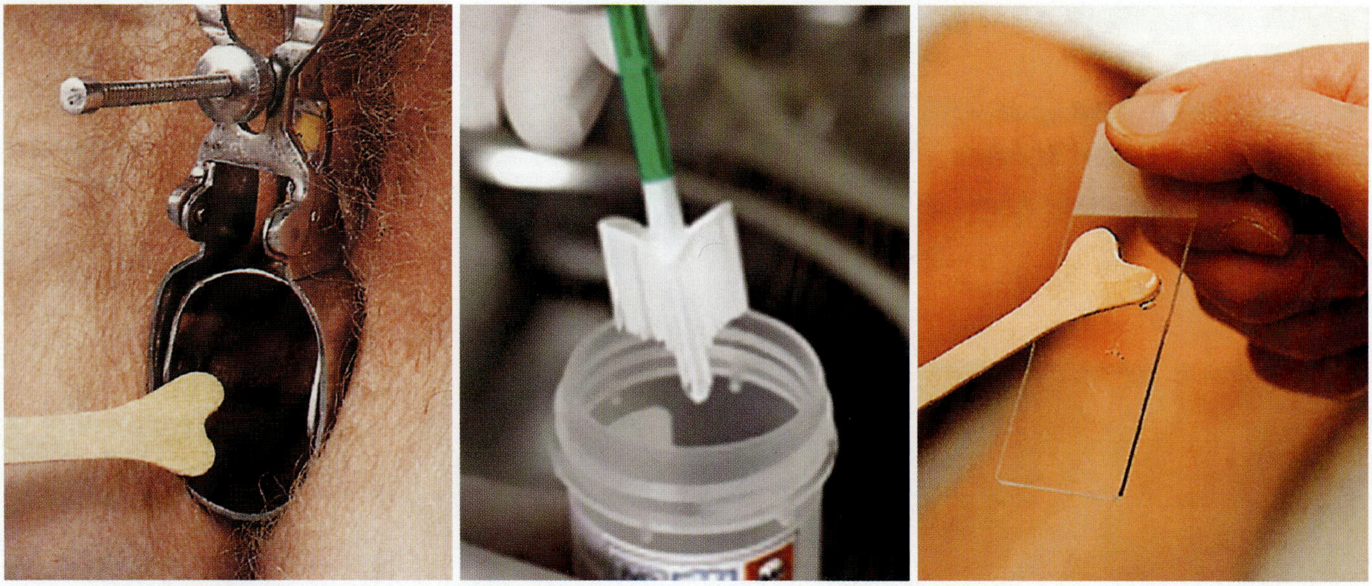

A B C

Fig. 19.24 (A) A cervical smear is taken using an Ayres spatula. (B) A sample being taken for liquid-based cytology examination using the broom-like device (cytobrush). (C) The material obtained is plated onto a glass slide and fixed. (Reused with permission from Symonds IM, Arulkumaran S: *Essential obstetrics and gynaecology*, ed 6, St. Louis, 2019, Elsevier.)

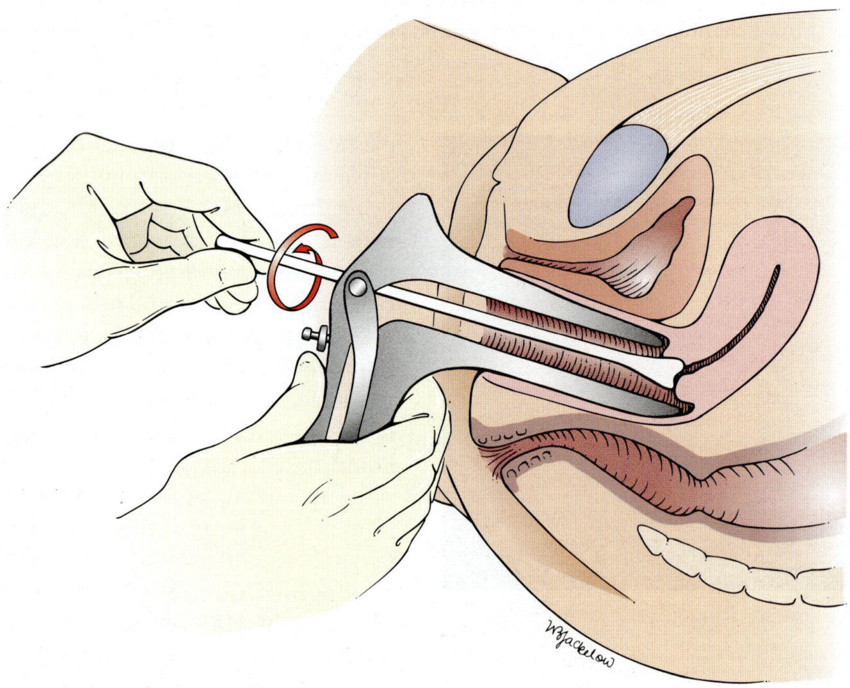

Fig. 19.25 Illustration of the Traditional Technique for Obtaining a Cervical Smear for the Papanicolaou Test. Note that the longer end of the wooden spatula is placed in the cervical os.

and ulcerations. The walls should be smooth and nontender. A moderate amount of colorless or white mucus is usually present. If a plastic speculum is used, carefully in a controlled fashion, unclip the two bills before removing and try to avoid pinching the sides of the vaginal wall.

Bimanual Palpation

See Video 19.7.

The bimanual examination is used to palpate the uterus and adnexa. Lower the head of the examination table to a 15-degree angle or flat, depending on the patient's preference. In this examination, the examiner's fingers are placed in the patient's vagina and on the abdomen, and the pelvic structures are palpated between the hands. In general, the right hand is inserted into the vagina and the left hand palpates the abdomen, but this is a matter of personal preference.

Technique

The examiner should be positioned between the patient's legs. If the examiner's right hand is to be used vaginally, a suitable jelly lubricant is held in the left hand, and a small amount is dropped from the tube onto the examiner's gloved right index and middle fingers. The examiner should not touch the tube of lubricant to the gloves, because such touching will contaminate the lubricant. The patient is told that the internal examination will now begin.

As the bimanual examination is being performed, the examiner should observe the patient's face. Their facial expression will quickly reveal whether the examination is painful. The labia are separated, and the examiner's lubricated right index and middle fingers are introduced vertically into the vagina. A downward pressure toward the perineum is applied. The right fourth and fifth fingers are flexed into the palm of the hand. The right thumb is extended. The area around the clitoris should not be touched. The examiner may now rest the right elbow on their right knee so that undue pressure is not placed on the patient. There is no need to palpate deeply with the "abdominal hand" if the uterus is sufficiently elevated with the "vaginal hand."

The correct positions of the examiner, assistant, and patient are demonstrated in Fig. 19.26.

The vaginal walls are palpated for nodules, scarring, and induration.

Once inserted into the vagina, the examiner's right (vaginal) hand is rotated 90 degrees clockwise so that the palm is facing upward. Some healthcare professionals prefer not to rotate the vaginal hand because this may decrease the depth of penetration. The left hand is now placed on the abdomen approximately one-third of the way to the umbilicus from the pubic symphysis. The wrist of the abdominal hand should not be flexed or supinated. The vaginal hand pushes the pelvic organs up out of the pelvis and stabilizes them while they are palpated by the abdominal hand. It is the abdominal, not the vaginal, hand that performs the palpation. The technique for the bimanual examination is shown in Fig. 19.27 and diagrammed in Fig. 19.28.

Palpate the Cervix and Uterine Body

The cervix is palpated. What is its consistency (soft, firm, nodular, friable)?

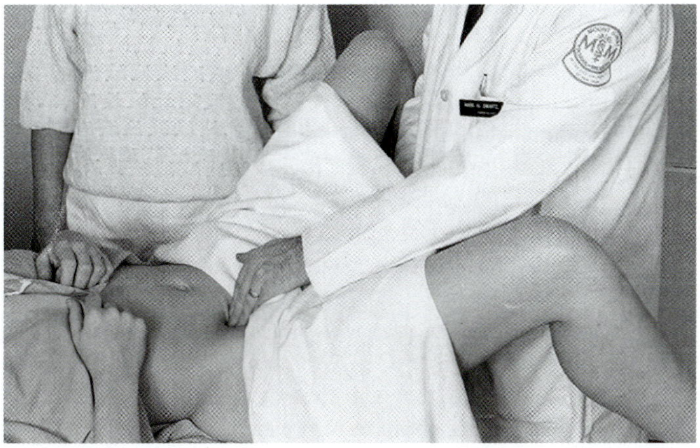

Fig. 19.26 Positions of the examiner *(right)*, assistant *(left)*, and patient *(bottom)* for the bimanual examination.

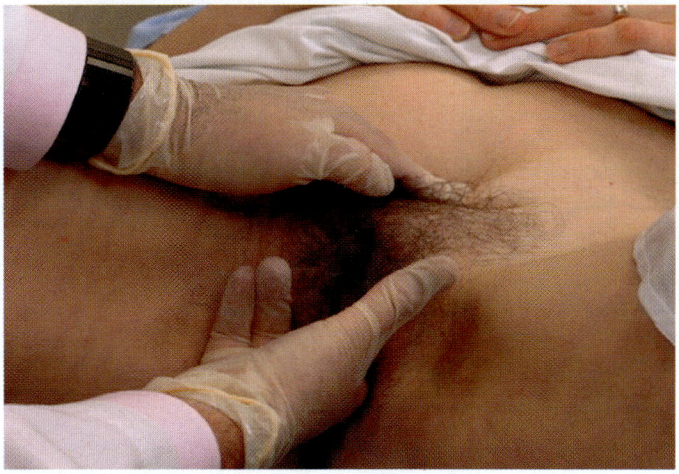

Fig. 19.27 Technique for the Bimanual Examination.

Tell the patient that they will now feel you move the cervix and uterus, but this should not be painful. The cervix can usually be moved 2 to 4 cm in any direction. The cervix is pushed backward and upward toward the abdominal hand as the abdominal hand pushes downward. Any restriction of motion or the development of pain on movement should be noted. Pushing the cervix up and back tends to tip an anteverted, anteflexed uterus forward into a position where it is more easily palpated. The uterus should then be felt between the two hands. Describe its *position, size, shape, consistency, mobility,* and *tenderness.* Determine whether the uterus is anteverted or retroverted. Is it enlarged, firm, or mobile? Are any irregularities felt? Is there any tenderness when the uterus is moved?

Palpation by the bimanual technique is easiest if the uterus is anteverted and anteflexed, which is the most common uterine position. A retroverted uterus is directed toward the spine and is therefore felt by the vaginal hand, rather than the abdominal hand in bimanual palpation.

Palpate the Adnexa

After the uterus has been evaluated, the right and left adnexa are palpated. If the patient is concerned of pain on one side, start the examination on the other side. The right hand should move to the left lateral fornix while the left (abdominal) hand moves to the patient's left lower quadrant. The vaginal fingers lift the adnexa toward the abdominal hand, which attempts to palpate the adnexal structures. This is illustrated in Fig. 19.29.

The adnexa should be explored for masses. Describe the *size, shape, consistency,* and *mobility,* as well as any *tenderness,* of the structures in the adnexa. The normal ovary is sensitive to pressure when pressure is applied. After the left side is examined, the right adnexa is palpated by moving the right (vaginal) hand to the right lateral fornix and the left (abdominal) hand to the patient's right lower quadrant.

In many patients, especially postmenopausal patients or those with greater central adiposity, the adnexal structures cannot be palpated. Adnexal tenderness or enlargement is relatively specific for a pathologic state.

After completion of the examination of the adnexa, the examining vaginal fingers move to the posterior fornix to palpate

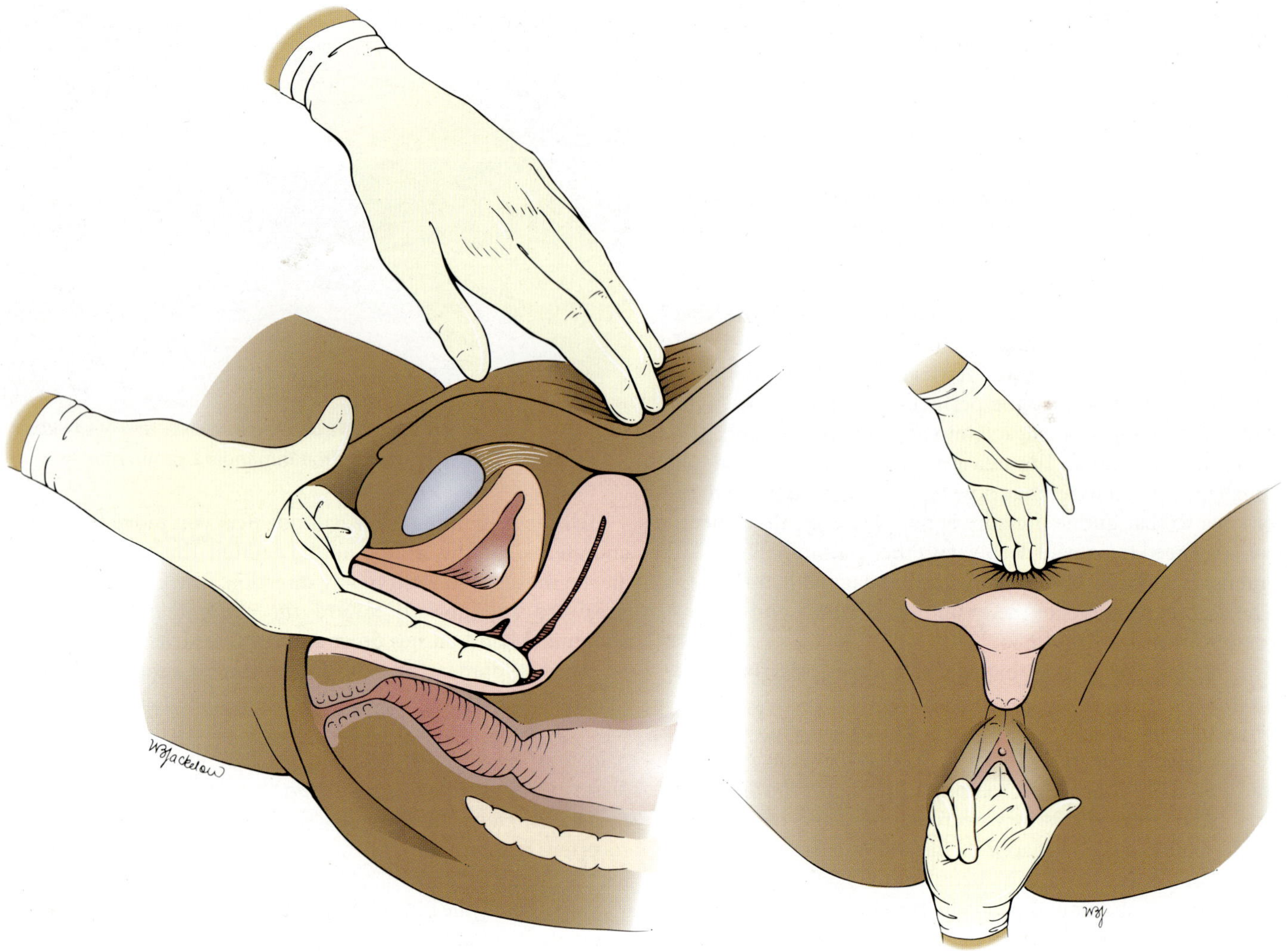

Fig. 19.28 Cross-Sectional View of the Bimanual Examination Through the Pelvic Organs. The uterus is positioned between the examining hands. Note the position of the right thumb, held away from the clitoris.

the uterosacral ligaments and the pouch of Douglas. Marked tenderness and nodularity are suggestive of endometriosis.

If the patient has experienced childbirth, the examiner should have no difficulty using the right index and middle fingers in the vagina for bimanual palpation. If the introitus is narrow, the examiner should introduce the right middle finger first and gently push downward toward the anus. This technique will allow for the subsequent insertion of the right index finger with minimal discomfort. Should the patient's vaginal muscles remain tense, the examiner can suggest contraction and relaxation of these muscles around a single finger prior to introducing the second. In scenarios where the patient is a virgin, solely the right middle finger should be utilized.

Rectovaginal Palpation

Palpate the Rectovaginal Septum

See Video 19.8.

Tell the patient that you will now examine the vagina and rectum. The rectovaginal examination allows for better evaluation of the posterior portion of the pelvis and the cul-de-sac than does the bimanual examination alone. The examiner evaluates for scarring or masses that may indicate cancer. Typically, this type of exam is performed to assess rectal symptoms, pelvic pain, or a pelvic mass. The examiner can often reach 1 to 2 cm higher into the pelvis with the rectovaginal examination. Remove your fingers from the vagina and change your glove. Explain to the patient that this examination may cause the sensation of having a bowel movement. Lubricate the gloved index and middle fingers. Inspect the anus for hemorrhoids, fissures, polyps, prolapse, or other growths. Insert the index finger back into the vagina while the middle finger is introduced into the anus. The examining right index finger is positioned as far up the posterior surface of the vagina as possible. This technique is shown in Fig. 19.30 and diagrammed in Fig. 19.31.

The rectovaginal septum is palpated. Is it thickened or tender? Are nodules or masses present? The right middle finger should feel for tenderness, masses, or irregularities in the rectum.

The patient is told that the internal examination is completed and that you are about to remove your fingers. When you withdraw your fingers, inspect them for discharge or blood. Offer the patient tissues to wipe off any excess lubricant.

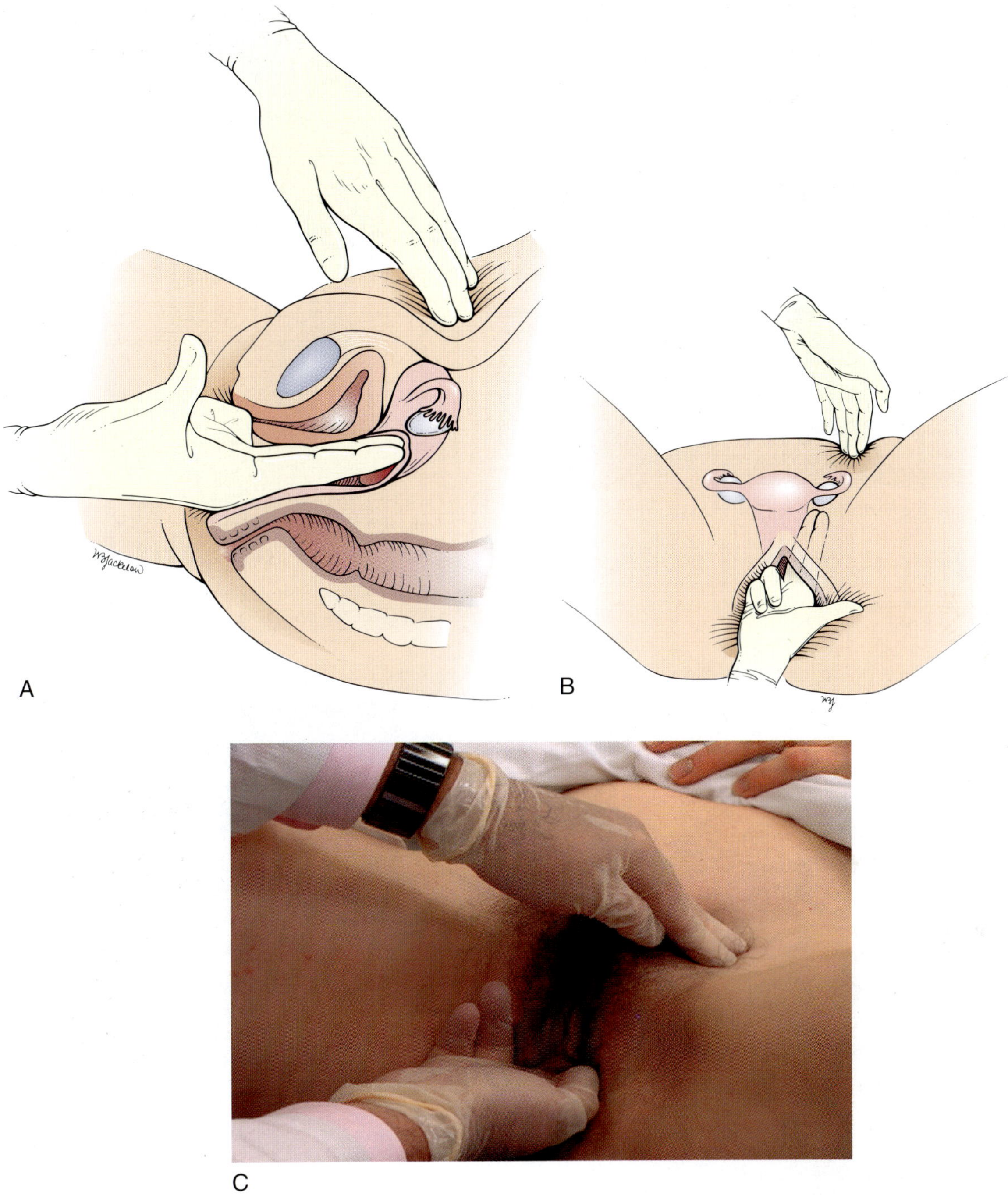

Fig. 19.29 Technique for Palpating the Left Adnexa. (A) Cross-sectional view through the pelvic organs. (B) Position of the ovary and fallopian tube between the examining hands. (C) Position of examiner's hands.

Completion of the Examination

Ask the patient to move back on the examination table, remove their legs from the heel rests, and then sit up slowly. Remove your gloves and wash your hands. This concludes the examination of the female genitalia.

CLINICOPATHOLOGIC CORRELATIONS

Vaginitis is a condition that causes inflammation of the vagina and vulva, resulting in pain, itching, and vaginal discharge. The normal vaginal discharge consists of mucous secretions from the cervix and vagina, along with exfoliated vaginal cells. A normal vaginal discharge is usually thin, transparent, and has little to no odor. However, when the bacteria in the vagina is disturbed, one or more organisms can multiply excessively, causing an imbalance in the normal bacterial flora. This change in the normal flora makes the vagina more vulnerable to other invading organisms. The rapid growth of these organisms produces an excess of waste products, which can irritate tissues, cause a burning sensation, and itching, and also produce a

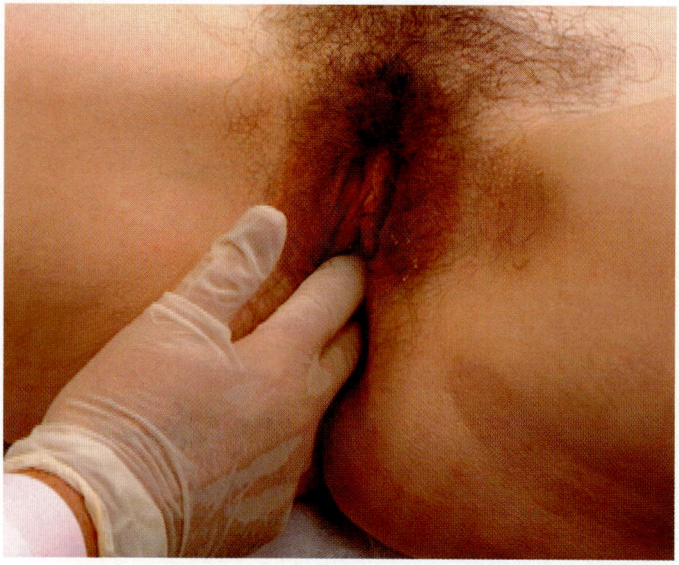

Fig. 19.30 Technique for Performing the Rectovaginal Examination.

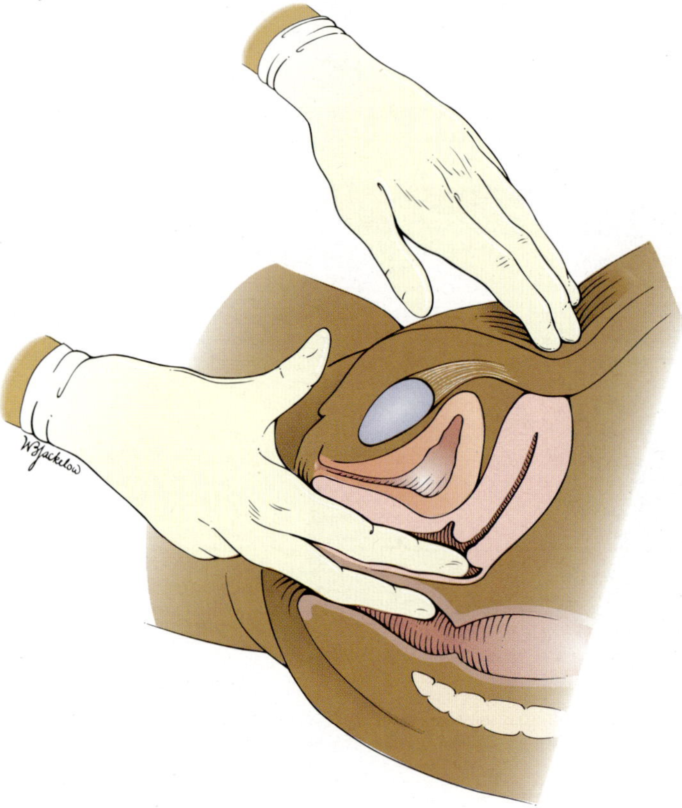

Fig. 19.31 Cross-Sectional View Illustrating the Rectovaginal Examination.

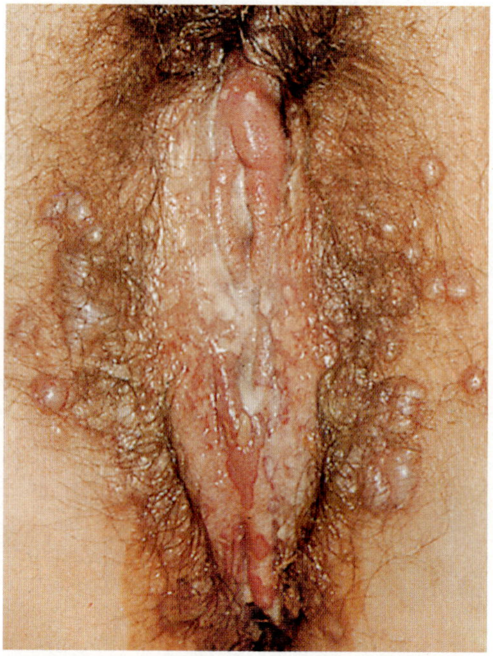

Fig. 19.32 Herpes Simplex Infection. (From Korting GW: *Practical dermatology of the genital region*, Philadelphia, 1980, WB Saunders.)

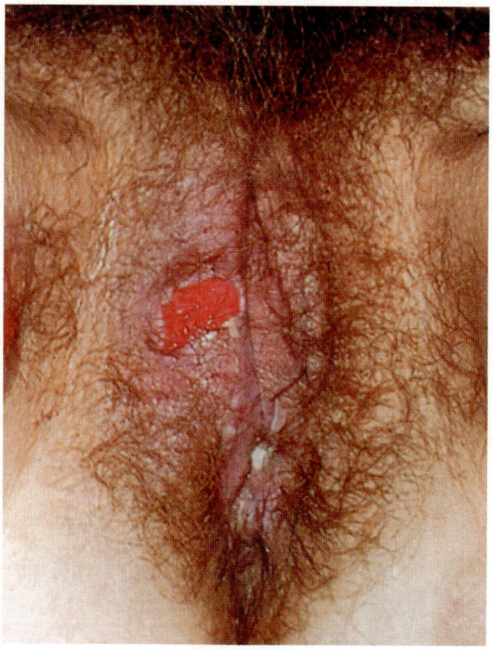

Fig. 19.33 Chancre of Primary Syphilis. (From Korting GW: *Practical dermatology of the genital region*, Philadelphia, 1980, WB Saunders.)

discharge with an unpleasant odor. Different organisms cause different types of discharges with varying appearances.

Lesions of the vulva are very common. Fig. 19.32 shows the vesicular stage of herpes simplex infection. Fig. 19.33 shows a chancre (generally painless) in a patient with primary syphilis. Chancroid is a disease in which 5 to 15 days after exposure small papules or vesicles appear that break down to form tender, nonindurated ulcers (generally painful); lymphadenopathy develops. Fig. 19.34 shows the classic ulceration of vulvar chancroid. Table 19.2 summarizes the clinical features of genital ulcerations.

Fig. 19.35 shows several of the common uterine positions.

Pelvic organ prolapse is a common problem. The consequences include cystocele, rectocele, and uterine prolapse. Fig. 19.36 illustrates these sequelae of relaxation of the pelvic floor.

A summary of AUB is illustrated in Fig. 19.37.

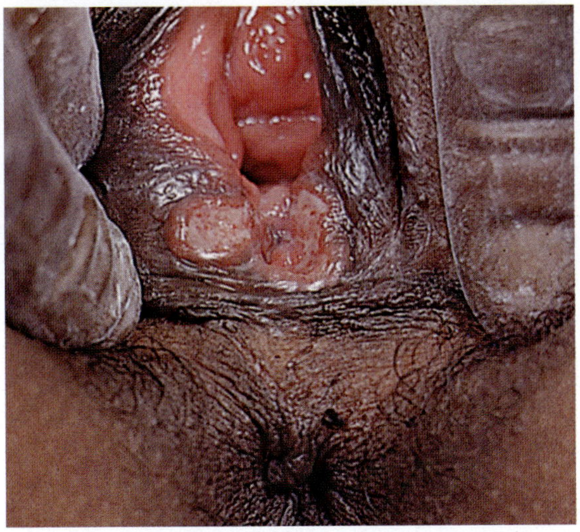

Fig. 19.34 Chancroid. (From Callen JP, Paller AS, Greer KE, et al: *Color atlas of dermatology*, ed 2, Philadelphia, 2000, WB Saunders.)

TABLE 19.2 Clinical Features of Genital Ulcerations

Feature	Genital Herpes (Fig. 19.32)	Primary Syphilis (Fig. 19.33)	Chancroid (Fig. 19.34)
Incubation period	3–5 days	9–90 days	1–5 days
Number of ulcers	Multiple	Single	Multiple
Appearance at onset	Vesicle	Papule	Papule/pustule
Later appearance	Small, grouped	Round, indurated	Irregular, ragged
Ulcer pain	Present	Absent	Present
Inguinal adenopathy	Present, tender	Present, painless	Present, painful
Healing	Within 2 weeks	Slowly for weeks	Slowly for weeks
Recurrence (even if not infected)	Common	Rare	Common

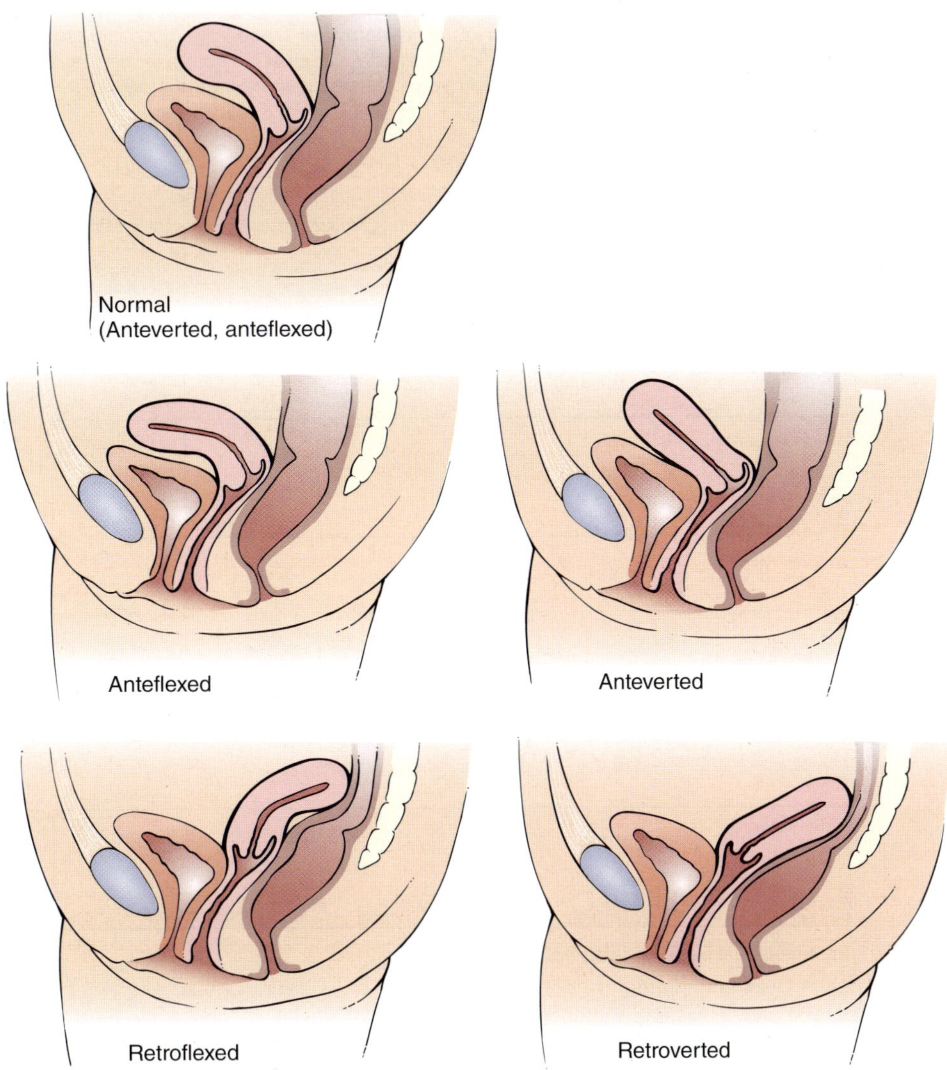

Fig. 19.35 Common Uterine Positions.

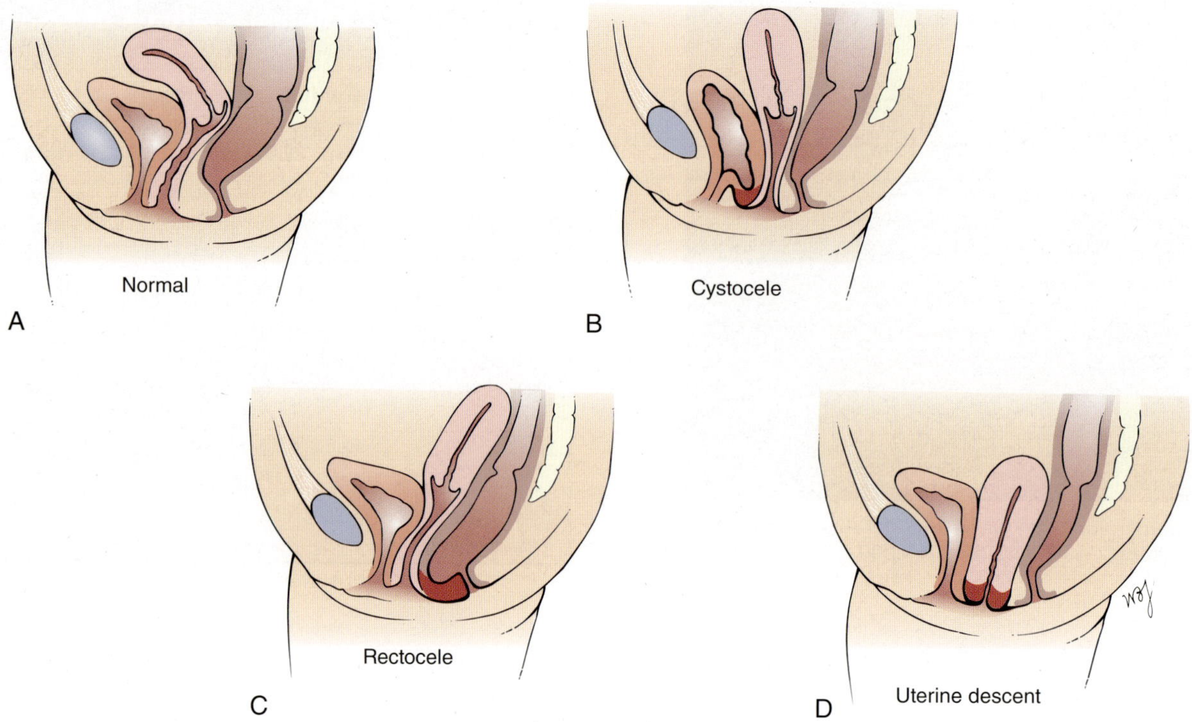

Fig. 19.36 Sequelae of Pelvic Organ Prolapse. (A) Normal anatomy. (B) Cystocele, which is a protrusion of the wall of the urinary bladder through the vagina. (C) Rectocele, which is a protrusion of the rectal wall through the vagina. (D) Uterine descent, which is a protrusion of the uterus through the vagina.

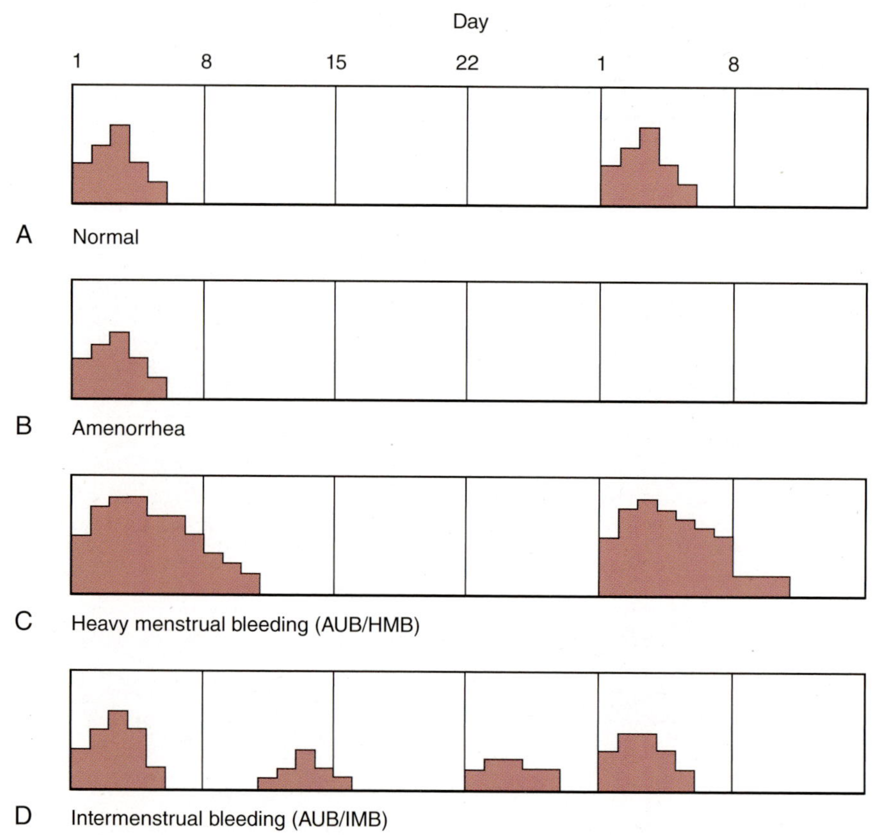

Fig. 19.37 Types of Uterine Bleeding. (A) Normal 28-day cycle. Note that menstrual flow occurs on day 1 and lasts for approximately 5 days. (B) Amenorrhea. After a menstrual flow of 5 days, the period does not recur. (C) Heavy menstrual bleeding. Note that the flow occurs at 28-day intervals, but the amount of flow is heavier, and its duration is longer than normal. (D) Intermenstrual bleeding. In this condition, flow is regular, but there is bleeding between the normal menstrual flow cycles.

While a pelvic examination can detect many cancers of the female reproductive system, including advanced uterine cancers, it is not very effective in identifying early-stage uterine cancer. The Pap test can detect some early endometrial cancers, but most cases are not detected by this test. On the other hand, the Pap test is highly effective in detecting early-stage cervical cancers. Currently, there are no recommended screening tests, either through sonogram or blood tests, that can effectively detect ovarian cancer.

Although there is often disagreement among various healthcare organizations regarding screening for various diseases, there has been a great deal of work to accomplish consensus recently regarding cervical cancer screening. In 2019, The American Cancer Society, the American Society for Colposcopy and Cervical Pathology, the American Society for Clinical Pathology, the U.S. Preventive Services Task Force, and the American College of Obstetricians and Gynecologists essentially all agreed on the new guidelines shown in Table 19.3.

TABLE 19.3 Cervical Cancer Guidelines for Average-Risk Females, 2019

When to start screening	Age 21 regardless of the age of onset of sexual activity
Annual screening	Cervical cancer screening should not be done annually. The annual visit is an opportunity to discuss other health problems and preventive measures.
Screening Method and Intervals	
21–29 years of age	Cytologic examination every 3 years HPV co-test[a] should not be performed in females aged <30 years
30–65 years of age	Cytologic examination every 3 years (acceptable) or Cytologic examination + HPV co-testing every 5 years (preferred)
When to stop screening	Aged >65 years with adequate screening history
Screening posthysterectomy	Not needed unless cervix still present (supracervical hysterectomy)

[a]Co-testing using the combination of Pap cytologic examination plus HPV DNA testing is the preferred cervical cancer screening method for females 30 to 65 years old.
HPV, Human papillomavirus; *Pap*, Papanicolaou.
Data from http://www.cdc.gov/cancer/cervical/pdf/guidelines.pdf. (Accessed December 26, 2018).

USEFUL VOCABULARY

Listed here are the specific roots that are important for understanding the terminology related to diseases of the female genitalia.

Root	Pertaining to	Example	Definition
amni(o)-	amnion	***amnio***rrhexis	Rupture of the amnion
colp(o)-	vagina	***colpo***scopy	Examination of vagina (and cervix)
-cyesis	pregnancy	pseudo***cyesis***	False pregnancy
gyn(e)-	female	***gyne***cology	Branch of medicine that deals with treating diseases of the genital tract in females
hyster(o)-	uterus	***hyster***ectomy	Surgical removal of the uterus
metro-	uterus	***metro***rrhagia	Uterine bleeding
oophor(o)-	ovary	***oophoro***tomy	Incision of an ovary
ov-	egg	***ov***ulation	Discharge of an egg from the ovary
salping(o)-	fallopian tube	***salping***itis	Inflammation of the fallopian tube

WRITING UP THE PHYSICAL EXAMINATION

Listed here are examples of the write-up for the examination of the female genitalia.

- Examination of the vulva is within normal limits. No lesions are present. The cervix appears pink, smooth, and nulliparous. There is no discharge from the external cervical os. The vaginal walls appear normal. Bimanual palpation reveals an anteverted, anteflexed uterus without masses or tenderness. The adnexa are unremarkable. Rectovaginal examination reveals a thin rectovaginal membrane without tenderness. Stool guaiac result is negative.
- Examination of the vulva reveals groups of tense vesicles and scattered erosions that are covered with exudate. The cervix is pink and multiparous. No cervical lesions are present. No discharge is present. The vagina is within normal limits. The uterus is anteverted and anteflexed. A 6 × 6 cm mass is felt within the uterus. The ovaries and tubes are unremarkable. Rectovaginal examination findings are within normal limits.
- The vulva appears within normal limits without masses or lesions. The cervix has an erosion, and there is a thick, white, cottage cheese–like discharge in the vagina. The discharge is adherent to the vaginal walls. The uterus is retroverted and cannot be adequately examined. A walnut-sized mass is felt in the left adnexa. It appears rubbery and is freely mobile. The rectovaginal examination findings are normal. Stool guaiac result is negative.
- The vulva is normal. On straining, a rectocele becomes apparent. The vagina is normal. The cervix is smooth, pink, and multiparous. The uterus is anteverted and anteflexed and is not enlarged. The adnexa are difficult to assess because of obesity of the patient. No tenderness is present.

FULL VIDEOS

- Video 19.9 Full video: Performing the speculum examination
- Video 19.10 Full video: Performing the bimanual examination
- Video 19.11 Full video: Performing the rectovaginal examination

REVIEW QUESTIONS

1. **Which female external genitalia structure is analogous to the scrotum in males?**
   A. Mons veneris
   B. Labia majora
   C. Labia minora
   D. Clitoris
   E. Perineum
2. **What is the primary function of the fallopian tube?**
   A. To produce estrogen and progesterone
   B. To provide a conduit for the egg from the ovary to the uterus
   C. To secrete lactic acid
   D. To regulate the menstrual cycle
   E. To drain lymphatic fluid from the vagina
3. **Which hormone is responsible for the rise in basal body temperature and is considered a reliable sign of ovulation?**
   A. Estrogen
   B. Luteinizing hormone
   C. Progesterone
   D. Follicle-stimulating hormone
   E. Gonadotropins
4. **What is the appropriate terminology to represent a female with two full-term children, one child born at 34 weeks, a history of one ectopic pregnancy, and two miscarriages in the first trimester, who is currently pregnant?**
   A. G6 P1232
   B. G4 P1112
   C. G7 P2133
   D. G3 P2102
   E. G4 P1122
5. **Which condition is characterized by uterine bleeding of normal amount at irregular, noncyclic intervals, particularly between normal menstrual cycles?**
   A. Dysmenorrhea
   B. Intermenstrual bleeding
   C. Mittelschmerz
   D. Amenorrhea
   E. Heavy menstrual bleeding
6. **What is the term for urinary incontinence that occurs with straining or coughing, is more common among females, and is often associated with a weakening of pelvic support?**
   A. Overflow incontinence
   B. Stress incontinence
   C. Neurologic incontinence
   D. Psychogenic incontinence
   E. Urge incontinence
7. **What position is commonly used for pelvic examinations in the United States?**
   A. Lying on the left side in bed
   B. Sitting upright in a chair with legs abducted
   C. Lying supine on an examining table
   D. Standing with legs apart
   E. Kneeling on the floor
8. **What is the purpose of the rectovaginal examination during a pelvic examination?**
   A. To evaluate the cervix
   B. To inspect the labia minora
   C. To palpate the adnexal structures
   D. To examine the vaginal walls
   E. To better evaluate the posterior portion of the pelvis
9. **Which type of speculum is often used for patients with a small introitus?**
   A. Metal Cusco speculum
   B. Plastic disposable bivalve speculum
   C. Graves speculum
   D. Pedersen speculum
   E. Liquid-based speculum
10. **Which of the following statements about cancer screening is true?**
    A. Pelvic examination is highly effective in detecting early cervical cancer.
    B. The Pap test is the most effective method for detecting ovarian cancer.
    C. There are no recommended screening tests for ovarian cancer.
    D. Cervical cancer screening guidelines have not seen any recent consensus among healthcare organizations.
    E. Early endometrial cancers are usually detected by the Pap test.

REFERENCES

Available online.

BIBLIOGRAPHY

Available online.

20

The Musculoskeletal System

Mark H. Swartz, Christine S. Williams, and Darwin Chen

The hand of the Lord was upon me...and set me down in the midst of the valley which was full of bones...behold, there were very many in the open valley; and, lo, they were very dry...Thus saith the Lord God unto these bones: Behold, I will cause breath to enter into you, and ye shall live. And I will lay sinews upon you, and will bring up flesh upon you, and cover with skin, and put breath in you, and ye shall live...there was a noise, and behold a commotion, and the bones came together, bone to bone...and skin covered them...and the breath came into them, and they lived, and stood up upon their feet.

Ezekiel 37:1–10

VIDEOS

Video 20.1	Performing the screening musculoskeletal examination.
Video 20.2	Evaluating gait
Video 20.3	Examining a patient with a trigger finger

GENERAL CONSIDERATIONS

Pathology of the musculoskeletal system ranks first among disease conditions that alter the quality of life.[1] This is related to limitation of activity, disability, and impairment. Musculoskeletal disorders are associated with high costs to employers due to decreased productivity or absenteeism, as well as healthcare costs, disability, and worker's compensation costs.

Musculoskeletal disorders are often more life-altering than other common injuries or illnesses. These disorders can affect muscles, nerves, tendons, joints, and cartilage in the extremities or spine. In the United States, 1 in every 4 persons suffers from a musculoskeletal disorder. Here are the facts:

- Musculoskeletal disorders account for nearly 70 million healthcare professional office visits in the United States annually and an estimated 130 million total healthcare encounters, including outpatient, hospital, and emergency room visits.
- The Institute of Medicine[2] estimates musculoskeletal disorders result in an economic burden of $45 to $54 billion annually, as measured by compensation costs, lost wages, and lost productivity.
- The Bureau of Labor Statistics reported 26,794 carpal tunnel syndrome cases involving days away from work.
- The Bureau of Labor Statistics reported 372,683 back injury cases involving days away from work.
- In 2013, the total medical cost for arthritis conditions was $140 billion. The national arthritis-associated lost wages were $164 billion.[3]
- Osteoarthritis (OA) affects more than 32.5 million adults in the United States. In 2013, OA was the second most costly health condition treated in a hospital, which accounted for $16.5 billion dollars, or 4.3%, of the combined costs for all hospitalizations.[4]
- Persons who are limited in their work by arthritis are said to have arthritis-attributable work limitations. These limitations affect 1 in 20 working-age adults (aged 18 to 64 years) in the United States, and 1 in 3 working-age adults with self-reported, healthcare professional-diagnosed arthritis.
- In 2004, the sum of the direct expenditures in healthcare costs and the indirect expenditures in lost wages has been estimated to be $849 billion, or 7.7% of the national gross domestic product.

Table 20.1 lists the most common musculoskeletal disorders.

Diseases of the musculoskeletal system are divided into two categories: *systemic* and *local.* Patients with systemic diseases, such as rheumatoid arthritis (RA), systemic lupus erythematosus, or polymyositis, may appear chronically ill with generalized weakness, pain, and episodic stiffness of the joints. Patients with local disease are otherwise healthy individuals who suffer restriction of motion and pain from a single area. This includes patients with back pain, tennis elbow, arthritis, or bursitis. Although these patients have localized symptoms, their ailment can significantly limit their work capacity, and the disease can have a severe effect on quality of life.

Diseases of the musculoskeletal system rank first in cost to workers' compensation insurance carriers. Liberty Mutual, the largest workers' compensation insurance provider in the United States, reports that musculoskeletal injuries related to overexertion cost employers $13.4 billion every year.[2]

TABLE 20.1 Common Musculoskeletal Disorders

Condition	Pathologic Findings	Symptoms	Typical Causes
Bursitis	Inflammation of the bursa between skin and bone, or bone and tendon, occurring at the hip, knee, elbow, or shoulder	Pain and swelling at the site of the injury	Kneeling, pressure at the elbow, repetitive shoulder movements, tight iliotibial (IT) band
Carpal tunnel syndrome	Pressure on the median nerve that passes up the wrist	Tingling, pain, and numbness in the thumb and fingers, especially at night	Repetitive work with a bent wrist, use of vibrating tools; sometimes follows tenosynovitis (see later in table)
Ganglion	A cyst at a joint or in a tendon sheath, usually on the back of the hand or wrist	Hard, small, round swelling; usually painless	Repetitive hand movements
Tendonitis	Inflammation of the area where muscle and tendon are joined	Pain, swelling, tenderness, and redness of hand, wrists, or forearm; difficulty in using the hand	Repetitive movements
Tenosynovitis	Inflammation of tendons or tendon sheaths	Aching, tenderness, swelling, extreme pain, difficulty in using the hand	Repetitive movements, often nonstrenuous; can be brought on by sudden increases in workload or by introduction of new processes
Tension neck or shoulder	Inflammation of the neck and shoulder muscles and tendons	Localized pain in the neck and shoulders	Having to maintain a rigid posture
Trigger finger	Inflammation of tendons or tendon sheaths of the fingers	Inability to move fingers smoothly, with or without pain	Repetitive movements; having to grip too long, too tightly, or too frequently

It has been estimated that musculoskeletal problems rank second (after cardiovascular disorders) in accounting for visits to healthcare professionals and third in terms of surgical procedures in hospitals (after gynecologic and abdominal surgery). According to a Gallup poll in 2014,[5] 77% of individuals older than 18 years had concerns of foot pain at some time. More than $300 million is spent annually on insoles, corn remedies, bunion removers, other foot care products, and over-the-counter medications for foot care. Despite this widespread problem, fewer than 50% of healthcare professionals know how to examine a foot correctly.

Musculoskeletal conditions, although not usually fatal, can significantly impact one's quality of life. Studies indicate that back pain is experienced by over 80% of Americans at some point in their lives. Additionally, those who suffer from back pain for more than 6 months are at risk of permanent disability, with more than 50% never returning to work. Arthritis affects more than 25 million Americans, ranking second only to cardiac disease as a cause of activity limitation. Table 20.2 provides a list of the most common musculoskeletal disorders in adults aged 45 years and older in the United States.

TABLE 20.2 The Most Common Musculoskeletal Disorders in Adults Aged 45 Years and Older: Prevalence in Adult Populations in the United States

Extremely Common (Prevalence >5%)
Low back pain
Osteoarthritis
Tendinitis or bursitis
Common (Prevalence 0.5%–5%)
Gout
Fibromyalgia
Rheumatoid arthritis

In the United States, at least 10% of the population experiences a bone fracture, dislocation, or sprain annually. Females older than 50 years sustain over 1.2 million fractures annually. There are more than 200,000 hip fractures annually, and these are associated with prolonged disability and significant mortality at 1 year. Age-related fractures are projected to increase nationally from 2.1 million in 2005 to over 3 million fractures in 2025, solely based on growth in the elderly population most at risk.[6] There is an estimated 12.1% and 4.6% lifetime risk of fragility hip fracture for females and males, respectively. The estimated worldwide annual incidence of hip fracture may increase from 1.6 million per year in 2000 to 4.5 million per year by 2050.[7]

Osteoporosis is a common musculoskeletal disorder that occurs when bones lose density and become less mineralized than usual. It is the second most common cause of morbidity in the elderly population, after arthritis. Osteoporosis related to menopause and aging increases the risk of fractures in the older population. In the United States, there are over 40 million females over the age of 50, and more than half of them have evidence of spinal osteoporosis. For females over the age of 75, 90% have significant radiographic evidence of osteoporosis.

Musculoskeletal disease is prevalent among older adults who need assistance, and it significantly impacts the U.S. economy. The annual nursing home care cost for patients with such illnesses is around $75 billion. Over 10 million Americans have some form of inflammatory arthritis, with RA being the most common, affecting approximately 7 million people.

Musculoskeletal problems have the most significant financial effect on the aged population. Medicare spends more than $1 billion annually for hospitalization of patients with these conditions. This represents 20% of all Medicare payments.

STRUCTURE AND PHYSIOLOGY

The principal functions of the musculoskeletal system are to support and protect the body and bring about movement of the extremities for locomotion and the performance of tasks. The parts of the musculoskeletal system are composed of variable forms of dense connective tissue, which include the following:

- Bone
- Skeletal muscle
- Ligaments
- Tendons
- Cartilage

Bone is composed of an organic matrix that consists of collagen fibers embedded in a cementing gel made up of calcium and phosphate. Bone is an actively changing tissue with constant *remodeling* while reappropriating its mineral stores and matrix according to mechanical stresses. Normal bone is composed of collagen fibers aligned parallel to the tension stresses to which the bone is exposed. The long bones in adults are composed of tubes of *cortical,* or compact, bone surrounding a medullary cavity of *cancellous,* or spongy, bone. Cortical bone exists in areas where support is necessary, whereas cancellous bone is found in areas where hematopoiesis and bone formation occur. In cortical bone, the bone cells, or *osteocytes,* are enclosed in lacunae, which are spaces in the sheets of bone tissue called *lamellae.* Several lamellae are arranged concentrically around a vascular channel and are termed a *haversian canal.* In cancellous bone, the lamellae are not arranged in haversian systems but are organized into a spongy network called *trabeculae.* These trabeculae align along lines of stress.

The ends of the long bones, called *epiphyses,* are expanded near the articular surfaces and are composed of spongy bone. The shaft of the long bone, the *diaphysis,* is covered with a layer of *periosteum.* The inner cavity of the long bone is lined with *endosteum* and is filled with marrow.

For a time, a layer of cartilage exists between the diaphysis and the epiphysis. This cartilage is known as the *growth plate* or *epiphyseal plate.* The purpose of the growth plate is to determine the longitudinal growth of the bone. The parts of a long bone are illustrated in Fig. 20.1.

Cells in the periosteum can develop into *osteoblasts,* which lay down new bone, or into *osteoclasts,* which resorb bone. Trauma, infection, and tumors stimulate the development of osteoblasts. Osteoblasts secrete the matrix that is refashioned into lamellae and arranged to endure the mechanical stresses to which the bone is subjected. Paget disease is a disease with pathologic process that interferes and disrupts the normal bone architecture. Patients with this condition are extremely susceptible to pathologic fractures.

Skeletal muscle is an organ, the contraction of which produces movement.

Ligaments attach bone to bone, and *tendons* attach muscle to bone. Both are dense connective tissues that offer great resistance to pulling forces. Ligaments appear as crisscross bands that help stabilize a joint. The anterior cruciate ligament (ACL) attaching the femur to the tibia is an example. Tendons are located at the end of a muscle and attach the muscle to a bone.

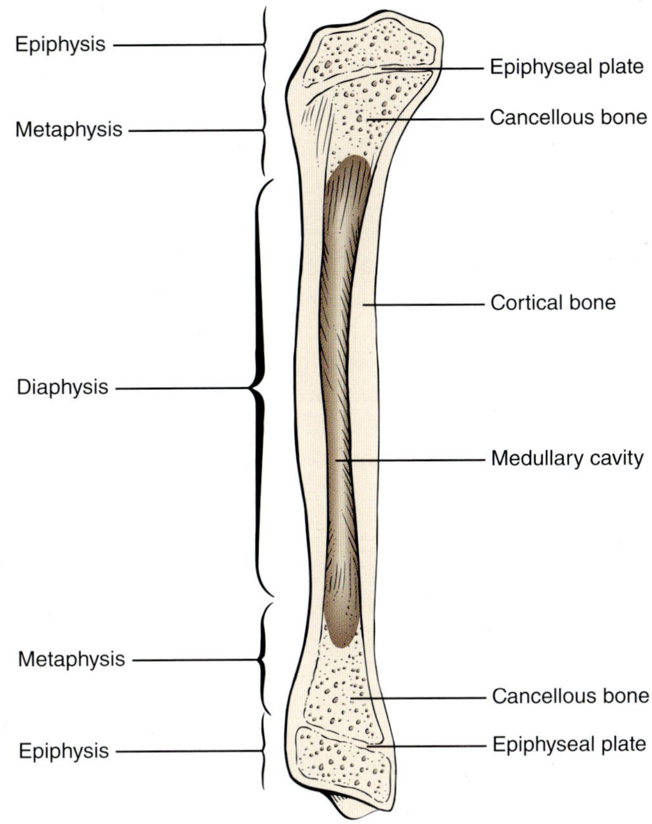

Fig. 20.1 Anatomy of a Long Bone.

The Achilles tendon attaches the gastrocnemius and soleus muscles to the calcaneus.

Cartilage is a type of connective tissue with great resilience. It plays an important role in joint function and in determining bone length. Cartilage allows our bones to move easily to glide over each other with very little friction. Unlike other types of tissue, cartilage does not have a blood supply. Because of this, damaged cartilage takes much longer to heal compared with other tissues that are supplied by blood.

The basic functional unit of the musculoskeletal system is the *joint.* A joint is comprised of two or more bones. There are several types of joints in the body:

- Immovable
- Slightly movable
- Movable

Immovable joints are fixed as a result of fibrous tissue banding. Examples of this type of joint are the sutures of the skull and the sacroiliac joints. *Slightly movable joints* are termed *symphyses.* In this type of joint, fibrocartilage joins the articulating bones. The pubic symphysis is an example of a slightly movable joint. The most common type of joint is the *movable joint.* The body has many different types of movable joints, also known as *synovial joints.* In synovial joints, the bone structures come in contact with each other and are covered with hyaline articular cartilage. A capsule surrounds the joint by attaching to the bones on either side of the joint. Within the capsule is a small amount of synovial fluid, which provides lubrication and nourishment of the articular cartilage. Synovial joints are classified according to the type of movement their structure permits. The classifications are as follows:

- Hinge joint
- Pivot joint
- Condyloid joint
- Saddle joint
- Ball-and-socket joint
- Plane joint

A *hinge joint* permits movement in only one axis, namely flexion or extension. The axis is transverse. An example of a hinge joint is the elbow. A *pivot joint* permits rotation in one axis. The axis is longitudinal along the shaft of the bone. One bone moves around a central axis without any displacement from that axis. An example of a pivot joint is the proximal radioulnar joint. A *condyloid joint* permits movement in two axes. The articular surfaces are oval; thus, these joints have been described as "egg-in-spoon" joints. One axis is the long diameter of the oval, and the other axis is the short diameter of the oval. The wrist joint is an example of a condyloid joint. A *saddle joint* is also a biaxial joint. The articular surfaces are saddle-shaped, with movements similar to those of a condyloid joint. The carpometacarpal joint of the thumb is an example of a saddle joint. The *ball-and-socket joint* is an example of a polyaxial joint; motion is possible in many axes. In a ball-and-socket joint, the articular surfaces are reciprocal segments of a sphere. The hip and shoulder joints are examples of ball-and-socket joints. A *plane joint* is also a polyaxial joint. In the plane joint, the articular surfaces are flat, and one bone merely rides over the other in many directions. The patellofemoral joint is an example of a plane joint. The different types of movable joints are shown in Fig. 20.2.

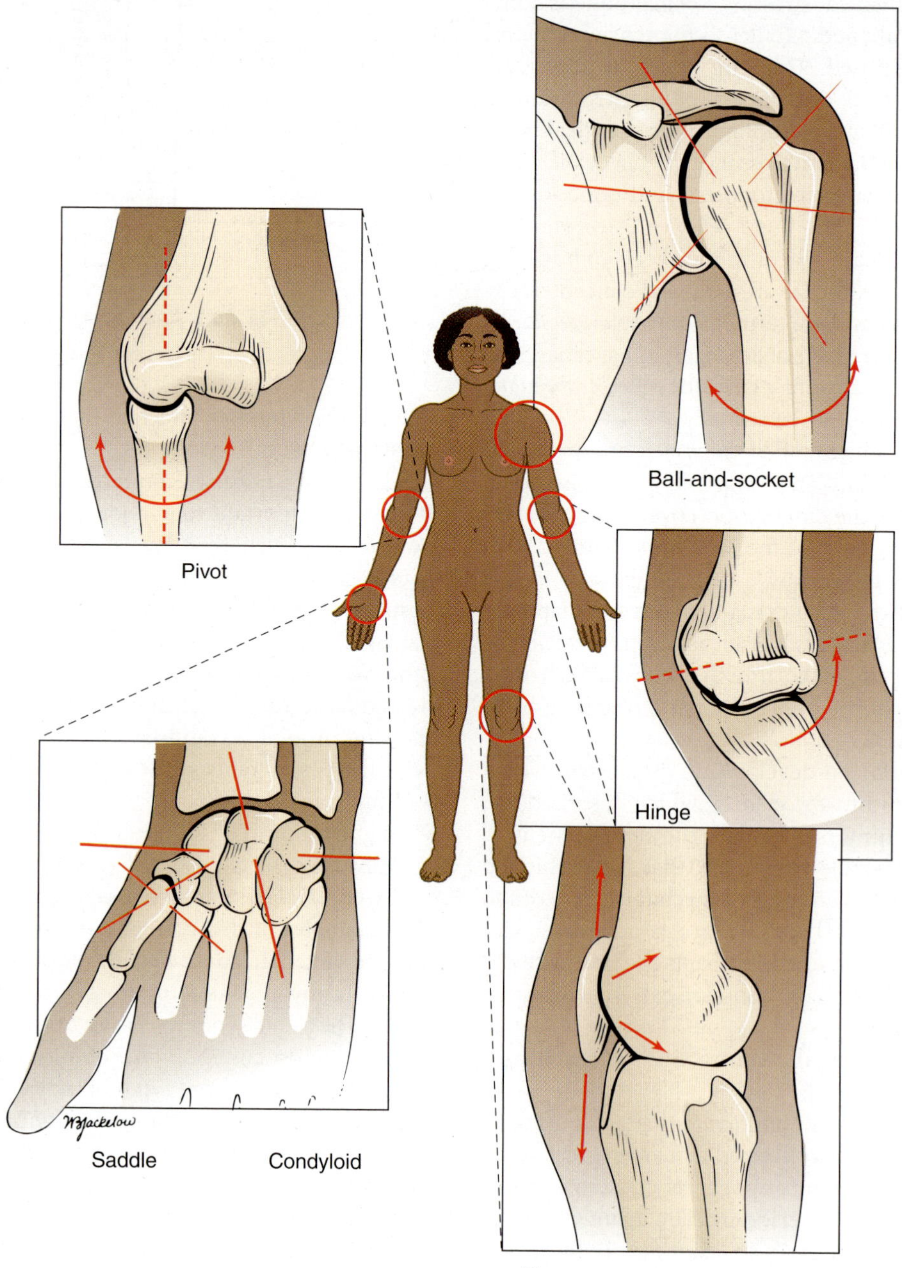

Fig. 20.2 Types of Movable Joints.

The stability of a joint depends on the following:

- Shape of the articular surfaces
- Ligaments
- Associated muscles

It is necessary to be familiar with certain anatomic terms that refer to position (Table 20.3). The *median plane* bisects the body into right and left halves. A plane parallel to the median plane is a *sagittal plane.* The terms *medial* and *lateral* are used in reference to the sagittal plane. A position closer to the median plane is medial; farther from the median plane, it is lateral. In the upper limb, the term *ulnar* is often used to denote medial, and *radial* to denote lateral. In the lower limb, *tibial* is used to denote medial, and *peroneal* or *fibular* denotes lateral. These anatomic terms are illustrated in Fig. 20.3.

TABLE 20.3 Anatomic Terms for the Upper and Lower Limb

Limb	Medial	Lateral
Upper	Ulnar	Radial
Lower	Tibial	Peroneal/Fibular

The front of the body is the *anterior,* or *ventral,* surface, and the back of the body is the *posterior,* or *dorsal,* side. The *palmar,* or *volar,* aspect of the hand is the anterior surface. The *dorsal aspect* of the foot faces upward, and the *plantar aspect* is the sole. *Proximal* refers to the part of an extremity that is closest to its root; *distal* refers to the part farthest from the root.

The most important terms relating to deformities of the bone structure are *valgus* and *varus.* In a valgus deformity, the distal portion of the bone is displaced away from the midline, and angulation is toward the midline. In a varus deformity, the distal portion of the extremity is displaced toward the midline, and angulation is away from the midline. The name of the deformity is determined by the joint involved. A valgus deformity of the knees, knock-knee, is termed *genu valgum.* A varus deformity of the knee, bowleg, is termed *genu varum.*

In the evaluation of a joint, assess the *range of motion.* Each joint has a characteristic range of motion that can be measured passively and actively. *Passive* range of motion is the motion elicited when the examiner moves the patient's body. *Active* range of motion is the motion the patient performs as a result of moving the musculature. The passive range of motion usually equals the active range of motion except in cases of paralyzed

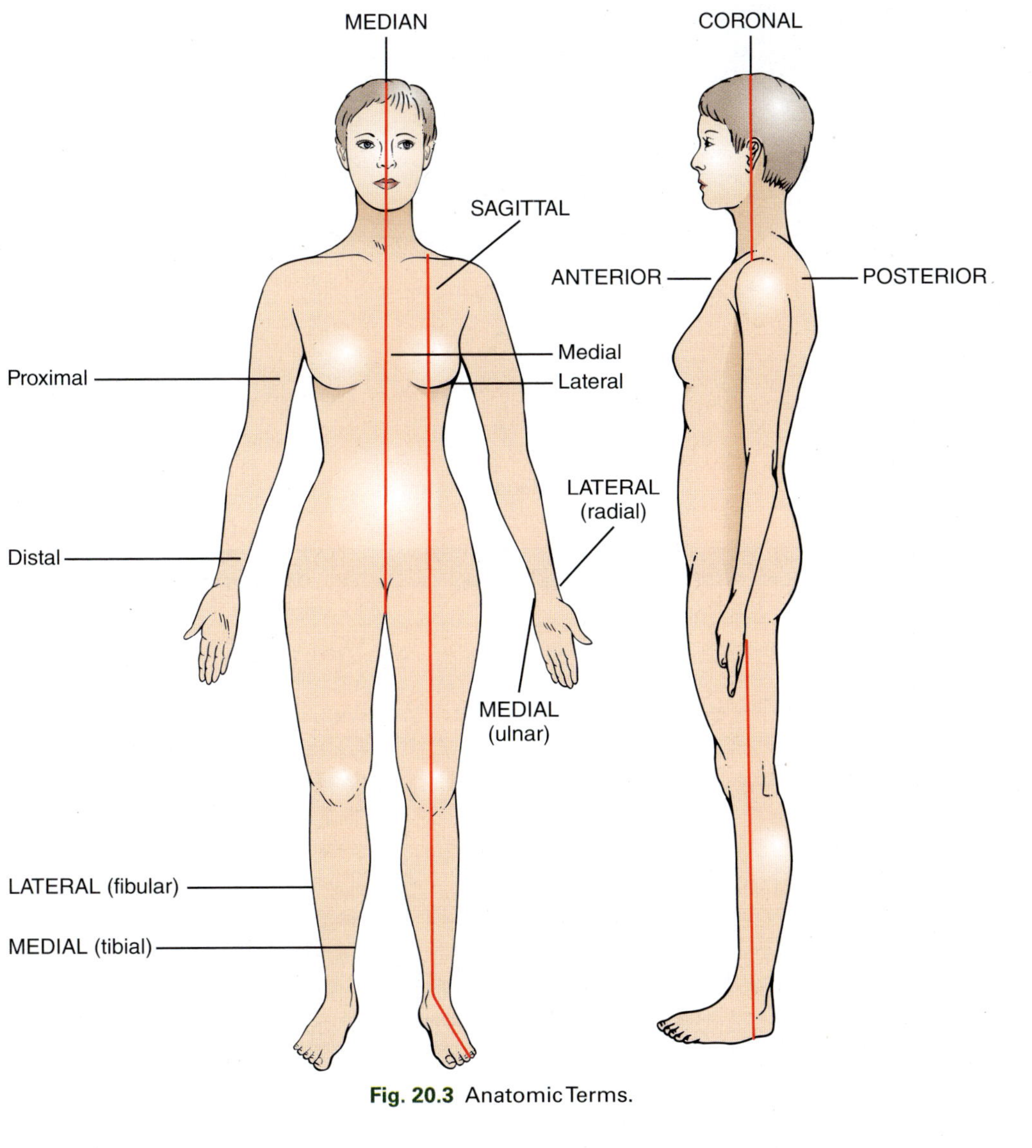

Fig. 20.3 Anatomic Terms.

muscles or ruptured tendons. The range of motion of individual joints is discussed later in this chapter. Joint motion is measured in degrees of a circle, with the joint at the center. If a limb is extended with the bones in a straight line, the joint is at *zero position*. The zero position is the neutral position of the joint. As the joint is flexed, the angle increases. The concept of range of motion is illustrated in Fig. 20.4.

The six basic types of joint motion are as follows:

- Flexion and extension
- Dorsiflexion and plantar flexion
- Adduction and abduction
- Inversion and eversion
- Internal and external rotation
- Pronation and supination

The definitions of these motions and the joints at which they occur are summarized in Table 20.4.

The anatomy of the *shoulder joint* is illustrated in Fig. 20.5. The joint movements at the shoulder are abduction and adduction, flexion and extension, and internal and external rotation. These motions are illustrated in Fig. 20.6.

The anatomy of the *elbow joint* is shown in Fig. 20.7. The joint movements at the elbow are flexion and extension, and supination and pronation. These motions are illustrated in Fig. 20.8.

The anatomy of the *wrist* and *fingers* is illustrated in Fig. 20.9. The joint movements at the wrist are dorsiflexion (or extension), palmar flexion, and supination and pronation. These motions are illustrated in Fig. 20.10. The joint movements at the fingers are abduction and adduction, and flexion and extension. These motions are illustrated in Fig. 20.11. The joint movements of the *thumb* are flexion and extension, abduction and adduction, and opposition. These motions are illustrated in Fig. 20.12.

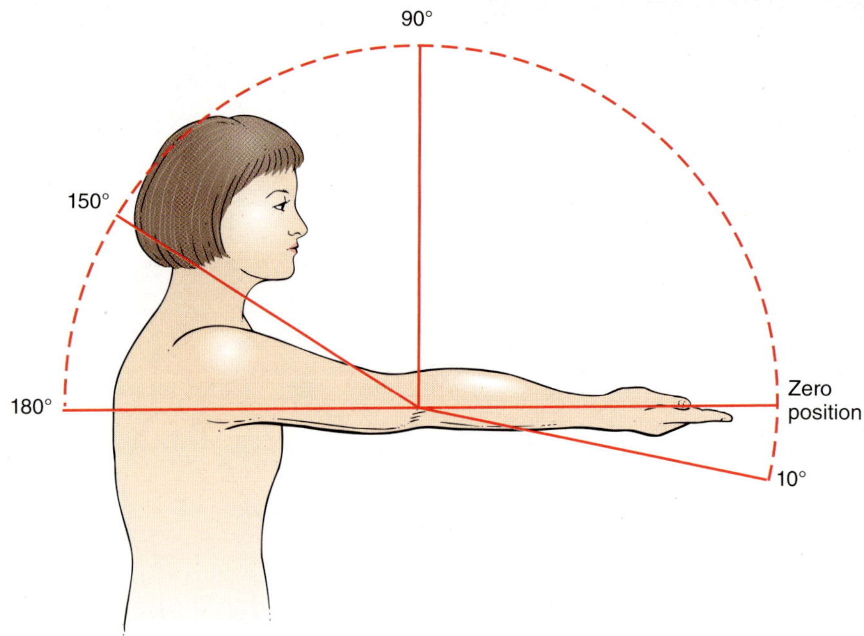

Fig. 20.4 Range of Motion.

TABLE 20.4 Joint Motion

Motion	Definition	Example
Flexion	Motion away from the zero position	Most joints
Extension	Return motion to the position[a]	Most joints
Dorsiflexion	Movement in the direction of the dorsal surface	Ankle, toes, wrist, fingers
Plantar (or palmar) flexion	Movement in the direction of the plantar (or palmar) surface	Ankle, toes, wrist, fingers
Adduction	Movement toward the midline[b]	Shoulder, hip, metacarpophalangeal, metatarsophalangeal joints
Abduction	Movement away from the midline	Shoulder, hip, metacarpophalangeal, metatarsophalangeal joints
Inversion	Turning of the plantar surface of the foot inward	Subtalar and midtarsal joints of the foot
Eversion	Turning of the plantar surface of the foot outward	Subtalar and midtarsal joints of the foot
Internal rotation	Turning of the anterior surface of a limb inward	Shoulder, hip
External rotation	Turning of the anterior surface of a limb outward	Shoulder, hip
Pronation	Rotation so that the palmar surface of the hand is directed downward	Elbow, wrist
Supination	Rotation so that the palmar surface of the hand is directed upward	Elbow, wrist

[a]Extension that goes beyond the zero position is called *hyperextension*.
[b]In the hand or foot, the midline is an imaginary line through the middle finger or middle toe, respectively.

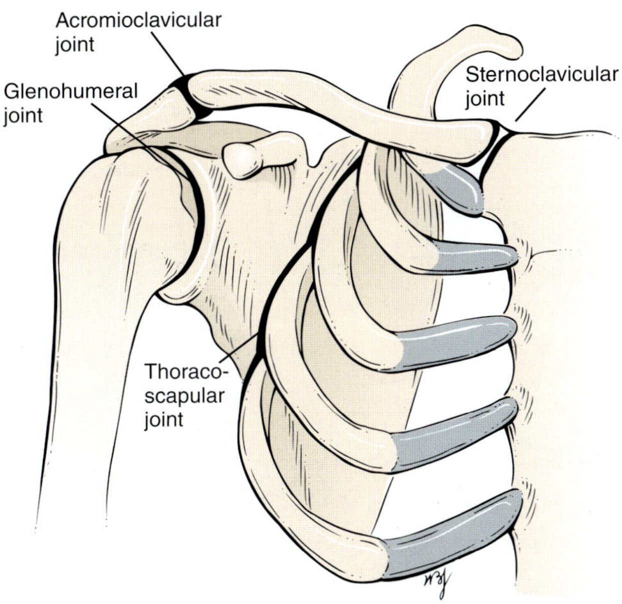

Fig. 20.5 Anatomy of the Shoulder Joint.

The anatomy of the *hip* is illustrated in Fig. 20.13. The joint movements at the hip are flexion and extension, abduction and adduction, and internal and external rotation. These motions are illustrated in Fig. 20.14.

The anatomy of the *knee* is shown in Fig. 20.15. The joint movements at the knee are flexion and extension. These motions are illustrated in Fig. 20.16.

The anatomy of the *ankle* and *foot* is illustrated in Fig. 20.17. There are 26 bones and 55 articulations in the foot. The bones can be divided into three regions: forefoot, midfoot, and hind foot. The *forefoot* is represented by the 14 bones of the toes and 5 metatarsals. The big toe (hallux) has two phalanges and one joint (interphalangeal [IP] joint) and two tiny and round *sesamoid bones* that enable it to move up and down. The sesamoid bones are about the size of a kernel of corn. These bones are embedded in the flexor hallucis brevis tendon, one of several tendons that exert pressure from the big toe against the ground and help initiate the act of walking: the propulsive phase of the gait cycle. The other four toes each have three bones and two joints. The phalanges are connected to the metatarsals by five

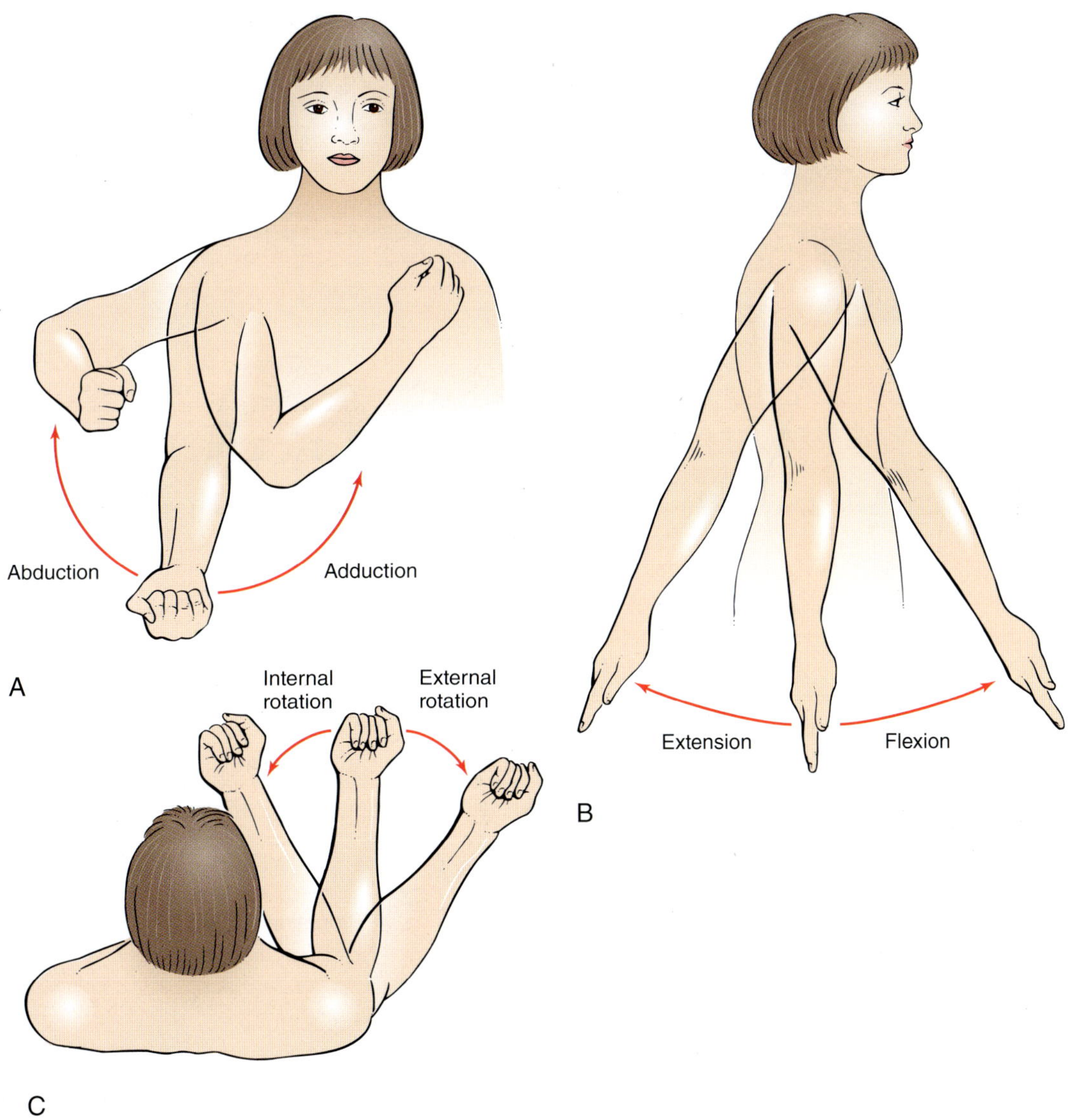

Fig. 20.6 Range of Motion at the Shoulder. (A) Abduction and adduction. (B) Flexion and extension. (C) Internal and external rotation.

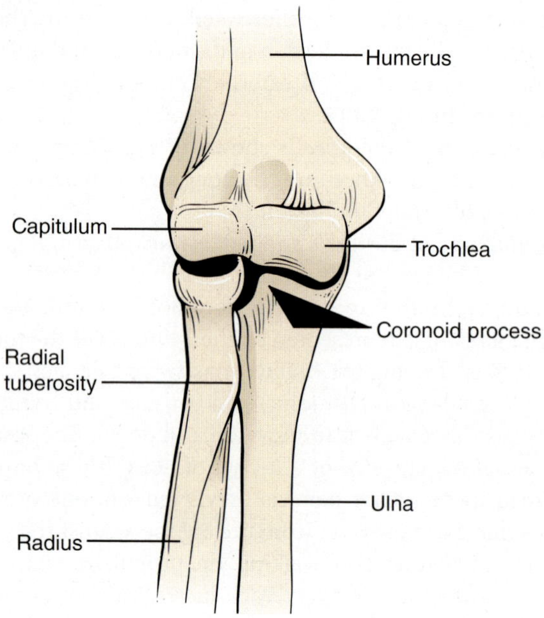

Fig. 20.7 Anatomy of the Elbow Joint.

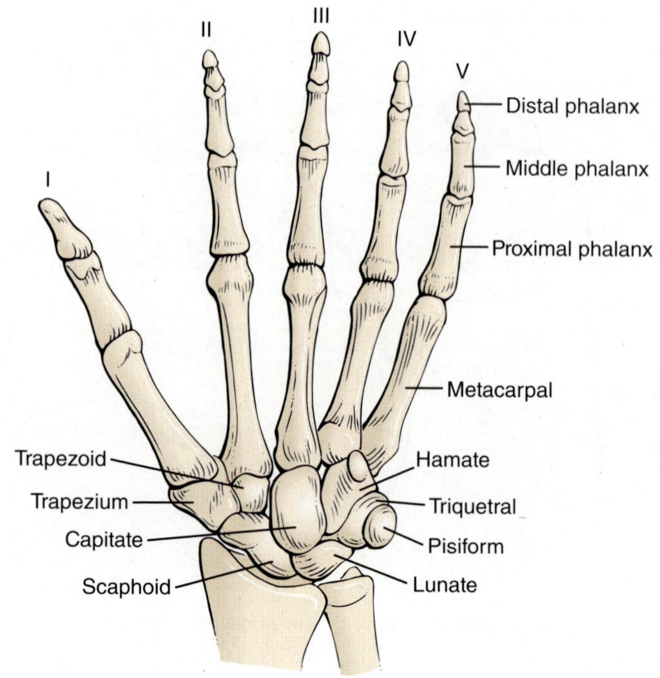

Fig. 20.9 Anatomy of the Wrist and Fingers.

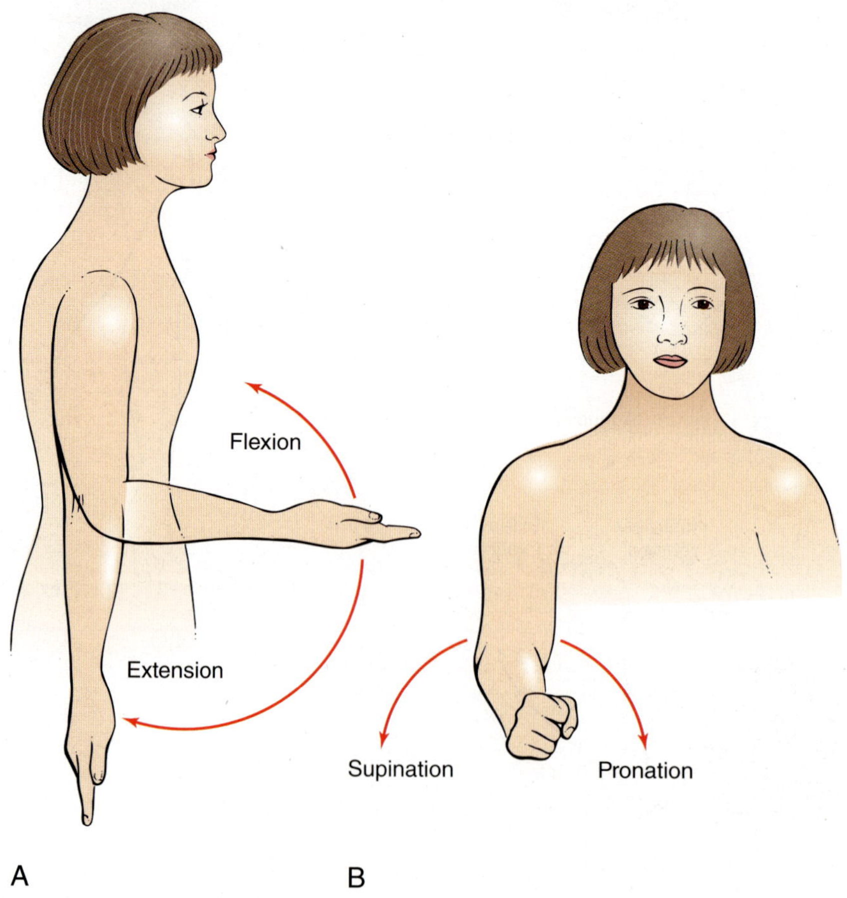

Fig. 20.8 Range of Motion at the Elbow Joint. (A) Flexion and extension. (B) Supination and pronation.

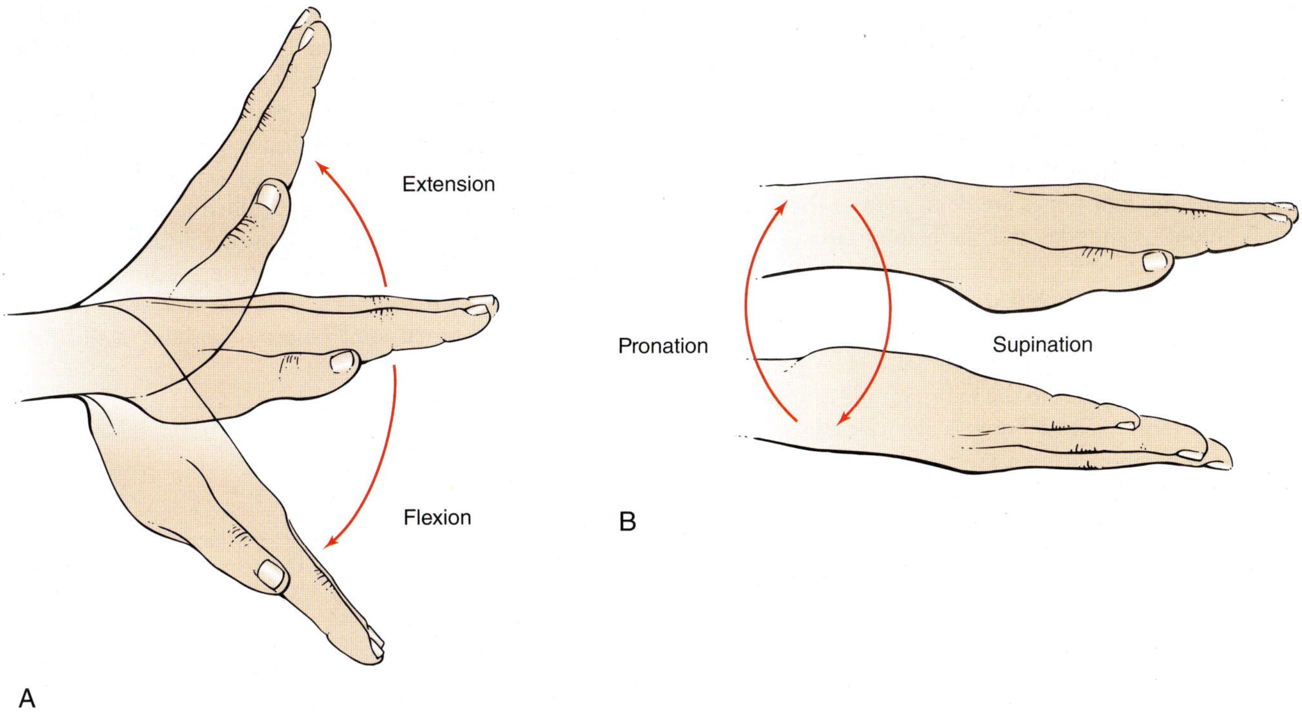

Fig. 20.10 Range of Motion at the Wrist Joint. (A) Dorsiflexion (extension) and palmar flexion. (B) Supination and pronation.

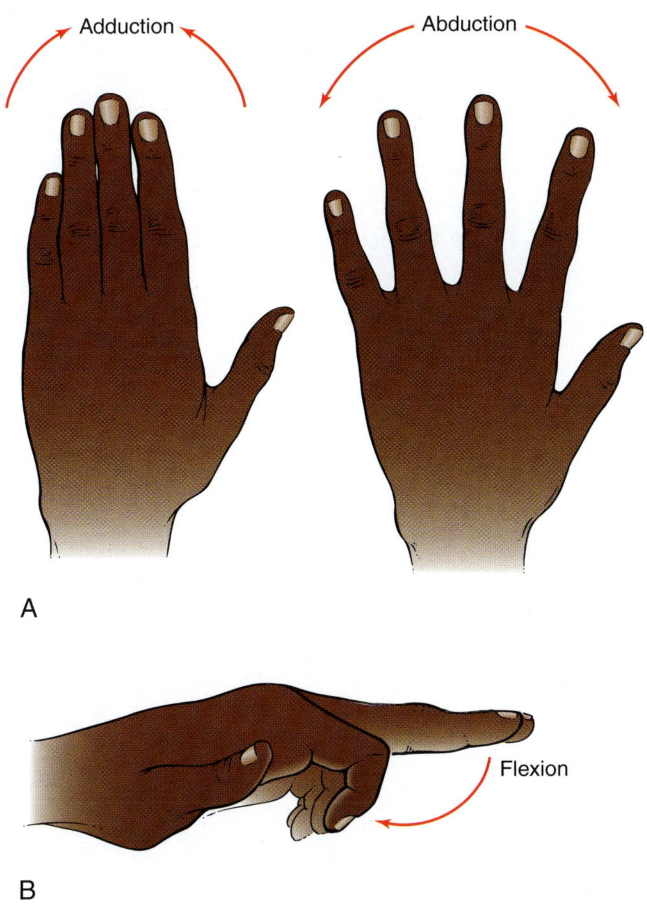

Fig. 20.11 Range of Motion at the Finger Joints. (A) Abduction and adduction. (B) Flexion.

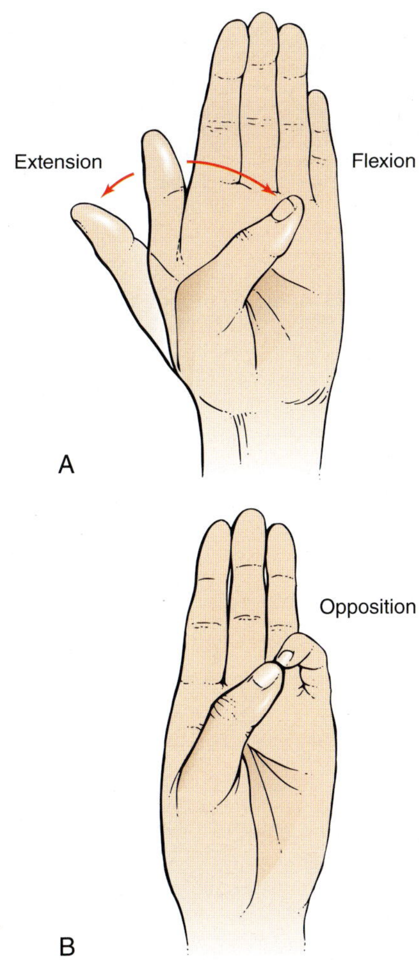

Fig. 20.12 Range of Motion of the Thumb. (A) Flexion and extension. (B) Opposition.

metatarsophalangeal (MTP) joints at the ball of the foot. The forefoot bears half the body's weight and balances pressure on the ball of the foot.

The *midfoot* consists of the three cuneiform bones, the cuboid, and the navicular. The midfoot has five irregularly shaped tarsal bones that form the foot's arch and serve as a shock absorber. The midfoot bones are connected to the forefoot and the hindfoot by muscles and the plantar fascia (arch ligament).

The *hind foot* is composed of the talus and the calcaneus. The foot contains two arches: the longitudinal in the midpart and the transverse in the forepart. The midtarsal joint is formed by the articulations of the navicular to the talus and the calcaneus to the cuboid. The largest tarsal bone is the calcaneus, the bottom of which is cushioned by a layer of fat. The attachment of the foot to the leg occurs through the talus. The joint movements at the ankle are dorsiflexion and plantar flexion. The motion of the subtalar joint is inversion and eversion. These motions are illustrated in Fig. 20.18.

The anatomy of the *cervical spine* is shown in Fig. 20.19. The joint movements of the neck are flexion and extension, rotation, and lateral flexion. These motions are illustrated in Fig. 20.20.

The anatomy of the *lumbar spine* is illustrated in Fig. 20.21. The joint movements of the lumbar spine are flexion and extension, rotation, and lateral extension. These motions are illustrated in Fig. 20.22.

A summary of normal joint ranges of motion is shown in Table 20.5.

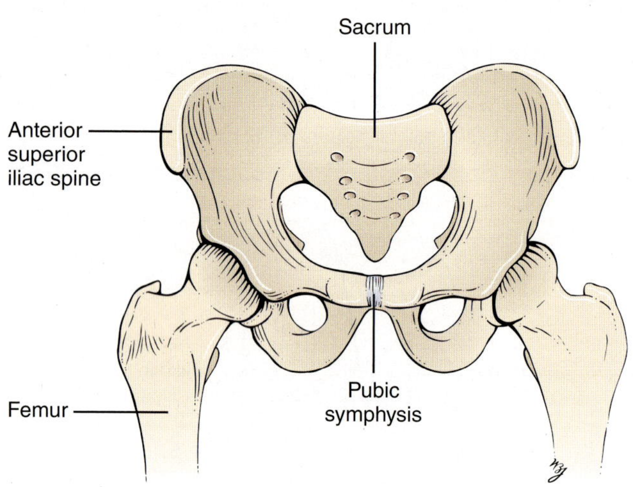

Fig. 20.13 Anatomy of the Hip Joint.

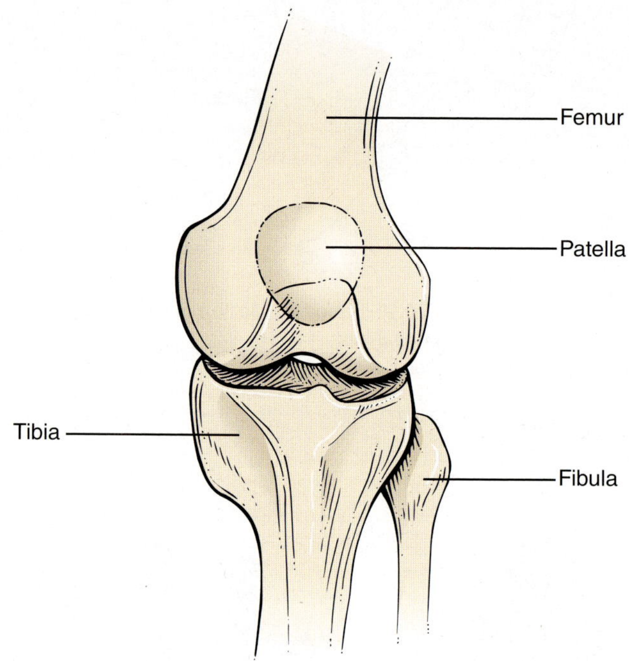

Fig. 20.15 Anatomy of the Knee Joint.

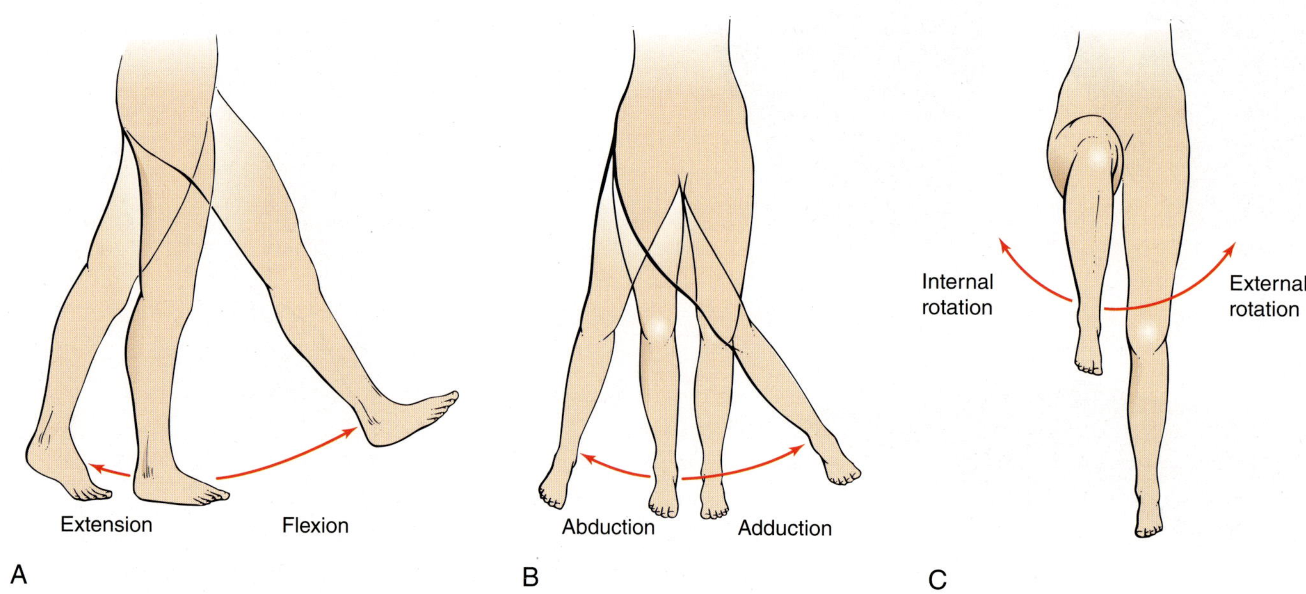

Fig. 20.14 Range of Motion at the Hip Joint. (A) Flexion and extension. (B) Abduction and adduction. (C) Internal and external rotation.

REVIEW OF SPECIFIC SYMPTOMS

The most common symptoms of musculoskeletal disease are as follows:

- Pain
- Weakness
- Deformity
- Limitation of motion
- Stiffness
- Swelling
- Crepitus

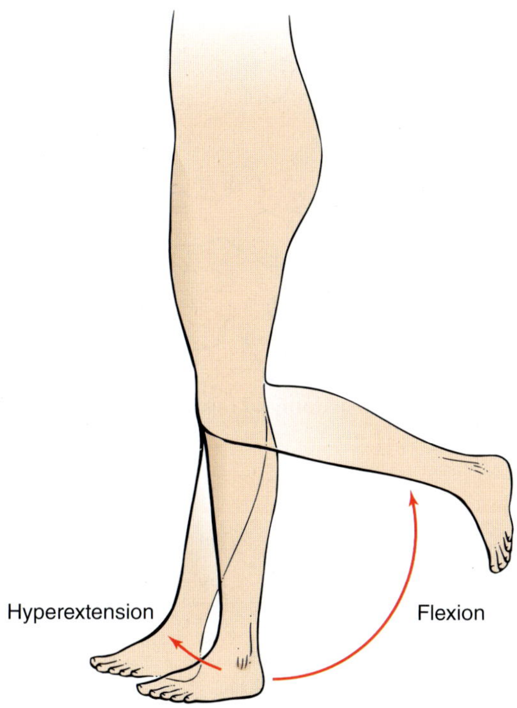

Fig. 20.16 Range of Motion at the Knee Joint: Flexion and Hyperextension.

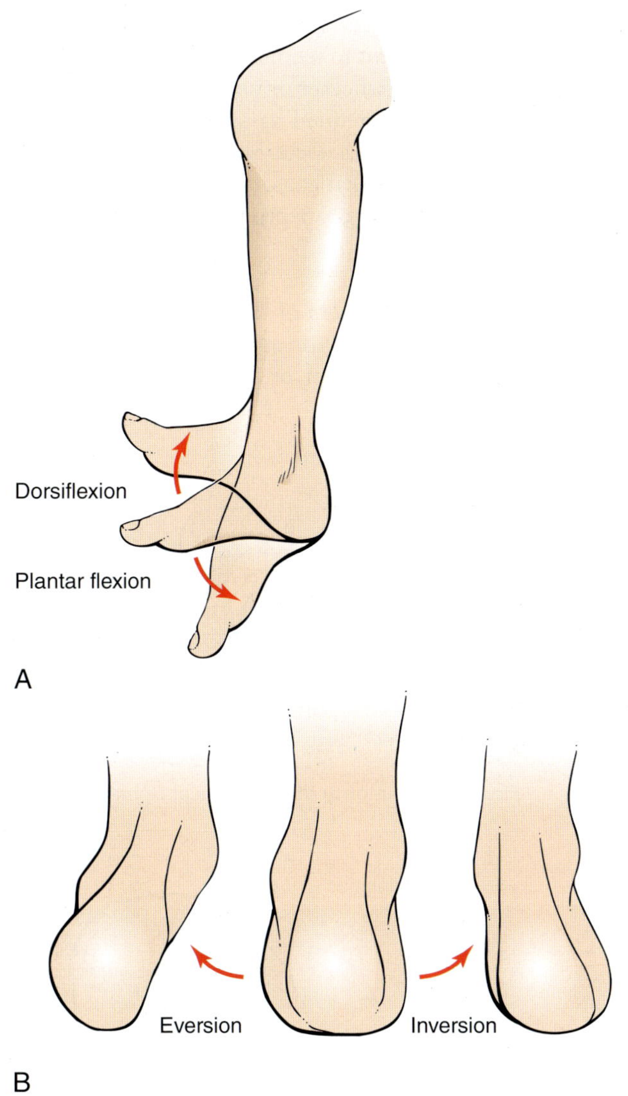

Fig. 20.18 Range of Motion at the Ankle and Foot Joints. (A) Dorsiflexion and plantar flexion. (B) Eversion and inversion.

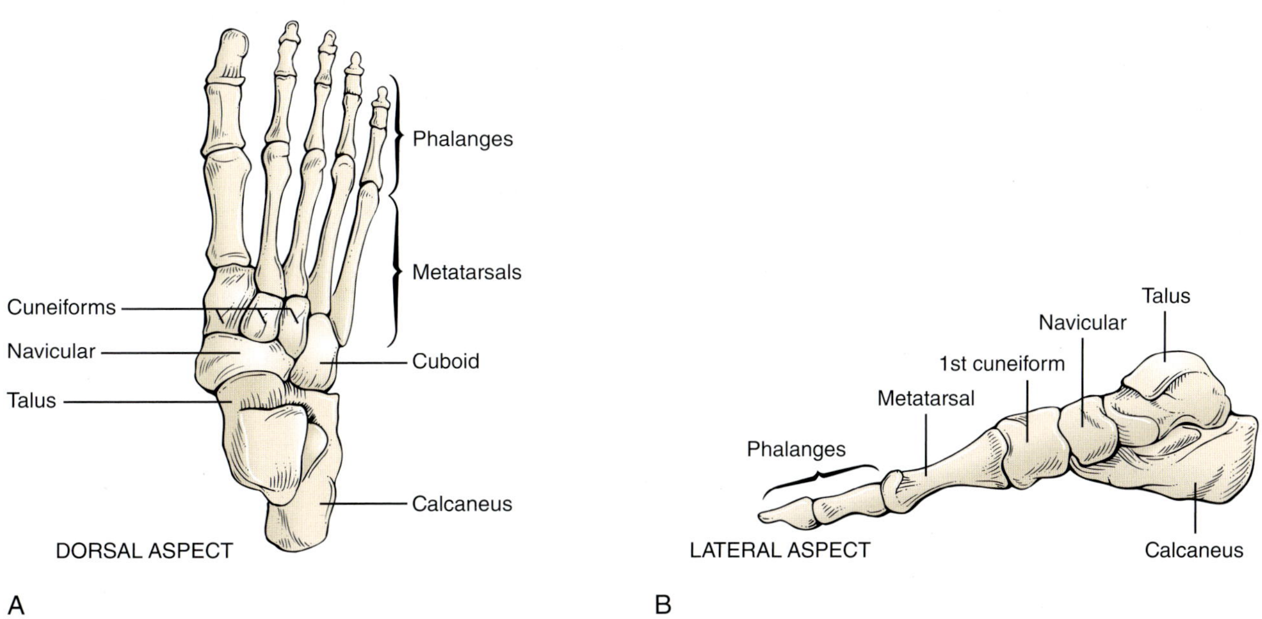

Fig. 20.17 Anatomy of the Ankle and Foot Joints. (A) View from above. (B) Medial view.

The location, character, and onset of each symptom must be ascertained. It is important to learn the specifics of the onset of the symptom, including whether or not the problem is acute or chronic. Acuity is often defined as symptoms occurring less than or greater than 6 weeks. Determine if there was a mechanism of injury or trauma that caused the symptom of concern as well as the symptom duration, progression, and severity.

Pain

Pain can result from disorders of the bone, muscle, or joint. Important considerations include quality of pain, severity (on a scale of 0–10), timing, radiation, or antecedent pain.

Ask the following questions:

"When did you first become aware of the pain?"

"Where do you feel the pain? Point to the most painful spot with one finger."

"Did the pain occur suddenly?"

"Does the pain occur daily?"

"During which part of the 24-hour day is your pain worse: Morning? Afternoon? Evening?"

"Did a recent illness precede the pain?"

"What makes the pain worse?"

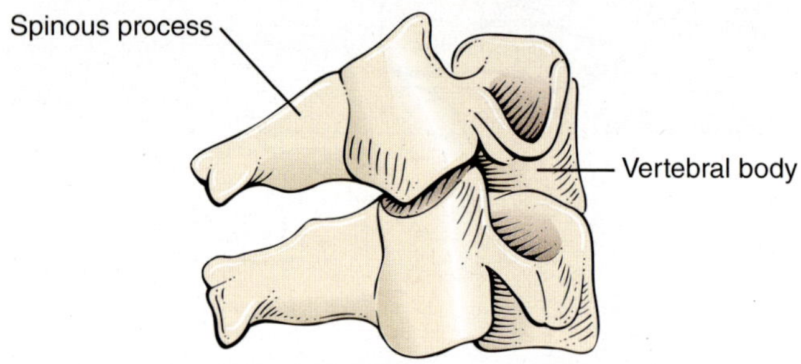

Fig. 20.19 Anatomy of the Cervical Spine.

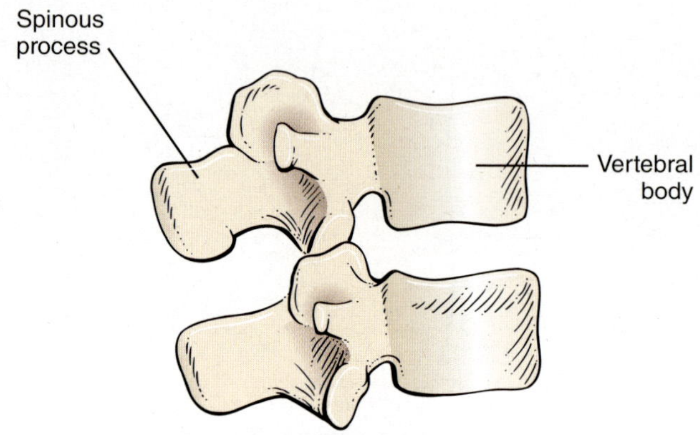

Fig. 20.21 Anatomy of the Lumbar Spine.

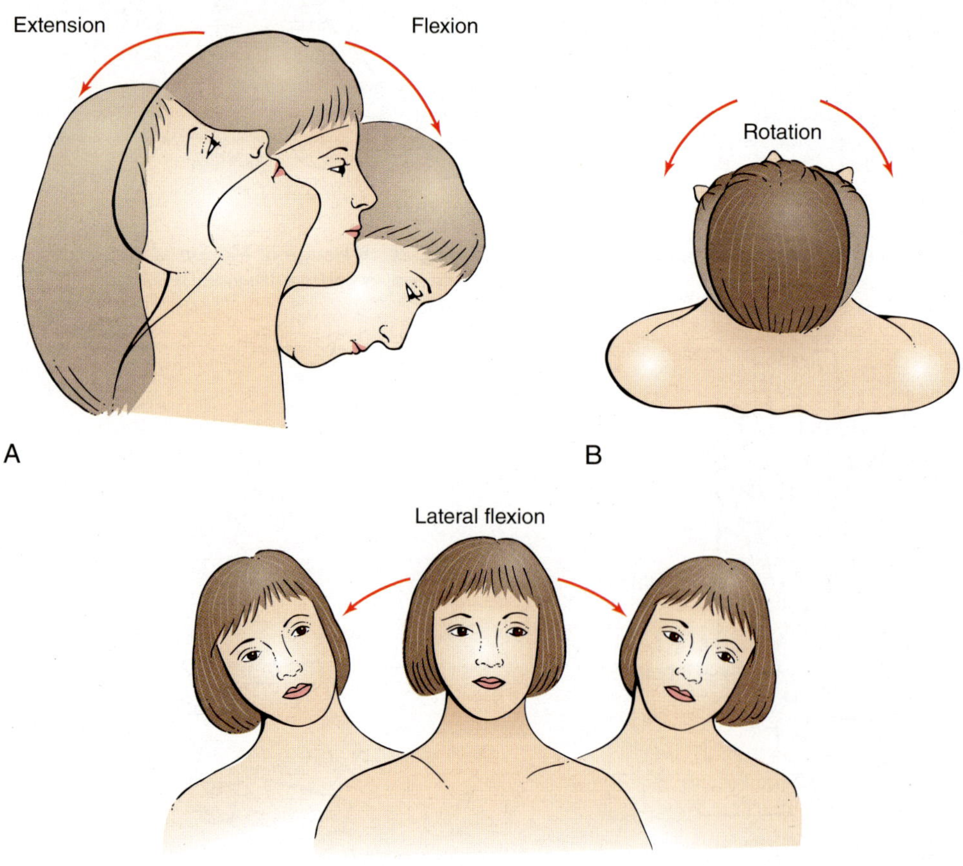

Fig. 20.20 Range of Motion at the Cervical Spine. (A) Flexion and extension. (B) Rotation. (C) Lateral flexion.

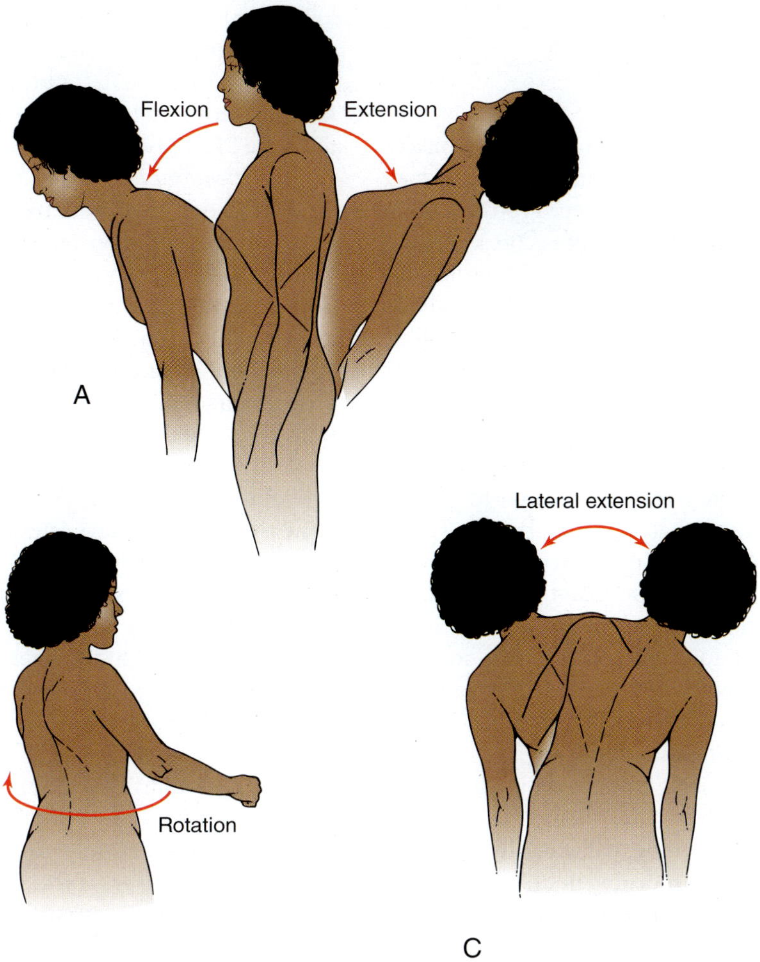

Fig. 20.22 **Range of Motion at the Lumbar Spine.** (A) Flexion and extension. (B) Rotation. (C) Lateral extension.

TABLE 20.5 Normal Joint Ranges of Motion

Joint	Flexion	Extension	Lateral Bending	Rotation
Cervical spine	45 degrees	55 degrees	40 degrees	70 degrees
Thoracic and lumbar spine	75 degrees	30 degrees	35 degrees	30 degrees
Shoulder	180 degrees	50 degrees	Abduction; 180 degrees	Adduction; 50 degrees
Elbow	150 degrees	180 degrees	Pronation; 80 degrees	Supination; 80 degrees
Wrist	80 degrees	70 degrees	Radial motion; 20 degrees	Ulnar motion; 55 degrees
Metacarpophalangeal joint	90 degrees	20 degrees	—	—
Hip	90 degrees with knee extended	30 degrees with knee extended	40 degrees	45 degrees
	120 degrees with knee flexed	—	Abduction; 45 degrees	Adduction; 30 degrees
Knee	135 degrees	0–10 degrees	—	—
Ankle	50 degrees	15 degrees	—	—
Subtalar	—	—	Inversion; 20 degrees	Eversion; 10 degrees
First metatarsophalangeal joint	40 degrees	65–75 degrees	—	—

"What do you do to relieve the pain?"
"Is the pain relieved by rest?"
"What kinds of medications have you taken to relieve the pain?"
"Have you noticed that the pain changes according to the weather?"
"Do you have any difficulty putting on your shoes or coat?"
"Does the pain ever awaken you from sleep?"
"Does the pain shoot to another part of your body?"
"Have you noticed that the pain moves from one joint to another?"

"Has there been any injury, overuse, or strain?"
"Have you noticed any swelling?"
"Are other bones, muscles, or joints involved?"
"Have you had a recent sore throat?"

Bone pain may occur with or without trauma. It is typically described as "deep," "dull," "boring," or "intense." The pain may be so intense that the patient is unable to sleep. Typically, bone pain is unrelated to movement unless a fracture is present. Pain from a fractured bone is often described as "sharp." Muscle pain is frequently described as "crampy." It may last only briefly or for longer periods. Muscle pain in the lower extremity on walking (described in Chapter 15, The Peripheral Vascular System) suggests ischemia of the calf or hip muscles. Muscle pain associated with weakness is suspicious for a primary muscular disorder. Joint pain is usually felt around or in the joint. It may also cause radiating pain in a region proximal or distal to the affected joint. In some conditions, the joint may be exquisitely tender. Movement usually worsens the pain, except with RA, in which movement often reduces the pain. Infection in the joint needs to be ruled out for acute onset pain. However, chronic infection with tuberculosis or fungal infections may smolder for years before the onset of pain. The severity of the pain can often be assessed by the time interval from pain onset to the time the patient seeks medical attention.

The time of day when the pain is worse may be helpful in diagnosing the disorder. The pain of many rheumatic disorders tends to be accentuated in the morning, particularly on rising. Tendinitis worsens during the early morning hours and eases by midday. OA worsens as the day progresses.

The sudden onset of pain in a MTP joint should raise suspicion for gout. Entrapment syndromes are apt to radiate pain distally. RA and tendinitis often cause early awakening because of pain, particularly when the patient lies on the affected limb.

Acute rheumatic fever, leukemia, gonococcal arthritis, sarcoidosis, and juvenile RA are commonly associated with *migratory polyarthritis,* in which one joint is affected, the disease subsides, and then another joint becomes involved.

Whether from an accident, sports injury, or general wear and tear, knee pain and knee injuries are very common concerns. Meniscal injuries may be the most common knee injury. The menisci are small, rubbery cartilaginous discs, located between the femur and tibia, which act to cushion the knee and allow the bones to glide smoothly against one another. Meniscus tears are common in contact sports such as football, as well as noncontact sports that require jumping and running such as volleyball and soccer. Meniscus tears can be painful and debilitating. Although commonly related to trauma, significant trauma is not necessary. A sudden twist or repeated squatting motion can tear the meniscus. Pain, swelling, a popping sensation during an injury, difficulty in bending and straightening the leg, and a tendency for the knee to get "stuck" are common symptoms of a meniscal tear. Meniscal tears can often occur with other knee injuries such as an ACL injury.

Injuries to the ACL occur typically due to a rotational movement or hyperextension of the knee. They commonly occur in female athletes but can occur during benign, non-sport-related activities. The ACL is one of the ligaments that stabilize the knee. Athletes who participate in sports that require sudden stopping and quickly changing directions while they are running are prone to ACL injuries. These sports include soccer, football, basketball, tennis, gymnastics, and volleyball. Symptoms are like those of a meniscal tear.

Patellofemoral arthritis is an overuse injury, often known as "runner's knee." It results from softening and deterioration of the cartilage on the posterior aspect of the patella. The condition can also be seen in older adults with arthritis. Manifestations of this form of arthritis range from no symptoms to vague anterior knee pain to severe difficulties with stair climbing and ambulation. Chondromalacia of the patella is used to describe the early manifestations of the articular cartilage that eventually lead to arthritis.

Viral illnesses are commonly associated with muscle aches and joint pain. A recent history of a sore throat, with joint pain occurring 10 to 14 days later, is suspect of rheumatic fever. If rest does not relieve the pain, a more serious musculoskeletal disease may be present. The interviewer should also keep in mind the possibility of *referred pain.* Pain from a hip disorder is frequently referred to the knee, especially in a child.

Weakness

Muscular weakness should always be differentiated from fatigue. Ascertain which functions the patient is unable to perform because of "weakness." Is the weakness related to proximal or distal muscle groups? *Proximal weakness* is usually a myopathy; *distal weakness* is usually a neuropathy. A patient with the symptoms of muscular weakness should be asked these questions:

"Do you have difficulty combing your hair?"
"Do you have difficulty lifting objects?"
"Have you noticed any problem with holding a pen or pencil?"
"Do you have difficulty turning doorknobs?"
"Do you have trouble standing up after sitting in a chair?"
"Do you find that, as the day goes on, there is a change in the weakness?" If yes, *"Does the weakness worsen or improve?"*
"Have you noticed any decrease in your muscle size?"
"Are the weak muscles stiff?"
"Do you have trouble with double vision? Swallowing? Chewing?"

A patient with proximal weakness of the lower extremity has difficulty walking and crossing the knees. A proximal weakness of the upper extremity is manifested by difficulty brushing the hair or lifting objects. Patients with *polymyalgia rheumatica* have proximal muscle weakness. This condition is discussed in Chapter 25, The Geriatric Patient. A distal weakness of the upper extremity is manifested by difficulty turning doorknobs or buttoning a shirt or blouse. Patients with myasthenia gravis have generalized weakness, diplopia, and difficulty swallowing and chewing.

Deformity

Deformity may be the result of a congenital malformation or an acquired condition. In any patient with a deformity, it is important to determine the following:

"When was the deformity first noticed?"
"Did the deformity occur suddenly?"

"Did the deformity occur as a result of trauma?"
"Has there been any change in the deformity with time?"

Limitation of Motion

Limitation of motion may result from changes in the articular cartilage, scarring of the joint capsule, or muscle contractures. Determine the types of motion the patient can no longer perform easily, such as combing the hair, putting on shoes, or buttoning a shirt or blouse.

Stiffness

Stiffness is a common symptom of musculoskeletal disease. For example, a patient with arthritis of the hip may have difficulty crossing their legs to tie shoes. Ask the patient whether the stiffness is worse at any particular time of day. Patients with RA tend to experience stiffness after periods of joint rest. These patients typically describe morning stiffness, which may take several hours to subside.

Swelling

Swelling occurs as a result of inflammation. Joint swelling can be a symptom of a chronic disease or an acute injury. There are many causes of swelling; these include but are not limited to inflammatory diseases (e.g., gout), Behçet disease, bursitis, juvenile arthritis, ankylosing spondylitis, reactive arthritis, sprains, tendonitis, RA, septic arthritis (e.g., gonococcal arthritis), torn ligaments, torn tendons, fractures, dislocations, bleeding disorders (e.g., hemophilia), OA, tendon sheath inflammation (e.g., tenosynovitis), and autoimmune disorders (e.g., systemic lupus erythematosus, psoriasis, and Sjögren syndrome).

Crepitus

Crepitus, commonly described by the patient as a "clicking" or "popping" sensation can be from a multitude of conditions. The most common condition that causes clicking is an arthritic joint due to an incongruent joint surface. In the hand, a clicking sensation of the finger is most often secondary to a trigger finger. Subluxation of a tendon about its tendon sheath can also cause a popping sensation, like an extensor tendon in the hand or wrist, or the biceps tendon from its groove in the shoulder. It is important to assess the joint affected and evaluate the motion of that joint to see if the described sensation is reproducible.

EFFECT OF MUSCULOSKELETAL DISEASE ON THE PATIENT

Musculoskeletal diseases have a significant impact on patients and their families. Disability and limitations on daily activities can be more devastating than the pain itself.

Diseases of the musculoskeletal system range from minor aches and pains to severe crippling disorders, often associated with premature death. RA is a crippling disorder that strikes many patients in the prime of life. In addition to having joint pain that limits activity, patients with RA fear the possibility of losing their independence as the disease progresses. Often, their self-image and self-esteem become altered due to the inability to live the life they previously lived before affected by the disease. There is also a component of deformity and altered body image that often causes patients to become withdrawn and isolated.

Musculoskeletal disease can have significant physical limitations, particularly when accompanied by joint or muscle pain. These limitations can have a profound impact on patients' social lives, leading to strain on marital and familial relationships as well as withdrawal from social activities. Such disabilities may also result in job loss or a need to change careers, leading to financial uncertainty. The loss of social status and financial stability can further strain personal relationships and contribute to anxiety and depression.

Rehabilitation is a crucial part of treatment for the physical and psychological improvement of a patient. The patient plays a pivotal role in the rehabilitation process. While caregivers can initially provide motivation, it is the patient's own attitude that ultimately determines the success of rehabilitation. Factors like self-image, psychological, social, and financial resources affect the patient's motivation to overcome the disability. It's important for healthcare professionals to build trust with the patient, set realistic expectations, and become a source of motivation to aid in their recovery.

PHYSICAL EXAMINATION

The musculoskeletal exam does not require special equipment. The healthcare professional's musculoskeletal examination is a screening examination to indicate or exclude functional impairment of the musculoskeletal system. The examination is not timely and should be included in a routine examination. If an abnormality is noted or the patient has symptoms localized to a specific joint, a joint-focused examination should be done. Detailed descriptions of the examination of specific joints follow the discussion of the screening examination.

Screening Examination

See Video 20.1.

In the screening examination, the healthcare professional should assess the following components:

- General inspection
- Palpation
- Passive and active range of motion
- Muscle strength
- Integrated function

General Principles

General inspection should start with the skin. One should note if there are any skin changes like swelling, redness, rashes, masses, nodules, or prior scars. Are there any signs of inflammation? *Swelling, warmth, redness,* and *tenderness* are suggestive of inflammation. To determine a difference in temperature, use the back of your hand to compare one side with the other. Asymmetry should also be assessed. It is important to note if there is any muscle wasting, deformity, or an abnormal contour of the joint, which could indicate a joint dislocation.

Palpation may reveal areas of tenderness or discontinuity of a bone. Is *crepitus* present? Crepitus is a palpable crunching sensation often felt in the presence of roughened articular cartilages or may even indicate a fracture.

The *assessment of range of motion* of specific joints is next. Remember that inflamed or arthritic joints may be painful, and one should take care when assessing motion.

Muscle strength and integrated function are usually evaluated during the neurologic examination, and these topics are discussed in Chapter 21, The Nervous System.

Evaluate Gait

See Video 20.2.

The first part of the screening examination consists of inspection of gait and posture. To determine any eccentricity of gait, ask the patient to disrobe down to underwear and walk barefoot. Have the patient walk away from you, then back to you on tiptoes, away from you on the heels, and finally back to you in tandem gait. If there is any gait difficulty, these maneuvers must be modified. The positions of the foot during the normal gait cycle are shown in Fig. 20.23.

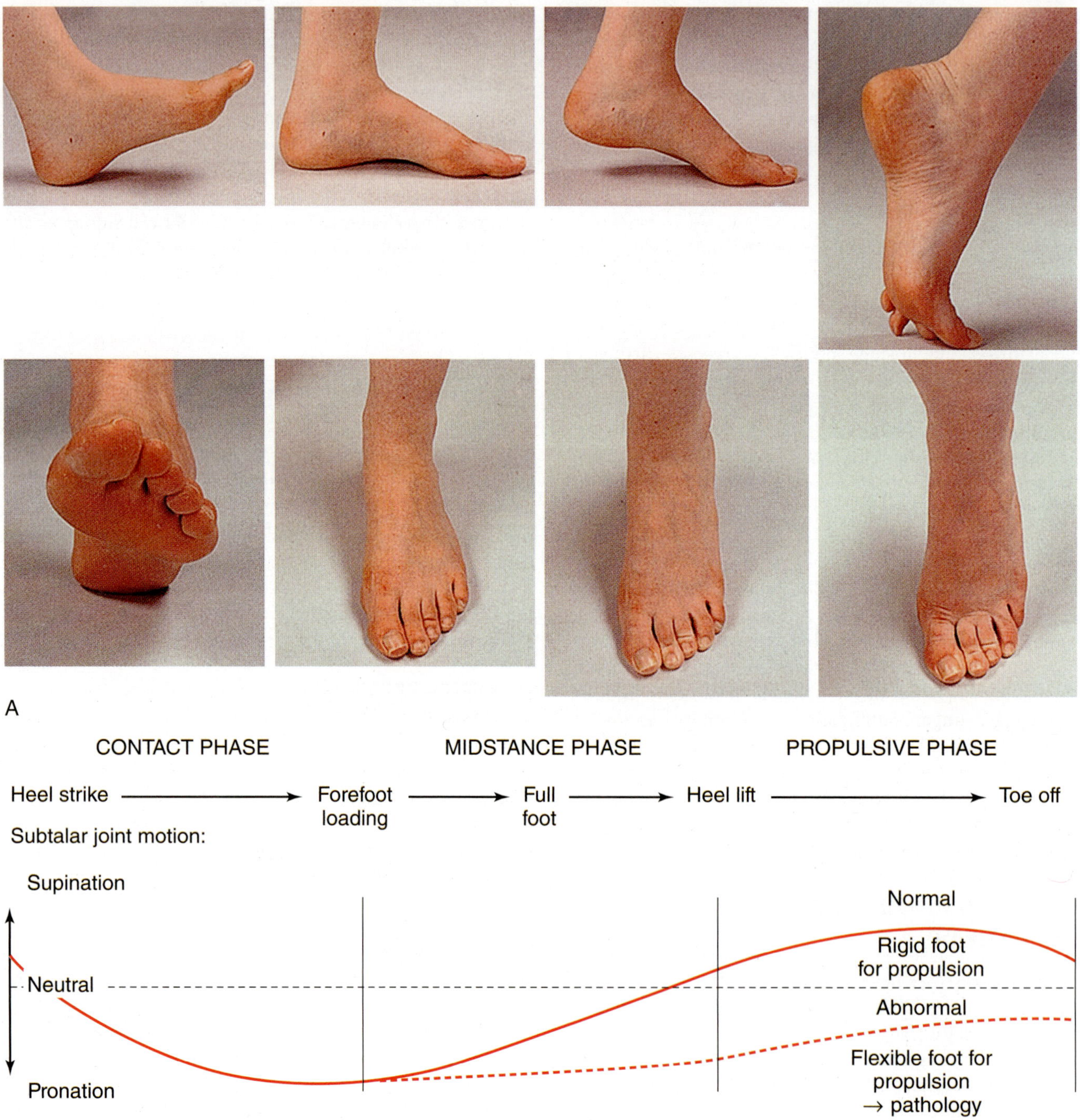

Fig. 20.23 (A and B) Positions of the foot in the normal gait cycle. (From Baran R, Dawber RPR, Tosti A, et al: *A text atlas of nail disorders: diagnosis and treatment*, St. Louis, 1996, Mosby.)

Observe the rate, rhythm, and arm motion used in walking. Does the patient have a staggering gait? Are the feet lifted high and slapped downward firmly? Does the patient walk with an extended leg that is swung laterally during walking? Are the steps short and shuffling? A complete discussion of gait abnormalities can be found in Chapter 21, The Nervous System. Fig. 21.59 illustrates common gait abnormalities.

Evaluate the Spine

Attention should then focus on the spine to detect any abnormal spinal curvatures. Have the patient stand erect and stand at the patient's side to inspect the profile of the patient's spine. Are the cervical, thoracic, and lumbar curves normal?

Move to inspect the patient's back. What is the level of the iliac crests? A difference may result from a leg length inequality, scoliosis, or flexion deformity of the hip. An imaginary line extending from the posterior occipital tuberosity should extend in line to the intergluteal cleft. Any lateral curvature is abnormal. Fig. 20.24 illustrates this point. Fig. 20.25A shows severe kyphoscoliosis. See also Fig. 13.6.

Ask the patient to bend forward, flexing at the trunk as far as possible with the knees extended. Note the smoothness of this action. This position is best for determining whether scoliosis is present. As the patient bends forward, the lumbar concavity should flatten. Fig. 20.25B shows the patient in Fig. 20.25A when bending forward.

Ask the patient to bend to each side from the waist and then bend backward from the waist to test *extension of the spine,* as shown in Fig. 20.26A.

To test *rotation of the lumbar spine,* sit on a stool behind the patient and stabilize the patient's hips by placing your hands on them. Ask the patient to rotate the shoulders one way and then reverse, as shown in Fig. 20.26B.

Evaluate Strength of the Lower Extremities

To assess the function of all major joints of the lower extremities, stand in front of the patient. Have the patient squat, with knees and hips fully flexed. Assist the patient by holding their hands to secure balance. This is shown in Fig. 20.27. Ask the patient to stand. Observing the manner in which the patient squats and then stands provides an excellent impression of the muscle strength and joint action of the lower extremities.

In addition, assessment of specific muscle groups can be performed and integrated into the arthrometric examination. Muscle strength can be graded according to the scale described in Chapter 21, The Nervous System.

Measure the strength of dorsiflexors and plantar flexors of the leg. With the patient seated, have the patient dorsiflex and

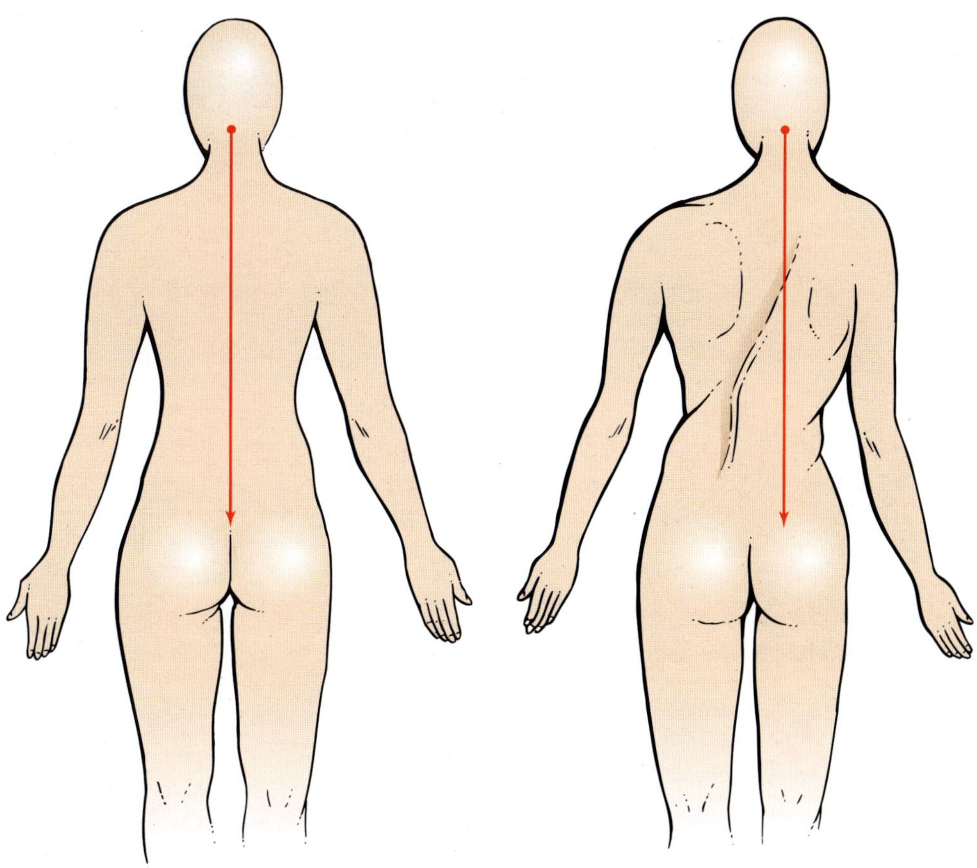

Fig. 20.24 Technique for Evaluating "Straightness" of the Spine. Lateral deviation of the spine may be related to a herniated disc or to a spasm of the paravertebral muscles. This functional deviation is often termed a *list*. True scoliosis may result from an actual deformity of the spine. In many cases, the spine twists in the opposite direction, so that a plumb line may actually be in the center.

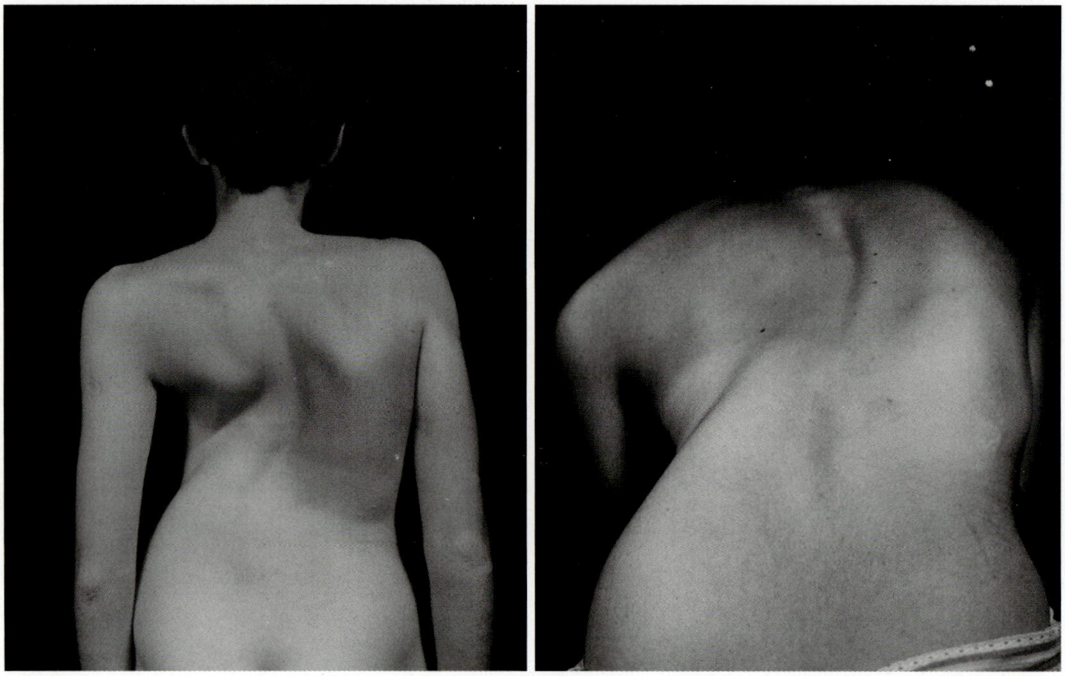

A B

Fig. 20.25 (A) Severe kyphoscoliosis. (B) Patient asked to bend forward.

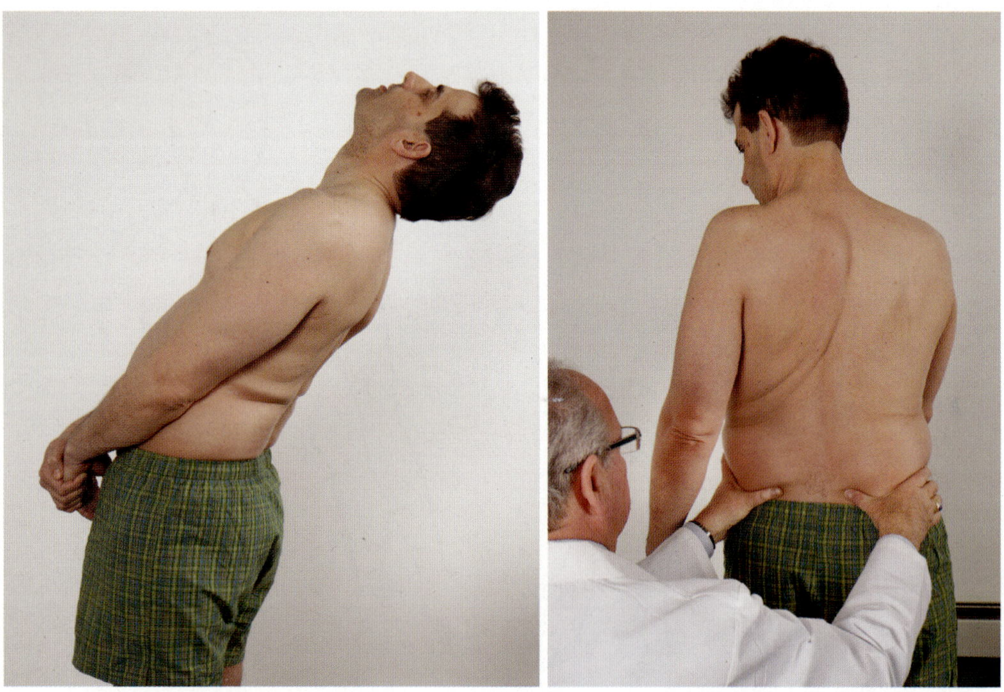

A B

Fig. 20.26 Technique for Evaluating Motion of the Lumbar Spine. (A) Test for extension of the spine. (B) Test for rotation of the spine.

plantarflex the foot against resistance. This can also be accomplished by asking the patient to walk toward and away from you on the heels and then on the toes. Injury to the common peroneal nerve causes weakness of the anterior muscle group, with a diminished capacity to dorsiflex the foot. Injury to the Achilles tendon or to the gastrocsoleus complex impairs plantar flexion.

Measure the invertors and evertors of the foot. With the patient seated, have the patient invert and then evert the foot against resistance.

Measure the quadriceps and hamstrings. With the patient seated, have the patient extend and then flex the knee against resistance.

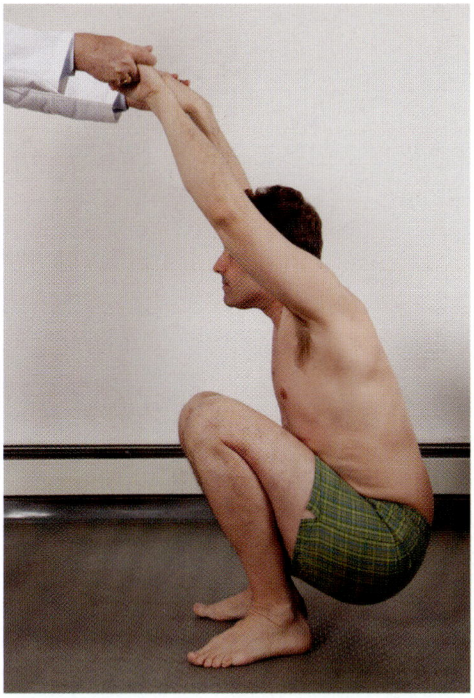

Fig. 20.27 Technique for Evaluating Strength of the Lower Extremities.

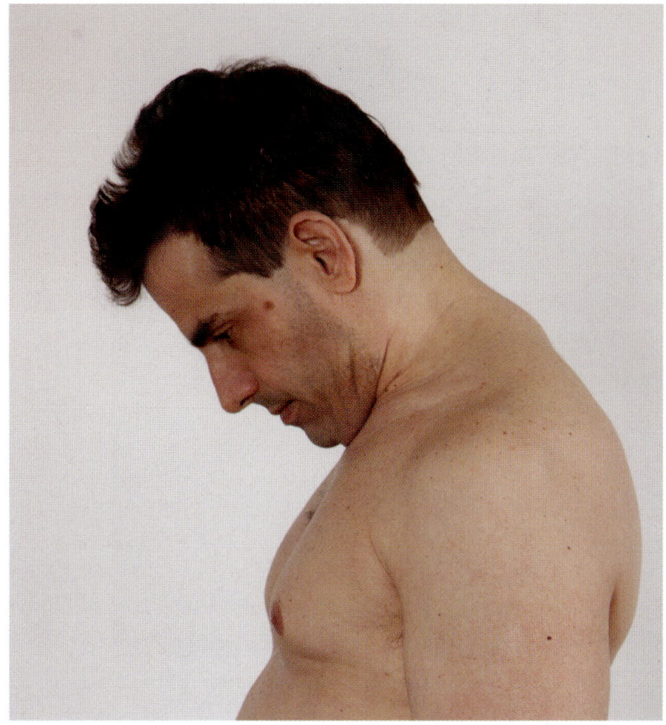

Fig. 20.28 Technique for Testing Flexion of the Neck.

Measure the hip abductors and adductors. With the patient seated, have the patient bring their knees together, then apart against the examiner's opposing force.

Measure the hip flexors and extensors. With the patient seated, have the patient raise the knee off the examination table against the examiner's downward, then upward, opposing force. Hip extensors can also be assessed by asking the patient to rise from a seated position unassisted.

Human immunodeficiency virus–related myopathy affects proximal muscle groups first, and patients may initially be concerned about difficulty rising from a chair or climbing stairs.

Evaluate Neck Flexion

The patient is instructed to sit, and the range of motion of the neck is assessed. The patient is asked to put their chin on the chest, with the mouth closed, as shown in Fig. 20.28. This tests full flexion of the neck.

Evaluate Neck Extension

To test full extension of the neck, place your hand between the patient's occiput and spinous processes of C7. Instruct the patient to trap your hand by extending the neck. This is shown in Fig. 20.29.

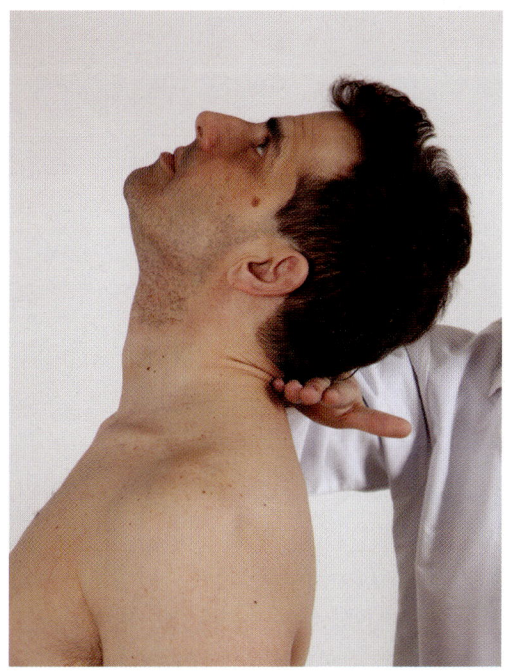

Fig. 20.29 Technique for Testing Extension of the Neck.

Evaluate Neck Rotation

Evaluate rotation of the neck by asking the patient to rotate the neck to one side and touch chin to shoulder. This is shown in Fig. 20.30. The examination is then repeated on the other side.

Evaluate Intrinsic Muscles of the Hand

The patient is instructed to stretch out the arms with the fingers spread. The examiner attempts to compress the fingers together against resistance, as shown in Fig. 20.31. This assesses the strength of the intrinsic muscles of the hand.

Evaluate External Rotation of the Arm

To test the functional range of rotation of the humerus and the *shoulder, acromioclavicular (AC),* and *sternoclavicular joints,* instruct the patient to abduct the arms fully and place the palms

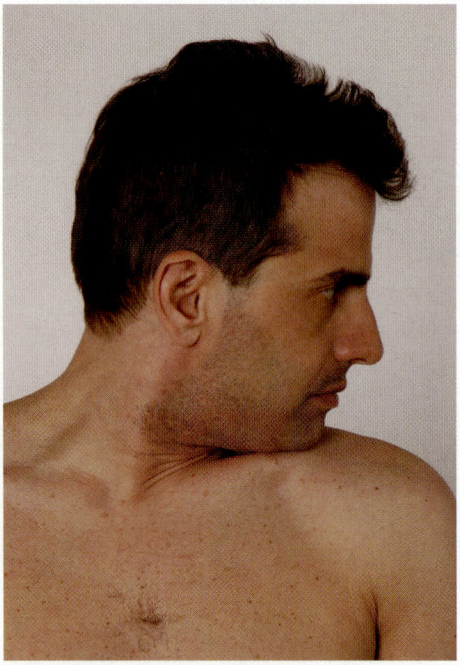

Fig. 20.30 Technique for Testing Rotation of the Neck.

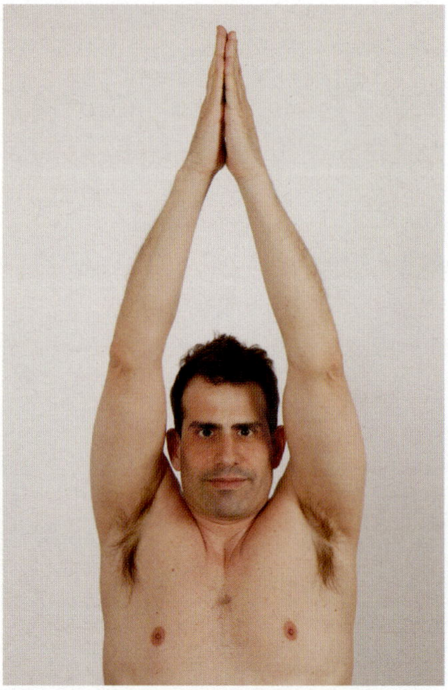

Fig. 20.32 Technique for Testing External Rotation of the Arm.

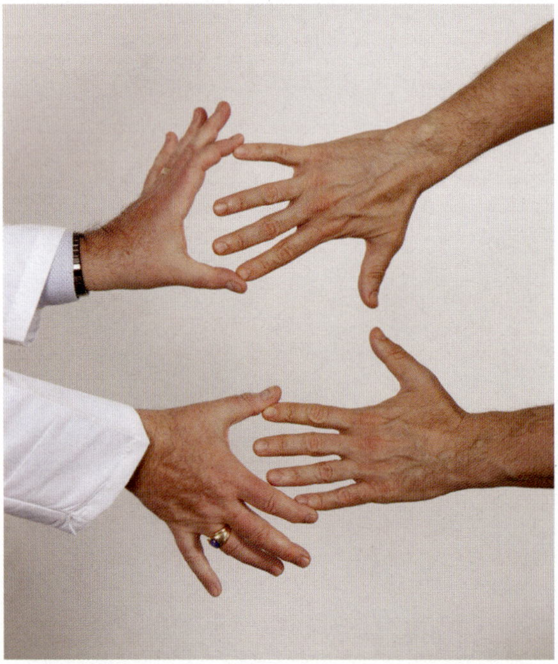

Fig. 20.31 Technique for Testing the Intrinsic Muscles of the Hand.

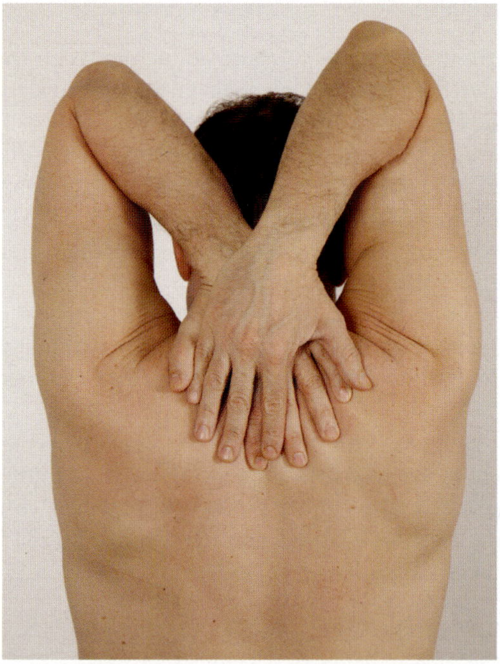

Fig. 20.33 Technique for Testing Internal Rotation of the Arm.

together above the head. The arms should touch the patient's ears with the head and cervical spine in the vertical position. This is shown in Fig. 20.32.

Evaluate Internal Rotation of the Arm

The patient is then asked to place their hands on the back between the scapulae. The hands should normally reach the level of the inferior angle of the scapulae. This is shown in Fig. 20.33. This maneuver tests the internal rotation of the humerus and range of motion at the elbow.

Evaluate Strength of the Upper Extremities

The final test of the screening examination assesses the power of the major groups of muscles in the upper extremities. The patient is asked to grasp the examiner's index and middle fingers in each hand. The patient is instructed to resist upward, downward, lateral, and medial movement by the examiner. This position is shown in Fig. 20.34.

This completes the basic musculoskeletal screening examination. The remainder of this section describes the symptoms and examination of specific joints.

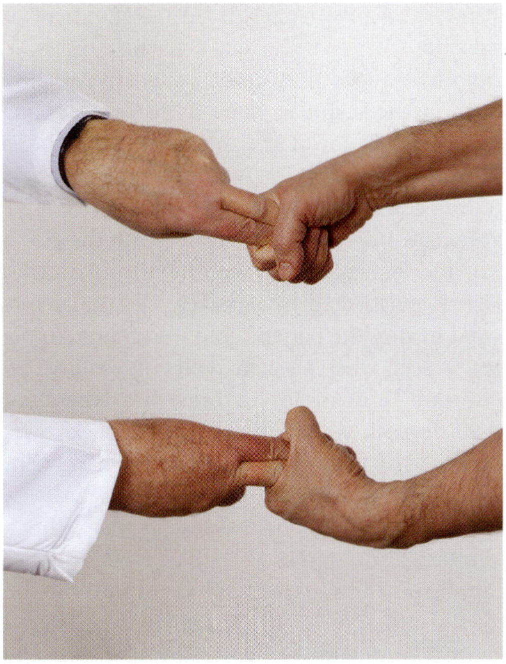

Fig. 20.34 Technique for Assessing Strength in the Upper Extremities.

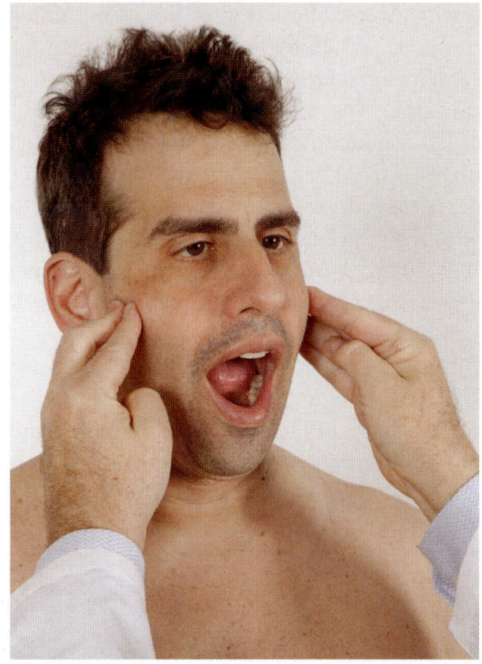

Fig. 20.35 Technique for Evaluating the Temporomandibular Joint.

Examination of Specific Joints

Any area must be inspected for evidence of swelling, atrophy, redness, and deformity, as well as palpated for swelling, muscle spasm, and local painful areas. The range of motion is assessed both actively and passively.

Temporomandibular Joint

Symptoms. A patient with temporomandibular joint problems may be concerned about unilateral or bilateral jaw pain. The pain is worse in the morning and after chewing or eating. The patient may also have concerns of "clicking" of the jaw.

Examination. To examine this joint, the examiner places their index fingers in front of the tragus and instructs the patient to open and close the jaw slowly. The examiner observes the smoothness of the range of motion and notes any tenderness. This is illustrated in Fig. 20.35.

Shoulder

Symptoms. Although shoulder pain may be related to a primary shoulder disorder, *always* consider the possibility that shoulder pain is referred from the chest, the abdomen, or cervical spine. Coronary artery disease, pulmonary tumors, and gallbladder disease are commonly associated with pain referred to the shoulder. Many cervical spine patients will have radiculopathy pain around the shoulder as well.

Pain is the main symptom of shoulder disorders. Inflammation of the *supraspinatus muscle* causes pain that is usually worse at night or when the patient lies on the affected shoulder. The pain often radiates down the arm as far as the elbow. The pain is commonly referred to the lower part of the deltoid area and is characteristically aggravated by combing the hair, putting on a coat, or reaching into the back pocket. Diffuse tenderness of the shoulder associated with pain on moving the humerus posteriorly is associated with disorders of the teres minor, infraspinatus, and subscapularis muscles. In this case, the pain usually does not radiate into the arm and is usually absent when the arm is dependent.

The movements of the shoulder occur at the *glenohumeral, thoracoscapular, AC,* and *sternoclavicular joints.* The glenohumeral joint is a ball-and-socket joint. In contrast to the hip joint, which is also a ball-and-socket joint, the glenohumeral joint has a very shallow glenoid socket. Therefore, the function of the joint depends on the muscles surrounding the socket for stability. These muscles and their tendons form the *rotator cuff* of the shoulder. For this reason, many shoulder problems are muscular, not bone or joint related, in origin.

Examination. Inspect the shoulder for deformity, wasting, swelling, and asymmetry. The shoulder should be palpated for local areas of tenderness. The range of motion for abduction, adduction, external and internal rotation, and flexion is evaluated and compared with that of the other side. Any pain is noted.

Special tests are necessary to determine specific diagnoses. The impingement syndrome, tears of the rotator cuff, bicipital tendinitis, and adhesive capsulitis are common. The examinations for these conditions are described in this section.

The *Apley scratch test* is a useful maneuver to assess shoulder range of motion. In this test, abduction and external rotation are measured by having the patient reach behind the head and touch the superior aspect of the opposite scapula. Internal rotation and adduction are tested by having the patient reach behind the back to touch the inferior aspect of the scapula. The presence of weakness and pain is a positive test.

Sudden onset of shoulder pain in the deltoid area 6 to 10 hours after trauma suggests a *rotator cuff tear* or *rupture.* Extreme tenderness over the greater tuberosity of the humerus and pain and restricted motion at the glenohumeral joint are usually present. Active abduction of the glenohumeral joint is markedly reduced. When the examiner attempts to abduct the arm, pain and a characteristic *shoulder shrug* result.

Supraspinatus. The *Jobe* or *empty can test* evaluates the rotator cuff. To conduct the Jobe test, have the patient stand and elevate both arms to 90 degrees of forward flexion in the scapular plane. Have the patient fully rotate the arms with the thumbs facing downward. The examiner applies downward pressure as shown in Fig. 20.36. A positive test is the development of pain on the injured side. The test has a sensitivity of 74% and a specificity of 38%.

The *full can test* evaluates the integrity of the supraspinatus tendon. To conduct the test, have the patient stand and elevate both arms to 90 degrees of forward flexion in the scapular plane with the thumbs facing upward. Ask the patient to hold while the examiner applies downward pressure. Fig. 20.37 illustrates the "full can test." A positive test is the development of pain on the injured side.

The *drop arm test* is performed by passively elevating the patient's arm in the scapular plane to 90 degrees, then asking the patient to slowly lower the arm to the side as shown in Fig. 20.38. A positive test is weakness or pain causing the patient to drop the arm suddenly to the side.

Infraspinatus. Infraspinatus is tested with the arm adducted at the body and externally rotating the arm. An *external rotation lag sign* is performed by passively externally rotating the shoulder and having the patient hold it to maintain position. A positive test is seen when the arm drifts into internal rotation.

Teres minor. Teres minor is tested with the shoulder abducted at 90 degrees. A *Hornblower sign,* also known as *Patte test,* is performed by flexing the elbow so the hand comes to the mouth, like blowing a horn (Fig. 20.39). Ask the patient to maintain the position. A positive test is seen when the arm drifts into internal rotation or with the development of pain.

Subscapularis. The subscapularis is responsible for internal rotation of the shoulder. A *lift off test* (Fig. 20.40) is useful in testing the inferior portion of the subscapularis. It is performed with the patient standing. Ask the patient to place the dorsum of their hand at the middle of the spine (palm facing outward) and lift the hand while the examiner watches for abnormal motion of the scapula. The examiner then asks the patient to push backward against resistance. The inability to perform this test suggests subscapularis pathology.

The *belly press test* assesses the superior portion of the subscapularis. Place your hand on the patient's abdomen with your palm facing outward. Ask the patient to press against your hand. The "belly press test" is illustrated in Fig. 20.41. Inability to perform this indicates weakness in internal rotation and suggests subscapularis pathology.

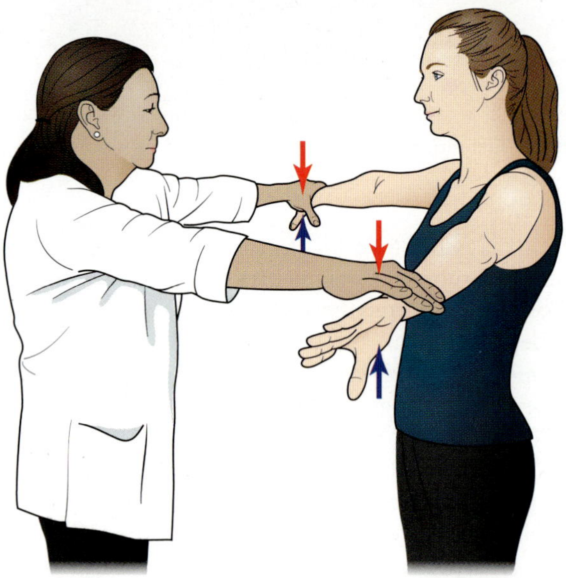

Fig. 20.36 The Jobe or "Empty Can Test" for Rotator Cuff Injury.

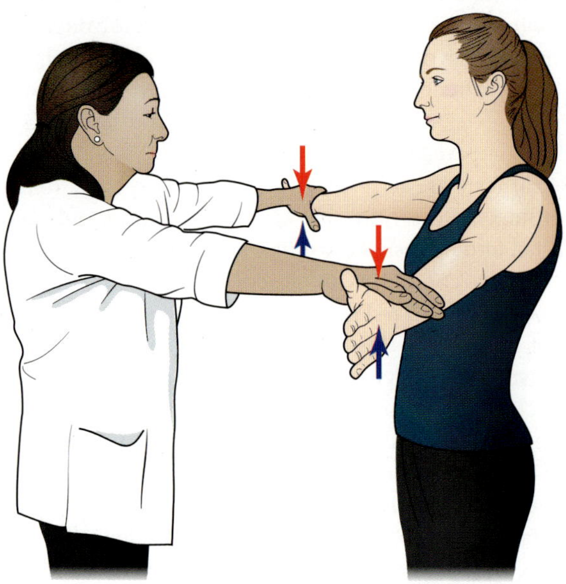

Fig. 20.37 The "Full Can Test" for Integrity of the Supraspinatus Tendon.

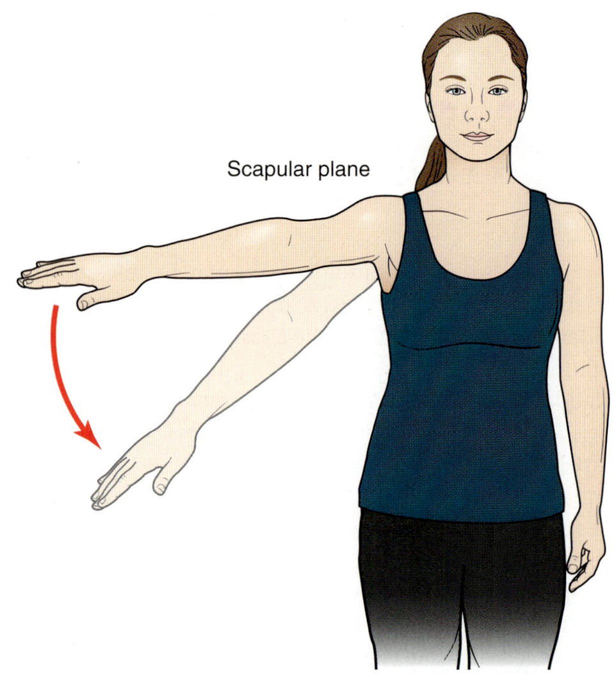

Fig. 20.38 The "Drop Arm Test" for Integrity of the Supraspinatus Tendon.

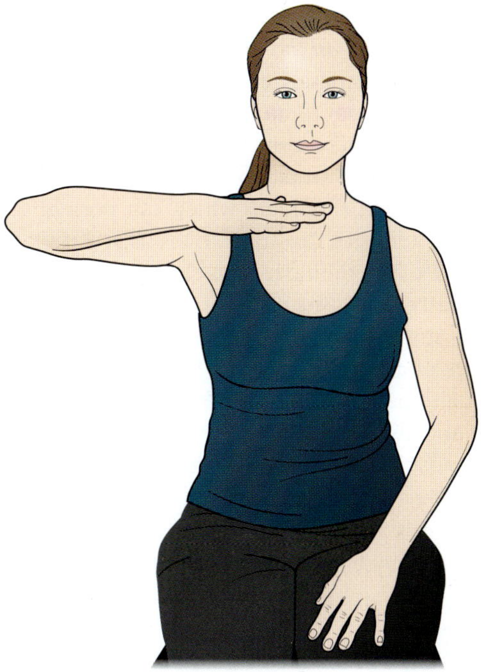

Fig. 20.39 The "Hornblower Test" for Integrity of Teres Minor.

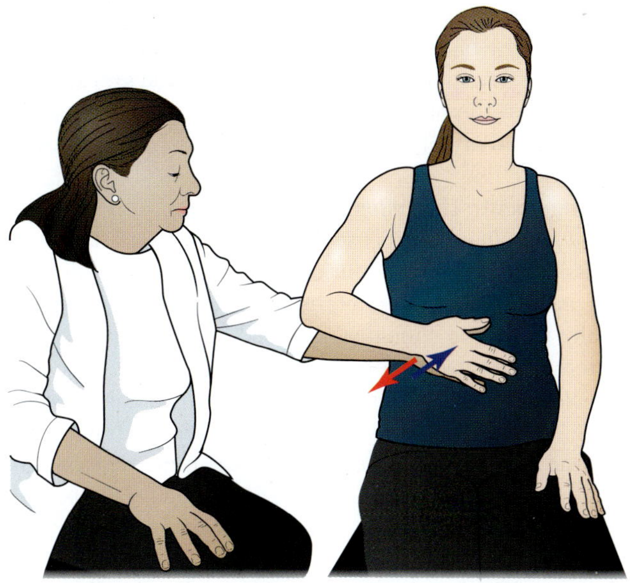

Fig. 20.41 The "Belly Press Test" for Integrity of the Superior Portion of the Subscapularis.

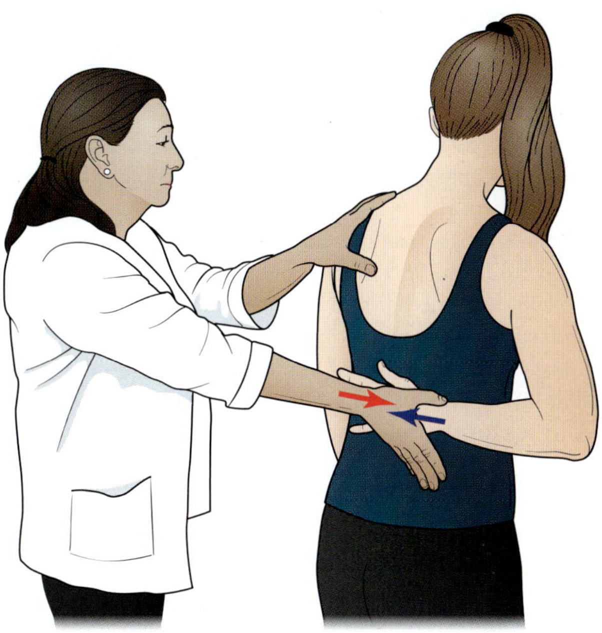

Fig. 20.40 The "Lift Off Test" for Integrity of the Inferior Portion of the Subscapularis.

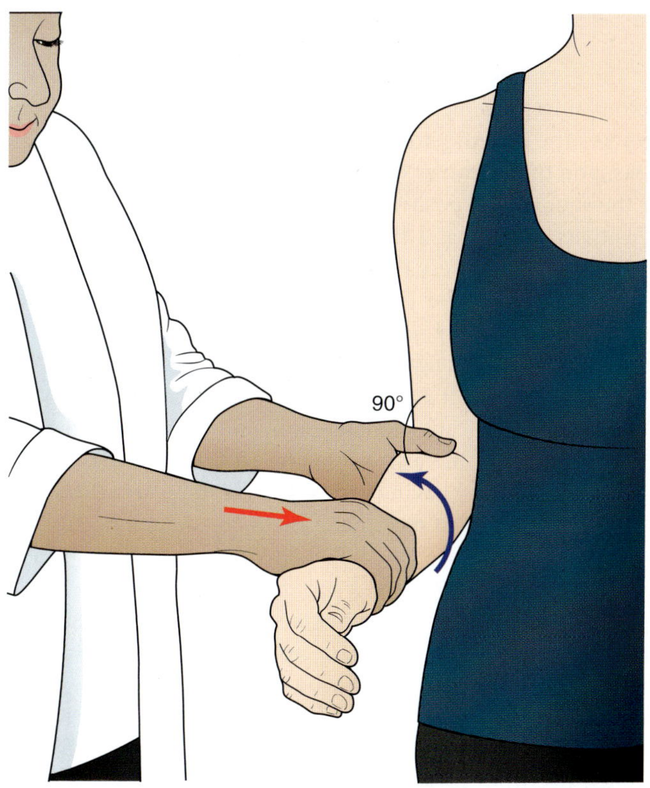

Fig. 20.42 The Yergason test for evaluating pathology of the long biceps tendon and superior labrum and posterior lesions.

Biceps. Generalized tenderness anteriorly over the long head of the biceps that is associated with pain, especially at night, should raise suspicion of *biceps tendinitis*, a common cause of shoulder pain. If you feel the biceps tendon popping out of the groove, a tear of the transverse humeral ligament is suggested. Tenderness or pain without popping is suggestive of biceps tendinitis. Although the sensitivity is low, the specificity is 87%.

The *Speed's test* is performed by having the patient supinate their forearm with an extended elbow. The patient is then asked to forward elevate the arm against resistance. A positive test is when pain is elicited in the bicipital groove. The sensitivity is 20% and the specificity is 78%.

The *Yergason test* (Fig. 20.42) is performed to evaluate pathology of the long biceps tendon and superior labrum and posterior (SLAP) lesions. Have the patient stand. Ask the patient to flex the forearm at 90 degrees with forearm pronated and stabilized against the body. Then ask the patient to perform supination against resistance at the same time while the examiner palpates the biceps tendon in the bicipital groove. A positive test is the development of pain in the bicipital groove or the popping out of the biceps tendon in the bicipital groove. The test has a sensitivity of 32% and a specificity of 88% for biceps pathology.

Impingement. The *impingement syndrome,* also known as *rotator cuff impingement,* is usually secondary to sports trauma. It results from mechanical impingement of the rotator cuff tendon beneath the anteroinferior portion of the acromion, especially when the shoulder is placed in the forward flexed and internally rotated position.

The *Neer test* is used for rotator cuff impingement. To perform the Neer test, have the patient seated. The examiner stands behind the patient. With one hand, the examiner depresses the scapula and with the other hand internally rotates the patient's arm. The examiner performs maximally forced forward flexion in the glenohumeral joint (the shoulder ball and socket joint). A positive test is the reproduction of shoulder pain. If the patient has a concern of anterior shoulder pain, this is likely to be subacromial impingement; if the patient experiences posterior shoulder pain, the diagnosis is more likely to be related to an internal impingement. The sensitivity of the Neer test is 72%, and the specificity is 60%.

The *Hawkins Kennedy test* is a commonly used test for subacromial impingement. Have the patient seated. The examiner elevates the patient's arm to 90 degrees of forward flexion and rests it on the examiner's arm. Perform passive internal rotation of the shoulder. A positive test is the development of pain. The sensitivity is 80%, and the specificity is 58%. The test will be negative with an internal impingement.

Acromioclavicular joint pathology. The AC joint is a very stable joint, and only slight motions occur there. Still, one can suffer a sprain of the ligaments that hold your AC joint together. When this occurs, it is called an *AC joint separation.* This will likely cause significant shoulder pain, and the patient may have difficulty moving the arm normally. The *cross-body adduction test* is performed by having patient elevate the arm to 90 degrees of flexion and then at maximal horizontal adduction across the body. It is positive when pain is elicited in the AC joint. The test has a sensitivity of 77% and a specificity of 79%.

The *O'Brien test,* or *active compression test* is performed with the patient forward flexing their shoulder to 90 degrees and adducting to 20 degrees with the elbow fully extended. The patient is then asked to resist downward pressure with either pronation or supination of the forearm. A positive test is when pain was elicited over the AC joint while the forearm was pronated but no pain when supinated.

Instability. The *sulcus sign* is used for diagnosing multidirectional instability. The test is performed with arms at the side while the examiner applies direct inferior force on the arm. The test is positive if a dimple, or sulcus, forms at the superior aspect of the humeral head.

The *apprehension test* is performed by having the patient lie supine with the shoulder at 90 degrees of abduction. The examiner then slowly externally rotates the arm to 90 degrees. The test is considered positive if the patient experiences feelings of instability. The *relocation test* is then performed by placing posterior force on the humeral head with the shoulder at 90 degrees abduction and external rotation. It is positive when the patient experiences reduction or elimination of a sense of instability.

Rotator cuff injury must be distinguished from *adhesive capsulitis,* or "frozen shoulder," which can present with similar symptoms. In adhesive capsulitis, there is scarring, thickening, and shrinkage of the shoulder joint capsule; it becomes inflamed and stiff, greatly restricting range of motion and causing chronic pain lasting months to years. The *coracoid pain test* evaluates for the presence of a frozen shoulder. The examiner stands behind the patient and palpates the AC joint, the anterolateral subacromial area, and the coracoid process with one digit. The test is considered positive when more intensive pain is produced in the coracoid process with respect to the other shoulder areas. The test has a sensitivity of 96% and a specificity of 89%; the test represents a cardinal test for adhesive capsulitis.

Elbow

Symptoms. The most common symptom of elbow disorders is well-localized elbow pain. Although it is a simple hinge joint, the elbow is the most complicated joint of the upper extremity. The distal end of the humerus articulates with the proximal ulna and radius. Flexion and extension of the elbow are affected through the humeroulnar portion of the joint. The radius plays little role in this action; its role is primarily in pronation and supination of the forearm. The ulnar nerve lies in a vulnerable position as it passes around the medial epicondyle of the humerus.

Examination. Palpate the elbow for swelling, masses, tenderness, and nodules. Specifically, palpate the olecranon process, radial head, and medial and lateral epicondyle to differentiate the tender points. Test flexion and extension.

To test for pronation and supination, the elbows should be flexed at 90 degrees and placed firmly on a table. The patient is asked to rotate the forearm with wrist down (pronation), as shown in Fig. 20.43A, and wrist up (supination), as shown in Fig. 20.43B. Any limitation of motion or pain is noted.

The biceps tendon is a relatively common source of pain in the anterior elbow. Although distal biceps tendon ruptures are rare, comprising 3% of all tendon ruptures, distal *biceps tendinopathy* is more common. This condition presents with an insidious course of vague anterior elbow pain, especially with resisted flexion and resisted supination of the forearm. The *hook test* is used to assess the continuity of the biceps tendon. The examiner's finger is used to hook under the distal biceps tendon. The distal biceps tendon is ruptured if the examiner's finger does not meet resistance.

Tennis elbow, also known as *lateral epicondylitis,* is a common condition characterized by pain in the region of the lateral epicondyle of the humerus. The pain radiates down the extensor surface of the forearm. Patients with tennis elbow often experience pain when attempting to open a door or when lifting a glass. This overuse tendinopathy occurs in 1% to 3% of the population annually, and although it is commonly called tennis elbow, only 5% to 10% of tennis players develop the condition.

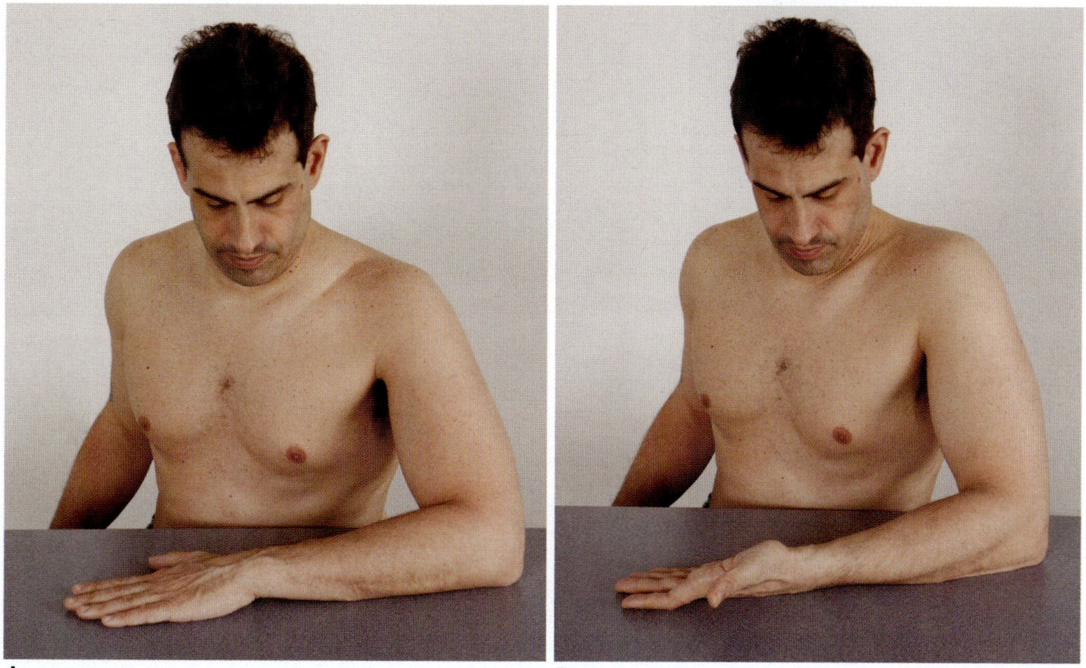

A B

Fig. 20.43 Technique for Evaluating Pronation and Supination at the Elbow. (A) Pronation. (B) Supination.

Most patients are in their 30s and 40s and develop lateral epicondylitis as a result of occupational rather than recreational activities. The lateral elbow is affected 4 to 10 times more often than the medial side. To test for tennis elbow, the examiner should flex the patient's elbow and fully pronate the hand. Pain over the lateral epicondyle while the elbow is extended is diagnostic of tennis elbow.

Another test for lateral epicondylitis is the *Mill test*. Have the patient in a standing position. The examiner fixates the humerus with one hand while pronating the patient's forearm, fully flexing the wrist, and extending the elbow. The test is positive if the patient experiences sudden pain at the lateral epicondyle. The test has a sensitivity of 53% and a specificity of 100%.

A third test for lateral epicondylitis is the *Cozen test,* also known as the *resisted wrist extension test.* The patient should be seated next to a table. The examiner stabilizes the elbow in 90 degrees of flexion with one hand while the other hand palpates over the lateral epicondyle with the thumb. Ask the patient to make a fist, pronate the forearm, radially deviate, and extend the wrist against manual resistance. The test is considered positive if the patient experiences sudden pain at the lateral epicondyle.

Golfer elbow, also known as *medial epicondylitis*, is a condition in which there is tenderness over the medial epicondyle and common flexor origin. It is much less common than lateral epicondylitis and typically occurs in athletes or workers who participate in activities that involve repetitive valgus stress and flexion at the elbow, as well as repetitive wrist flexion and pronation. It is a tendinopathy of the common flexor tendon. To test for medial epicondylitis, have the patient stand. The examiner fixates the humerus and palpates the medial epicondyle at the same time. Support the elbow with one hand, while the other hand passively supinates the patient's forearm and fully extends the elbow, wrist, and fingers. The test is considered positive if sudden pain or discomfort is reproduced along the region of the medial epicondyle.

Wrist

Symptoms. The symptoms of wrist disorders include pain in the wrist or hand, numbness or tingling in the wrist or fingers, loss of movement, stiffness, and deformities. Pain in the hand may be referred from the neck or elbow.

The wrist is composed of the articulation of the distal end of the radius with the proximal row of the carpal bones. The stability of the wrist is caused by the banding together of these bones by strong ligaments. The distal ulna does not articulate with any of the carpal bones. On the volar aspect of the wrist, the carpal bones are connected by the carpal ligament. The passage under this ligament is the *carpal tunnel,* through which the median nerve and all the flexor tendons of the wrist pass. Entrapment of the nerve, known as *carpal tunnel syndrome,* produces symptoms of numbness and tingling. Severe cases could lead to motor impairments.

Examination. Palpate the patient's wrist joint between your thumbs and index fingers, noting tenderness, swelling, or redness (Fig. 20.44).

The range of motion of dorsiflexion and palmar flexion is noted. With the forearms fixed, the degree of supination and pronation is evaluated. Is ulnar or radial deviation present?

When the diagnosis of carpal tunnel syndrome is suspected, a sharp tap or pressure directly over the median nerve may reproduce the paresthesias of carpal tunnel syndrome, called *Tinel sign*. Another useful test is for the examiner to stretch the

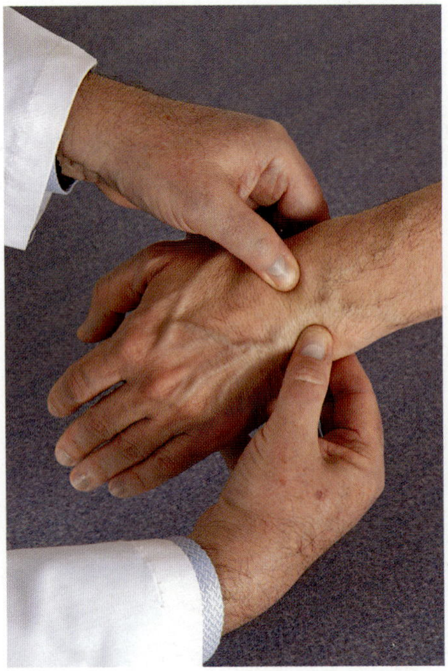

Fig. 20.44 Technique for Palpation of the Wrist Joint.

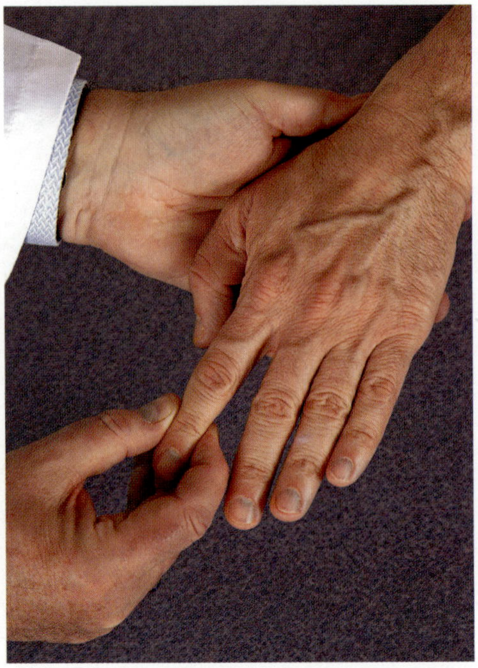

Fig. 20.46 Technique for Palpation of the Interphalangeal Joints.

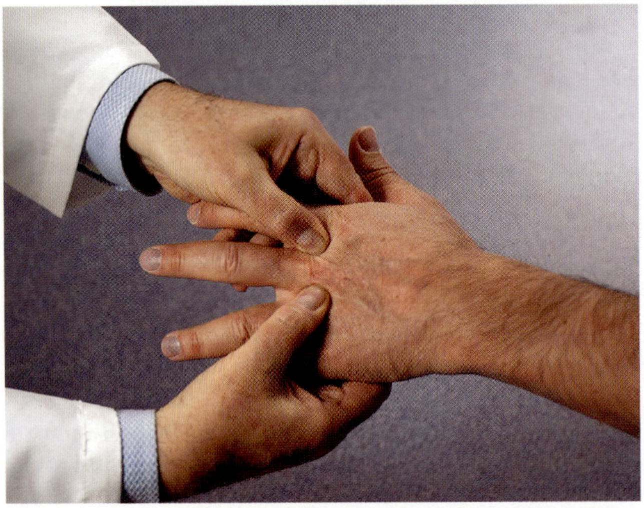

Fig. 20.45 Technique for Palpation of the Metacarpophalangeal Joints.

median nerve by extending the patient's elbow and dorsiflexing the wrist. The development of pain or paresthesias is suggestive of the diagnosis. A third test entails the patient holding both wrists in a fully palmar-fixed position for 2 minutes. The development or exacerbation of paresthesias is suggestive of carpal tunnel syndrome.

Hand

Symptoms. Pain and swelling of joints are the most important symptoms of disorders of the hand.

Examination. Palpate the patient's metacarpophalangeal (MCP) joints and note swelling, redness, or tenderness, as demonstrated in Fig. 20.45. Palpate the medial and lateral aspects of the proximal and distal IP joints between your thumb and index finger, as shown in Fig. 20.46. Again, note swelling, redness, or tenderness.

The range of motion of the fingers includes movements at the distal IP joint, the proximal IP joint, and the MCP joints of the fingers and the thumb.

Ask the patient to make a fist with the thumb across the knuckles and then extend and spread the fingers. Normally, the fingers should flex to the distal palmar crease. The thumb should oppose to the distal metacarpal head. Each finger should extend to the zero position in relation to its metacarpal.

Tenosynovitis of the thumb abductors and extensors is known as *de Quervain disease.* The patient has concerns about weakness of grip and pain at the base of the thumb that is aggravated by certain movements of the wrist. To confirm the diagnosis, ask the patient to flex the thumb and close the fingers over it. You should now attempt to move the hand into ulnar deviation. Excruciating pain will accompany this maneuver if de Quervain tenosynovitis is present.

Spine

Symptoms. The most common symptom of disorders of the spine is pain. Pain from the thoracic spine often radiates around the trunk along the lines of the intercostal nerves. Pain from the upper lumbar spine may be felt in the front of the thighs and knees. Pain originating in the lower lumbar spine can be felt in the coccyx, hips, and buttocks, as well as shooting down the back of the legs to the heels and feet. The pain is often intensified by movement. Patients with herniated vertebral discs may be concerned of pain that is exacerbated by sneezing or coughing. Determine whether there is associated numbness or tingling in the lower extremity, which is related to nerve root lesions.

Examination. The cervical spine can be examined with the patient seated. You should inspect the cervical spine from the front, back, and sides for deformity and unusual posture. Test range of motion of the cervical spine. Palpate the paravertebral muscles for tenderness and spasm.

The thoracolumbar spine is examined with the patient standing in front of you. Inspect the spine for deformity or swelling. Inspect the spine from the side for abnormal curvature. Test ranges of motion. Palpate the paravertebral muscles for tenderness. Percuss each spinous process for tenderness.

The ranges of motion tested in the spine are forward flexion, extension, lateral flexion, and rotation.

The presence of a *cervical rib* may cause coldness, discoloration, and trophic changes as a result of ischemia to an upper extremity. To test for a cervical rib, palpate the radial pulse. Move the arm through its range of motion. Obliteration of the pulse by this maneuver suggests the presence of a cervical rib. Ask the patient to turn the head toward the affected side and take a deep breath while you are palpating the radial pulse on the same side. Obliteration of the pulse by this maneuver also suggests a cervical rib. Often, auscultation over the subclavian artery reveals a bruit suggestive of mechanical obstruction by a cervical rib. Repeat any of these tests on the opposite side. Cervical ribs are rarely bilateral.

Pain from entrapment of the sciatic nerve is called *sciatica.* Patients with sciatica describe pain, burning sensation, or aching in the buttocks radiating down the posterior thigh to the posterolateral aspect of the calf. Pain is worsened by sneezing, laughing, or straining at stool. One of the tests for sciatica is the straight leg-raising test. The patient is asked to lie supine while the examiner flexes the extended leg to the trunk at the hip. The presence of pain is a positive test result. The patient is asked to plantarflex and dorsiflex the foot. This stretches the sciatic nerve even more. If sciatica is present, this test reproduces pain in the leg. The test is illustrated in Fig. 20.47.

Another test for sciatica is the sitting knee–extension test. The patient sits off the side of the bed and flexes the neck, placing the chin on the chest. The examiner fixes the thigh on the bed with one hand while the other hand extends the leg. If sciatica is present, pain is reproduced as the leg is extended. This test is demonstrated in Fig. 20.48.

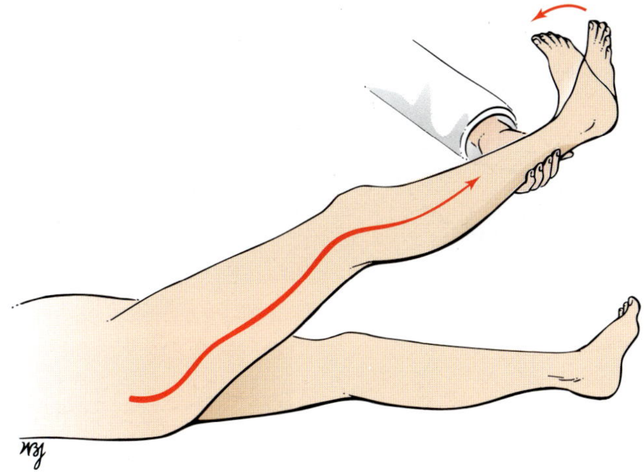

Fig. 20.47 Straight Leg Raising Test.

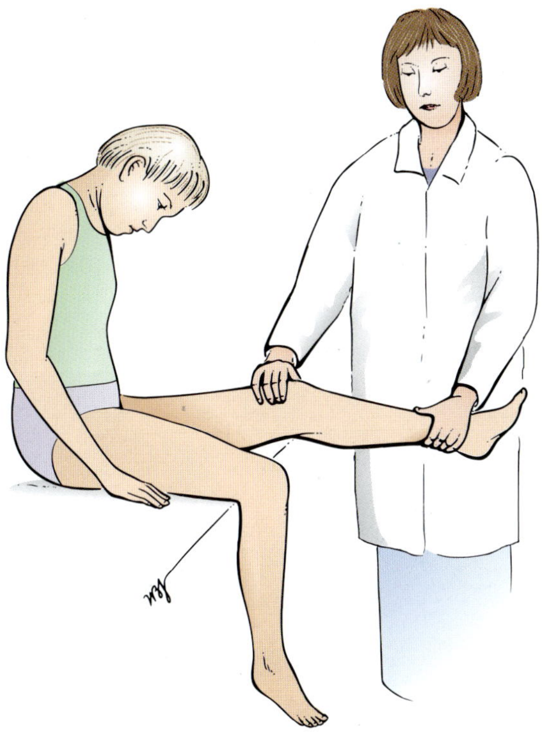

Fig. 20.48 Sitting Knee Extension Test.

Hip

Symptoms. The main symptoms of hip disease are pain, stiffness, deformity, and a limp. Hip pain may be localized to the groin or may radiate down the medial aspect of the thigh. Stiffness may be related to periods of immobility. An early symptom of hip disease is difficulty putting on shoes. This requires external rotation of the hip, which is the first motion to be lost with degenerative disease of the hip. This is followed by loss of abduction and adduction; hip flexion is the last movement lost.

Examination. The examination of the hip is performed with the patient standing, walking, and lying supine. Inspection of the hips and gait has already been described. Leg length measurements are useful in evaluating hip disorders. The distance between the anterosuperior iliac spine and the tip of the medial malleolus is measured on each side, and the two measurements are compared. A difference in leg length may be caused by hip joint disorders.

The following tests are performed with the patient supine:

Evaluate range of motion: abduction, adduction, extension, and internal and external rotation. As indicated previously, loss of rotation of the hip is an early finding in hip disease. To test this movement, ask the patient to lie supine. Flex the patient's hip and knee to 90 degrees, and rotate the ankle inward for external rotation as illustrated in Fig. 20.49A, and outward for internal rotation as shown in Fig. 20.49B.

The *FABER,* or *Patrick, test* is a test for intra-articular pathology. It is performed by the examiner moving the patient's leg into 45 degrees of **f**lexion, then externally rotating and **ab**ducting the leg so that the ankle rests proximal to the knee of the contralateral leg (**e**xternal **r**otation). Restriction of this motion or pain is a sensitive sign of degenerative disease at the hip, lumbar, or the sacroiliac region. The FABER test is

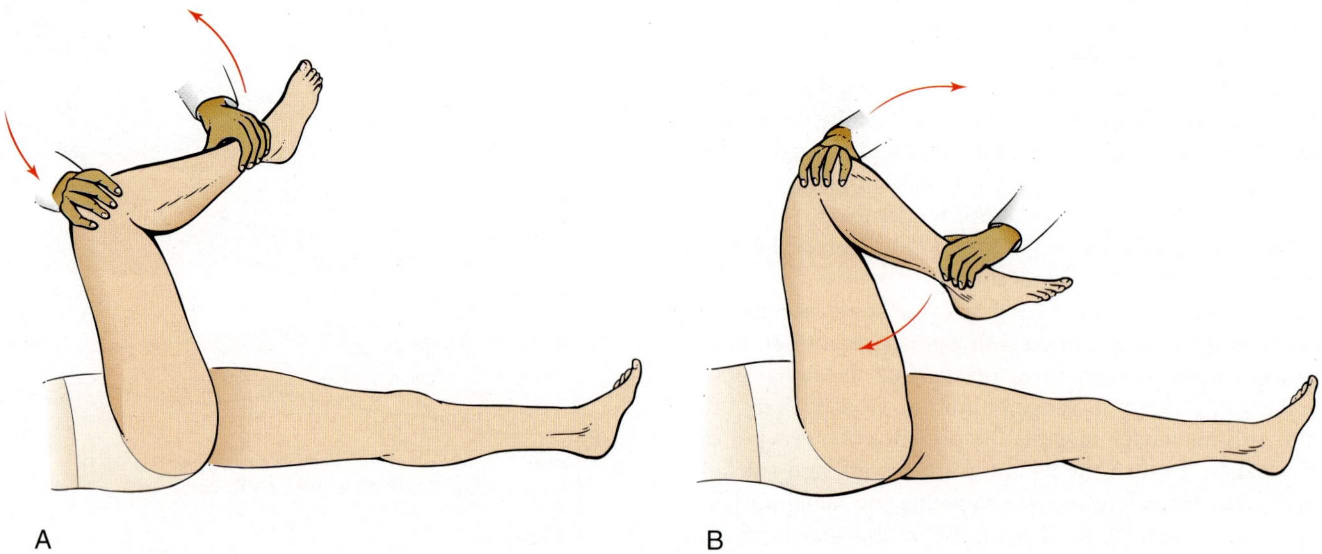

Fig. 20.49 **Testing the Range of Motion at the Hip.** The examiner flexes the patient's hip and knee to 90 degrees and rotates the ankle inward for external rotation (A) and outward for internal rotation (B).

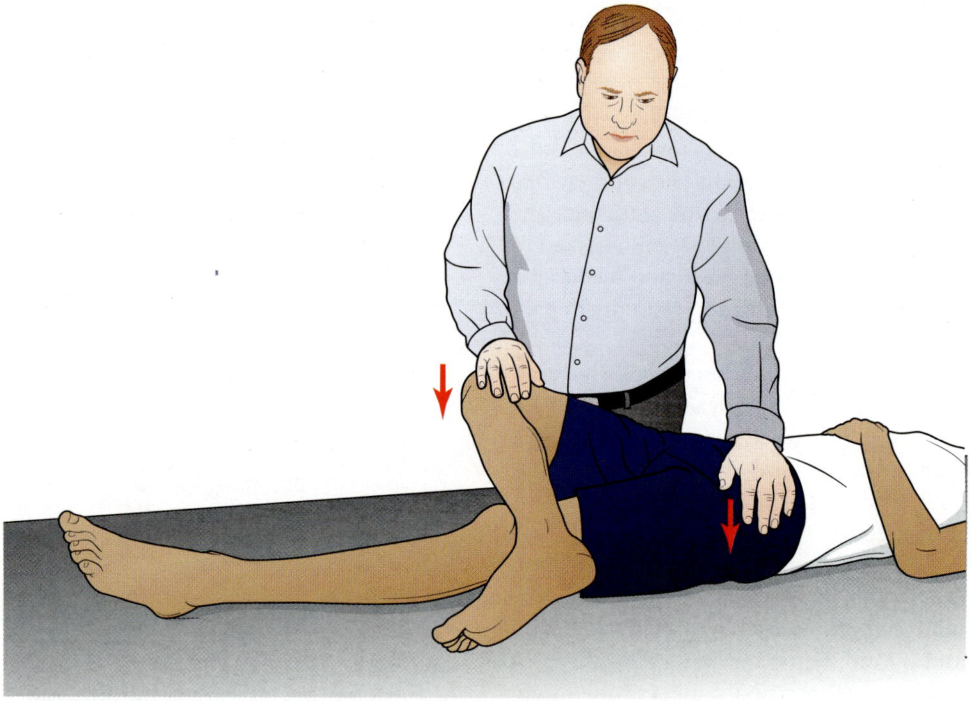

Fig. 20.50 FABER Test for Degenerative Disease of the Hip, Lumbar, or Sacroiliac Region.

illustrated in Fig. 20.50. It is important to note that the FABER test can be positive for hip or back depending on the location of pain when the maneuver is performed. If the patient reports pain in the groin or hip, then pathology is in the hip; however, if the patient reports pain in the lower back, then the pathology is sacroiliitis.

The *FADIR test*, or *hip impingement test*, is performed by the examiner passively moving the patient's leg into full **f**lexion, and then into **ad**duction and **i**nternal **r**otation. Hip impingement,[8] also known as femoroacetabular impingement (FAI), is the abutment of the acetabular rim against the proximal femur. The FADIR is the most sensitive physical examination test for FAI. The development of the patient's anterolateral pain or restriction of movement is a positive test.

The *Freiberg test* is a log roll test in which the patient's leg is extended while the examiner internally and externally rotates the leg back and forth. The development of pain or restricted movement is a positive test.

Another useful test is the *Stinchfield test*. For this maneuver, the patient lifts the straight leg 45 degrees while the examiner applies downward pressure on the thigh. Weakness to resistance or pain is a positive test.

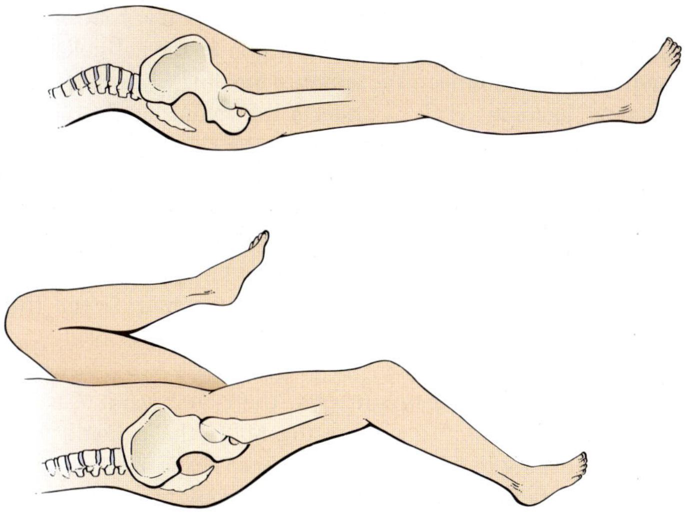

Fig. 20.51 Thomas Test for Flexion Deformity of the Hip.

To measure the flexibility of the hip flexors, which includes the iliopsoas, rectus femoris, pectineus, gracilis, and sartorius muscles, one can perform the *Thomas test*, also known as the *iliopsoas test*. First check for lumbar lordosis that is usually a predictor of a tight iliopsoas muscle. The patient is then asked to acutely flex the hip on the abdomen (bringing the knee as far to the chest as possible) to flatten the lumbar spine and to hold it afterward. This will cause the lumbar lordosis to straighten out. Flexion of the opposite thigh is suggestive of a fixed flexion deformity of that hip. Fig. 20.51 illustrates the technique. If the patient has bilateral hip flexion deformities, the Thomas test cannot be used.

To assess iliotibial (IT) band tightness, one can perform the *Ober test*. The IT band is a lateral thickening of the fascia lata in the thigh. Proximally the band splits into superficial and deep layers, enclosing tensor fasciae lata and anchoring this muscle to the iliac crest. It also receives most of the tendon of the gluteus maximus. The patient is asked to turn to the lateral position, with the lower (uninvolved) leg in flexion at the hip and the knee for stability. Stand behind the patient and firmly stabilize the pelvis to prevent movement in any direction. Grasp the distal end of the patient's affected leg with your other hand and flex the leg to 90 degrees at the knee. Extend and abduct the hip joint. Then slowly lower the upper leg (adduct the hip) all the way down to the examination table. The knee support is then released. If a contraction is present in the IT band, the hip remains in the abducted position and does not adduct past anatomic neutral; this indicates a positive test. The patient may also experience lateral knee pain.

Failure of knee adduction is a positive test for IT band tightness.

The patient is now asked to stand.

The *Trendelenburg test* is used to evaluate hip abductor strength, primarily the gluteus medius. The patient is asked to stand on the "good" leg, as illustrated in Fig. 20.52A. The patient may be allowed to hold onto something if balance is a problem. The examiner should note if the pelvis on the opposite side elevates, demonstrating that the gluteus medius is working efficiently. When the patient is asked to stand on the "bad" leg, as shown in Fig. 20.52B, the pelvis on the opposite side falls. This is a positive Trendelenburg test result that usually indicates weakness in the gluteus medius or gluteus minimus. The Trendelenburg test is fairly accurate, but it is not necessarily specific to any one structure.

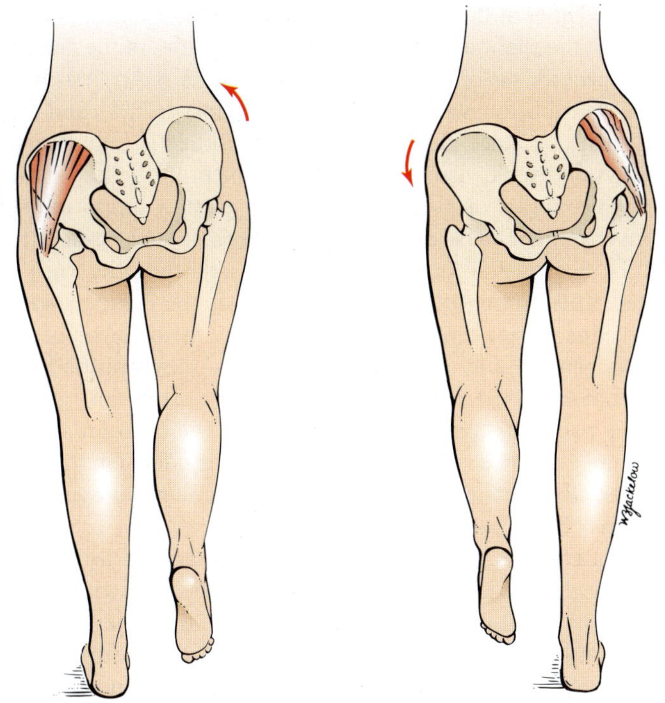

A B

Fig. 20.52 Trendelenburg Test. (A) Position of the hips when standing on the *normal* left leg. Note that the right hip elevates as a result of contraction of the left hip abductor musculature. (B) Position of the hips when standing on the *abnormal* right leg. Note that the left hip falls as a result of lack of adequate contraction of the right hip abductor muscles.

Knee

Symptoms. Although the knee is the largest joint in the body, it is not the strongest. The knee is a hinge joint between the femur and the tibia and enables flexion and extension. When it is flexed, a small degree of lateral motion is also normal. As with the shoulder, the knee depends on the strong muscles and ligaments around the joint for its stability.

Pain, swelling, joint instability, and limited movement are the main symptoms of knee disorders. Knee pain is exacerbated by movement and may be referred to the calf or thigh. Swelling of the knee indicates a synovial effusion or bleeding into the joint, also known as *hemarthrosis*. Knee trauma may result in hemarthrosis and limitation of joint motion. *Locking* of the knee results from small pieces of broken cartilage lodged between the femur and the tibia, blocking full extension of the joint. Patients with arthritis of the knee often have concerns of pain when walking down stairs.

Examination. The examination of the knee is performed with the patient standing and lying supine.

While the patient is standing, any varus or valgus deformity should be noted. Is there wasting of the quadriceps muscle? Is there swelling of the knee? An early sign of knee joint swelling is loss of the slight depressions on the lateral sides of the patella.

Inspect for swelling in the popliteal fossa. A *Baker cyst*[9] may be responsible for swelling in the popliteal fossa (76%), and calf and posterior knee pain (32%) when the knee is fully flexed. The cyst is usually associated with a problem in the knee joint such as arthritis or a cartilage tear related to a sports injury. Gout is another cause of a Baker cyst. If palpable, the cyst often will be firm in full knee extension and soft when the knee is flexed. This finding is commonly known as the *Foucher sign*[10] and is due to cyst compression between the medial head of the gastrocnemius and semimembranosus as they approximate each other and the joint capsule during knee extension.

The patient is then asked to lie supine. The contours of the knee are evaluated. The patella is palpated in extension for tenderness. By stressing the patella against the femoral condyles, pain may be elicited. This occurs in OA.

Joint effusion. Testing for *knee joint effusion* is performed by pressing the fluid out of the suprapatellar pouch down behind the patella. Start approximately 15 cm above the superior margin of the patient's patella and slide your index finger and thumb firmly downward along the sides of the femur, milking the fluid into the space between the patella and the femur. While you maintain pressure on the lateral margins of the patella, tap on the patella with the other hand. This technique is termed *ballottement.* In the presence of an effusion, a distinct bump is felt in response to your tap, and the transmitted impulse is felt by the fingers on either side of the patella. This technique is shown in Fig. 20.53.

Joint line tenderness. *Joint line tenderness* test is used to screen for sensitivity related to meniscal injuries. The joint line position lies about 3 cm distal to the medial femoral epicondyle and 15 mm above the fibular head. Place the index, middle, and ring fingers of your left hand along the lateral joint line. Gently extend and flex the knee. If the lateral meniscus has been injured, you may feel a "click" or "pop" with the hand palpating the joint line. Pain may also be elicited.

Meniscal damage. The test that is commonly performed as part of the routine knee examination to test for the presence of meniscal damage is the *McMurray test.*[11] To test the right lateral meniscus, grasp the heel of the patient's right foot with your right hand. With the right knee fully flexed, rotate the tibia medially and bring the knee into extension with your left hand on the joint line. Repeat this motion several times with a different degree of knee flexion. If there is a meniscal injury, you will feel a "click" with the hand on the knee as it is extended, or most often, patient will report pain at the joint line. To test the right medial meniscus, hold the patient's right heel with your right hand and bring the knee into full flexion while laterally rotating the tibia with your left hand on the joint line. The McMurray test is illustrated in Fig. 20.54. The test attempts to trap the meniscus between the tibia and femur. The McMurray test has been shown to have a 78% specificity and an 80% sensitivity in diagnosing meniscal tears.

Collateral ligament damage. Next evaluate the ligaments of the knee. There are four primary knee ligaments. The cruciate ligaments cross each other to form an "X" with the ACL in front and the posterior ligament in back. They control the back-and-forth movement of the knee. The medial collateral ligament (MCL) connects the femur to the tibia while the lateral collateral ligament (LCL) connects the femur to the fibula. These two collateral ligaments control the sideways motion of the knee. Injuries to the collateral ligaments are generally caused by a force that pushes the knee sideways. An injury to the MCL is the more common of the two and occurs by being struck on the outside of a partially flexed knee, as in a football tackle. Listen to the patient's description of the injury event. The force vector of injury to the knee indicates the most likely site of pathology.

Medial collateral ligament tests. There are several tests for evaluating the MCL. To palpate the MCL, the patient's foot should be resting on the bed, with the knee flexed at 90 degrees. Grasp the patient's leg and, using your thumbs, try to elicit tenderness over the patellar tendon beneath the femoral epicondyles at the joint line. This technique and a *left medial collateral ligament* rupture are illustrated in Fig. 20.55.

Another test for MCL rupture is the valgus stress test. Have the patient in supine position with the legs fully extended. Standing at the side of the patient, the examiner should place one hand just above the ankle and the other hand at or above the knee to fixate the femur. Slightly externally rotate the tibia and perform passive abduction at the knee joint, thus putting stress on the MCL. The test is illustrated in Fig. 20.56A. Look for excessive gapping on the medial side of the knee and/or the development of pain. Repeat the same test now with the knee at 20 to 30 degrees of flexion (Fig. 20.56B). The result should be compared with that on the other side. Performing this test in full extension (A) tests the MCL as well as the cruciate ligaments. Doing the exam in 20 to 30 degrees of flexion (B) is the maneuver that isolates the collateral ligaments. Abnormal lateral motion is seen in rupture of the right MCL, as illustrated in Fig. 20.57.

Lateral collateral ligament tests. The varus stress test is used to test for LCL injury. Have the patient in supine position with the legs fully extended. Standing at the side of the patient, the examiner should place one hand just above the ankle and fixate with the other hand on the medial side of the femur. Apply lateral rotation of the knee joint and perform passive adduction on the knee joint to put stress on the LCL. The test is illustrated in Fig. 20.58A. Look for excessive gapping on the lateral side of the knee and/or the development of pain. Repeat the same test now with the knee at 20 to 30 degrees of flexion (see Fig. 20.58B). The result should be compared with that on the other side. Performing this test in full extension (A) tests the LCL as well as the cruciate ligaments. Doing the exam in 20 to 30 degrees of flexion (B) is the maneuver that isolates the collateral ligaments.

Cruciate ligament damage. The cruciate ligaments are the ACL and the posterior cruciate ligament (PCL). They extend from the head of the tibia to the intercondyloid notch of the femur. The ACL is lateral, and the PCL is medial. The ACL is the most commonly injured ligament in the knee. PCL injuries occur far less often than ACL injuries.

The *Lachman test* is a test for ACL rupture. With the patient supine, make sure that the patient's hip muscles, quadriceps, and

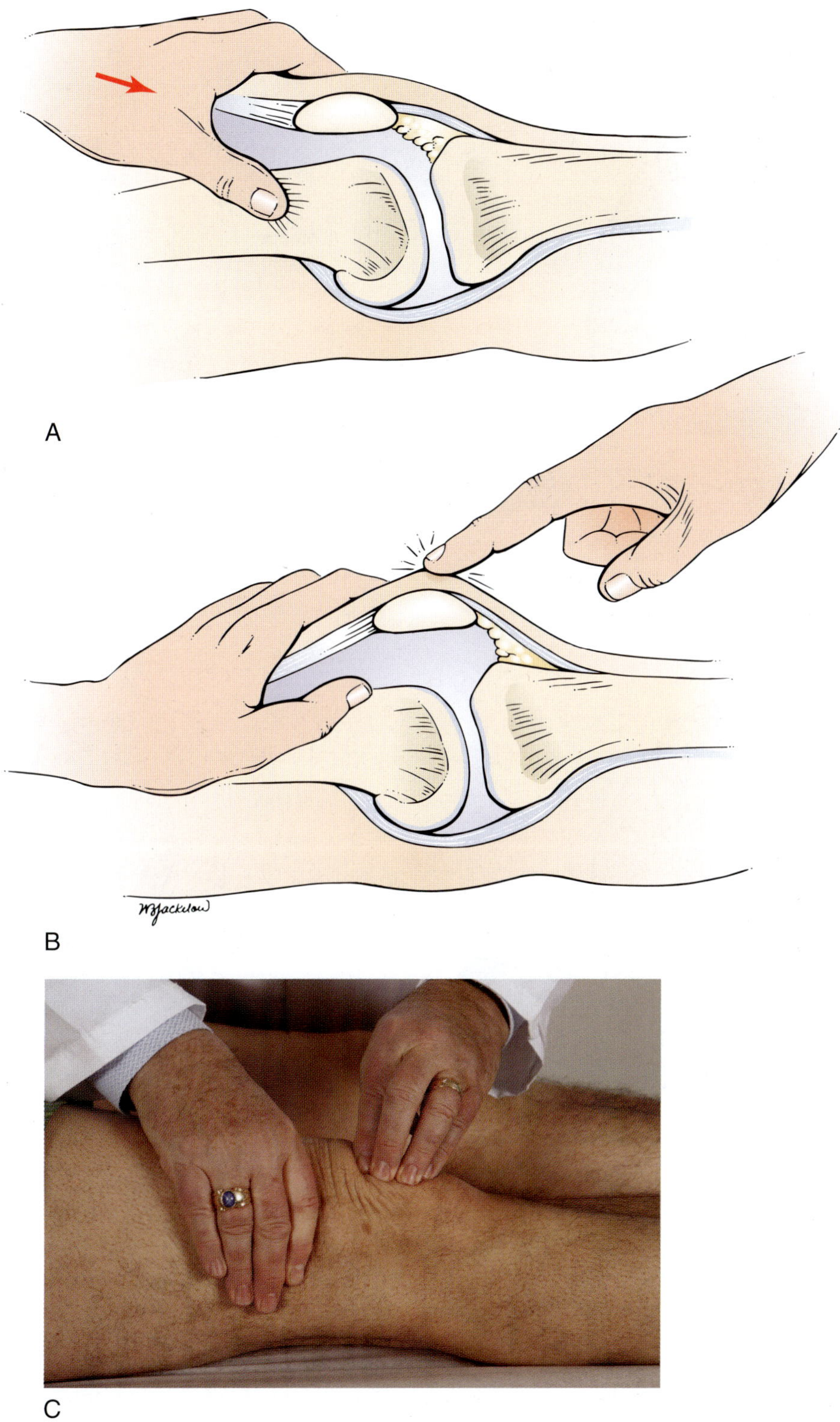

Fig. 20.53 Technique for Testing for Knee Joint Effusion. (A) Position of the hand when pushing fluid out of the bursae. (B and C) Position for tapping the patella.

hamstring muscles are all relaxed. Passively flex the knee to 20 to 30 degrees while the heel rests on the examination table. Stabilize the femur with your left (or nondominant) hand to prevent movement of the femur. Then grasp the proximal end of the lower leg and pull the tibia anteriorly and posteriorly against the femur. With an intact ACL, as the tibia is pulled forward, you should feel a firm endpoint. If the endpoint is lax, the examination will feel softer with no endpoint, and the Lachman test is considered positive. Fig. 20.59 illustrates the Lachman test. The Lachman test is the most sensitive examination for ACL injury.

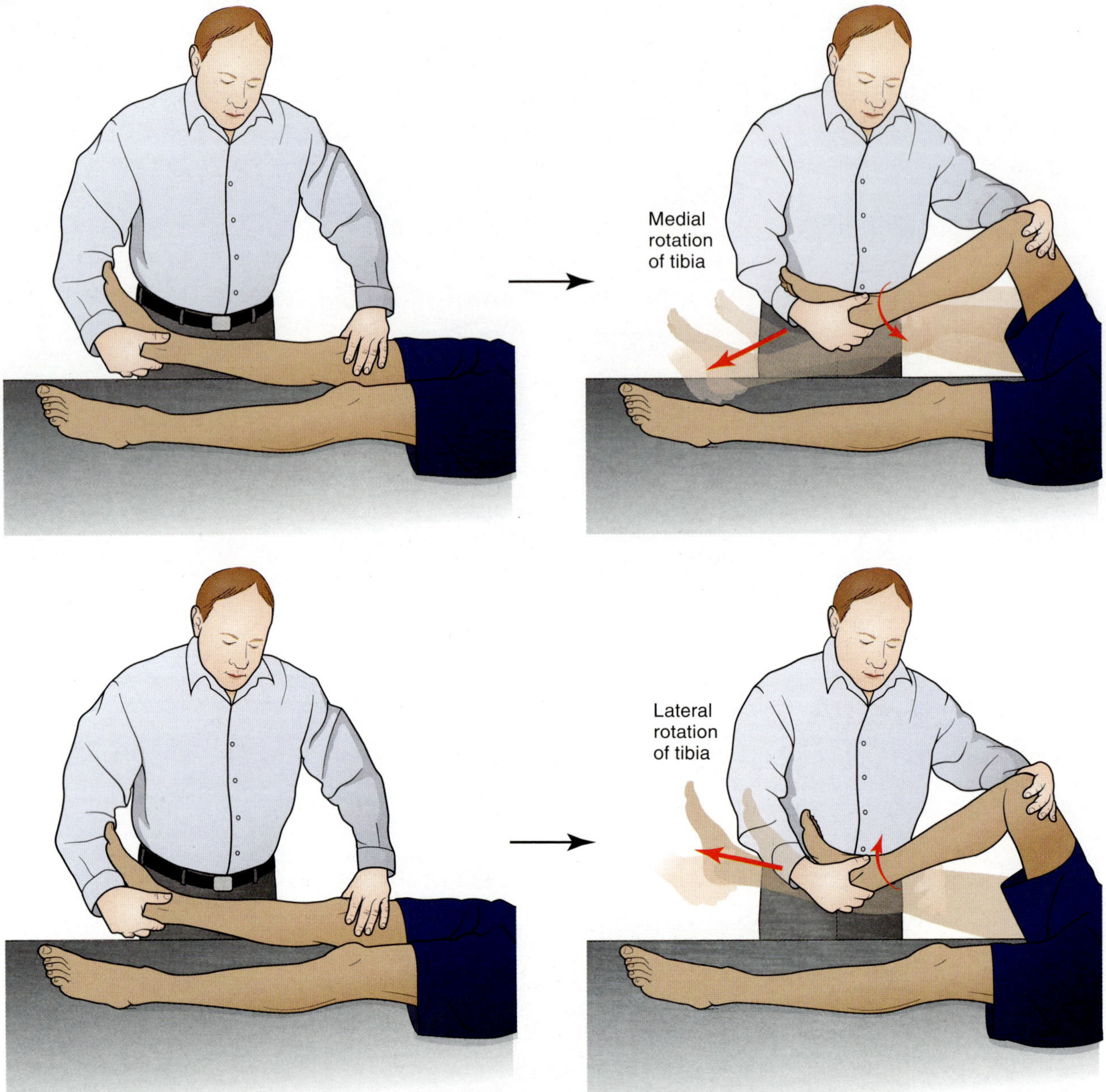

Fig. 20.54 McMurray Test. (A, *above*) Position of the hands for evaluating right lateral meniscus. (B, *below*) Position of the hands for evaluating right medial meniscus.

The *drawer test* is used to test for rupture of the *cruciate ligaments.* The *anterior drawer test* is performed with the patient lying supine and instructed to flex one knee to 90 degrees. The examiner should sit on the foot to steady it. The examiner then grasps the leg at the joint line with both hands and pulls the tibia forward with an explosive movement, as illustrated in Fig. 20.60. The thumbs of both hands are on the superior-anterior aspect of the tibia. Abnormal forward mobility of 6 cm or more is suggestive of rupture of the ACL. The sensitivity of the test is 92%, and the specificity of the test is 91%. This maneuver can be used to test the PCL by flexing the knee to 90 degrees, steadying the foot, and attempting to push the leg backward quickly: the *posterior drawer test.* Abnormal backward motion of 6 cm or more indicates rupture of the PCL.

The *lateral pivot shift test* is another useful exam to determine ACL integrity. The patient needs to be fully relaxed with knee flexed around 30 degrees. The tibia is held in internal rotation with axial load. A valgus force is then applied while flexing the knee. The examiner should feel the knee reduced at around 30 degrees of knee flexion. This maneuver reproduces the injury mechanism and the giving away event. The test has a sensitivity of 24% and a specificity of 98%.

Ankle and Foot

Symptoms. The ankle is a hinge joint between the lower end of the tibia and the talus. Although symptoms in the ankle and foot usually have a local cause, they can also be secondary to systemic disorders. Symptoms may include pain, swelling, and deformities.

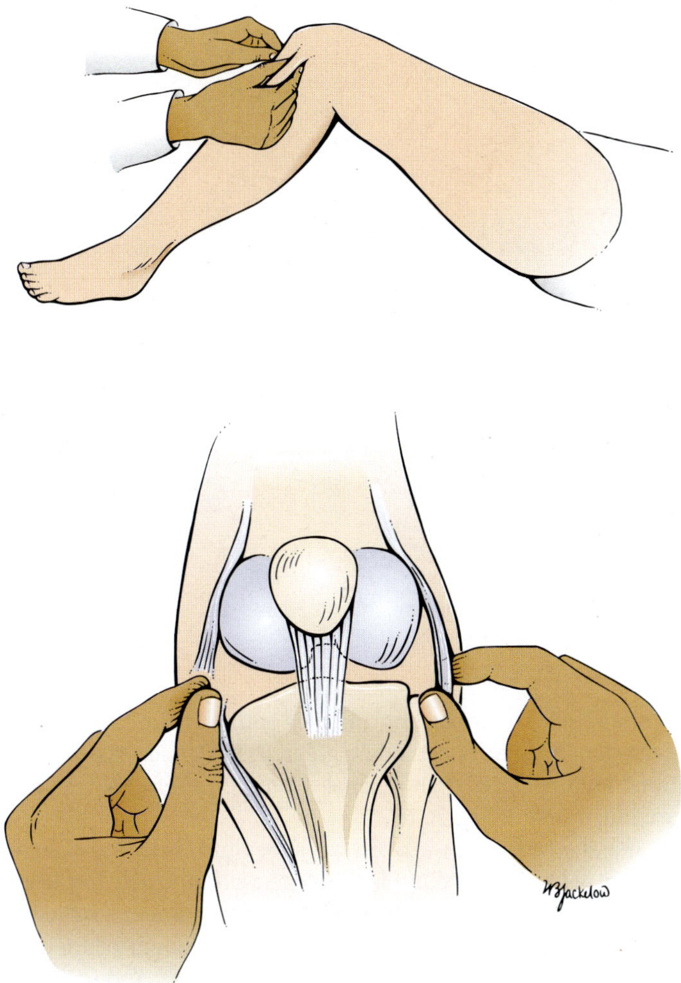

Fig. 20.55 *Top,* Technique for testing the left medial collateral ligament. *Bottom,* Rupture of the left medial collateral ligament.

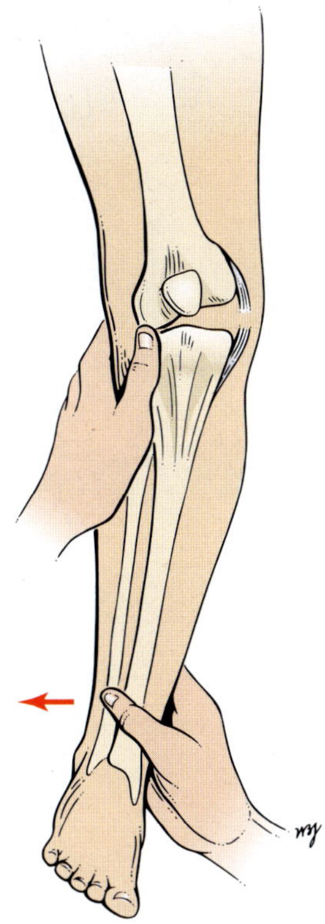

Fig. 20.57 Abnormal Lateral Motion Due to Rupture of Right Medial Collateral Ligament.

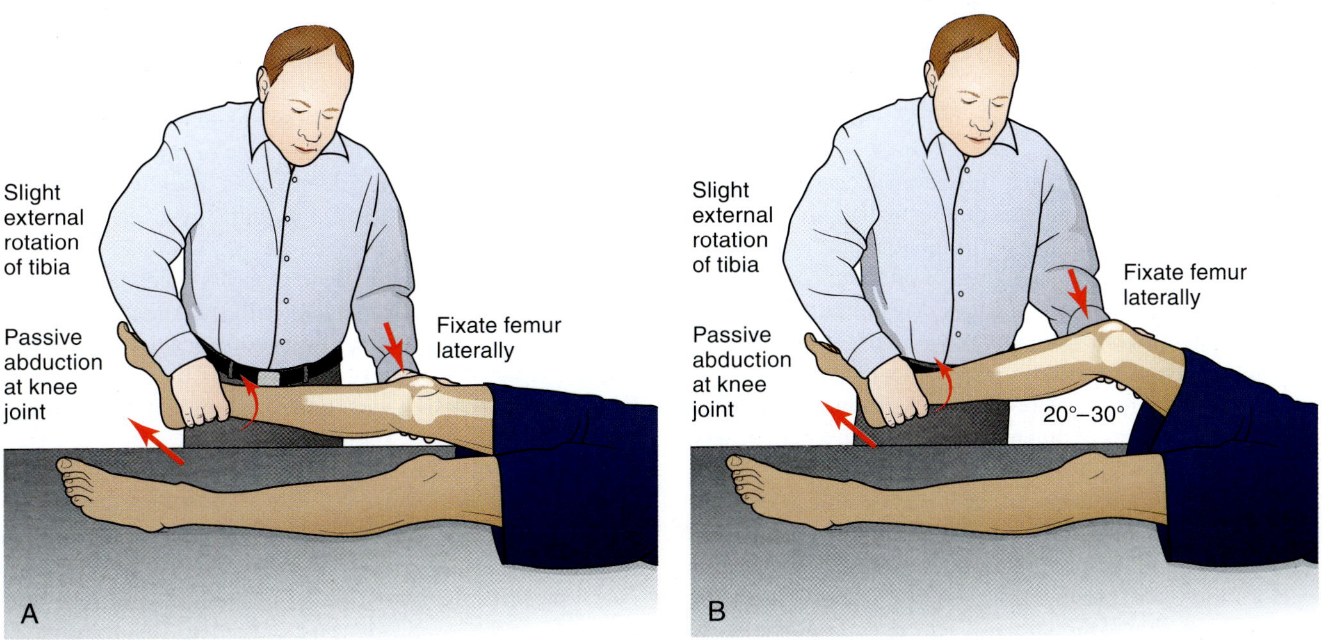

Fig. 20.56 Valgus Stress Test for Medial Collateral Ligament Injury. (A) At 0 degrees. (B) At 30 degrees.

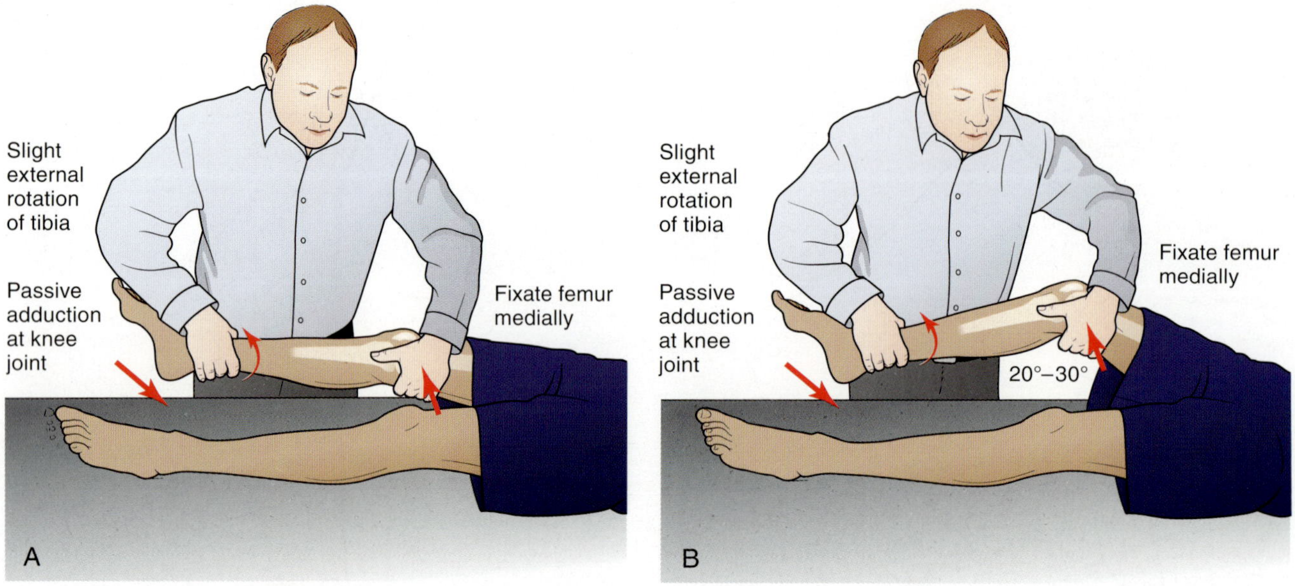

Fig. 20.58 Varus Stress Test for Lateral Collateral Ligament Injury. (A) At 0 degrees. (B) At 30 degrees.

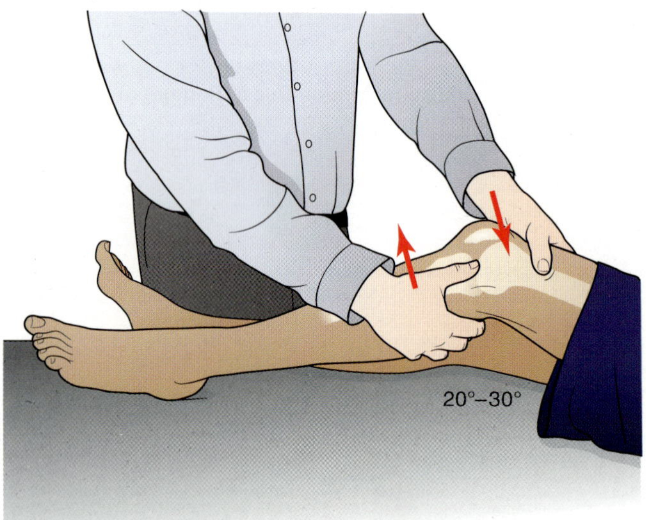

Fig. 20.59 Lachman Test for Anterior Cruciate Ligament Rupture.

The patient's only concern may be uneven shoe wear. Patients with flatfoot wear down their soles on the medial side extending to the tip of the shoe. The outer portion of the heel is also worn out early. Scuff marks are usually present on the medial sides of the heels. Excessive wear under the toes may indicate an equinus foot type or a tight Achilles tendon. Asymmetric shoe wear may result from a difference in limb length. Isolated areas of wear under the ball of the foot may result from a plantar-flexed metatarsal and indicate areas of potential ulceration in a patient with diabetes and neuropathy.

Examination. The examination of the ankle and foot is performed with the patient standing, walking, and then sitting. Ask the patient to stand. Inspect the ankles and feet for swelling and deformities. The number and position of toes should be noted. The toes should be straight, flat, and proportional to one another in comparison with the other foot. Compare one foot with the other with regard to symmetry. Are any toes overlapping? Describe abnormalities of the longitudinal arch. A *cavus foot* has an abnormally high arch. In *flatfoot,* the longitudinal arch is flatter than normal. Common foot abnormalities are illustrated in Fig. 20.61.

Ask the patient to walk without shoes and socks and observe the gait. The patient should be able to walk normally on heels, on toes, and one foot in front of the other (tandem walking). Note any deformities such as the width or length of the feet, heel varus or valgus, calf atrophy, varicose veins, and in-toeing or out-toeing. Take note of the patient's posture and any shuffling or other abnormality.

Ask the patient to sit with their feet dangling off the side of the bed. Normally, there is mild plantar flexion and inversion of the feet. Palpate the medial and lateral malleoli. The distal portion of the fibula constitutes the lateral malleolus. It extends more distally than the medial malleolus. Palpate the Achilles tendon. Are any nodules present? Is tenderness present?

Test the range of motion at the ankle, which includes dorsiflexion and plantar flexion. The range of motion necessary for normal gait is 10 degrees dorsiflexion and 20 degrees plantar flexion. Ankle joint dorsiflexion with the knee flexed should approach 15 degrees.

If dorsiflexion at the ankle joint is less than 10 degrees, measurement should be taken again with the knee flexed. If dorsiflexion is less than 10 degrees in both positions, limitation of motion is usually caused by an osseous block at the ankle. If dorsiflexion increases with knee flexion, a tight gastrocsoleus complex is probably responsible.

Test the range of motion at the subtalar joint, which includes eversion and inversion. With the patient lying prone on the examination table, hold the patient's leg in one of your hands, and move the heel with your other hand into inversion and eversion. Measure the excursion of the heel with regard to the bisection of the lower one-third of the leg. This technique is illustrated in Fig. 20.62. The average range of motion of the subtalar joint is 20 degrees of inversion and 10 degrees of eversion.

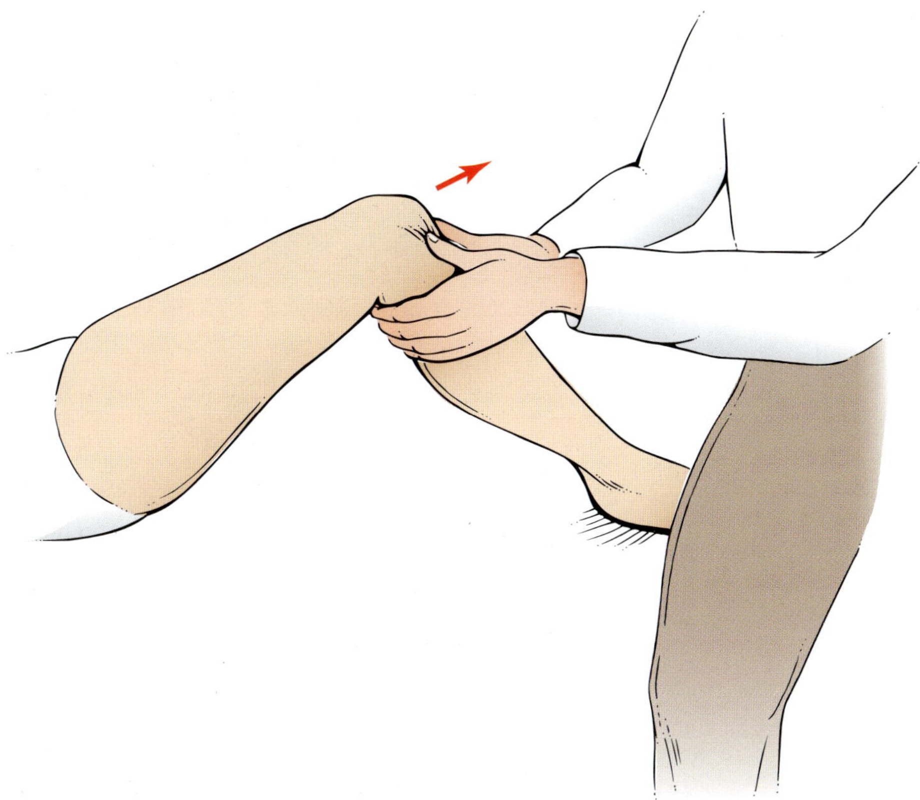

Fig. 20.60 Technique for Testing the Anterior Cruciate Ligament: Anterior Drawer Test.

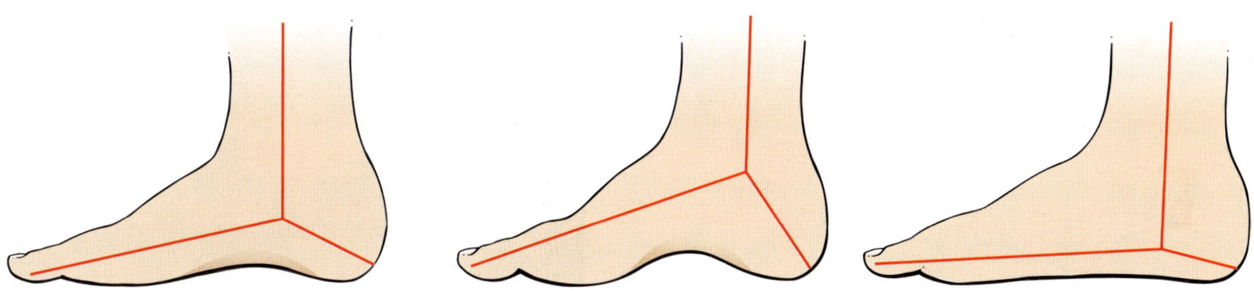

Fig. 20.61 Common Foot Abnormalities.

Test the range of motion at the midtarsal joint, which includes eversion and inversion. With the patient in the prone position, stabilize the heel with one of your hands, and rotate the forefoot into inversion and eversion. Measure excursion of the plane of the metatarsal heads with regard to the bisection of the heel. This technique is illustrated in Fig. 20.63.

The movements of the MTP joints are tested individually. Palpate the head of each metatarsal and the base of each proximal phalanx, as well as the groove between them. Is tenderness or joint effusion present?

The Achilles tendon, which is the combined tendon of the gastrocnemius and soleus muscles, may rupture. You can test for its integrity by direct observation and having the patient jump up and down on the balls of the feet or walk on the toes. Another test for its integrity is known as the *Thompson-Doherty squeeze test.* This test is performed by squeezing the calf while you observe the motion of the foot. Normally, squeezing produces plantar flexion; a ruptured tendon produces little or no motion. When examining the tendon for continuity, remember that the most common place for rupture is 1 to 2 inches (2.5 to 5 cm) proximal to its insertion on the calcaneus. This lies within a region of poorest blood supply that is often referred to as the "watershed area."

Describe abnormalities of the joints, including hallux abducto valgus (HAV), commonly known as a *bunion*, and deformities and flexion contractures of the lower digits *(hammertoes)*. Fig. 20.64 shows a patient with bilateral bunions and hammertoes. Note the medial deviation of the first metatarsal and the lateral deviation of the hallux at the first MTP joints bilaterally. The hammertoe is best seen on the right second toe.

Palpate the soft tissue over the first MTP joint. Is bursal inflammation caused by pressure, friction, or urate deposition? Measure the range of motion of the joint. Dorsiflexion of the hallux is measured against the bisection of the first metatarsal.

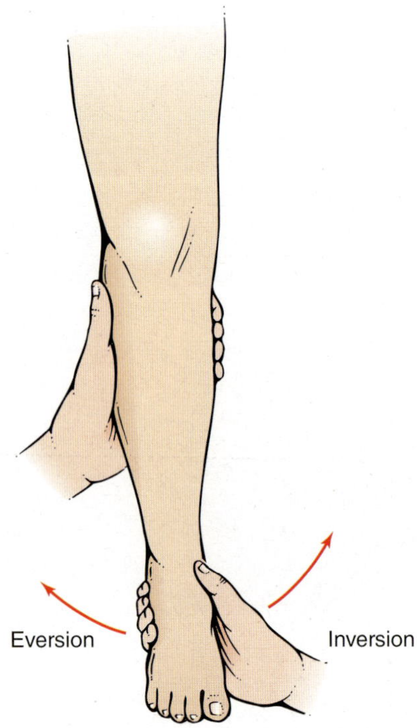

Fig. 20.62 Evaluating the Range of Motion at the Subtalar Joint.

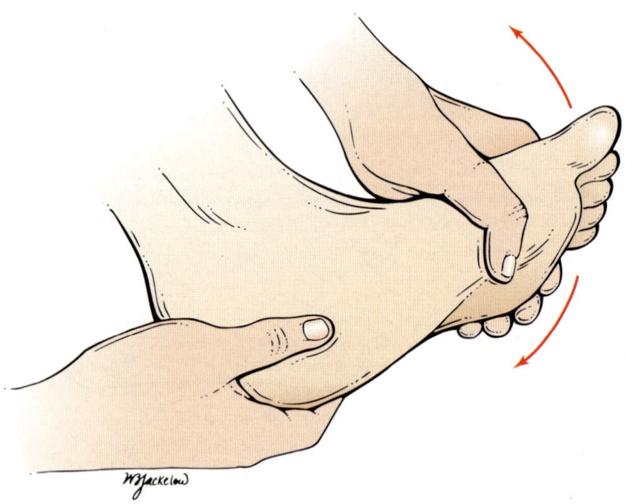

Fig. 20.63 Evaluating the Range of Motion at the Midtarsal Joint.

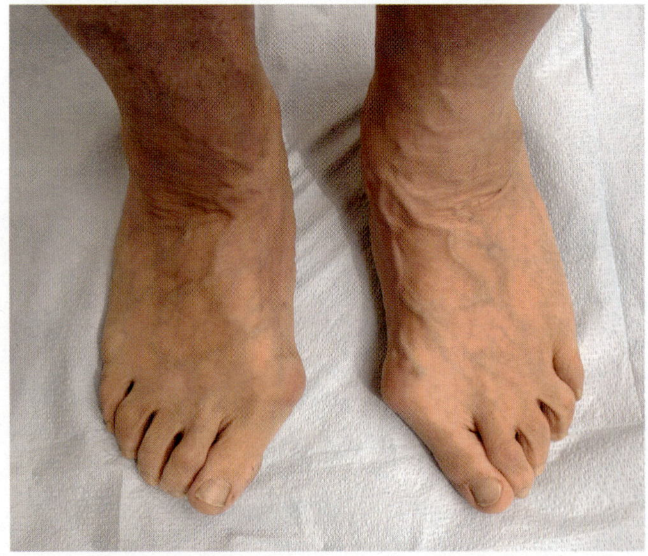

Fig. 20.64 Bunions and Hammer Toes. Note the medial deviation of the first metatarsal and a lateral deviation of the hallux at the first metatarsophalangeal joints bilaterally. The hammertoe is best seen on the right second toe.

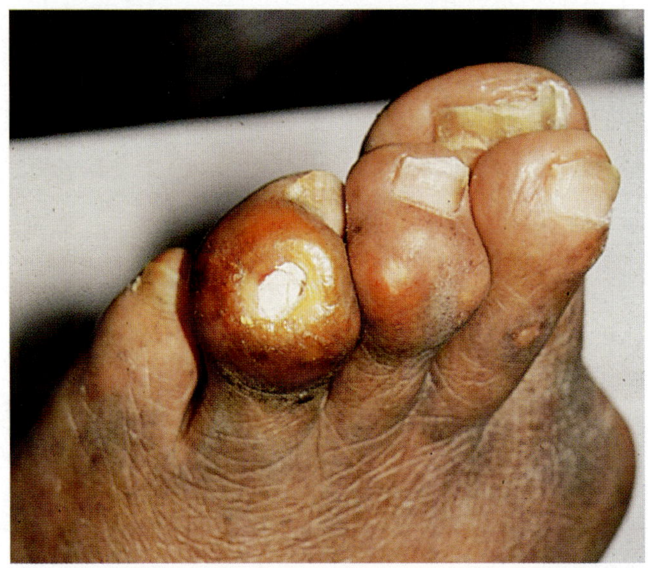

Fig. 20.65 Gout of the Lesser Metatarsophalangeal Joints.

The normal dorsal range of motion is 65 degrees to 75 degrees. Limitation of motion of this joint is termed *hallux limitus* and is most commonly caused by OA (see next section).

Fig. 20.65 depicts ulceration over the distal IP joint of the fourth toe of a patient with chronic tophaceous gout. Note the bunion deformity and underlapping hallux. An acute attack of gout commonly manifests with severe pain, swelling, and inflammation in the first MTP joint, a condition termed *podagra*. Podagra in a patient with acute gout is illustrated in Fig. 20.66. Notice the erythema of the left hallux and the generalized swelling of the left foot.

Examine the lesser MTP joints. Grasp the MTP joints between your thumb and index finger and attempt to compress the forefoot. Pain elicited by this maneuver is often an early sign of RA. This test is demonstrated in Fig. 20.67.

CLINICOPATHOLOGIC CORRELATIONS

Rheumatoid arthritis (RA) is a common musculoskeletal disorder and is the most destructive and disabling of the principal joint diseases. It is an autoimmune disease that causes chronic inflammation of the joints and of many other organs such as the skin, heart, kidneys, lungs, digestive tract, blood vessels, nervous system, and eyes. However, the joints display the most marked destructive changes. RA is a progressive illness that can cause significant functional disability as a result of pain, swelling, and stiffness of the involved joints. More than 2 million Americans suffer from RA. It is 2 to 3 times more common in females than in males. Although RA generally occurs between the ages of 40 and 60 years, it can also affect young children and older adults.

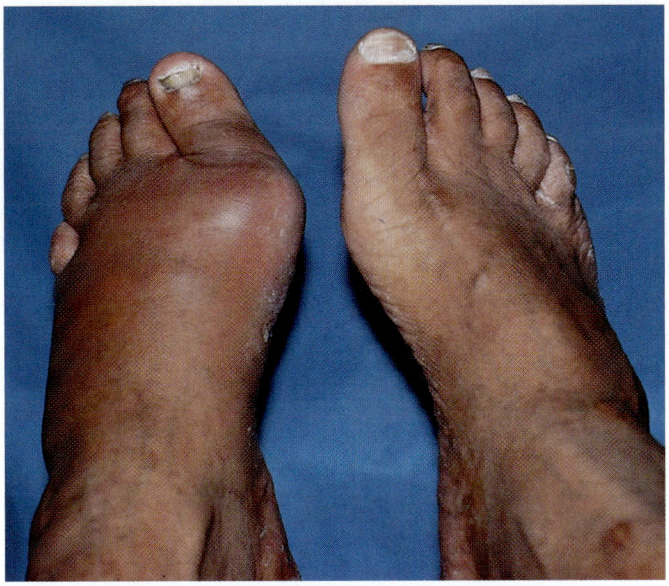

Fig. 20.66 Acute Gout and Podagra, Left Big Toe.

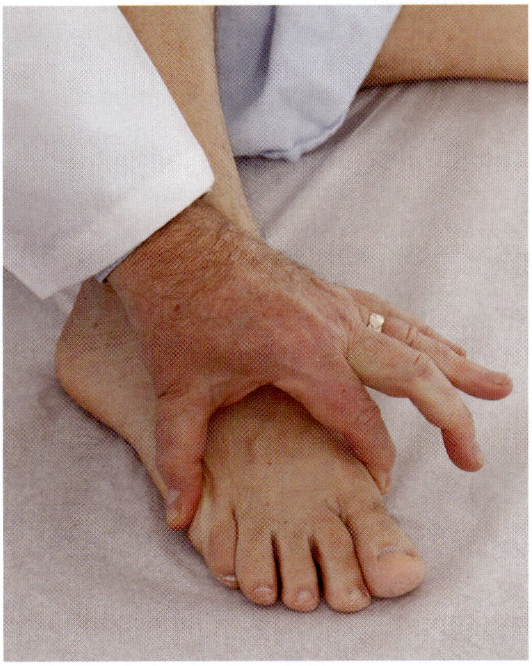

Fig. 20.67 Technique for Evaluating the Metatarsophalangeal Joints.

One of the most noticeable symptoms of RA is changes in the hands. In the initial stages, there may be inflammation and swelling in the proximal IP, MCP, and wrist joints. As the illness progresses, bone erosion occurs, leading to the typical signs of the disease. The most common finger deformity is ulnar deviation at the MCP joints. The two primary IP joint deformities are the swan-neck and the boutonnière deformities.

The *swan-neck deformity* is a condition that occurs when the interosseous muscles shorten, causing the MCP joints to flex, the proximal IP joints to hyperextend, and the distal IP joints to flex. On the other hand, the *boutonnière deformity* is a flexion deformity of the proximal IP joints, which results in the hyperextension of the distal IP joints. In Fig. 20.68, you can see the hands of a female with RA, where the MCP joints are notably deviated toward the ulnar side. Fig. 20.69 depicts the characteristic swan-neck deformity.

Osteoarthritis (OA), also known as *degenerative joint disease*, is a common condition that affects more than 20 million people in the United States. It is usually associated with aging. Males are more likely to develop OA before the age of 45, while females are more prone to it after the age of 55. The incidence of OA is similar across all races in the United States, although the Japanese population has a higher incidence of the disease while black people from South Africa, people from the East Indies, and people from southern China have lower rates.

OA is a type of arthritis that is caused by the breakdown and eventual loss of the cartilage of one or more joints. In most cases, the inflammatory response is minimal compared to that of RA. OA causes pain, swelling, and reduced motion in the joints. The form of OA depends on the joints involved. OA commonly affects the hands, feet, spine, and large weight-bearing joints, such as the hips and knees. The lifetime risk of developing OA of the knee is about 46%, and the lifetime risk of developing OA of the hip is 25%.[12] The joints of the hand are the third most common joints affected by OA. OA of the distal IP joint is called *Heberden nodes*. As the disease progresses, the

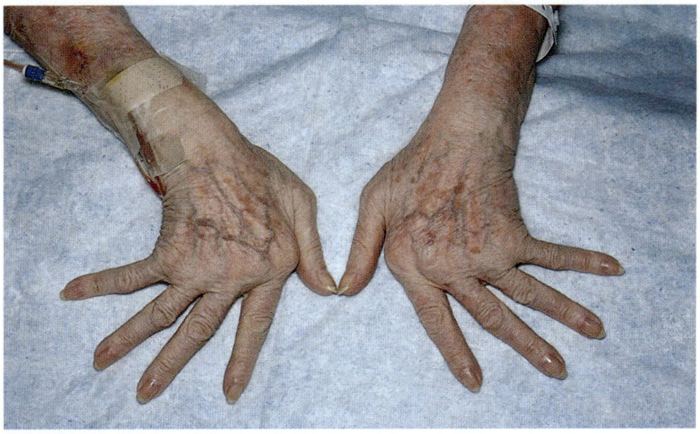

Fig. 20.68 Rheumatoid Arthritis. Note the marked ulnar deviation of the wrists.

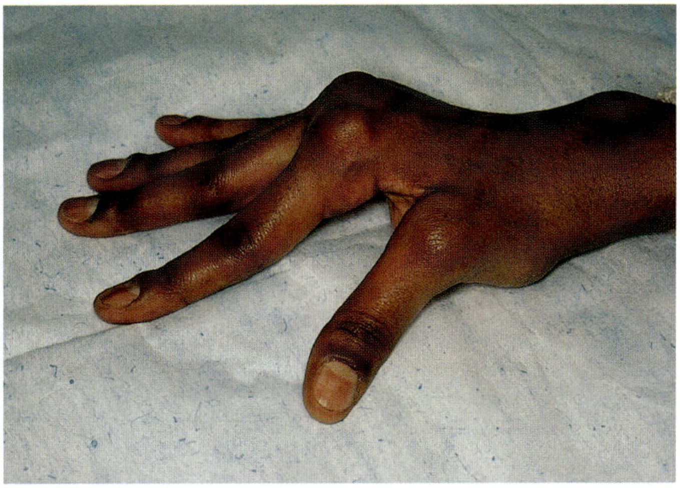

Fig. 20.69 Rheumatoid Arthritis. Note the swan-neck deformity.

proximal IP joints may become involved, resulting in *Bouchard nodes*. Fig. 20.70 shows the hands of a female with OA.

A *trigger finger* is a common, painful condition caused by inflammation and narrowing of the tendon sheath in the affected finger. In trigger finger, also known as *stenosing tenosynovitis,* one of the fingers or thumbs get stuck in a bent position and then straightens with a snap or pop, similar to a trigger being pulled and released. In severe cases, the finger may become locked in a bent position. Individuals whose work or hobbies require repetitive gripping actions are more susceptible. Trigger finger is more common in females, in patients with diabetes, and in individuals who are between 40 and 60 years of age. It is generally diagnosed by physical examination of the hand and fingers.

See Video 20.3.

Another common podiatric concern is an exostosis at the metatarsocuneiform joint, which produces a painful dorsal lesion. Fig. 20.71A depicts this type of problem; Fig. 20.71B is an x-ray film of the foot showing the bony abnormality.

As discussed in Chapter 8, The Skin, psoriasis is among the most common skin diseases in the United States. The pustular variant is characterized by pustules localized to the palms and soles. The patient may be quite ill, with fever and leukocytosis. Fig. 20.72 shows pustular psoriasis of the soles. Note the hyperkeratosis on an erythematous base.

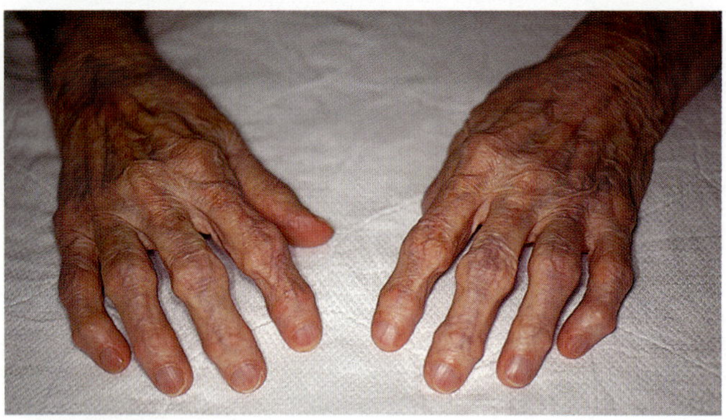

Fig. 20.70 Osteoarthritis. Note Heberden and Bouchard nodes.

Joint disease develops in approximately 7% of patients with psoriasis. The most common form of *psoriatic arthritis* (70%) is asymmetrical arthritis involving only two or three joints at a time. *Arthritis mutilans* is the most deforming type of psoriatic arthritis. In the most severe cases, there is osteolysis of the phalangeal and metacarpal joints, resulting in "telescoping of the digits," also known as the *opera-glass deformity*. The hands of a patient with this deforming type of psoriatic arthritis are shown in Fig. 20.73.

Table 20.6 lists the most common disorders associated with heel pain. *Plantar fasciitis* is an inflammation of the plantar fascia, usually caused by excessive, repetitive stretching. The plantar fascia is a broad band of fibrous tissue that runs along the bottom surface of the foot, attaching at the bottom of the calcaneus and extending to the forefoot. The pain is often most severe with the first steps in the morning or when rising from a chair. When the plantar fascia is excessively stretched, plantar fasciitis can occur, leading to arch pain, heel pain, and heel spurs. The most common causes of plantar fasciitis are:

- Overpronation (flatfoot), which results in the arch's collapsing with weight bearing
- A foot with an unusually high arch
- A sudden increase in physical activity
- Excessive weight on the foot, usually attributed to obesity or pregnancy
- Improperly fitting footwear

Gout is a metabolic disease characterized by high uric acid levels, recurrent attacks of acute arthritis, and deposition of urate crystals in and around the joints. The initial manifestation is frequently acute pain in the first MTP joint, often waking the patient from sleep. Even at rest, the pain is severe, but the slightest movement of the joint is agonizing. Within a few hours, the joint becomes swollen, shiny, and red. The higher the uric acid level, the more likely the patient is to develop *tophi,* which are subcutaneous and periarticular deposits of urate crystals. The commonly involved sites are over the first MTP joint, the finger, the ear, the elbow, and the Achilles tendon. Fig. 20.74 shows a gouty deposit on the big toe. Fig. 20.75 shows the arms of a

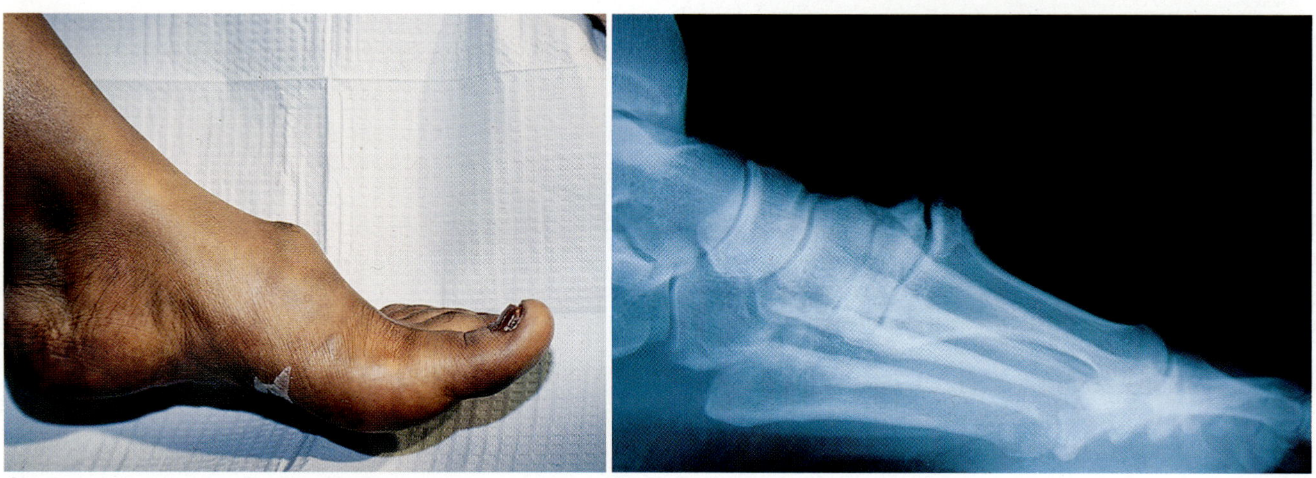

A B

Fig. 20.71 (A) Exostosis at the metatarsocuneiform joint. (B) X-ray film of the affected metatarsocuneiform joint.

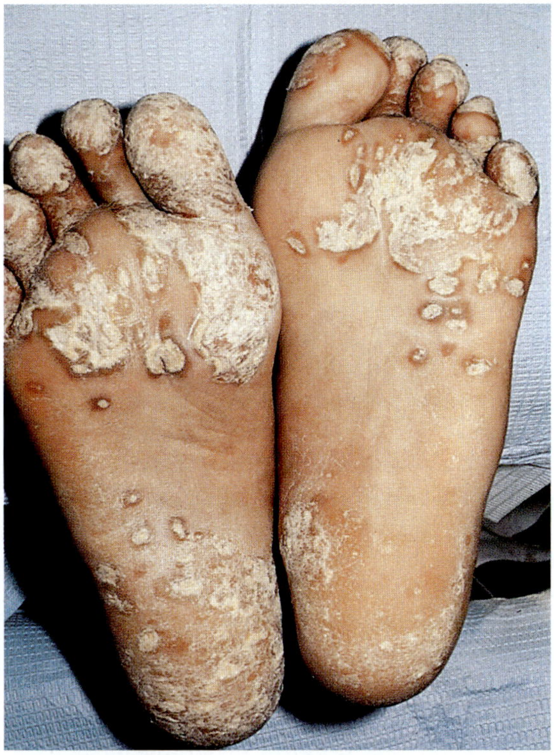

Fig. 20.72 Pustular Psoriasis.

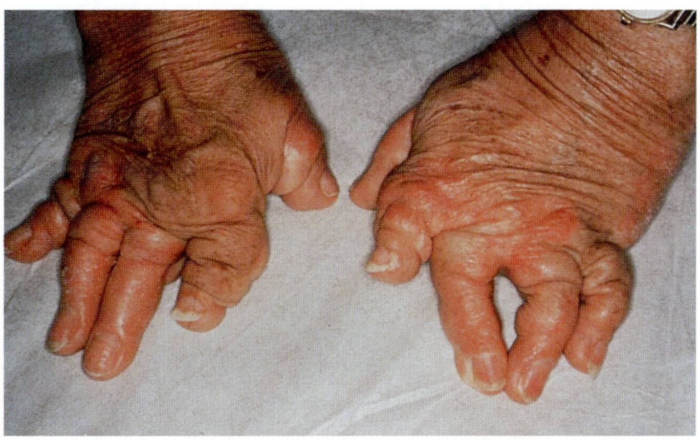

Fig. 20.73 Psoriatic Arthritis. (From Lebwohl MG, editor: *Atlas of the skin and systemic disease*, New York, 1995, Churchill Livingstone.)

TABLE 20.6 **Disorders Causing Heel Pain**
Plantar calcaneal spur (enthesopathy)
Plantar fasciitis
Inferior calcaneal bursitis
Atrophy of plantar fat pad
Rheumatoid arthritis
Ankylosing spondylitis
Reiter syndrome
Gout
Fracture
Neoplasm
Foreign body
Nerve entrapment

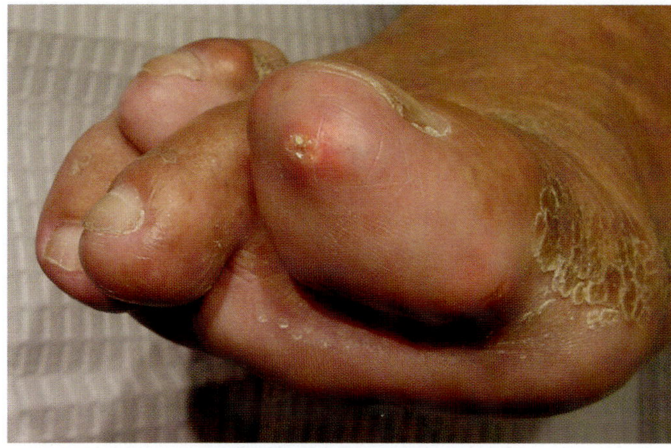

Fig. 20.74 Gout Affecting Big Toe.

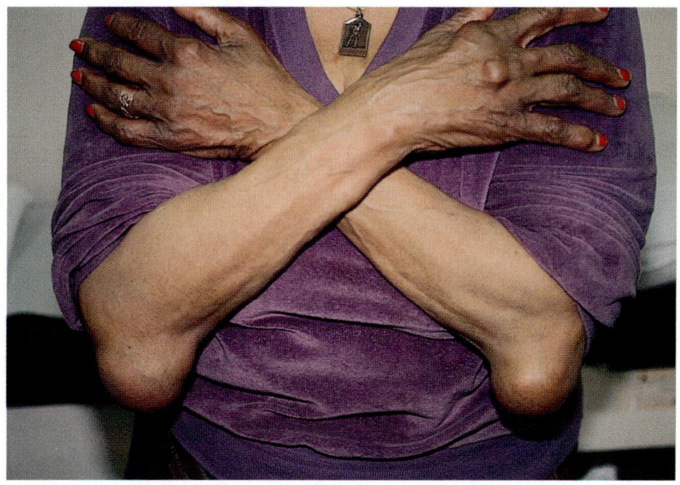

Fig. 20.75 Gout. Note tophi on the elbows and hands.

patient with chronic tophaceous gout who has large tophi on her elbows, as well as smaller tophi on her hands. Tophi frequently develop over the distal IP joints of the fingers and in the olecranon and prepatellar bursae. Fig. 20.76 shows the hands of a patient with tophi on her fingers.

Ankle sprains are a common musculoskeletal injury, especially among those who participate in sports. The most common type of ankle sprain is the inversion sprain. These sprains most commonly involve a complete or partial tear of the anterior talofibular ligament. In more severe injuries, it is important to rule out tibia, fibula, and talar dome fractures. A useful maneuver is the Potts test, in which the heel of each hand is used to compress the tibia against the fibula at a point midway up the leg. Pain in the ankle or at the proximal aspect of the fibula constitutes a positive test. A high fibular spiral fracture *(Maisonneuve fracture)* resulting from external rotation of the ankle is another frequently overlooked consequence of an ankle sprain and should always be screened for by examining the proximal fibula as well. An x-ray of the leg is used to make the diagnosis. A fracture of the base of the fifth metatarsal can accompany an ankle sprain and should be evaluated for on examination.

A sudden onset of pain along the midshaft of the lesser metatarsals should alert the healthcare professional to the

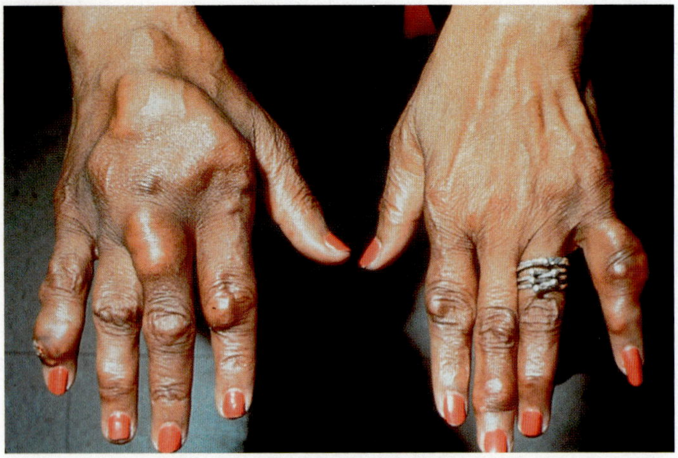

Fig. 20.76 Gout. Note tophi on the fingers.

possibility of a *stress fracture.* The pain is usually pinpoint and can occur spontaneously even without overt trauma. Early diagnosis is often based on clinical suspicion because x-ray examinations may appear normal. With continued weight bearing and in the absence of treatment, the hairline fracture may widen and cause symptoms to become more severe.

Pain and swelling on the medial aspect of the ankle, along the course of the posterior tibial tendon, may indicate *posterior tibial tendon dysfunction (PTTD).* This condition is usually worsened by activity and may be accompanied by an inability to perform a single limb heel raise on the affected side. PTTD is one of the most common causes of acquired flatfoot in adults.

Table 20.7 lists disorders associated with first MTP joint pain. *Metatarsalgia* is a common ailment that affects the plantar forefoot, typically occurring in young people who engage in physical activities such as dancing or jogging. Patients with high-arch foot types are particularly susceptible. Any activity that places force on the ball of the foot—even walking—can cause metatarsalgia. *Sesamoiditis* is a general description of any inflammatory condition affecting the sesamoid bones. The sesamoids are tiny bones within the flexor tendons that run to the big toe. With repetitive stress, they can eventually become inflamed and even fractured. Sesamoiditis can be distinguished from other forefoot conditions by its gradual onset and location. The pain usually begins as a mild ache under the first metatarsal head and increases gradually as the aggravating activity is continued; the pain may build to an intense throbbing.

TABLE 20.7 **Disorders Causing Pain in the First Metatarsophalangeal Joint**
Osteoarthritis
Bursitis and capsulitis
Fracture
Sesamoiditis
Gout
Rheumatoid arthritis
Reiter syndrome
Septic arthritis

Morton neuroma is a common foot problem associated with pain, swelling, and inflammation of an intermetatarsal nerve, usually between the third and fourth metatarsal heads. The digital nerve traveling between the adjacent metatarsal heads becomes entrapped or pinched during the push-off phase of gait. Symptoms of this condition include sharp pain, burning, cramping, and even a lack of feeling in the toes supplied by that nerve. Symptoms of Morton neuroma can occur during or after application of significant pressure on the forefoot area while walking, standing, jumping, or sprinting. A patient may also be concerned that it feels as if a marble or pebble were inside the ball of the foot. Constricting shoes can worsen the condition by pinching the nerve between the toes, causing discomfort and extreme pain.

To evaluate a patient with a suspected Morton neuroma, try to reproduce the pain by gently pushing the adjacent metatarsal heads together. Next, try to palpate the neuroma by pressing your thumb into the third interspace. Finally, hold the patient's first, second, and third metatarsal heads with one of your hands and the fourth and fifth metatarsal heads in the other, and push half the foot up while pushing half the foot down slightly. In a patient with Morton neuroma, this maneuver may elicit an audible click, known as the *Mulder sign.* Local injections, shoe gear modification, and orthoses may prove helpful; however, surgery may also be necessary.

Bunions are one of the most frequently encountered musculoskeletal pathologic conditions seen in the foot. Also referred to as an *HAV* (hallux abductovalgus) *deformity,* a bunion is characterized by a medial deviation of the first metatarsal and a lateral deviation of the hallux at the first MTP joint (Fig. 20.77). Bunions are commonly caused by forefoot adductus and excess pronation of the subtalar joint. Due to excessive pronation, forces load the medial forefoot. This increased adductory load on the first metatarsal shaft causes rotation of the shaft, which then requires the hallux to compensate by abducting. Degenerative arthritis, limitation of motion, and pain can develop as the articular cartilage is slowly worn away by joint malalignment. Occasionally, the laterally deviated hallux encroaches on the second toe, causing it to either under- or overlap. This can cause pain not only to the bunion but to the second toe as well. Symptoms can become worse due to pressure within the toe box of a narrow or high-heeled shoe.

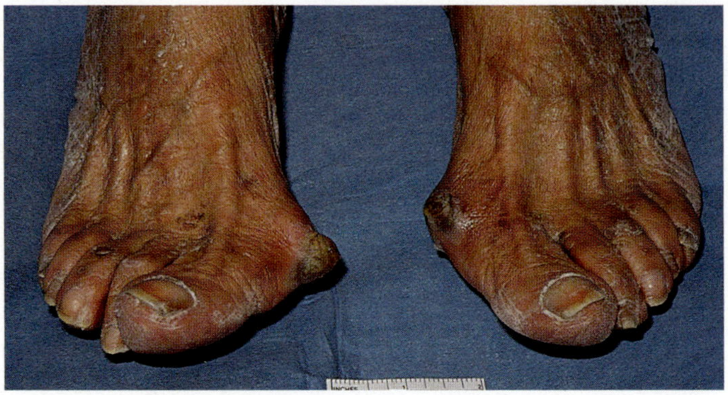

Fig. 20.77 Hallux Abductovalgus Deformity and Hammer Toes. Notice the bowstringing of the extensor tendons.

Fig. 20.77 shows HAV deformity, flexion contractures of the IP joints, and bowstringing of the extensor tendons. This is a typical presentation in the geriatric age group. Note the hyperkeratotic lesion over the right bunion from shoe pressure. Bunion deformities can be a source of undue pressure in diabetic patients, leading to ulceration and infection. A large pressure ulceration over the medial eminence of the first MTP joint resulting from shoe irritation in a diabetic patient is shown in Fig. 20.78.

Hammertoes are characterized by a flexion contracture of the proximal IP joint of one or more of the lesser toes, resulting in a dorsal prominence. Hammertoes are deformities of the second, third, fourth, or fifth toes in which the toe becomes bent at the middle joint, resembling a hammer. The most common cause of a hammertoe is a muscle/tendon imbalance. Shoe pressure may lead to a reactive hyperkeratosis or "corn" to form on the top of the toe. Bowstringing of the extensor tendons may also be seen. The patient shown in Fig. 20.64 has both bunion and hammertoe deformities.

Hallux limitus and *hallux rigidus* are common conditions characterized by pain and a limitation of motion at the first MTP joint. *Limitus* is a term that refers to the decreased motion of a joint; this is the early stage. *Rigidus* denotes a joint that has very little, if any, motion available; this is the later stage. As the condition progresses from hallux limitus to rigidus, a bone spur may develop at the first MTP joint and prevent the big toe from bending as much as it needs to during gait. Pain and stiffness of the first MTP joint during activities such as walking or running are common symptoms of both conditions. The patient in Fig. 20.79 has hallux rigidus and a large dorsal-medial bump. Notice the callus on the bump caused by increased pressure and rubbing on shoes. Fig. 20.80 is an x-ray examination of a patient with bilateral hallux rigidus. Note the bony spurs. OA of the first MTP joint is evident with narrowing of the joint space and periarticular spurring.

Ankylosing spondylitis (AS), a spondyloarthropathy, is a chronic, lifelong, multisystem inflammatory disorder involving primarily the sacroiliac joints and the axial skeleton. It causes inflammation of the vertebrae that can lead to severe, chronic pain and discomfort. Although symptoms usually start to appear in late adolescence or early adulthood (ages 15 to 40), symptoms can occur in childhood or much later in life.

As part of the body's reaction to inflammation, calcium is laid down where the ligaments attach to the vertebrae. This reduces the flexibility of the back and causes new bone to grow at the sides of the vertebrae. Eventually, the individual bones of the spine may fuse, a condition known as *ankylosis*. This fusing makes the spine less flexible and can result in a hunched-forward posture. If the ribs are affected, the patient may have difficulty breathing.

The severity of AS varies greatly from person to person. Almost all cases of AS are characterized by acute, painful episodes, which are followed by periods of pain-free remission.

Although the exact cause of AS is unknown, genetics does play a key role in this disease. Most individuals who have AS also have a gene that produces a "genetic marker" protein, HLA-B27. This protein is found in more than 95% of people in the

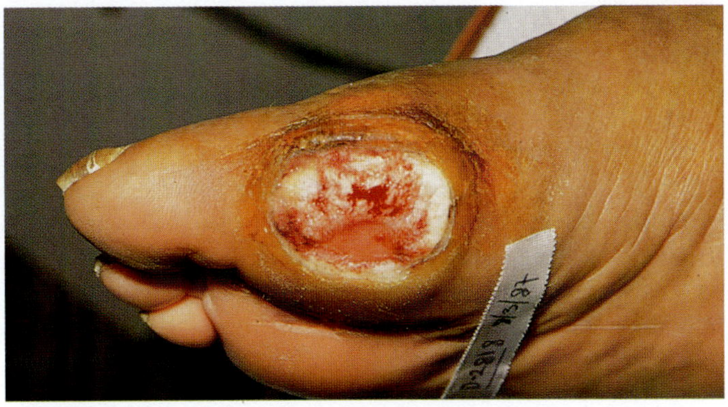

Fig. 20.78 Hallux Abductovalgus Deformity and Ulceration.

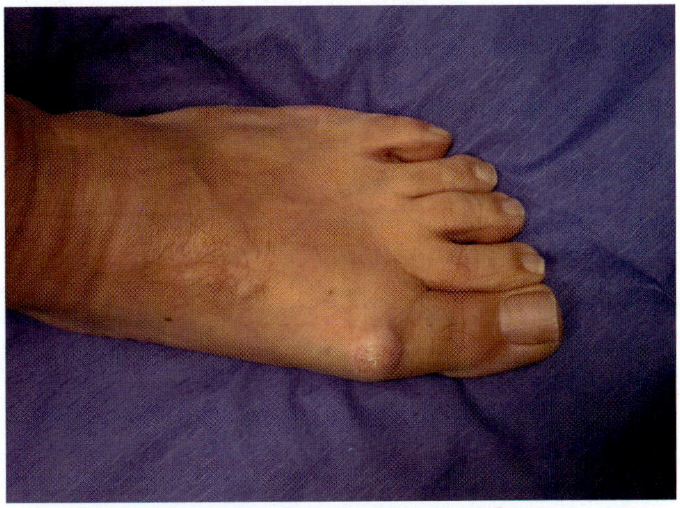

Fig. 20.79 Hallux Rigidus. Note the large dorsal-medial bump on the first metatarsophalangeal joint.

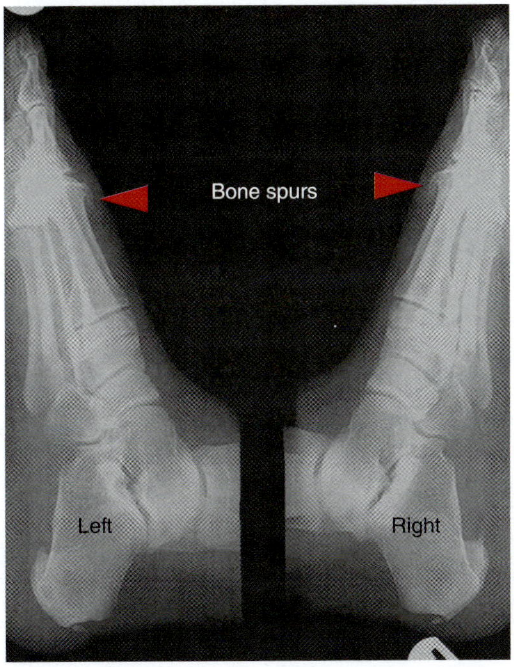

Fig. 20.80 Hallux Rigidus. X-ray examination showing the bone spurs on the first metatarsophalangeal joints bilaterally.

White population with AS. It is important to note, however, that many people with AS are not HLA-B27 positive. Also, many people with this marker never develop AS.

Uveitis, reactive arthritis, aortitis, and inflammatory bowel disease are also commonly associated with AS.

The Schöber test is a test for AS; it evaluates the lumbar range of motion during flexion. The patient is asked to stand with their back toward the examiner. The examiner determines the location of the lumbosacral junction by pressing on the location of the dimples of Venus. The intersection of the top of the dimples of Venus is marked by drawing a horizontal line. This line acts as the landmark. A second line is marked 10 cm above the first, and a third line is marked 5 cm below the first line, for a total of 15 cm in distance. The patient is asked to touch their toes while keeping the knees straight. If the distance of the two points does not increase by at least 5 cm (with the total distance greater than 20 cm), then this is a sign of restriction in the lumbar flexion and suggestive of AS. The Schöber test is illustrated in Fig. 20.81.

Table 20.8 summarizes the clinical features that differentiate RA from OA. Table 20.9 summarizes some of the features of diseases affecting the hands and wrists. Table 20.10 outlines the clinical features that differentiate common musculoskeletal disorders affecting the elbow. Table 20.11 lists the clinical features that differentiate significant diseases affecting the knee. Table 20.12 lists the clinical features differentiating diseases of the foot.

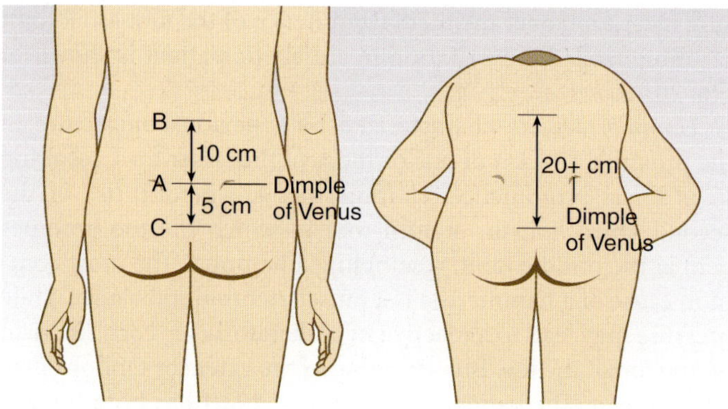

Fig. 20.81 **Schober's Test.** When the patient bends forward maximally with the knees straight, distance BC should increase by at least 5 cm. (Reprinted from Gibson J, Brenkel I: The musculoskeletal system. In Innes JA, Dover, AR, Fairhurst K, editors: *Macleod's clinical examination*, ed 14, 2017, Elsevier, pp 251–282, with permission from Elsevier.)

TABLE 20.8 Clinical Features Differentiating Rheumatoid Arthritis from Osteoarthritis

Clinical Feature	Rheumatoid Arthritis (see Figs. 20.68 and 20.69)	Osteoarthritis (see Fig. 20.70)
Patient's age (years)	3–80	Older than 45
Morning stiffness	More than 1 h	Less than 1 h
Disability	Often great	Variable
Joint distribution		
• Distal interphalangeal joint	Rare	Very common
• Proximal interphalangeal joint	Very common	Common
• Metacarpophalangeal joint	Very common	Absent
• Wrist	Very common	Absent
Soft tissue swelling	Very common	Rare
Interosseous muscle wasting	Very common	Rare
Swan-neck deformity	Common	Rare
Ulnar deviation	Common	Absent

TABLE 20.9 Clinical Features Differentiating Diseases Affecting the Hands and Wrists

Clinical Feature	Rheumatoid Arthritis	Psoriatic Arthritis[a]	Acute Gout (see Fig. 20.66)	Osteoarthritis	Carpal Tunnel Syndrome
Age (years)	3–80	10–60	30–80	50–80	40–80
Sex	Female	Male	Male	Female	Male, female
Pain onset	Gradual	Gradual	Abrupt	Gradual	Gradual
Stiffness	Very common	Common	Absent	Common	Absent
Swelling	Common	Common	Common	Common	Common
Redness	Absent	Uncommon	Common	Uncommon	Absent
Deformity	Flexion of PIP and MCP; swan-neck (see Fig. 20.69), boutonnière deformities; ulnar deviation (see Fig. 20.68)	Frequent DIP, PIP, and MCP involvement; "sausage-shaped" digits (see Fig. 20.73)	None in acute stage; resembles rheumatoid arthritis if deposits occur in tendon sheaths in chronic gout	Flexion and lateral deviation of DIP and PIP (see Fig. 20.70)	Thenar muscle atrophy

[a]Needlepoint pitting of the nails is often associated with psoriatic arthritis. See Figs. 8.14 and 8.16.
DIP, Distal interphalangeal joint; *MCP*, metacarpophalangeal joint; *PIP*, proximal interphalangeal joint.

TABLE 20.10 Clinical Features Differentiating Diseases Affecting the Elbow

Clinical Feature	Rheumatoid Arthritis	Psoriatic Arthritis	Acute Gout	Osteoarthritis	Tennis Elbow
Age (years)	3–80	10–60	30–80	50–80	20–60
Sex	Female	Male	Male	Female	Male, female
Pain onset	Gradual	Gradual	Abrupt	Gradual	Gradual
Stiffness	Very common	Common	Absent	Common	Occasional
Swelling	Common	Common	Common	Common	Absent
Redness	Absent	Uncommon	Common	Absent	Absent
Deformity	Flexion contractures, usually bilateral	Flexion contractures, usually bilateral	Flexion contractures only in chronic state[a]	Flexion contractures	None

[a]See Fig. 20.75, which shows a patient with chronic tophaceous gout and painless tophi on the elbows.

TABLE 20.11 Clinical Features Differentiating Diseases Affecting the Knee

Clinical Feature	Rheumatoid Arthritis	Psoriatic Arthritis	Acute Gout	Osteoarthritis	Torn Meniscus
Age (years)	3–80	10–60	30–80	50–80	20–60
Sex	Female	Male	Male	Female	Male
Pain onset	Gradual	Gradual	Abrupt	Gradual	Abrupt
Stiffness	Very common	Common	Absent	Common	Occasional
Swelling	Common	Common	Common	Common	Common
Redness	Absent	Uncommon	Common	Absent	Absent
Deformity	Flexion contractures	Flexion contractures	Flexion contractures only in chronic state	Flexion contractures	None

TABLE 20.12 Clinical Features Differentiating Diseases Affecting the Foot

Clinical Feature	Rheumatoid Arthritis	Psoriatic Arthritis	Acute Gout	Osteoarthritis	Reiter Syndrome
Age (years)	3–80	10–60	30–80	50–80	10–80 (peak, 30s)
Sex	Female	Male	Male	Female	Male
Pain onset	Gradual	Gradual	Abrupt	Gradual	Gradual
Stiffness	Very common	Common	Common	Common	Common
Swelling	Common	Common	Very common	Uncommon	Common
Redness	Uncommon	Uncommon	Very common	Uncommon	Common
Joint predilection and deformity	Abductovalgus deformity of MTP	Fusiform swelling of DIP	First MTP (may also have hallux abductovalgus deformity)	Hallux abductovalgus deformity	Ankle, heel, toes ("sausage" swelling of digits)

DIP, Distal interphalangeal joint; *MTP,* metatarsophalangeal joint.

USEFUL VOCABULARY

Listed here are the specific roots that are important for understanding the terminology related to musculoskeletal diseases.

Root	Pertaining to	Example	Definition
ankyl(o)-	stiff	***ankylo**sis*	Immobility or stiffness of a joint
arthr(o)-	joint	***arthro**gram*	Radiograph of a joint
chir(o)-	hand	***chiro**spasm*	Writer's cramp
dactyl(o)-	finger or toe	***dactylo**spasm*	Cramping of a digit
myo-	muscle	***myo**pathy*	Disease of muscle
oste(o)-	bone	***osteo**malacia*	A condition marked by softening of the bones
pod-	foot	***pod**iatrist*	Specialist in conditions of the foot
scolio-	twisted	***scolio**sis*	Lateral deviation of the spine
spondyl(o)-	vertebrae	***spondyl**itis*	Inflammation of vertebrae
teno-	tendon	***teno**tomy*	Surgical cutting of a tendon

WRITING UP THE PHYSICAL EXAMINATION

Listed here are examples of the write-up for the examination of the musculoskeletal system.

- All the joints have full range of motion. No deformities, tenderness, or abnormalities are detected.
- There is marked ulnar deviation of both hands in association with a flexion deformity of all the proximal interphalangeal (IP) joints and hyperextension of all the distal IP joints. Marked tenderness of both wrists is present.
- There is abnormal forward mobility of the knee. There is 3 to 4 cm of motion detected.
- The left first metatarsophalangeal (MTP) joint is markedly erythematous and painful. The joint is shiny and edematous.
- No joint deformities are noted. There is marked reduction of hip internal and external rotation. No pain is produced by these movements. Pain is produced by abduction of the right shoulder against resistance. The range of right shoulder abduction is reduced. The range of motion of the hands, wrists, spine, knees, and ankles is normal.

REVIEW QUESTIONS

1. Which of the following is an example of a common musculoskeletal disorder?
- **A.** Osteoarthritis
- **B.** Carpal tunnel syndrome
- **C.** Trigger finger
- **D.** Lumbar disc herniation
- **E.** All of the above

2. Which of the following motions is correctly described below?
- **A.** Pronation is rotation of the palm upward.
- **B.** Supination is rotation of the palm downward.
- **C.** Internal rotation is turning the anterior surface of a limb inward.
- **D.** Adduction is movement away from the midline.
- **E.** Abduction is movement toward the midline.

3. All of the following are sources of heel pain *except:*
- **A.** Plantar fasciitis
- **B.** Sesamoiditis
- **C.** Plantar calcaneal spur
- **D.** Nerve entrapment
- **E.** Calcaneus fracture

4. Rheumatoid arthritis differs from osteoarthritis in that:
- **A.** The distal interphalangeal joint is rarely involved
- **B.** It does not cause ulnar deviation deformity
- **C.** It does not result in disability
- **D.** It does not cause morning stiffness
- **E.** It is not an autoimmune disease

5. All of the following are clinical features of carpal tunnel syndrome *except:*
- **A.** Hand pain
- **B.** Hand numbness
- **C.** Stiffness
- **D.** Muscle atrophy
- **E.** Pins and needles or tingling

6. Osteoarthritis is a degenerative joint disease that:
- **A.** Affects more than 20 million people in the United States
- **B.** Causes pain, swelling, and reduced joint range of motion
- **C.** Most commonly affects weight-bearing joints like the hip and knee
- **D.** Can result in the formation of Heberden nodes in the distal interphalangeal joint
- **E.** All of the above

7. All of the following are exam maneuvers to assess the integrity of the cruciate ligaments of the knee *except:*
- **A.** Posterior drawer test
- **B.** Lachman test
- **C.** Hornblower test
- **D.** Anterior drawer test
- **E.** Pivot shift test

8. Which of the following statements regarding shoulder pathologies is false?
- **A.** The sulcus sign is a test for multidirectional instability.
- **B.** Adhesive capsulitis or "frozen shoulder" causes inflammation and stiffness in the joint, severely restricting range of motion.
- **C.** A positive Neer test is indicative of rotator cuff impingement.
- **D.** Speed's test is used to assess the rotator cuff.
- **E.** The cross-body adduction test is used to assess the AC joint.

9. All of the following muscle tendons make up the rotator cuff *except:*
- **A.** Subscapularis
- **B.** Teres major
- **C.** Supraspinatus
- **D.** Infraspinatus
- **E.** Teres minor

10. The joint movements of the thumb include:
- **A.** Flexion
- **B.** Abduction
- **C.** Adduction
- **D.** Opposition
- **E.** All of the above

REFERENCES

Available online.

BIBLIOGRAPHY

Available online.

21

The Nervous System

Mark H. Swartz

As the debility increases and the influence of the will over the muscles fades, the tremulous agitation becomes more vehement. It now seldom leaves him for a moment; but even when exhausted nature seizes a small portion of sleep, the motion becomes so violent as not only to shake the bed-hangings, but even the floor and sashes of the room. The chin is now almost immovably bent down upon the sternum. The slops with which he is attempted to be fed, with the saliva, are continually trickling from the mouth. The power of articulation is lost. The urine and feces are passed involuntarily; and at the last, constant sleepiness, with slight delirium, and other marks of extreme exhaustion, announce the wished-for release.

James Parkinson (1755–1824)

VIDEOS

Video 21.1	Assessing mental status
Video 21.2	Testing cranial nerve V (trigeminal)
Video 21.3	Testing cranial neve VII (facial)
Video 21.4	Testing cranial nerve VIII (vestibulocochlear)
Video 21.5	Testing cranial nerve IX (glossopharyngeal) and cranial nerve X (vagus)
Video 21.6	Testing cranial nerve XI (spinal accessory)
Video 21.7	Testing cranial nerve XII (hypoglossal) and motor function
Video 21.8	Testing the biceps tendon reflex
Video 21.9	Testing the brachioradialis tendon reflex
Video 21.10	Testing the triceps tendon reflex
Video 21.11	Testing the patellar tendon reflex
Video 21.12	Testing the Achilles tendon reflex
Video 21.13	Testing for abnormal reflexes–Babinski reflex
Video 21.14	Testing light touch
Video 21.15	Testing pain sensation
Video 21.16	Testing vibration sense
Video 21.17	Testing proprioception
Video 21.18	Performing the finger-to-nose test
Video 21.19	Performing the Romberg test
See also,	
Video 10.1	Assessing visual acuity (CN II—optic)
Video 10.4	Evaluating the cardinal positions of gaze (CN III—oculomotor; CN IV—trochlear; CN VI—abducens)
Video 20.2	Evaluating gait

GENERAL CONSIDERATIONS

By the 2nd century CE, Galen had already described the cerebral ventricles, 7 of the 12 cranial nerves, and the cerebral convolutions. There was, however, little further interest in the anatomy and physiologic characteristics of the neurologic system until the 16th century. In 1543, Andreas Vesalius illustrated the basal ganglia, and in 1552, Bartolomeo Eustachius described the cerebellar peduncles and the pons.

During the 17th century, Thomas Willis provided detailed explanations and images of the cerebral circulation, the "striate body," and the internal capsule. While some people, like Caspar Bartholin, believed that the function of the cerebral cortex was to protect blood vessels, others thought that the cerebrum had higher functions. François Pourfour du Petit emphasized that the cortex was responsible for motor activity, but this idea was not widely accepted until the late 19th century.

Scientists from the 18th and early 19th century provided detailed descriptions of the tracts, nuclei, and gyri of the brain. Johann Christian Reil and Karl Friedrich Burdach named many of the gross anatomic structures that had previously been illustrated by others. Reil named the insula, capsule, uncinate and cingulate fasciculi, and tapetum, while Burdach named the uncus, lenticular nucleus, pulvinar, and gyrus cinguli. During this period, Samuel von Soemmering, Felix Vicq d'Azyr, Franz Josef Gall, Louis Gratiolet, and Luigi Rolando created many detailed illustrations of the cerebral convolutional patterns.

During the early 19th century, there were several disease states that were described for the first time. James Parkinson wrote an essay in 1817 where he described the "shaking palsy," which is now known as Parkinson disease. In 1829, Charles Bell wrote:

The next instance was in a man wounded by the horn of an ox. The point entered under the angle of the jaw and came out before the ear. … He remains now a singular proof of the effects of the loss of function in the muscles of the face by this nerve being divided. The forehead of the corresponding side is without motion, the eyelids remain open, the nostril has no motion in breathing, and the mouth is drawn to the opposite side.

This is the classic description of facial nerve (seventh cranial nerve) palsy, also known as Bell's palsy.

During the mid-19th century, there was a growing fascination with microscopic neuroanatomy. Many neuroanatomists, such as Jan Purkinje, Theodor Schwann, and Hermann von Helmholtz, made significant contributions to our knowledge of the nervous system. However, it was not until the late 19th century that specific staining techniques were developed by Camillo Golgi, Vittorio Marchi, and Franz Nissl. These techniques led to our current understanding of neuronal disease and the discovery of the nerve cell.

In the 20th century, there were significant discoveries made in the understanding of the cerebral cortex, anterior commissure, thalamus, and hypothalamus. One key breakthrough was made in 1904 by Santiago Ramón y Cajal, whose research helped clarify the complexities of the neuron. However, it wasn't until 1925 that the connections between the hypophyseal and hypothalamic areas were fully described, and even today, the function of the hypothalamus remains not completely understood.

Research has shown that over 40% of patients who visit healthcare professionals have symptoms related to neurologic disease. It is important for these professionals to be able to recognize the early signs and symptoms of neurologic disease and provide appropriate treatment. Unfortunately, subtle signs and symptoms are frequently overlooked, leading to a delayed diagnosis and advanced disability.

Cerebrovascular disease is a devastating condition and is currently the fifth leading cause of death in the United States. Every year, over 795,000 Americans suffer from a stroke, which is the primary cause of disability. In 2021, one in six deaths from cardiovascular disease was due to a stroke.[1] Unfortunately, more than 3 million Americans live with permanent brain damage resulting from a stroke. Shockingly, every 40 seconds, someone in the U.S. experiences a stroke,[2] and every 3 minutes, someone dies from it. Currently, around 6.2 million noninstitutionalized adults have had a stroke, which has severe consequences on their lives. The impact of stroke is not just on individuals but also on society, leading to significant economic effects. Stroke-related costs in the United States came to nearly $56.5 billion between 2018 and 2019.[2] The total cost of stroke includes healthcare services, medications, and lost workdays. Stroke is a major contributor to long-term disability, with more than half of survivors over 65 experiencing reduced mobility.

The primary healthcare professional plays a crucial role as patients with neurological issues usually approach them first. Having a comprehensive understanding of basic neuroanatomy and physiology is fundamental to making accurate neurological diagnoses.

STRUCTURE AND PHYSIOLOGIC CHARACTERISTICS

The brain is the central organ of the nervous system, enclosed in the cranium and surrounded by protective membranes called meninges. It consists of the cerebral hemispheres (divided into two parts), basal ganglia, diencephalon (including the thalamus and hypothalamus), brainstem, and cerebellum.

The brain's largest portion is made up of two cerebral hemispheres. These hemispheres can each be divided into four major lobes—frontal, parietal, occipital, and temporal—named after the cranial bones they lie under. The cerebral surface is divided by fissures and sulci, with a deep longitudinal fissure separating the two hemispheres. The convolutions, or gyri, are found between the sulci. A lateral view of the left cerebral hemisphere is pictured in Fig. 21.1. Fig. 21.2 is a medial view of the right cerebral hemisphere. A basal view of the cerebral hemispheres is pictured in Fig. 21.3.

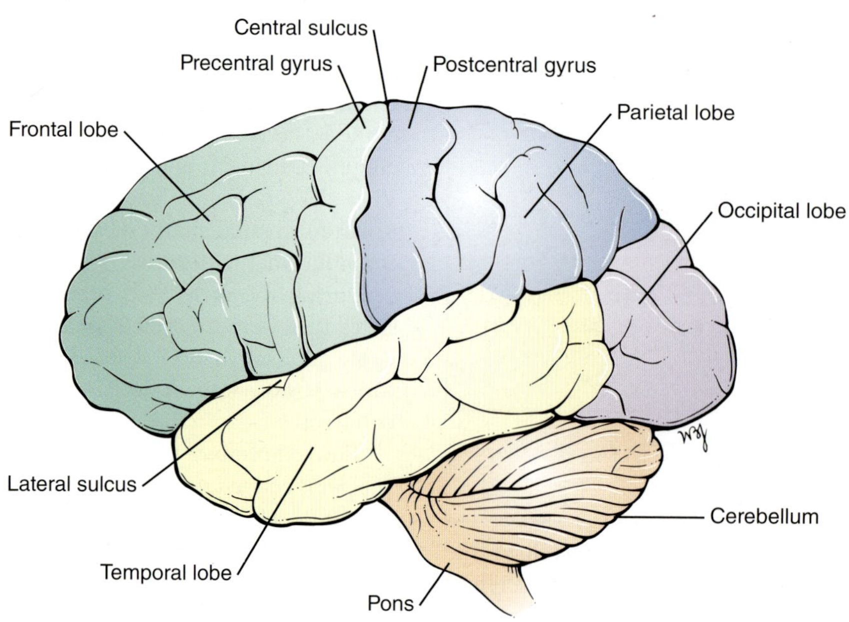

Fig. 21.1 Lateral View of the Left Cerebral Hemisphere.

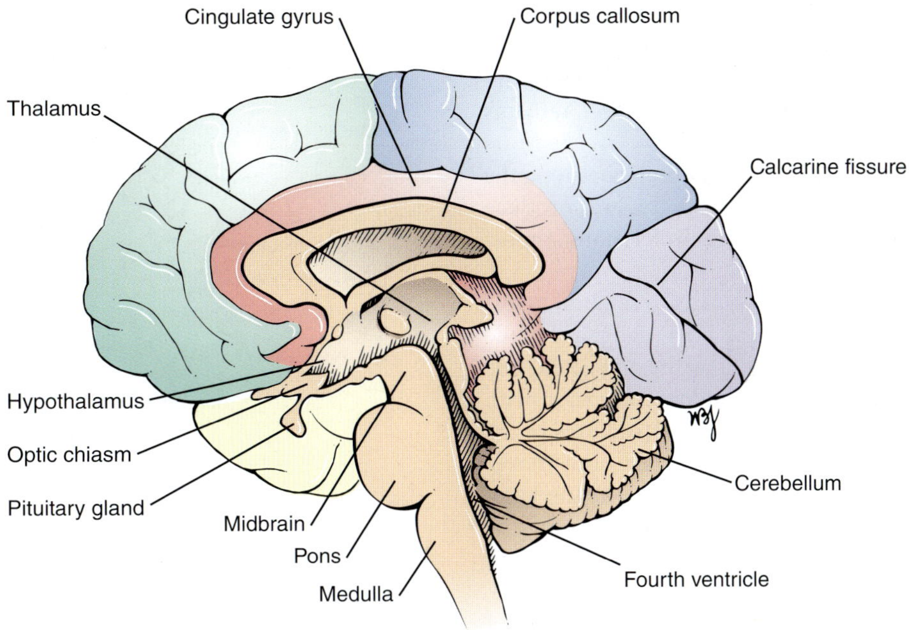

Fig. 21.2 Medial View of the Right Cerebral Hemisphere.

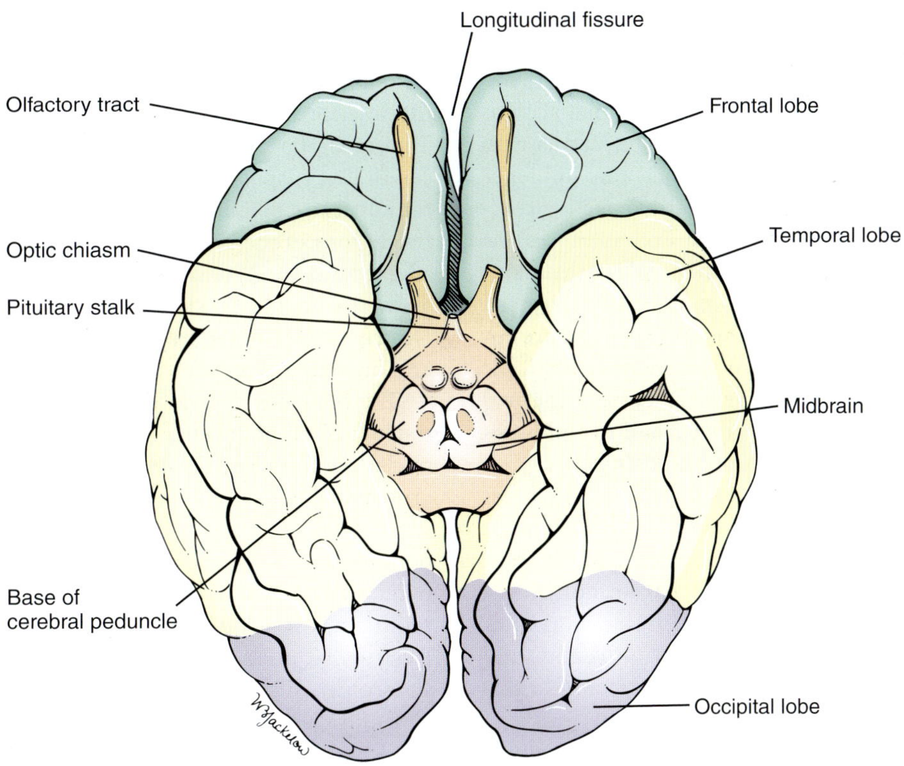

Fig. 21.3 Basal View of the Cerebral Hemispheres.

The *cerebrum* is responsible for motor, sensory, associative, and higher mental functions. The primary *motor cortex* is in the precentral gyrus. Neurons in this area control voluntary movements of the skeletal muscles on the opposite side of the body. An irritative lesion in this area may cause seizures or changes in consciousness. Destructive lesions in this area can produce contralateral flaccid paresis or paralysis.

The primary *sensory cortex* is in the postcentral gyrus. Irritative lesions in this area may produce paresthesias ("numbness" or a "pins-and-needles" sensation) on the opposite side. Destructive lesions produce impairment in cutaneous sensation on the opposite side.

Located in the occipital lobe along the calcarine fissure, the primary *visual cortex* is divided into the cuneus and the lingual gyri. If this area experiences irritative lesions, it can cause visual symptoms like flashes of light or rainbows. On the other hand, destructive lesions can lead to homonymous hemianopsia on the opposite side. However, central macular vision remains unaffected.

The primary *auditory cortex* is in the temporal lobe along the transverse temporal gyrus. Irritative lesions in this area produce a buzzing or ringing in the ears. Destructive lesions almost never produce deafness.

The *basal ganglia* are situated deep within the cerebral hemispheres. The structures constituting the basal ganglia include the caudate and lenticular nuclei, as well as the amygdala. The amygdala is part of the limbic system and is concerned with emotion. All other components are important structures in the extrapyramidal system, which modulates voluntary body movements, postural changes, and autonomic integration. The basal ganglia are especially involved with fine movements of the extremities. Disturbances of the basal ganglia can result in tremors and rigid movements.

The *thalamus* is a large nuclear mass located on each side of the third ventricle. The thalamus is the chief sensory and motor integrating mechanism of the neuraxis. All sensory impulses, except olfactory ones, and the major output from systems that modulate and modify motor function (i.e., the cerebellum and corpus striatum) terminate in the thalamus, from which they are projected to specific areas of the cerebral cortex. The thalamus is involved in certain emotional connotations that accompany most sensory experiences. Through its connections with the hypothalamus and striatum, the thalamus can influence visceral and somatic effectors serving primarily affective reactions. Through its control of the electrical excitability of the cerebral cortex, the thalamus plays a dominant role in the maintenance and regulation of the state of consciousness, alertness, and attention. The thalamus may be the critical structure for pain perception and thermal sense, which remain after the complete destruction of the primary sensory cortex. Thermal sense endows sensation with discriminative faculties and is not concerned with recognizing crude sensory modalities.

The *hypothalamus* is located below the thalamus. It includes the optic chiasm and the neurohypophysis. The hypothalamus is responsible for many regulatory mechanisms, such as temperature regulation; neuroendocrine control of catecholamines, thyroid-stimulating hormone, adrenocorticotropic hormone, follicle-stimulating and luteinizing hormones, prolactin, and growth hormones; thirst; appetite; water balance; and sexual behavior.

The *brainstem* consists of the midbrain, pons, and medulla. Fig. 21.4 shows the external anatomy of the brainstem. The brainstem is responsible for relaying all messages between the upper and lower levels of the central nervous system. Cranial nerves III to XII also arise from the brainstem. The brainstem contains the reticular formation, a network that provides constant muscle stimulation to counteract the force of gravity. In addition to its antigravity effects, this area of the brain is essential for the control of consciousness. The neurons in the reticular activating system can wake and arouse the entire brain.

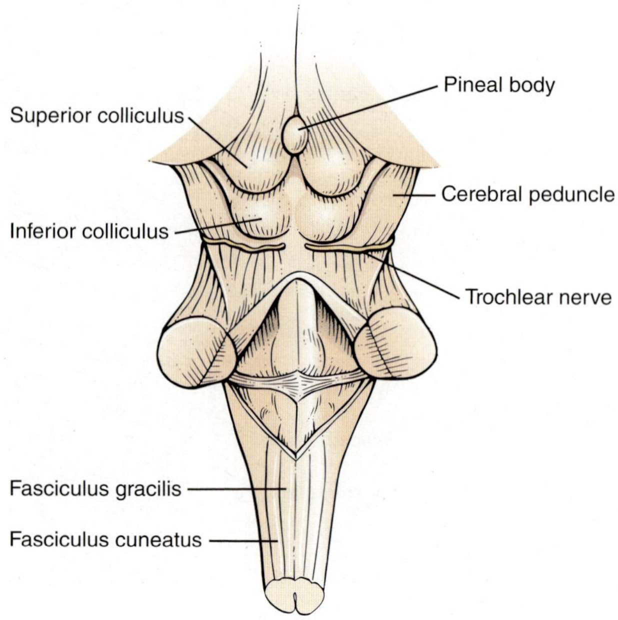

Fig. 21.4 Anatomy of the Brainstem.

The *midbrain* contains the superior and inferior colliculi, the cerebral peduncles, and the motor nuclei of the trochlear (cranial nerve IV) and oculomotor (cranial nerve III) nerves. The superior colliculi are associated with the visual system, and the inferior colliculi are associated with the auditory system. The cerebral peduncles converge from the inferior aspect of the cerebral hemispheres and enter the pons. A destructive lesion of the superior colliculi causes paralysis of upward gaze. Destructive lesions of the cranial nerve nuclei produce paralysis of the affected nerve. A destructive lesion of the cerebral peduncle gives rise to spastic paralysis on the other side of the body. Destruction of other tracts in the midbrain results in rigidity and involuntary movements.

The *pons* lies ventral to the cerebellum and rostral to the medulla. The abducens, facial, and acoustic (and vestibular) nuclei are found in the pons, and their nerves exit through a groove that divides the pons from the medulla. The motor and sensory nuclei of the trigeminal nerve are also located in the pons. At this level, the corticospinal tracts (also known as the pyramidal tracts) have not yet crossed, and a lesion at this level produces loss of voluntary movement on the opposite side. Destructive lesions of the pons may produce a variety of clinical syndromes, such as the following:

- Contralateral hemiplegia with ipsilateral trigeminal hemiplegia (paralysis of the jaw muscles and loss of sensation over the same side of the face)
- Contralateral hemiplegia with ipsilateral facial palsy (Bell palsy)
- Contralateral hemiplegia with ipsilateral facial palsy and ipsilateral abducens palsy (paralysis of the lateral rectus muscle on the same side of the face)
- Contralateral hemiplegia with ipsilateral abducens palsy
- Quadriplegia and nystagmus

The *medulla* is the portion of the brainstem between the pons and the spinal cord. The nuclei of the hypoglossal, vagus, glossopharyngeal, and spinal accessory nerves are in the medulla. It is within the medulla that most of the fibers in the corticospinal tracts cross to the opposite side. Destructive lesions in the medulla produce symptoms that refer to the tracts interrupted by the lesion. Some clinical syndromes are as follows:

- Contralateral hemiplegia with ipsilateral hypoglossal palsy[a]
- Ipsilateral vagal palsy[b] with contralateral loss of pain and temperature sense
- Ipsilateral vagal palsy with ipsilateral spinal accessory palsy[c]
- Ipsilateral vagal palsy with ipsilateral hypoglossal palsy
- Ipsilateral vagal palsy, ipsilateral spinal accessory palsy, and ipsilateral hypoglossal palsy

The *cerebellum* is in the posterior fossa of the skull and is composed of a small midline vermis and two large lateral hemispheres. The cerebellum acts to keep the individual oriented in space and to halt or check motions. The cerebellum is also responsible for the fine movements of the hands. Essentially, the cerebellum coordinates and refines the action of muscle groups to produce steady and precise movements. Destructive lesions of the cerebellum cause swaying, staggering, intention tremors,[d] and inability to change movements rapidly.

Of the blood supply to the brain, 80% is through the internal carotid arteries and 20% is through the vertebral basilar arteries. Each internal carotid artery terminates at the anterior cerebral and middle cerebral arteries. The posterior cerebral artery arises from the basilar artery, which joins with the posterior communicating artery, a branch of the internal carotid artery. The two anterior cerebral arteries are joined by the anterior communicating artery. This vascular network forms the circle of Willis, located at the base of the brain. This is illustrated in Fig. 21.5.

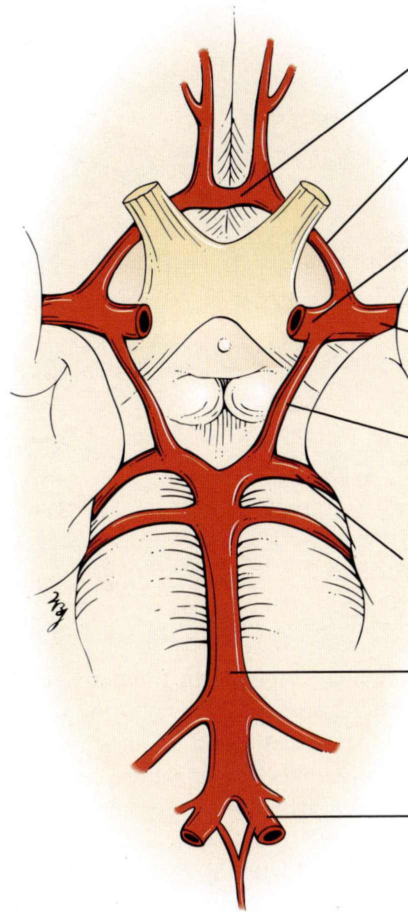

Fig. 21.5 Circle of Willis.

Continuous with the medulla is the *spinal cord,* a cylindric mass of neuronal tissue measuring 40 to 50 cm in length in adults. Its distal end attaches to the first segment of the coccyx. The spinal cord is divided into two symmetric halves by the anterior median fissure and the posterior median sulcus. Each half contains white and gray matter, which can be further subdivided. This is illustrated in Fig. 21.6.

In the center of the spinal cord is the *gray matter.* The anterior gray matter, or the *anterior horn,* is the motor portion of the spinal cord and contains multipolar cells of origin of the *anterior roots* of the peripheral nerves. The *lateral horn* (sympathetic preganglionic neurons) is found at the T1 to L2 spinal levels. The posterior gray matter, or the *posterior horn,* is the receptor portion of the spinal cord.

The *white matter* of the spinal cord consists of tracts that link segments of the spinal cord and connect it to the brain. There are three main columns (funiculi). Between the anterior median fissure and the anterolateral sulcus is the *anterior white column,* which contains the descending fibers of the *ventral corticospinal tract* and the ascending fibers of the *ventral spinothalamic tract.* The ventral corticospinal tract is involved with voluntary motion, and the ventral spinothalamic tract carries impulses related to light touch.

The *lateral white column* is located between the anterolateral and posterolateral sulci and contains the descending fibers of the *lateral corticospinal tract* and the ascending *spinocerebellar* and *lateral spinothalamic tracts.* The lateral corticospinal tract is responsible for voluntary movement; the spinocerebellar tracts, for reflex proprioception; and the lateral spinothalamic tract, for pain and temperature sensation.

The *posterior white column* is located between the posterolateral and posterior median sulci. The most important fibers in this column are the ascending fibers of the *fasciculus gracilis* and *fasciculus cuneatus.* These tracts are involved with vibration sense, passive motion, joint position, and two-point discrimination.

There are 31 pairs of spinal nerves, each with a ventral (motor) and dorsal (sensory) root. The ventral root consists

---

[a]Paralysis of the tongue muscles on the same side as the lesion. The tongue deviates to the side of the lesion when the patient is asked to stick out the tongue.

[b]Paralysis of the soft palate and difficulty speaking termed *dysarthria.*

[c]Paralysis of the sternocleidomastoid or trapezius muscle, or both. This results in the inability to turn the head to the side opposite the lesion and to shrug the shoulder. There are many more clinical syndromes that are beyond the scope of this text. The reader is advised to review the neuroanatomy further to understand the complexities of these neurologic syndromes.

[d]Tremors that result when the individual moves their hands to do something but may not be present at rest.

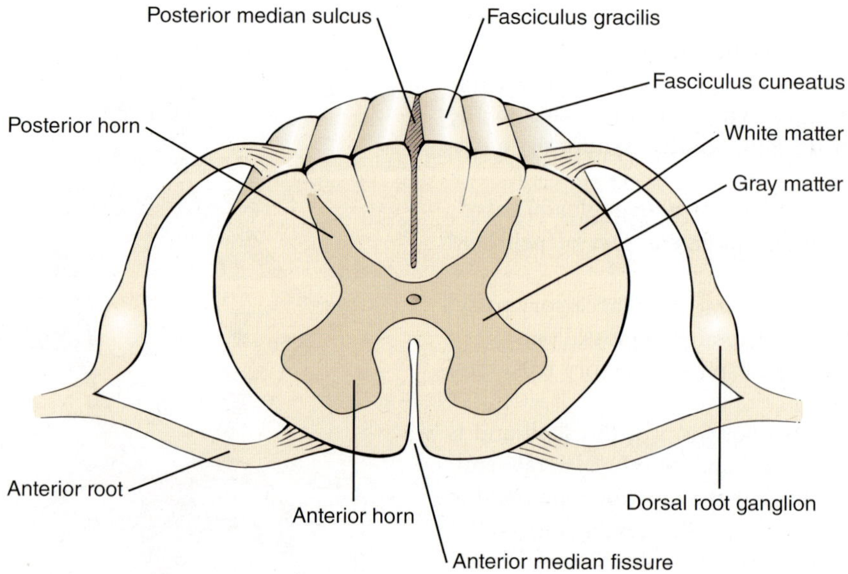

Fig. 21.6 Cross-Sectional View Through the Spinal Cord.

of *efferent* nerve fibers, which originate in the anterior and lateral gray matter (T1 to T2 only) and travel to the peripheral nerve and muscle, which constitute the motor root. The dorsal root consists of *afferent* nerve fibers whose cell bodies are in the *dorsal root ganglion*, which is the sensory root.

The spinal nerves are grouped into 8 cervical (C1 to C8), 12 thoracic (T1 to T12), 5 lumbar (L1 to L5), 5 sacral (S1 to S5), and 1 coccygeal nerve. These nerves are illustrated in Fig. 21.7.

A *spinal reflex* involves an afferent neuron and an efferent neuron at the same level in the spinal cord. The basis for this reflex arc is an intact sensory limb, functional synapses in the spinal cord, an intact motor limb, and a muscle capable of responding. The afferent and efferent limbs travel together in the same spinal nerve. When a stretched muscle is suddenly stretched further, the afferent sensory limb sends impulses through its spinal nerve that travel to the dorsal root of that nerve. After reaching a synapse in the gray matter of the spinal cord, the impulse is transmitted to the ventral nerve root. These impulses are then conducted through the ventral root to the neuromuscular junction, where a brisk contraction of the muscle completes the reflex arc. Fig. 21.8 illustrates a reflex spinal arc.

The afferent sensory limb is important not only in the reflex arc but also in the conscious appreciation of sensation. Nerve fibers carrying pain and temperature sensation enter the spinal cord and cross to the other side within one or two spinal segments. They ascend in the contralateral *lateral spinothalamic tract,* travel through the brainstem and the thalamus, and end in the postcentral gyrus of the parietal lobe, as illustrated in Fig. 21.9A. Fibers carrying *proprioceptive* sensation from muscles, joints, and tendons enter the dorsal root and participate in the reflex arc. Other fibers carrying proprioceptive sensation pass directly into the *posterior columns* and ascend in the fasciculi gracilis and cuneatus to their ipsilateral nuclei, cross in the medial lemniscus, reach a synapse in the thalamus, and end in the postcentral gyrus of the parietal lobe. Still, other proprioceptive fibers ascend crossed and uncrossed in the spinocerebellar tracts to the cerebellum. These additional pathways are illustrated in Fig. 21.9B.

REVIEW OF SPECIFIC SYMPTOMS

The most common symptoms of neurologic disease are as follows:

- Headache
- Loss of consciousness
- "Dizziness"
- Ataxia
- Changes in consciousness
- Visual disturbance
- Dysphasia
- Dementia
- Cerebrovascular accident
- Gait disturbance
- Tremor
- "Numbness"
- "Weakness"
- Pain

Headache

Headaches are a prevalent neurologic symptom with over 35 million individuals in the United States experiencing recurrent headaches. Typically, these headaches are linked to migraines, muscle contractions, or tension. If a patient has been experiencing the same headache pattern for several years, it is unlikely to be related to their current illness. Patients who have experienced a recent change in the frequency or severity of their headaches should have several points clarified to determine the cause. Ask the following questions:

"How long have you been having headaches?"

"When did you notice a change in the pattern or severity of your headaches?"

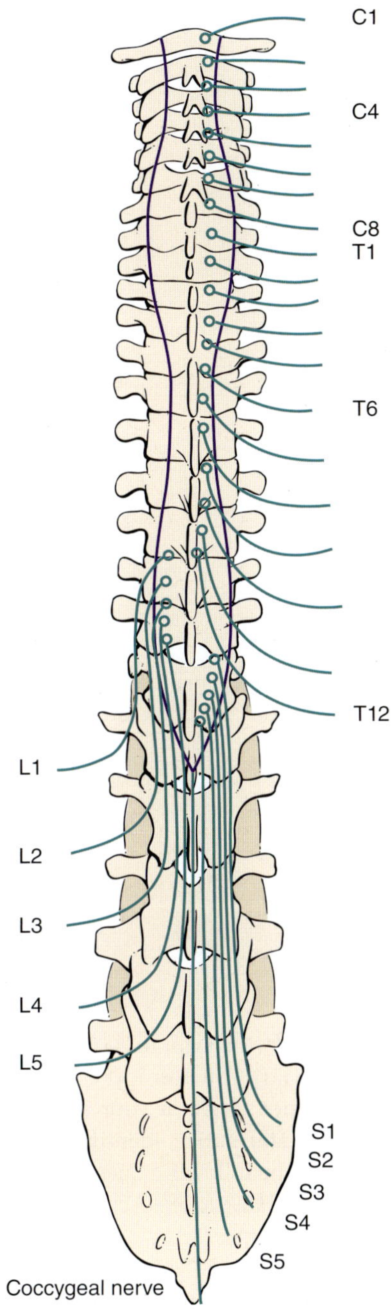

Fig. 21.7 Spinal Nerves.

"How has the pattern of your headaches changed?"
"How often do your headaches occur?"
"How long does each headache last?"
"Which part of your head aches?"
"What does the headache feel like?"
"How quickly does the headache reach its maximum?"
"When you get headaches, do you have any other symptoms?"
"Are you aware of anything that produces the headaches?"
"Are there any warning signs?"
"Does anything make the headaches worse?"
"What makes the headaches better?"

When patients experience a *sudden* onset of headache, it could indicate a more serious illness than those with chronic headaches. A *continuous* headache may be due to muscle spasms, while a *recurrent* headache may be from a migraine or cluster headache. A *throbbing* headache is often due to a vascular cause. Some headaches come with visual disturbances, nausea, or vomiting. Patients with increased intracranial pressure may experience worsened headaches from certain maneuvers like coughing or bending. If a patient experiences a severe and sudden headache, it's important to consider the possibility of a stroke.

Migraine is a biphasic type of severe headache often associated with a prodromal phase, called the *aura,* followed by the headache phase. During the aura, one or more physiologic events may occur. These include transient experiences of autonomic, visual, motor, or sensory phenomena. Common visual symptoms are photophobia, blurred vision, and scotomata. Other common aural symptoms include increased sensitivity to light, noise, and odors; nausea; and vomiting. As the aura fades, the headache begins. It is usually unilateral and is often described as severe throbbing and pulsating; untreated attacks can last for hours to days.

Migraines can have four stages for certain people: prodrome, aura, headache attack, and postdrome. The prodrome stage may happen 1 or 2 days prior to the migraine, during which the patient may notice changes that indicate a migraine is coming, such as constipation, mood changes, food cravings, neck stiffness, increased urination, or frequent yawning. Next is the aural stage, which is then followed by the headache attack. The postdrome stage, after the headache, concludes the migraine, leaving the patient often feeling drained, confused, and washed out for a day or more.

Migraines commonly occur in the morning, especially upon waking up. Some people may experience migraines at particular times, such as before their menstrual cycle or on weekends following a stressful workweek. Migraines can affect children and adults, although they tend to occur more frequently in adult females, occurring three times more often than in males. Migraine affects 29.5 million Americans.

Migraine headaches can be caused by various factors such as stress, anxiety, hormonal changes, and the use of birth control pills. In some cases, excitement or hunger can trigger these headaches as well. Certain foods like chocolate, cheese, cured meats, and highly spiced foods can also be a trigger. Other factors that may cause migraines include sudden changes in weather, inadequate or excessive sleep, overexertion, loud noises, hypoglycemia, bright or flashing lights, and tobacco. Genetics can also play a role in migraines, as many sufferers have a family history of the disorder.

Cluster headache is a type of primary headache disorder and is the most prevalent in the group of headache disorders known as *trigeminal autonomic cephalalgias,* affecting approximately 1 in 1000 people.[3] The name "cluster headache" is derived from the fact that these attacks usually occur in groups or "clusters." They commonly affect middle-aged males who experience repeated episodes of pain near the eye. The pain, usually during sleep, lasts between 15 and 180 minutes and occurs every day or every other day up to eight times per day, typically in cycles lasting weeks to months. Cluster headaches are known to be the most excruciating type of headache. Sufferers often describe the

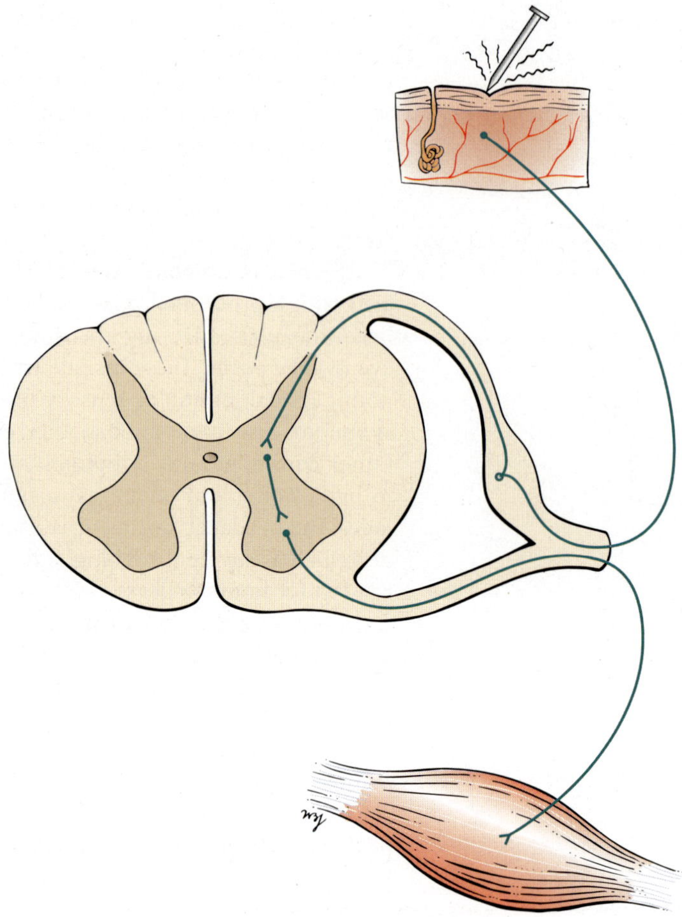

Fig. 21.8 Reflex Spinal Arc.

pain as "boring," "burning," or akin to "a hot poker in the eye." Symptoms during a cluster headache include ipsilateral miosis, ptosis, swelling of the conjunctiva, tearing, and a stuffy nose. It is believed that alcohol consumption, smoking, changes in altitude, bright light, cocaine use, and foods containing nitrates, such as bacon or lunch meat, can trigger these attacks. Fortunately, cluster headaches are rare and not life-threatening.

Cluster headaches can be caused by various other factors such as sinus infections, ocular disease, dental disease, viral infections, chronic obstructive pulmonary disease, and poisoning. It is important to identify if the patient is taking any medication that could be causing the headache. (See Table 21.3 later in this chapter, which provides an approach to patients with the symptom of headache.)

Loss of Consciousness

Fainting or *syncope* can be caused by issues with the heart or nervous system. More information about cardiovascular causes can be found in Chapter 14, The Heart, and Chapter 15, The Peripheral Vascular System. It's important to note that the term "blackout" can mean different things to different people. If a patient uses this term, it's best to ask for clarification. They may be referring to impaired vision, or decreased awareness of their surroundings without losing consciousness, or to an actual loss of consciousness,

A useful way to clarify the symptom of loss of consciousness is to ask the patient, "Have you ever lost consciousness, fainted, or felt that you were not aware of your surroundings?" If the patient answers in the affirmative, identify the cause of the loss of consciousness. Ask the following questions:

"Can you describe the attack to me—every event as it occurred until you lost consciousness?"

"Did anyone witness the attack?"[e]

"Were there any symptoms that preceded the attack?"

"Were you told that there were body movements?"

"Can you describe everything you remember after the attack until you felt completely normal?"

"Was there a period of sleepiness that followed?" If yes, *"For how long did this period last?"*

"How did you feel after the attack? Were you confused?"

"Did you notice afterward that you had urinated or had a bowel movement during the attack?"

Seizures caused by the sudden, excessive, and disorderly discharge of neurons can result in a loss of consciousness. To address this symptom, it's important to first determine the type of seizure. If the discharge is *focal*, the seizure will impact the specific body area affected by the excessive discharge. For

[e]Document a history with an observer, if possible.

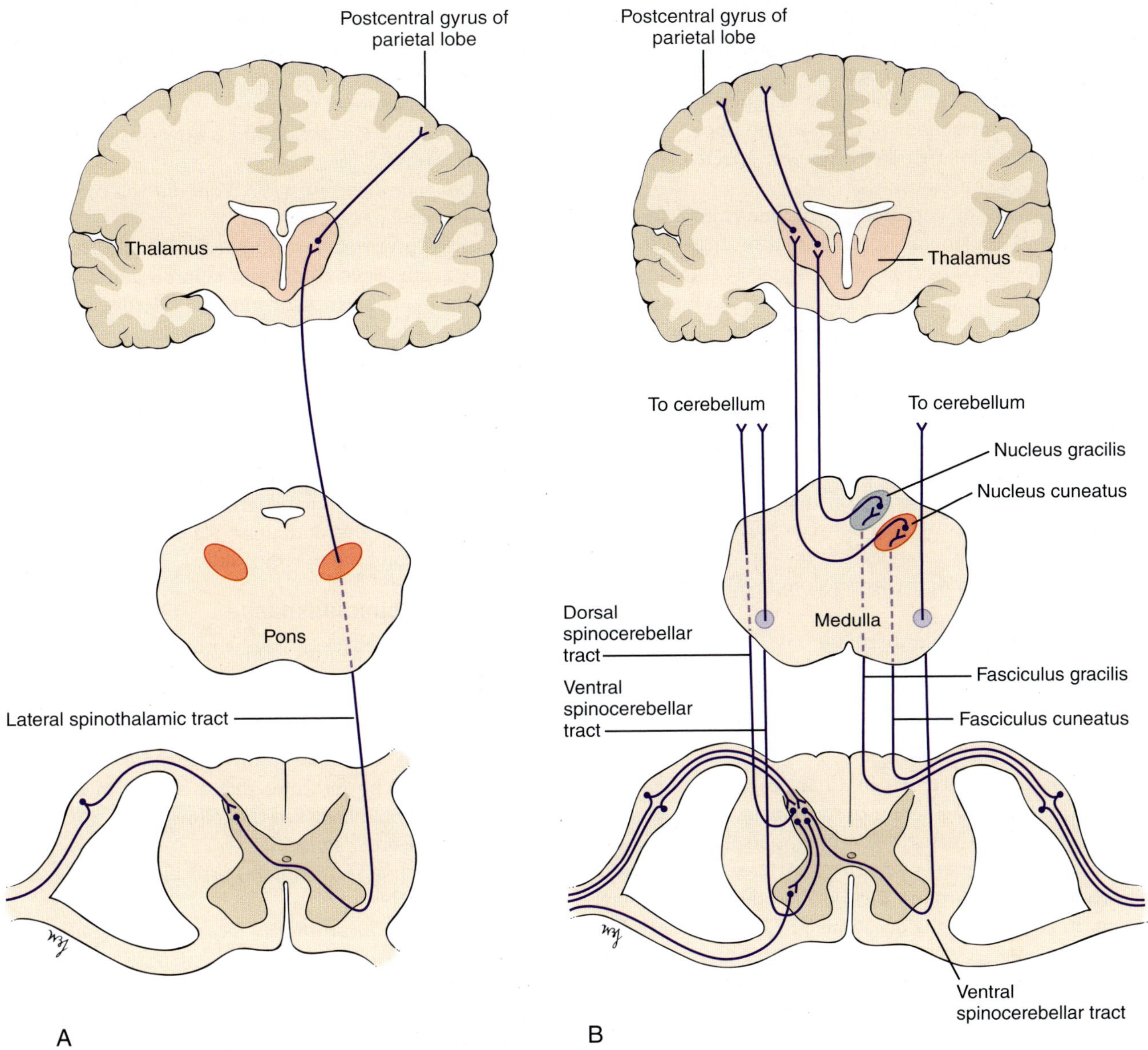

Fig. 21.9 Conscious Appreciation of Sensation. (A) Nerve pathways for pain and temperature sensation through the lateral spinothalamic tracts. (B) Pathways of the fibers carrying proprioceptive sensation through the posterior columns and in the spinocerebellar tracts.

instance, if the discharge happens in the inferior precentral gyrus, which is responsible for hand and arm movements, the seizure will cause involuntary movements of the hand and arm. On the other hand, a *generalized* seizure is a result of a discharge in the subcortical structures, such as the thalamocortical radiations, which have widespread bilateral cortical connections. There are three main types of generalized seizures:

- Petit mal (absence seizure)
- Grand mal (generalized tonic-clonic)
- Myoclonic

A *petit mal* seizure is characterized by a sudden attack of unconsciousness lasting only about 10 seconds, usually without warning. During the petit mal seizure, the patient appears to be staring or daydreaming. There is no associated falling or involuntary limb motion. The patient rapidly returns to normal activity without being aware of the attack. These seizures are most common in children between 5 and 15 years of age. On occasion, they may persist into adulthood.

A *grand mal* seizure is a generalized major motor convulsion. Affected patients lose consciousness, and many fall rigidly. In 50% of patients with grand mal seizures, there is an aura of giddiness, involuntary twitching, change in mood, confusion, or epigastric discomfort as the seizure begins. Some patients may cry out initially. During this *tonic* phase, there is an increase in muscle tone, resulting in a rigid, flexed posture and then a rigid, extended posture. The patient may become apneic and cyanotic. The eyes may open and stare or may be deviated to one side. The *clonic* phase follows, with involuntary movements of the body. These are often associated with salivation, eye-rolling, and incontinence. Biting the tongue is common. After the clonic phase, the individual passes into a phase resembling sleep from which she or he cannot be easily awakened.

Postictally, or after the seizure, the patient may be confused and often falls into a deep sleep that lasts for hours. Accompanying muscle pain and headache are common.

A *myoclonic* seizure is a minor motor seizure characterized by sudden muscle contractions of the face and upper extremities. The eyelids and forearms are commonly affected. There is no detectable loss of consciousness.

Febrile convulsions are common in children from 6 months to 6 years old and are similar to grand mal seizures. When a child has a high fever, a seizure lasting less than 10 minutes may occur. The younger the child is at the time of the first febrile seizure, the greater is the likelihood that seizures will recur.

"Dizziness"

Dizziness is a term used frequently by patients and should be avoided by the interviewer. When a patient reports feeling "dizzy," it is important to clarify if they are experiencing vertigo, ataxia, or lightheadedness, as each of these can have different underlying causes. To distinguish between vertigo and ataxia, the interviewer should ask targeted follow-up questions. If a patient mentions feeling dizzy, it is recommended to ask the following questions:

"How would you describe your dizziness?"

"Would you describe the dizziness as a strange spinning sensation in your head?"

"Did the room spin, or did it feel like you were spinning?"

"Were you unsteady while walking?"

Vertigo is partially discussed in Chapter 11, The Ear and Nose. Vertigo is the hallucination of movement. Acute vertigo may be associated with nausea, vomiting, perspiration, and a sense of anxiety. Ask patients whether they have the sensation that objects are moving around them or that they are spinning or moving. In addition to the questions in Chapter 11, ask the following:

"During the attack, did you experience any nausea or vomiting?"

"Have you noticed any problem with your hearing or ringing in your ears?"

"Have you ever been given an antibiotic called gentamicin?"

Ménière disease can result in protracted attacks of severe vertigo associated with vomiting. Many patients with Ménière disease also have the symptoms of tinnitus and hearing loss. During the attack, the patient is unsteady, with horizontal nystagmus directed away from the affected ear. Certain drugs (such as gentamicin or the diuretic, ethacrynic acid) are associated with changes in the labyrinth of the ear and can cause vertigo and deafness. See Chapter 11, The Ear and Nose, for more information.

Dizziness and stumbling are commonly associated with a stroke.

Ataxia

When the vestibular-ocular-cerebellar control mechanism is disrupted, it can lead to ataxia, which is an ongoing unsteadiness while standing upright. It's important to check if a patient experiencing dizziness has any issues with their vestibular, visual, proprioceptive, or cerebellar systems. Maintaining balance relies on the combination of sensory input and motor output, which work together as reflexes. The ears, eyes, and connections in the brainstem and cerebellum are intimately involved with balance. Any patient with ataxia should be asked the following questions:

"Are you unsteady when you walk?"

"Have you noticed that the dizziness is worse when your eyes are open or closed?"

"What does your diet consist of? What did you eat yesterday?"

"Have you ever had syphilis?"

Abnormal proprioceptive input from the lower extremities can cause ataxia. Severe posterior column damage from syphilis, vitamin B_{12} deficiency, or multiple sclerosis may produce a "sensory" ataxia, resulting in a wide-based, high-stepping gait. The gait is worsened by having the patient close the eyes and is improved by having the patient observe the feet. Vitamin B_{12} deficiency may result from pernicious anemia or inadequate intake, although poor nutrition is a rare cause. "Motor" ataxia results from an abnormality in the cerebellum and central vestibular pathways. It is characterized by wide-based, irregular placement of the feet and poor placement of the center of gravity, with a lurching to either side.

Changes in Consciousness

Changes in consciousness may be related to changes in attention span, perception, arousal, or a combination. In *confusional states,* the patient can receive information normally, but the processing is disturbed. In *delirium,* the individual perceives the information abnormally. Any patient or member of the patient's family who indicates that a change in consciousness has occurred should be asked the following:

"Did the change occur suddenly?"

"Have there been other symptoms associated with the change in consciousness?"

"Do you use any medications? Depressants? Insulin? Alcohol? Recreational drugs?"

"Is there a history of psychiatric illness?"

"Is there a history of kidney disease? Liver disease? Thyroid disease?"

"Have you ever had an injury to your head?"

Many factors can produce changes in consciousness. The acuteness of the change in consciousness is often helpful in making a diagnosis. Hemiparesis, paresthesia, hemianopsia, garbled speech, and arm and leg weakness are commonly associated symptoms of supratentorial lesions. Brainstem lesions are often associated with changes in consciousness and with nystagmus, vomiting, double vision, nausea, and excessive yawning. Drugs of any type can produce acute changes in consciousness. A history of earlier psychiatric illness is important. Toxic and metabolic changes are frequently associated with changes in consciousness. Liver or kidney failure, myxedema, and diabetic ketoacidosis are common causes of metabolic abnormalities. A history of head trauma may result in a subdural hematoma and produce a gradual change in consciousness.

Visual Disturbance

Visual disturbances are common neurologic presenting symptoms. The most important symptoms are acute visual loss,

chronic visual loss, and double vision. Ask any patient concerned with visual disturbances the following questions:
"How long have you noticed these visual changes?"
"Is the visual loss associated with pain?"
"Did it occur suddenly?"
"Do you have a history of glaucoma?"
"Have you ever been told that you had a thyroid problem?"
"Do you have diabetes?"

Acute painless visual loss is caused by either a vascular accident or a retinal detachment. Painless vision loss over a longer period occurs with compression of the optic nerve or tract or radiation. Glaucoma is often the cause of chronic, insidious, painless loss of vision. Acute narrow-angle glaucoma, however, may be responsible for transient loss of vision associated with intense ocular pain. Episodes of migraine may produce transient episodes of visual loss before developing the headache. *Amaurosis fugax* is transient visual loss lasting up to 3 minutes and is a feature of internal carotid artery disease.

Double vision, or *diplopia,* is discussed in Chapter 10, The Eye. Ocular motor palsies, thyroid abnormalities, myasthenia gravis, and brainstem lesions are well-known causes of diplopia. Ocular motor palsies can occur in trauma, multiple sclerosis, myasthenia gravis, aneurysms of the circle of Willis, diabetes, and tumors. Ask the following questions of any patient concerned with diplopia:
"Are you diabetic?"
"In which field of gaze do you have double vision?"
"Did the double vision occur suddenly?"
"Was there any pain associated with the double vision?"
"Has there been any injury to your head or eye?"
"Have you ever been told that your blood pressure was elevated?"
"Does the double vision get worse when you are tired?"
"Have you been exposed to the AIDS (acquired immune deficiency syndrome) virus?"

When a cranial nerve is affected, resulting in an extraocular muscle palsy, the patient may be concerned of diplopia in one field of gaze when the affected eye cannot move conjugately with the other. Ocular palsies involve the third, fourth, and sixth cranial nerves. A complete third (oculomotor) nerve palsy causes ptosis, mydriasis, and loss of all extraocular movements except abduction. Trauma, multiple sclerosis, tumors, and aneurysms are the most frequent causes. Aneurysms of the posterior communicating artery can involve the third nerve, which passes near the artery on its way to the cavernous sinus. Cavernous sinus thrombosis, not infrequently seen in patients with AIDS, may also produce a complete third nerve palsy. Pupil-sparing third nerve, fourth (trochlear) nerve, and sixth (abducens) nerve palsies are seen in diabetic patients and in patients with long-standing hypertension. Patients with myasthenia gravis often have diplopia in the later part of the day as the muscles tire and weaken.

Visual disturbances, including blocked vision or loss of vision in one eye, blurry vision, or "graying out" are seen frequently in stroke patients.

Dysphasia

Speech abnormalities, or dysphasia, may be either nonfluent (expressive) or fluent (receptive). In *expressive aphasia,* the speech pattern is hesitant and labored, with poor articulation. The patient has no problem with comprehension. When asked to say, "*no ifs, ands, or buts,*" the patient has great difficulty. In *receptive aphasia,* the speech is rapid and appears fluent but is full of syntax errors, with the omission of many words. Handwriting changes are nonspecific but indicate an impairment of neuromuscular control. Ask the following questions:
"Have you noticed any recent change in your speech pattern, such as slurring of your words?"
"Do you have trouble understanding things that are said to you?"
"Have you had any difficulty finding the right word in conversation?"
"Has your handwriting changed recently?"

Language problems, as well as slurred speech, are found commonly in patients suffering from a stroke.

Dementia

One significant indication of neurologic illness is a decline in memory. Dementia refers to the gradual deterioration of cognitive abilities such as orientation, memory, judgment, and other intellectual functions. It is not a specific disease, but rather a symptom. The most common cause of dementia is *Alzheimer disease.* There are various factors that can contribute to cognitive impairment such as Parkinson disease, vascular and metabolic disorders, tumors, drug usage, vitamin B_{12} deficiency, tertiary syphilis, and normal-pressure hydrocephalus. Patients with early onset of dementia often experience difficulty in understanding written information. People with dementia may recognize their cognitive impairment but may not want to admit it to their friends and family. The condition can be so subtle that family members may not notice it, even when the person with dementia lives with them for years. Additionally, loved ones may not want to accept that the person's mental abilities are declining.

Ask the patient and their friends and family the following:
"Have you noticed any change in your memory lately?"
"Do you have difficulty reading or understanding what you have read?"
"What was the patient's personality like a few years ago?"
"When was the last time the patient seemed normal?"
"What does the patient's diet consist of? Do they eat well?"
"Can the patient live alone?"

Cerebrovascular Accident

Strokes, or cerebrovascular accidents, are common. Most are thromboembolic (80%), but some are hemorrhagic (20%). Thirty percent of patients who sustain a stroke die within the first month. Most patients with strokes have paresis of at least one limb. *Transient ischemic attacks* (TIAs) are short episodes manifested by focal neurologic dysfunction. They usually last only a few minutes, after which complete recovery occurs. The importance of TIAs is that, in 30% of affected patients, a stroke occurs within 4 to 5 years.

Gait Disturbance

There are many reasons why someone might experience difficulty with their gait. Pain in the foot or joint, hip or leg claudication, bone disease, vestibular issues, and extrapyramidal disorders can all cause changes in gait. Additionally, after a stroke, interruption of the corticospinal tracts in the cerebrum can lead to spastic weakness in the opposite leg. This can cause the foot to drag and the leg to seem stiff and extended. Lesions in the spinal cord may also result in spastic paralysis that affects both legs. Patients with Parkinson disease tend to walk with a slow and stiff gait, taking small steps and appearing stooped over. They may also shuffle their feet quickly. See Fig. 21.59 for common gait abnormalities. If a patient has a gait disturbance, it's important to ask them the following questions:

"Do you have pain in your leg or hip when you walk?"
"Do you have diabetes?"
"Have you ever had syphilis?"
"What do you eat? Tell me everything you ate yesterday."

Patients with vascular occlusive disease of the hip or leg may experience pain while walking and may alter their gait. Diabetes, syphilis, and pernicious anemia may produce a sensory loss, and each condition can result in gait abnormalities.

Tremor

A tremor is a rhythmic motion of the distal parts of the limbs or head. A physiologic tremor oscillates 10 to 12 cycles per second and is more obvious after exercise. A pathologic tremor is slower. *Parkinson disease* is the most frequently encountered extrapyramidal movement disorder. In this condition, the tremor is present at rest and is decreased with action. It has a frequency of 3 to 6 cycles per second and is worsened by anxiety. An intention, or *ataxic,* tremor is slow (2 to 4 cycles per second) and worsens on attempted movement. Multiple sclerosis is one of the many causes of intention tremor. Metabolic problems from liver or kidney failure are frequently responsible. Withdrawal from alcohol or caffeine is often a precipitating factor. Any patient with the symptom of tremor should be asked these questions:

"Does the tremor worsen when you try to do something?"
"Is there a history of thyroid disease?"
"Have you ever been told about any problems with your liver or kidneys?"
"What is your daily consumption of alcoholic beverages?"
"How much coffee or tea do you drink?"
"How much chocolate do you eat?"

Chorea is involuntary jerky motions of the face and limbs. A common cause is *Huntington disease,* in which chorea is accompanied by personality changes and progressive mental deterioration terminating in dementia.

Huntington disease is a genetic disorder that leads to the gradual deterioration of nerve cells in the brain. It is inherited in an autosomal dominant pattern and can have serious effects on a person's cognitive, movement, and psychiatric abilities. Symptoms of this condition can start at any age but are typically noticed in individuals who are in their 30s or 40s.

The early symptoms of Huntington disease include irritability, depression, poor coordination, and difficulty learning or making decisions. Individuals with the disease may experience involuntary jerking or twitching movements called chorea. As the disease advances, these movements become more pronounced, and people may experience trouble with walking, speaking, and swallowing.

"Numbness"

Patients often use the term *numbness* to describe different sensations like a "pins-and-needles" feeling, coolness, pain, or clumsiness. It's important for the interviewer to clarify the specific meaning. During the physical examination, the examiner must check for arterial insufficiency by palpating the distal pulses in patients concerned with numbness. Lower extremity numbness is commonly caused by diabetes mellitus, while multiple sclerosis can cause numbness in any extremity.

"Weakness"

Weakness may be a symptom of the motor system. A patient with a *proximal arm* motor weakness will be concerned of difficulty brushing hair, shaving, or reaching up to shelves. A patient with *distal arm* motor weakness will have concerns of difficulty putting a button through a buttonhole, using keys, or writing with a pen or pencil. *Proximal leg* motor weakness is characterized by difficulty climbing stairs or getting into bed or the bathtub. Foot drop is a classic sign of *distal leg* motor weakness. Chapter 20, The Musculoskeletal System, reviews some of the important questions related to weakness.

Face droop and weakness are common signs of a stroke, as is the presence of numbness or clumsiness in one arm or hand.

Pain

Pain is an infrequent symptom of neurologic disease, but it merits mention. *Trigeminal neuralgia,* also known as *tic douloureux,* is the occurrence of severe, jabbing pain lasting only seconds most commonly in the distribution of the maxillary or mandibular divisions of the trigeminal nerve (Fig. 21.10). It is frequently provoked by motion, touch, eating, or exposure to cold temperatures. Another cause of facial pain is cluster headache, already discussed. *Herpes zoster* infection of a sensory nerve root, also known as *shingles,* manifests with intense pain along the distribution of that nerve root. The classic linear, vesicular skin eruption develops 3 to 4 days later along the distribution of the nerve. Figure 8.70A shows the classic dermatologic manifestations of herpes zoster infection of spinal nerve T3.

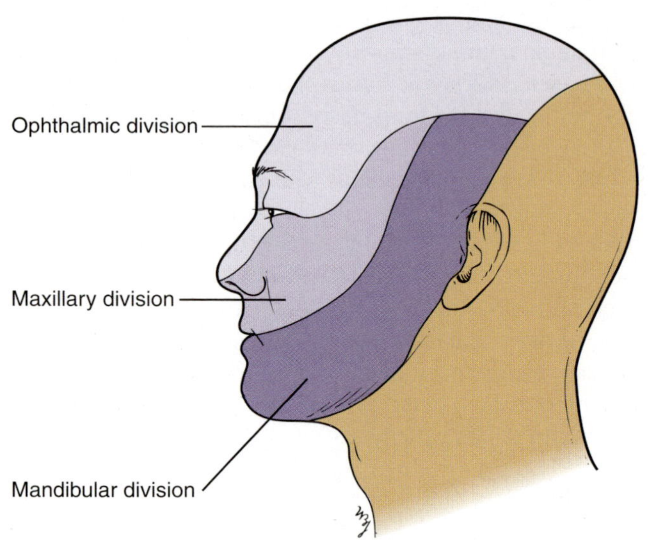

Fig. 21.10 Areas Innervated by Divisions of the Trigeminal Nerve.

Sciatica is intense pain shooting down the leg in the distribution of the sciatic nerve. In this condition, there is impingement of portions of the sciatic nerve by the vertebrae. Arthritis of the lumbosacral spine is frequently the cause.

Sometimes the paresthesias associated with demyelinating diseases are so intense that the patient may describe them as pain.

Patients with *inflammation of the meninges* are often concerned with pain in the neck and resistance to flexion of the neck. If *meningitis* is suspected, have the patient lie on their back. Place your hand behind the patient's neck and flex until the chin touches the sternum. In patients with meningitis, there is neck pain and resistance to motion. This is called the *Brudzinski sign*. There may also be flexion of the patient's hips and knees. Jósef Brudzinski described at least five different physical signs indicative of meningeal irritation. This sign is the best-known and most reliable sign. Another sign of meningeal irritation can be elicited while the patient lies on the back, and you flex one of the patient's legs at the hip and knee. If pain or resistance is elicited as the knee is extended, a positive *Kernig sign* is present.

EFFECT OF CHRONIC NEUROLOGIC DISEASE ON THE PATIENT

Chronic neurologic disease has significant effects on both the patient and their family. As the disease progresses, family members experience emotional distress while witnessing the patient's decline. Additionally, the family is tasked with a heavy responsibility in helping the patient adapt to their disability.

One example of a progressive neurologic condition is Alzheimer disease. A devastating chronic disorder of unknown cause, Alzheimer disease is the most common diffuse brain degeneration causing brain failure. This condition is characterized by progressive and widespread brain degeneration with a hopeless prognosis.

Alzheimer disease mainly affects memory and intellectual function, resulting in symptoms such as forgetfulness and cognitive impairment. Depression is also common among patients. This can affect their ability to navigate their surroundings, leading to forgetting where they live or leaving a gas burner on the stove or cigarette unattended. In some cases, patients may wander aimlessly outdoors.

Alzheimer disease can cause a range of symptoms, from mild cognitive impairment to severe dementia. Some patients may even lose touch with reality. In interviews with these patients, it may become apparent that they have difficulty recalling their medical history.

In the early stages of the disease, patients with Alzheimer disease may use alternative words when they can't find the right ones. They may also become confused about their whereabouts or the time. Seeing things that aren't there is a frequent occurrence. Losing interest in sexual activity is typical. As consciousness deteriorates, motor skills decrease. A significant symptom is the emergence of strange thoughts and imaginations that control their mind. Frequently, individuals experience delusions, particularly of being persecuted.

During the initial phases of the illness, when individuals can still perceive their surroundings but have begun to experience memory loss, they may commonly exhibit mild depression, anxiety, and irritability. As the disease advances, the primary characteristic becomes apathy. Patients may appear indifferent and emotionally withdrawn. Some people with increased motor activity may experience common symptoms of anxiety and fear. They may also have terror and panic attacks, as well as develop hostility and paranoia quickly. These individuals may also exhibit regression and sudden displays of intense emotions due to their frequent hallucinations.

In less severe cases, individuals with Alzheimer disease may experience symptoms such as depression, hypochondria, and phobias. They may also have hysterical conversion reactions, such as hysterical blindness. Losing social interaction, sudden outbursts of anger, anxiety, or tears are also common. As the disease progresses, suicide attempts become more frequent. Individuals may exhibit extreme emotional changes, with periods of laughter followed by crying. With the advancement of the disease, they may lose their ability to express emotions and develop gross neurologic disability. In the later stages, severe body wasting and profound brain failure may occur.

PHYSICAL EXAMINATION

To perform a neurologic examination, you will need safety pins, cotton-tipped applicators, a 128-Hz tuning fork for testing vibration sense, a 512-Hz tuning fork for hearing, gauze pads, common objects like coins and keys, and a reflex hammer.

The neurologic examination consists of an assessment of the following:

- Mental status
- Cranial nerves
- Motor function
- Reflexes
- Sensory function
- Cerebellar function

Mental Status

See Video 21.1.

In the interview, the healthcare professional has already learned a lot about the patient's mental state. They may have assessed the patient's remote memory, affect, and judgment. To begin the formal mental status portion of the neurologic examination, the examiner will tell the patient, "I am going to ask you a few routine questions. Some will be easy, others more difficult. Just do your best."

The mental status examination consists of the evaluation of the following:

- Level of consciousness
- Speech
- Orientation
- Knowledge of current events
- Judgment
- Abstraction
- Vocabulary
- Emotional responses

- Memory
- Calculation ability
- Object recognition
- Praxis

Assess Level of Consciousness

The level of consciousness can be assessed as soon as you introduce yourself to the patient. Is the patient awake? Alert? Do exogenous or endogenous insults cloud the patient's sensorium? Does the patient appear confused? If the patient does not respond to your introduction, hold the patient's hand, and softly say, "Hello, _______. Can you hear me? If you hear me, squeeze my hand." If there is no response, try gently shaking the patient. If there is still no response and the patient appears obtunded, squeezing the nipple or applying pressure with your thumb to the bony ridge under the eyebrow is a painful maneuver that may rouse the patient. If these maneuvers fail to awaken the patient, the patient is in a *coma*. When a person is in a coma, they are completely unconscious and cannot be awakened even by painful stimuli. If you need to use a painful stimulus, be cautious not to pinch or bruise the patient's skin. If there are friends or family members present, be sure to explain what you are doing. See Chapter 27, The Acutely Ill or Injured Patient.

Evaluate Speech

If the patient is awake and alert, you have already observed their speech. The patient should be asked to recite short phrases such as "no ifs, ands, or buts." Is dysarthria, dysphonia, dysphasia, or aphasia present? *Dysarthria* is difficulty in articulation. In general, lesions of the tongue and palate are responsible for dysarthria. *Dysphonia* is difficulty in phonation. The result is an alteration in the volume and tone of the voice. Lesions of the palate and vocal cords are often responsible. *Dysphasia* is difficulty comprehending or speaking as a result of cerebral dysfunction. Patients with a total loss of speech have *aphasia.* Different areas of the brain are responsible for the different types of aphasia. A motor, expressive, nonfluent aphasia is present when patients know what they want to say but have a motor impairment and cannot articulate properly. They understand written and verbal commands but cannot repeat them. A frontal lobe lesion is often the cause. A sensory, receptive, fluent aphasia is present when the patient articulates spontaneously but uses words inappropriately. The patient has difficulty understanding written and verbal commands and cannot repeat them. A temporoparietal lesion is frequently the cause.

Evaluate Orientation

The patient's orientation to person, place, and time must be established. *Orientation* refers to the person's awareness of self in relation to other persons, places, and times. Disorientation occurs in association with impairment of memory and attention span. The patient should be asked these questions:

"What is today's date?"
"What is the day of the week?"
"What month is this?"
"What is the season now?"
"What is the name of this hospital (or building)?"

When assessing orientation, avoid asking questions that cannot be confirmed, such as if the patient knows if they have children. Those with early cognitive impairment may be hesitant to provide a response if they are unsure of the correct answer. They may hope that you will accept their response and not inquire further. For instance, if asked where they currently are and the patient cannot recall the address, they may respond with something like, "I'm in your office." To clarify, ask a follow-up question such as, "Can you tell me where my office is located?"

Evaluate Knowledge of Current Events

To determine a patient's knowledge of current events, one can ask them to name the last three presidents of the United States, or the name of their local mayor or governor. If the patient is not from America or is not familiar with American news, asking about more general current events can be helpful. Being able to recall current events indicates that the patient has an intact orientation, recent memory, and the ability to think abstractly.

Assess Judgment

Judgment evaluation is performed by asking the patient to interpret a simple problem. Ask the patient the following:

"What would you do if you noticed an addressed envelope with an uncanceled stamp on it on the street near a mailbox?"
"What would you do if you were in a crowded movie theater and a fire started?"

A correct response to the first question would be to pick up the letter and mail it. An example of an incorrect response might be, "I'd throw it in the trash." Judgment requires higher cerebral function.

Assess Abstraction

The ability to understand and make judgments about abstract concepts is a complex cognitive function. Proverbs are often used to assess one's abstract reasoning skills. To test this ability, patients may be asked to interpret the following statements:

"People who live in glass houses shouldn't throw stones."
"A rolling stone gathers no moss."

A patient with an abnormality in abstract reasoning might respond to the first quotation with a *concrete* interpretation, such as, "The glass will break if you throw a stone through it." A concrete interpretation of the second proverb might be "Moss grows only on rocks that don't move and not on a rolling stone." Concrete responses are common in patients with mental retardation or brain failure. Schizophrenic patients often answer with concrete interpretations, but bizarre assessments are common. Be careful when assessing abstraction in patients whose mother tongue is not English. They may also provide concrete answers as they literally translate the words of the proverb.

Another method of testing abstract reasoning is to ask the patient how two items are similar or dissimilar. You might ask, "What is similar about a dog and a cat?" "What is similar about a church and a synagogue?" or "What is dissimilar about an apple and a chicken?"

Assess Vocabulary

Assessing someone's vocabulary can be challenging as it is influenced by various factors such as education, background, work, environment, and cerebral function. However, it is a crucial aspect of measuring intellectual capacity. Individuals with mental challenges typically have a restricted vocabulary, while those with mild brain impairment tend to have a well-preserved vocabulary. To evaluate vocabulary, patients can be asked to define words or use them in sentences. It is recommended to use words in increasing difficulty to gauge their proficiency. The following list is an example:

- Car
- Ability
- Dominant
- Voluntary
- Telescope
- Reticent
- Enigma

Assess Emotional Responses

Although the emotional response has probably been informally observed already, inquire specifically whether the patient has noticed any sudden mood changes. It is appropriate to ask, "How are your spirits?" During the interview, the interviewer has already noticed the patient's *affect,* which is the emotional response to an event. The response may be *appropriate, abnormal,* or *flat.* An appropriate response to a loved one's death may be to cry. An inappropriate response is to laugh. A flat response shows little emotion. Patients with bilateral cerebral damage lose control of their emotions.

Assess Memory

Memory is a complex ability that involves the recall and recognition of previous experience. The formation of new memory involves recognition and registration of the initial sensory input, retention, and storage of information, and recall or retrieval of stored information. Memory functions have traditionally been divided into three areas: *immediate, recent, and remote memory.* Immediate memory can be checked by asking the patient to repeat six digits forward and backward. Recent memory can be checked by asking the patient about their appetite and then about what they had for their breakfast or for dinner the previous evening. In the end, remote memory can be tested by asking patients for information about their childhood that can be later verified.

To test memory, have the patient recall the *immediate, recent,* and the *remote past. Immediate* memory is easily tested by presenting three words to the patient and asking them to repeat them 5 minutes later. For example, tell the patient, "Repeat these words after me and remember them. I will ask for them later: necklace, thirty-two, barn." Continue with the mental status examination. Five minutes later, ask the patient, "What were those words I asked you to remember?"

A test of *recent* memory is to have the patient recall as many elements in a category as possible. Request that the patient do one of the following:

"Name as many flowers as you can."

"Name as many occupations as you can."

"Name as many tools as you can."

A neurological cause of recent memory problems could be a lesion in the temporal lobe.

There are many common things that can cause memory loss such as medications,[f] alcohol, smoking,[g] drug use, sleep deprivation,[h] depression, stress, nutritional deficiency,[i] head injury, and stroke.

To assess a patient's remote past memory, inquire about widely recognized events from the past. Avoid asking about events that cannot be confirmed. Remote past memory pertains to recollections from years or even decades ago. The memories provide detailed accounts of events in the patient's life, almost like chapters in their biography. They cover different types of memory, including autobiographical, personal semantic, and general semantic memory, and include historical people and events.

Neuropsychologists refer to memories of events that happened a long time ago as remote past memory, but most people mistakenly call it long-term memory. During clinical interviews, patients may claim that their long-term memory is good because they can recall events from their childhood or early adulthood. However, they often have trouble with short-term memory, such as forgetting what they ate for dinner the night before. The terms long-term and short-term memory are commonly used incorrectly and actually refer to memories that are years or decades old and memories that are only hours, days, weeks, or months old, respectively.

Assess Calculation Ability

To determine a patient's ability to calculate, it is important to consider both the integrity of their dominant cerebral hemisphere and their intelligence. One way to test this is to ask the patient to perform simple arithmetic problems, such as subtracting 7 from 100 and repeating the process several times. This is known as the *serial sevens test.* If the patient struggles with this test, you can also ask them to add or subtract several numbers, such as "What is 5 plus 7?" or "What is 27 minus 9?"

Assess Object Recognition

The term for recognizing objects is called gnosia, while *agnosia* refers to the inability to recognize a sensory stimulus despite

[f]There are various medications, both prescription and over-the-counter, that can affect memory function. These may include antidepressants, antihistamines, anti-anxiety drugs, muscle relaxants, tranquilizers, sleeping pills, and pain relievers.

[g]Studies have shown that smoking can harm memory by reducing the amount of oxygen reaching the brain. As a result, smokers may find it more challenging to associate faces with names compared to nonsmokers.

[h]Both the amount and quality of sleep play a vital role in memory retention. Insufficient sleep or frequent awakenings can result in tiredness, which hinders the brain's ability to store and recall information effectively.

[i]Having a balanced diet with sufficient high-quality proteins and fats is crucial for optimal brain function. It's worth noting that a deficiency in vitamins B_1 and B_{12} can specifically impact memory.

normal primary sensation. To test for visual agnosia, show the patient a series of familiar objects like coins, pens, eyeglasses, or pieces of clothing, and ask them to name them. If the patient has normal vision but cannot recognize the object, they have visual agnosia. On the other hand, tactile agnosia is the inability to recognize an object by touch without a sensory deficit, which occurs with a lesion in the nondominant parietal lobe. Autotopagnosia is another condition where the patient is unable to recognize their own body part, like the hand or leg.

Assess Praxis

Praxis refers to the ability to perform a motor activity, while apraxia is the inability to perform a voluntary movement despite having no deficits in motor strength, sensation, or coordination. Dyspraxia, on the other hand, is a decreased ability to perform an activity, wherein the patient cannot integrate the motor activities required to complete an action. For instance, if you ask the patient to pour water from the pitcher into a glass and drink it, a patient with dyspraxia may drink the water straight from the pitcher or try to drink from an empty glass. This disorder is often caused by a deep frontal lobe lesion.

Constructional apraxia is a type of apraxia where the patient is unable to create or draw basic designs. During examination, the patient may be asked to replicate a shape or draw a clock face, but they will struggle to do so. This condition is often caused by a lesion in the posterior part of the parietal lobe.

Cranial Nerves

The examination of the cranial nerves should be carried out in an orderly manner. Several cranial nerves have already been evaluated. Table 21.1 lists the cranial nerves, their functions, and the clinical findings when a lesion exists.

Cranial Nerve I: Olfactory

The olfactory nerve supplies nerve endings to the superior nasal concha and upper one-third of the nasal septum. The olfactory nerve is not routinely tested. However, in any patient with a suspected frontal lobe disorder, the olfactory nerve should be evaluated.

Test olfaction. During the test, the patient is required to close one nostril and their eyes while the examiner holds a test substance close to the patient's other nostril. The patient must then sniff the substance, which should be non-irritating and volatile, such as cloves, vanilla beans, freshly ground coffee, or lavender. It's important to avoid using an irritating substance such as alcohol since it may affect the accuracy of the test results by involving both cranial nerve V and cranial nerve I.

During the smell test, each nostril is tested individually. The examiner requests the patient to identify the test material. It is more significant to detect unilateral *anosmia,* which is the loss of smell in only one nostril, as it suggests a potential issue with the olfactory nerve or tract on that side, compared to a bilateral loss.

Cranial Nerve II: Optic

See Video 10.1.

The optic nerve ends in the retina. The examinations for visual acuity and the ophthalmoscopic examination are discussed in Chapter 10, The Eye.

Cranial Nerve III: Oculomotor

See Video 10.4.

The oculomotor nerve controls the movements of the eyes through the medial, superior, and inferior rectus muscles, as well as the inferior oblique muscle. Additionally, it also controls the pupillary constriction and accommodation through the intrinsic muscles.

Extraocular muscle movements are discussed in Chapter 10. A patient with a right oculomotor palsy is shown in Fig. 10.150. The pupillary light reflex depends on the function of cranial nerves II and III (see Chapter 10). Visual fields are part of both the eye examination and the neurologic examination. The technique for visual field testing is discussed in Chapter 10.

TABLE 21.1 Cranial Nerves

Cranial Nerve	Function	Clinical Findings With Lesion
I: Olfactory	Smell	Anosmia
II: Optic	Vision	Amaurosis
III: Oculomotor	Eye movements, papillary constriction, accommodation	Diplopia, ptosis, mydriasis, loss of accommodation
IV: Trochlear	Eye movements	Diplopia
V: Trigeminal	General sensation of face, scalp, and teeth; chewing movements	"Numbness" of face; weakness of jaw muscles
VI: Abducens	Eye movements	Diplopia
VII: Facial	Taste; general sensation of palate and external ear; lacrimal gland and submandibular and sublingual gland secretion; facial expression	Loss of taste on anterior two thirds of tongue, dry mouth, loss of lacrimation, paralysis of facial muscles
VIII: Vestibulocochlear	Hearing; equilibrium	Deafness, tinnitus, vertigo, nystagmus
IX: Glossopharyngeal	Taste, general sensation of pharynx and ear, elevation of palate, parotid gland secretion	Loss of taste on posterior one third of tongue, anesthesia of pharynx, partially dry mouth
X: Vagus	Taste; general sensation of pharynx, larynx, and ear; swallowing; phonation; parasympathetic innervation to heart and abdominal viscera	Dysphagia, hoarseness, palatal paralysis
XI: Spinal accessory	Phonation; head, neck, and shoulder movements	Hoarseness; weakness of head, neck, and shoulder muscles
XII: Hypoglossal	Tongue movements	Weakness and wasting of tongue

Cranial Nerve IV: Trochlear

See Video 10.4.

The trochlear nerve is responsible for the movement of the superior oblique muscle. Extraocular muscle movements are discussed in Chapter 10.

Cranial Nerve V: Trigeminal

See Video 21.2.

The trigeminal nerve is responsible for supplying sensation to the face, the nasal and buccal mucosa, and the teeth. The motor division supplies the muscles of mastication. The three major subdivisions of the trigeminal nerve are the ophthalmic, the maxillary, and the mandibular. These divisions are illustrated in Fig. 21.10.

The *ophthalmic division* supplies sensation to the frontal sinuses, the conjunctiva, the cornea, the upper eyelid, the bridge of the nose, the forehead, and the scalp as far as the skull vertex. The *maxillary division* supplies sensation to the cheek, the maxillary sinus, the lateral aspects of the nose, the upper teeth, the nasal pharynx, the hard palate, and the uvula. The *mandibular division* supplies sensation to the chin, the lower jaw, the anterior two-thirds of the tongue, the lower teeth, the gums and floor of the mouth, and the buccal mucosa of the cheek. The motor division innervates the muscles of mastication and the tensor tympani.

The examination of the trigeminal nerve consists of the following:

- Testing the corneal reflex
- Testing the sensory function
- Testing the motor function

Test corneal reflex. The corneal reflex depends on the function of cranial nerves V and VII. To evaluate the corneal reflex, the examiner uses a cotton-tipped applicator, the tip of which has been pulled into a thin strand about 1.3 cm in length. The examiner stabilizes the patient's head by placing a hand on the patient's eyebrow and head. The patient is asked to look straight ahead or to the left side as the cotton tip is brought in from the right side to touch the right cornea gently. This is demonstrated in Fig. 21.11. A prompt bilateral reflex closure of the eyelids is the normal response. The examination is repeated on the other side by reversing the directions.

The responses on the two sides are compared. The sensory limb of the corneal reflex is the ophthalmic division of the trigeminal nerve; the motor limb is conducted through the facial nerve.

When doing the corneal reflex test, make sure to only touch the cornea and avoid touching the eyelashes or conjunctiva. Touching these areas can result in an inaccurate test result.

Test sensory function. The sensory function of the trigeminal nerve is tested by asking the patient to close the eyes and to respond when a touch is felt. A piece of gauze is brushed against one side of the forehead and then the corresponding position on the other side. This test is then performed on the cheeks and the jaw, so that all three subdivisions of the nerve are tested. The patient is also asked whether one side feels the same as or different from the other side. The examination is demonstrated in Fig. 21.12 using a cotton-tipped applicator stick.

Test motor function. The motor function of the trigeminal nerve is tested by having the patient bite down or clench the teeth while the masseter and temporalis muscles are palpated bilaterally. This is demonstrated in Fig. 21.13. Unilateral weakness causes the jaw to deviate toward the side of the lesion.

Cranial Nerve VI: Abducens

See Video 10.4.

The abducens nerve is responsible for the movement of the lateral rectus muscle. Extraocular muscle movements are discussed in Chapter 10, The Eye.

Cranial Nerve VII: Facial

See Video 21.3.

The facial nerve innervates the facial muscles and enables taste on the anterior two thirds of the tongue. A small component also supplies general sensation to the external ear. The facial nerve carries parasympathetic motor fibers to the salivary

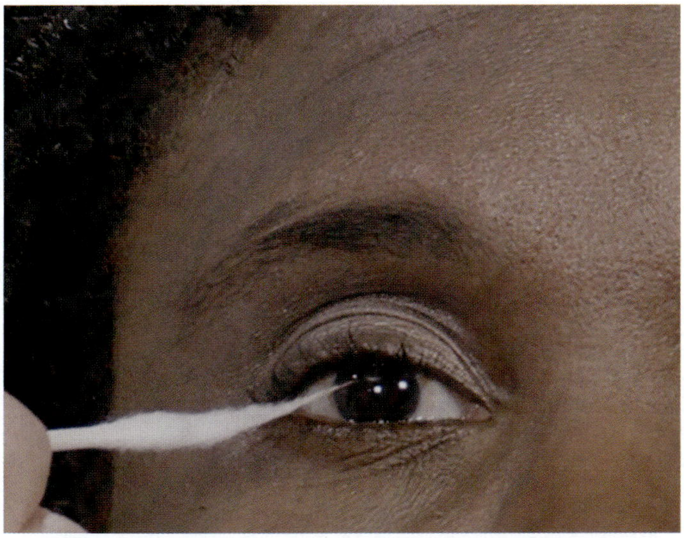

Fig. 21.11 Technique for Evaluating the Corneal Reflex.

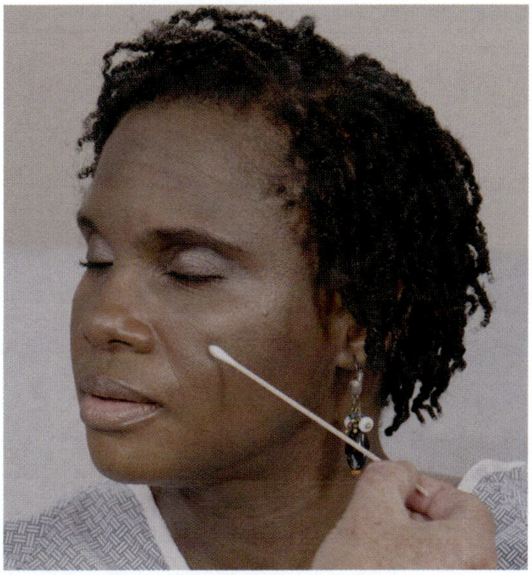

Fig. 21.12 Technique for Testing the Sensory Function of the Trigeminal Nerve, Maxillary Division.

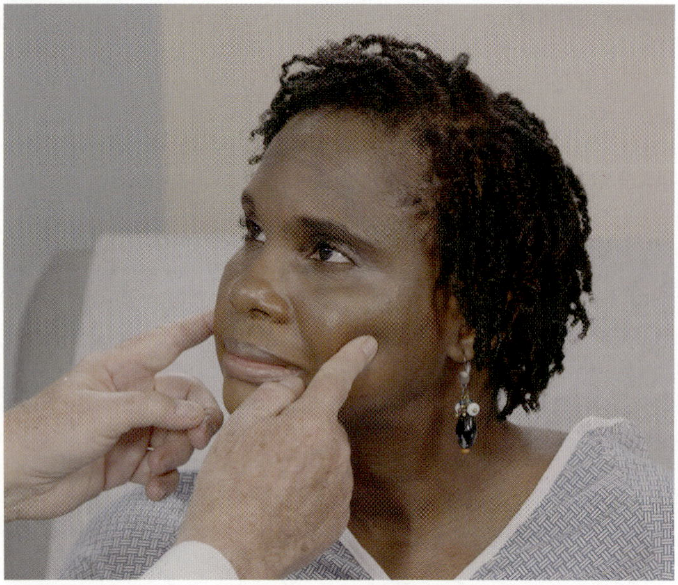

Fig. 21.13 Technique for Testing the Motor Function of the Trigeminal Nerve.

glands and chorda tympani. Testing for abnormalities of taste is usually not performed by a healthcare professional.

Test motor function. The patient is asked to bare the teeth while the examiner observes for asymmetry. The patient is asked to puff out the cheeks against resistance and then to wrinkle the forehead. It is helpful if the examiner first demonstrates these maneuvers for the patient. These maneuvers are demonstrated in Fig. 21.14.

The patient is then asked to close the eyes as tightly as possible while the examiner tries to open them. The examiner can say, "Don't let me open them." This procedure is demonstrated in Fig. 21.15A. Each eye is examined separately, and the strengths are compared. Normally the examiner should not be able to open the patient's eyes. The patient in Fig. 21.15B had marked weakness of the left orbicularis oculi muscle as a result of a stroke involving the facial nucleus.

The innervations of the facial nerve are illustrated in Fig. 21.16. There are two types of facial weakness. Upper motor neuron lesions such as a stroke involving the corticobulbar pathways produce contralateral weakness of the lower face, with

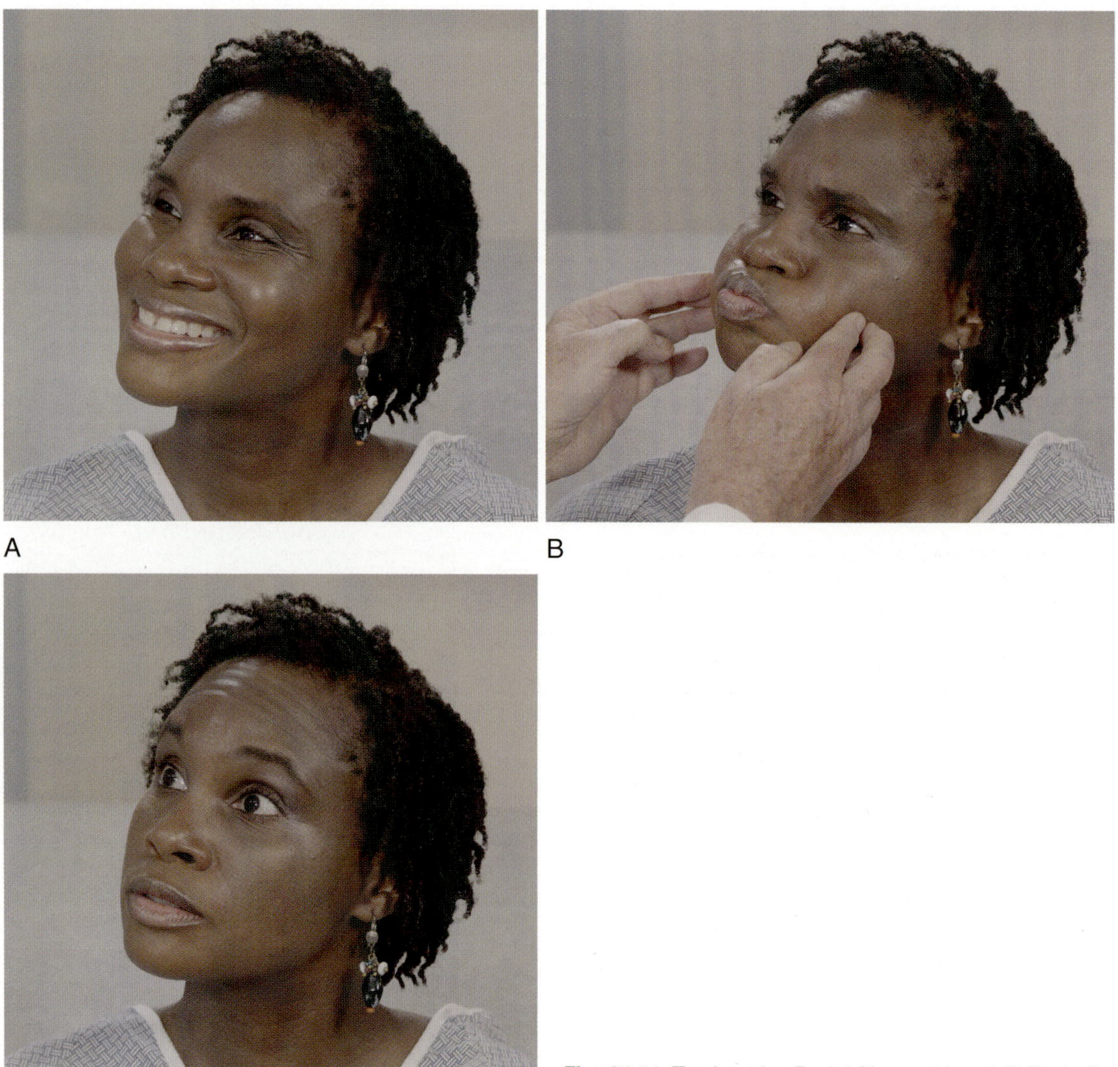

A

B

C

Fig. 21.14 Testing the Facial Nerve. (A and B) Tests for the lower division. (C) Test for the upper division.

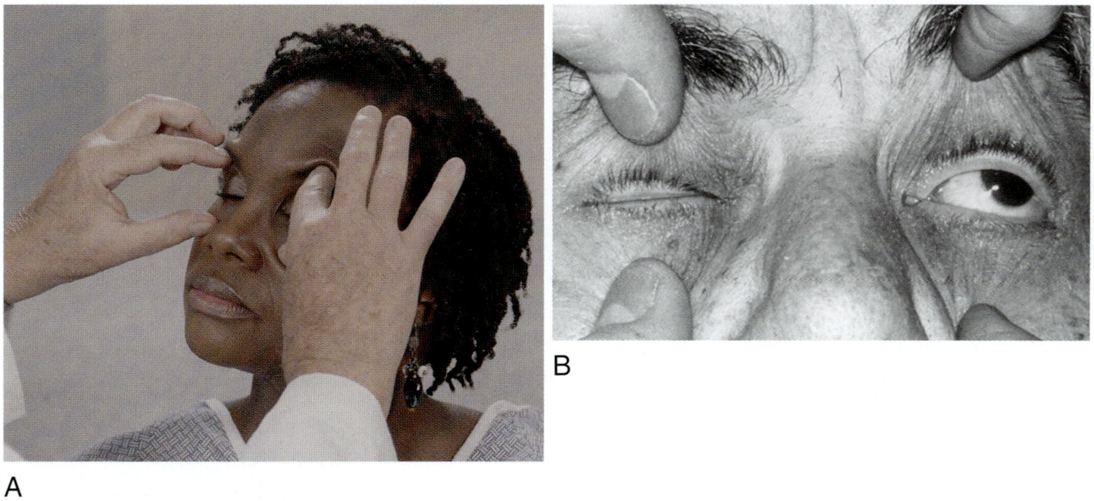

Fig. 21.15 Testing the Strength of Eyelid Closure. (A) Normal response. Note that the eyelids cannot be opened by the examiner. (B) Test in a patient with a stroke that involved the facial nerve nucleus. Note the loss in strength of the muscle around the left eye.

normal function of the upper face. The patient is still able to wrinkle the forehead. This is related to the bilateral innervation of the upper face by the corticobulbar fibers. The lower face has only unilateral innervation from contralateral cortical centers. This type of upper motor neuron lesion is illustrated by lesion A in Fig. 21.16. The second type of facial weakness produces total involvement of the ipsilateral facial muscles, with no area being spared. This may result from lesions of the nerve as it exits from the skull or from involvement of the facial nucleus in the pons, as illustrated by lesion B in Fig. 21.16.

When the patient in Fig. 21.17 was asked to smile, the right side of his face was drawn to the left. This patient has right facial palsy, also known as *right Bell palsy.* Further maneuvers revealed that the entire right side of his face was involved because of a lesion affecting the right facial nucleus.

Cranial Nerve VIII: Vestibulocochlear

See Video 21.4.

The vestibulocochlear nerve is responsible for hearing, balance, and awareness of position. Auditory testing is discussed in Chapter 11, The Ear and Nose. Tests for the vestibular function of cranial nerve VIII usually are not performed.

Cranial Nerve IX: Glossopharyngeal

See Video 21.5.

The glossopharyngeal nerve supplies sensation to the pharynx, posterior one-third of the tongue, and tympanic membrane, as well as secretory fibers to the parotid gland.

Test sensory function. When examining the glossopharyngeal nerve, the healthcare professional will check the gag reflex. This can be done by touching the back of the tongue, the soft palate, or the back of the throat with either a tongue blade or applicator stick. The glossopharyngeal nerve is responsible for the sensory part of the reflex, while the vagus nerve controls the motor part.

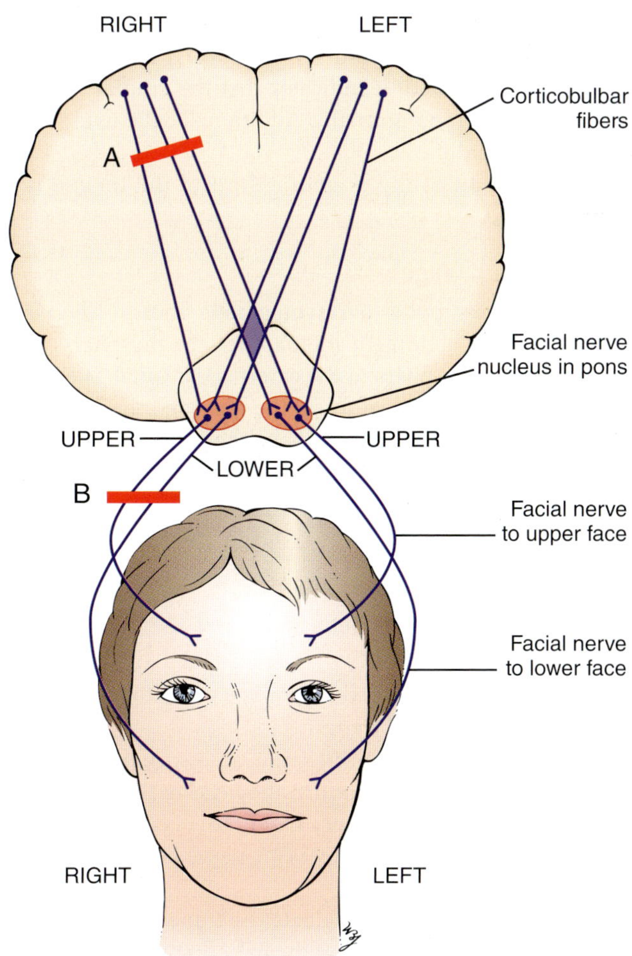

Fig. 21.16 Innervations of the Facial Nerve and Types of Facial Weakness. Lesion *A* produces an upper motor nerve palsy that causes contralateral weakness of the lower face but spares the contralateral forehead. Lesion *B* produces a lower motor nerve palsy that causes total paralysis of the ipsilateral face.

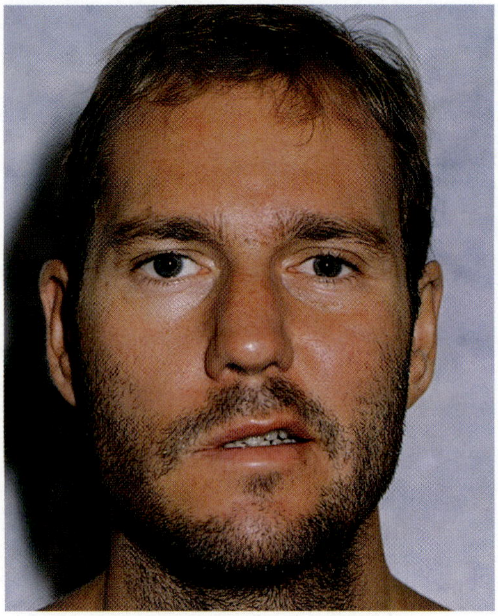

Fig. 21.17 Right Facial Palsy.

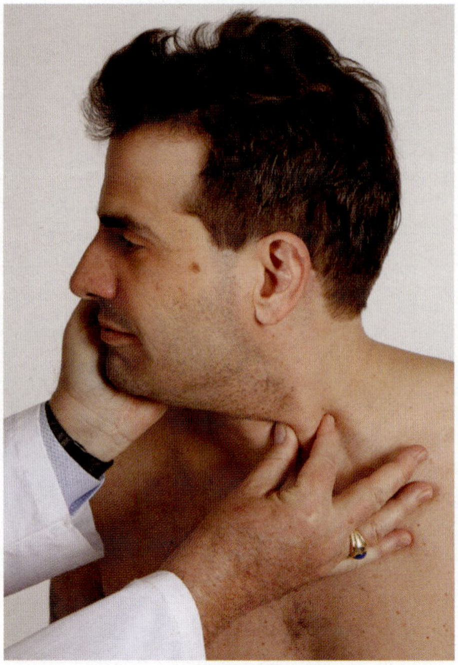

Fig. 21.18 Technique for Evaluating the Spinal Accessory Nerve.

Another way to test the IX cranial nerve is to ask a patient to open their mouth widely and say *"Ah...ah."* If the soft palate is symmetrically elevated, it indicates that the cranial nerves IX and X are functioning normally. Additionally, the uvula should remain in the midline.

Taste sensation of the posterior third of the tongue is not routinely tested.

Cranial Nerve X: Vagus

The vagus nerve supplies parasympathetic fibers to the viscera of the chest and abdomen; motor fibers to the pharynx and larynx; and sensory fibers to the external ear canal, the meninges of the posterior cranial fossa, the pharynx, the larynx, and the viscera of the body cavities above the pelvis.

Examination of the vagus nerve was performed during the evaluation of the glossopharyngeal nerve.

Dysphonia or dysarthria may result from paralysis of the vagus nerve.

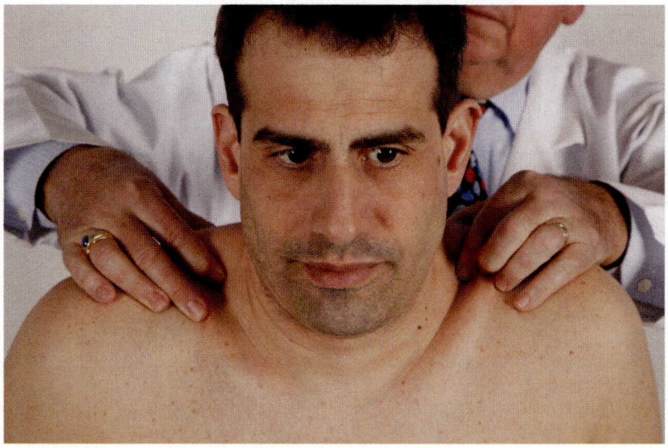

Fig. 21.19 Alternative Technique for Evaluating the Spinal Accessory Nerve.

Cranial Nerve XI: Spinal Accessory

See Video 21.6.

The spinal accessory nerve is a motor nerve that supplies the sternocleidomastoid and trapezius muscles.

Test motor function. The left spinal accessory nerve is examined by asking the patient to turn the head to the right against the resistance of the examiner's hand. This is demonstrated in Fig. 21.18. The right spinal accessory nerve is examined by reversing the directions.

An alternative test is to evaluate the trapezius muscles. The examiner places both hands on the patient's trapezius muscles. Both muscles are palpated between the examiner's thumbs and index fingers. The patient is then asked to shrug the shoulders against the resistance of the examiner's hands. Both sides should move equally. This technique is demonstrated in Fig. 21.19.

Cranial Nerve XII: Hypoglossal

See Video 21.7.

The hypoglossal nerve supplies motor fibers to the muscles of the tongue. The examination of the hypoglossal nerve is performed by asking the patient to open the mouth, with the tongue resting quietly on the floor of the mouth. Inspection for *fasciculations*[j] is performed. Fasciculations are indicative of a hypoglossal lower motor neuron lesion.

Test motor function. Ask the patient to open the mouth and stick out the tongue. Normally, the tongue is protruded and lies in the midline. This is demonstrated in Fig. 21.20. Deviation of the tongue to either side is abnormal. Because the tongue muscles push rather than pull, weakness of one side results in

[j]Spontaneous contractions of groups of muscles that are visible on inspection.

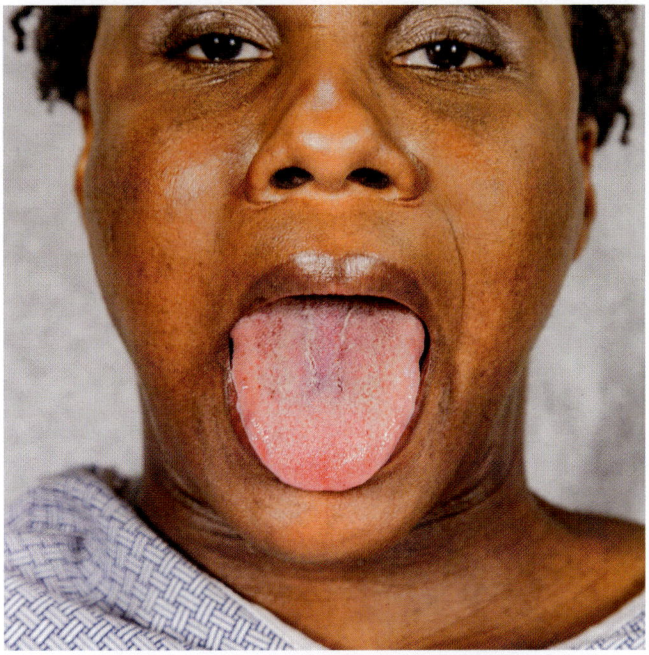

Fig. 21.20 Technique for Evaluating the Hypoglossal Nerve.

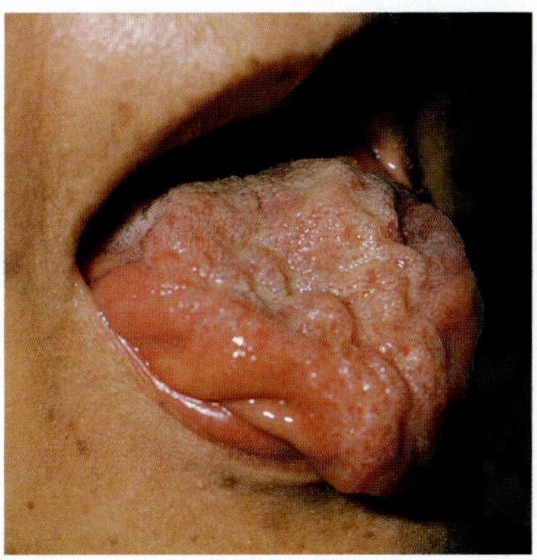

Fig. 21.21 Amyotrophic Lateral Sclerosis. Note the scalloping of the tongue.

the tongue being pushed by the normal side to the side of the lesion.

In Fig. 21.21, notice the marked scalloping of the tongue's surface. The patient has a chronic neurologic disease known as *amyotrophic lateral sclerosis (ALS)*[k] characterized by progressive degeneration of motor neurons. The patient has the typical features of a lower motor neuron bulbar palsy affecting the hypoglossal nucleus: wasting of the tongue with fasciculations.

[k]Lou Gehrig disease, also known as ALS, affects motor neurons responsible for controlling voluntary muscles. Sadly, when these cells perish, people living with ALS experience a gradual loss of muscle control and movement, leading to weakness and disability. Eventually, they may lose the ability to move their arms, legs, and body, and even breathe on their own. Despite this, their minds usually remain sharp and alert. Unfortunately, the average life expectancy for people diagnosed with ALS is between 2 to 5 years.

TABLE 21.2 Muscle Strength Grading

0, absent:	No muscle activation
1, Trace:	Trace muscle activation, such as a twitch, without achieving full range of motion
2, Weak:	Muscle activation with gravity eliminated, achieving full range of motion
3, Fair:	Muscle activation against gravity, full range of motion
4, Good:	Muscle activation against some resistance, full range of motion
5, Normal:	Muscle activation against examiner's full resistance, full range of motion

Grading originally developed by The Medical Research Council of the United Kingdom.

Motor Function

Basic Principles

The motor system is evaluated for the following:

- Muscle bulk
- Muscle strength
- Muscle tone

The motor examination begins with inspection of each area being tested. The contours of symmetric *muscle masses* in both the upper and lower extremities are compared. Inspection is used to detect muscle atrophy and the presence of fasciculations.

Muscle strength should be graded. Test muscle strength by having the patient move actively against your resistance. This method involves testing key muscles from the upper and lower extremities against the examiner's resistance and grading the patient's strength on a 0 to 5 scale accordingly. The following modified scale, originally developed by The Medical Research Council of the United Kingdom, is now used universally (see Table 21.2). The difficulty with this and similar scales is the large range in strength possible between grades 4 and 5.

Commonly chosen muscles include proximal upper, distal upper, proximal lower, and distal lower muscles. Additional muscles may be tested to evaluate individual peripheral nerves. In general, proximal weakness is related to muscle disease; distal weakness is related to neurologic disease. George Newman, MD, PhD, from the Albert Einstein Medical Center suggested the following.[4] Functional testing often provides a better picture of the relationship between strength and disability. As the patient does various maneuvers, deficiencies are noted and quantified as much as possible (e.g., number of squats done or steps climbed). Rising from a squatting position or stepping onto a chair tests proximal leg strength; walking on the heels and on tiptoe tests distal strength. Pushing with the arms to get out of a chair indicates quadriceps weakness. Swinging the body to move the arms indicates shoulder girdle weakness. Rising from the supine position by turning prone, kneeling, and using the hands to climb up the thighs and slowly push erect (Gowers sign) suggests pelvic girdle weakness.[l]

[l]Neurologist Sir William Richard Gowers coined the term "Gowers sign" in 1879 to describe a pattern often seen in patients with Duchenne muscular dystrophy. This involves using their hands to climb up their thighs to compensate for the weakness in their pelvic and lower limb muscles.

Muscle tone can be defined as the slight residual tension in a voluntarily relaxed muscle. Muscle tone is an unconscious low-level contraction of muscles while they are at rest. Tone is assessed by resistance to passive movement. Ask the patient to relax a muscle. Perform passive motion of the muscle. Compare one side with the other. The degree of resistance is determined to be less than normal (hypotonic), normal, or more than normal (hypertonic). The latter may be referred to as *spasticity.* Hypotonia usually occurs with lower motor neuron disease, whereas upper motor neuron lesions produce spasticity,[m] hyperreflexia, clonus,[n] and Babinski sign.[o]

Lower motor neuron lesions produce atrophy, fasciculations, decreased tone, and hyporeflexia. Both types of lesions result in weakness. Fasciculations may become more apparent by gently tapping the muscle with a reflex hammer.

It is impractical to test all muscles during the neurologic examination. By testing key muscle groups, the examiner can determine whether a gross deficit exists. Further testing of specific muscles and nerve roots may then be necessary. The student is referred to the many textbooks on neurology for these detailed examinations.

Examine Upper Extremities

In the assessment of motor function, the upper extremities are examined first.

Inspect the upper extremities for symmetry. Ask the patient to sit on the side of the bed facing you. Inspect both arms and hands for size differences, paying special attention to the size of the thumbs and the small muscles of the hands. Is muscle wasting present?

Test flexion and extension of the arm. Test flexion and extension strength of the upper extremity by having the patient pull and push against your resistance. You might say, "Push down … relax," "Push up … relax," "Push back … relax," and "Push forward … relax." Say "relax" after each direction so that the patient does not continue to push or pull after you have removed your hands. After one side is tested, the other is tested, and the results of the two sides are compared. In other clinical situations, NEVER tell a patient to relax!

Test arm abduction. Ask the patient to extend the arms with palms facing down. Place your hands at the lateral aspect of the patient's arms. Instruct the patient to abduct the arms against resistance. This is a test of abduction of the arm by the *axillary nerve* from roots C5 to C6. This test is demonstrated in Fig. 21.22.

Test forearm flexion. Have the patient make a fist and flex the forearm. Hold the patient's fist or wrist. Ask the patient to pull the arm in against your resistance. This is a test of flexion of the forearm by the *musculocutaneous nerve* from roots C5 to C6. This test is demonstrated in Fig. 21.23.

Test forearm extension. Ask the patient to abduct the arm and hold it midway between flexion and extension. Support the patient's arm by holding the wrist. Instruct the patient to extend the arm against your resistance. This is a test of extension of the forearm by the *radial nerve* from roots C6 to C8. This test is demonstrated in Fig. 21.24.

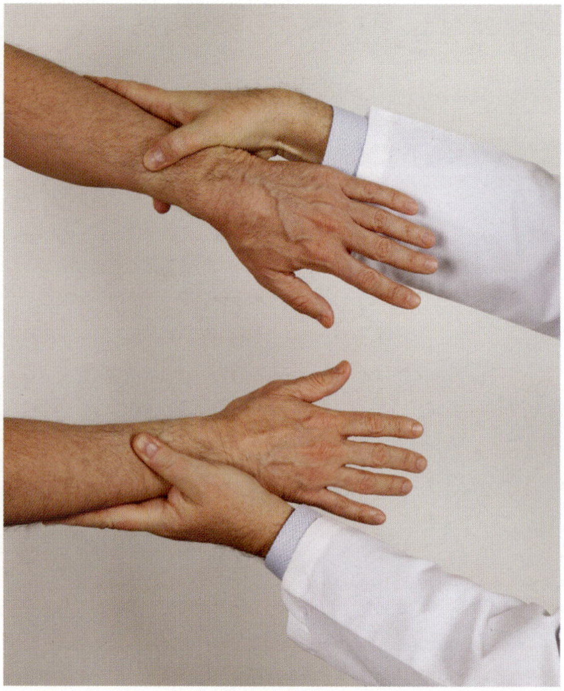

Fig. 21.22 Technique for Testing Abduction of the Arm.

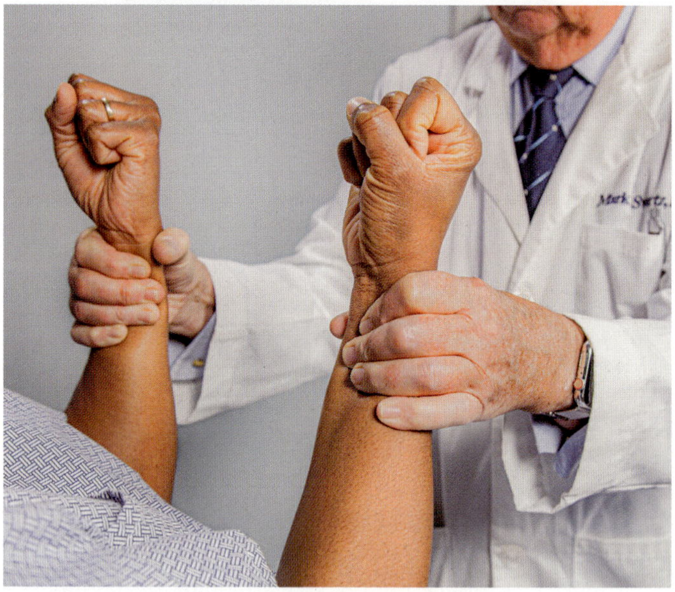

Fig. 21.23 Technique for Testing Flexion of the Forearm.

Test wrist extension. Instruct the patient to make a fist and extend the wrist while you attempt to push it up. This is a test of extension of the wrist by the *radial nerve* from roots C6 to C8. This test is demonstrated in Fig. 21.25.

Test wrist flexion. Ask the patient to make a fist and flex the wrist while you attempt to pull it down. This is a test of flexion of the wrist by the *median nerve* from roots C6 to C7. This test is demonstrated in Fig. 21.26.

[m]An increase in muscle tone that results in continuous resistance to stretching. Spasticity is usually worse at extremes of range.

[n]Spasm in which rigidity and relaxation alternate in rapid succession.

[o]Dorsiflexion of the big toe on stimulation of the sole of the foot (see Fig. 21.46).

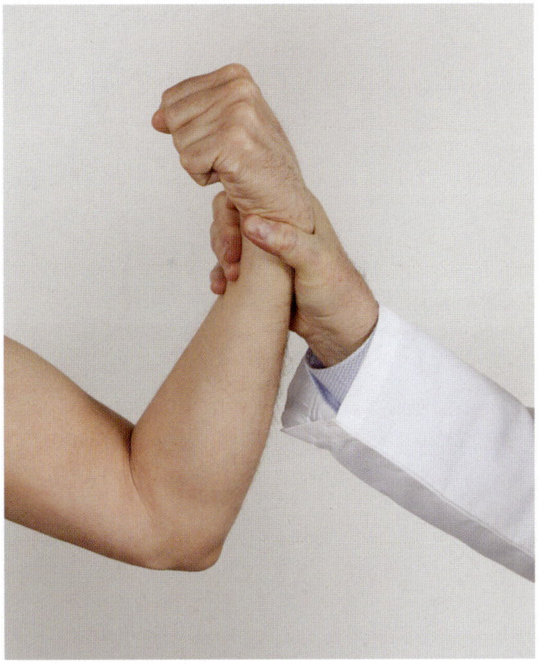

Fig. 21.24 Technique for Testing Extension of the Forearm.

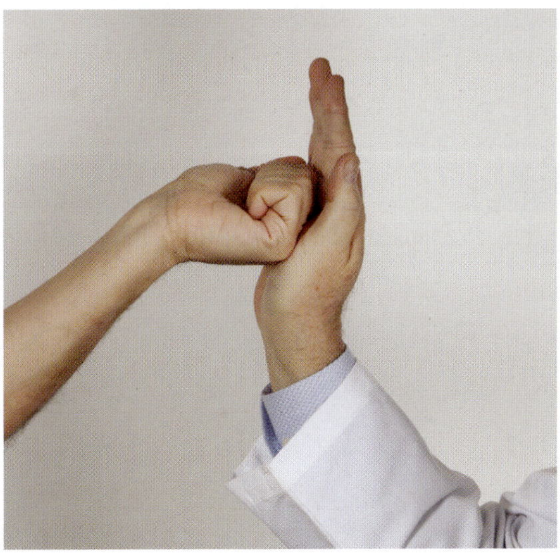

Fig. 21.25 Technique for Testing Extension of the Wrist.

Test finger adduction. Ask the patient to grasp your extended index and middle fingers and to squeeze them as hard as possible. Compare the strengths of both hands. (It is important for you to remove any rings, which may produce discomfort.) This is a test of adduction of the fingers by the *median nerve* from roots C7 to T1. This test is demonstrated in Fig. 21.27.

Test finger abduction. Ask the patient to extend the hand with the palm down and to spread the fingers as widely as possible. Tell the patient to resist your attempt to bring the fingers together. This is a test of abduction of the fingers by the *ulnar nerve* from roots C8 to T1. This test is demonstrated in Fig. 21.28.

Test thumb adduction. Instruct the patient to touch the base of the little finger with the tip of the thumb against resistance

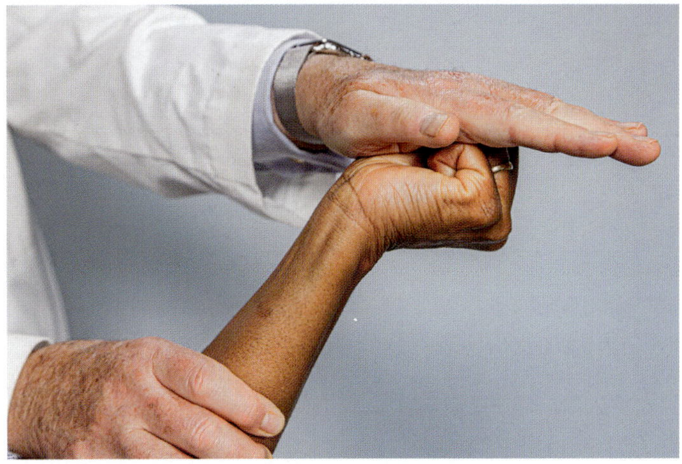

Fig. 21.26 Technique for Testing Flexion of the Wrist.

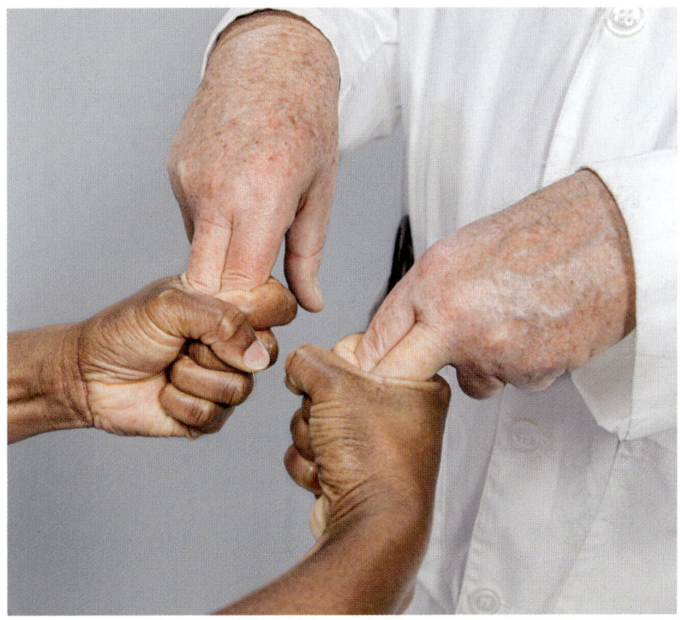

Fig. 21.27 Technique for Testing Finger Adduction.

while the thumbnail remains parallel to the palm. This is a test of adduction of the thumb by the *median nerve* from roots C8 to T1. This test is demonstrated in Fig. 21.29.

Assess upper extremity tone. Tone is assessed in the patient's upper limbs by passively flexing and extending the limbs to determine the amount of resistance to the examiner's movements. Increased resistance, such as that in muscle rigidity or spasticity, means increased muscle tone. Decreased resistance, such as that in limpness or flaccidity, means decreased muscle tone. Normal tone has a smooth sensation. In extrapyramidal disease, palpation of a proximal muscle during passive movement detects the presence of *cogwheeling,* which is a ratchet jerkiness to the motion.

Examine Lower Extremities

Inspect the lower extremities for symmetry. The lower extremities are now examined for muscle bulk and muscle wasting. This examination is performed with the patient lying

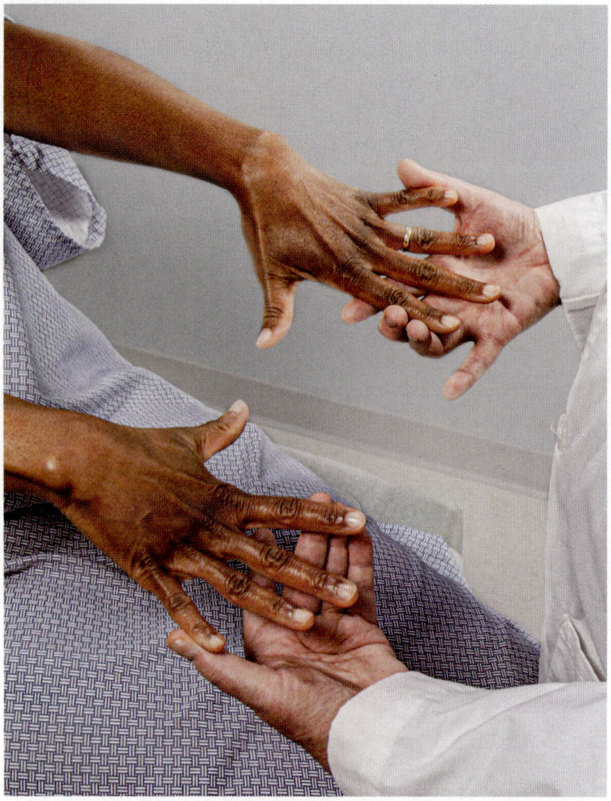

Fig. 21.28 Technique for Testing Finger Abduction.

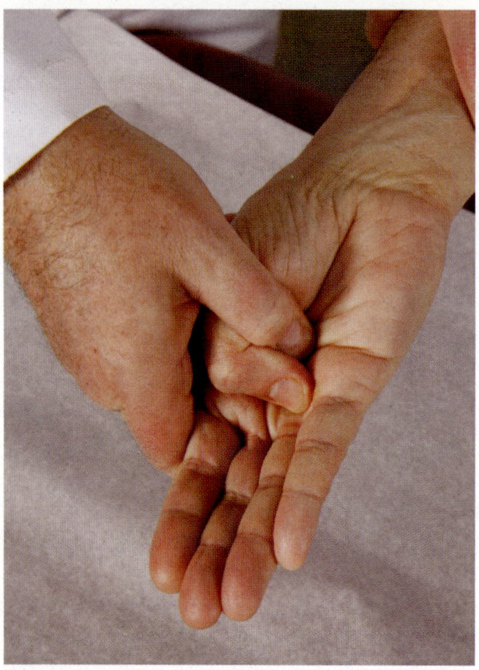

Fig. 21.29 Technique for Testing Thumb Adduction.

on their back in bed. As with the upper extremities, proximal and distal muscle strengths are compared as are the legs for symmetry.

Test hip adduction. Ask the patient to move the legs apart. Place your hands on the medial aspect of the patient's knees. Instruct the patient to close the legs against your resistance.

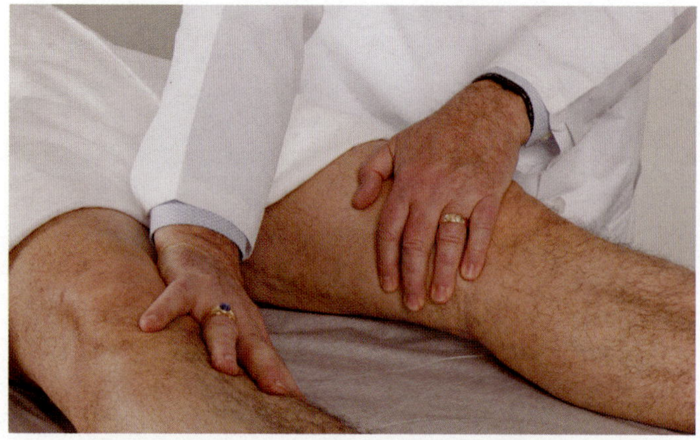

Fig. 21.30 Technique for Testing Hip Adduction.

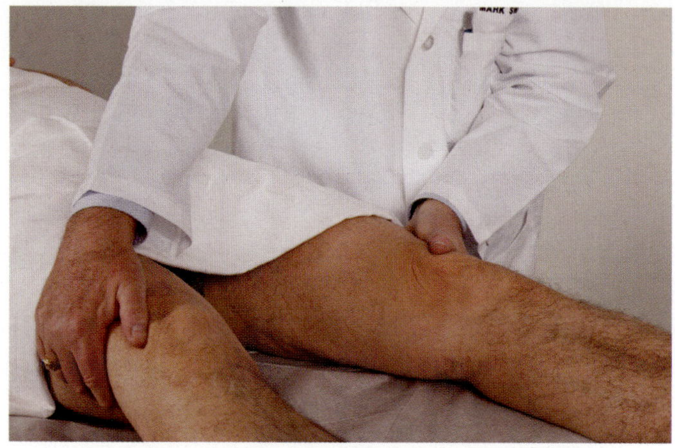

Fig. 21.31 Technique for Testing Hip Abduction.

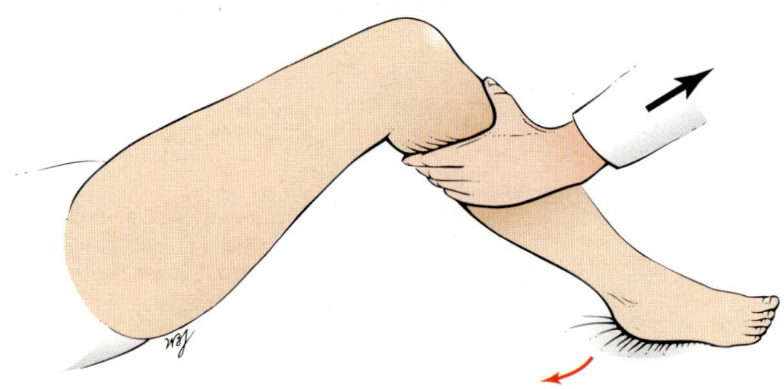

Fig. 21.32 Technique for Testing Knee Flexion.

This is a test of adduction of the hips by the *obturator nerve* from roots L2 to L4. This test is demonstrated in Fig. 21.30.

Test hip abduction. Place your hands on the lateral margins of the patient's knees. Ask the patient to open the legs against your resistance. This is a test of abduction of the hips by the *superior gluteal nerve* from roots L4 to S1. This test is demonstrated in Fig. 21.31.

Test knee flexion. Ask the patient to elevate a knee, with the foot resting on the bed. Instruct the patient to hold the foot down as you try to extend the leg. This is a test of flexion of the knee by the *sciatic nerve* from roots L4 to S1. This test is illustrated in Fig. 21.32.

Test knee extension. Instruct the patient to elevate the knee, with the foot resting on the bed. Place your left hand under the knee. Ask the patient to straighten the leg against the resistance of your right hand, which is placed on the patient's shin. This procedure tests extension of the knee by the *femoral nerve* from roots L2 to L4. This test is illustrated in Fig. 21.33.

Test ankle dorsiflexion. Place your hands on the dorsum of the foot and ask the patient to dorsiflex the foot at the ankle against your resistance. This is a test of dorsiflexion of the ankle by the *deep peroneal nerve* from roots L4 to L5. This maneuver is demonstrated in Fig. 21.34.

Test ankle plantar flexion. Place your hand on the sole and ask the patient to plantarflex the foot at the ankle against your resistance. This is a test of plantar flexion of the ankle by the *tibial nerve* from roots L5 to S2. This test is demonstrated in Fig. 21.35.

Test great toe dorsiflexion. Place your hand on the dorsal aspect of the patient's big toe. Ask the patient to dorsiflex the big toe against your resistance. This is a test of dorsiflexion of the big toe by the *deep peroneal nerve* from roots L4 to S1. This test is demonstrated in Fig. 21.36.

Test great toe plantar flexion. Place your hand on the plantar surface of the patient's big toe. Ask the patient to plantarflex the great toe against your resistance. This is a test of plantar flexion of the great toe by the *posterior tibial nerve* from roots L5 to S2. This test is demonstrated in Fig. 21.37.

Assess lower extremity tone. Tone in the lower extremities is assessed in the same way as in the upper extremities.

Grasp the foot and passively dorsiflex and plantarflex it several times, ending with dorsiflexion of the foot. If a sudden rhythmic involuntary dorsiflexion and plantar flexion occur, *ankle clonus* is present. This frequently occurs in conditions of increased tone.

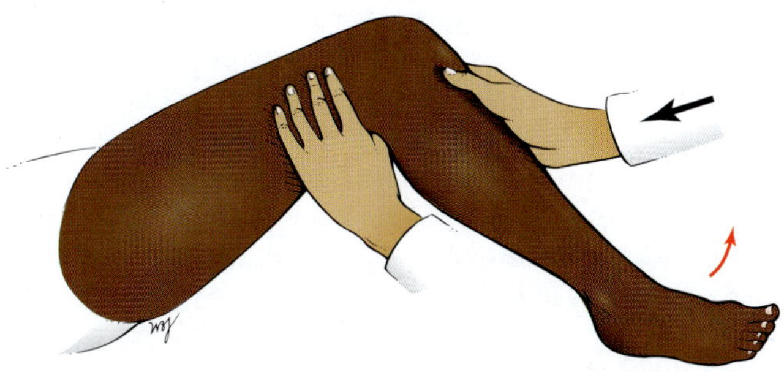

Fig. 21.33 Technique for Testing Knee Extension.

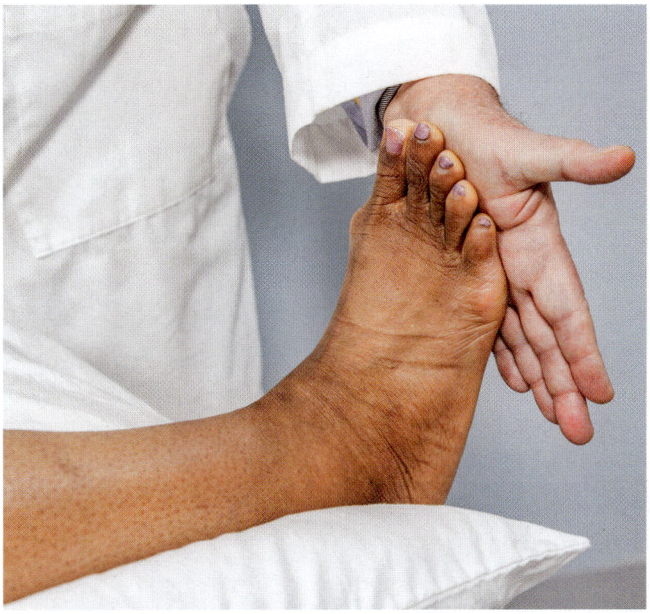

Fig. 21.35 Technique for Testing Plantar Flexion.

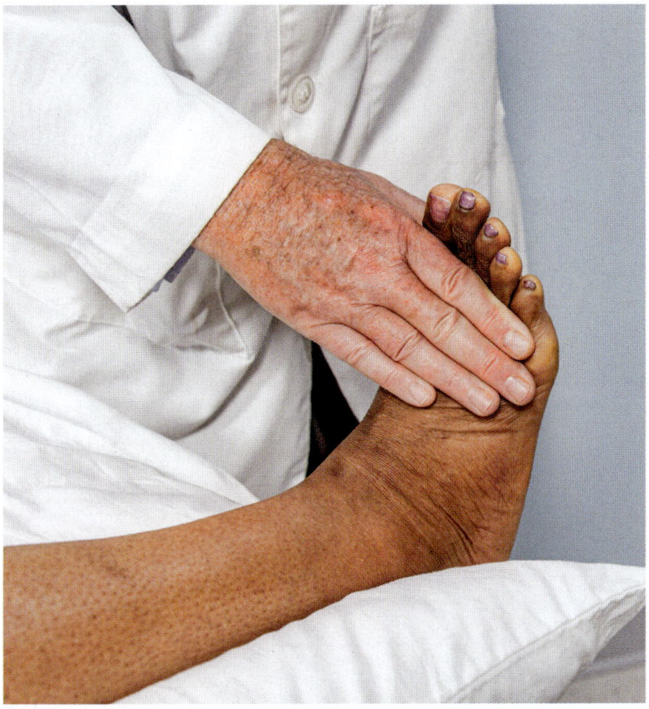

Fig. 21.34 Technique for Testing Ankle Dorsiflexion.

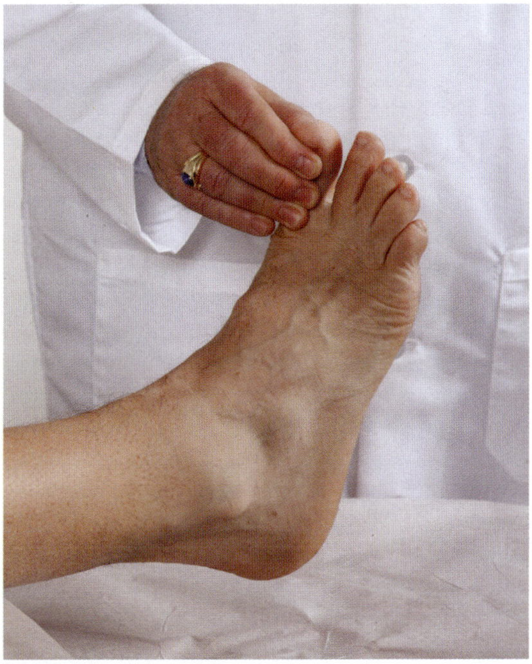

Fig. 21.36 Technique for Testing Great Toe Dorsiflexion.

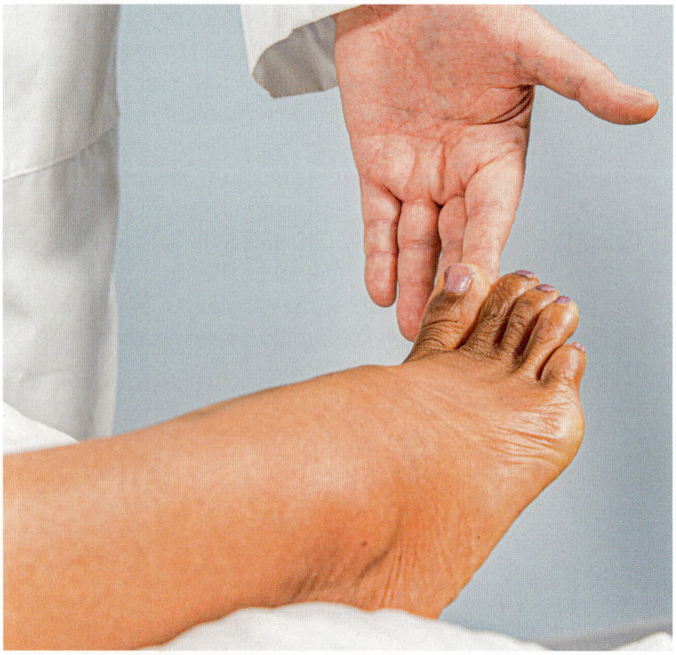

Fig. 21.37 Technique for Testing Great Toe Plantar Flexion.

If any abnormality is noted in the motor strength of the upper or lower extremity, a more detailed examination should be performed. See Table 21.7 for a list of the muscle innervations and their actions.

Reflexes

Basic Principles

During a neurologic exam, there are two main types of reflexes that are tested: stretch, or *deep tendon*, reflexes and *superficial* reflexes. Testing reflexes helps differentiate between upper and lower motor neuron lesions. There are five deep tendon reflexes and a few superficial reflexes that are examined.

There are several different types of reflex hammers. The Taylor, or tomahawk, reflex hammer is the most well-known reflex hammer in the United States. It consists of a triangular rubber component that is attached to a flat metallic handle (see Fig. 21.41). The hammer is held at the end, and the entire device is swung in an arc-like motion onto the tendon being evaluated. Another commonly used reflex hammer is the Buck reflex hammer. It is a "T" design dual mallet-type hammer (see Fig. 21.39).

To elicit a deep tendon reflex, support the joint being tested so that the muscle is relaxed. The extremity being tested must be in a relaxed position. A quick, precise tap on the tendon with a reflex hammer should elicit the response. Hold the reflex hammer between your thumb and index finger and swing it by motion at the wrist, not the elbow. In general, the flat end of a triangular reflex hammer is used. A gentle tap over the tendon being tested should produce muscle contraction. To assess muscle contraction, it is often necessary both to palpate and to observe the muscle. Test each reflex and compare it with the other side. Reflexes should be symmetrically equal.

There is individual variation in the reflex response. Only with experience is the examiner able to make an adequate assessment of normal reflexes. Reflexes are commonly graded on a scale from 0 to 4+ as follows:

0: No response, always abnormal
1+: Diminished response, may or may not be normal
2+: Brisk response, normal
3+: Very brisk response, may or may not be normal
4+: Hyperactive, tap elicits a repeating reflex (clonus), always abnormal

If a patient has *hyperactive* reflexes, it could be a sign of pyramidal tract disease, as well as electrolyte abnormalities, hyperthyroidism, or other metabolic issues. On the other hand, *diminished* reflexes could indicate anterior horn cell disorders or myopathies. It's important for the examiner to consider the size of the muscle mass in relation to the strength of the reflex. Sometimes, a patient's reflexes may appear diminished because of decreased muscle bulk. One specific symptom of hypothyroidism is reduced relaxation following a deep tendon reflex known as a "hung up reflex" or Woltman sign. Although not commonly observed, the hung up reflex is distinct and typically manifests in the ankle jerk. This reflex is named after Henry Woltman, an American neurologist.

If a patient has a reduced reflex, the reinforcement technique can be helpful. By contracting other muscles, the overall reflex activity may be increased. To test reflexes in the upper limbs, instruct the patient to clench their teeth or push down on the bed using their thighs. For testing reflexes in the lower limbs, ask the patient to interlock their fingers and attempt to pull them apart during the examination. This technique, also known as the *Jendrassik maneuver,* is illustrated in Fig. 21.38 for the testing of the knee jerk.

Test the Deep Tendon Reflexes

The five deep tendon reflexes that are routinely tested are as follows:

- Biceps
- Brachioradialis
- Triceps
- Patellar
- Achilles

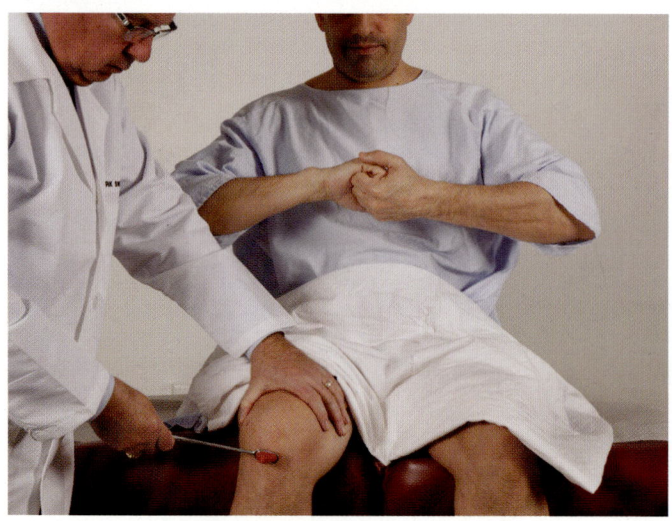

Fig. 21.38 Jendrassik Maneuver.

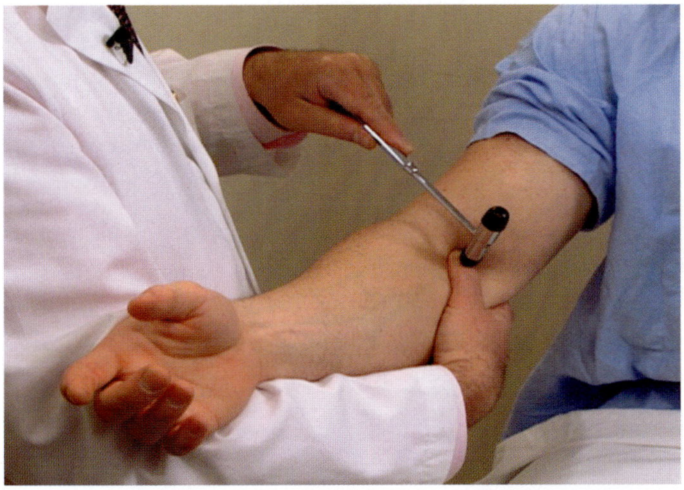

Fig. 21.39 Technique for Testing the Biceps Tendon Reflex.

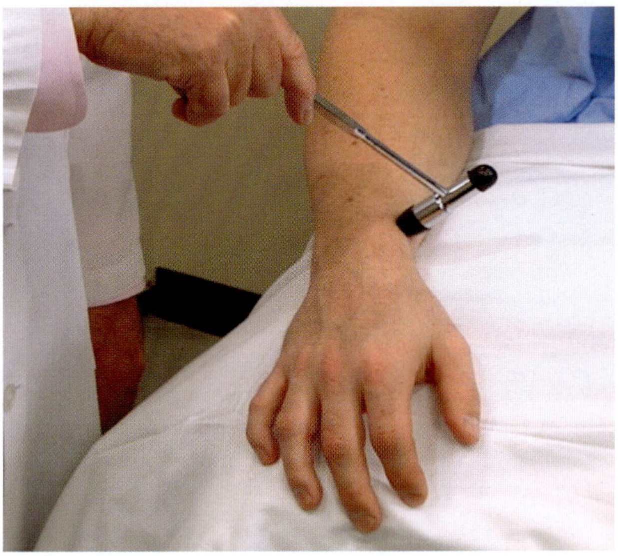

Fig. 21.40 Technique for Testing the Brachioradialis Tendon Reflex.

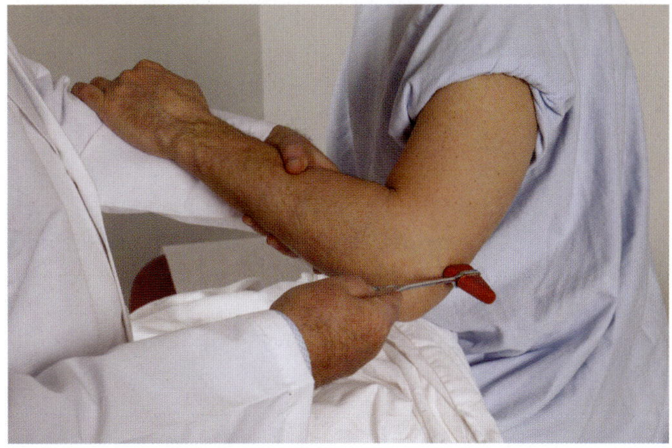

Fig. 21.41 Technique for Testing the Triceps Tendon Reflex.

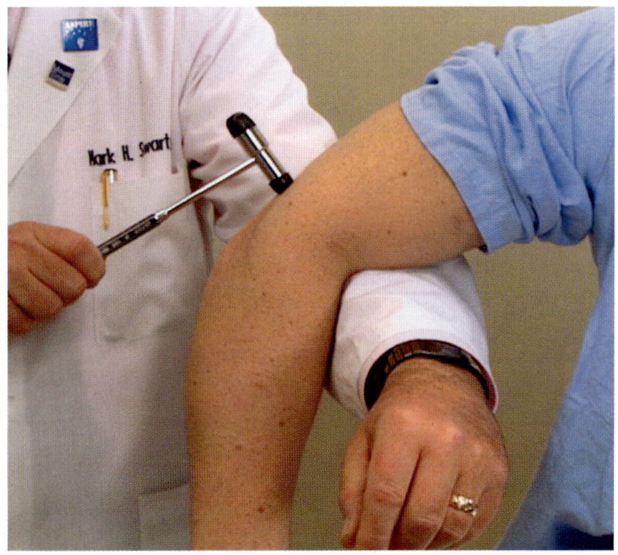

Fig. 21.42 Another Test of the Triceps Tendon Reflex.

Test the biceps tendon reflex. See Video 21.8.

The *biceps tendon* reflex is assessed by having the patient relax the arm and pronate the forearm midway between flexion and extension. The examiner should place a thumb firmly on the biceps tendon. If a triangular reflex hammer is used, the pointed end of the hammer is then struck on the examiner's thumb. Testing the biceps tendon reflex is demonstrated in Fig. 21.39. The examiner should observe for contraction of the biceps tendon, followed by flexion at the elbow. The examiner may also palpate the contraction of the muscle. This procedure is a test of the nerves at roots C5 to C6.

Test the brachioradialis tendon reflex. See Video 21.9.

The *brachioradialis tendon reflex* is performed by having the patient's forearm in semiflexion and semipronation. The arm should be rested on the patient's knee. If a triangular reflex hammer is used, the flat end should strike the styloid process of the radius approximately 2.5 to 5 cm above the wrist. The examiner should observe for flexion at the elbow and simultaneous supination of the forearm. The position is demonstrated in Fig. 21.40. This procedure tests the nerves at roots C5 to C6.

Test the triceps tendon reflex. See Video 21.10.

The *triceps tendon reflex* is tested by flexing the patient's forearm at the elbow and pulling the arm toward the chest. The elbow should be midway between flexion and extension. If the triangular reflex hammer is used, tap the triceps tendon above the insertion of the ulna's olecranon process approximately 2.5 to 5 cm above the elbow with the flat end of the hammer. Do not use the pointed end of the hammer, as it could hit the ulnar nerve and cause pain. There should be a prompt contraction of the triceps tendon with extension at the elbow. This technique is demonstrated in Fig. 21.41. This procedure is a test of the nerves at roots C6 to C8.

If the triceps tendon reflex cannot be elicited by this maneuver, try to hang the patient's arm over your arm, as demonstrated in Fig. 21.42. Tapping the triceps tendon in this position often elicits the reflex.

Test the patellar tendon reflex. See Video 21.11.

Perform the *patellar tendon reflex,* also known as the *knee jerk,* by having the patient sit with their legs dangling off the side of the bed. Place your hand on the patient's quadriceps muscle. Strike the patellar tendon firmly with the flat end of the reflex hammer. A contraction of the quadriceps should be felt, and extension at the knee should be observed. This technique is demonstrated in Fig. 21.43. It is a test of the nerves at roots L2 to L4.

Test the Achilles tendon reflex. See Video 21.12.

The *Achilles tendon reflex,* also known as the *ankle jerk,* is elicited by having the patient sit with their feet dangling off the side of the bed. The leg should be flexed at the hip and the knee. The examiner places a hand under the patient's foot to dorsiflex the ankle. The Achilles tendon is struck just above its insertion on the posterior aspect of the calcaneus with the flat end of the reflex hammer. The result is plantar flexion at the ankle. This technique is demonstrated in Fig. 21.44. It is a test of the nerves at roots S1 to S2.

Another method of testing for the Achilles reflex is to have the patient lie in bed. Flex one of the patient's legs at the hip and knee and rotate the leg externally so that it lies on the opposite shin. Dorsiflex the ankle as the tendon is struck. This test is demonstrated in Fig. 21.45A.

A patient with a depressed Achilles reflex should be asked to kneel, if possible, on the bed with the feet hanging off the side, as shown in Fig. 21.45B. Tap the Achilles tendon with the flat end of the triangular reflex hammer and observe the reflex response in this position.

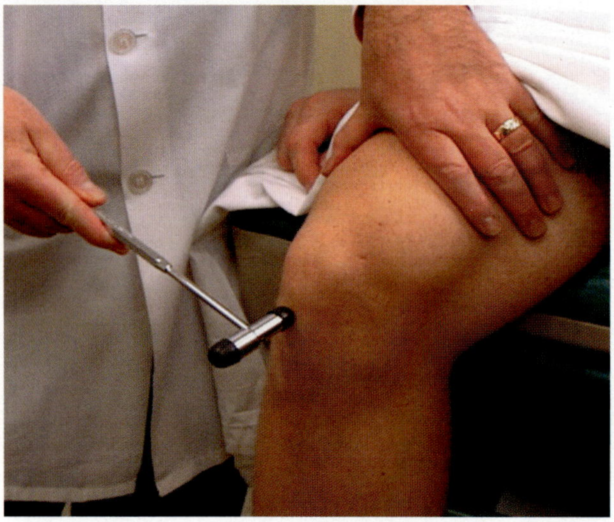

Fig. 21.43 Technique for Testing the Patellar Tendon Reflex.

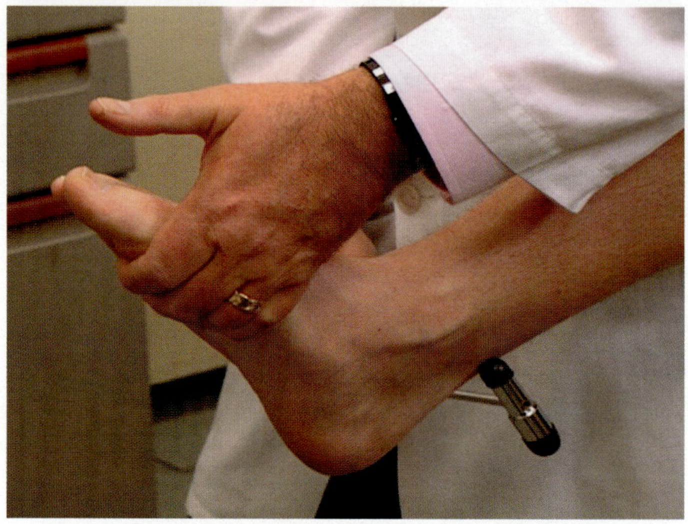

Fig. 21.44 Technique for Testing the Achilles Tendon Reflex.

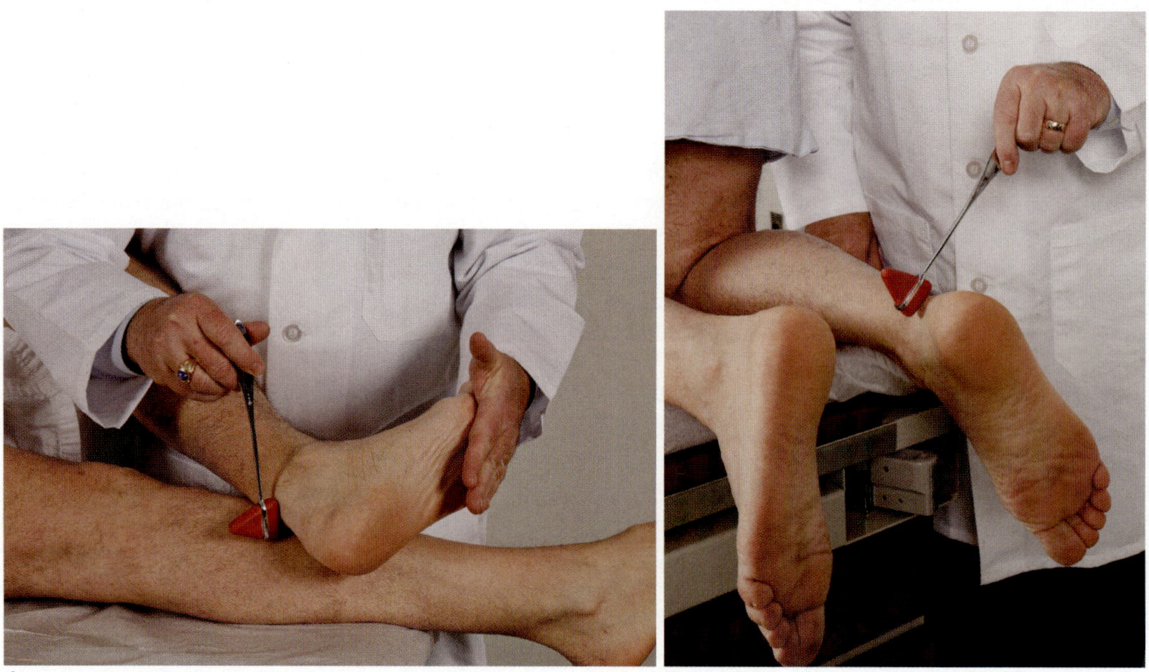

A B

Fig. 21.45 (A) Alternative technique for evaluating the Achilles tendon reflex. (B) Technique for assessing the Achilles tendon reflex when the reflex appears to be depressed.

Test the Superficial Reflexes

Superficial reflexes are motor responses to scraping of the skin and are graded simply as "present" or "absent" The most tested superficial reflexes are the abdominal and the cremasteric. The *abdominal* superficial reflex is elicited by having the patient lie on their back. An applicator stick or tongue blade is quickly stroked horizontally, laterally, and medially toward the umbilicus. The result is a contraction of the abdominal muscles, with the umbilicus deviating toward the stimulus. The abdominal reflex is frequently not seen in obese individuals. The *cremasteric* superficial reflex in males is elicited by lightly stroking the inner aspect of the thigh with an applicator stick or tongue depressor. The result is a rapid elevation of the testicle on the same side. Although the superficial reflexes are absent on the side of a corticospinal tract lesion, there is little clinical significance to their presence or absence because they are absent in 20% of normal individuals, more in the elderly population. They are described here for completeness only.

Test for Abnormal Reflexes

See Video 21.13.

Babinski sign or *reflex* is a pathologic reflex in an adult. It is normal in infants (see Chapter 24, The Pediatric Patient). Normally, when the lateral aspect of the sole is stroked from the heel to the ball of the foot and curved medially across the heads of the metatarsal bones, there is plantar flexion of the big toe. This is a test of the nerve roots at L5 to S2. The foot should be stroked with a stimulus such as a key. A pin should *never* be used. In the presence of pyramidal tract disease, when the described movement is performed, there is *dorsiflexion* of the big toe, with fanning of the other toes. This is Babinski reflex. Because the Babinski sign is an abnormal reflex, the examiner should note it only when it is present. It is correct to describe the plantar reflex as either plantar flexion (normal) or dorsiflexion (abnormal, Babinski sign). The technique for evaluating the plantar reflex is shown in Fig. 21.46.

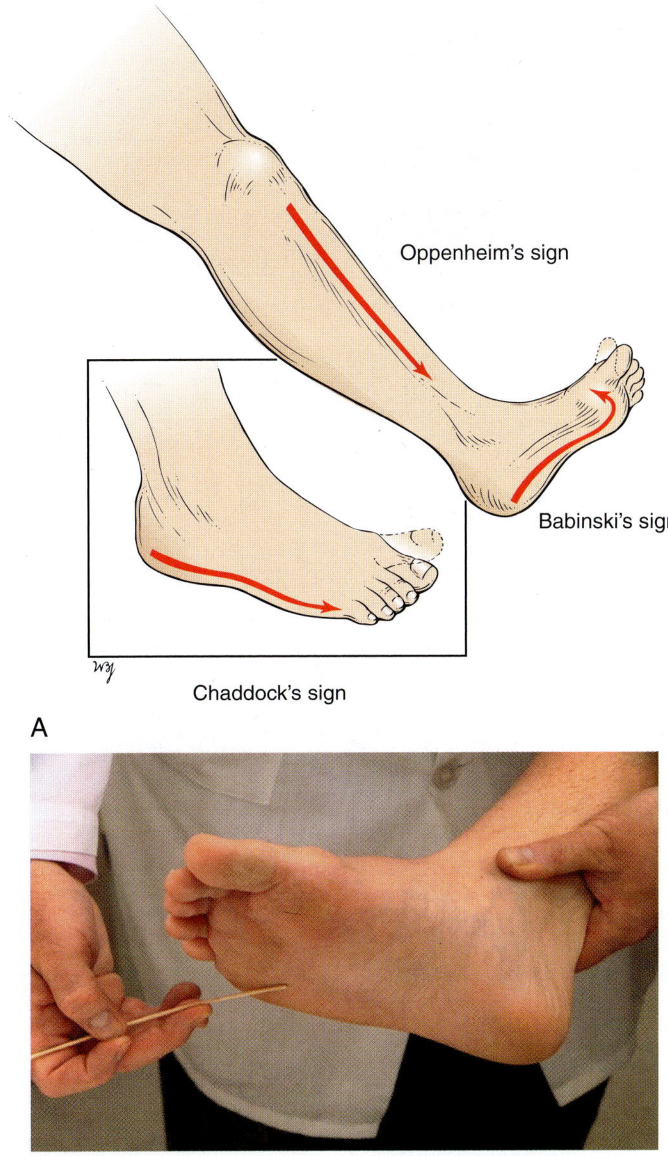

Fig. 21.46 (A and B) Techniques for evaluating the plantar reflex.

Pyramidal tract disease is also suggested when the big toe dorsiflexes on stroking the lateral aspect of the foot. This is the *Chaddock sign.* In the presence of pyramidal tract disease, downward pressure along the shin causes the big toe to dorsiflex. This is the *Oppenheim sign.* The elicitation of these signs is less sensitive than stroking the plantar surface.

Another abnormal reflex associated with pyramidal tract disease is *Hoffmann sign.* To elicit this sign, the patient's hand is pronated, and the examiner grasps the terminal phalanx of the middle finger between the index finger and thumb. With a sharp jerk, the phalanx is passively flexed and suddenly released. A positive response consists of adduction and flexion of the thumb as well as flexion of the other fingers.

Sensory Function

Basic Principles

The sensory examination consists of testing for the following:

- Light touch
- Pain sensation
- Vibration sense
- Proprioception
- Tactile localization
- Discriminative sensations (two-point discrimination, stereognosis, graphesthesia, and point localization)

In a patient without any symptoms or signs of neurologic disease, the examination for sensory function can be performed by quickly assessing the presence of normal sensation on the distal fingers and toes. The examiner can choose to test for light touch, pain, and vibration sense. If these are normal, the rest of the sensory examination is not required. If symptoms or signs refer to a neurologic disorder, complete testing is indicated.

As with the motor examination, the examiner compares side with side and proximal with distal aspect. Neurologic disorders usually result in a sensory loss that is first seen more distally than proximally.

The hand is supplied by the median, ulnar, and radial nerves. The median nerve is the chief nerve of sensation because it supplies the palmar surfaces of the digits, the parts of the hand

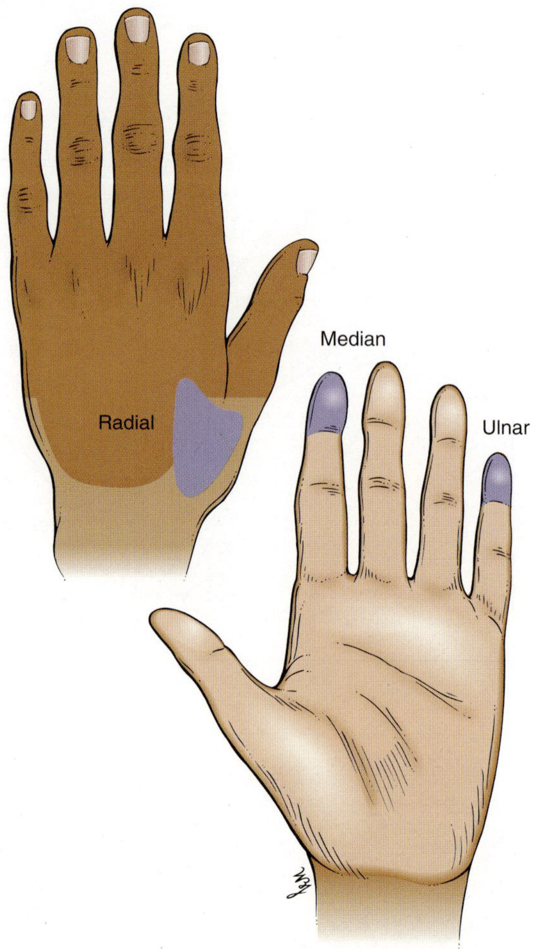

Fig. 21.47 Most Reliable Cutaneous Areas for Testing Hand Sensation.

most used for feeling. The ulnar nerve supplies sensation only to the ulnar one and a half fingers. The radial nerve has its sensory distribution to the dorsum of the hand. There is considerable overlap in innervation. The most reliable cutaneous areas for testing these nerves are illustrated in Fig. 21.47. These areas have the least likelihood of overlapping innervation.

Test Light Touch

See Video 21.14.

Light touch is evaluated by lightly touching the patient with a small piece of gauze. Ask the patient to close their eyes and to tell you when the touch is felt. Try touching the patient on the toes and fingers. This is demonstrated in Fig. 21.48. If sensation is normal, continue with the next test. If sensation is abnormal, work proximally until a *sensory level* can be determined. A sensory level is a spinal cord level below which there is a marked decrease in sensation. Fig. 21.49 illustrates the segmental distribution of the spinal nerves that transmit sensation to the spinal cord.

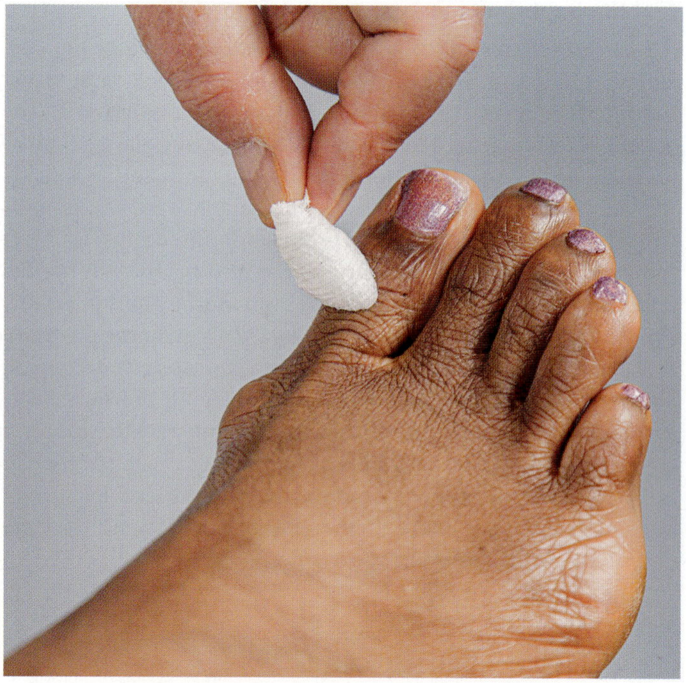

Fig. 21.48 Technique for Testing Light Touch.

Test Pain Sensation

See Video 21.15.

Pain sensation is tested by using a broken applicator stick. Ask the patient to close their eyes. Touch the patient with its pointed, sharp tip. Tell the patient, "This is sharp." Now touch the patient with the blunt, cotton end and say, "This is dull." This is demonstrated in Fig. 21.50. Start testing pain sensation on the toes and fingers and say, "What is this, sharp or dull?" If there is a sensory loss to pain, continue proximally to determine the sensory level.

Test Vibration Sense

See Video 21.16.

Vibration sense is tested using a 128-Hz tuning fork. Tell the patient what you are going to do. Ask the patient to close their eyes. Tap the tuning fork on the heel of your hand. Place the tuning fork on a patient's finger or toenail with your own finger under the patient's finger, as demonstrated in Fig. 21.51A. Instruct the patient to inform you when the vibration is no longer felt. In this manner, you will be able to feel the vibration through the patient's finger to determine the accuracy of the patient's response. After the fingers are tested, test the big toes, as demonstrated in Fig. 21.51B. If there is no loss of vibration sense, proceed with the next examination. If a loss is present, determine the level.

Test Proprioception

See Video 21.17.

Position sense, or proprioception, is tested by moving the distal phalanx. Hold the distal phalanx at its *lateral* aspects, and move the digit up while telling the patient, "This is up." Move the distal phalanx down and tell the patient, "This is down." With the patient's eyes closed, move the distal phalanx up and down and finally stop and ask, "What is this, up or down?" This is demonstrated in Fig. 21.52A. Grasp only the *sides* of the digit so that the patient cannot be clued by the pressure exerted on the digit. It is routine to test the terminal phalanx of a finger on each hand and the terminal phalanx of the toes

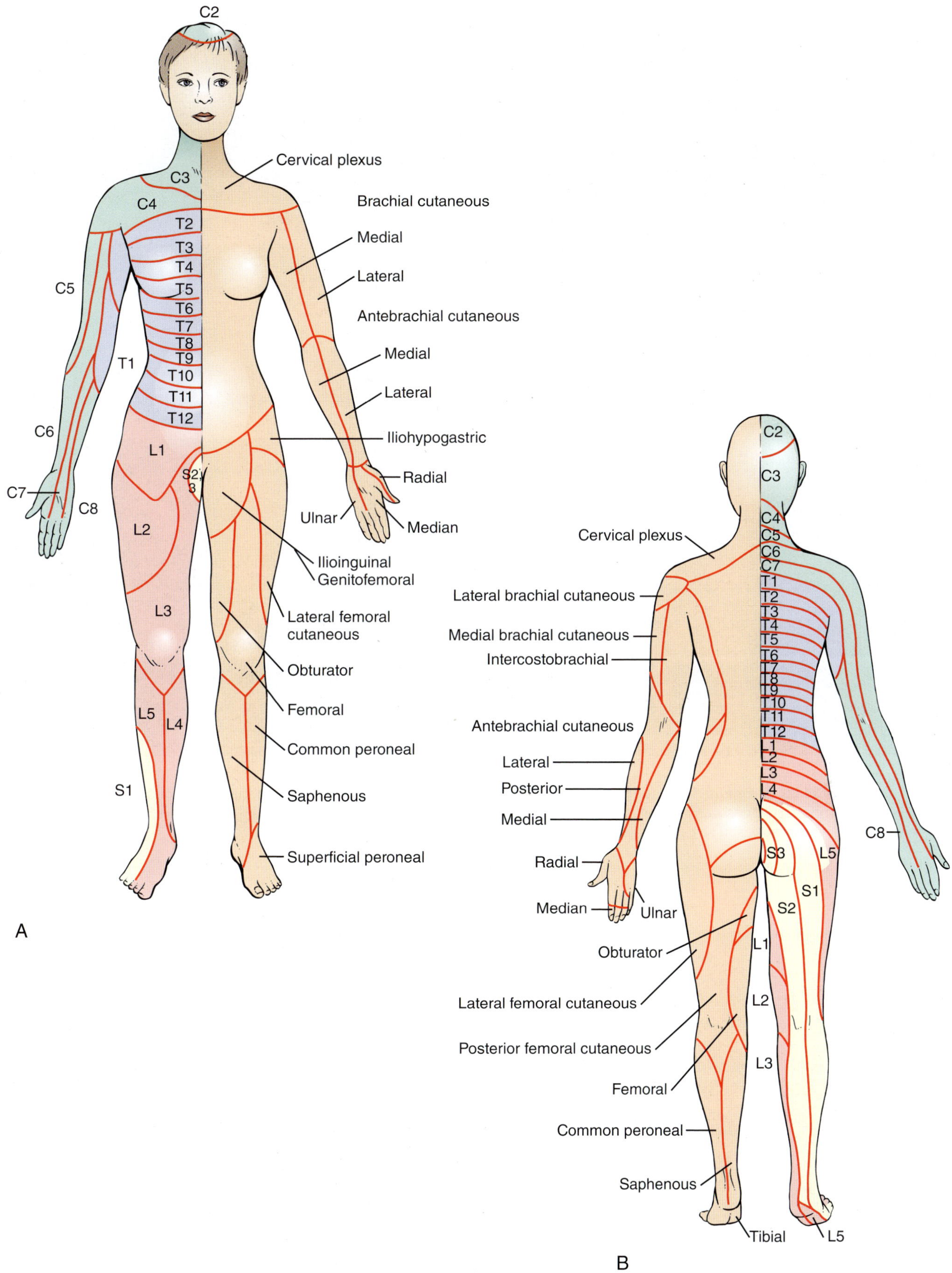

Fig. 21.49 Segmental Distribution of the Spinal Nerves. (A) Distribution in the front. (B) Distribution in the back.

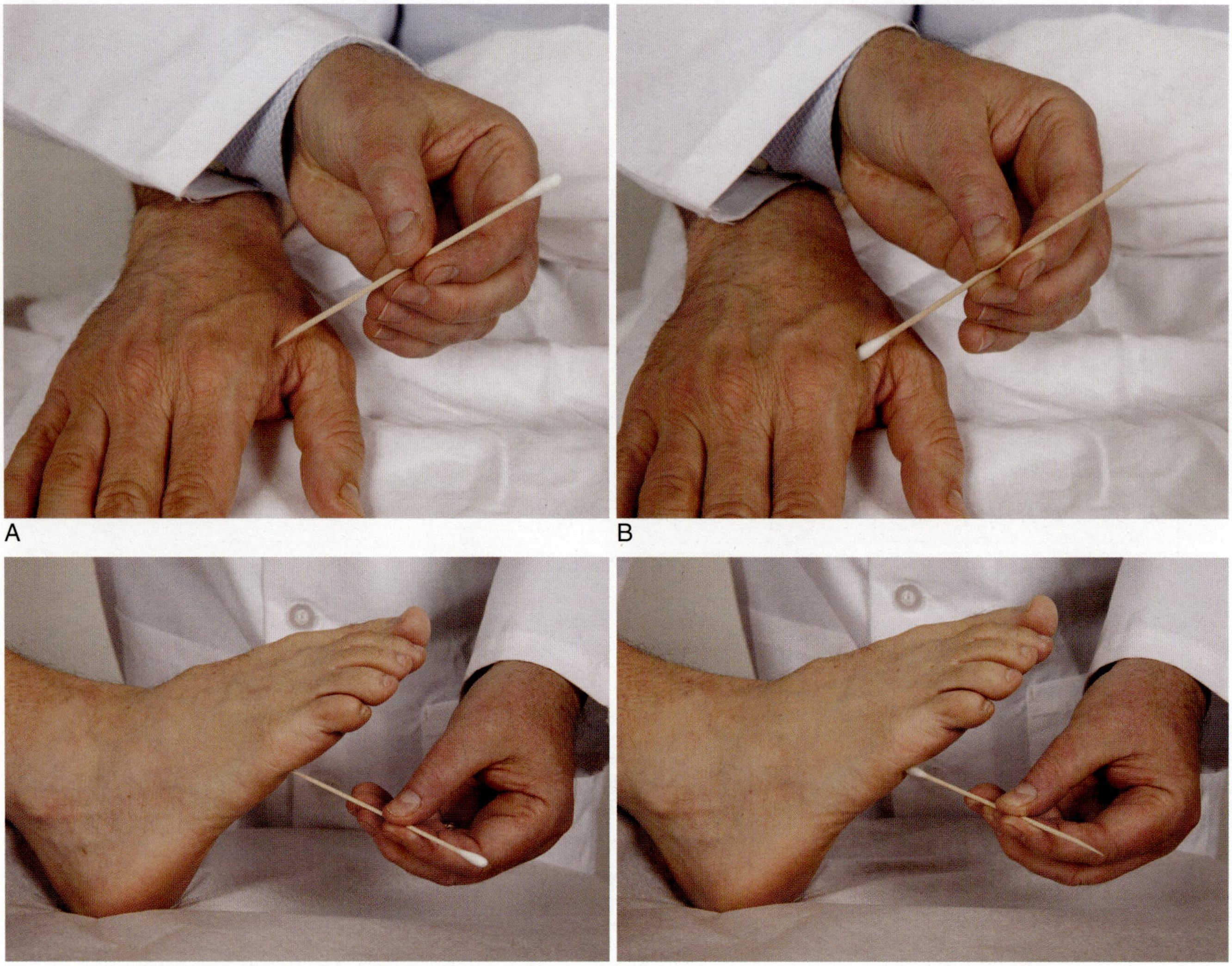

A B C D

Fig. 21.50 Technique for Testing Pain Sensation. (A and C) The examiner should hold the applicator stick as demonstrated and say, "This is sharp." (B) and in (D) The examiner should hold the blunt (cotton) end of the applicator stick and say, "This is dull."

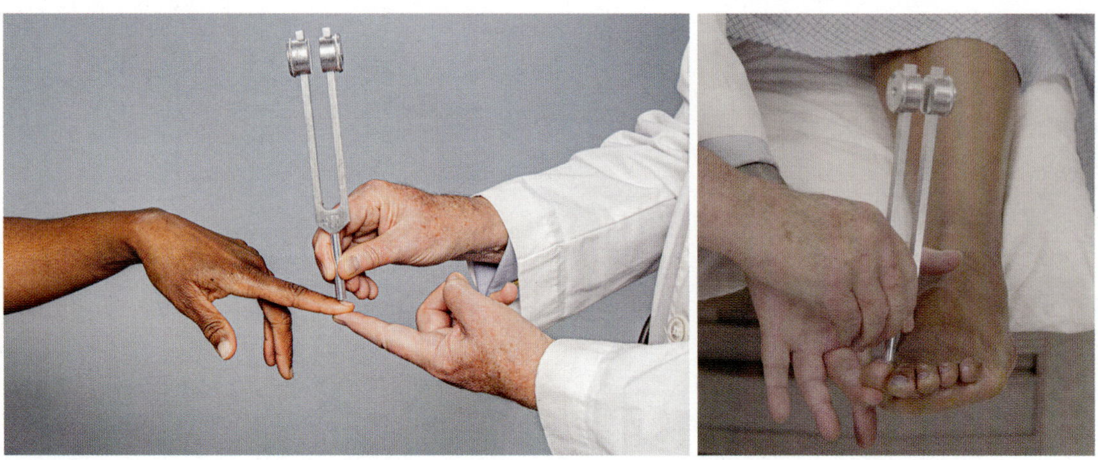

A B

Fig. 21.51 Technique for Testing Vibration Sensation. (A) Correct position for evaluating vibration sensation in the finger. (B) Technique for the toe.

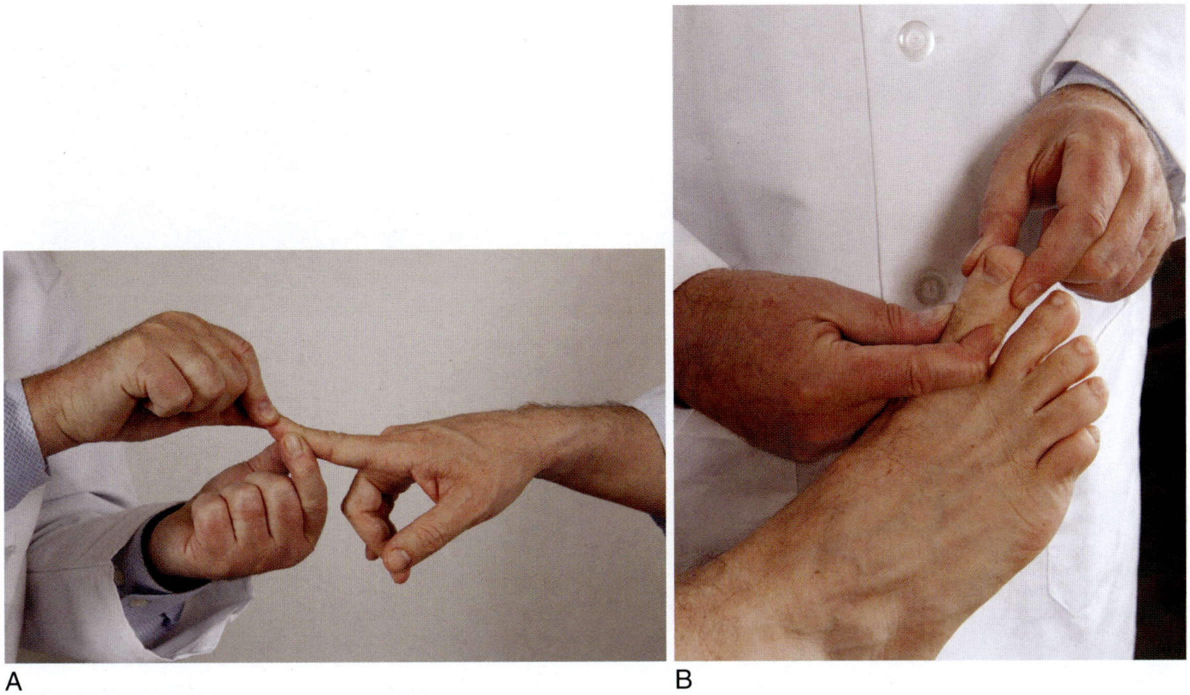

Fig. 21.52 Technique for Testing Proprioception. (A) Correct manner of holding the finger. (B) Technique for holding the toe.

(see Fig. 21.52B). If no loss of position sense is detected, continue with the rest of the examination. A loss of proprioception necessitates further evaluation to determine the level of loss.

Test Tactile Localization

Tactile localization, also known as *double simultaneous stimulation,* is assessed by having the patient close their eyes and identify where your touch was felt. Touch the patient on the right cheek and the left arm. The patient is then asked, "Where did I touch you?" This is demonstrated in Fig. 21.53. Normally, patients have no problem identifying both areas. A patient with a lesion in the parietal lobe may feel the individual touches but may "extinguish" the sensation on the side contralateral to the side of the lesion. This is the phenomenon termed *extinction.*

Test Two-Point Discrimination

Two-point discrimination tests the patient's ability to differentiate one stimulus from two. Gently hold two pins 2 to 3 mm apart and touch the patient's fingertip. Ask the patient to state the number of pins felt. This is demonstrated in Fig. 21.54. Compare this finding with that from the corresponding area on the fingertip of the other hand. Because different areas of the body have different sensitivities, you must know these differences. At the fingertips, two-point discrimination is 2 mm apart. The tongue can discriminate two objects 1 mm apart; the toes, 3 to 8 mm apart; the palms, 8 to 12 mm apart; and the back, 40 to 60 mm apart. A lesion in the parietal lobe impairs two-point discrimination.

Test Stereognosis

Stereognosis is the integrative function of the parietal and occipital lobes. It is tested by having the patient attempt to identify an object placed in the hands. Have the patient close their eyes. Place a key, pencil, paper clip, or coin in the palm of the patient's hand and ask what it is. Test the other hand and compare the findings.

Test Graphesthesia

Graphesthesia is the ability to identify a number "written" in the palm of one's hand. Ask the patient to close their eyes and extend the hand. Use the blunt end of a pencil to "write" numbers from 0 to 9 in the palm. *The numbers should be oriented facing the patient*, as shown in Fig. 21.55. Normally, the patient should be able to identify the numbers. Compare one hand with the other. The inability to identify the numbers is a sensitive sign of parietal lobe disease.

Test Point Localization

Point localization is the ability of a person to point to an area where they were touched. Have the patient close their eyes. Touch the patient. Ask the patient to open the eyes and point to the area touched. Abnormalities of the sensory cortex impair the ability to localize the area touched.

Cerebellar Function

Cerebellar function is tested by the following:

- Finger-to-nose test
- Heel-to-knee test
- Rapid alternating movement
- Romberg test
- Gait assessment

Perform the Finger-to-Nose Test

See Video 21.18.

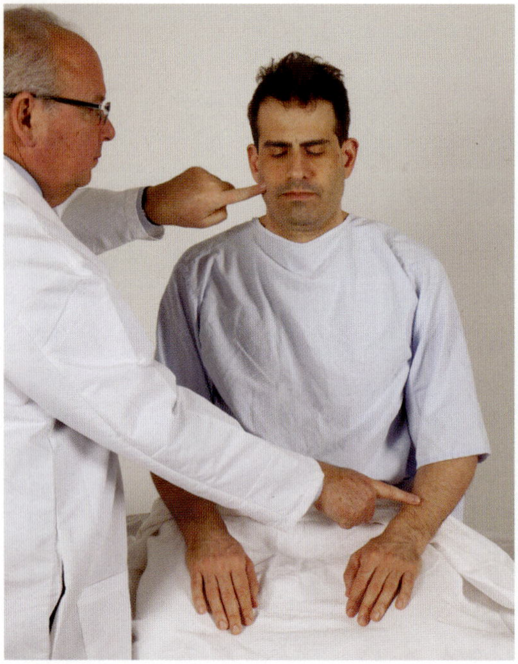

Fig. 21.53 Technique for Testing Tactile Localization.

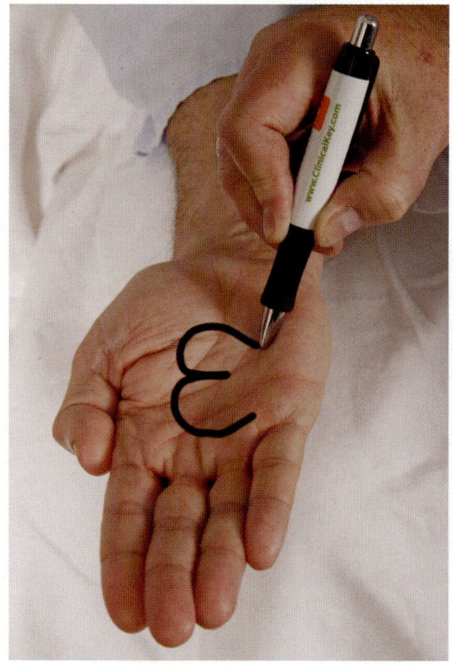

Fig. 21.55 Technique for Testing Graphesthesia.

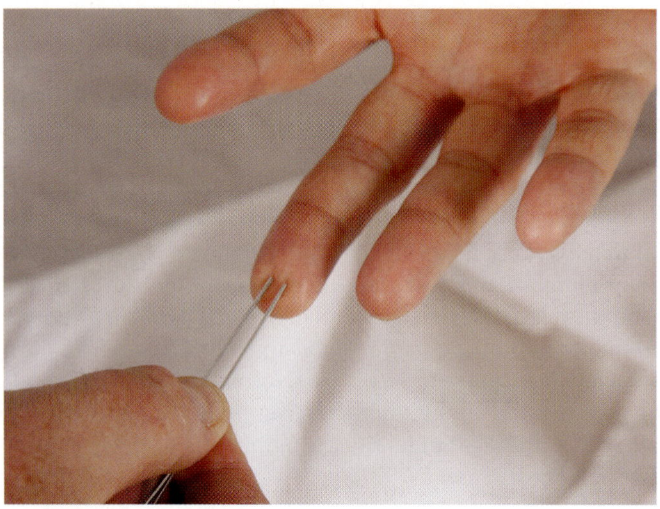

Fig. 21.54 Technique for Testing Two-Point Discrimination.

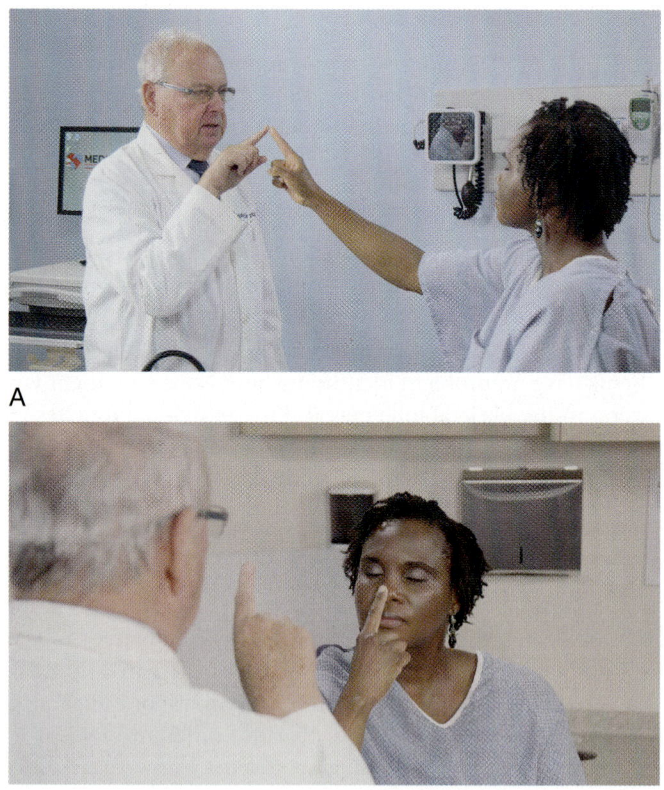

A

B

Fig. 21.56 (A and B) Finger-to-Nose Test.

The finger-to-nose test is performed by asking the patient to touch their own nose and the examiner's finger alternately as quickly, accurately, and smoothly as possible. The examiner holds a finger at arm's length from the patient. The patient is instructed to touch the finger and then the nose. This is repeated several times, after which the patient is asked to perform the test with eyes closed. This is demonstrated in Fig. 21.56. Patients with cerebellar disease persistently overshoot the target, a condition known as *past pointing*. They may also have a tremor as the finger approaches the target.

Perform the Heel-to-Knee Test

The heel-to-knee test is performed by having the patient lie on their back. The patient is instructed to slide the heel of one lower extremity down the shin of the other, starting at the knee. This is demonstrated in Fig. 21.57. A smooth movement should be seen, with the heel staying on the shin. In patients with cerebellar disease, the heel wobbles from side to side.

Assess Rapid Alternating Movements

The ability to perform rapid alternating movements is called *diadochokinesia.* These motions may be tested in the upper extremity or the lower extremity. The patient can be asked to pronate and supinate one hand on the other hand rapidly. Another technique involves having the patient touch the thumb to each finger as quickly as possible. The patient may also be asked to slap the thigh, raise the hand, turn it over, and slap the thigh again rapidly. This pattern is repeated over and over as quickly as possible. These techniques are illustrated in Fig. 21.58. An abnormality in performing rapid alternating movements is called *adiadochokinesia.*

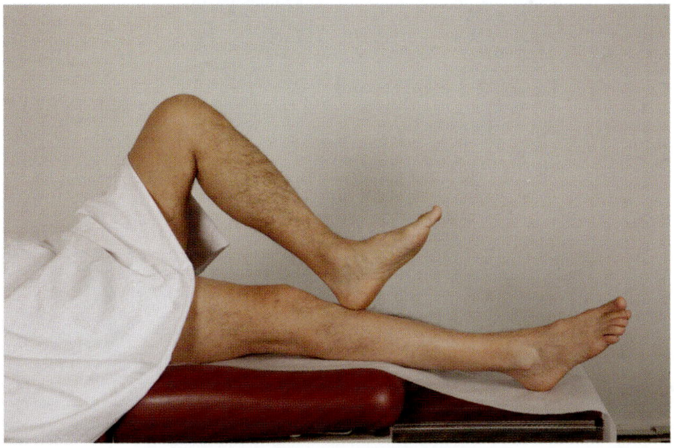

Fig. 21.57 Heel-to-Knee Test.

Perform the Romberg test. See Video 21.19.

The *Romberg test* is performed by having the patient stand in front of the examiner with feet together so that the heels and toes are touching. The examiner instructs the patient to extend the arms with palms facing upward and to close the eyes. If the patient can maintain this posture without moving, the test result is negative. The result is positive if the patient begins to sway and must move their feet for balance. The Romberg test examines the posterior columns rather than actual cerebellar function. The examiner should be at the patient's side during this test because an occasional patient may suddenly sway and fall if assistance is not provided.

Another way to evaluate upper motor function in an awake and responsive patient is by conducting the *pronator drift* test. This can be done with the patient sitting or standing. To perform the test, ask the patient to close their eyes and extend both

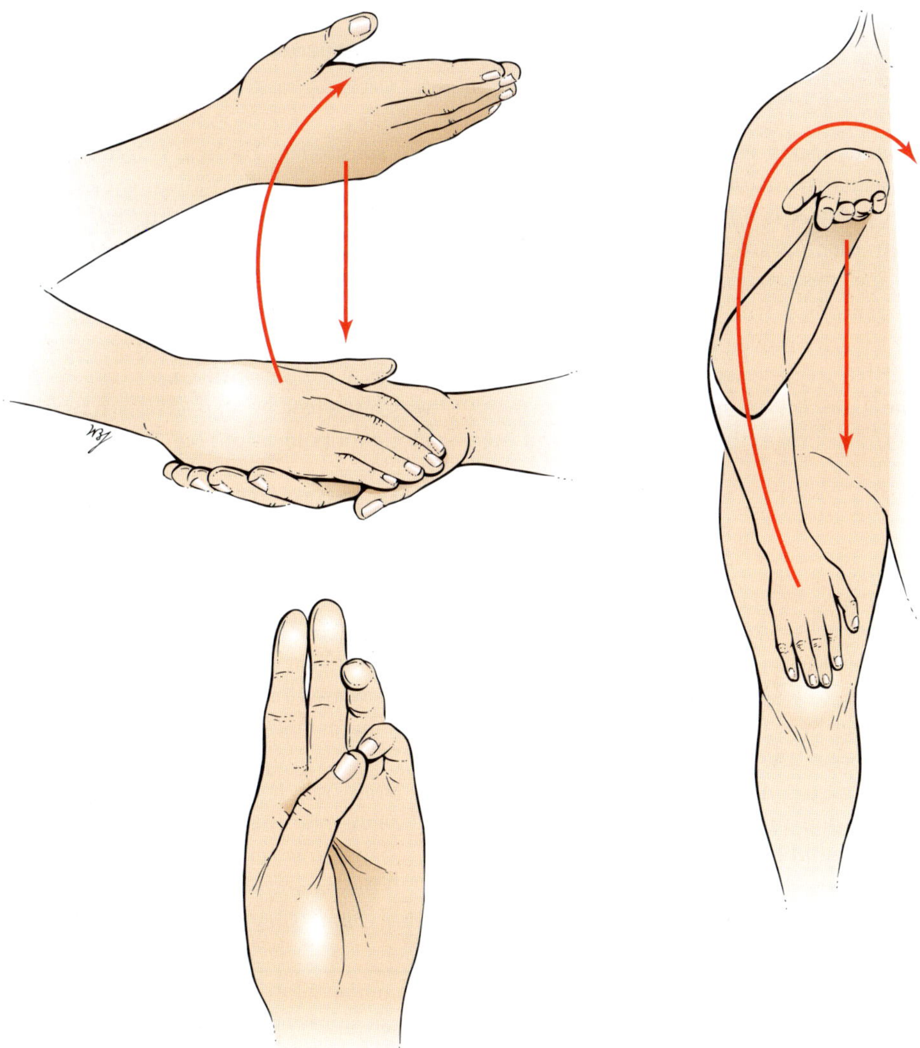

Fig. 21.58 Techniques for Testing Rapid Alternating Movements.

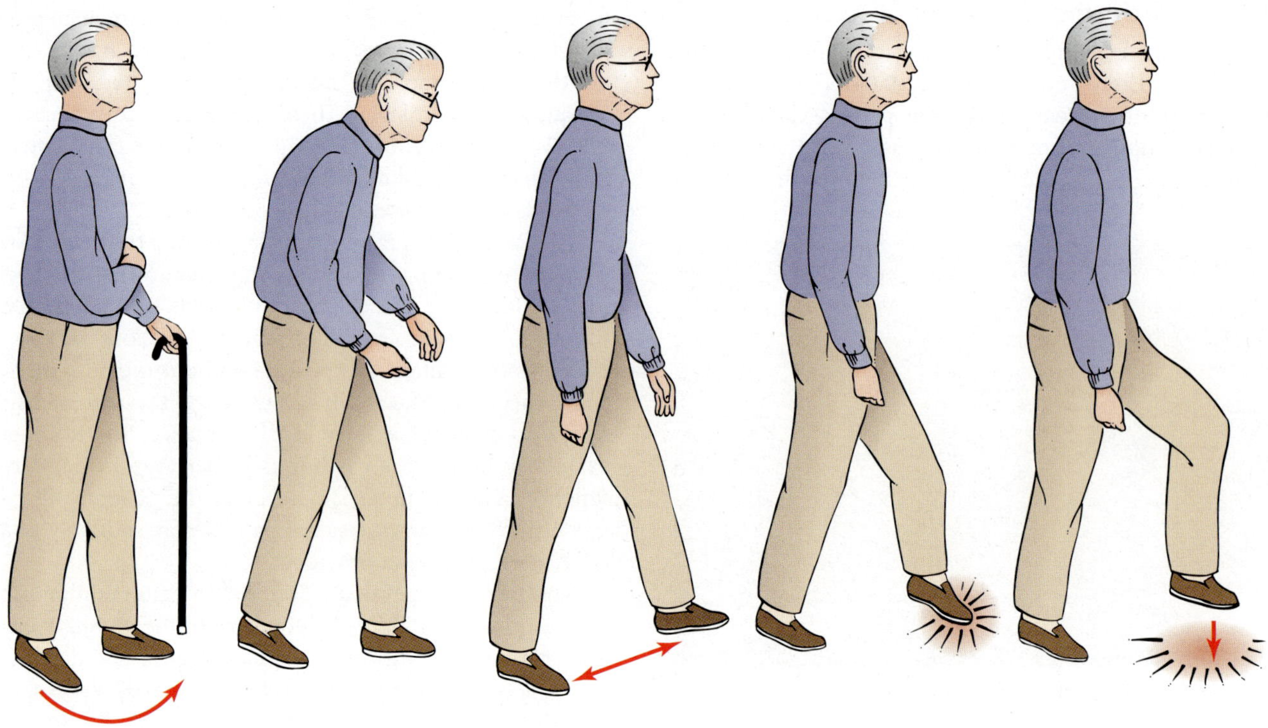

Fig. 21.59 Common Types of Gait Abnormalities.

arms straight out with palms facing up. Observe the arms for 20 to 30 seconds. If both arms are maintained at the same level, it suggests that the motor pathway is unimpaired. On the other hand, if one arm and palm turn inward and downward, it indicates muscle weakness and dysfunction of the corticospinal tract (the upper motor neurons in the brain and spinal cord that control voluntary muscle movement) in the opposite hemisphere. Pronator drift can be caused by conditions like stroke, subdural hematoma, or cervical spinal injury. Be sure to document any signs of pronator drift, the affected arm, and the direction of the drift.

Assess Gait

See Video 20.2.

Foremost in the examination of cerebellar function is the observation of gait. The patient is asked to walk straight ahead while the examiner observes the gait. The patient is then instructed to return on tiptoes, to walk away again on the heels, and to return to the examiner by walking in tandem gait—one foot placed in front of the other, the heel of one foot touching the toes of the other on each step. The examiner may need to demonstrate this gait for the patient. The patient should have a normal posture, and there should be normal associated movements of the arms. The examiner should pay special attention to the way in which the patient turns around. These maneuvers often accentuate cerebellar ataxia, as well as indicate weakness in the lower extremities.

Many neurologic disorders produce striking and characteristic gaits. A *hemiplegic* patient tends to drag or circumduct a weak and spastic leg. The arm is frequently flexed at the elbow across the abdomen as the patient walks. A patient with *Parkinson disease* shuffles with short, hurried steps. The head is bowed, with the back bent over. A patient with *cerebellar ataxia* walks with a wide-based gait. The feet are very far apart as the patient staggers from side to side. A patient with *footdrop* has a characteristic slapping gait resulting from weakness of the dorsiflexors of the ankle. A patient with *sensory ataxia* has a high-stepping gait in which the feet are slapped down firmly as if the person is unsure of the foot's location. Fig. 21.59 illustrates these gaits.

CLINICOPATHOLOGIC CORRELATIONS

The Comatose Patient

Coma is the state in which the patient is unable to respond to any stimuli. The causes of coma include the following:

- Meningeal infection
- Increased intracranial pressure of any cause
- Subarachnoid hemorrhage
- Focal cerebral lesion
- Brainstem lesion affecting the reticular system
- Metabolic encephalopathy[P]
- Status post seizure activity

If the patient's friends or family members are available, speak with them. They can help in the evaluation of the patient by

[P]Common causes include electrolyte abnormalities, endocrine disorders, liver or kidney failure, vitamin deficiencies, poisoning, intoxications, and marked changes in body temperature.

giving valuable information. Is there a history of hypertension, diabetes, epilepsy, substance abuse, or recent head trauma?

If there is any evidence of head trauma, radiographs of the cervical spine must be taken before the examiner moves the patient's neck.

The physical examination of the comatose patient should start with an inspection. The clothing, age, and evidence of chronic illness provide valuable clues as to the cause of the coma. Does the patient have gingival enlargement consistent with antiepileptic medical therapy?[q]

Is there a characteristic odor to the breath? The sweet smell of ketones may be present in diabetic ketoacidosis. An odor of alcohol may be present. Is fetor hepaticus[r] present? Breath that smells of ammonia or urine is known as *azotemia*. This condition is typically caused by severe renal disease. The inability to metabolize three types of amino acids (i.e., leucine, isoleucine, and valine) can cause maple syrup urine disease, in which a person's breath or urine smell like maple syrup or caramelized sugar.

What is the *posture* of the patient? Patients with cerebral hemispheric dysfunction or a destructive lesion of the pyramidal tracts maintain a *decorticate* posture, whereas those patients with a midbrain or pons lesion maintain a *decerebrate* posture. In decorticate rigidity, the arms are adducted, and the elbows, wrists, and fingers are flexed. The legs are internally rotated. In decerebrate rigidity, the arms are also adducted but they are rigidly extended at the elbows, and the forearms are pronated. The wrists and fingers are flexed. In both postures, the feet are plantarflexed. The positions of the arms and hands are shown in Fig. 21.60.

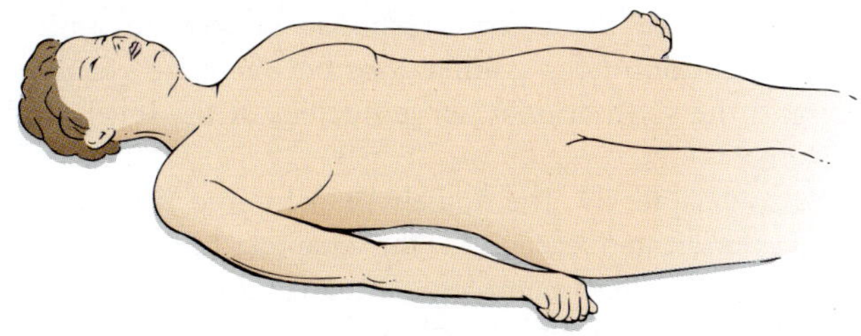

Decerebrate posture

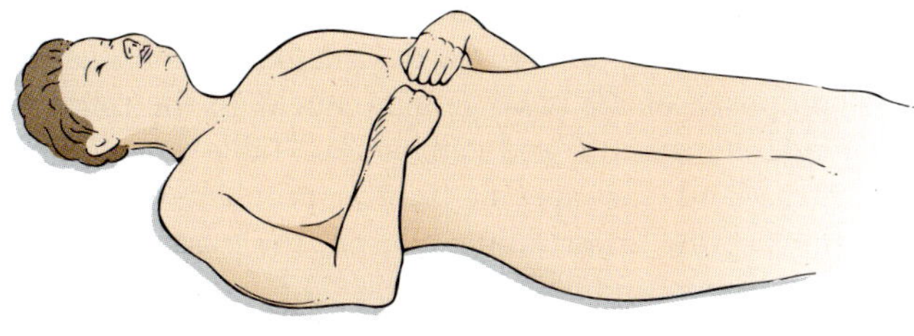

Decorticate posture

Fig. 21.60 Postures of Comatose Patients.

The head should be evaluated for any areas of depression, as in a depressed skull fracture. Does the nose appear broken? Are there any broken teeth? Is there any clear, watery discharge from the nose or ear, suggestive of a leakage of cerebrospinal fluid? Is orbital discoloration (i.e., raccoon eyes) present, suggestive of a basilar skull fracture (see Fig.10.32)?

The *respiratory pattern* should be evaluated. Central neurogenic hyperventilation is seen in lesions of the midbrain or pons. This type of respiration consists of rapid, deep, regular breathing. *Cheyne-Stokes* breathing is characterized by rhythmic changes in the breathing pattern. Periods of rapid breathing are separated by periods of apnea. Cheyne-Stokes breathing is associated with brainstem compression or bilateral cerebral dysfunction and is discussed in Chapter 13, The Chest, as well.

The neurologic examination of the comatose patient is largely based on pupillary size and light reflexes. The pupils are small and reactive in bilateral cerebral dysfunction. They are dilated after an overdose of hallucinogenic agents or central nervous system stimulants. A unilateral fixed and dilated pupil is suggestive of pressure on the ipsilateral oculomotor nerve. Pupillary dilation precedes paralysis of the extraocular muscles; this is because the pupillary nerve fibers are superficial to the fibers innervating the extraocular muscles and are more vulnerable to extrinsic stresses. This is an important sign of uncal herniation. In the presence of normally reactive pupils with an absence of corneal reflexes and absence of extraocular movement, a metabolic abnormality may be the cause of the coma.

The fundus of the eye may provide a clue as to the cause of the coma.

If there is no evidence of a fracture of the cervical spine, *oculocephalic reflexes* should be tested. If a comatose patient's head is rapidly turned to one side while the eyelids are held open, the eyes should move conjugately to the other side. This is the *doll's eyes reflex.* In a patient with a lesion in the brainstem, the doll's eyes reflex is absent. The doll's eyes reflex can be elicited only in a comatose patient because alert individuals fixate on an object and override this reflex.

Caloric stimulation is used to enhance the doll's eyes reflex or to test movements in an individual with a fractured cervical spine. The patient should be placed with the head flexed at 30 degrees. This orients the semicircular canal in a horizontal position. A large-bore syringe is filled with 20 to 30 mL of ice water, and the water is squeezed into one of the external auditory canals. The normal response is the development of nystagmus. Slowly the eyes move conjugately to the ipsilateral side and then move rapidly (nystagmus) back to the midline. The use of cold water causes nystagmus to the opposite side. If warm water is used, the eyes move rapidly toward the side being irrigated. This can easily be remembered by using the mnemonic *COWS*, which stands for "*c*old *o*pposite, *w*arm *s*ame."

[q]Commonly related to phenytoin (Dilantin®) therapy.

[r]Fetor hepaticus is the characteristic breath of patients with severe parenchymal liver disease, which has been said to resemble the odor of a mixture of rotten eggs and garlic. The distinctive smell is produced by volatile organic compounds that build up in the body when the liver is not functioning properly. Dimethylsulfide is believed to be chiefly responsible for the musty smell.

An absence of the caloric response is seen in patients with a disruption of the connections between the vestibular nuclei and the sixth cranial nerve nucleus at the level of the brainstem.

See also Chapter 27, The Acutely Ill or Injured Patient.

As was indicated earlier in the chapter, headache is an important symptom of neurologic disease. Table 21.3 provides a differential diagnosis of headaches.

The correct assessment of a patient's motor activity can help localize the site of a lesion. The term *extrapyramidal* refers to those parts of the motor system that are not directly involved with the pyramidal tracts. The extrapyramidal system is composed of the basal ganglia, nuclei of the midbrain and reticular formation, and cerebellum. Table 21.4 lists the major areas and the specific motor problems associated with lesions of the lower motor neuron, the pyramidal tract, and the extrapyramidal tract. Table 21.5 summarizes the important signs and symptoms in five common chronic neurologic disorders.

A comparison of the effects of upper and lower motor neuron lesions is shown in Table 21.6.

Paraplegia and *quadriplegia* are upper motor neuron defects. They can also involve lower motor neurons. Injury of the spinal cord can produce partial or complete paralysis. In patients with cervical or thoracic lesions, spasticity is present below the level of the lesion, and flaccidity is present in all muscles supplied from reflex arcs at the level of the lesion. In the presence of sacral lesions, a flaccid paralysis results. Table 21.7 summarizes motor involvement in spinal cord lesions.

Often a patient may be concerned of a decreased ability to perform a task. Physical examination may reveal decreased motor strength. Table 21.8 summarizes the major actions of the more common muscles and their corresponding cord segments.

TABLE 21.3 Differential Diagnosis of Headache

Type	Epidemiology	Location	Signs and Symptoms
Migraine	Family history Young adults Female	Bifrontal	Nausea Vomiting Possible neurologic deficits
Cluster	Adolescent male	Orbitofrontal Unilateral	Unilateral nasal congestion Lacrimation
Tension	Female	Bilateral Generalized or occipital	
Hypertensive	Family history	Variable	Hypertensive retinopathy Possible papilledema
Increased intracranial pressure		Variable	Nausea Vomiting Papilledema
Meningitis		Bilateral Often occipital	Nuchal rigidity Fever
Temporal arteritis (see Chapter 25, The Geriatric Patient)	Older adults	Unilateral Over temporal artery	Tender temporal artery Loss of vision in ipsilateral eye

TABLE 21.4 Effects of Various Lesions

Feature	Lower Motor Neuron	Pyramidal Tract	Extrapyramidal Tract
Major effect	Flaccid paralysis	Spastic paralysis Hyperactive reflexes	No paralysis
Muscle appearance	Atrophy Fasciculations	Mild atrophy from disuse	Rest tremor
Muscle tone	Decreased	Increased	Increased
Muscle strength	Decreased or absent	Decreased or absent	Normal
Coordination	Absent or poor	Absent or poor	Slowed

TABLE 21.5 Common Neurologic Conditions and Their Signs and Symptoms

Condition	Age at Onset (Year)	Sex	Signs and Symptoms
Multiple sclerosis	30–35	Female	• Nystagmus • Diplopia • Slurring of speech • Muscular weakness • Paresthesias • Poor coordination • Bowel and bladder dysfunction
Amyotrophic lateral sclerosis	50–80	Male	• Irregular twitching of involved muscles • Muscular weakness • Muscle atrophy (see Fig. 21.21) • Absence of sensory or mental deficits
Parkinson disease	60–80	Male	• Rigidity • Slowing of movements • Involuntary tremor • Difficulty swallowing • Tremor in upper extremities • Jerky, "cogwheel" motions • Slow, shuffling gait with loss of arm swing • Mask-like facial expression • Body in moderate flexion • Excessive salivation
Myasthenia gravis	20–50	Female	• Generalized muscular fatigue • Bilateral ptosis (see Fig. 10.16) • Diplopia • Difficulty swallowing • Voice weakness
Huntington disease	35–50	Both sexes	• Choreiform movements • Dementia • Rapid movements • Facial grimacing • Dysarthria • Personality change

TABLE 21.6 Comparison of Effects of Upper and Lower Motor Neuron Lesions

Effect	Upper Motor Neuron Lesion	Lower Motor Neuron Lesion
Voluntary control	Lost	Lost
Muscle tone	Spastic, increased	Flaccid, decreased
Reflex arcs	Present	Absent
Pathologic reflexes	Present	Not present
Muscle atrophy	Little or none	Significant

TABLE 21.7 Motor Involvement in Spinal Cord Lesions

Affected Cord Segment	Motor Involvement
C1–C4	Paralysis of neck, diaphragm, intercostals, and all four extremities
C5	Spastic paralysis of trunk, arms, and legs; partial shoulder control
C6, C7	Spastic paralysis of trunk and legs; upper arm control; partial lower arm control
C8	Spastic paralysis of trunk and legs; hand weakness only
T1–T10	Spastic paralysis of trunk and legs
T11–T12	Spastic paralysis of legs
L1–S1	Flaccid paralysis of legs
S2–S5	Flaccid paralysis of lower legs; bowel, bladder, and sexual function affected

TABLE 21.8 Motor Function According to Cord Segments

Area of Body	Action Tested	Cord Segment
Shoulder	Flexion, extension, or rotation of neck	C1–C4
Arm	Adduction of arm Abduction of arm Flexion of forearm Extension of forearm Supination of forearm Pronation of forearm	C5–T1 C4–C6 C5–C6 C6–C8 C5–C7 C6–C7
Hand	Extension of hand Flexion of hand	C6–C8 C7–C8, T1
Finger	Abduction of thumb Adduction of thumb Abduction of little finger Opposition of thumb	C7–C8, T1 C8, T1 C8, T1 C8, T1
Hip	Flexion of hip Extension of leg Flexion of leg Adduction of thigh Abduction of thigh Medial rotation of thigh Lateral rotation of thigh Flexion of thigh	L1–L3 L2–L4 L4–L5, S1–S2 L2–L4 L4–L5, S1–S2 L4–L5, S1 L4–L5, S1–S2 L4–L5
Foot	Dorsiflexion of foot Plantar flexion of foot	L4–L5, S1 L5, S1–S2
Toe	Extension of great toe Flexion of great toe Spreading of toes	L4–L5, S1 L5, S1–S2 S1–S2

USEFUL VOCABULARY

Listed here are the specific roots that are important for understanding the terminology related to neurologic diseases.

Root	Pertaining to	Example	Definition
esthe-	feeling	an***esthe***sia	Loss of feeling
-gnosia	recognition	ag***nosia***	Loss of the power to recognize sensory stimuli
myelo-	spinal cord	***myelo***gram	Radiographic study of the spinal cord
-paresis	weakness	hemi***paresis***	Muscular weakness affecting half the body
-plegia	paralysis	ophthalmo***plegia***	Paralysis of the eye muscles
radicul(o)-	spinal nerve root	***radiculo***pathy	Disease of a spinal nerve root

WRITING UP THE PHYSICAL EXAMINATION

Listed here are examples of the write-up for the examination of the neurologic system.

- The patient is oriented to person, time, and place. Cranial nerves II to XII are intact. Motor examination reveals normal gait, normal heel-to-toe movement, and normal strength bilaterally. Reflexes are equal bilaterally and are within normal limits. The sensory examination results are normal, with pain, light touch, and stereognosis intact. Cerebellar function is normal.
- The mental status examination results are within normal limits. There is a marked weakness of the lower half of the right side of the face. The right nasolabial fold is flat, and the mouth droops downward on the right. There is no other cranial nerve abnormality. The motor and sensory examination results are within normal limits. Reflexes are normal. Romberg test result is negative.
- The patient has an expressive aphasia and a right hemiplegia with ipsilateral trigeminal hemiplegia. Reflexes in the right lower extremity are hyperactive in comparison with the left. Sensory examination is difficult to assess. Babinski sign is present on the right side.
- Mental status is within normal limits. Motor examination results and reflexes are equal bilaterally. There is a sensory level at L2 on the right and at L4 on the left. Vibration sense is impaired more on the right than on the left, as is position sense. Romberg test result is positive.

REVIEW QUESTIONS

1. The most common symptoms of neurologic disease include all the following *except:*
 A. Vomiting
 B. Headache
 C. Visual disturbance
 D. Dementia
 E. Pain

2. Regarding loss of consciousness, which statement is most correct?
 A. "Did anyone witness the attack?"
 B. "Were there any symptoms that preceded the attack?"
 C. "Were you told that there were body movements?"
 D. "Can you describe everything you remember after the attack until you felt completely normal?"
 E. All the above

3. All the following diseases can cause "sensory" ataxia *except:*
 A. Syphilis
 B. Vitamin B_{12} deficiency
 C. Multiple sclerosis
 D. Posterior column disease
 E. Hyperthyroidism

4. Which of the statements is correct about tremor?
 A. A tremor is a rhythmic motion of the proximal parts of the limbs or head.
 B. A physiologic tremor oscillates 15–20 cycles per second.
 C. Parkinson disease is the most frequently encountered extrapyramidal movement disorder.
 D. An intention tremor is faster than a physiologic tremor and worsened by exercise.
 E. Multiple sclerosis is not associated with an intention tremor.

5. The mental status exam consists of:
 A. Level of consciousness; speech; orientation
 B. Knowledge of current events; judgment; praxis
 C. Abstraction; vocabulary; emotional responses
 D. Memory; calculation ability; object recognition
 E. All the above

6. "What would you do if you noticed an addressed envelope with an uncanceled stamp on it on the street near a post office?" This question would be a test of:
 A. Judgment
 B. Abstraction
 C. Object recognition
 D. Praxis
 E. Orientation

7. Which pair of cranial nerves and clinical findings is incorrect?
 A. Cranial nerve I – amaurosis
 B. Cranial nerve III – diplopia, ptosis, mydriasis, and loss of accommodation
 C. Cranial nerve IV – diplopia
 D. Cranial nerve VII – loss of taste on anterior 2/3 of tongue; dry mouth; loss of lacrimation
 E. Cranial nerve XII – weakness and wasting of tongue

8. Which of the following statements about reflexes is incorrect?
 A. A 2+ reflex is a brisk response and normal.
 B. The triceps tendon reflex is assessed with the pointed end of the triangular reflex hammer.

C. Contraction of the quadriceps muscle and extension at the knee is a normal patellar tendon reflex.
D. A patient with a depressed Achilles tendon reflex should be asked to kneel on the bed with their feet hanging off the side.
E. The cremasteric superficial reflex has limited clinical significance as it may be absent in 20% of normal males, more in the elderly population.

9. **Cerebellar function is tested by:**
A. Finger-to-nose test
B. Heel-to-shin test
C. Rapid alternating movements
D. Romberg test
E. All of the above

10. **In the differential diagnosis of headache, which of the following pairs is incorrect?**
A. Migraine – bifrontal in location
B. Cluster – adolescent males
C. Tension – bilateral in location
D. Meningitis – nuchal rigidity and fever
E. Increased intracranial pressure – nausea and vomiting

REFERENCES

Available online.

BIBLIOGRAPHY

Available online.

22

Putting the Examination Together

Mark H. Swartz

A physician is not only a scientist or a good technician. He must be more than that—he must have good human qualities. He has to have a personal understanding and sympathy for the suffering of human beings.

Albert Einstein (1879–1955)

THE TECHNIQUES

In the previous chapters, we discussed the various organ systems and the relevant history and physical examinations for each of them. This chapter aims to assist you in combining all the individual examinations into one seamless and comprehensive examination.

To ensure a successful physical examination, it is best to conduct it in an organized and thorough fashion, with minimal movement required from the patient. Mistakes during the examination typically occur due to a lack of organization and thoroughness rather than a lack of knowledge. Mistakes can occur during physical examinations, especially in certain areas. The most common areas where mistakes occur include:

- Technique
- Omission
- Detection
- Interpretation
- Recording

Errors in *technique* are related to a lack of order and organization during the examination, faulty equipment, and poor bedside etiquette. Errors of *omission* are common in examinations of the eye and nose; auscultation of the neck vessels, chest, and heart; palpation of the spleen; rectal and genital examinations; and the neurologic examination. Errors of *detection* are those in which the examiner fails to find abnormalities that are present. The common errors in this category include identifying thyroid nodules, tracheal deviation, abnormal breath sounds, diastolic murmurs, hernias, and abnormalities in the extraocular muscles. Errors in the *interpretation* of findings occur most commonly with tracheal deviation, venous pulses, systolic murmurs, fremitus changes, abdominal tenderness, liver size, eye findings, and reflexes. *Recording* errors often involve inaccurate descriptions of heart size and murmurs, the use of improper terminology, and the use of obscure abbreviations.

Here is a commonly used complete physical examination sequence, but there is no one right way to do the complete examination. Feel free to develop your approach as long as you ensure that a thorough examination is completed by the end of your chosen technique.

When you arrive to see a hospitalized patient, they will likely be lying in bed. After you introduce yourself and gather their medical history, let them know you are ready to begin the physical examination. Remember to always start by washing your hands or using hand sanitizer for hygiene.

To gain a better understanding of the complete physical examination of male and female patients, it is recommended that you watch the video presentations. These videos will assist you in putting the entire examination together.

Patient Lying Supine in Bed

General Appearance

Inspect the patient's facial expression (see Chapter 13, The Chest; Chapter 14, The Heart; Chapter 17, The Abdomen; and Chapter 21, The Nervous System).

Vital Signs (Chapter 14, the Heart)

1. Palpate blood pressure in the right arm.
2. Auscultate blood pressure in the right arm.
3. Auscultate blood pressure in the left arm.[a]

Have Patient Sit Up in Bed

Vital Signs

Check for orthostatic changes in the left arm (see Chapter 14, The Heart).

Have Patient Turn and Sit With Legs Dangling Off Side of Bed

Vital Signs

1. Palpate the radial pulse for rate and regularity (see Chapter 15, The Peripheral Vascular System).
2. Determine the respiratory rate and pattern (see Chapter 13, The Chest).

[a]To rule out coarctation of the aorta, it's important to check the blood pressure in both the upper and lower extremities if the patient is found to be hypertensive in the upper extremities. The patient should be asked to lie face down, and blood pressure is measured in the popliteal fossa (see Chapter 14, The Heart).

Head (Chapter 9, The Head and Neck)

1. Inspect the cranium.
2. Inspect the scalp.
3. Palpate the cranium.

Face (Chapter 8, The Skin, and Chapter 9, The Head and Neck)

1. Inspect the face.
2. Inspect the skin on the face.

Eyes (Chapter 10, The Eye)

1. Assess visual acuity in both eyes.
2. Check visual fields in both eyes.
3. Determine eye alignment in both eyes.
4. Test extraocular muscle function in both eyes.
5. Check the pupillary response to light in both eyes.
6. Test for convergence.
7. Inspect the external eye structures in both eyes.
8. Perform the ophthalmoscopic examination of both eyes.

Nose (Chapter 11, The Ear and Nose)

1. Inspect the nose.
2. Palpate the nasal skeleton.
3. Palpate the sinuses (frontal, maxillary), both sides.
4. Inspect the nasal septum on both sides.
5. Inspect the turbinates on both sides.

Ears (Chapter 11, The Ear and Nose)

1. Inspect the external ear structures on both sides.
2. Palpate the external ear structures on both sides.
3. Evaluate auditory acuity on both sides.
4. Perform the Rinne test on both sides.
5. Perform the Weber test.
6. Perform the otoscopic examination on both sides.
7. Inspect the external canal on both sides.
8. Inspect the tympanic membrane on both sides.

Mouth (Chapter 12, The Oral Cavity and Pharynx)

1. Inspect the outer and inner surfaces of the lips.
2. Inspect the buccal mucosa.
3. Inspect the gingivae.
4. Inspect the teeth.
5. Observe Stensen and Wharton ducts on both sides.
6. Inspect the hard palate.
7. Inspect the soft palate.
8. Inspect the tongue.
9. Test for hypoglossal nerve function (see Chapter 21, The Nervous System).
10. Palpate the tongue.
11. Inspect the floor of the mouth.
12. Palpate the floor of the mouth.
13. Inspect tonsils on both sides.
14. Inspect the posterior pharyngeal wall.
15. Observe the uvula as the patient says "Ah" (see Chapter 21, The Nervous System).
16. Test the gag reflex (see Chapter 21, The Nervous System).

Neck (Chapter 9, The Head and Neck)

1. Inspect the neck on both sides.
2. Palpate the neck on both sides.
3. Palpate the lymph nodes of the head and neck on both sides.
4. Palpate the thyroid gland with the anterior approach.
5. Evaluate the position of the trachea (see Chapter 13, The Chest).

Neck Vessels (Chapter 14, The Heart)

Inspect the height of the jugular venous pulsation on the right side.

Neck[b] (Chapter 9, The Head and Neck)

1. Palpate the thyroid gland with the posterior approach.
2. Palpate for the presence of supraclavicular lymph nodes on both sides.

Posterior Chest (Chapter 13, The Chest)

1. Inspect the back on both sides.
2. Palpate the back for tenderness on both sides.
3. Evaluate chest excursion on both sides.
4. Palpate for tactile fremitus on both sides.
5. Percuss the back on both sides.
6. Evaluate diaphragmatic excursion on the right side.
7. Auscultate the back on both sides.
8. Palpate for the presence of costovertebral angle tenderness on both sides (see Chapter 17, The Abdomen).

Sacrum (Chapter 14, The Heart)

Test for edema.

Anterior Chest[c] (Chapter 13, The Chest)

1. Inspect the patient's posture.
2. Inspect the configuration of the chest.
3. Inspect the chest on both sides.
4. Palpate the chest for tactile fremitus on both sides.

Female Breast (Chapter 16, The Breast)

1. Inspect the breast on both sides.
2. Inspect the breast during maneuvers to tense the pectoral muscles on both sides.

Heart (Chapter 14, The Heart)

1. Inspect for abnormal chest movements.
2. Palpate for the point of maximum impulse.
3. Auscultate for heart sounds in all four positions.

Axilla (Chapter 16, The Breast)

1. Inspect the axilla on both sides.
2. Palpate the axilla on both sides.

[b]The examiner should now go behind the patient while the patient remains seated with legs dangling off the side of the bed.

[c]The examiner should now go in front of the patient while the patient remains seated with legs dangling off the side of the bed.

3. Palpate for epitrochlear nodes on both sides (see Chapter 15, The Peripheral Vascular System).

Have Patient Lean Forward

Heart (Chapter 14, The Heart)

Auscultate with the diaphragm at the cardiac base.

Have Patient Lie Supine With Head of Bed Elevated Approximately 30 Degrees

Neck Vessels (Chapter 14, The Heart)

1. Inspect the jugular venous waveform on the right side.
2. Auscultate the carotid artery on both sides.
3. Palpate the carotid artery, each side separately.

Breasts, Male and Female (Chapter 16, The Breast)

1. Inspect the breast on both sides.
2. Palpate the breast on both sides.
3. Palpate the subareolar area on both sides.
4. Palpate the nipple on both sides.

Chest (Chapter 13, The Chest)

1. Inspect the chest on both sides.
2. Evaluate chest excursion on both sides.
3. Palpate for tactile fremitus on both sides.
4. Percuss the chest on both sides.
5. Auscultate breath sounds on both sides.

Heart (Chapter 14, The Heart)

1. Inspect for movements.
2. Palpate for localized motion in all four positions.
3. Palpate for generalized motion in all four positions.
4. Palpate for thrills in all four positions.
5. Auscultate the heart sounds in all four positions.
6. Time the heart sounds to the carotid pulse.

Have Patient Turn on Left Side

Heart (Chapter 14, The Heart)

Auscultate with the bell at the cardiac apex.

Have Patient Lie Supine With Bed Flat

Abdomen (Chapter 17, The Abdomen)

1. Inspect the contour of the abdomen.
2. Inspect the skin of the abdomen.
3. Inspect for hernias.
4. Auscultate the abdomen for bowel sounds in one quadrant.
5. Auscultate the abdomen for bruits on both sides.
6. Palpate the abdomen lightly in all quadrants.
7. Palpate the abdomen deeply in all quadrants.
8. Percuss the abdomen in all quadrants.
9. Percuss the liver.
10. Percuss the spleen.
11. Test for the superficial abdominal reflex (see Chapter 21, The Nervous System).
12. Check for rebound tenderness.
13. Check for hepatic tenderness.
14. Evaluate for the hepatojugular reflux (see Chapter 14, The Heart).
15. Palpate the liver.
16. Palpate the spleen.
17. Palpate the aorta.
18. Check for shifting dullness if ascites is suspected.

Pulses (Chapter 15, The Peripheral Vascular System)

1. Palpate the radial pulse on both sides.
2. Palpate the brachial pulse on both sides.
3. Palpate the femoral pulse on both sides.
4. Palpate the popliteal pulse on both sides.
5. Palpate the dorsalis pedis pulse on both sides.
6. Palpate the posterior tibial pulse on both sides.
7. Time the radial and femoral pulses on the right side.
8. Perform heel-to-knee test (part of the neurologic examination; see Chapter 21, The Nervous System).

Male Genitalia (Chapter 18, Male Genitalia and Hernias)

1. Inspect the skin and hair distribution.
2. Instruct the patient to bear down and observe the inguinal area.
3. Inspect the penis.
4. Inspect the scrotum.
5. Palpate for inguinal nodes on both sides.
6. Elevate the scrotum and inspect the perineum.

Have Male Patient Stand in Front of Seated Examiner

Male Genitalia (Chapter 18, Male Genitalia and Hernias)

1. Inspect the penis.
2. Inspect the external urethral meatus.
3. Palpate the shaft of the penis.
4. Palpate the urethra.
5. Inspect the scrotum.
6. Palpate the testicle on both sides.
7. Palpate the epididymis and vas deferens on both sides.
8. Instruct the patient to bear down and observe the inguinal area.
9. Test for superficial cremasteric reflex (see Chapter 21, The Nervous System).
10. Transilluminate any masses.
11. Palpate for hernias on both sides.

Have Male Patient Turn Around and Bend Over Bed

Rectum (Chapter 17, The Abdomen)

1. Inspect the anus.
2. Inspect the anus while the patient strains.
3. Palpate the anal sphincter.
4. Palpate the rectal walls.
5. Palpate the prostate gland.
6. Test the stool for occult blood.

Help Female Patient to Lithotomy Position

Female Genitalia (Chapter 19, Female Genitalia)

1. Inspect the skin and hair distribution.
2. Inspect the labia majora.
3. Palpate the labia majora.
4. Inspect the labia minora, clitoris, urethral meatus, and introitus.

5. Inspect the area of Bartholin glands on both sides.
6. Inspect the perineum.
7. Test for pelvic organ prolapse.
8. Perform the speculum examination.
9. Inspect the cervix.
10. Obtain a Pap smear.
11. Inspect the vaginal walls.
12. Perform the bimanual examination.
13. Palpate the cervix and uterine body.
14. Palpate the adnexa, both sides.
15. Palpate the rectovaginal septum.
16. Test the stool for occult blood.

Have Patient Sit on Bed With Legs Off Side

Mental Status

Ask routine questions (see Chapter 1, The Interviewer's Questions; Chapter 21, The Nervous System; and Chapter 25, The Geriatric Patient).

Face (Chapter 21, The Nervous System)

1. Test motor function of the trigeminal nerve on both sides.
2. Test sensory function of the trigeminal nerve on both sides.
3. Test the corneal reflex in both eyes.
4. Test the facial nerve on both sides.
5. Test the spinal accessory nerve on both sides.
6. Test double simultaneous stimulation on both sides.
7. Perform the finger-to-nose test.

Neck

Test the range of motion (see Chapter 20, The Musculoskeletal System).

Hands and Wrists (Chapter 20, The Musculoskeletal System, and Chapter 21, The Nervous System)

1. Inspect the hand and wrist on both sides.
2. Inspect the nails on both sides (see Chapter 8, The Skin).
3. Palpate the shoulder joint on both sides.
4. Palpate the interphalangeal joints on both sides.
5. Palpate the metacarpophalangeal joints on both sides.
6. Test light touch sensation on both sides.
7. Test vibration sense on both sides.
8. Test position sense on both sides.
9. Test object identification on both sides.
10. Test graphesthesia on both sides.
11. Test two-point discrimination on both sides.
12. Assess rapid alternating movements on both sides.

Elbows (Chapter 20, The Musculoskeletal System)

1. Inspect the elbow on both sides.
2. Test range of motion on both sides.
3. Palpate the elbow on both sides.
4. Test the upper extremity strength on both sides.
5. Test the biceps tendon reflex on both sides (see Chapter 21, The Nervous System).
6. Test the triceps tendon reflex on both sides (see Chapter 21, The Nervous System).

Shoulders (Chapter 20, The Musculoskeletal System)

1. Inspect the shoulder on both sides.
2. Test range of motion on both sides.
3. Palpate the shoulder joint on both sides.

Shins

1. Inspect the skin on both sides.
2. Test for edema on both sides (see Chapter 14, The Heart).

Feet and Ankles (Chapters 20, The Musculoskeletal System, and Chapter 21, The Nervous System)

1. Inspect the feet and ankles.
2. Test range of motion on both sides.
3. Palpate the Achilles tendon on both sides.
4. Palpate the metatarsophalangeal joints on both sides.
5. Palpate the metatarsal heads on both sides.
6. Palpate the ankle and foot joints on both sides.
7. Test light touch sensation on both sides.
8. Test vibration sense on both sides.
9. Test position sense on both sides.
10. Test lower extremity strength on both sides.
11. Test ankle reflex on both sides.
12. Test plantar response on both sides.

Knees (Chapters 20, The Musculoskeletal System, and Chapter 21, The Nervous System)

1. Inspect the knee on both sides.
2. Test range of motion on both sides.
3. Palpate the patella on both sides.
4. Perform ballottement of patella if effusion is suspected.
5. Test patellar reflex on both sides.

Have Patient Stand With Back to Examiner

Hips (Chapter 20, The Musculoskeletal System)

1. Inspect the hips.
2. Test range of motion.

Spine (Chapters 20, The Musculoskeletal System, and Chapter 21, The Nervous System)

1. Inspect the spine.
2. Palpate the spine.
3. Test range of motion.
4. Assess gait.
5. Perform the Romberg test.

THE WRITTEN PHYSICAL EXAMINATION

Once the examination has been completed, it is important for the examiner to record all findings of inspection, palpation, percussion, and auscultation in an objective manner. It is recommended to be precise when noting abnormalities, providing specific locations, and, if necessary, using small drawings to better describe shape and location. When expressing the size of a finding, it is best to state it in millimeters or centimeters instead of comparing it to a fruit or nut, as these items can vary significantly in size.

Most abbreviations[d] should be avoided, as they could have different meanings for different readers. However, the abbreviations used in the following write-ups are standard and can generally be used.

Finally, it is advised not to include diagnostic statements in the write-up and instead save them for the summary at the end. For instance, it is better to indicate that "a grade III/VI holosystolic murmur at the apex with radiation to the axilla" is present rather than stating "a murmur of mitral insufficiency" is heard.

Patient: John Michaelson[e]

General appearance: The patient is a 65-year-old male who is lying in bed on two pillows and is in no acute distress. He is well-developed, thin, and appears slightly older than his stated age. The patient is well-groomed, alert, and cooperative.

Vital signs: Blood pressure (BP), 185/65/55 right arm (lying), 180/60/50 left arm (lying), 175/65/50 left arm (sitting); heart rate, 90 and regular; respirations, 16.

Skin: Pink, with small hyperkeratotic papules over the face; nail beds slightly dusky; hair thin on head; hair absent on lower portion of lower extremities; normal male escutcheon (distribution of pubic hair).

Head: Normocephalic without evidence of trauma; no tenderness present.

Eyes: Visual acuity with glasses using near card: right eye (OD), 20/80, left eye (OS) 20/40; visual fields full bilaterally; extraocular movements (EOMs) intact; pupils are equal, round, and reactive to light and to accommodation (PERRLA); xanthelasma present bilaterally, L > R; eyebrows normal; bilateral arcus senilis present; conjunctivae without injection; opacities present in both lenses, R > L; left disc sharp with normal cup-disc ratio; normal arteriovenous (AV) ratio OS; no AV nicking present OS; there is a flame-shaped hemorrhage at the 6 o'clock position OS; several cotton-wool spots are also present at the 1 and 5 o'clock positions OS; right fundus not well visualized as a result of lenticular opacity.

Ears: Pinnae in normal position; no tenderness present; a small amount of cerumen in the left external canal; canals without injection or discharge; Rinne test, BC > AC right ear, AC > BC left ear; Weber test, lateralization to the right ear; both tympanic membranes are gray without injection; normal landmarks seen bilaterally.

Nose: Nose straight without masses; patent bilaterally; mucosa pink with a clear discharge present; inferior turbinate on the right slightly edematous.

Sinuses: No tenderness detected over frontal and maxillary sinuses.

Throat: Lips slightly cyanotic without lesions; patient wears an upper denture; buccal mucosa pink without injection; all lower teeth are present and are in fair condition; no obvious caries; gingivae normal; tongue midline without fasciculations; no lesions seen or palpated on tongue; mild injection of the posterior pharynx with yellowish-white discharge present on posterior pharynx and tonsils; tonsils minimally enlarged; uvula elevates in the midline; gag reflex intact.

Neck: Supple with full range of motion; trachea midline; small (1- to 2-cm) lymph nodes are present in superficial cervical and tonsillar node chains; thyroid borders palpable; no thyroid nodules or enlargement noted; no abnormal neck vein distention present; neck veins flat while the patient is sitting upright.

Chest: Anteroposterior (AP) diameter increased; symmetrical excursion bilaterally; tactile fremitus normal bilaterally; chest resonant bilaterally; vesicular breath sounds bilaterally; coarse breath sounds with occasional crackles present at the bases.

Breasts: Mild gynecomastia, L > R; no masses or discharge present.

Heart: Point of maximum impulse, sixth intercostal space (PMI 6ICS) 2 cm lateral to midclavicular line (MCL); normal physiologic splitting present; no heaves or thrills are present; S_1 and S_2 distant; a grade II/VI high-pitched holodiastolic murmur is heard at the 2ICS at the right upper sternal border; a grade I/VI medium-pitched systolic crescendo-decrescendo murmur is heard in the aortic area; the systolic murmur is mid-peaking (Fig. 22.1).

Vascular: A carotid bruit is present on the right; no bruits are heard over the left carotid, renal, femoral, or abdominal

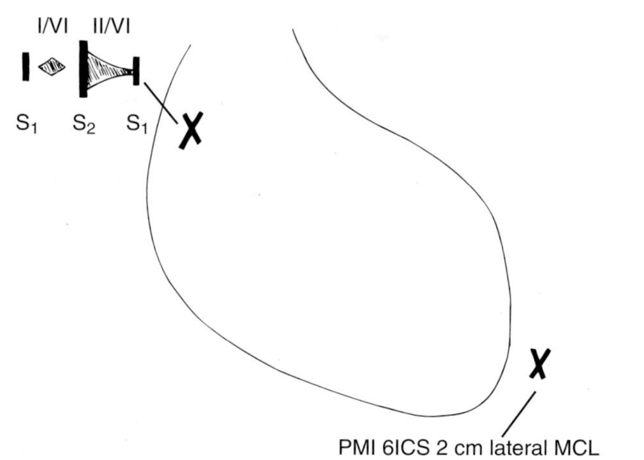

Fig. 22.1 Location of Cardiac Physical Signs. *MCL*, Midclavicular line; *PMI 6ICS*, point of maximum impulse, sixth intercostal space.

---

[d]The widespread use of medical abbreviations is a growing concern as it may endanger patient safety. Medical abbreviations have been in use for almost two centuries, initially limited to prescriptions but are now commonly used in all forms of medical documentation. The practice of using medical abbreviations has become so deeply ingrained in healthcare that even novice healthcare students are accustomed to using them. One of the problems is that healthcare professionals in different fields of medicine may use the same abbreviations to mean different things, leading to misunderstandings and potential harm to patients. For example, "*PND*" is commonly used to mean paroxysmal nocturnal dyspnea, but it is also used to mean post-nasal drip! To address this issue, The Joint Commission, which is the nation's oldest and largest standards-setting and accrediting body in healthcare, now mandates healthcare institutions to create a list of approved and not approved medical abbreviations. To ensure patient safety, **it is always best to write out medical terms in full.**

[e]This name is fictitious. Any similarity to any person living or dead with this name is purely coincidental.

arteries; lower extremities are slightly cool in comparison with upper extremities; 1+ pretibial edema is present on the right lower extremity; 2+ pretibial edema is present on the left; mild venous varicosities are present from midthigh to calf bilaterally; no ulceration or stasis changes are present; no calf tenderness is present.

Abdomen: The abdomen is scaphoid; a right lower quadrant (RLQ) appendectomy scar and a left lower quadrant (LLQ) herniorrhaphy scar are present; both scars are well healed; a 3 × 3 cm mass is seen in the RLQ after coughing or straining; no guarding, rigidity, or tenderness is present; no visible pulsations are present; bowel sounds are present; percussion note is tympanitic throughout the abdomen except over the suprapubic region, where the percussion note is dull; liver span is 10 cm from top to bottom in the MCL; spleen percussed in left upper quadrant but not palpated; kidneys not felt; no costovertebral angle tenderness (CVAT) present; an easily reducible right indirect inguinal hernia is felt at the external ring.

Rectal: Anal sphincter normal; no hemorrhoids present; nontender prostate enlarged symmetrically; prostate firm without nodules felt; no luminal masses felt in rectum; stool negative for blood.

Genitalia: Circumcised male with normal genitalia; penis without induration; left hemiscrotum 4 to 5 cm below the right; palpation of left hemiscrotum reveals dilation of the pampiniform plexus; soft testes 2 × 3 × 1 cm bilaterally.

Lymphatic: Nodes in anterior triangle chains already noted; two firm, 1- to 2-cm, rubbery, freely mobile nodes in left femoral area; no epitrochlear, axillary, or supraclavicular nodes felt.

Musculoskeletal: Distal interphalangeal joint enlargement on both hands, causing pain on making a fist, L > R; no tenderness or erythema present; proximal joints normal; neck, arms, hips, knees, and ankles with full range of active and passive motion; muscles appear symmetrical; mild kyphosis present.

Neurologic: Oriented to person, place, and time; cranial nerves I to XII intact; gross sensory and motor strength intact; cerebellar function normal; plantar reflexes down; gait normal; deep tendon reflexes as shown in Table 22.1.

Summary: Mr. Michaelson is a 65-year-old male in no acute distress. Physical examination reveals systolic hypertension, retinal changes suggestive of sustained hypertension, a mild cataract in his right eye, a conductive hearing loss in his right ear, tonsillopharyngitis, and gynecomastia. Cardiac examination reveals aortic insufficiency. Peripheral vascular examination reveals possible atherosclerotic disease of the right carotid artery and mild venous disease of the lower extremities. The patient has a right, easily reducible inguinal hernia. A left-sided varicocele is present. Mild osteoarthritis of the hands is also present.

TABLE 22.1 Deep Tendon Reflexes of Patient John Michaelson

Side	Biceps	Triceps	Knee	Achilles
Right	1+	0	2+	1+
Left	2+	1+	3+	2+

Patient: Martha Green[f]

General appearance: The patient is a 51-year-old female in bed with moderate respiratory distress. She is overweight and appears to be her stated age. She is well-groomed and alert, but she is constantly concerned about her shortness of breath.

Vital signs: BP, 130/80/75 right arm (lying), 125/75/70 left arm (lying), 120/75/70 (sitting); heart rate, 100 and regular; respirations, 20.

Skin: Upper extremities slightly dusky compared to lower extremities; good tissue turgor; patient is wearing a wig to cover her marked total baldness; normal female escutcheon.

Head: Normocephalic without evidence of trauma; face appears edematous; no tenderness noted.

Eyes: Visual acuity using the near card: OD, 20/40, OS, 20/30; visual fields full bilaterally; EOMs intact; PERRLA; eyebrows thin bilaterally; conjunctivae red bilaterally with injection present; lenses clear; both discs appear sharp with some nasal blurring; the cup-disc ratio is 1:3 bilaterally, and the cups are symmetrical; the retinal veins appear dilated bilaterally.

Ears: Pinnae in normal position; no mastoid or external canal tenderness; canals without injection or discharge; Rinne test, AC > BC bilaterally; Weber test, no lateralization; both tympanic membranes clearly visualized; normal landmarks seen bilaterally.

Nose: Straight without deviation; mucosa reddish-pink; inferior turbinates within normal limits.

Sinuses: No tenderness detected.

Throat: Lips cyanotic; all teeth present except for all third molars, which have been extracted; occlusion normal; no caries seen; gingivae normal; tongue midline with markedly dilated tortuous veins on undersurface; no fasciculations of tongue noted; posterior pharynx appears within normal limits; uvula midline and elevates normally; gag reflex intact.

Neck: Full with normal range of motion; trachea midline; neck veins distended to the angle of the jaw while sitting upright; no neck adenopathy noted.

Chest: AP diameter normal; symmetrical excursion bilaterally; increased tactile fremitus at right base posteriorly corresponds to area of bronchial breath sounds; percussion note in this area is dull, all other chest areas are resonant; bronchophony and egophony present in area of bronchial breath sounds; crackles and wheezes present in area at right posterior base.

Breasts: Left mastectomy scar; right breast without masses, dimpling, or discharge.

Heart: PMI 5ICS MCL; normal physiologic splitting present; no heaves or thrills present; S_1 and S_2 within normal limits; no murmurs, gallops, or rubs present.

Vascular: There are no bruits present over the carotid, renal, femoral, or abdominal arteries; the extremities are without clubbing or edema.

[f]This name is fictitious. Any similarity to any person living or dead with this name is purely coincidental.

Abdomen: The abdomen is obese without guarding, rigidity, or tenderness; no visible pulsations are present; bowel sounds are normal; percussion note is tympanitic throughout the abdomen; liver span is 15 cm in the MCL; spleen not percussed or palpated; kidneys not palpated; no CVAT present.

Rectal: Refused.

Pelvic: Deferred until the patient is more stable.

Lymphatic: No adenopathy felt in the neck chains or in the epitrochlear, axillary, supraclavicular, or femoral regions.

Musculoskeletal: Marked edema of both upper extremities, L > R; neck, arms, knees, and ankles with full range of active and passive motion; muscles appear symmetrical except for upper extremities.

Neurologic: Oriented to person, place, and time; cranial nerves I to XII intact; gross sensory and motor strength intact; cerebellar function normal; plantar reflex down bilaterally; deep tendon reflexes as shown in Table 22.2.

TABLE 22.2 **Deep Tendon Reflexes of Patient Martha Green**

Side	Biceps	Triceps	Knee	Achilles
Right	2+	2+	2+	1+
Left	2+	1+	2+	2+

Summary: Ms. Green is a 51-year-old female, status post left mastectomy, in moderate respiratory distress. She is cyanotic and has evidence of vascular engorgement of the upper half of her body. Her trachea is fixed to the mediastinum. Chest examination reveals evidence of consolidation of the right lower lobe of her lung.

BIBLIOGRAPHY

Available online.

SECTION 4

Evaluating Specific Patients

23

The Pregnant Patient

Mark H. Swartz and Barbara Deli

My mother groaned, my father wept, into the dangerous world I leapt.

William Blake (1757–1827)

GENERAL CONSIDERATIONS

Patients often seek healthcare professionals for pregnancy confirmation and diagnosis. At some point in their reproductive years, the vast majority of females will be pregnant and give birth. The percentage of females in the United States who have ever given birth has been increasing. In 2015–19, 84% of females have given birth over their lifetime compared with 80% in 2006. The average number of children born per 1000 females aged 15–44 years old in the United States has been decreasing from 68.5 in 2006 to 56.1 in 2022. In the United States, 45% of pregnancies in 2011 were unintended. Although this number has decreased from 51% in 2008, it is still relatively high. Due to this high rate of unplanned pregnancy, many patients may not have received preconception care. It is ideal for patients to visit their healthcare professional prior to conceiving to optimize their health and increase the chances of a successful pregnancy outcome. However, due to the high rate of unintended pregnancy, patients may seek medical care after discovering they are pregnant or before realizing they are pregnant.

When interviewing a patient of reproductive age, always consider pregnancy. **With any reproductive-aged patient who is sexually active, pregnancy should always be considered.** It's important to keep in mind that pregnancy should be considered as a possibility in any patient at risk for pregnancy, even if they have had recent menses, since up to 25% of pregnant patients may experience bleeding during their first trimester. Thus, when evaluating reproductive-aged patients, always keep ***Think pregnancy*** as your motto. It's crucial to be mindful of this as the diagnosis and treatment of medical or surgical problems in a pregnant patient can have an impact on the developing fetus. As discussed later in this chapter, many of the symptoms of pregnancy are nonspecific and can be interpreted erroneously if pregnancy is not recognized. During early pregnancy, urinary frequency can be easily mistaken for cystitis, which can lead to an incorrect diagnosis and the patient receiving an antibacterial agent that is not ideal for the developing fetus, such as sulfonamide or quinolone. If the urinary symptoms persist despite the medication, the patient may be referred for intravenous pyelography, which can result in unnecessary tests, wasteful spending on healthcare, and increased radiation risk during early pregnancy.

When discussing a patient's pregnancy and reproductive history, it is crucial to respect their privacy. While it is common for patients to bring their partner or family member to prenatal appointments, it is important to have a one-on-one conversation with the patient to gather their gynecologic and social history. This conversation requires trust and privacy between the healthcare professional and the patient. During the discussion, topics such as prior pregnancy histories and outcomes, possible history of sexually transmitted infections, history of abuse, mental health issues, and ambivalence about the pregnancy may come up. As the discussion can uncover complex and unresolved issues, it is necessary to have resources for support such as social workers and therapists readily available.

GENDER-INCLUSIVE LANGUAGE

It is crucial to understand how to use gender-inclusive language when caring for pregnant patients, as many individuals with a uterus, including females, transgender males, and non-binary individuals, can and do become pregnant. Assuming that gender identity aligns with the sex recorded at birth *(cisnormativity)* can lead to discomfort and systemic discrimination against transgender individuals.

An increasing number of transgender and non-binary individuals are choosing to become gestational parents. An article published in 2021 in the *International Journal of Transgender Health* reported that out of 1694 eligible transgender, nonbinary, and gender-expansive people who responded to a survey in the United States, 210 (12%) had been pregnant. Of these, 115 (55%) had one prior pregnancy, 47 (22%) had two prior pregnancies, and 48 (23%) had three or more prior pregnancies.[1]

Mainstream institutions in the United States, such as the American Civil Liberties Union and the Centers for Disease Control and Prevention, are increasingly adopting gender-neutral language when referring to pregnancy. Terms like "pregnant people" or "birthing parents" are being used instead of "women" or "females" to be inclusive of transgender and non-binary individuals who become pregnant. This shift in language reflects an effort to acknowledge and affirm the diverse identities and experiences of people and families. It is important to use inclusive language when discussing pregnancy as it recognizes that not only cisgender females can become pregnant. Inclusive language is about accepting and validating the experiences of others.

See Chapter 26, The Transgender Patient, for more information on this subject.

STRUCTURE AND PHYSIOLOGIC CHARACTERISTICS

The anatomy and the physiologic changes related to the menstrual cycle that occur in the nonpregnant patient have already been discussed. This chapter reviews the physiologic alterations resulting from pregnancy and the functional pelvic anatomy.

Basic Physiologic Characteristics of Reproduction

After ejaculation, sperm travels through the cervix and uterus and into the fallopian tubes. If an egg is present, fertilization may occur. However, most of the sperm die within 1 to 2 hours due to the normal acidic environment of the vagina. The sperm are helped in their journey by uterine and tubal contractions and favorable mucous conditions.

The fertilized ovum, or zygote, remains in the fallopian tube for approximately 3 days. While in the tube, the fertilized ovum divides repeatedly to form a round mass of cells called the *morula.* If there is an obstruction in the fallopian tube, the fertilized ovum may become trapped in the tube and attach itself to the lining of the tube, giving rise to an *ectopic,* or *tubal, pregnancy.* In a normal pregnancy, approximately 6 to 8 days after fertilization, the morula becomes a *blastocyst,* which migrates through the tube into the uterus, where it attaches itself to the endometrium *(implantation),* with the inner cell mass adjacent to the endometrial surface. Substances that destroy the surface epithelial cells are released, allowing the blastocyst to burrow into the endometrium. The endometrium then grows over the invading blastocyst.

The primitive *chorion,* the combination of *trophoblast* and primitive *mesoderm,* secretes a luteinizing hormone known as *human chorionic gonadotropin (hCG),* which controls the corpus luteum and inhibits pituitary gonadotropic activity. Quickly thereafter, as the invasion proceeds, maternal venous blood vessels are tapped to form lakes of blood, and *chorionic villi* develop. These can be identified as early as the 12th day after fertilization. These villi develop a leafy appearance and are called the *chorion frondosum.* By the 15th day after fertilization, the maternal arterial vessels are tapped, and by the 17th to 18th day, a functioning placental circulation is established. At term, the uteroplacental blood flow is estimated to be approximately 550 to 705 mL/minute. Fig. 23.1A illustrates the path of sperm, fertilization, and implantation.

Decidua is the name given to the endometrium of pregnancy. There are three types, distinguished by location with regard to the growing embryo. The *decidua capsularis* is the overlying endothelium that covers the conceptus, and the *decidua basalis* is the decidual tissue lying between the blastocyst and the myometrium. The decidua of the remainder of the endometrial cavity is the *decidua vera.* A cross-section through the pregnant uterus and the different types of decidua in early pregnancy are illustrated in Fig. 23.1B and C.

One of the first placental hormones produced by the developing trophoblastic tissue is *hCG.* This hormone is present as early as the 8th day after fertilization has taken place. The titers increase to a maximal level by about the 60th to 70th days after fertilization and then decrease. The primary function of hCG is to maintain the corpus luteum during the first 2 months of pregnancy until the placenta can produce enough progesterone by itself. Other hormones, such as human placental lactogen, human chorionic thyrotropin, adrenocorticotropic hormone, and estrogens are also produced by the placenta. It is beyond the scope of this book to discuss the actions of these hormones; the reader is referred to the references for this chapter for further information.

Functional Anatomy of Birth

The pelvic cavity is bounded above by the plane of the *brim* (the inner sacral promontory to the upper and inner borders of the symphysis pubis), below by the plane of the *outlet* (the lower and inner borders of the symphysis pubis to the end of the sacrum or coccyx), posteriorly by the sacrum, laterally by the sacrosciatic ligaments and ischial bones, and anteriorly by the pubic rami.

The birth canal, through which the fetus is delivered, may be thought of as a cylindrical passage with walls composed partially of hard parts (the bony pelvis) and partially of soft parts (the muscles of the pelvic floor and the pelvic ligaments). The cross-section of the cylinder is oval, rather than circular, to accommodate the oval cross-section of the entering fetal part (e.g., the head) as it descends through the pelvis as a result of the expulsive effect of uterine contractions.

This mechanism for delivery and its corresponding anatomy would be easily understood were it not for the fact that the long axis of the schematic oval, which lies transversely at the entrance to the pelvis, comes to lie in the anteroposterior axis in the midpelvis. The entering fetal part must therefore descend in a spiral path as it progresses through the birth canal.

The process of birth varies greatly, depending on the relationships—lie, presentation, attitude, and position—of the fetus to the maternal anatomy. It is important to define these relationships accurately to understand the birth process.

The term *lie* refers to the relation of the long axis of the fetus to that of the patient. In more than 99% of full-term pregnancies, the lie is in the same plane as or parallel to the long axis of the patient; this is called a *longitudinal lie.* In rare instances, the long axis of the fetus is perpendicular to the maternal pelvis; this is called a *transverse lie.*

The term *presentation* refers to the part of the fetus in the lower pole of the uterus overlying the pelvic brim (e.g., cephalic or vertex, breech, shoulder) that can be felt through the cervix. The fetus is in the cephalic or vertex presentation (head first) in approximately 95% of all labors. In most cases, the occipital fontanelle is the *presenting part.*

The *attitude* of the fetus is the posture of the fetus: flexion, deflexion, or extension. Fig. 23.2 illustrates these postures.

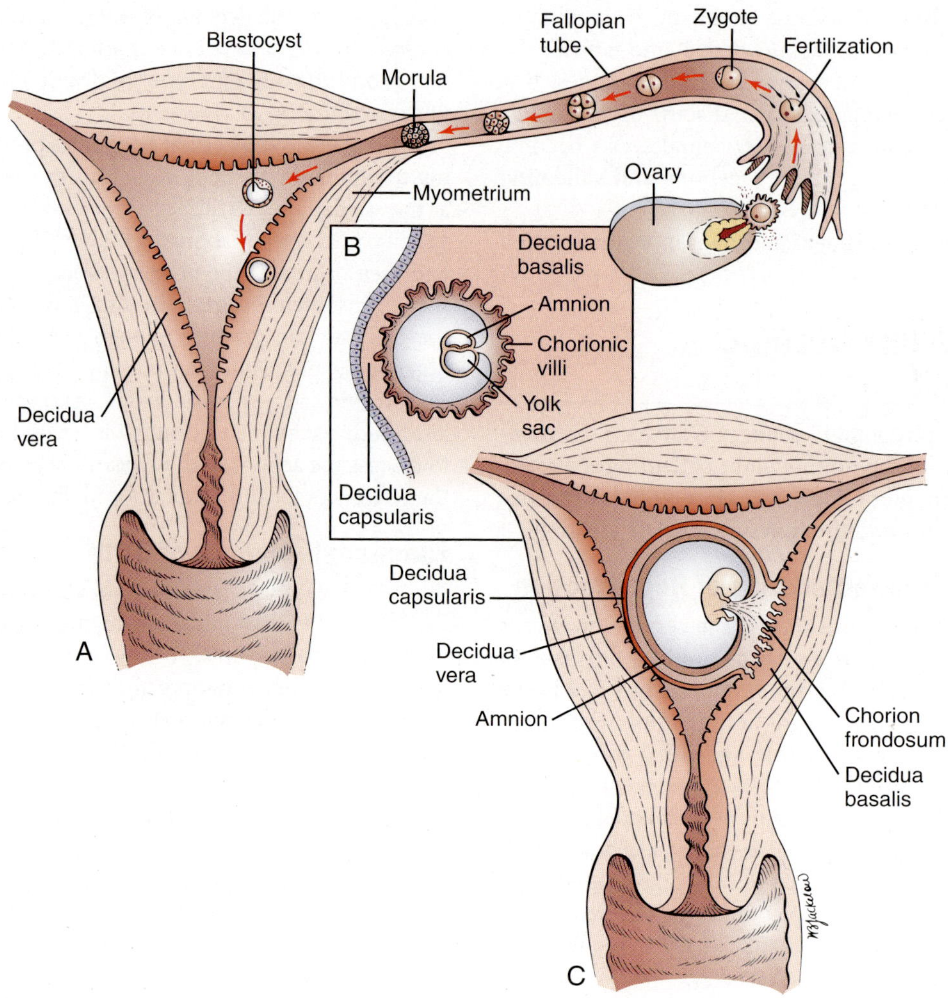

Fig. 23.1 (A) Fertilization and implantation. Cross-sectional view through the pregnant uterus at approximately 8 days (B) and 20 days (C).

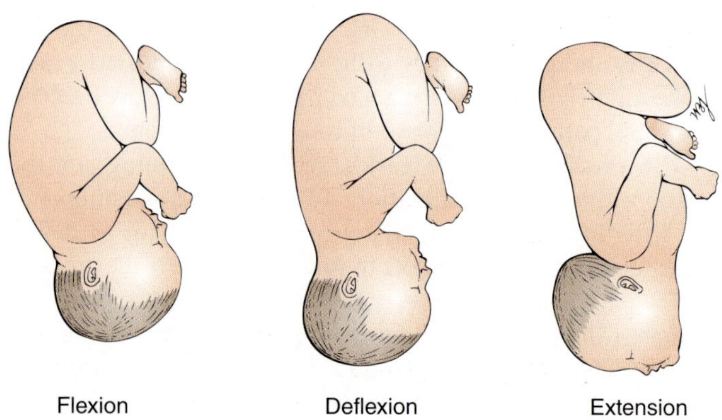

Fig. 23.2 Types of Fetal Positions.

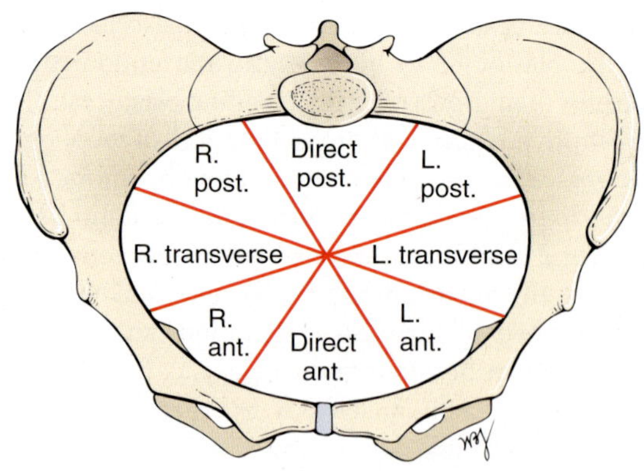

Fig. 23.3 Divisions of maternal pelvis as seen from above. *ant.,* Anterior; *L.,* left; *post.,* posterior; *R.,* right.

In most cases, the fetus becomes bent over so that the back is convex, the head is sharply flexed on the chest, the thighs are flexed over the abdomen, and the legs are bent at the knees. This is the description of the fetal attitude of flexion.

The *position* is the relationship of an arbitrarily chosen portion of the presenting part of the fetus to the maternal pelvis. For example, in a vertex presentation, the chosen portion is the fetal *occiput;* in a breech presentation, it is the *sacrum;* and in a face presentation, it is the chin, termed the *mentum.* The maternal pelvis is divided into eight parts for the purpose of further defining position. These divisions are shown in Fig. 23.3.

Because the arbitrarily chosen portion of the presenting part may be either left or right, the portion can be described as

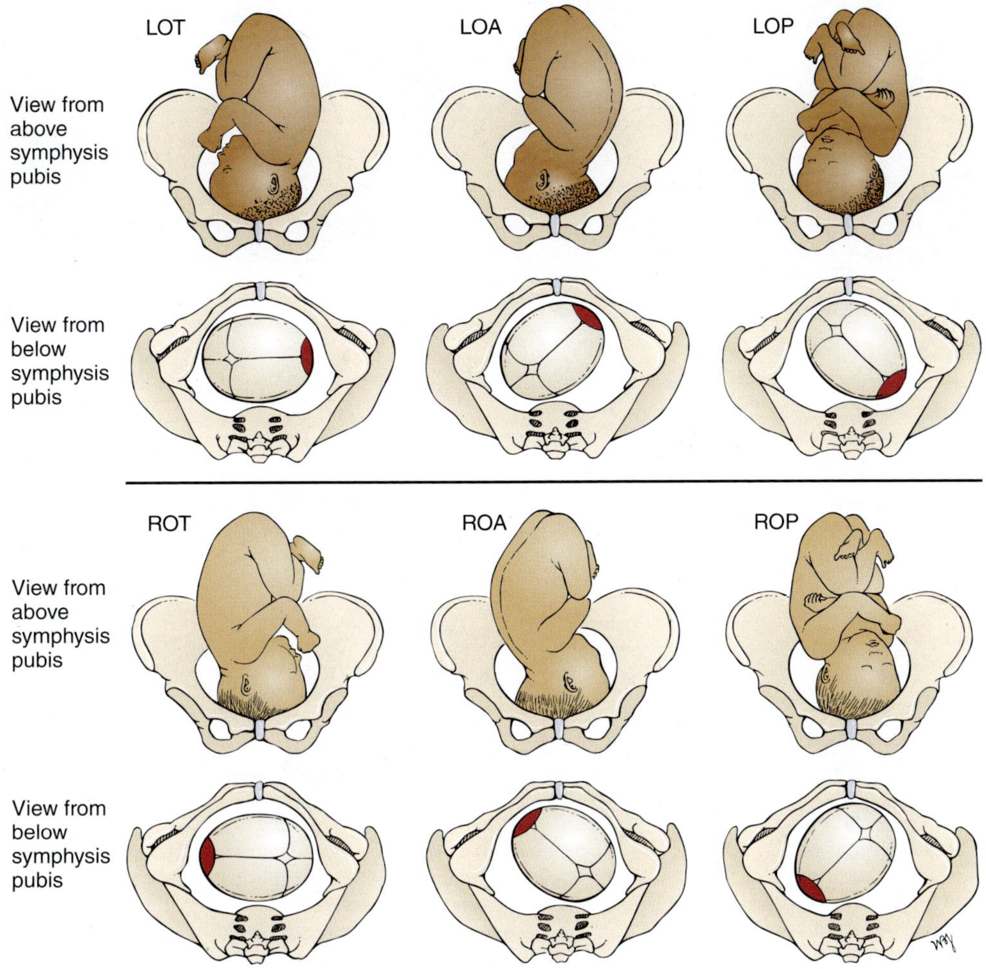

Fig. 23.4 Common Clinical Vertex Positions. For each position shown, the top diagram is the view from above the symphysis pubis; the bottom is the view from below the symphysis pubis. *Right* and *left* refer to the patient's side. *Anterior, posterior,* and *transverse* refer to the maternal pelvis. *Red area* is the fetal occiput. *LOA,* Left occiput anterior; *LOP,* left occiput posterior; *LOT,* left occiput transverse; *ROA,* right occiput anterior; *ROP,* right occiput posterior; *ROT,* right occiput transverse.

left occiput (LO), right occiput (RO), left sacral (LS), right sacral (RS), left mental (LM), or *right mental (RM).* This part is also directed *anteriorly (A), posteriorly (P),* or *transversely (T).* For each of the three presentations (vertex, breech, and face), there are therefore six varieties of position. For example, in a vertex presentation, if the occiput is in the left anterior segment of the maternal pelvis, the position is described as *left occiput anterior (LOA),* which is the most common of all vertex presentations. The common clinical vertex positions are illustrated in Fig. 23.4. *Left* and *right* always denote the side of the patient. Likewise, *anterior, posterior,* and *transverse* refer to the patient's pelvis.

The term *station* characterizes the level of descent of the presenting part of the fetus; "0 station" signifies that the fetal occiput has reached the level of the maternal ischial spines and that the widest transverse part of the infant's head *(biparietal diameter)* is at the level of the pelvic brim. This is also known as *engagement.* If the vertex is at "−1 station," it means that the fetal occiput is at a plane 1 cm above the level of the maternal ischial spines (and that the biparietal diameter is therefore 1 cm above the pelvic brim), and the infant's head is therefore not engaged.

The cardinal movements of labor are engagement, descent, flexion, internal rotation, extension, external rotation, and expulsion. These cardinal movements are illustrated in Fig. 23.5.

There are four basic pelvic configurations: *gynecoid, anthropoid, android,* and *platypelloid.* These are based on the shape of the brim, midpelvis, and outlet. Any pelvis is likely to combine features of more than one configuration. Fig. 23.6 illustrates these basic types and summarizes the differences in pelvic anatomy.

REVIEW OF SPECIFIC SYMPTOMS

The most common symptoms of pregnancy are the following:

1. Amenorrhea
2. Nausea
3. Breast changes
4. Heartburn
5. Backache

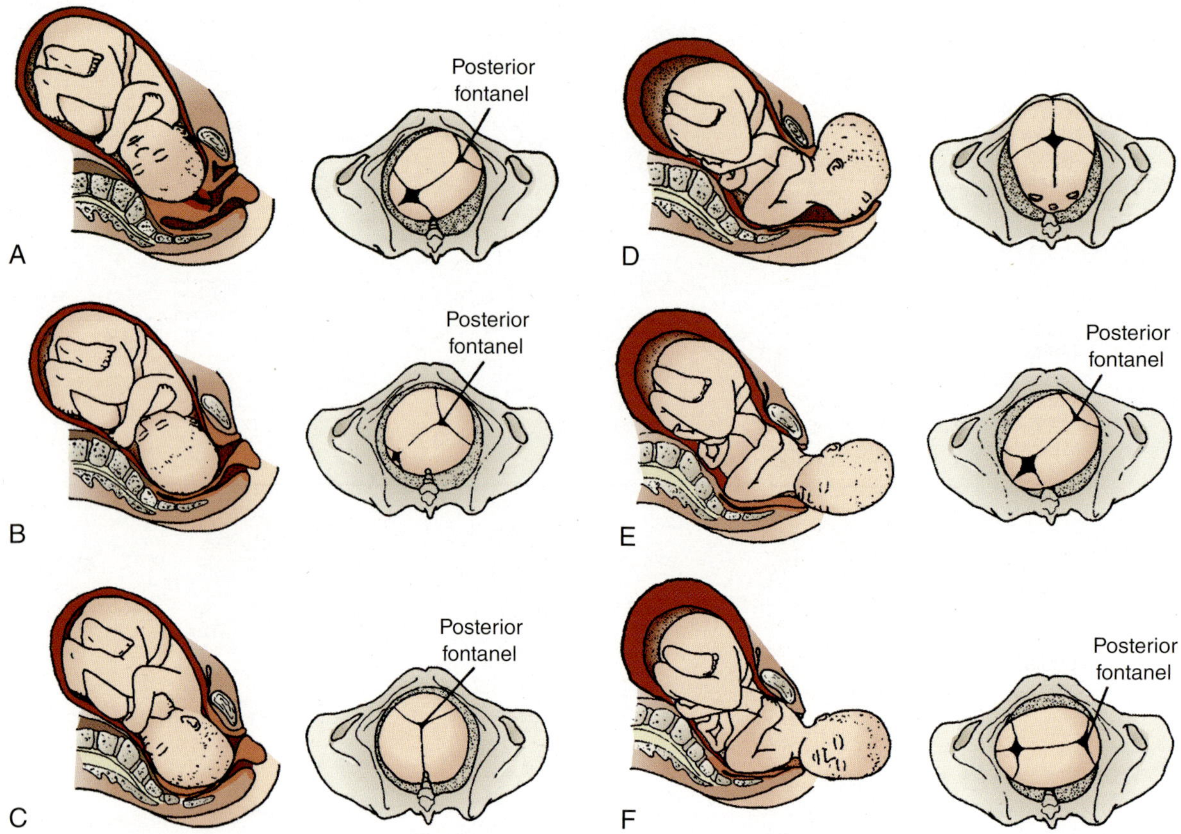

Fig. 23.5 Cardinal Movements of the Mechanism of Labor. Left occipitoanterior (LOA) position. Pelvic figures show the position of the fetal head as seen by the birth attendant. (A) Engagement and descent. (B) Flexion. (C) Internal rotation to occipitoanterior (OA) position. (D) Extension. (E) External rotation beginning (restitution). (F) External rotation. (From Cashion K: Labor and birth processes. In Perry SE, Hockenberry MJ, Lowdermilk DL, et al. editors: *Maternal child nursing care*, ed 6, Philadelphia, 2018, Elsevier.).

6. Abdominal enlargement
7. Quickening
8. Skin changes
9. Changes in urination
10. Vaginal discharge
11. Fatigue

Amenorrhea

Amenorrhea, or absence of menses, results from the high levels of estrogen, progesterone, and hCG, which increase and alter *(decidualize)* the uterine endometrium and do not allow the endometrium to slough as in menstrual bleeding.

Nausea

Nausea, with or without vomiting, is the so-called *morning sickness of pregnancy.* As the name implies, the symptom is usually worse during the early part of the day and usually passes in a few hours, although it may last longer. More than 50% of pregnant patients in their first trimester have gastrointestinal symptoms. Although the cause is unknown, high levels of estrogen and hCG have been implicated in its development. Pregnant patients can also be hypersensitive to odors, and they may experience alterations in taste. Morning sickness usually improves after 12 to 16 weeks, when the hCG levels fall. Severe vomiting may occur, resulting in dehydration and ketosis, but this is uncommon, occurring in fewer than 2% of pregnancies.

Breast Changes

Several changes in the breast occur with pregnancy. One of the earliest symptoms is an increase in the vascularity of the breast, associated with a sensation of heaviness, almost pain. This occurs at approximately the sixth week. By the eighth week, the nipple and areola have become more pigmented, and the nipple becomes more erectile. The Montgomery tubercles become prominent as raised pinkish-red nodules on the areola. By the 16th week, a clear fluid called *colostrum* is secreted and may be expressed from the nipple. By the 20th week, further pigmentation and mottling of the areola have developed. Fig. 23.7 illustrates the changes in the nipple and areola.

Heartburn

Heartburn in pregnancy occurs because progesterone causes relaxation of the gastroesophageal sphincter. Another cause of heartburn in the third trimester is the upward pressure of the enlarged uterus. This upward displacement exerts pressure on the stomach. There is also a decrease in gastric motility, as well as a decrease in gastric acid secretion, which delays digestion.

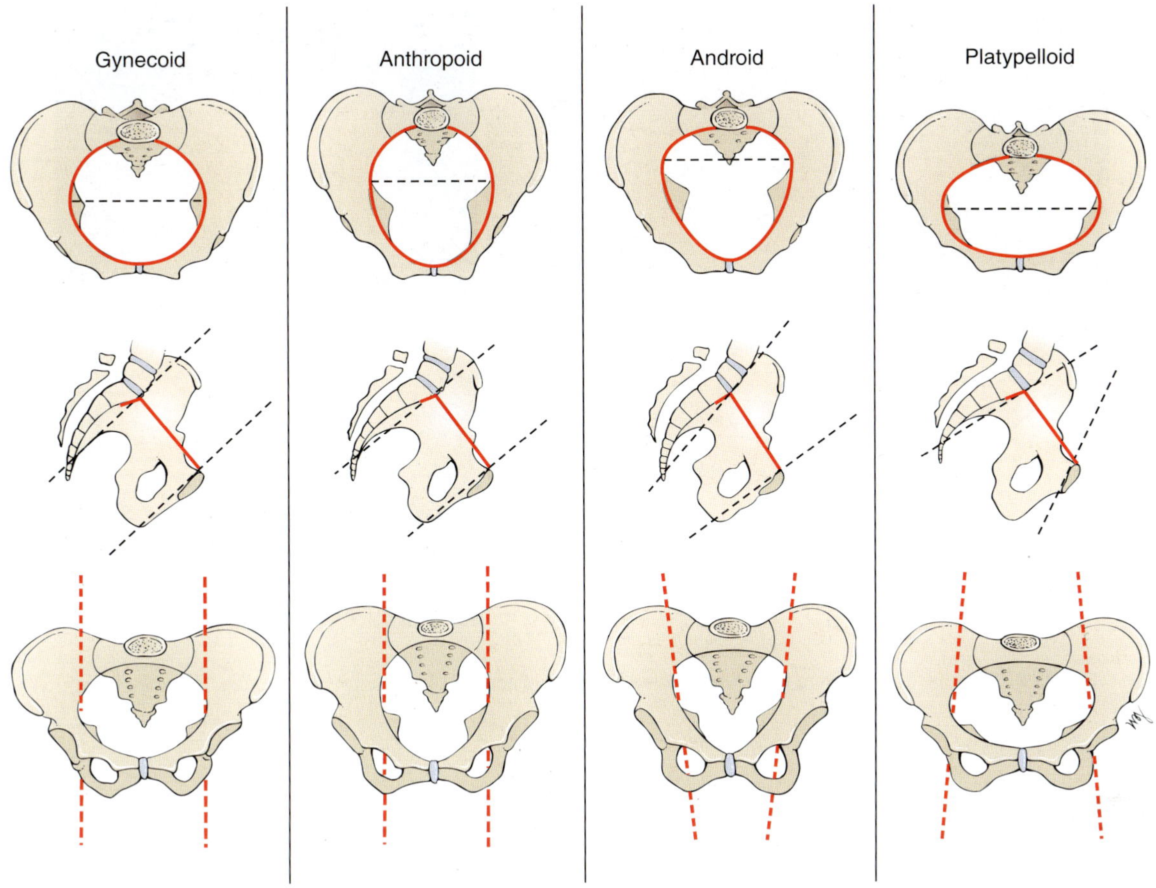

Fig. 23.6 Basic Types of Pelvic Anatomy. *Top view* is from above, looking down at the inlet; *middle view* is from the side; *bottom view* is from the front.

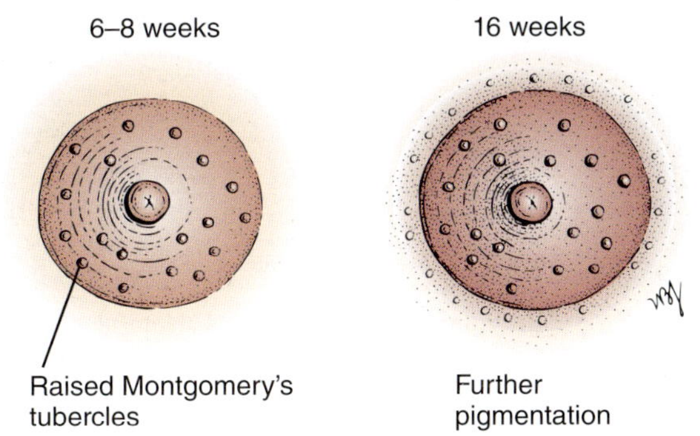

Fig. 23.7 Nipple and Areola Changes During Pregnancy.

Backache

As a result of the secretion of estrogen and progesterone, the pelvic joints relax, and the increased uterine weight accentuates lordosis. The abdominal muscles stretch and lose tone.

Abdominal Enlargement

The uterus rises out of the pelvis and into the abdomen by the 12th week of gestation, and an increase in abdominal girth is usually apparent by the 15th week. This enlargement is usually more apparent earlier in multiparous patients, whose abdominal muscles have lost some of their tone during previous pregnancies.

Quickening

Quickening is the sensation of fetal movement. It is a faint sensation initially. Quickening usually begins at approximately 20 weeks in the first pregnancy but is usually felt 2 to 3 weeks earlier in the multiparous patient.

Skin Changes

In addition to the skin changes of the breast already discussed, hyperpigmentation is common, especially in patients with dark hair and a dark complexion. The linea alba darkens to become the *linea nigra,* as shown in Fig. 23.8A. Areas prone to friction (e.g., medial thighs, axilla) also tend to darken. New pigmentation on the face, called *chloasma,* also commonly develops on the cheeks, forehead, nose, and chin. These skin changes are caused by the presence of high levels of ovarian, placental, and pituitary hormones. A pregnant patient with chloasma appears in Fig. 23.8B.

"Stretch marks," or *striae gravidarum,* are irregular, linear, pinkish-purple lesions that develop on the abdomen, breasts, upper arms, buttocks, and thighs. They are caused by tears in the connective tissue below the stratum corneum. Figs. 23.9 and 23.10 show striae gravidarum of the abdomen and breasts, respectively. Fig. 23.11 illustrates the common skin changes seen in pregnancy.

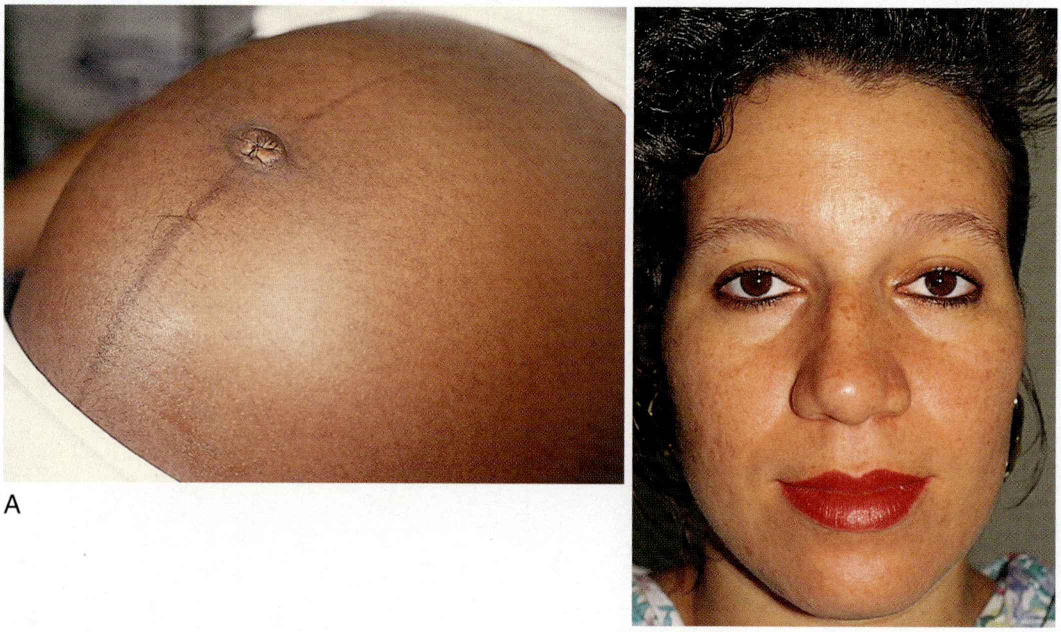

A

B

Fig. 23.8 Skin changes resulting from high levels of ovarian, placental, and pituitary hormones. (A) Linea nigra. (B) Chloasma.

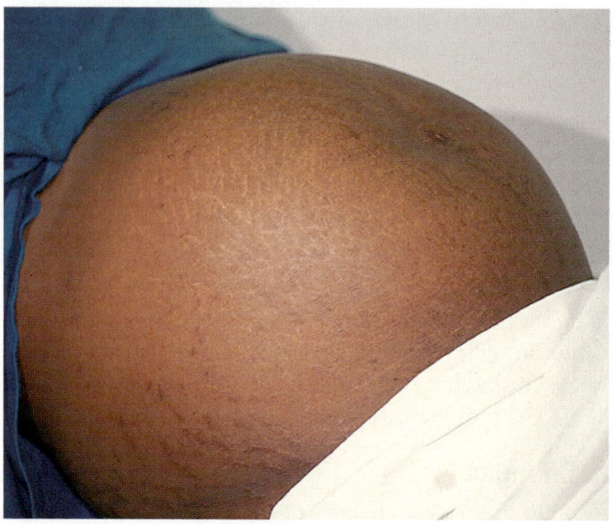

Fig. 23.9 Striae Gravidarum of the Abdomen. Note also the linea nigra.

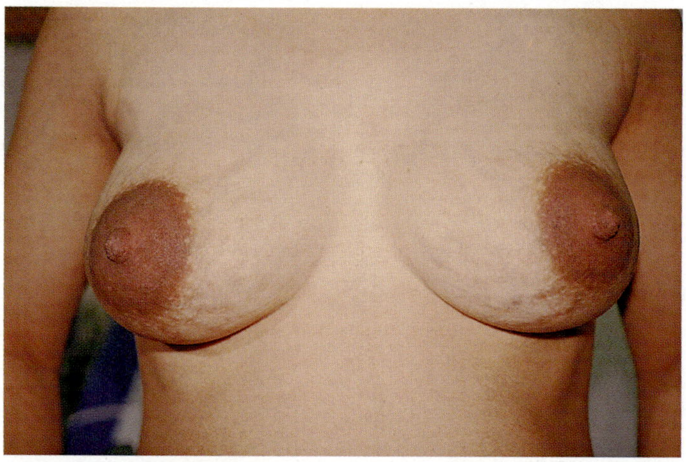

Fig. 23.10 Striae Gravidarum of the Breasts. Note also the marked pigmentation of the areolae.

Transverse grooving, as well as increased brittleness or softening, of the nails, may occur. Eccrine sweating progressively increases throughout pregnancy, whereas apocrine gland activity decreases. Hirsutism, caused by increased androgen secretion, may also occur on the face, arms, legs, and back.

Changes in Urination

Beginning at the sixth week, urinary bladder symptoms are common. Increased frequency of urination is thought to be caused by increased vascularity of the bladder, as well as by pressure of the enlarging uterus on the bladder. As the uterus rises above the pelvis, the symptoms tend to remit. Near term, however, urinary symptoms recur as the fetal head settles into the maternal pelvis and impinges on the volume capacity of the urinary bladder.

Vaginal Discharge

An asymptomatic, white, milky vaginal discharge is common as the elevated estrogen levels increase the production of cervical mucus and secretions from the vaginal walls.

Fatigue

Easy fatigability is common during early pregnancy. Some patients feel that progesterone makes them feel drowsy and contributes to fatigue.

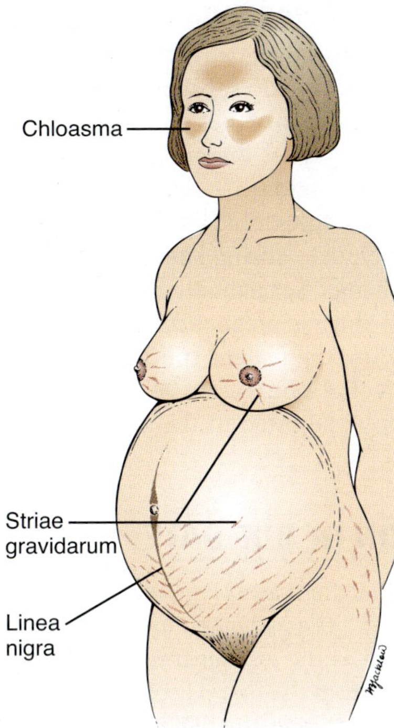

Fig. 23.11 Common Skin Changes During Pregnancy.

Other Symptoms

Several other symptoms are common in pregnant patients. These include varicose veins, headache, leg cramps, swelling of the legs and hands, constipation, bleeding gums, nosebleeds, insomnia, and "dizziness."

OBSTETRIC RISK ASSESSMENT

Documentation of the medical history of the pregnant patient is similar to that of the nonpregnant patient. In addition, the interviewer must assess obstetric risk. The following major risk factors must be evaluated:

- Age
- Parity and obstetric history
- Height
- Pre-pregnancy weight
- Diabetes, hypertension, and renal disease
- Hemoglobinopathy and isoimmunization
- Sexually transmitted infections
- Other infections
- Family history to screening for risk of inherited conditions
- Tobacco, alcohol, and drug use

Age

As maternal age increases, the risk of conceiving a fetus with a chromosomal abnormality increases. The chance of having a child with a chromosomal abnormality is approximately 1 per 200 at age 35 years and increases to approximately 1 per 20 at age 44 years. Pregnant patients younger than 20 years are at increased risk of having a preterm birth or low-birth-weight baby when compared with patients aged 25 to 35 years.

Parity and Obstetric History

The outcomes of previous pregnancies are important predictors of outcomes in subsequent pregnancies. For instance, in patients who have had a prior ectopic pregnancy, there is a 10% risk of recurrent ectopic pregnancy. Patients who have had previous cesarean sections are at increased risk of abnormal implantation of the placenta such as *placenta previa* (placenta covering the cervix) and *placenta accreta* (abnormally adherent placenta with invasion beyond the normal boundaries.) These placental abnormalities confer a significant risk of bleeding during pregnancy and hemorrhage at delivery. For patients who have undergone previous cesarean section, exact information about the reason for the procedure and the type of uterine incision used are needed to determine whether the patient is a candidate for a vaginal birth.

Height

Patients who are less than 5 feet (152.5 cm) tall may have small pelves and may be prone to *cephalopelvic disproportion*[a] requiring cesarean section.

Pre-pregnancy Weight

The perinatal mortality rate is increased among patients whose initial pre-pregnancy weight is less than 120 pounds, especially if their weight gain during pregnancy is less than 11 pounds. Having obesity also puts the patient and fetus at increased risk of obstetric complications, including early miscarriage, gestational hypertension, preeclampsia, gestational diabetes, fetal macrosomia, cesarean delivery, and operative complications such as increased operative time, increased blood loss, infection, and anesthetic complications. Therefore, patients who are significantly underweight or overweight should undergo medical and nutritional evaluation, as well as support and counseling to attain a healthy weight before becoming pregnant.

Diabetes, Hypertension, or Renal Disease

In patients with diabetes, hypertension, or renal disease, there is an increased risk of fetal intrauterine growth restriction, preterm labor, preeclampsia, and abruptio placentae (see Clinicopathologic Correlations at the end of this chapter). Diabetes mellitus occurs in 2% to 3% of all pregnancies and is thus the most common medical complication of pregnancy. Screening for gestational diabetes is routine during pregnancy because the rate of gestational diabetes may be as high as 30% of births. Chronic hypertension is present in 0.9% to 1.5% of pregnancies. Blood pressure screening is an important component of prenatal care as 2% to 8% of previously normotensive patients will develop preeclampsia in pregnancy, and 16% of pregnancy-related deaths are the result of hypertensive disease.

[a]Cephalopelvic disproportion (CPD) is a disparity between the size of the maternal pelvis and the fetal head, resulting in "failure to progress" in labor for mechanical reasons. This can happen when the fetus is too large, the pelvis is too small, the fetus is in an incorrect position, or the relationship between the fetus and the pelvis is incorrect. It is estimated that CPD occurs in 1 out of 250 pregnancies.

Hemoglobinopathy and Isoimmunization

It is crucial to determine the presence of any hemoglobinopathy because pregnancy can precipitate an exacerbation of the anemia. Hemoglobinopathy history may be elicited, but screening via laboratory analysis is done in most practices. Patients who are Rh-negative must be monitored closely throughout pregnancy if they have Rh antibodies from isoimmunization because severe hemolytic anemia may develop in the fetus before delivery.

Sexually Transmitted Infections

A thorough screening for sexually transmitted infections by history, and laboratory analysis, if applicable, is routinely offered to all pregnant patients. Because medical therapy for a pregnant patient who is human immunodeficiency virus (HIV)–positive can reduce transmission of the infection to the fetus by more than two-thirds, determination of HIV status is essential. Although HIV testing cannot be required of the patient, it is mandatory that they be counseled about the value of testing. Screening for HIV is routinely offered and is usually (>90%) accepted. For patients with a history of genital herpes, prophylaxis with antivirals can prevent recurrences near the time of delivery that would necessitate cesarean delivery to prevent transmission to the neonate. Screening for gonorrhea, chlamydia, and syphilis is routinely offered.

Other Infections

Routine screening tests are conducted to check for immunity and exposure to rubella, as well as hepatitis B, to ensure overall health and well-being. Rubella infection and exposure pose a significant threat to fetal health and can even lead to severe morbidity and mortality. Fortunately, rubella exposure is rare, and most patients have immunity from previous vaccination. For hepatitis B, at-risk neonates can be protected from transmission by administering immune globulin and early vaccination. Pregnant patients are screened for group B streptococcus colonization in the third trimester, as this is a common but asymptomatic condition in adults that can be dangerous for neonates if they are exposed during birth. Antibiotic prophylaxis is initiated to prevent neonatal exposure. Additionally, high-risk populations are screened for tuberculosis.

Family History to Screening for Risk of Inherited Conditions

A thorough family history and review of prior poor pregnancy outcomes aid in screening for inherited conditions.

If a patient has a history of adverse pregnancy outcomes or if there is a family history of miscarriage, preterm birth, newborn screening test abnormalities, or birth defects, they may be at a higher risk for these disorders. Both genetic and environmental factors can play a role in these outcomes. Informing a patient of their increased risk based on family history may motivate them to take steps to reduce their environmental risk factors. For example, quitting smoking or achieving a healthy weight can help reduce the risk of adverse pregnancy outcomes.

It is important to regularly update family history information and consider further evaluation for positive responses with referral to genetic services as needed.

Tobacco, Alcohol, and Drug Use

Determinations must be made regarding tobacco, alcohol, and drug use; exposure to toxic substances in the workplace or at home; and exposure to other teratogenic agents. Patients who smoke cigarettes place their pregnancies at a higher risk of complications and should be encouraged to stop smoking. The fetus is more likely to exhibit intrauterine growth restriction and to become hypoxic during labor as a result of a reduction in placental exchange. Special note must be made of *any* drugs or alcohol used during pregnancy. Ideally, this issue should be discussed before the patient conceives so that treatment of substance or alcohol abuse can be initiated and prescribed medications can be adjusted to the safest possible medication for pregnancy.

CALCULATION OF DUE DATE

After learning that they are pregnant, most patients will ask, "When am I due?" The *estimated date of delivery (EDD)*, also known previously as the *estimated date of confinement (EDC)*, can be calculated from the first day of the last menstrual period (LMP) by the *Naegele rule*. The EDD is estimated by subtracting 3 months, adding 1 year, and adding 7 days to the LMP. For example:

LMP	8/29/2023
Subtract 3 months	5/29/2023
Add 1 year	5/29/2024
Add 7 days	6/4/2024 = EDD

EDD, Estimated date of delivery; *LMP,* last menstrual period.

Alternatively, the EDD can be calculated by adding 9 months and 7 days to the first day of the patient's LMP.

By knowing the EDD, the examiner can predict the size of the uterus on physical examination, provided that the LMP is correct, and that conception occurred during the cycle after the presumed LMP. If the size of the uterus differs significantly from that expected according to the EDD, the causes must be determined. Early ultrasonography can be helpful in dating a pregnancy.

EFFECT OF PREGNANCY ON THE PATIENT

Pregnancy is a wonderful experience, but it can also come with its own set of challenges. Even if a patient is excited about being pregnant, they may still experience stress and anxiety during this time. Common questions that pregnant patients ask themselves include, "Will my baby be healthy?", "How will I handle labor?", "How will having a baby change my life?", and "Will I ever be able to lose the weight I've gained?"

It's important to note that pregnancy can exacerbate preexisting psychiatric conditions. Studies have shown that approximately 20% of pregnant patients experience some form of mental health issue during their pregnancy. Furthermore, a severe psychotic episode can occur in 1 to 2 out of every 1000 live births.

It's common for pregnant people to experience depression, with around 14% of all pregnant patients being affected. And of those, 40% will experience it after giving birth. Postpartum blues can be caused by a range of issues, including losing the excitement of delivery, not getting enough sleep during labor, anxiety about taking care of the baby, perineal pain, difficulties with feeding, and concerns about appearance. The good news is that these blues usually go away on their own within a few weeks. All patients should be screened for depression and anxiety using standardized, validated instruments before during and after pregnancy. Patients who experience persistent symptoms of depression in the postpartum period should seek medical evaluation because psychotherapy and medications are effective in treating postpartum depression.

PHYSICAL EXAMINATION

The equipment necessary for the examination of the pregnant patient is the same as for the nonpregnant patient. In addition, specialized instruments such as an ultrasonic Doppler scanner or fetoscope may be used to listen to the fetal heart. The ultrasonic scanner can detect the fetal heartbeat as early as gestational weeks 6 to 7; an ultrasonic Doppler scanner is used at about week 10; and a fetoscope or stethoscope can be used after the 20th week to auscultate the fetal heartbeat.

Always try to make the patient as comfortable as possible. They should be examined in comfortable surroundings, with attention to privacy. Discuss with them all the procedures that you will perform. The patient's gown should be opened in the front for ease of examination. The patient is draped in the same way as discussed in previous chapters and as shown in Fig. 19.26. If the patient is in advanced pregnancy, avoid having them lie for a long period on her back, because the gravid uterus diminishes venous return and produces supine hypotension. It is useful for the patient to urinate before the pelvic examination. As always, wash your hands before beginning the examination. Make sure that your hands are gloved, warm, and dry.

Because the examination of the pregnant patient is identical to the examinations described in the other chapters of this book, only special techniques and modifications for pregnancy are discussed here.

Initial Comprehensive Evaluation

There are three main goals of the initial evaluation:

1. Determine the health of the pregnant patient and fetus.
2. Determine the gestational age of the fetus.
3. Initiate a plan for continuing care.

The physical examination must include the following:

- Determination of height and weight
- Assessment of blood pressure
- Inspection of the teeth and gums
- Palpation of the thyroid gland
- Auscultation of the heart and lungs
- Examination of the breasts and nipples
- Examination of the abdomen
- Examination of the legs for varicosities and edema
- Inspection of the vulva, vagina, and cervix
- Cytologic study (Pap smear) and testing for HPV if indicated
- Swab for *Chlamydia* and gonorrhea screening
- Palpation of the cervix, uterus, and adnexa, including physical assessment of uterine size in terms of gestational age

Whenever possible, ultrasonography should be performed at the first prenatal visit to verify the presence of an intrauterine pregnancy with a fetal heartbeat, to confirm or adjust the gestational age, and to check for multiple fetuses. Another sonographic examination is usually performed at about 16 to 20 weeks to evaluate the fetal anatomy and identify any structural anomalies.

Head, Eyes, Ears, Nose, Throat, and Neck

Inspect the face. Is chloasma present? What is the texture of the hair and skin? Inspect the mouth. What is the condition of the teeth and gums? Palpate the thyroid. Is it enlarged symmetrically?

Chest

Inspect, palpate, and auscultate the chest. Is there any evidence of labored breathing?

Heart

Palpate for the point of maximum impulse. Is it displaced laterally? During the later stages of pregnancy, the gravid uterus pushes up on the diaphragm, and the point of maximum impulse is displaced laterally. Auscultate the heart. Systolic ejection murmurs are common during pregnancy as a result of the hyperdynamic state. They are termed "flow murmurs" and occur in about 93% of all pregnant patients. The murmurs are located predominantly at the second left intercostal space or along the left sternal border, although they may radiate widely. Diastolic murmurs are always indicative of a pathologic condition.

Breasts

Inspect the breasts. Are they symmetric? Notice the presence of vascular engorgement and pigmentary changes. Are the nipples everted? An inverted nipple may present difficulties during breastfeeding. Palpate the breasts. The normal nodularity of breast tissue is accentuated during pregnancy, but *any discrete mass should be considered indicative of a pathologic condition until proven otherwise and should be evaluated.*

Abdomen

Inspect for the linea nigra and striae gravidarum. Notice the contour of the abdomen. Palpate the abdomen. Fetal movement may be felt by the examiner after 24 weeks. Are there uterine contractions? Hold your hand on the abdomen as the uterus relaxes.

Use a tape measure to assess the fundal height. The measurement should be taken from the top of the symphysis pubis in a straight line to the top of the fundus, with the bladder empty. The technique is demonstrated in Fig. 23.12. Between 20 and 32 weeks, the superior-inferior measurement in centimeters should approximately equal the number of weeks of gestation. The uterus rises up and enters the abdomen at 12 weeks. It reaches the umbilicus at approximately 20 weeks and is just under the costal margin by 36 weeks. The reduction in fundal

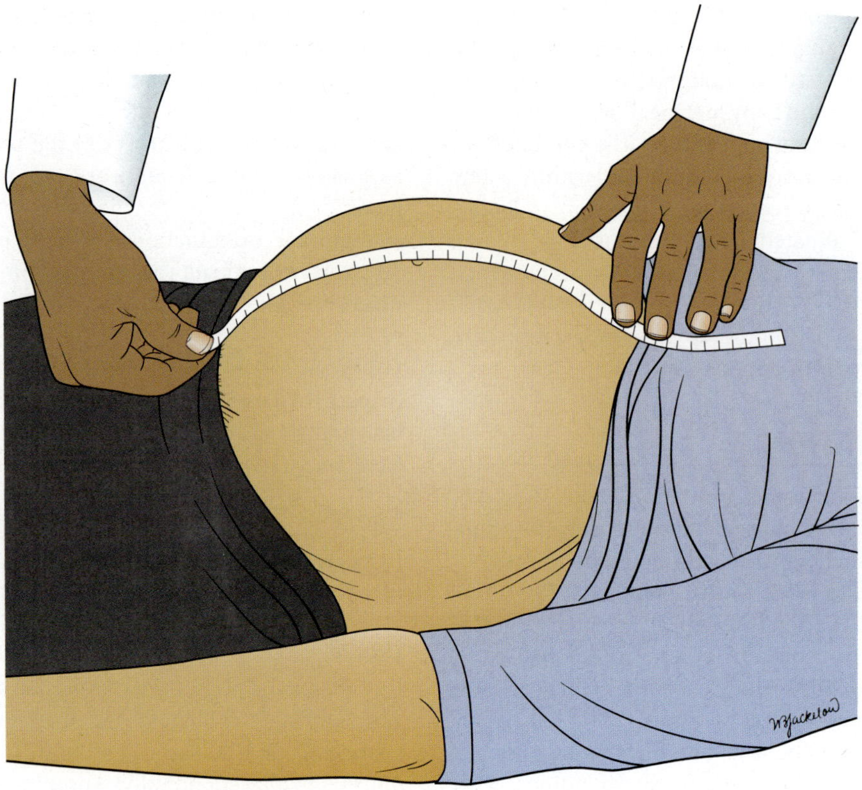

Fig. 23.12 Technique for Measuring Fundal Height.

height that usually occurs between the 38th and 40th weeks is called *lightening* and results from the descent of the fetus into the pelvis, or "dropping." Fig. 23.13 illustrates the approximate size of the uterus by weeks.

Auscultate the fetal heart, determine the *fetal heart rate* (FHR) and note its location. Throughout pregnancy, the FHR is approximately 120 to 160 beats per minute. From weeks 12 to 18, the FHR is usually detected in the midline of the patient's lower abdomen. After 30 weeks, the FHR is best heard over the fetal chest or back. Knowing the location of the fetal back is helpful in determining where to listen for the FHR.

Genitalia

Inspect the patient's external genitalia. Are any lesions present? Inspect the anus. Are varicosities present?

With gloves on, perform a speculum examination as described in Chapter 19, Female Genitalia. Inspect the cervix. A dusky blue color is characteristic of pregnancy and occurs by weeks 6 to 8. Is the cervix dilated? If so, fetal membranes may be seen within. Note the character of the vaginal secretions. Obtain cytologic studies for a Pap test and human papillomavirus, and a swab for *Chlamydia* and gonorrhea screening. As the speculum is removed, inspect the vaginal walls. The vaginal walls are commonly violaceous in pregnancy. Withdraw the speculum carefully.

Perform a digital bimanual examination, paying special attention to the consistency, length, and dilation of the cervix; the fetal presenting part (in advanced pregnancy); the structure of the pelvis; and any abnormalities of the vagina and perineum. Is the cervix closed? Prior to the last few weeks of pregnancy, a nulliparous cervix should be closed, whereas a multiparous cervix may allow the tip of a finger through the external os. Estimate the length of the cervix by palpating the lateral side of the cervix from the cervical tip to the lateral fornix. Only at term should the cervix shorten or efface. The normal length of the palpable (vaginal) portion of the cervix is 1.5 to 2 cm.

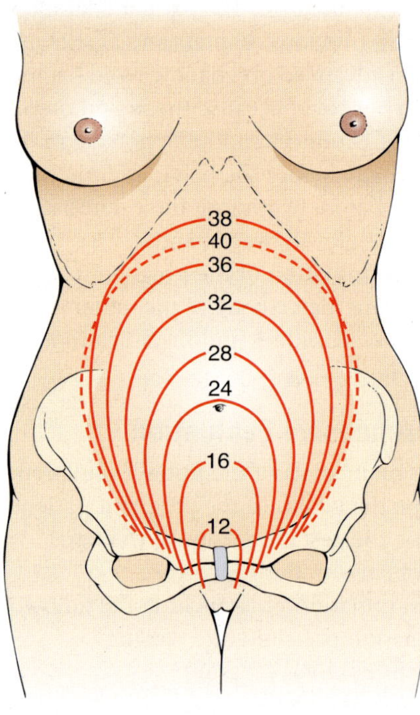

Fig. 23.13 Approximate Uterine Size by Week.

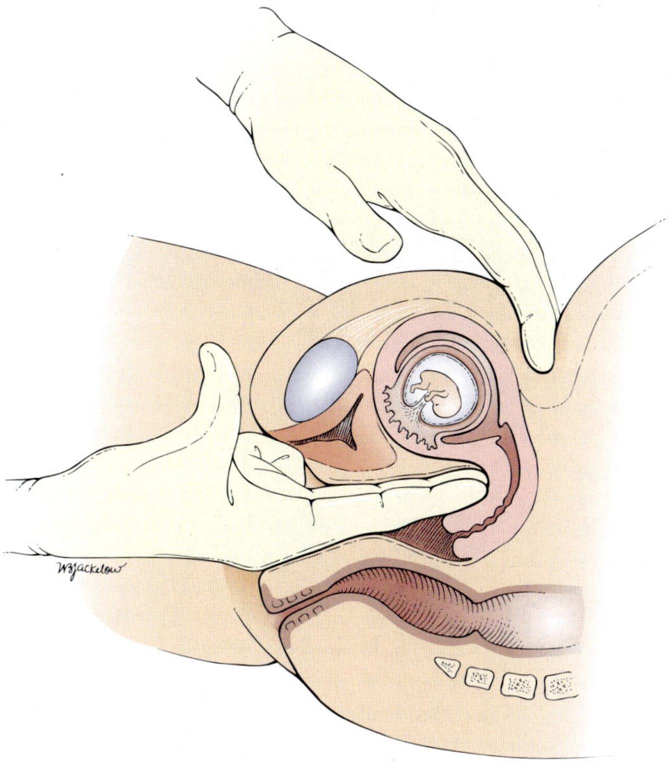

Fig. 23.14 Technique for Evaluating the Presence of Hegar's Sign.

Palpate the uterus for size, consistency, and position. An early sign of pregnancy, at approximately 6 to 12 weeks, is the softening of the entire isthmus of the cervix; this is known as *Hegar's sign*.[b] During the bimanual examination of the uterus, the examiner will notice an extreme softening of the lower uterine segment. This produces a sensation of the close proximity of the fingers of the hand in the vagina (internal) and in the abdomen (external). The technique for evaluating the presence of Hegar's sign is illustrated in Fig. 23.14. Bimanual palpation of the uterus is useful up to about 12 to 14 weeks' of pregnancy. After that, the uterus can be palpated abdominally. Fetal parts are usually palpated from about 26 to 28 weeks' gestation by abdominal examination (described later).

Palpate the adnexa. Early in pregnancy, the corpus luteum may be palpable as a cystic mass on one ovary. As you withdraw your hand from the vagina, evaluate the pelvic muscles.

A rectovaginal examination allows evaluation of the rectum and can identify if the patient has a retroverted, retroflexed uterus.

[b]Hegar's sign, first described by Ernst Ludwig Alfred Hegar, a German gynecologist in the late 19th century, has historical significance in the field of obstetrics and gynecology. It reflects early attempts to diagnose pregnancy based on physical examination. Modern blood and urine pregnancy tests are more accurate and reliable methods. It is important to know that Hegar's sign is a non-sensitive indication of pregnancy; its absence does not exclude pregnancy. Softening and compressibility of the uterine isthmus can also be present in other conditions unrelated to pregnancy, such as certain benign uterine conditions or hormonal fluctuations. Therefore, Hegar's sign, although useful, should not be relied upon as the sole indicator of pregnancy.

Extremities

Inspect for varicosities. Is edema present? This completes the routine initial examination.

Subsequent Antenatal Examinations

Subsequent antenatal examinations are important for screening for impaired fetal growth, malpresentation, anemia, preeclampsia, and other problems. In the absence of specific concerns by the patient or of abnormal findings on the initial examination or initial laboratory and sonographic studies, only a few parts of the physical examination outlined above are routinely performed during each visit. These include weight, blood pressure, and examination of the abdomen. This section concerns the abdominal examination.

The physical examination should confirm that fetal growth is consistent with gestational age. Attention should then be given to assessing the lie and presentation of the fetus. From the 28th week of gestation to term, the following four maneuvers, known as *Leopold's maneuvers,* provide vital information for the examiner about these important questions. The patient lies supine for these maneuvers.

The *first maneuver* is used to evaluate the upper pole and defines the fetal part in the fundus of the uterus. Stand facing the patient at their side, and gently palpate the upper uterine fundus with your fingers to ascertain which fetal pole is present. This technique is demonstrated in Fig. 23.15. Usually, the fetal buttocks are felt at the upper pole. They feel firm but irregular. In a breech presentation, the head is at the upper pole. The head feels hard and round and is usually movable.

The *second maneuver* is used to locate the position of the fetal back. Standing in the same place as in the first maneuver, place the palms of your hands on either side of the patient's abdomen, and apply gentle pressure to the uterus to identify the fetal back and limbs, as shown in Fig. 23.16. On one side, the fetal back is felt: rounded, smooth, and hard. On the other side are the limbs, which are nodular or bumpy, and kicking may be felt.

The *third maneuver* is to palpate the lower pole of the fetus. From the same position as in the first two maneuvers, use your thumb and fingers of one hand to grasp the lower portion of the maternal abdomen just above the symphysis pubis. This maneuver is illustrated in Fig. 23.17. If the presenting portion is not engaged, a movable part, usually the head of the fetus, is felt. If the presenting portion is engaged, this maneuver indicates that the lower pole of the fetus is fixed in the pelvis.

The *fourth maneuver* is performed to confirm the presenting portion and to locate the side of the fetus's cephalic prominence. You should now stand beside the patient, facing their feet. Place your hands on either side of their lower abdomen. With the tips of your fingers, exert a deep pressure in the direction of the pelvic inlet, as indicated in Fig. 23.18. If the presenting portion is the head and the head is flexed normally, one hand will be stopped by the cephalic prominence as the other hand descends farther down on the pelvis. In a vertex presentation, the cephalic prominence is on the same side as the fetal small parts. In a vertex presentation with the head extended, the prominence is on the side of the back.

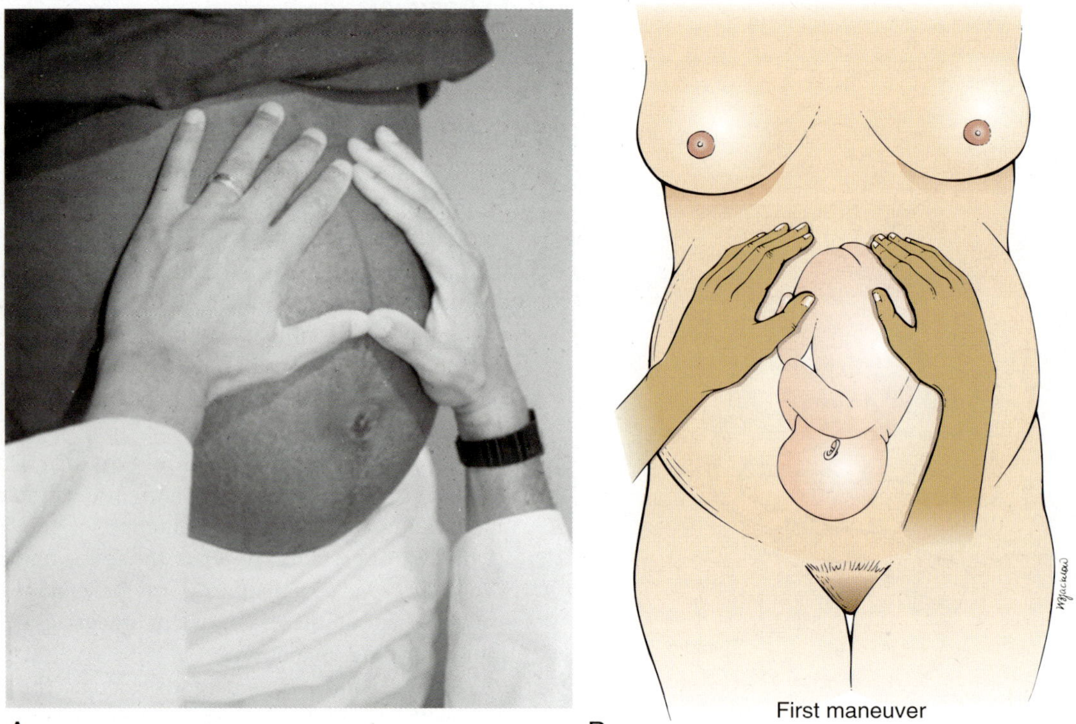

A B

Fig. 23.15 **Leopold's First Maneuver.** (A) Position of healthcare professional's hands on patient's abdomen. (B) Illustration of the relationship of the examiner's hands and fetus.

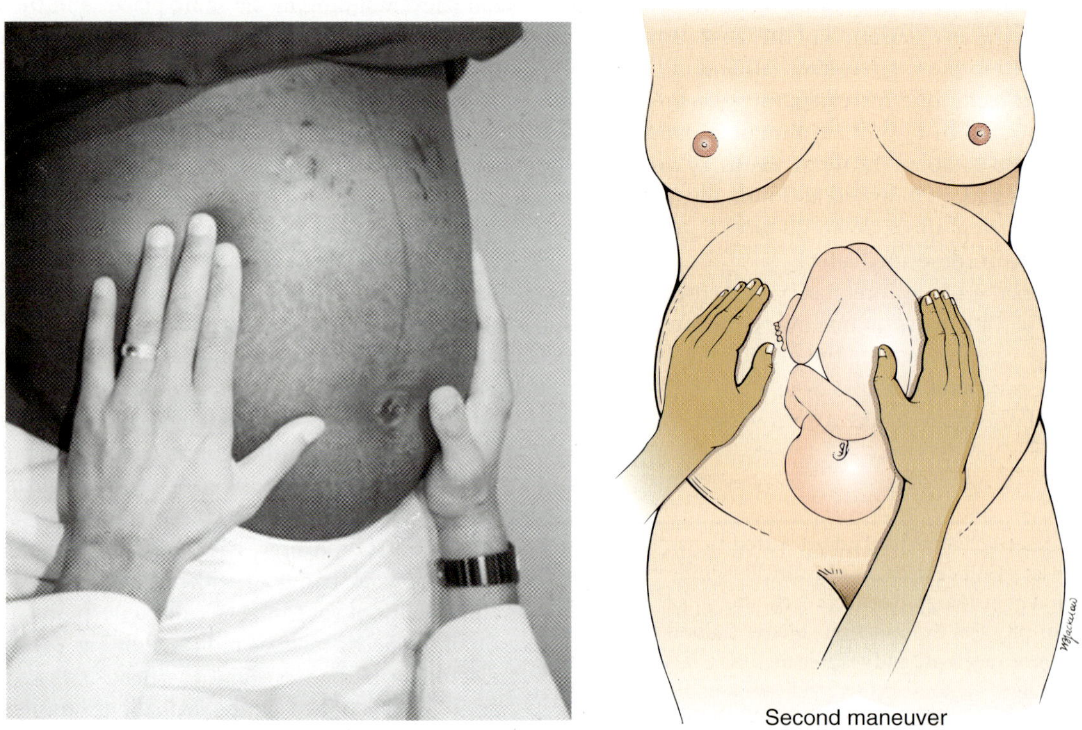

A B

Fig. 23.16 **Leopold's Second Maneuver.** (A) Position of healthcare professional's hands on patient's abdomen. (B) Illustration of the relationship of the examiner's hands and fetus.

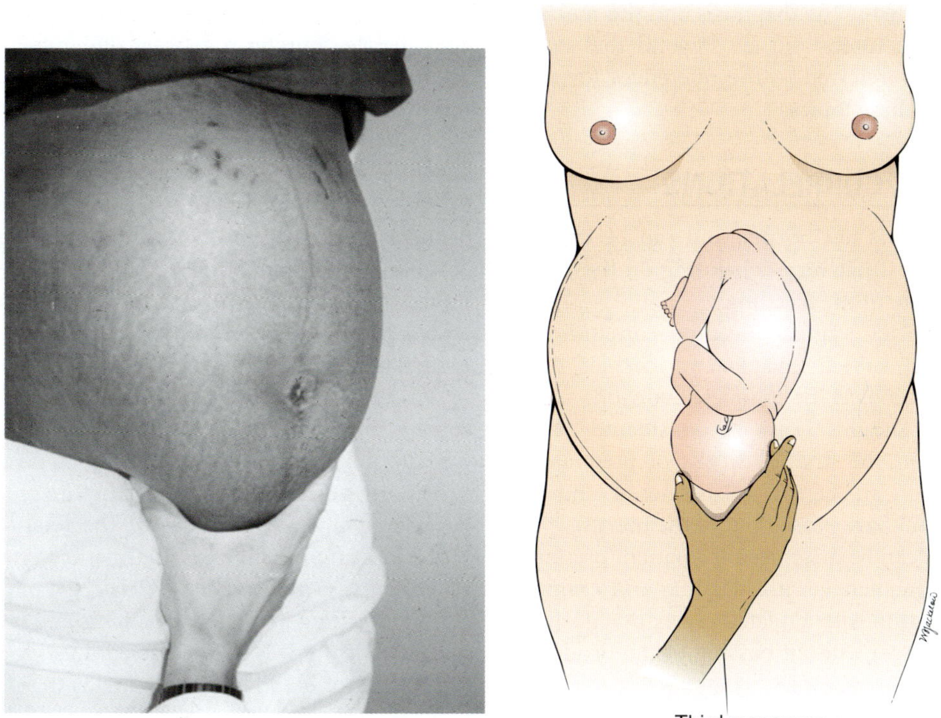

A B

Fig. 23.17 **Leopold's Third Maneuver.** Relationship of the healthcare professional's hand and fetal presenting part. (A) Position of the examiner's hand on patient's abdomen. (B) Illustration of the relationship of the examiner's hand and fetus.

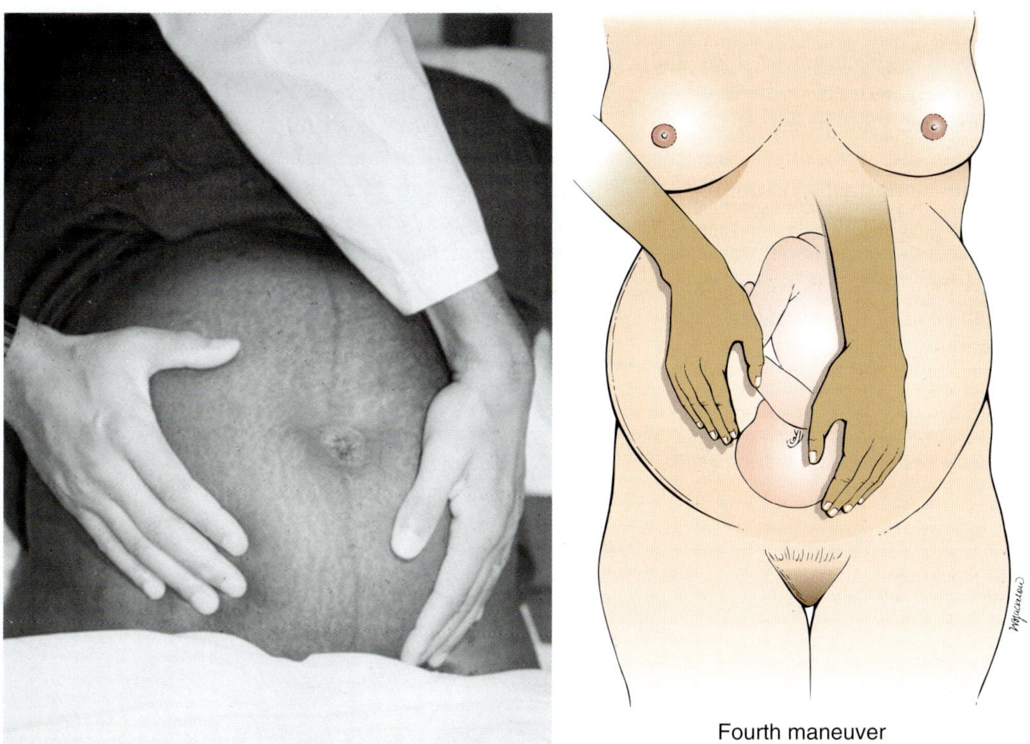

A B

Fig. 23.18 **Leopold's Fourth Maneuver.** Relationship of the healthcare professional's hands and fetal presenting part. (A) Position of examiner's hands on patient's abdomen. (B) Illustration of the relationship of examiner's hands and fetus. Note that the examiner's right hand is stopped higher by the fetus's cephalic prominence.

Labor is the process of birth. The diagnosis and the mechanism of labor are complex topics and are beyond the scope of this book. The reader is referred to the references for this chapter for discussions of these topics.

CLINICOPATHOLOGIC CORRELATIONS

Bleeding during pregnancy is not normal and can be caused by benign or serious factors that vary depending on the stage of pregnancy and the nature of the bleeding.

During the first trimester, vaginal bleeding can indicate implantation of the ovum, cervicitis, vaginal varicosities, or a threatened, inevitable, incomplete, or complete abortion.

A *threatened abortion* should always be considered when vaginal bleeding occurs in the first 20 weeks of pregnancy. With a threatened abortion, the cervix will be closed, and no products of conception will have passed out of the uterus.

An *inevitable abortion* can be diagnosed if a patient presents during the first half of pregnancy with bleeding and crampy abdominal pain in association with a dilated cervix or a gush of fluid (rupture of membranes) without passing of the products of conception.

An *incomplete or complete abortion* occurs when part or all the products of conception are extruded through the cervix and into the vagina and are passed out of the body.

Second- or third-trimester bleeding occurs in approximately 3% of all pregnancies. Approximately 60% of these bleeding episodes result from placenta previa or abruptio placentae. Both of these conditions may gravely endanger the patient and fetus.

Placenta previa is a condition that affects about 1 in 250 deliveries, and it is more common in patients who have had multiple pregnancies than in those who are pregnant for the first time. Placenta previa can take different forms, but the symptoms always arise from the abnormal positioning of the placenta near or over the internal os of the cervix. The most common presentation of placenta previa is painless vaginal bleeding, often accompanied by a soft, nontender uterus. Hemorrhage typically occurs at the end of the second trimester or later, and up to 90% of patients with placenta previa have at least one antepartum hemorrhage. Furthermore, there is a 20% chance of preterm delivery due to hemorrhage.

Abruptio placentae is the premature separation of a normally situated placenta. It has an incidence of 1 per 75 to 225 deliveries. The symptoms include mild to severe pain with or without external bleeding in association with increasing uterine tone and tenderness. Fetal distress may or may not occur. Hypertension is, by far, the most commonly associated condition. Cigarette smoking and cocaine use have also been linked to an increased risk of abruptio placentae. Patients with a history of abruptio placentae are at significant risk of recurrence in subsequent pregnancies.

Vasa praevia is another serious but rare condition in which some of the fetal vessels in the membranes cross the region of the internal os. These vessels occupy a position in front of the presenting portion of the fetus. Rupture of the membranes may be accompanied by rupture of the fetal vessel, causing fetal blood loss and possible exsanguination.

Postpartum hemorrhage (PPH) is the most common cause of serious bleeding in obstetric patients and is the leading cause of maternal death. It is defined as cumulative blood loss in excess of 1000 mL or blood loss combined with signs and symptoms of hypovolemia during the first 24 hours after delivery. The most common cause of PPH is uterine atony, and it is responsible for 70% to 80% of PPH. There are many other causes for PPH: lacerations, retained placenta, abnormally adherent placenta, coagulation defects, uterine inversion, and infection. It has been estimated that PPH occurs in 1% to 5% of all deliveries.

SUMMARY

As we conclude this chapter on "The Pregnant Patient," it is clear that pregnancy is a profound and transformative journey for both the patient and the healthcare professional. It is a time marked by unique challenges and opportunities, where the delicate balance between birthing parent and fetal well-being takes center stage. By fostering a compassionate, informed, and patient-centered approach, healthcare professionals can navigate the complexities of care for the pregnant patient with skill and empathy.

USEFUL VOCABULARY

Listed here are the specific roots that are important for understanding the terminology related to the pregnant patient.

Root	Definition	Example	
ante-	before	***ante***partum	Before birth
nulli-	none	***nulli***parous	Having never given birth before
multi-	many	***multi***parous	Having given birth before
-par/o	to give birth	multi***parous***	Having given birth before
-gravid	pregnancy	primi***gravida***	Pregnant for the first time
puer-	childbirth	***puer***perium	Time period around childbirth
-cyesis	pregnancy	pseudo***cyesis***	False pregnancy
-tocia	labor	dys***tocia***	Abnormal labor
-natal	birth	pre***natal***	Before birth
lochi-	postpartum	***lochi***orrhea	Abnormally profuse discharge of vaginal lochia

WRITING UP THE PHYSICAL EXAMINATION

Listed here are examples of the write-up for the assessment of the pregnant patient.

- The patient is a 32-year-old healthy, cisgender[c] female, gravida 3, para 2-0-0-2 (see Chapter 19, Female Genitalia) LMP = 8/29/23, EDD = 6/5/24 at 32 weeks of gestation presenting for routine prenatal care. She has no concerns and reports no contractions, leaking of fluid, or vaginal bleeding. She reports normal fetal movement. Her obstetric history is unremarkable with 2 normal, spontaneous vaginal deliveries (NSVD) with the largest infant weighing 7 pounds, 4 ounces. Blood pressure is 125/80. Findings of examination of the head, eye, ear, nose, throat, and neck are unremarkable except for the presence of chloasma. Breasts are symmetrically enlarged with visible venous pattern. No dominant masses were palpated. Chest is clear to percussion and auscultation. Heart rate is 100 and regular. Heart sounds are normal. A grade II/VI midsystolic murmur is heard in the aortic area. No gallops are present. Examination of the abdomen reveals a 32-week-sized gravid uterus which is appropriate for dates. There are reddish, slightly depressed streaks on the lower abdomen. 1+ pretibial edema is present bilaterally. Movement of the fetus is felt. The fetus is in a longitudinal lie in a vertex presentation, with its back to the left. Fetal heart rate is 150 beats per minute and is heard through the back of the fetus, 2 cm to the left of midline in the lower left quadrant.
- The patient is a 29-year-old healthy, cisgender female, para 2-1-1-3 with LMP = 9/3/23 and EDD = 6/10/24 at 16 weeks presenting for routine prenatal care. She reports no cramping, vaginal bleeding, or leakage of fluid. She has not felt any fetal movement yet. Her first pregnancy was preterm (at 35 weeks) and delivered by cesarean section because of preterm labor with a double footling breech presentation; weight, 6 pounds 2 ounces. Her next two pregnancies were full-term, vaginal deliveries after cesarean section (VBAC). The first infant weighed 7 pounds, 7 ounces, and the second one weighed 6 pounds 9 ounces. She had one elective termination of pregnancy at 8 weeks between her first and second children. Blood pressure is 135/75. Thyroid is mildly enlarged symmetrically without nodularity. Multiple spider angiomas are present over the face, neck, upper chest, and arms. Breasts are symmetrically enlarged, with increased pigmentation of the areolae present. Striae gravidarum are present on the breasts. Chest is clear to percussion and auscultation. Heart rate is 90 and regular. S_1 and S_2 are normal. No murmurs, gallops, or rubs are heard. Uterus is felt in the abdomen at about a 16-week gestation, which is consistent with dates. Fetal heart rate is 160 by Doppler and is located in the midline of the lower abdomen. Bimanual examination reveals a soft lower uterine segment. External os admits a fingertip with a closed internal os. Cervix is approximately 2 cm in length. Uterus is globular and smooth. Adnexa are unremarkable. Rectovaginal examination not performed. No edema present. Mild varicosities of both lower extremities are present.

[c]This current terminology recognizes that everyone has gender identity and not all people who become pregnant are females, as described earlier in this chapter. See Chapter 26, The Transgender Patient, for more information.

REVIEW QUESTIONS

1. A change that is NOT normal in the pregnant patient's chest is:

A. Breast enlargement
B. Increased vascularity of the breasts
C. Breast tenderness
D. Bleeding from the nipples
E. Increased pigmentation of the areola

2. One of the most important infections to screen for in pregnancy is:

A. Strep pharyngitis
B. Syphilis
C. Trichomoniasis
D. Influenza
E. HPV

3. Patients with chronic hypertension have:

A. A decreased risk for preterm labor
B. A decreased risk of growth restriction of the fetus
C. An increased risk of developing preeclampsia
D. No change in their risk of abruptio placentae
E. A universal need for antihypertensive medication

4. Shortly (3 days) after fertilization, the fertilized egg develops into a:

A. Blastocyst
B. Morula
C. Embryo
D. Ectopic pregnancy
E. Fetus

5. Common characteristics of the postpartum blues include all of the following *EXCEPT:*

A. Difficulty sleeping
B. Anxiety about stresses of parenting
C. Concern about appearance
D. Increased excitement about birth and parenting
E. Self-limited nature

6. Which term characterizes the level of descent of the presenting part of the fetus?

A. Presentation
B. Station
C. Flexion
D. Lie
E. Effacement

7. Which has been associated with placental abruption?

A. Drinking alcohol
B. Thyroid disease
C. Smoking cigarettes
D. Opioid use
E. Aspirin use

8. Unintended pregnancy rates in the U.S. are:

A. Less than 10%
B. Lower than other developed nations
C. 25%
D. Rising
E. 45%

9. Which is NOT common in pregnancy?

A. Heartburn
B. Backache
C. Chest pain
D. Urinary frequency
E. Increased vaginal discharge

10. The term for the sensation of fetal movement is:

A. Contractions
B. Descent
C. Parity
D. Quickening
E. Rotation

REFERENCES

Available online.

BIBLIOGRAPHY

Available online.

24

The Pediatric Patient

Miriam Schechter and Hai Jung Helen Rhim

"There can be no keener revelation of a society's soul than the way in which it treats its children."

—Nelson Mandela, Former President of South Africa (1918–2013)

VIDEOS

Video 24.1 Full video: Examining the newborn
Video 24.2 Full video: Examining the toddler
Video 24.3 Full video: Performing the neurologic examination
Video 24.4 Conducting a telephone interview with a parent of a sick toddler

GENERAL CONSIDERATIONS

The field of pediatrics is quite extensive and covers the period from birth to adolescence, which is often defined as up to the age of 22. During this time, children experience significant changes in their emotional, social, cognitive, and physical development, and all of these aspects must be thoroughly evaluated. While previous chapters focused on the history and physical examination in the context of adult patients, this chapter will examine the differences related to physical diagnosis in the pediatric age group.

Role of the Pediatric Healthcare Professional

The role of pediatric healthcare professionals (including, but not limited to, pediatricians, pediatric nurse practitioners, and physician assistants) is multifaceted and includes taking care of children while they are well and when they are ill, recognizing the importance of the behavioral and social aspects of a child's health. At well-child checks, pediatric healthcare professionals screen for any problems or abnormalities, monitor growth and development to detect any delays, and provide anticipatory guidance to families so they know what to expect at every stage of childhood. In addition, pediatric healthcare professionals provide care to children when they are sick with minor illnesses and major conditions. However, an added dimension to the pediatric healthcare professional's role is the one that partners with families and caregivers to foster a healthy and productive life for a child. Pediatric healthcare professionals take great care in considering the caregiver–child relationship and the interactions within that dyad. This is reflected in the approach to family-centered care that is at the heart of every encounter.

Cultural Effectiveness

It is critical for the pediatric healthcare professional to provide culturally effective healthcare and to be sensitive to differences in culture, beliefs, and values. According to the American Academy of Pediatrics (AAP), "culturally effective healthcare can be defined as the delivery of care within the context of appropriate physician knowledge, understanding, and appreciation of all cultural distinctions leading to optimal health outcomes."[1] No matter the background of the patient, their family, or the healthcare professional, everyone has culturally based beliefs about health and illness. It is important for pediatric healthcare professionals to recognize these differences and cultivate the knowledge, skills, and attitudes that will help them to achieve culturally effective healthcare.

Children and Youth with Special Healthcare Needs

Pediatric healthcare professionals take care of pediatric patients with a variety of acute and chronic conditions, including children and youth with special healthcare needs (CYSHCN). These children have a chronic physical, developmental, behavioral, and/or emotional condition. They need healthcare more often and services that are generally not needed by the majority of children. CYSHCN makes up about 18% of children in the United States.[2] Children with complex medical problems make up a subset of CYSHCN, and they often have multiple chronic conditions and multisystem diseases and may be technology-dependent. They also have frequent admissions to the hospital and require care coordination across several subspecialists. This can lead to a greater use of services and resources. Having a medical home is important for all patients; however, this need is even more critical for children with medical complexity.

Unique Considerations of the Pediatric History

One unique aspect of history taking in pediatrics is the common use of multiperson history source. When the patient is an infant, the primary source of the history is the caregiver. As children grow, they can provide progressively more of their history. Even when pediatric patients can provide their own account, oftentimes the history is supplemented by caregivers to get the full extent of the story.

An infant communicates by crying and, in so doing, indicates the existence of an unmet need. Although older children can communicate through language, they also often use crying as a response to pain or to express emotional unrest. This mode of communication merits attention. Newborns can also communicate by cooing and babbling, which indicates contentment. Three-year-olds can give the healthcare professional a good idea of what hurts, where, and how it feels. The 6-year-old can give some idea of how and when the concern started. The examiner must pay attention to everything children say because the words used may give insight into the child's physical, emotional, and developmental state; their home situation; and other factors in their environment.

Another distinction is in regard to the social history that, while important for all patients, is of utmost importance in the pediatric history. This underscores the significance of the psychosocial context of a child's existence and how it can profoundly impact a child's health and development. Pediatric healthcare professionals take it beyond the usual social history questions and inquire about the housing situation, financial security of the family, availability of health insurance, pets, and other exposures. Social and structural determinants of health impact health outcomes and health equity.

In addition, there are specific unique aspects of the pediatric history depending on the child's age. For example, in the newborn period, the prenatal and birth histories are of paramount importance, whereas these become less pertinent in adolescence. For infants and toddlers, the focus tends to be on feeding, growth, and development. In school-age children, academics and the social aspects of school play a large role. Lastly, for teenagers, confidentiality and the age-appropriate aspects of an adolescent social history are highlighted.

Purpose of the Pediatric Physical Exam

While, like the adult exam, the purpose of the physical exam in children is to assess health, uncover new or changing findings, and help make diagnoses, the physical examination in pediatrics has some unique goals that vary over time. In the newborn period, it is crucial to identify major malformations, such as congenital heart defects, that may impact the neonate's transition to extrauterine life. Additionally, there may be important physical findings that need less immediate but significant intervention, such as developmental dysplasia of the hips (DDH). Finally, there are countless minor malformations or benign findings, such as molding of the head, that need to be noted to educate the caregivers on their natural history and just require expectant management.

For the infant age group, the physical exam becomes an essential component of every patient encounter as the patient is not verbal and cannot express concerns. Healthcare professionals must become detectives and rely heavily on what is uncovered during the exam to make a diagnosis. Identifying the source of a fever for example is much easier when older children can tell you they have severe ear pain. Furthermore, the physical exam in an infant includes important observations and findings in regard to development. Monitoring of social/emotional, language/communication, cognitive, and movement/physical milestones of development starts in infancy and continues straight through toddler- and preschool-aged children. Toddlers are actually a challenging group due to their severe stranger anxiety that often impedes a comprehensive physical. The goal in these patients is to use a variety of techniques, including distraction, doing an exam in a caregiver's lap, and informed observation to assess health and identify abnormalities in the most efficient, complete manner possible in light of these limitations.

Preschool- and school-aged children begin to not only cooperate but truly participate in the exam. As a healthcare professional, a large part of the exam is engaging the child in the techniques and meaning of exam components and giving them more of a role in the visits overall. The adolescent exam carries a unique purpose too, as patients progress through puberty. Without a caregiver in the room, the healthcare professional is expected to explore psychosocial issues with the teen in a confidential manner and monitor the physical stages of sexual maturity, also known as Tanner stages. Finally, in late adolescence, the exam becomes identical to the adult exam, and the patient is prepared to mature into adulthood and in many cases care by a new primary care professional. In summary, it is clear that healthcare professionals must take into consideration the age and developmental level of the pediatric patient when embarking on the physical examination.

Unique Considerations of the Pediatric Physical Examination

It is a well-known saying in pediatrics that "*children are not just small adults*," and this is certainly true when it comes to performing the physical exam. The breadth of unique age groups, spanning newborns through young adulthood, warrants individualized approaches unique from that of the adult examination. In pediatrics, the power of observation cannot be overemphasized. Children are by nature interested in their environment and paying close attention to those who are interacting and those who are not is a key distinguishing factor between a well and a worrisome child. Watching the breathing pattern of an infant with bronchiolitis,[a] including presence of tachypnea, retractions, and nasal flaring, can determine the disposition between hospitalization and home management. Furthermore, observation of the child's nutritional status, color, skin findings, tone, developmental milestones, dysmorphic features, and orthopedic deformities can all be done without even touching the patient. Indirect observation, barely noticed by the child, can be done from the moment one steps into the room and can continue throughout the history-taking process, whether the child is in a stroller, on a caregiver's lap, in a crib, or exploring around an exam room. A tremendous amount of clinically relevant

[a]Bronchiolitis is a common viral infection of the lungs in infants and in young children under 2 years of age. It causes inflammation and congestion of the bronchioles, resulting in wheezing and respiratory distress. Typically, the peak time for bronchiolitis is during the winter months.

information is obtained through this process of informed observation.

Another unique aspect of the pediatric exam is in the approach. Unlike the physical exam of an adult that generally progresses in a head-to-toe sequence, the exam in young children does not. In young patients up until school age, the sequence generally goes from least invasive to the more invasive or uncomfortable. Listening gently to the heart and lungs will always precede the ear and throat exam, which should come last. As children age and become more cooperative and involved in the exam, going from head to toe will become the routine. Importantly, flexibility by the healthcare professional in the exact sequence of the exam is essential and will likely vary from patient to patient. For example, if a newborn's eyes are open at the start of the exam, immediately do the red reflex exam; however, if the eyes remain closed until the end, the red reflex exam may be the last part of the exam. If a toddler starts screaming when approached, grab a light to get a great look in the oropharynx. Always be ready to jump around in the exam of infants and toddlers to get the most out of the exam.

Another skill often necessary for a successful exam of young infants and children is to ally with the adult caregiver in the room. They know how to soothe a crying infant to allow for a good lung and heart exam once the child quiets. Toddlers who may have stranger anxiety may not be happy separating from their caregiver to sit on an exam table and are much better off being examined in the comfort of the caregiver's lap. Using a caregiver to tightly hold the flailing arms and moving head of a young child during an ear exam will be a huge assistance to the healthcare professional in getting an optimal look.

Being playful and innovative when it comes to examining a child can also be a huge help in successfully completing an exam and also make it fun. Whether it's making a game using the instruments, singing songs, asking about their toys, or blowing bubbles, distractions will go a long way with young children. Often pediatric healthcare professionals will have small attractive toys in their pockets or hanging off their stethoscope: toys that light up or make noise will distract a toddler long enough to get a good lung and cardiac exam. Gaining the trust and cooperation of a preschool- or school-aged child by asking about their school, family, or interests will make the exam much easier than if the child feels scared or mistrustful. Similarly, building rapport with preteens and teens will always result in a more mutually comfortable interaction.

Even vital signs vary for children of different ages, with newborns having much higher heart and respiratory rates and lower blood pressures (BP) than older children, which then gradually change throughout childhood until they reach adult levels. A baby could be breathing very comfortably 55 times a minute, whereas this would indicate respiratory failure in an adult. Being aware of norms for different ages is necessary to use vital signs to make appropriate assessments.

Also different from the adult exam are some of the unique maneuvers that must be completed for different age groups that do not exist as part of the adult exam. For example, in infants, check for open fontanelles and hip dislocation; in adolescents, check for scoliosis and the physical changes of puberty. The hip and back exams of a newborn will be rather different than those of the adolescent and adult. There are distinct maneuvers that must be learned and will be delineated in the corresponding portion of this chapter.

This chapter will first review the basics of the pediatric history and physical examination. It will then highlight the differences in various age groups, including neonatal, infancy, early childhood, middle childhood, and adolescence.

PEDIATRIC HISTORY

The pediatric history, like the adult history, is obtained before the examination is performed. During this period, the child can get accustomed to the healthcare professional. Much of the pediatric history is taken from the caregiver, but it can be helpful to include the child in the process. If children are able to provide history, interview them as well.

Effective relationships with children begin by engaging with them. Ways to make a child feel more comfortable include admiring the child's toy, sharing a book, asking about their friends or school, or offering praise. Some examiners may choose not to wear a white coat to potentially alleviate some of the child's fears.

It is important not to talk down to children. The examiner must assess the developmental level of the child and choose words that are appropriate to that child's level of understanding. This is especially important in dealing with a preadolescent. It is essential to give an adolescent private time with the healthcare professional. Laws in most states entitle adolescents to *confidential care* for reproductive health, mental health, and misused substances.

The pediatric history format is similar to the general adult history; however, special attention is paid to development and psychosocial issues and also to the unique aspects, which change with the age of the child. In addition, there are sections in the pediatric history that do not exist in the adult format (i.e., birth history, immunizations, development, adolescent social history, when appropriate).

Sections of a Pediatric History

Chief Concern

This should be a brief statement of the presenting concern (no matter the clinical setting). The chief concern is usually best presented as a direct quote from the patient or informant explaining why the child was brought to medical attention.

Informant

Identify each person who is providing the history, state whether an interpreter was used, and make an assessment of the reliability of the informant(s).

History of Present Illness

Start with identifying data (i.e., age and sex recorded at birth) and then relate history chronologically. Be as complete as possible by including the seven dimensions of a symptom (i.e., timing, location, quality, quantity, setting, aggravating/alleviating factors, and associated manifestations). The history of present illness (HPI) should include information about the effect of an acute illness on the child's oral intake, activity level, hydration status, and ability to sleep. If the illness is chronic, include information about initial presentation, course, response to medications, impact on the child's growth and development, etc. For inpatient cases, a brief summary of the emergency department course can be provided after the HPI, including a clear statement as to the reason for admission.

Past Medical History

Include information about all significant illnesses, operations, accidents, common childhood diseases, and hospitalizations. Ask about chronic health problems, such as asthma, eczema, recurrent ear infections, or developmental delays. Verify if the child is receiving routine healthcare and, if so, the name of the healthcare professional.

Medications

List all medicines that the child is taking, including over-the-counter medications and herbal remedies/complementary medicines. Be sure to include medication names, dosages, route of administration, frequency, and indications.

Allergies

Include allergies to medications, foods, and environmental allergens. Ask about specific reactions. If it was a rash, try to clarify if it was urticarial, which is likely to be a true allergy, rather than a nonspecific eruption that may have occurred coincidentally.

Birth History

Note sex recorded at birth, birth weight, gestational age, type of delivery, and place of delivery. Include age and parity[b] of the mother, maternal medications or substance use, and prenatal complications (e.g., gestational diabetes, hypertension, abnormal maternal labs or studies). Record duration of ruptured membranes, Apgar scores (as described in the newborn physical exam section), and resuscitation measures, if performed. Comment on nursery or neonatal intensive care unit (NICU) course/complications and baby's age at discharge. Include information on common nursery screening tests. Note the order of these questions: they begin with the prenatal course, then focus on the actual birth, and then turn to the postnatal course. In general, little detail is needed here for teens unless there were complications. In contrast, more detail is needed for infants less than 2 months of age or born prematurely, as the birth history has more relevance.

Box 24.1 contains a list of maternal/prenatal tests, screens, and procedures. Some of these are universal; others are selective. Box 24.2 demonstrates the shorthand notation for maternal pregnancy history. See also Chapter 23, The Pregnant Patient. Box 24.3 lists the tests, screens, and procedures performed on newborns before discharge from the nursery.

[b]Parity, or "para," indicates the number of pregnancies reaching viable gestational age (including live births and stillbirths).

BOX 24.1 Typical Prenatal Testing/Screening

Serologies/Infectious Disease Screening
Chlamydia
Gonorrhea
Group B strep
Hepatitis B
Hepatitis C
HIV
Measles
Parvovirus
Rubella
Syphilis (RPR)
Varicella

Genetic Testing
Amniocentesis
Chorionic villus sampling
Noninvasive prenatal screening (NIPS; cell free DNA testing)
Quad screen (AFP, hCG, Estriol, and Inhibin-A)

Other Labs
Blood type
Glucose testing
Hemoglobin electrophoresis
Lead level

Ultrasound
Initial dating/viability scan
Early anatomy/sequential screen scan (depends on maternal age)
Detailed anatomy scan at 18–20 weeks
36-week scan for size, position, fluid level

AFP, alpha fetoprotein; *hCG,* human chorionic gonadotropin; *RPR,* rapid plasma reagin.

BOX 24.2 Shorthand for Maternal Pregnancy History

Gravida = # of pregnancies
Para = outcomes of pregnancies
4 numbers FPAL
- **F**ull-term deliveries
- **P**reterm deliveries
- **A**bortions or miscarriages
- **L**ive children

Example 1:
G3P1102. This is the 3rd pregnancy for this female who already has 2 live children, one born at term, one born preterm
Example 2:
G4P1022. This is the 4th pregnancy for a female who had 2 miscarriages or terminations and had twins born at term.[a]

[a]*Note that a twin pregnancy carried to viable gestational age is counted as 1. The number of fetuses does not determine the parity.*

Diet History

Nutrition is central to the child's well-being. Getting a complete *nutritional history* not only helps in monitoring the child's nutritional health but may also help you make the diagnosis of an acute problem. For newborns and young infants, ask about the methods of feeding (i.e., breast or formula), as

BOX 24.3 Routine Care in the Nursery

Bilirubin (transcutaneous or serum)
Blood type and Coombs
Critical congenital heart disease (CCHD) screen
Hearing screen
Measurements (i.e., weight, length, head circumference)
State-based newborn screening
Routine administration of medications/vaccines:
 Erythromycin eye ointment (prevention of gonorrhea conjunctivitis)
 Hepatitis B vaccine, dose #1
 RSV monoclonal antibody
 Vitamin K (prevention of hemorrhagic disease of the newborn)

RSV, respiratory syncytial virus
Universal newborn hearing screening is performed in the nursery through either evoked otoacoustic emissions (EOAE) or auditory brainstem response (ABR) testing. These are noninvasive, easily performed evaluations of physiologic activity that underlie normal auditory function.
Critical congenital heart defect (CCHD) screening is part of the recommended newborn universal screening panel. It is performed in the nursery after 24 hours of age using pulse oximetry to measure oxygen saturation in the right hand and one foot. Readings of ≥95% in right hand and foot and ≤3% difference between the two is considered passing.
Universal newborn screening tests performed on newborn blood samples for early identification of treatable congenital conditions before symptoms begin. These conditions include a variety of inborn errors of metabolism, endocrine disorders, hemoglobinopathies, immunodeficiencies, and genetic disorders. There is a core set of recommended tests and others that are U.S. state-specific.

well as amount and frequency of feedings. For older infants and toddlers, document when and which solids were started and describe the child's present diet, including what the child is drinking. In school-aged children and older, find out what the child eats in and out of the home, including during and between meals. Specify what the child drinks, including water, juice, milk, and sweetened beverages. For more details, see individual sections later for each age group.

Growth and Development

Describe the child's general pattern of growth, weight gain, and any concerns or abnormalities. Inquire if the caregiver is worried about poor weight gain, overweight or obesity, unexpected change in growth, short stature, and abnormal head growth.

If meeting a patient for the first time beyond the neonatal period, obtain a developmental history. Note when the child first smiled, rolled over, reached for objects, sat up, walked with and without support, spoke their first words and sentences, was toilet trained, etc. Often caregivers will not remember the exact age at the time of these milestones but will be able to state if milestones were met on time or if they or their healthcare professionals ever had concerns about the child's development. Ask if there was ever an evaluation or services provided by Early Intervention.

For children under the age of 6, assess current achievement of age-appropriate developmental milestones in four domains: movement/physical development, language/communication, social/emotional, and cognitive. This can be done through a combination of healthcare professional observations, parental report, and a wide array of developmental surveillance and screening questionnaires. There are many tools available for identifying developmental milestones.[c] Tailor this to the child's age. Adolescents do not need in-depth developmental histories.

See Table 24.1 that summarizes developmental milestones for developmental surveillance at preventive care visits.

School History

Progress and achievement in school is a key component of a child's well-being. Unsatisfactory school performance can be indicative of learning disabilities, psychosocial problems, or medical conditions. Identify what school the child attends and if they are in the appropriate grade. If behind a grade level, has the child been evaluated, or do they receive special education services (e.g., small class, speech, occupational or physical therapy, counseling)? Ask about the child's performance both academically and behaviorally. It is important to find out if the child likes school, has friends, or is the victim of bullying.

Immunization History

Vaccines are one of the major successes of 20th-century medicine; healthcare professionals are unlikely to see many vaccine-preventable diseases such as polio, rubella, chickenpox, or diphtheria. It is essential to review the child's immunization history from birth through adolescence as there are recommended vaccines for all age groups. Ask to see the child's vaccine record if the caregiver has one. State registries are also a good resource for determining immunization status. Compare the child's vaccines with the most up-to-date Centers for Disease Control and Prevention (CDC) recommended immunization schedule (available at https://www.cdc.gov/vaccines/).

If immunizations have been delayed, state the reason. If caregivers have declined vaccines, address their concerns, explain the rationale, and continue to encourage catch-up immunizations. If the child is missing one or more vaccines, consider the possibility the child is suffering from a vaccine-preventable illness. Note that the immunization schedule offers instructions for providing "catch-up" vaccinations for children who have fallen behind.

Menstrual History (if Appropriate)

Note age at menarche, regularity, length, associated symptoms, character of menses, and date of last menstrual period (LMP).

Social History/Social and Structural Determinants of Health

It is essential to obtain a thorough social history for pediatric patients, as many social factors in their life, beyond what is apparent at the point of a medical visit, can affect their health and have a large influence on their overall well-being. It has become increasingly clear that the environment in which a child grows up has a tremendous impact on their physical and mental health in potentially positive and negative ways. These family and com-

[c]For example, the "CDC Milestones" app is a milestone tracker for parents that also has age-based checklists with videos demonstrating each milestone.

TABLE 24.1 CDC Developmental Milestones[a]

Age	Social/Emotional Milestones	Language/Communication Milestones	Cognitive Milestones	Movement/Physical Development Milestones
2 MONTHS	Calms down when spoken to or picked up Looks at your face Seems happy to see you when you walk up to them Smiles when you talk to or smile at them	Makes sounds other than crying Reacts to loud sounds	Watches you as you move Looks at a toy for several seconds	Holds head up when on tummy Moves both arms and both legs Opens hands briefly
4 MONTHS	Smiles on their own to get your attention Chuckles (not yet a full laugh) when you try to make them laugh Looks at you, moves, or makes sounds to get or keep your attention	Makes sounds like "oooo", "aahh" (cooing) Makes sounds back when you talk to them Turns head toward the sound of your voice	If hungry, opens mouth when they see breast or bottle Looks at their hands with interest	Holds head steady without support when you are holding them Holds a toy when you put it in their hand Uses their arm to swing at toys Brings hands to mouth Pushes up onto elbows/forearms when on tummy
6 MONTHS	Knows familiar people Likes to look at themself in a mirror Laughs	Takes turns making sounds with you Blows "raspberries" (sticks tongue out and blows) Makes squealing noises	Puts things in the mouth to explore them Reaches to grab a toy they want Closes lips to show they don't want more food	Rolls from tummy to back Pushes up with straight arms when on tummy Leans on hands to support themself when sitting
9 MONTHS	Is shy, clingy, or fearful around strangers Shows several facial expressions, like happy, sad, angry, and surprised Looks when you call their name Reacts when you leave (looks, reaches for you, or cries) Smiles or laughs when you play peek-a-boo	Makes different sounds like "mama mama" and "baba baba" Lifts arms up to be picked up	Looks for objects when dropped out of sight (like a spoon or toy) Bangs two things together	Gets to a sitting position by themself Moves things from one hand to the other hand Uses fingers to "rake" food towards themself Sits without support
12 MONTHS	Plays games with you, like pat-a-cake	Waves "bye-bye" Calls a parent "mama" or "dada" or another special name Understands "no" (pauses briefly or stops when you say it)	Puts something in a container, like a block in a cup Looks for things they see you hide, like a toy under a blanket	Pulls up to stand Walks, holding on to furniture Drinks from a cup without a lid, as you hold it Picks things up between thumb and pointer finger, like small bits of food
15 MONTHS	Copies other children while playing, like taking toys out of a container when another child does Shows you an object they like Claps when excited Hugs stuffed doll or other toy Shows you affection (hugs, cuddles, or kisses you)	Tries to say one or two words besides "mama" or "dada," like "ba" for ball or "da" for dog Looks at a familiar object when you name it Follows directions given with both a gesture and words. For example, they give you a toy when you hold out your hand and say, "Give me the toy." Points to ask for something or to get help	Tries to use things the right way, like a phone, cup, or book Stacks at least two small objects, like blocks	Takes a few steps on their own Uses fingers to feed themself some food

TABLE 24.1 CDC Developmental Milestones—cont'd

Age	Social/Emotional Milestones	Language/Communication Milestones	Cognitive Milestones	Movement/Physical Development Milestones
18 MONTHS[b,c]	Moves away from you, but looks to make sure you are close by Points to show you something interesting Puts hands out for you to wash them Looks at a few pages in a book with you Helps you dress them by pushing arm through sleeve or lifting up foot	Tries to say three or more words besides "mama" or "dada" Follows one-step directions without any gestures, like giving you the toy when you say, "Give it to me."	Copies you doing chores, like sweeping with a broom Plays with toys in a simple way, like pushing a toy car	Walks without holding on to anyone or anything Scribbles Drinks from a cup without a lid and may spill sometimes Feeds themself with their fingers Tries to use a spoon Climbs on and off a couch or chair without help
2 YEARS[c]	Notices when others are hurt or upset, like pausing or looking sad when someone is crying Looks at your face to see how to react in a new situation	Points to things in a book when you ask, like "Where is the bear?" Says at least two words together, like "More milk." Points to at least two body parts when you ask them to show you Uses more gestures than just waving and pointing, like blowing a kiss or nodding yes	Holds something in one hand while using the other hand; for example, holding a container and taking the lid off Tries to use switches, knobs, or buttons on a toy Plays with more than one toy at the same time, like putting toy food on a toy plate	Kicks a ball Runs Walks (not climbs) up a few stairs with or without help Eats with a spoon
30 MONTHS[b,c]	Plays next to other children and sometimes plays with them Shows you what they can do by saying, "Look at me!" Follows simple routines when told, like helping to pick up toys when you say, "It's clean-up time."	Says about 50 words Says two or more words together, with one action word, like "Doggie run" Names things in a book when you point and ask, "What is this?" Says words like "I," "me," or "we"	Uses things to pretend, like feeding a block to a doll as if it were food Shows simple problem-solving skills, like standing on a small stool to reach something Follows two-step instructions like "Put the toy down and close the door." Shows they know at least one color, like pointing to a red crayon when you ask, "Which one is red?"	Uses hands to twist things, like turning doorknobs or unscrewing lids Takes some clothes off by themself, like loose pants or an open jacket Jumps off the ground with both feet Turns book pages, one at a time, when you read to them
3 YEARS	Calms down within 10 minutes after you leave them, like at a childcare drop off Notices other children and joins them to play	Talks with you in conversation using at least two back-and-forth exchanges Asks "who," "what," "where," or "why" questions, like "Where is mommy/daddy?" Says what action is happening in a picture or book when asked, like "running," "eating," or "playing" Says first name, when asked Talks well for enough for others to understand, most of the time	Draws a circle when you show them how Avoids touching hot objects, like a stove, when you warn them	Strings items together, like large beads or macaroni Puts on some clothes by themself, like loose pants or a jacket Uses a fork
4 YEARS	Pretends to be something else during play (teacher, superhero, dog) Asks to go play with children if none are around, like "Can I play with Alex?" Comforts others who are hurt or sad, like hugging a crying friend Avoids danger, like not jumping from tall heights at the playground Likes to be a "helper" Changes behavior based on where they are (place of worship, library, playground)	Says sentences with four or more words Says some words from a song, story, or nursery rhyme Talks about at least one thing that happened during their day, like "I played soccer." Answers simple questions like "What is a coat for?" or "What is a crayon for?"	Names a few colors of items Tells what comes next in a well-known story Draws a person with three or more body parts	Catches a large ball most of the time Serves themself food or pours water, with adult supervision Unbuttons some buttons Holds crayon or pencil between fingers and thumb (not a fist)

Continued

TABLE 24.1 CDC Developmental Milestones—cont'd

Age	Social/Emotional Milestones	Language/Communication Milestones	Cognitive Milestones	Movement/Physical Development Milestones
5 YEARS	Follows rules or takes turns when playing games with other children Sings, dances, or acts for you Does simple chores at home, like matching socks or clearing the table after eating	Tells a story they heard or made up with at least two events. For example, a cat was stuck in a tree and a firefighter saved it Answers simple questions about a book or story after you read or tell it to them Keeps a conversation going with more than three back-and-forth exchanges Uses or recognizes simple rhymes (bat-cat, ball-tall)	Counts to 10 Names some numbers between 1 and 5 when you point to them Uses words about time, like "yesterday," "tomorrow," "morning," or "night" Pays attention for 5 to 10 minutes during activities. For example, during story time or making arts and crafts (screen time does not count) Writes some letters in their name Names some letters when you point to them	Buttons some buttons Hops on one foot

[a]Developmental milestones are intended for discussion with caregivers for the purposes of surveillance of a child's developmental progress and for developmental promotion for the child. They are not intended or validated for use as a developmental screening test in the pediatric medical home or in early childhood day care or educational settings. Milestones are also commonly used for instructional purposes on early child development for pediatric and child development professional trainees. These milestones generally represent the age at which 75% or more of children would be expected to perform the skills.
[b]AAP recommends that a standardized developmental screening tool be used at the 18 and 30 months visits or whenever there is a concern related to development.
[c]AAP recommends that a standardized autism screening tool be used at the 18 and 24 months visits or whenever there is a concern. CDC recommends an additional autism screen at the 30 months visit.
Adapted from Centers for Disease Control and Prevention https://www.cdc.gov/ncbddd/actearly/milestones/index.html

munity strengths and challenges make up social determinants of health. Assessing social determinants will provide context for the child's surroundings and help identify protective factors as well as potentially harmful factors, which can then be addressed.

Ask about family makeup (i.e., family members, caregivers, their relationships, and dynamics), living situation (e.g., type of home, household members), living conditions (e.g., presence of heat, hot water, peeling paint, window guards), childcare arrangements (e.g., primary caretakers, home care, daycare, after school care), caregivers' occupations, etc. Find out about play habits, friends, hobbies, activities (e.g., sports, digital media use), and family life. The presence of environmental exposures in the home such as cigarette smoke, allergens (e.g., mold, roaches, dust, pets), and lead should be elicited. Find out about potential safety risks in or near the home (e.g., stairs, animals, machinery, firearms, violence).

Other important social determinants of health to ask about include legal problems (e.g., housing, immigration status, child support) and food insecurity. Find out about health insurance status and access to entitlements such as Special Supplemental Nutrition Program for Women, Infants, and Children (WIC); Supplemental Nutrition Assistance Program (SNAP) or food stamps; and Supplemental Security Income for patients with disabilities (SSI).

The IHELLP questionnaire in Table 24.2 is a good framework to approach the assessment of social determinants in the pediatric population.

Structural determinants of health, which are upstream societal factors that impact health and well-being, should also be recognized. Problems such as racism have been shown to adversely affect the health of children, adolescents, and their families. Although progress has been made toward racial equality and equity, evidence to support the continued negative impact of racism on health and well-being through implicit and explicit biases, institutional structures, and interpersonal relationships is clear.[3] See Chapter 5, Anti-Racist and Anti-Oppressive Clinical Skills, and Chapter 33, Clinical Ethics and Professionalism.

Constant reassessment of the social history at every health maintenance visit is essential as it can change often and have potentially positive or negative effects on the child. Reviewing areas such as childcare arrangements, changes in the household, the physical and mental health of caregivers, social determinants of health and their impact, environmental exposures, and access to needed services must not be overlooked.

Furthermore, questions about culture and spirituality need to be explored to understand the unique contexts in which children and families view their health and illness. Kleinman's explanatory model[4] frames questions to elicit responses from children and families about their illnesses that are influenced by their beliefs. See also Chapter 5, Anti-Racist and Anti-Oppressive Clinical Skills.

TABLE 24.2 IHELLP Social Questions History

Domain	Example Questions
Income	
General	Do you ever have trouble making ends meet?
Food income	Do you ever have a time when you don't have enough food? Do you have WIC? Food stamps?
Housing	
Housing	Is your housing ever a problem for you?
Utilities	Do you ever have trouble paying your electric/heat/telephone bill?
Education	
Appropriate education placement	How is your child doing in school? Are they getting the help to learn what they need?
Early childhood program	Is your child in Head Start, preschool, or early childhood enrichment?
Legal Status	
Immigration	Do you have questions about your immigration status? Do you need help accessing benefits or services for your family?
Literacy	
Child literacy	Do you read to your child every night?
Parent literacy	How happy are you with how you read?
Personal Safety	
Domestic violence	Have you ever taken out a restraining order? Do you feel safe in your relationship?
General safety	Do you feel safe in your home? In your neighborhood?

WIC, Women, infants, and children.
From the National Center for Medical-Legal Partnership https://downloads.aap.org/AAP/PDF/IHELLPPocketCard.pdf

For adolescents, a special format is utilized to obtain a detailed social history, called the *HEEADSSS exam*. This is an acronym for **H**ome, **E**ducation, **E**ating, **A**ctivities, **D**rugs, **S**exuality, **S**uicide/Depression, and **S**afety. The history is obtained directly from the teenager in a private setting and is confidential. Details of the HEEADSSS exam are provided in the adolescence section of this chapter.

Family History

The pediatric family history is basically the same as in the adult history but may play a more significant role in identifying genetic disorders and inborn errors of metabolism. Information about three generations should be obtained: that is, the child and their siblings, the parents and their siblings, and the grandparents. For each individual, the following information should be obtained:

- If alive, name and current age; if deceased, age at and cause of death
- Presence of any illnesses, such as asthma, coronary artery disease, diabetes, hypertension, stroke, cancer, or mental health disorders
- Presence of congenital malformations, developmental problems, or genetic disorders

Updating the family medical history should be done routinely as this too may change with time and can be influential on the evolution of the child's medical conditions.

Review of Systems

The review of systems (ROS) needs to be age-appropriate; for the school-aged child and adolescent, it may be similar to that of the adult, whereas for younger children, it will vary. Be complete, but tailor your questions to the age of the child and what the caregiver can report. For example, to elicit a history of congestive heart failure in an infant, it is useless to ask about two-flight dyspnea or exertion. Instead, ask whether the infant appears short of breath or sweaty when they feed. Also think about which symptoms can and cannot be reported based on the child's age or developmental level (i.e., realize that infants and young children cannot report dizziness, nausea, headache, or cold intolerance). Age-appropriate ROSs will be elaborated in each following respective section.

Screening Questionnaires and Tools

Screening questionnaires and tools are used as part of history taking to assess additional aspects of the child's well-being. Tools can be administered verbally, in writing, or online before or during a visit. The AAP and Bright Futures Guidelines for Health Supervision of Infants, Children, and Adolescents recommend validated tools and/or questionnaires to assess exposure to lead and tuberculosis; adverse childhood experiences (ACEs); motor, language, and social-emotional development; mental health; and oral health. A summary of validated tools is available from Bright Futures.[5]

Developmental surveillance should be performed at every health maintenance visit based on parental concerns and reports, examiner observations, and identification of risk factors. More formal developmental screenings using a standardized test is recommended at 9, 18, and 30 months.[6] Additionally, sensory screening of hearing and vision is done routinely per the Bright Futures periodicity schedule.

Sample questionnaires are shown in Boxes 24.4 and 24.5; the American Academy of Pediatrics Oral Health Risk Assessment Tool is available at https://downloads.aap.org/AAP/PDF/oralhealth_RiskAssessmentTool.pdf (Accessed December 2023).

Setting-Specific Pediatric History

Lines of questioning also must be adapted to the type of encounter. The sections provided above encompass a full history; however, it may need to be tailored depending on visit type or setting, such as for an emergency department or sick visit, a hospital admission, in the newborn nursery, or during a well-child visit in the primary care office.

For acute care visits, the questions will be symptom-/concern-based and should include a specific reason for presentation. Related questions and looking for pertinent positive and negative findings are essential for an accurate assessment. For example, one must ask about oral intake and urine output for a child with vomiting and diarrhea, activity level for a child with fever, or the presence of a limp for a child with leg pain. In the case of a hospital admission, the course of action in the

BOX 24.4 Lead Exposure Questionnaire

1. Does your child live in or regularly visit a building built before 1978 with potential lead exposures, such as peeling or chipping paint, recent or ongoing renovation or remodeling, or high levels of lead in the drinking water?
2. Has your child spent any time outside the United States in the past year?
3. Does your child live or play with a child who has an elevated blood lead level?
4. Does your child have developmental disabilities, put nonfood items in their mouth, or peel or disturb painted surfaces?
5. Does your child have frequent contact with an adult who may bring home traces of lead from a job or hobby such as: house painting, plumbing, renovation, construction, auto repair, welding, electronics repair, battery recycling, lead smelting, jewelry, stained glass or pottery making, fishing (weights, "sinkers"), firearms, or collecting lead or pewter figurines?
6. Does your family use traditional medicines, health remedies, cosmetics, powders, spices, or food from other countries?
7. Does your family cook, store, or serve food in crystal, pewter, or pottery from other countries?
8. Did your child miss a lead test? New York State requires all children be tested for lead at age 1 and again at age 2.

Data from New York State Department of Health https://www.health.ny.gov/publications/6670.pdf

BOX 24.5 Questions for Determining Risk of Tuberculosis in Children

1. Has a family member or contact had tuberculosis disease?
2. Has a family member had a positive tuberculin skin test result?
3. Was your child born in a high-risk country (countries other than the United States, Canada, Australia, New Zealand, or Western and North European countries)?
4. Has your child travelled to a high-risk country? How much contact did your child have with the resident population?

emergency department should be elicited, along with the final reason for admission.

In the newborn nursery, a detailed prenatal history of the mother and the details of labor and delivery must be reviewed very carefully. Any one of these details can potentially impact the neonate in the short or long term, or may inform neonatal care regarding specific testing or treatments. See the neonatal section of this chapter.

For well-child visits, there are additional areas to inquire about to help assess the patient's well-being. For these visits, ask detailed questions about diet, elimination, and sleep habits. Ask about behavioral concerns and, of course, details about the child's development or school progress. Although these categories remain constant from neonates through young adults, the actual questions will certainly vary. Sample questions will be provided in the appropriate age-related sections that follow.

Another crucial component of well-child visits is providing anticipatory guidance. This means giving advice to parents about topics such as feeding, safety, and developmental expectations based on the anticipated or next stage of development of the child. The goal is to prepare parents to be well-equipped to manage the next stage of their child's development. As children grow, advice is intended to guide them to lead safe, healthy lives. Common domains to cover with age-appropriate advice at each well visit include social determinants of health, behavior and development, feeding and nutrition, and safety. Other areas depending on age may include oral health, school readiness, media use, and reproductive health. Samples of such advice will be provided in each age-specific section to follow.

The Bright Futures/AAP Guidelines (https://downloads.aap.org/AAP/PDF/periodicity_schedule.pdf) tabulate all the elements of healthcare maintenance visits into a periodicity schedule to guide healthcare professionals as to the timing of various history and physical exam components, screenings, testing, and procedures.

Physical Exam

For all patients, the healthcare professional should make sure to explain the portions and scope of the exam to the caregiver and/or child, often talking through the exam as it proceeds. The physical examination of an infant, toddler, or child is always done in the presence of a caregiver. Partner with the caregiver who can be a helpful assistant during the exam of young patients. The infant or toddler should be undressed, and as children develop more of a sense of modesty, a gown should be worn and drapes used to help ensure privacy during the exam. If the adolescent or young adult patient requires an examination of their breasts or genitals, a chaperone is recommended. The use of a chaperone should be a shared decision between the patient and healthcare professional.

It is imperative for the protection of both the patient and the examiner that the examiner washes their hands thoroughly with soap or use a hand sanitizer product both before and after every single examination or patient. This is the most effective way to prevent the spread of infections. Another important safety measure is to never leave an infant or toddler unattended on the exam table. If it is necessary to reach for equipment, use the caregiver to stand near the table or keep a hand on the child. On an inpatient unit, make sure to raise up a lowered crib or bedside rail after the exam or if stepping away. Finally, do not leave any small objects on the table that can lead to choking in a young patient.

There is undoubtedly a great deal of overlap in the body part components of the physical exam in the pediatric and adult populations, yet within these areas, there are also components specific to various age groups. Like adults, all children should have the following areas examined, though the extent of an exam will be dependent on the purpose of the visit and diagnostic possibilities raised by the preceding history.

- General appearance and nutritional status
- Anthropometrics[d]
- Vital signs
- Head
- Eyes
- Ears
- Nose

[d]Weight, length, and head circumference for children <2 years of age. Weight, height, and body mass index for children >2 years of age.

- Oropharynx
- Neck
- Nodes
- Lungs
- Heart
- Abdomen
- Back
- Musculoskeletal
- Genitourinary
- Skin
- Neurologic

Special attention is paid to unique findings, for example, fontanelles, red reflex, hip exam, and primitive reflexes in newborns and infants; strabismus in toddlers/preschoolers and school-age children; and pubertal changes and scoliosis in older school-age, preteens, and adolescents.

Much of the exam of the preschool- and school-age child, preteen, and adolescent is the same as the adult. Listening to the heart and lungs, for example, will be performed in a similar manner even though the chest wall and back may be smaller. As there are some portions of the exam that will be unique to different age groups and the technique may vary in some cases; we will discuss those distinctive features of the exam in the age-based sections to follow. This means, unless otherwise specified, the technique for the component being reviewed will be the same as in the adult, as described in prior chapters.

Anthropometrics

A crucial and unique component of the pediatric examination is assessment of growth, also known as anthropometrics. This is accomplished through careful measurements of growth parameters, then plotting of values on a standardized, gender-specific growth chart. For children under the age of 2 years, measurement of weight, length, and head circumference is a routine part of the well-child examination. Weight alone is usually measured for sick visits. Weight should be obtained on either an infant scale (lying down or sitting) or adult scale when willing and able to stand alone, which is first zeroed and measured without clothes or diaper. Length should be measured with the child lying down, using a special measuring stick with the upper extension arm flush with the top of the head and the lower one flush with the bottom of the feet. Head circumference is measured with a measuring tape wrapped around the head like a crown, just above the attachment of the ears, around the occiput and forehead. For children above the age of 2 years, weight is measured standing up without outer clothes. Height is measured standing up using a stadiometer.[e] Body mass index (BMI) should then be calculated and plotted.

To monitor growth of children in the United States, the CDC recommends using the World Health Organization (WHO) growth charts for children under 2 years of age[7] and the CDC growth charts for children above the age of 2 years.[8]

[e]A stadiometer is used for measuring height. It is commonly constructed out of a ruler and a sliding horizontal headpiece that is adjusted to rest on the top of the patient's head.

After the measurements are plotted, the charts should be assessed for changes over time. This should be done at every well-child visit. Growth in children should ideally follow along an expected trajectory, along a percentile line for that patient. This reflects varying degrees of expected growth and weight gain at different ages. Growth charts can reveal problems such as obesity (BMI >95 percentile), overweight (BMI >85 percentile), short stature, microcephaly, or macrocephaly. Looking at trends is important as crossing percentile lines may indicate too rapid or inadequate weight gain or growth, or lack of or excessive growth of the head, all of which can be cause for concern.

There are specialized growth charts for certain populations of children. Specific growth charts exist for patients with trisomy 21; Turner, Williams, and Marfan syndromes;[f] and some other genetic syndromes. There are also growth charts for newborns, including those born prematurely.[9] Babies born preterm should have their measurements plotted at their corrected age (adjusted by subtracting gestational age in weeks from 40 weeks) until 2 years of age for most, and 3 years for those with birth weight <1000 g. However, if the child's growth catches up to the chronologic age-appropriate growth before 24 to 36 months of age, chronologic age is subsequently used. Additionally, the CDC has published extended BMI for age growth charts.[10]

Vital Signs

Vital signs, like in adults, include temperature, heart rate, respiratory rate, and BP. Which vital signs are measured may depend on the type of visit and the age of the patient. Temperature is measured with a digital rectal thermometer in infants and is most important to measure in young infants with suspicion of an infection. A temperature above 100.4°F (38°C) will warrant further investigation for the source of the fever. While often measured for older children at sick visits, the actual number may not be as significant as the presence or absence of a fever or how the child appears clinically. Rectal temperatures will be the closest approximation of core body temperature. Other means of measuring temperature include oral or axillary thermometer or tympanic membrane device.

Heart rate in infants is most easily counted with a stethoscope on the chest at the apex. For older children, it can be measured at the radial pulse. The rate can be counted for 15 seconds and multiplied by 4. Respiratory rate in infants should be counted for a full

[f]*Trisomy 21*, also known as Down Syndrome, is the most common chromosomal abnormality among live born infants due to an extra chromosome 21. Most common features include intellectual disabilities, heart defects, and characteristic physical features. *Turner syndrome*, a condition that affects only females, results when one of the X chromosomes is missing. Turner syndrome can cause a variety of medical and developmental problems, including short height, failure of the ovaries to develop, and cardiac defects. *Williams syndrome* is caused by a gene deletion that results in patients having distinctive facial appearance, cognitive and developmental disabilities, and variable abnormalities in the cardiac, renal, and endocrine systems. *Marfan syndrome* is an inherited connective tissue disorder of varying severity involving the ophthalmologic, cardiac, and musculoskeletal systems.

TABLE 24.3 Vital Signs in Children

Heart Rate (rate/min)	
Age	**Awake Rate/Sleeping Rate**
Newborn to 3 months	85 to 205/80 to 160
3 months to 2 years	100 to 190/75 to 160
2 to 10 years	60 to 140/60 to 90
>10 years	60 to 100/50 to 90
Respiratory Rate (breaths/min)	
Age	**Rate**
Infant	30 to 60
Toddler	24 to 40
Preschooler	22 to 34
School-age child	18 to 30
Adolescent	12 to 16
Definition of Hypotension by Systolic Blood Pressure and Age	
Age	**Systolic Blood Pressure**
Term neonates (0 to 28 days)	<60 mm Hg
Infants (1 to 12 months)	<70 mm Hg
Children 1 to 10 years (5th BP percentile)	<70 mm Hg + (age in years × 2) mm Hg
Children >10 years	<90 mm Hg

Source: https://chemm.hhs.gov/pals.htm

minute as young infants have periodic breathing which means it speeds up and slows down in waves. It can be measured by watching the chest rise and fall or auscultating with a stethoscope on the chest. The respiratory rate in older children can similarly be counted by observation or auscultation but for a shorter period of time. It is important to know that normal ranges for heart rate and respiratory rate vary by age. They start very high and decrease as the child gets older, until they reach adult norms. See Table 24.3 for general vital signs and guidelines by age.

Routine measurement of BP starts at age 3, but it is done earlier for children with high-risk conditions such as history of prematurity <32 weeks gestation, small for gestational age, very low birth weight, other neonatal complications requiring intensive care, or umbilical artery line.

BP measurement must be done with proper cuff size and technique to obtain an accurate measurement. The child should be quietly seated with feet uncrossed and BP should be measured in the right arm, supported at heart level. The bladder length within the cuff should be 80% to 100% of the arm circumference and the width at least 40% of the arm circumference. Initial measurements can be done with a calibrated oscillometric machine or by auscultation. To measure BP in the legs, use an appropriately sized cuff at mid-thigh with the patient in the prone position. If the initial BP is >90th percentile, perform two more oscillometric or auscultatory measurements at the same visit and average them.

BP norms vary by age, sex, and height and are based on measurements from over 50,000 children. Percentile should be noted according to the current BP tables.[11] An online BP calculator will be of assistance in obtaining appropriate percentiles and subsequent course of action, if indicated.[12] Classification of normal and elevated BPs is found in Table 24.3.

NEONATAL: UNDER 1 MONTH OF AGE

Neonatal History

In the newborn nursery and at the initial newborn office visit, a detailed prenatal and birth history as well as postnatal nursery course should be obtained or reviewed. Any finding during these periods may have an impact on the infant's successful transition to extrauterine life. The neonate's history begins with the mother's history. It is important to obtain a full past medical history and pregnancy history of the mother. Next obtain a detailed history of the peripartum period including labor and delivery. Now, the infant's history follows, from the time of birth through the nursery stay.

See the sample write-up of a newborn's history and physical at the end of this chapter.

Maternal/Prenatal History

- Age
- Medical problems before the pregnancy (e.g., asthma, obesity, diabetes, epilepsy, hypertension, mental health issues, surgeries)
- Number and outcome of prior pregnancies (i.e., term vs. preterm births, miscarriage or termination, delivery complications)
- Use of assisted reproductive technology (e.g., in vitro fertilization, donor egg or sperm, surrogate)
- Location and duration of prenatal care
- Complications during the pregnancy (e.g., gestational diabetes or hypertension, bleeding, infections, treatment for preterm labor)
- Medications (including supplements) taken during the pregnancy
- Lab results (e.g., serologies, genetic testing, blood type, other labs) (see Box 24.1)
- Ultrasound results
- Cigarette, alcohol, and/or substance use

Birth History

- Gestational age at time of delivery (<37 weeks = preterm; 34 to 37 weeks = late preterm; 37 to 42 weeks = term; >42 weeks = postterm)
- Induced or natural labor and duration of labor
- Duration of rupture of membranes (i.e., less than or greater than 18 hours)
- Intrapartum complications (e.g., fever, bleeding, high BP, pre-eclampsia)
- Medications administered to mother (e.g., antibiotics, magnesium sulfate, anesthesia)
- Type of delivery (i.e., normal spontaneous vaginal delivery [NSVD], cesarean section [C/S], vacuum-assisted, forceps-assisted)
- Position of the baby at delivery
- Complications of delivery (e.g., meconium, shoulder dystocia, placental abruption, birth trauma)
- Complications in the postpartum period (e.g., infection, bleeding)

Postnatal History

- Birth weight
- Birth length and head circumference

BOX 24.6 Importance of Breastfeeding

When it comes to neonatal and infant nutrition, the adage "breast is best" is grounded in evidence that shows both short- and long-term health benefits for both the mother and child. For the breastfed baby, they include reduced incidence of respiratory tract infections and otitis media, gastrointestinal tract infections, necrotizing enterocolitis, sudden infant death syndrome and infant mortality, allergic disease, celiac disease, inflammatory bowel disease, obesity, childhood leukemia, and lymphoma. The American Academy of Pediatrics recommends exclusive breastfeeding for about 6 months, with complementary food introduction at about 6 months, and as mutually desired by mother and child, supports continued breastfeeding until 2 years or beyond.[a]

The AAP recommends that birth hospitals or centers implement maternity care practices that improve breastfeeding initiation, duration, and exclusivity, such as those in the WHO Ten Steps to Successful Breastfeeding, as monitored by the CDC.

[a]Meek JY, Noble L, Section on Breastfeeding: Policy statement: breastfeeding and the use of human milk, *Pediatrics* 150(1): e2022057988, 2022. doi:10.1542/peds.2022-057988.

- Resuscitation maneuvers administered (e.g., suction, oxygen, respiratory support)
- Evidence of birth trauma
- Apgar score
- Skin-to-skin[g] done?

Nursery History

- Feeding (e.g., breast, formula, any problems); see Box 24.6 for breastfeeding recommendations
- Weight change, weight at discharge (i.e., infants can lose up to 10% of birth weight in first few days)
- Abnormal physical exam findings (and treatment if indicated)
- Results of screenings (hearing, critical congenital heart defects); see Box 24.3
- Blood type and Coombs test
- Bilirubin result and recommended intervention or follow-up based on updated AAP guidelines (AAP guidelines[13])
- Complications in the nursery (e.g., respiratory distress, concern for sepsis, neonatal abstinence syndrome/neonatal opioid withdrawal syndrome, hypoglycemia)
- Receipt of routine medications (e.g., vitamin K, erythromycin, hepatitis B vaccine)
- Administration of other medications
- Was the state-specific newborn screening performed and are results available?
- Was a circumcision performed?
- Age at discharge
- Primary care follow-up

If the baby spent time in the NICU, the history will be more expansive. Get a detailed history of the NICU course by systems. Infants in the NICU have a unique set of conditions which are beyond the scope of this chapter. Review complications, studies, treatments, and length of stay.

It is also important to obtain a family history to be alerted to inheritable medical conditions that may affect the baby. One must also obtain a full social history for the neonate early on. What is the family makeup, and how are the living conditions in the home to which this baby will go? Who will be the primary caretaker, and is there a support system?

During the first month of life, the main focus is on appropriate feeding and physical growth as well as the bonding of the caregiver-infant dyad. Furthermore, bringing home a newborn is an exciting yet intimidating experience for new caregivers and providing thorough anticipatory guidance and answering all their questions about newborn care, no matter how trivial, is essential. For well-child visits during this neonatal period, obtain an interval history, asking about caregiver concerns and well-being, the infant's diet, elimination, and sleep habits. Inquire about or observe developmental milestones.

- Diet: What is the infant drinking?
  - If breastfeeding:
    - How is breastfeeding going?
    - How many times does the baby feed in a day? (expect 8 to 12 feeds/day)
    - How is the baby's latch? Is it painful?
    - Is the baby receiving vitamin D supplementation?
    - Is the baby taking any formula?
  - If formula feeding:
    - How much is the baby taking each feed?
    - How often is the baby feeding? (expect 6 to 8 feeds/day)
    - How is the formula being prepared (i.e., is it ready to feed, concentrated liquid, or powder)?
  - Elimination
    - How many wet diapers per day? (expect 1 per day of age until 1 week then 6 to 8 per day)
    - What is the consistency of the stool? (expect transition from the dark green-black tarry meconium stools to seedy soft yellow or green stools by a few days of age)
  - Sleep
    - Where is the infant sleeping? (i.e., crib or bassinet; co-sleeping not recommended) Is the infant in the caregiver's room?
    - Is the baby sleeping supine?
    - Is there anything in the crib? There should be no pillows, blankets, toys, stuffed animals, bumpers, or positioners.
  - Development/Behavior (see Table 24.1)
    - Movement/Physical Development (e.g., lifts head briefly when prone, moves all extremities, hands in a fist)
    - Language/Communication (e.g., responds to sounds, calms to voice)
    - Social/Emotional (e.g., fixates on face, follows with eyes)
    - Is the baby fussy?
  - Social
    - How has the family adapted to the newborn?
    - How is the mother's mood? Does she have a support system?

[g]Skin-to-skin is a term used to describe the placement of the naked newborn on the mother's bare chest immediately after delivery. This procedure helps stabilize the baby's breathing, temperature, and heart rate; promotes breastfeeding; and is routine in uncomplicated deliveries.

TABLE 24.4 Apgar Score

Sign	SCORE 0	1	2
Color	Blue pale	Pink body with blue extremities	Completely pink
Heart rate	Absent	Below 100	Over 100
Reflex irritability	No reaction	Grimace	Sneeze, cough or vigorous cry
Muscle tone	Flaccid	Some flexion of the extremities	Good flexion of the extremities
Respiratory effort	Absent	Weak, irregular	Good, crying

  - Do they have provisions and services in place for the baby? (WIC, baby care supplies)
- Screenings: Check state newborn screen results
- Anticipatory guidance (here are some examples)
  - Wash hands often, avoid sick contacts
  - Keep cord dry until it falls off
  - Use rear-facing car seat in back seat of car
  - Don't shake or hit the baby
  - Avoid exposure to second- or third-hand smoke

Newborn Physical Exam

See Video 24.1.

The newborn is assessed in the delivery room immediately after birth to determine the integrity of the cardiopulmonary system. Gloves are worn for this initial examination because the newborn is coated with the mother's vaginal secretions and blood.

The initial assessment consists of the evaluation of five signs:

1. Color
2. Heart rate
3. Reflex irritability
4. Muscle tone
5. Respiratory effort

Dr. Virginia Apgar developed a scale for rating these signs 1 and 5 minutes after birth. The Apgar score is shown in Table 24.4. Each of the signs is scored from 0 to 2. At 1 minute, a total score of 3 to 4 indicates severe cardiopulmonary depression, and the infant requires immediate resuscitative measures; a score from 5 to 6 indicates mild depression. The tests are repeated at 5 minutes; if the infant is still mild or moderately depressed at that point, a 10-minute Apgar score can also be given. A score of 8 or more indicates grossly normal findings of the cardiopulmonary examination.

When examining the newborn, try to answer three questions:

1. How well is this infant making the transition to extrauterine life?
2. Is there any evidence of birth trauma?
3. Does this infant have any evidence of congenital malformations?

General Assessment

The gestational age is important to determine as it will impact the expectations of the newborn's maturity, appearance, and ability to transition in the delivery room. Gestational age is generally determined based on last menstrual date and sonographic dating during pregnancy. If this information is not available, it is important to make an objective determination of the gestational age. A more formal assessment can be done using a standardized scoring tool, the *Ballard Maturational Assessment*. This is based on signs of neuromuscular and physical maturity. The total scores of the neurologic and external signs are summed. The sum is then correlated with the gestational age, according to the graph shown. See Table 24.5 for the Ballard scoring system.

The newborn infant is also weighed, but weight alone does not determine maturational age. The birth weight is correlated with gestational age using the Fenton growth charts.[9] By this method, the infant is classified as being small for gestational age (SGA), when the birth weight is lower than the 10th percentile; appropriate for gestational age (AGA), when the birth weight is between 10th and 90th percentile; or large for gestational age (LGA), when the birth weight is above the 90th percentile.

The value of the weight for gestational age determination lies in its ability to predict certain risk groups. Many babies who are LGA are infants of diabetic mothers. Such infants are at risk for a number of complications, both in the immediate neonatal period and later in life. These infants must be carefully monitored for hypoglycemia and polycythemia; they are more likely to have hyperbilirubinemia in the first 3 days after birth, and they are 3 to 5 times more likely to have a congenital malformation than are infants in the general population. In infants who are SGA, major considerations include the presence of a chromosomal abnormality or exposure to a teratogenic agent, such as alcohol, or a congenital infection, including cytomegalovirus, during gestation. Newborns who are SGA must also be monitored for hypoglycemia during the immediate neonatal period.

The remainder of the examination is usually performed within 24 hours after birth. The comprehensive examination begins with inspection. If the infant has achieved temperature stability, then they should be undressed except for the diaper. The following description of the examination is in a head-to-toe sequence. However, the examiner must usually vary the order when actually performing the examination, using the infant's quiet state to listen to the heart and lungs, catching glimpses of the eyes when the infant opens them, and taking advantage of crying spells to examine the mouth.

Vital Signs and Anthropometrics

The *respiratory rate* and degree of *respiratory effort* are carefully assessed while the infant is undressed. The respiratory rate of a newborn usually averages from 30 to 60 breaths/min. Observe the respiratory rate for 1 minute because periods of apnea and periodic breathing are common, especially among preterm infants. Look for grunting respirations and for chest retractions, each of which is evidence of respiratory distress.

Determine the *pulse* by auscultation of the heart. The average heart rate of a newborn ranges from 85 to 205 beats/min while awake. There are wide fluctuations; the rate increases to as fast as 200 during crying and decreases to as low as 80 during sleep. A heart rate lower than 80 is of concern.

TABLE 24.5 Ballard Scoring System

NEUROMUSCULAR MATURITY

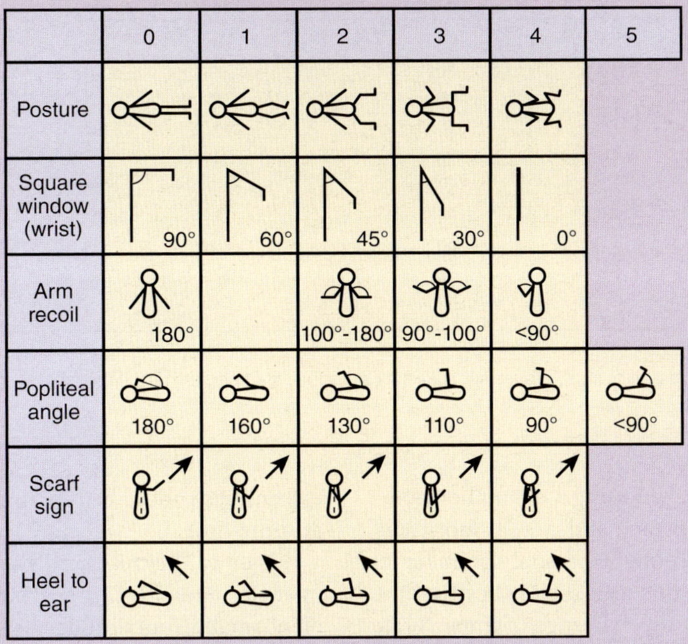

Ballard Clinical Assessment. Following are some notes on techniques for assessing the neurologic criteria: Posture: Observed with infant quiet and in supine position. Score *0*, arms and legs extended; *1*, beginning of flexion of hips and knees, arms extended; *2*, stronger flexion of legs, arms extended; *3*, arms slightly flexed, legs flexed and abducted; *4*, full flexion of arms and legs. Square window: The hand is flexed on the forearm between the thumb and index finger of the examiner. Enough pressure is applied to get as full a flexion as possible, and the angle between the hypothenar eminence and the ventral aspect of the forearm is measured and graded according to the diagram. (Care is taken not to rotate the infant's wrist while performing this maneuver.) Arm recoil: With the infant in the supine position, the forearms are first flexed for 5 seconds, then fully extended by pulling on the hands, and then released. The sign is fully positive if the arms return briskly to full flexion (score 2). If the arms return to incomplete flexion or the response is sluggish, it is scored as 1. If they remain extended or show only random movements, the score is 0. Popliteal angle: With the infant supine and the pelvis flat on the examining couch, the thigh is held in the knee-to-chest position, with the examiner's left index finger and thumb supporting the knee. The leg is then extended by gentle pressure from the examiner's right index finger behind the ankle, and the popliteal angle is measured. Scarf sign: With the infant supine, the examiner takes the infant's hand and tries to put it around the neck and as far posteriorly as possible around the opposite shoulder. This maneuver is assisted by lifting the elbow across the body. How far the elbow goes across is measured and graded according to the illustrations. Score *0*, elbow reaches opposite axillary line; *1*, elbow reaches between midline and opposite axillary line; *2*, elbow reaches midline; *3*, elbow does not reach midline. Heel-to-ear maneuver: With the infant supine, the examiner draws the infant's foot as near to the head as it will go without forcing it. The examiner observes the distance between the foot and the head, as well as the degree of extension at the knee, and grades according to the diagram. Note that the knee is left free and may draw down alongside the abdomen. (Reprinted with permission from Ballard J, Novak K, Driver M. A simplified score for assessment of fetal maturation of newly born infants. J Pediatr. 1979;95:769–774.)

	SCORE					
Physical Maturity	**0**	**1**	**2**	**3**	**4**	**5**
Skin	Gelatinous red, transparent	Smooth, pink, visible veins	Superficial peeling and/or rash, few veins	Cracking pale area, rare veins	Parchment deep cracking, no vessels	Leathery, cracked, wrinkled
Lanugo	None	Abundant	Thinning	Bald areas	Mostly bald	
Plantar creases	No crease	Faint red marks	Anterior transverse crease only	Creases anterior ⅔	Creases cover entire sole	
Breast	Barely perceptible	Flat areola, no bud	Stippled areola, 1–2 mm bud	Raised areola, 3–4 mm bud	Full areola, 5–10 mm bud	
Ear	Pinna flat, stays folded	Sl. curved pinna; soft c̄ slow recoil	Well-curved pinna; soft but ready recoil	Formed and firm c̄ instant recoil	Thick cartilage ear stiff	
Genitals (male)	Scrotum empty, no rugae		Testes descending, few rugae	Testes down, good rugae	Testes pendulous, deep rugae	
Genitals (female)	Prominent clitoris and labia minora		Majora and minora equally prominent	Majora large, minora small	Clitoris and minora completely covered	

Continued

TABLE 24.5 Ballard Scoring System—cont'd

MATURITY RATING	
Score	**Weeks**
5	26
10	28
15	30
20	32
25	34
30	36
35	38
40	40
45	42
50	44

c̅, with

(Reprinted with permission from Ballard J, Novak K, Driver M: A simplified score for assessment of fetal maturation of newly born infants, *J Pediatr* 95:769–774, 1979.)

The *temperature* should be checked using a rectal thermometer. The infant's buttocks are spread, and a well-lubricated thermometer is inserted slowly through the anal sphincter to approximately 2.5 cm. Note that this also establishes that the anus is patent, thereby ruling out the existence of imperforate anus. Newborn infants often have relative thermal instability, and for this reason the ambient temperature should also be determined. Achieving temperature stability is one of the early adaptational challenges for a term infant and takes much longer for preterm infants.

Basic *measurements* are taken next. The infant's length is measured from the top of the head to the bottom of the feet; the length is usually between 47 and 52 cm. The head is measured at its greatest circumference around the occipitofrontal area. The head circumference is usually 34 to 37 cm. These and all other measurements performed during the physical examination should be plotted on appropriate growth curves, correcting for the gestational age.

General Appearance

There is a lot to be learned by simple observation of the newborn. At first glance, the examiner can assess the infant's activity level, coloring, and respiratory status to help determine immediate next steps. If the newborn is limp, cyanotic, or in respiratory distress, urgent attention is needed as opposed to proceeding with routine care. In addition, the general appearance of the baby can reveal dysmorphic features or congenital anomalies, such as cleft lip, or orthopedic deformities, findings that will be addressed later but are still important to note.

Note the *posture*. A normal term newborn keeps the arms and legs symmetrically flexed. Relaxation of the limbs is suggestive of neurologic depression and necessitates further evaluation. The finding of one side flexed while the other side is relaxed is abnormal; such posture is suggestive of an injury, either neurologic or musculoskeletal, that occurred before or during the birthing process.

Note the *movements*. Normally, all four limbs should be moving in a random and asymmetric manner. Fine movements of the face and fingers are usually present. Abnormal movements include jerky, symmetric, coarse movements. All extremities should be moving, with a full range of motion seen at some time.

Listen to the *child's cry*. Evaluate the cry for its nature, pitch, intensity, and effort. A healthy child has a strong cry, indicative of normally functioning airways. The cry varies in intensity with breathing. The cry is high-pitched and shrill in diseases associated with increased intracranial pressure. Children born to mothers with substance misuse often have high-pitched cries. A low-pitched, hoarse cry that is infrequent and low in intensity is often associated with hypothyroidism, hypocalcemic tetany, or Williams syndrome. A sound that resembles a cat mewing suggests a condition known as *cri du chat syndrome*. Absence of crying is suggestive of severe illness or central nervous system dysfunction.

Skin

Inspect the newborn's skin from head to toe looking for color changes, rashes, birthmarks, lesions, or signs of breakdown in the skin barrier. Are there any skin findings from *birth trauma*, manifested by petechiae, ecchymoses, or lacerations?

Skin color in newborns is related partially to the amount of fat present. In addition, the newborn has vasomotor instability, and the color of the skin may vary greatly from moment to moment and from one area of the body to another. It is sometimes noted that when the infant is lying on one side for a time, a sharp color demarcation appears: The dependent half of the body becomes darker and the upper half paler. Seen more commonly in preterm than in term infants, this has been termed the *harlequin color change* and is benign. The episodes may persist from 30 seconds to 30 minutes.

Inspect for *cyanosis* or *acrocyanosis*. Acrocyanosis is a benign condition in which the hands and feet are cyanotic and cool, but the trunk is pink and warm. See Fig. 24.1. This condition is common among newborns. In central *cyanosis*, the tongue and gums are also blue. Persistent central cyanosis can be suggestive of respiratory abnormalities or the presence of cyanotic congenital heart disease.

Is *plethora* present? Plethora is a condition marked by an excess of blood and a marked redness of the complexion. Plethora in the newborn usually indicates high levels of hemoglobin. Is

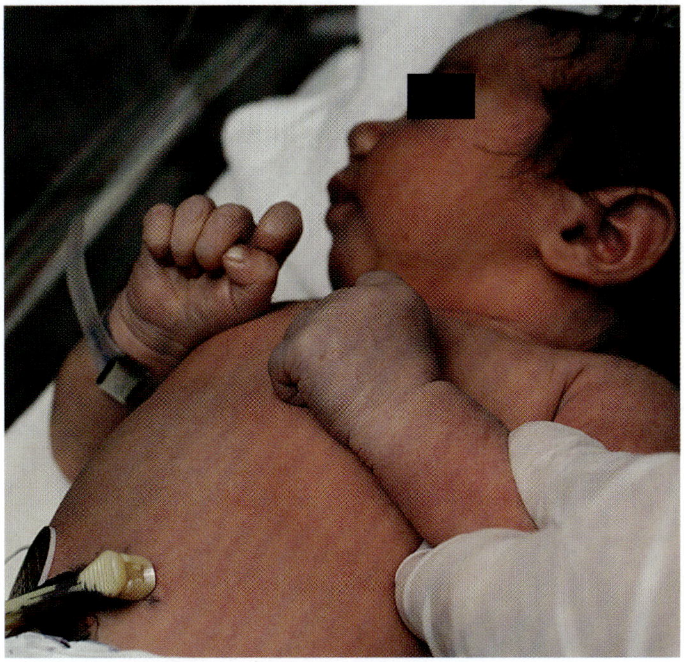

Fig. 24.1 Acrocyanosis of Hands of a Newborn. (From Ball JW, Dains JE, Flynn JA, et al: *Seidel's guide to physical examination*, 2018, Elsevier [chapter 9].)

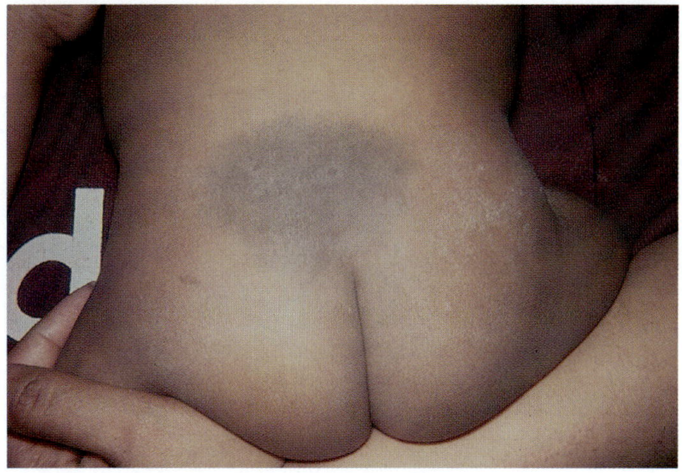

Fig. 24.2 Dermal Melanocytosis. (From Shah BR, Laude TA: *Atlas of pediatric clinical diagnosis*, Philadelphia, 2000, WB Saunders.)

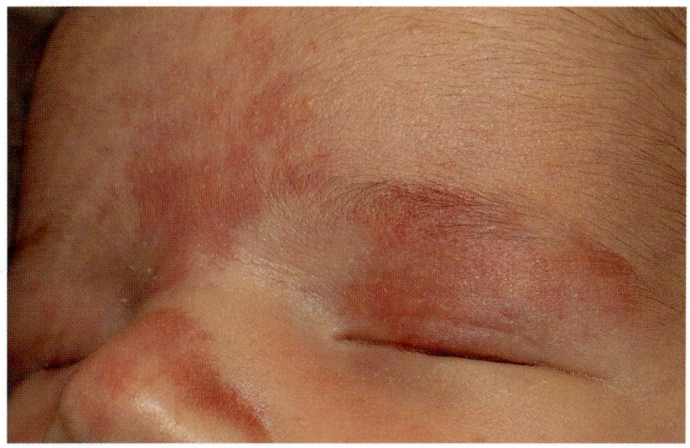

Fig. 24.3 Nevus Simplex on the Glabella, Nose, and Eyelids on a Newborn. (From Gupta D, Sidbury R: *Avery's diseases of the newborn*, 2017, Elsevier [chapter 104].)

pallor present? Pallor may be associated with anemia or, more commonly, with cold stress and peripheral vasoconstriction. Pallor may also reflect asphyxia, shock, sepsis, or edema. It should be recognized that the presence of pallor may mask cyanosis in a newborn with circulatory failure.

Physiologic jaundice is found in almost 50% of all term newborns by the third or fourth day after birth. This finding, which is even more prevalent among preterm infants, results from delay in the maturation of enzymatic processes in the liver. In most cases, jaundice is a self-limited condition, resolving after 96 hours of age. However, very high levels of bilirubin in the newborn's serum can lead to a condition known as *kernicterus*, in which permanent neurologic damage may occur. As such, it is important to monitor the serum bilirubin level and to treat elevated levels with phototherapy.

Icterus appearing before the third day may indicate a pathologic condition. Disorders that must be considered are hemolytic anemia, caused by blood group incompatibility or by bacterial or viral infections, and galactosemia, an inborn error of galactose metabolism. Visible jaundice in newborns does not appear until the serum bilirubin is approximately 5 mg/dL. When the level exceeds this threshold, the jaundice spreads in an orderly manner, from the top of the head to the soles of the feet. A transcutaneous bilirubinometer is used prior to discharge to facilitate recognizing potentially dangerous levels of jaundice.

Observe the *pigmentation*. Large, slate-blue, well-demarcated areas of pigmentation in the sacrogluteal area or elsewhere are called *congenital dermal melanocytosis* and are normal variants. Ninety percent of all dermal melanocytosis are in the buttock area, but they can also be found along the back, extremities, or even the face. These spots fade and disappear by 5 to 6 years of age in 98% of children who have them. Dermal melanocytosis is present in more than 85% of Asian newborns, greater than 60% of Black newborns, and greater than 45% of Hispanic newborns, but in fewer than 10% of White newborns. Fig. 24.2 shows a classic dermal melanocytosis.

Telangiectasias in the dermis on the eyelids, glabella, or nape of the neck are common and known as *nevus simplex* or salmon patches as seen in Fig. 24.3. They appear as pink patches with irregular, feathery borders. They are often referred to as "stork bites" or "angel kisses." Since they are due to dilated blood vessels beneath thin skin, they can darken with crying or lighten with pressure. Those on the face tend to fade as the skin thickens and disappear while those on the back of the neck may become permanent.

Vascular lesions, which encompass vascular neoplasms and vascular malformations, are common, generally benign, and usually will involute. However, some may be more serious, resulting in serious complications, or may be associated with complex syndromes. Vascular lesions have undergone changes in terminology, originally featuring descriptive characteristics (such as port wine stain or strawberry birthmark). Now the nomenclature is based on clinical characteristics, such as cellular makeup and natural clinical progression. The International

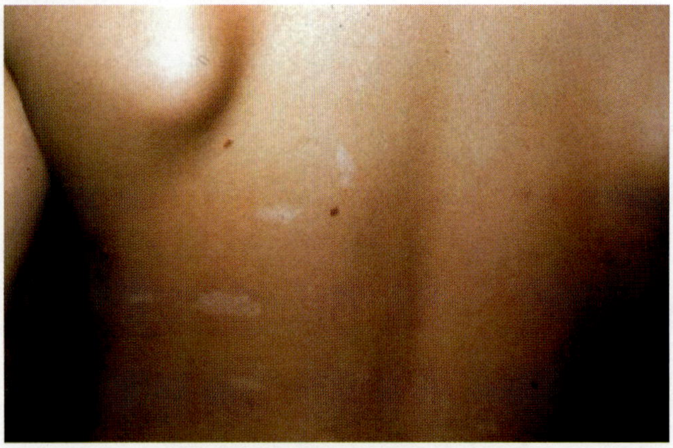

Fig. 24.4 Ash Leaf Macules in a Patient With Tuberous Sclerosis. (From Wofford J, Fenves AZ, Jackson JM, et al: The spectrum of nephrocutaneous disease and associations: genetic causes of nephrocutaneous disease, *J Am Acad Dermatol* 74:231–244, 2016.)

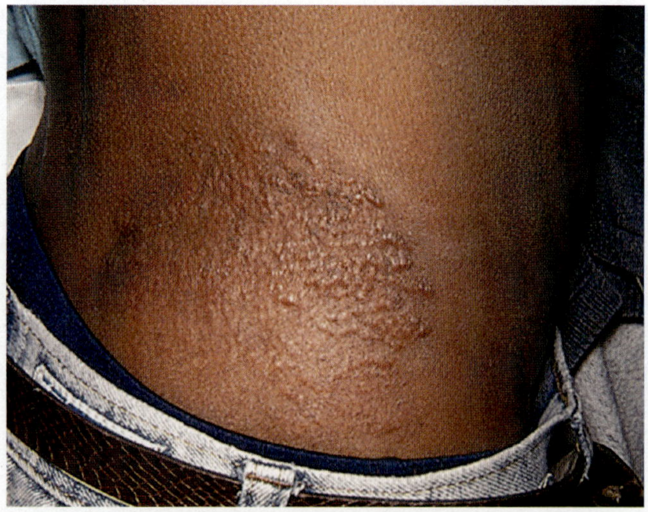

Fig. 24.5 Shagreen Patch.

Society for the Study of Vascular Anomalies (ISSVA) classifies vascular lesions into broad categories: vascular tumors, simple malformations, combined vascular malformations, anomalies of major named vessels, and vascular malformations associated with other anomalies. For more information on different types of vascular nevi, refer to the Clinicopathologic Correlations section at the end of this chapter.

Other birthmarks that may suggest the presence of an underlying genetic disorder include *café-au-lait spots* (see Fig. 8.46) and *hypopigmented macules.* One or two café-au-lait spots, the color of coffee with milk, are not uncommon in the newborn. In dark-skinned individuals, the macule is darker than the surrounding skin and should be described as "café sans lait" (coffee without milk). The presence of more than six of these spots, measuring greater than 0.5 cm, is the hallmark of *neurofibromatosis type I,* an autosomal dominantly inherited condition that combines café-au-lait spots, axillary (see Fig. 8.49) or inguinal freckles pigmented hamartomas in the iris *(Lisch nodules),* and bony abnormalities such as scoliosis and pseudarthrosis with benign tumors of the Schwann cells called *neurofibromas.* In this condition, multiple café-au-lait spots are frequently the presenting feature.

The presence of *hypopigmented macules* suggests a condition known as *tuberous sclerosis complex.* In this disorder, the hypomelanotic macules (Fig. 24.4) are often described as ash-leaf shaped, with one side smooth and the other side jagged, and are associated with other dermatologic manifestations (e.g., facial angiofibromas known as *adenoma sebaceum,* and shagreen patches,[h] as seen in Fig. 24.5), the presence of benign tumors in the brain (cortical "tubers," subependymal nodules), kidney (angiomyolipomas and cysts), and heart (rhabdomyomas), seizures, and developmental delay. Because of the significance of some of these findings, the presence of multiple hypomelanotic ash-leaf spots noted during an initial evaluation should trigger a full evaluation for associated features.

[h]An elevated cluster of closely set skin-colored papules often present on the back and lumbosacral area.

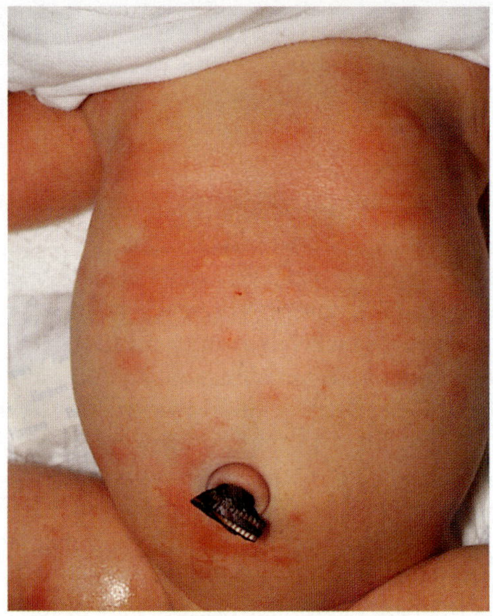

Fig. 24.6 Erythema Toxicum Neonatorum. (Reused with permission from Moon M, Guerrero AM, Li X, et al: Dermatology. In Zitelli BJ, McIntire SC, Nowalk AJ, et al, editors: *Zitelli and Davis' atlas of pediatric physical diagnosis*, ed 8, 2023, Elsevier.)

Is a *rash* present? *Erythema toxicum neonatorum* is a common rash among newborns. The condition is seen in 40% of otherwise healthy term newborns; it is not seen in premature newborns. It is a self-limited, benign eruption of unknown cause, consisting of individual papules or pustules on an erythematous base. Sometimes they are clustered. The lesions may appear anywhere on the body except on the palms and soles and have the appearance of flea bites. It is mostly seen during the first 1 to 3 days after birth but may be present at birth. The lesions tend to be transient, coming and going even up to a couple of weeks of life. Erythema toxicum is pictured in Fig. 24.6.

Milia on the face is seen in almost 50% of all newborns. Milia appears as tiny whitish papules on the cheeks, nose, chin, and forehead and usually disappear by 3 weeks of age.

Bullous lesions may be present at birth. One or two blisters on the lips or hands may represent "sucking blisters." Blisters that first appear at 3 to 4 days of life may be *staphylococcal pustulosis,* which manifests as pustular or bullous skin lesions found mainly around the groin and umbilicus. The vesicular lesions of herpes simplex also usually appear after the third day after birth, up to the third week, and require immediate treatment due to the very serious nature of herpes infection in neonates.

Widespread small pustules, many of them ruptured and leaving a collarette of scale with underlying pigmentation, represent *transient neonatal pustular melanosis,* which is benign. This condition, present at birth, is of unknown origin and is most commonly found on the trunk and extremities. It is seen most commonly in Black newborns and infants with darkly pigmented skin. Fig. 24.7 shows the stages of transient neonatal pustular melanosis in a newborn. Notice the intact pustule and the ruptured pustule with a collarette of scale. The pustules last 48 to 72 hours, and the pigmented macules may last 3 weeks to 3 months.

Prenatal or transplacental infections of the fetus may manifest with cutaneous symptoms. If a pregnant female contracts rubella in the first trimester, there is a 20% chance that the infant may have the congenital rubella syndrome. A cutaneous sign of congenital rubella is the *blueberry muffin* lesion. Such lesions, which represent sites of extramedullary hematopoiesis, are bluish-red macular or papular lesions ranging in size from 2 to 8 mm. They are noted at birth or within the first 24 hours and appear on the face, neck, trunk, or extremities. Other features of the congenital rubella syndrome include eye defects (especially cataracts), cardiac defects (e.g., ventricular septal defects and valvular defects), deafness, bone lesions, hepatosplenomegaly, jaundice, thrombocytopenia, interstitial pneumonitis, and later, developmental delay.

Congenital syphilis may present as an erythematous maculopapular rash that later turns brown or becomes a hemorrhagic vesicular rash. This is a rash that commonly affects the palms and soles.

Is *hair* present? A newborn's skin may be covered with fine, soft, immature hair, known as *lanugo hair.* Lanugo hair frequently covers the scalp and brow in premature infants but is usually absent in term infants, except perhaps on the ears and shoulders. Inspect the lumbosacral area for tufts of hair. Tufts of hair (hypertrichosis) in this area are suggestive of the presence of an occult spina bifida or a sinus tract, anomalies that may be an external sign of tethering of the spinal cord. Fig. 24.8 shows sacral hypertrichosis in a child who had a tethered spinal cord. Examine the *fingernails.* In a post-term infant, the fingernails are long and may be stained yellow if meconium was present in the amniotic fluid.

Head

Examination of the head involves a thorough assessment of its shape, symmetry, and fontanelles. The skull may be *molded,* especially if the labor was prolonged and the head was engaged for a long period. The head may appear elongated or egg- or cone-shaped. The head shape returns to normal in the ensuing

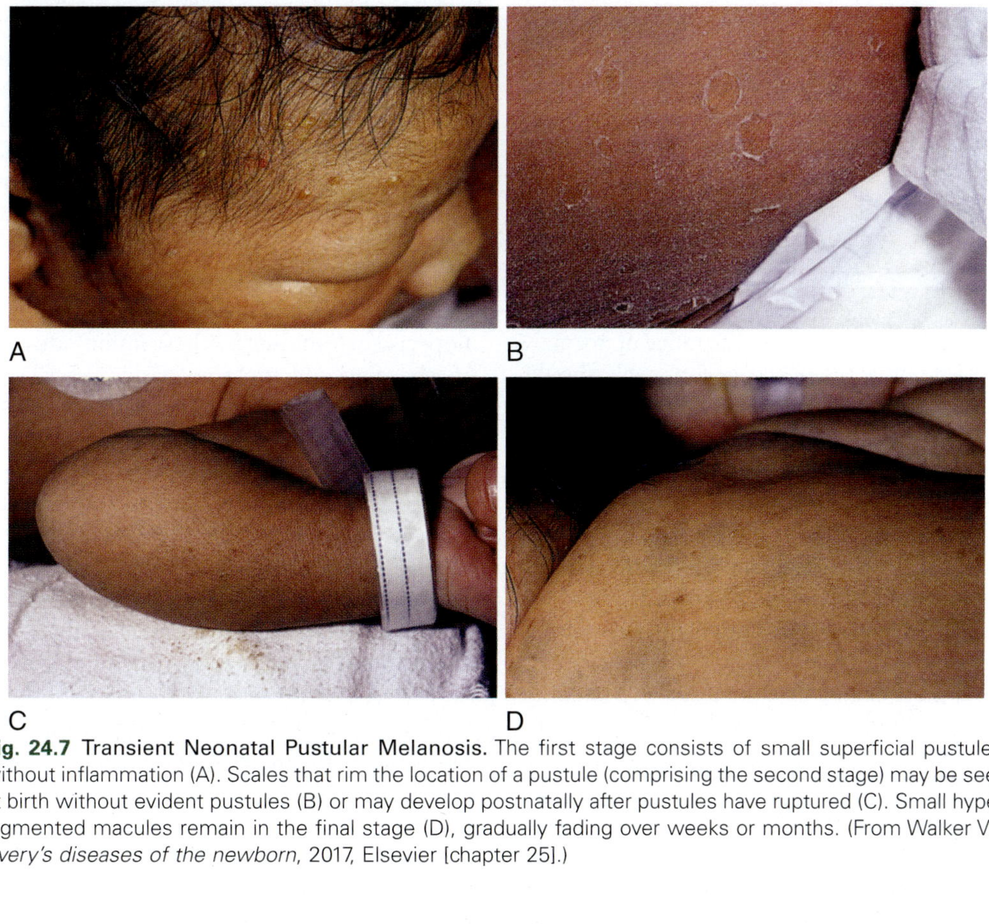

Fig. 24.7 Transient Neonatal Pustular Melanosis. The first stage consists of small superficial pustules, without inflammation (A). Scales that rim the location of a pustule (comprising the second stage) may be seen at birth without evident pustules (B) or may develop postnatally after pustules have ruptured (C). Small hyperpigmented macules remain in the final stage (D), gradually fading over weeks or months. (From Walker VP: *Avery's diseases of the newborn,* 2017, Elsevier [chapter 25].)

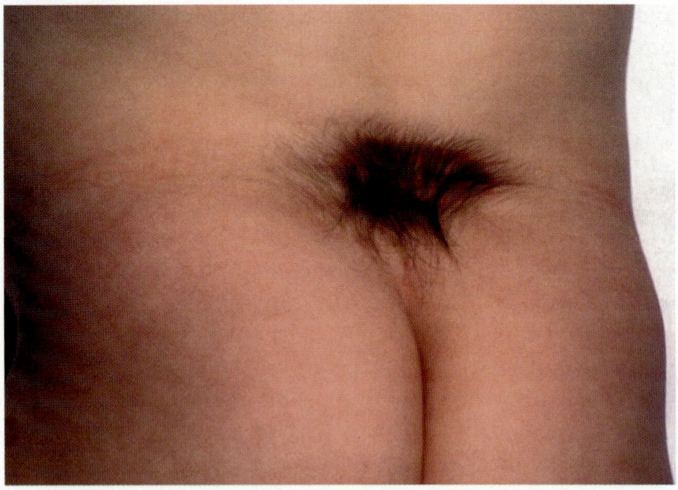

Fig. 24.8 Sacral Hypertrichosis. (Reused with permission from Kos L, Drolet BA: Developmental abnormalities. In Eichenfield LF, Frieden IJ, Esterly NB, editors: *Neonatal dermatology*, ed 2, Philadelphia, 2008.)

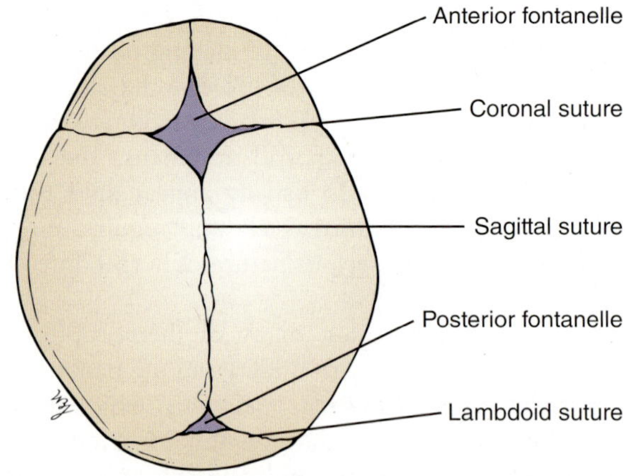

Fig. 24.9 Sutures of the Skull and Location of Fontanelles.

days to weeks. The skull of a child born by primary C/S without preceding labor has a characteristic roundness.

In the newborn, the *sutures* are frequently felt as ridges as a result of the overriding of the cranial bones by molding as the skull passes through the vaginal canal. The sutures may also separate due to shifting of the bones, called split sutures, which feel like spaces between the bones. Palpate the fontanelles, or "soft spots." The *anterior fontanelle* is located at the junction of the frontal (metopic), coronal, and sagittal sutures; is usually 3 to 6 cm in diameter; and is diamond-shaped. The triangular *posterior fontanelle* is located at the junction of the sagittal and lambdoid sutures and measures 1 to 2 cm in diameter. Normally, the fontanelles are flat. While the size may vary, they must be open, otherwise craniosynostosis[i] may be suspected. A bulging fontanelle may be indicative of increased intracranial pressure; a depressed fontanelle may be seen in dehydration. Normally while crying, the fontanelles bulge. Pulsations of the fontanelles reflect the pulse. The anterior fontanelle normally closes by 18 months of age, but there is a wide range of normality between 10 and 24 months; the posterior fontanelle should be closed by 2 months of age and may already be closed in the neonatal period. The locations of the fontanelles and suture names are shown in Fig. 24.9.

Caput succedaneum is edema of the soft tissues over the vertex of the skull that is related to the birth process during a vertex delivery. The normal movement of the fetal head through the birth canal produces a marked molding of the very soft fetal skull and scalp edema. This swelling, which is present at delivery, crosses the sutures and resolves in the first few days. In a face presentation, there can be discoloration, and swelling of the newborn's face.

Caput succedaneum should be differentiated from a *cephalohematoma,* which is a subperiosteal hemorrhage limited to one cranial bone, often the parietal. There is no discoloration of the overlying scalp, and the swelling does not cross the suture line. The swelling is usually not visible until several hours or days after birth, inasmuch as subperiosteal bleeding is generally a slow process. Approximately 15% of cephalohematomas are bilateral, and each is palpably distinct from the other side. No treatment is required for cephalohematomas, which are generally resorbed by 2 to 12 weeks, depending on the size; however, breakdown of the extravasated blood may contribute to jaundice. Fig. 24.10 shows a newborn with a caput succedaneum; Fig. 24.11 shows a child with a cephalohematoma. Note in Fig. 24.11 that the swelling stops in the midline at the sagittal suture; this is characteristic of a cephalohematoma.

Inspect the scalp for lesions from *fetal scalp electrodes,* used for monitoring fetal well-being during difficult labors, and for areas of alopecia. A 1- to 2-cm well-demarcated area of smooth shiny skin with no hair may represent *aplasia cutis congenita,* an abnormality of fetal development of unknown cause, which is usually an isolated finding in an otherwise well newborn. *Nevus sebaceous,* a benign hamartoma of the skin that is noted at birth or soon after, is most commonly found on the scalp or face. When on the scalp, the lesion has a clearly demarcated area of alopecia surrounding it. These lesions are caused by overgrowth of sebaceous and apocrine glands as well as the epidermis and immature hair follicles. They appear as well-defined yellow, pink, or tan plaques that vary in shape (round, oval, or linear) and ranging in size from one to several centimeters. In older children, they can appear thickened, verrucous, or nodular.

Inspect the *face* for symmetry. The eye creases should be equal. Observe the infant as they suck or cry. The mouth should remain on a level plane. If it is asymmetric, suspect a facial paralysis or a congenital anomaly of one or more facial muscles, a condition known as *asymmetric crying facies syndrome.*

The face may reveal abnormal features such as *epicanthal folds, widely spaced eyes,* or *low-set ears,* each of which may be associated with congenital or genetic syndromes.

Eyes

Several attempts to evaluate the eyes of the newborn may be necessary. Eyelid edema related to the birth process, infections,

[i]Craniosynostosis is a condition in which one or more of the sutures close too early, causing problems with normal brain and skull growth. This premature closure of the sutures may cause increased intracranial pressure resulting in asymmetry of the skull or facial bones.

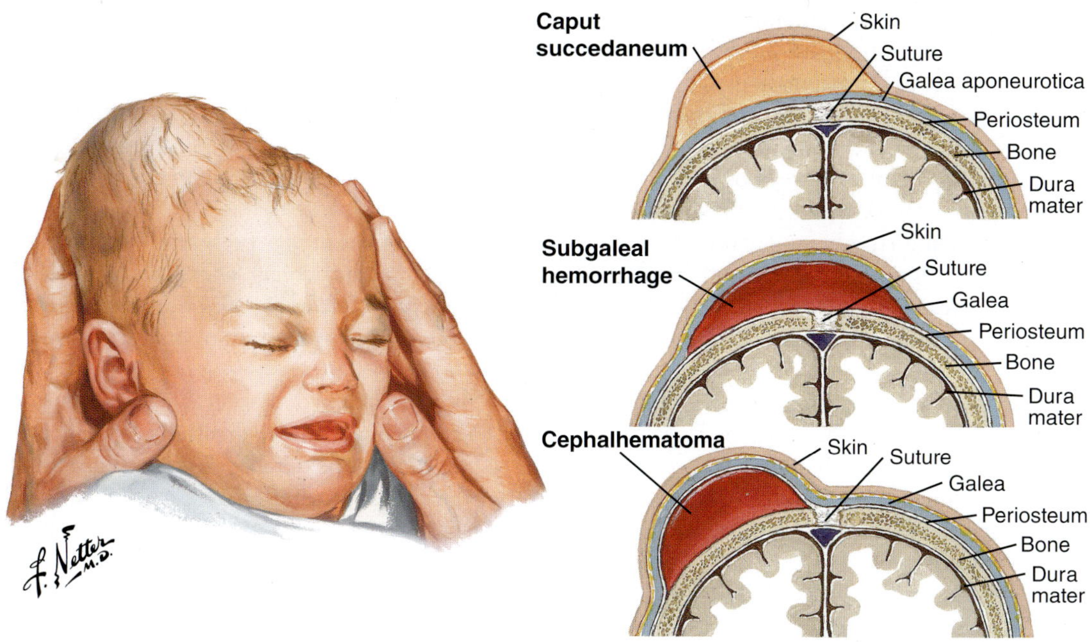

Fig. 24.10 Caput Succedaneum. (Reused with permission from Smith RP: *Netter's obstetrics and gynecology*, ed 4, 2024, Elsevier.)

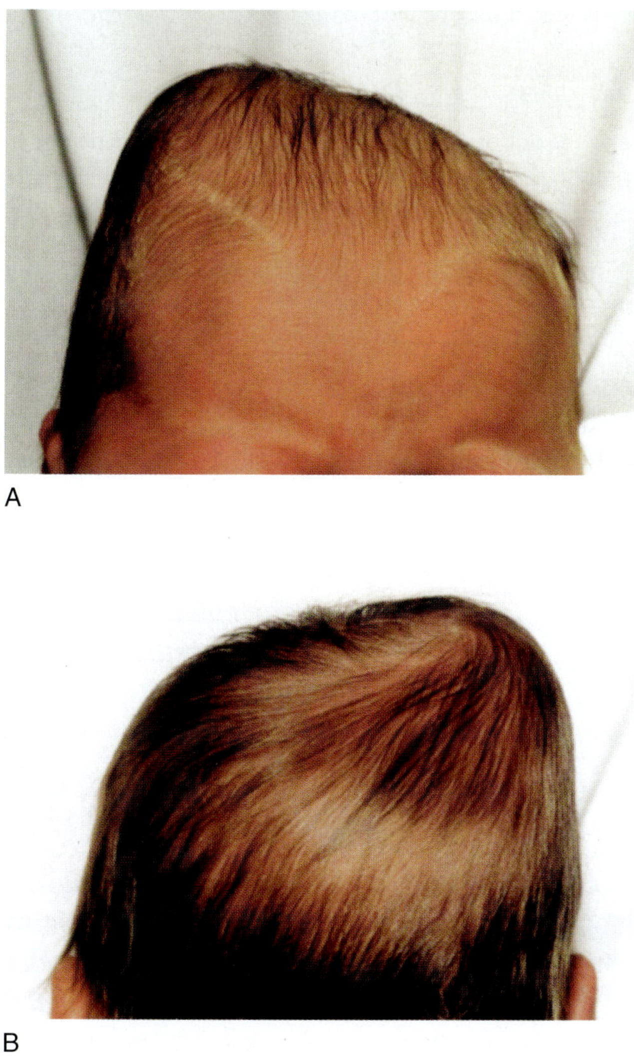

Fig. 24.11 Cephalohematoma. (From Walker VP: *Avery's diseases of the newborn*, 2017, Elsevier [chapter 25].)

or medications used to prevent infections may make this part of the examination difficult. The best method of evaluating the eyes of a newborn is to hold the infant upright at arm's length while slowly rotating them in one direction. The infant's eyes usually open spontaneously. If not, talking to the infant or dimming the lights may help. If necessary, the eyelids can be carefully held open.

Inspect the eyes for *symmetry.* The eyes should be the same size and should be at the same depth in the orbits. Assess whether the eyes are normal distance from one another or if they are too close together *(hypotelorism)* or too far apart *(hypertelorism).*

Inspect the *eyelids* for evidence of trauma. Newborns rarely have eyebrows, but long eyelashes are frequently present. Medial epicanthal folds, flaps of skin covering the inner canthus of the eye, are seen frequently in individuals with midface hypoplasia. This condition occurs in a number of disorders, including trisomy 21 and fetal alcohol spectrum disorder, but may be seen in individuals without syndromes as well.

Inspect the *sclerae.* In newborns, the sclerae may be icteric as a result of physiologic jaundice (described earlier). When icterus is absent, the sclerae of a young infant may appear bluish.

Inspect the *cornea.* The cornea should be clear. Cloudiness or a corneal diameter that is greater than 1 cm may be indicative of congenital glaucoma. Enlargement of the orbit, a condition known as *buphthalmos,* may also be seen in individuals with congenital glaucoma.

Inspect the *iris.* The iris of a newborn may be pale because full pigmentation does not occur before 10 to 12 months of life. Is an abnormal ventral cleft present in the iris? This cleft, known as a *coloboma,* is associated with defects in the iris and/or retina. See Fig. 10.66. A coloboma may occur in isolation but is commonly associated with some chromosomal abnormalities such as trisomy 13 or 18 and *CHARGE* syndrome (i.e., *c*oloboma, *h*eart disease, *a*tresia choanae, *r*etardation of growth or development, genitourinary tract anomalies, and *e*ar anomalies). In rare cases, the irides are absent; this condition, known as *aniridia,* is associated with the susceptibility to development of Wilms tumor.

Inspect the *conjunctivae.* Small subconjunctival hemorrhages are common, a result of the forces involved in the birth process. They appear as small red areas of blood. They heal without any effect on the child's vision. As a result of the erythromycin drops instilled at birth, there may be some inflammation of the conjunctivae, as well as edema of the eyelids.

The *pupils* of neonates are usually constricted until approximately the third week after birth. Pupillary reflexes are present but hard to interpret in this age group.

Rotate the infant slowly to one side. The eyes should turn in the direction to which they are being turned. At the end of the motion, the eyes should quickly look back in the opposite direction after a few quick, unsustained nystagmoid movements. This is termed the *rotational response,* and its presence establishes that the motor control of the eyes is intact.

Place the infant back on their back. To test for *visual acuity* in the newborn, the examiner must rely on indirect methods such as the response to a bright light, known as the *optical blink reflex.* This reflex is normally observed when a bright light is shined on each eye: the newborn blinks and dorsiflexes the head. The visual acuity of newborns has been estimated to be approximately 20/100 to 20/150, according to their ability to fixate on and imitate the adult face.

In all newborns, the presence of the *red reflex* bilaterally suggests grossly normal eyes and the absence of glaucoma, cataract, or intraocular disorders, such as a tumor. To determine the presence of the red reflex, start by turning off the lights in the room to dilate the newborn's pupils. Set the ophthalmoscope lens power to "0" and hold it close to the examiner's eye. Project the ophthalmoscope light onto both eyes of the patient simultaneously from approximately 18 inches away (distance of arm's length from the patient). When the child looks at the light, a red reflex should emanate from both eyes and be symmetric in character. For a confirmatory look, move closer and examine each eye separately. The presence of the red reflex indicates that there is no serious obstruction to light between the cornea and the retina. It should also be noted that the red reflex color can vary in children due to differences in ocular fundus pigmentation. In darkly pigmented brown eyes, the red reflex can be a dark red, but in lightly pigmented eyes, it can be orange-yellow. If there is a white reflex, known as *leukocoria*, or there are dark spots in the red reflex, or if the red reflex is diminished, absent, or asymmetrical, a referral to an ophthalmologist is indicated for a funduscopic examination. A frequent cause of leukocoria, as shown in Fig. 10.142, is a retinoblastoma, which is a malignant tumor of the retina. A referral to an ophthalmologist is also indicated if any of the intrauterine infections associated with chorioretinitis, such as toxoplasmosis, congenital rubella, or cytomegalovirus are suspected.

Ears

Inspect the *external ear.* Frequently, the ears are misshapen as a result of intrauterine positioning. Such misshaping usually resolves within 1 to 2 days after birth. In rare instances, one ear is malformed and reduced in size. This condition, *microtia,* is often associated with genetic syndromes or other anomalies on the ipsilateral side of the face. An imaginary line from the inner and outer canthus of the eye toward the vertex should be at or below the level of the superior attachment of the ear. Low-set ears are often associated with congenital kidney defects or chromosomal disorders.

Are any *skin tags* present? A skin tag or cleft in front of the tragus (preauricular) often represents a remnant of the first branchial cleft and may be an isolated anomaly or part of a more widespread group of malformations.

Nose

Newborns are nasal breathers, and obstruction to nasal flow can cause considerable distress; the infant with nasal obstruction is cyanotic and distressed at rest, but the cyanosis diminishes when they cry. If there is concern about the patency of the nasopharynx, pass a soft, sterile, 6-French catheter through each external naris, and advance it into the posterior nasopharynx. This test rules out the presence of unilateral or bilateral *choanal atresia,* which is a cause of severe respiratory distress in newborns. Choanal atresia may occur as an isolated anomaly (in which case, more than 90% of affected individuals are female), or it may be part of the *CHARGE syndrome.*

Oropharynx

Assess the lips and philtrum. Is there a cleft of the lip? This may be to the left or the right of the midline and may be unilateral or bilateral. Is the philtrum well formed, with normal architecture? Flattening of the philtrum is seen in infants with fetal alcohol spectrum disorder.

Inspect the *oral cavity.* The gums should be raised, smooth, and pink. Is there a *cleft palate* (see Fig. 12.32). A *bifid uvula* may be associated with a submucosal cleft palate. Is the palate *high-arched?* Pinhead, whitish-yellow, rounded papules on either side of the raphe on the hard palate are *Epstein pearls.* These are mucous-retention cysts and disappear within the first few weeks after birth as seen in Fig. 24.12. Similar cysts may be present on the gingivae. Inspect for *neonatal teeth.* These teeth have poor root systems and may have to be removed to prevent accidental aspiration.

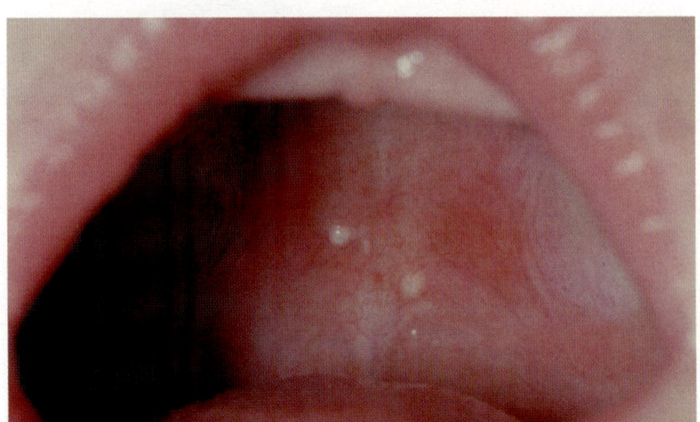

Fig. 24.12 Epstein Pearls. (From Neville BW, Damm DD, Allen CM: *Oral and maxillofacial pathology*, 2016, Elsevier [chapter 1].)

Inspect the *tongue.* The normal frenulum may be short or may extend almost to the tip of the tongue. Because the production of saliva is limited in the first few months of life, the presence of excessive saliva in the mouth is suggestive of *esophageal atresia.*

Test the *sucking reflex.* Put on a glove and insert your index finger into the newborn's mouth. A strong sucking reflex should be present. The sucking reflex is usually strong by 34 weeks' gestation and disappears at 9 to 12 months of age. Feel for any submucosal clefts in the palate.

Inspect the *pharynx.* This can be performed while the infant is crying. Tonsillar tissue is not visible in the newborn. Small ulcers or clusters of small, whitish-yellow follicles on an erythematous base are sometimes seen on the anterior tonsillar pillars and are known as *Bednar aphthae.* The cause is unknown, and they disappear within the first week after birth.

Assess the *mandible.* Is it hypoplastic, small, and recessed? Occurring in isolation or in association with a U-shaped cleft of the palate in the Pierre Robin malformation sequence, micrognathia may be associated with life-threatening obstructive apnea, a medical emergency that necessitates immediate attention.

Neck

The neck of a newborn appears relatively short. Is the neck *symmetric* with regard to the midline? Rotate the infant's head. Normally, the infant's head should be easily rotated to either side so that the chin can touch either shoulder. *Torticollis* is a condition in which the head is tilted to one side while the chin is rotated to the other shoulder. In the newborn, a hematoma of the sternocleidomastoid muscle as a result of a birth injury may produce this condition. Palpate for a mass in the area of the sternocleidomastoid muscle if torticollis is present.

Palpate for *masses.* A midline mass may be a thyroglossal cyst or thyromegaly. A lateral mass may be a cystic hygroma or branchial cleft cyst.

Is *webbing* of the neck present? Webbing is a feature of *Turner syndrome, Noonan syndrome,*[j] and other congenital abnormalities.

Palpate the *clavicles* to rule out a fracture. Palpate along the entire length of the clavicles with the index fingers, feeling for crepitus, present with a fractured clavicle. Swelling or a discontinuity of the clavicle may also be felt. Clavicular fractures as a result of a birth injury usually occur at the junction of the middle and outer thirds of the bone. Decreased motion in the upper extremity may be associated with a clavicular fracture. Clavicular fracture is a rather common injury even during uneventful births and usually heals without any sequelae.

Chest

Inspect the *respiratory pattern.* The breathing pattern of newborns is almost entirely diaphragmatic. Irregular shallow respirations are common in newborns. *Periodic breathing* is characterized by periods of pauses in breathing lasting 5 to 15 seconds and is not associated with bradycardia. *True apnea* has a duration of more than 20 seconds and is associated with bradycardia. The latter is more commonly found in premature infants with pulmonary disease. Infants with true apnea are thought to be at higher risk for sudden infant death syndrome (SIDS). The presence of an *expiratory grunt, retractions* of the chest, or *flaring* of the nostrils is indicative of respiratory distress. Note the location of retractions: below the ribcage (subcostal), between the ribs (intercostal), or above the sternum (suprasternal).

Inspect for *deformities.* The most important chest deformity in newborns is asymmetry owing to unequal chest expansion on one side. Other deformities seen in adults, such as pectus excavatum and pectus carinatum, are rarely seen in newborns. Sometimes the xyphoid process is protruding due to the relative thin musculature of the chest wall. In addition, asymmetry of the chest wall may be a normal variant or may represent hypoplasia of the pectoralis minor and major muscles.

Auscultate the anterior and posterior chest with either the bell or the small diaphragm of the stethoscope. Bronchovesicular breath sounds should be easily heard throughout the lung fields and are higher in pitch than those in adults. Absence of breath sounds on one side may be indicative of pneumothorax or a diaphragmatic hernia. Pneumothorax can occur in newborns as a result of the large transpulmonary pressures involved in inflation of the lungs for the first time. Crackles may be heard in infants with transient tachypnea of the newborn (TTN) due to residual fluid in the lungs often seen after cesarean delivery, or breath sounds can be clear. The hallmark of TTN is tachypnea at birth with a respiratory rate greater than 60 breaths/min, and there are often signs of respiratory distress. Cyanosis can also be present. Although TTN is benign and usually self-resolves within 12 to 24 hours, occasionally symptoms can last for as long as 3 days. Management is supportive care.

Another cause of respiratory distress in the newborn is *meconium aspiration syndrome (MAS),* which can occur when there is meconium-stained amniotic fluid (MSAF) at the time of delivery. Aspiration of this MSAF can lead to pulmonary disease, resulting in hypoxemia and acidosis. Signs of MAS span mild respiratory distress to acute hypoxic respiratory failure. Rales and rhonchi are typically heard on auscultation. In severe cases, there can be a pneumothorax or pneumomediastinum.

Breasts

Inspect the breasts. The breasts of both male and female newborns are enlarged. A milky discharge from the nipple, may be present. This is the effect of maternal estrogen and may persist for 1 to 2 weeks after birth.

Supernumerary nipples may be present along the milk line as shown in Fig. 24.13. They may or may not have areolae. They are often mistaken for congenital nevi and have no clinical significance.

Heart

Inspect the patient for *cyanosis.* If central cyanosis is present within the first hours or days after birth, suspect atresia of one

[j]Noonan syndrome is a genetic disorder that prevents normal development in various parts of the body. These include unusual facial characteristics, short stature, cardiac defects, other physical problems, and possible developmental delays.

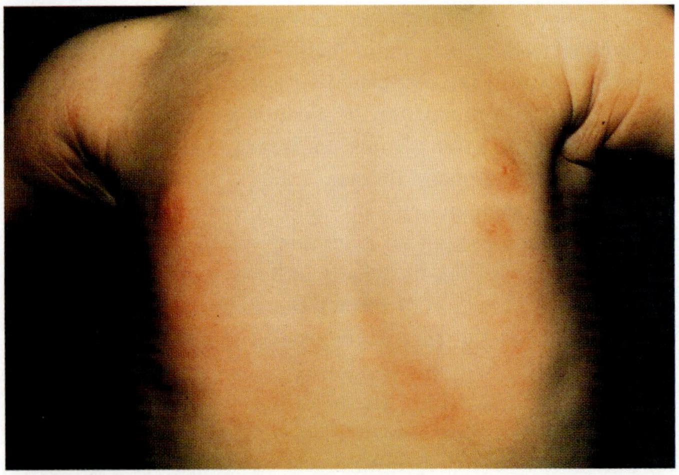

Fig. 24.13 Supernumerary Nipple Remnant on the Left Chest of an Infant. (From Moore KL, Persaud TVN, Torchia M: *The developing human*, 2015, Elsevier [chapter 19].)

of the right heart valves, transposition of the great vessels, or persistent fetal circulation.

Inspect for evidence of *congestive heart failure.* In newborns, the most important signs of heart failure are poor feeding, persistent tachycardia of up to 200 beats/min, tachypnea, pallor, and an enlarged liver. Crackles are not sensitive indicators of heart failure in newborns. Heart failure during the first few days after birth is frequently caused by hypoplastic left heart syndrome.

Palpate for the *point of maximum impulse.* In newborns younger than 48 hours old, the point of maximum impulse is often in the xiphoid region. After this period and for several years, the point of maximum impulse should be in the fourth left intercostal space just lateral to the midclavicular line. A right-sided point of maximum impulse is suggestive of *dextrocardia,* a left-sided pneumothorax, or a diaphragmatic hernia (which is usually on the left side, so that the herniated abdominal contents displace the heart to the right.)

Auscultate the heart in the same locations as in adults by using the small diaphragm and bell of the stethoscope. Because the respiratory rate is so rapid in newborns, it is often difficult to distinguish respiratory from cardiac events. Auscultation in newborns has a low degree of sensitivity in detecting congenital heart disease. Many "normal" murmurs heard in the early neonatal period are related to the marked changes in circulation after birth. A systolic murmur at the upper left sternal border from a *patent ductus arteriosus* is commonly heard at birth but disappears by the second or third day after birth as the ductus spontaneously closes. In contrast, many severe congenital heart lesions, such as transposition of the great vessels, produce no murmur in the neonatal period. If any murmurs are present, they should be noted and described as indicated in Chapter 14, The Heart. See Tables 24.10 and 24.11 at the end of this chapter for additional details.

Pulses

To palpate the femoral pulses, remove the diaper to expose the groin on both sides and extend and hold down both legs. This will make palpation easier by reducing leg movement and exposing the inguinal canals. With the tips of your index and middle fingers, find the femoral pulses at the midpoint of the inguinal ligament between the symphysis pubis and the iliac crest. Apply gentle pressure on both sides at the same time to compare them. Both sides should have equal and strong pulses. Spend enough time to be sure you are feeling the arterial pulsations and not the movement of the abdominal wall with respiration. Diminished pulses indicate poor cardiac output or ineffective vasoconstriction. Poor or unequal pulses suggest possible interruption of the thoracic aorta or other circulatory problems. Compare the femoral pulse to the infant's brachial pulse. Delayed or weakened femoral pulses as compared to brachial pulses should raise the suspicion of coarctation of the aorta. In hypoplastic left heart syndrome or preductal coarctation of the aorta, the femoral pulses may be present for the first 24 to 48 hours and disappear as the ductus closes. Repeated examinations of the newborn are important to be sure that the femoral pulses remain strong after ductal closure.

Abdomen

Inspect the abdomen. The abdomen of a newborn is protuberant as a result of the poor development of the abdominal musculature. If the abdomen is scaphoid, there should be a high index of suspicion that a diaphragmatic hernia is present and that the abdominal organs may be located in the chest.

Inspect the *umbilical cord stump.* The normal umbilical cord contains two thick-walled arteries and one thin-walled vein. Is there evidence of yellow staining by meconium as a result of fetal distress? This examination needs to be performed early before the stump starts to dry. Newborns with a single artery may have congenital abnormalities of the kidneys and spine. Drainage of a clear discharge from the umbilicus is suggestive of the presence of a patent urachus, which is a canal in the fetus that connects the urinary bladder to the allantois or possibly an omphalomesenteric duct.

In healthy infants, the umbilical cord stump falls off before the end of the second week after birth. Persistence of the stump past this period suggests the presence of white cell adhesion defect or a patent urachus. After the umbilical cord stump has fallen off, the examiner must check for an *umbilical granuloma,* which is granulation tissue ranging in size from 3 to 10 mm, and is soft, moist, and friable. If present, it can be cauterized with silver nitrate.

Is an *umbilical hernia* present? An umbilical hernia is a protrusion of abdominal contents (part of the abdominal lining, fluid, or intestines) through the umbilicus when the umbilical ring fails to close. Umbilical hernias are common in premature infants. Many umbilical hernias will resolve on their own by the time the child turns 3 or 4 years old. However, this is less likely to occur if the underlying fascial defect is larger than 1.5 cm, there is an excessive amount of overlying skin, or the infant has a predisposing condition, such as trisomy 21, hypothyroidism, Ehlers-Danlos, Beckwith-Wiedemann syndrome, and others.

Although uncommon, two major defects in the abdominal wall are well known. *Omphaloceles* are severe umbilical hernias in which some of the abdominal contents are located outside the body. Omphaloceles, which always involve the umbilicus and, as such, are always in the midline, may be isolated anomalies or may be associated with additional anomalies, such as in the *Beckwith-Wiedemann syndrome. Gastroschisis,* which results from an embryonic vascular deficiency, is similar to omphalocele in that abdominal contents are located outside the abdominal cavity. However, gastroschisis is never midline, is never covered by a membrane, and usually is located in the right upper quadrant.

Auscultate the abdomen. The abdomen of a newborn infant is tympanitic, with metallic tinkling sounds being heard every 15 to 20 seconds.

Palpate the abdomen. To relax the abdomen, use your left hand to hold the infant's hips and knees in a flexed position while the child is sucking, and palpate with your right hand. In general, the liver edge may be felt as much as 2 cm below the right costal margin in the newborn. A liver edge more than 3 cm below the right costal margin is suggestive of hepatomegaly. The liver span can be measured by percussion, and this measurement is more accurate than abdominal measurements because respiratory conditions could hyperinflate the lungs and push a normal liver down into the abdominal cavity. Palpation of the spleen tip is less common.

Palpate the *kidneys.* Place your left hand under the right side of the child's back and lift upward. At the same time, place your right hand in the child's right upper quadrant, and palpate for the right kidney. Reverse hands to palpate the left kidney.

Inspect the location of the *anus.* Unless it is clinically indicated, the *rectum* is not examined. In infants with *imperforate anus,* a blind dimple may be present; in infant girls, a rectovaginal fistula may allow passage of stool vaginally. In infant boys, an imperforate anus may be associated with a rectovesical fistula and no passage of meconium. Note that patency of the anus is established when the infant's temperature is taken rectally or with passage of meconium through the anus.

Genitalia

Inspect the *external genitalia.* In the term male infant, the scrotum is relatively large and rugate. The foreskin of the penis is tight and adherent to the glans penis. Never forcefully retract the foreskin. Inspect the glans for the location of the external urethral meatus. *Hypospadias* is a condition in which the meatus is located in an abnormal ventral position, anywhere from the lower glans of the penis to the scrotum. It is important to detect hypospadias in the neonatal period because it represents a contraindication to circumcision. The penis may look partially circumcised because in this defect, the foreskin usually does not cover the entire glans. See Fig. 24.14 for various locations and terminology for hypospadias. Penile erections are common, often preceding the voiding of urine.

Inspect the scrotum for symmetry and rugae. The testicles should be descended into the scrotum or the inguinal canals. Undescended testes are relatively common, especially in premature babies, as the testes usually descend from the abdominal cavity into the scrotum during the third trimester of pregnancy. Palpate the testicles by putting your index and/or middle finger over the posterior part of the scrotum and your thumb anteriorly

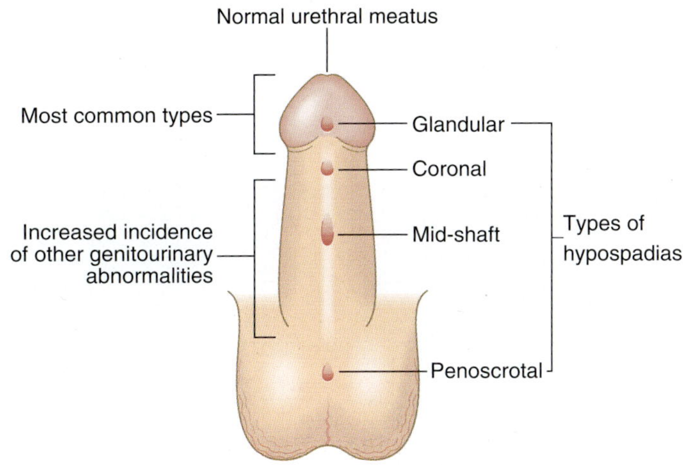

Fig. 24.14 Varieties of Hypospadias. (From Stenson B, Cunningham S: *Macleod's clinical examination,* 2018, Elsevier [chapter 15].)

and palpate with a downward movement, which counteracts the active cremasteric reflex. Placing a finger at the top of the scrotum will help prevent the testicle from being pushed upward. If the scrotal sac is empty, check the inguinal canal. If the testicle is there *(retractile testicle),* try to push it down into the scrotal sac using steady, gentle pressure. If a testicle is not palpable anywhere, it may be intraabdominal and will need further evaluation.

Look for asymmetry or enlargement of the scrotal sacs. Palpate for any masses. *Hydroceles* or *hernias* are common in newborns. A hydrocele is a fluid collection in the scrotum, which can be transilluminated. Hold an otoscope or penlight up to the scrotum and see if the light is transmitted and lights up the sac. Hydroceles can be monitored as they usually resolve on their own, but if still present by 6 months of age will need to be repaired. Inguinal hernias are not uncommon, especially in premature babies. A bulge will be seen, and a mass will be palpable in the scrotum or inguinal canal which does not transilluminate. Often bilateral, when they occur in isolation, a right-sided hernia is more common than one on the left. Because indirect inguinal hernias can lead to incarceration of abdominal contents, a hernia should be repaired as soon as possible. Fig. 24.15 shows a unilateral hernia in both a female (A) and male (B) infant.

To examine the female genitalia, take the diaper off and place the infant in frog-leg position. In the term female infant, the labia majora should cover the labia minora and clitoris, whereas in premature girls, the labia minora and clitoris are more prominent. There should be a fingertip space between the vagina and the anus. If not, the possibility of sexual ambiguity exists. A vaginal discharge that is white mucus is common during the first few days after birth and is an effect of estrogen; the discharge may become bloody later in the first week from withdrawal of maternal estrogen. The examiner should inspect the *urethral meatus* and *vaginal orifice* by placing a gloved thumb and index finger on the child's perineum while pressing downward and laterally on the buttocks. The vaginal opening should be fully visible.

In a male or female infant born vaginally after a breech presentation, the external genitalia are often erythematous and edematous as a result of the trauma related to the birth process.

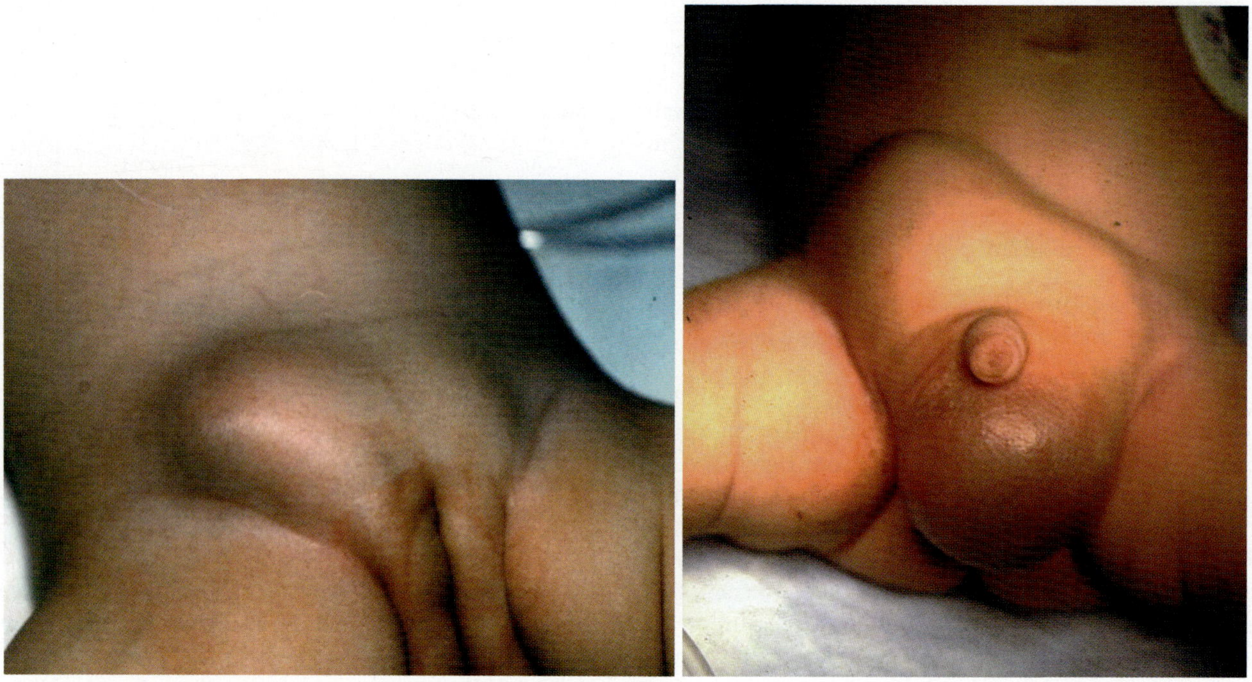

A B

Fig. 24.15 Unilateral inguinal hernias in a female (A) and male (B) infant. (From Ledbetter DJ, Chabra S, Javid PJ: *Avery's diseases of the newborn*, 2017, Elsevier [chapter 73].)

Difference of sex development (DSD) encompasses a wide range of conditions and etiologies that result in external genitalia that are difficult to assess as male or female, or the appearance of the external genitalia is not consistent with the chromosomal sex of the infant. DSD typically presents in the newborn period and is both a psychological emergency for the parents and possibly a medical emergency for the child. Signs of atypical genitalia in females include enlarged clitoris that looks like a small penis; urethral opening anywhere along the clitoris; labia that are fused and look like a scrotum; lump of tissue within the fused labia, further making it look like a scrotum with testicles. The most common cause is *congenital adrenal hyperplasia* resulting from 21-hydroxylase deficiency in a female infant. Affected children have a large clitoris or phallus and possibly fused labia but no palpable gonads in the *labioscrotal folds.* The child should be assessed immediately with appropriate blood tests because many infants with 21-hydroxylase deficiency manifest *salt loss* and Addisonian crisis, and can go into shock and die in the first week or two after birth.

If 21-hydroxylase deficiency has been ruled out, other causes of DSD must be explored. During this workup, management of the parents may be as important as management of the child. The evaluation should be conducted by a team, which includes a psychologist as well as a pediatric urologist, endocrinologist, geneticist, and neonatologist.

Musculoskeletal Examination

The purpose of the musculoskeletal examination of the newborn is to detect gross abnormalities. The appearance of the extremities at birth usually reflects the positioning of the child within the uterus, known as *intrauterine packing.*

Inspect the *extremities* and *digits.* Are all four extremities and 20 digits present? Polydactyly, the presence of one or more extra digits, occurs in approximately 1% of all newborns. It may be inherited as an autosomal dominant trait or may be part of a more complex multiple malformation syndrome. Most polydactyly is postaxial (on the small digit side of the hand or foot), and the extra digit is represented by a skin tag (called a *postminimus*). Hypodactyly, the absence of one or more digits, is never considered a normal variant. The absence of digits should always trigger an evaluation for associated anomalies.

Check for *brachial plexus palsy.* Injury to the *brachial plexus* may cause paralysis of the upper arm. This injury may result from lateral traction on the head and neck during delivery of the shoulder. *Erb palsy* produces an inability to spontaneously abduct the arm at the shoulder, rotate the arm externally, flex the elbow, and supinate the forearm. This injury to the fifth and sixth cervical nerves results in a characteristic position of arm adduction, with elbow extension, forearm pronation, and arm internal rotation known as the "waiter's tip" position. The grasp reflex is usually preserved. *Klumpke paralysis* is much rarer and results from injury to the seventh and eighth cervical nerves, producing paralysis of the hand and forearm. The grasp reflex is absent. Involvement of the first thoracic nerve with Klumpke paralysis may also result in ipsilateral ptosis and miosis, or *Horner syndrome.* The prognosis of any brachial plexus palsy depends on whether the nerve or nerves were lacerated or only bruised. If the palsy is related only to edema of the nerve fibers and not to actual injury, function usually returns within a few months with the help of physical therapy.

The most important part of the musculoskeletal examination of the newborn is the evaluation of the lower extremities. The *hips* are examined for the possibility of developmental dysplasia, in which a hip either is dislocated from the acetabulum or can be dislocated. Inspect the contours of the legs while the child is lying prone. The presence of asymmetric skin folds on the medial aspect of the thigh is suggestive of a proximally dislocated femur. The perineum should not be visible when the child is in this position because the normal position of the thighs should cover most of it. If the perineum is visible, you must suspect *bilateral* hip dislocations.

With the child lying supine, place the infant's feet side by side with the soles on the examination table, allowing the hips and knees to flex. Observe the relative height of the knees. If one knee is at a lower level, you should suspect that the shortness of that knee is secondary to a dislocation of the hip on that side, a congenitally short femur, or both. This is known as *Galeazzi sign.* If both knees are at the same height, either both hips are normal or both hips are dislocated.

After inspection of the knee heights, each hip is examined to determine joint stability. Two maneuvers are useful in detecting hip instability. First perform the *Barlow maneuver.* Flex the newborn's legs 90 degrees at the hip. Hold the legs by placing the thumbs over the mid-thigh medially and the index fingers over the greater trochanters, as shown in Fig. 24.16 *(right)*. Test one hip at a time. Adduct the knee to midline and gently press down posteriorly toward the examination table. Feel for a "clunk" as an unstable femoral head slips past the posterior rim of the acetabulum and dislocates from the socket. Now perform the *Ortolani maneuver,* which is a sign of relocating the femoral head into the acetabulum. Abduct the hip (knee goes outward) while you apply gentle upward pressure over the greater trochanter and push the femoral head anteriorly, as shown in Fig. 24.16 *(left)*. A "clunk" indicates that the hip is relocating in the socket. Repeat with the other leg. If a clunk is felt in either hip, avoid repeat examinations of the hip until an expert examination or ultrasound can be done: Movement of the femoral head in and out of the socket can damage the articular cartilage. It is common to feel clicks, which are benign ligamentous sounds under the examining fingers; when in doubt, ask for expert evaluation. These tests should be performed on a relaxed infant. After the neonatal period, the Ortolani maneuver may yield a false-negative result.

Inspect the *feet.* Observe the foot at the sole. An imaginary line from the center of the heel through the center of the metatarsal-tarsal line should bisect either the second toe or the space between the second and third toes. If the line crosses more laterally, the forefoot is adducted (turned inward) in relation to the hindfoot. This is the common condition known as *metatarsus adductus* and is often the result of intrauterine packing. The lateral aspect of the foot will curve inward, instead of being straight. It is considered flexible metatarsus adductus if the forefoot can be rotated laterally into an aligned position and usually resolves spontaneously within the first few years of life, especially with the aid of stretching exercises. Early casting or exercises for passive correction may be required if the foot is in a fixed position.

A common, but benign, foot abnormality is *talipes calcaneovalgus,* a condition where the foot excessively dorsiflexes, such that the dorsum of the foot touches the lower shin. It is thought to be caused by the crowding and positioning of the foot in utero. Most of the time, no treatment is necessary besides simple stretching exercises at home, and the condition will improve in several weeks. This condition is seen in Fig. 24.17.

The most serious foot deformity at birth is the *clubfoot,* also known as *talipes equinovarus.* The entire foot is deviated toward the midline. There is forefoot adduction, fixed inversion of the hindfoot, and fixed plantar flexion. The Achilles tendon is foreshortened, and the foot assumes the position of a horse's hoof, hence the prefix *equino-*. The calf muscles on the affected side are also smaller than those on the unaffected side. Therapy should begin within the first few days after birth. Manipulation is vital. If the deformity is not corrected by retention casting or splinting, surgical release may be necessary at a later date. The

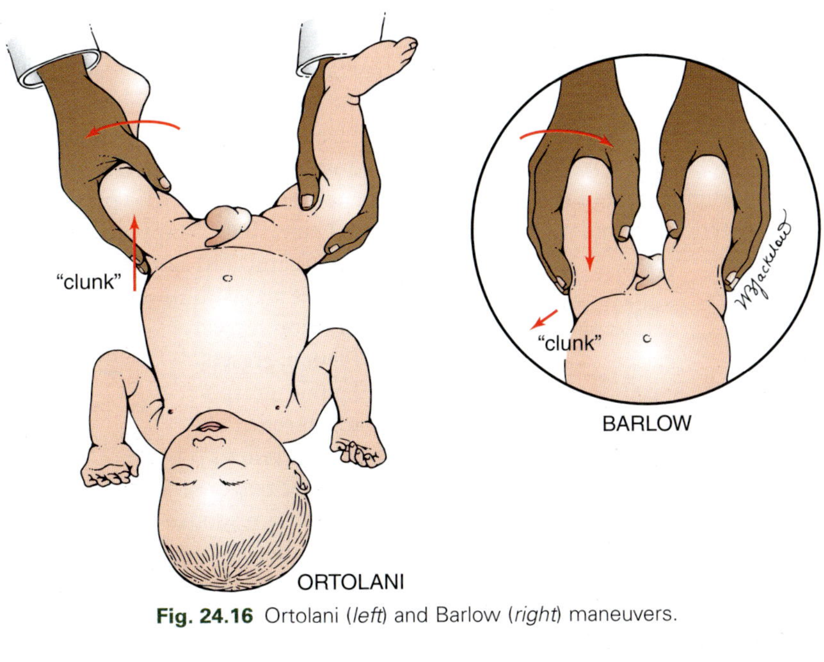

Fig. 24.16 Ortolani (*left*) and Barlow (*right*) maneuvers.

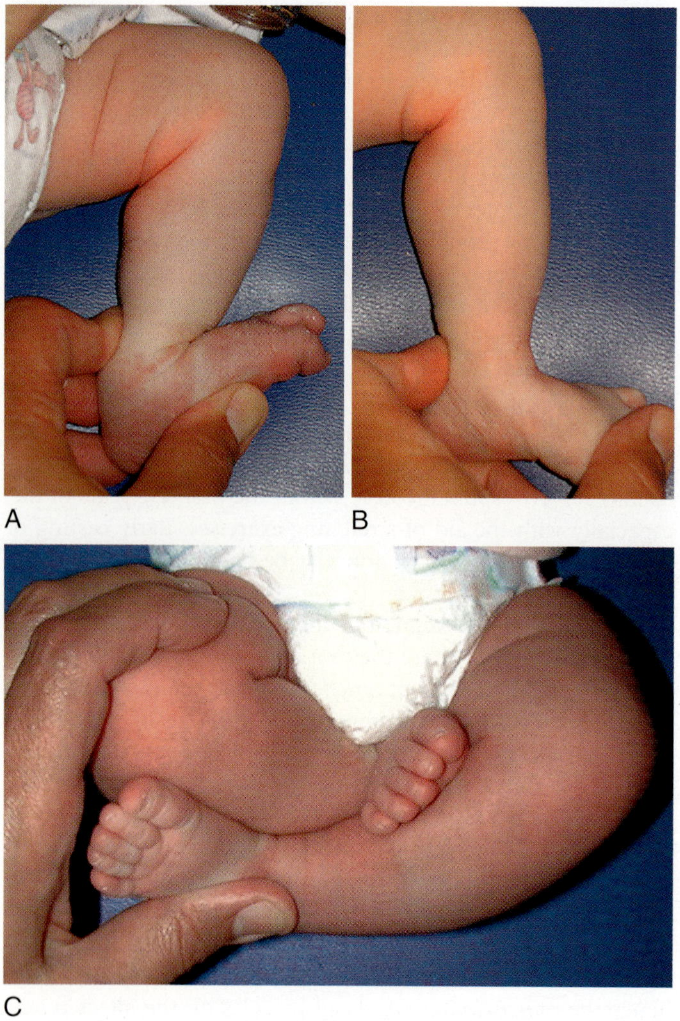

Fig. 24.17 Calcaneovalgus foot (A) which is passively correctable (B) and due to intrauterine position (C). (From Winell JJ, Davidson RS: *Nelson textbook of pediatrics*, Chapter 674, 2016, Elsevier, pp. 3247–3257.e1.)

3-week-old infant pictured in Fig. 24.18 was born with bilateral clubfoot and bilateral hip dislocations. Multiple musculoskeletal deformities may be a clue to a neuromuscular problem in utero.

Neurologic Examination

Careful inspection is the most important aspect of the neonatal neurologic examination. The inspection should include the following:

- Posture
- Symmetry of extremities
- Spontaneous movements
- Facial expressions and symmetry
- Eye movements and symmetry

Notice the *position* of the newborn. Healthy newborns have flexor tone of the upper and lower extremities. Extension of the extremities while awake may indicate hypotonia, which would be a concerning finding. Is hyperextension of the neck present? This sign is frequently found in infants with severe meningeal or brainstem irritation.

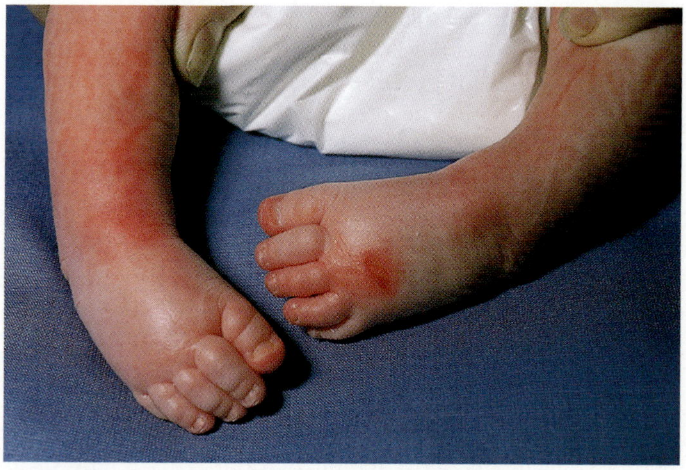

Fig. 24.18 Talipes Equinovarus.

The *motor* examination consists of testing the *range of motion* of all joints. Assess muscle tone and compare one side with the other. Compare the muscle sizes and strengths. Compare the resistance to passive stretch.

The *sensory* examination is performed only if a nerve palsy or spina bifida is suspected. Usually, pain is the only sensation tested; the object is to elicit a grimace or cry, which indicates cortical perception of pain, and not just withdrawal of the limb, which can be a spinal reflex. Testing the *cranial nerves* is also difficult in newborns, but the presence of facial symmetry and of the *rotational response* indicate that cranial nerves III, IV, VI, and VII are grossly intact. Observing a feeding for coordination of sucking, swallowing, and breathing is a good test of cranial nerves IX and X. A simple test for cranial nerve XII consists of pinching the nostrils of the newborn. A reflex opening of the mouth with extension and elevation of the tongue in the midline is the normal response. Deviation of the tongue to one side indicates a lesion of the cranial nerve on that side.

Because the corticospinal tracts are not fully developed in newborns, the response to testing of the deep tendon reflexes is variable and is neither sensitive nor specific. *Babinski reflex* (see Chapter 21, The Nervous System) is usually present in newborns, meaning the toes will be upgoing when the bottom of the foot is stroked. Babinski reflex may be present in normal children until the first birthday.

Test for *infantile automatisms*. These are primitive reflex phenomena that may be present at birth, depending on gestational age, but disappear soon thereafter. There are many automatisms, and not all have to be tested. The most important ones are as follows:

- Rooting response
- Plantar grasp
- Palmar grasp
- Moro reflex
- Galant reflex
- Placing response
- Stepping response
- Asymmetric tonic neck reflex

The rotational response and sucking response are also automatisms and are discussed earlier in this chapter.

The following reflexes are elicited while the newborn infant is lying supine on the examination table.

The *rooting response* is elicited by having the infant lie in a quiet state with hands held against the chest. The examiner then strokes the corner of the infant's mouth or cheek. The normal response is turning of the head to the same side and opening of the mouth to grasp the finger. If only the upper lip is touched, the head normally retroflexes; if only the lower lip is touched, the jaw normally drops. The rooting response is present by 32 weeks' gestation and usually disappears after 3 to 4 months after birth. This primitive response facilitates nursing. It is absent in infants with severe central nervous system disease.

The *plantar grasp* is elicited by placing the examiner's thumb on the plantar surface of the foot directly under the toes. The normal response is plantar flexion of the toes over the thumb. This response disappears by 9 to 12 months.

The *palmar grasp* is elicited by stabilizing the infant's head in the midline. Place a thumb or index finger into the newborn's palm from the ulnar side. The normal response is flexion of all the fingers to grasp the index finger. If the reflex is sluggish, allow the child to suck, which normally facilitates the grasp response. The palmar grasp is usually established by 32 weeks' gestation and usually disappears after 3 to 5 months after birth. The absence of this response in a newborn or its persistence after 5 months is suggestive of cerebral disease. The newborn commonly holds the hand in a fist. After 2 months, however, the presence of this sign might suggest neurologic disease.

The infant is now picked up and held supine in the examiner's hands.

The Moro reflex, or the *startle reflex,* is elicited by supporting the infant's body in the right hand and supporting the head with the left hand. The head is suddenly allowed to drop a few centimeters, with immediate resupport by the examiner's hand. The Moro reflex consists of symmetric abduction of the upper extremities at the shoulders and extension of the fingers. Adduction of the arm at the shoulder completes the reflex. The infant usually then emits a loud cry. The Moro reflex is one of the most important motor automatisms. The normal response, which appears in an incomplete form at 28 weeks' gestation, indicates an intact central nervous system. The reflex normally disappears by 3 to 5 months of age. Persistence past 6 months may indicate neurologic disease. An asymmetric Moro may indicate a brachial plexus palsy or clavicular or humerus fracture on one side.

The infant is now turned over to the prone position.

Galant reflex is elicited by stroking one side of the back along a paravertebral line 2 to 3 cm from the midline going from the shoulder to the buttocks. The normal response is lateral curvature of the trunk toward the stimulated side, with the shoulder and hip moving toward the side stroked. Galant reflex normally disappears after 2 to 3 months. This reflex is absent in newborns with transverse spinal cord lesions.

The child is now laid supine on the examination table and then picked up by the examiner, who holds the infant upright. The examiner's hands should be under the arms around the infant's chest, with the head supported by the fingers extended up the infant's back.

The *placing response* is elicited by allowing the dorsum of one of the infant's feet to touch the undersurface of a tabletop lightly. The normal placing response is for the infant to flex the knee and hip, then place the stimulated foot on top of the table. This response is then tested with the other foot. Placement of the soles of both feet on top of a table should elicit the *stepping response,* which is the alternating movement of both legs. Both these responses are best observed 4 to 5 days after birth and disappear after 2 to 5 months. If paresis of the lower extremities is present, these responses are absent.

At approximately 2 weeks of age, the *asymmetric tonic neck reflex* or "fencer's response" appears. When the child's head is turned to one side, the arm on the face side extends and the leg on that side flexes. On the occipital side, the arm flexes, and the leg usually extends. This reflex may last until 6 months of age and may affect the assessment of upper extremity tone if the head is not in the midline.

INFANCY: 1 MONTH TO 12 MONTHS

Infant History

During the first year of life, a major focus is on the gross motor development of an infant. In one short year infants should transition from lying to rolling over, to maintaining head control while upright to sitting independently by about 6 months of age. They then progress to bearing weight on their legs, pulling to stand, standing alone briefly, and finally taking their first steps. As infants start to gain some independence and mobility, ensuring a safe environment is an area of emphasis. Additionally, as solid foods are added to the diet, there is the opportunity to help parents establish healthy eating habits for their child from the start.

- Diet: What is the infant drinking?
  - If breastfeeding:
    - How many times a day is the baby nursing?
    - Is the baby taking vitamin D drops?
  - If formula feeding:
    - How much is the baby taking each feed?
    - How often is the baby feeding?
    - How is the formula prepared?
  - What foods are the baby eating?
    - Pureed baby foods? Store-bought or home-cooked? (Recommend starting at 4 to 6 months of age.)
    - Baby cereal by spoon? (Good source of iron starting at 4 to 6 months of age.)
    - Soft table foods? Soft finger foods? (Recommend starting at 9 to 12 months of age.)
  - What else is the baby drinking? (Encourage water by cup after 6 months, no cow's milk before 1 year of age, and juice is not recommended.)
- Elimination
  - Any concerns about stool consistency or frequency? (Hard pebbly stools indicate constipation.)
- Sleep
  - Where is the infant sleeping?
  - Is there anything in the crib? (There should be nothing in the crib.)

- Is the baby being put to sleep supine?
- Is the baby sleeping for a longer stretch at night? Through the night? (This may start at 4 to 6 months of age.)
- What is the baby's nap schedule?
- Development/behavior (see Table 24.1)
  - Social/Emotional (e.g., smiles, laughs, turns to name, has stranger anxiety, points)
  - Language/Communication (e.g., babbles, says mama/dada nonspecifically, then specifically, 1 other word)
  - Cognitive (e.g., puts things in mouth to explore, bangs two things together, looks for hidden objects)
  - Movement/Physical Development (e.g., rolls over, sits alone, transfers objects, pulls to stand, stands alone, has pincer grasp, walks independently)
  - Excessive crying? (colic)
- Social
  - What are the childcare arrangements?
  - Are social support services needed?
  - How are the caregivers managing?
  - Are there dangerous environmental exposures in the home?
- Screenings: Maternal depression, ACEs,[k] development, lead, anemia, tuberculosis, oral health
- Anticipatory guidance (here are some examples)
  - Use rear-facing car seat in back seat
  - Provide supervised tummy time
  - Avoid screens and other digital media
  - Never leave alone in a bath or car
  - Avoid direct sun exposure
  - Put small objects, medications, cleaning fluids out of reach or locked up and have poison control center phone number handy
  - Remove firearms from home; if necessary, store unloaded and locked
  - Use gates to block stairs or rooms with danger
  - Once teeth erupt, brush twice a day

Until an infant is 1 year of age, breast milk or infant formula should be their main drink. Cow's milk may be fine for older children, but it may irritate the infant's digestive system, which is not fully developed. There are some major differences between cow's milk and breast milk or formula: Cow's milk has too much protein and sodium and too little iron, vitamin C, copper, and zinc for a developing infant. Giving cow's milk to children under the age of 1 can lead to iron deficiency anemia.

For infants, differentiate diarrhea from normal liquid stools. If the child is breastfed, the stools are usually a yellow or mustard-colored liquid and may follow each feeding. If the child is formula-fed, the stools are more likely to be yellowish-tan and firmer. Infants frequently have green, brown, or grayish stools, and normal stools may be loose or liquid in consistency. With diarrhea, the stools are more frequent, all liquid, and watery rings stain the infant's diaper. Minor changes in the stool are common. Normal infants may have several bowel movements a day but may go 1 or more days without a bowel movement. Small, hard, pebble-like stools indicate constipation. Blood in the stool warrants further evaluation.

Age-Appropriate Review of Systems

The information for the ROS for an infant comes entirely from the caregiver. Infants cannot verbalize that they have pain except by crying or being irritable; thus, a major challenge in examining an infant is to localize the pain. In addition, infants cannot report symptoms such as dizziness, nausea, or dysuria, nor can their caretakers assess this. However certain symptoms are universally useful to get a sense of the infant's overall state of being, such as activity level and changes in sleeping pattern to assess mental status, and oral intake and urine output to assess hydration status. Otherwise, the remaining ROS should be guided by the chief concern to explore associated symptoms or to differentiate possible diagnoses. The following list provides examples of symptoms to inquire about for each system.

- **General:** Assess fever, activity level, sleeping, and feeding.
- **Head, eyes, ears, nose, and throat:** Assess bulging or sunken fontanelle, nasal discharge, stuffiness, drooling, ear pulling or rubbing, and ear discharge. Does the child see? Hear? Have crossed eyes? Is there excessive or decreased tearing? Any discharge from the eye? Does the infant tend to hold the head to a particular side (i.e., torticollis)?
- **Cardiovascular:** Assess history of murmur and cyanosis, trouble feeding, sweating during feedings, and squatting.[l]
- **Respiratory:** Assess cough, difficulty breathing (i.e., fast or labored breathing, flaring of nostrils, use of accessory muscles), noisy breathing, and hoarseness.
- **Gastrointestinal:** Assess feeding pattern, stool pattern, vomiting, diarrhea, distention, mass, jaundice. Crying and drawing up legs are characteristic of *intussusception.*[m]
- **Genitourinary:** Assess frequency of voids and wet diapers; strength of urinary stream; and crying with voiding, vaginal discharge, and skin irritation in diaper area.
- **Skin:** Is there a rash? Itching? Easy bruising? Change in birthmarks?
- **Musculoskeletal:** Is there equal use of both hands? Of both legs? Is there swelling or deformity of an extremity?
- **Neurologic:** Is there any seizure activity or other abnormal movements? How is the infant's developmental progress? Has there been loss of previously attained milestones?

[k]Adverse Childhood Experiences (ACEs) including childhood mistreatment, household dysfunction, and other social factors have been linked to poor physical and mental health outcomes in adults. https://www.cdc.gov/violenceprevention/aces/index.html. Accessed October 12, 2023.

[l]In older infants and toddlers, squatting is a symptom or tetralogy of Fallot because squatting increases peripheral resistance and decreases the right-to-left shunting across the ventricular septal defect. Tetralogy of Fallot consists of pulmonic stenosis, an overriding aorta, a ventricular septal defect, and right ventricular hypertrophy; these conditions, conotruncal defects, arise from an abnormal septation of the truncus arteriosus. Tetralogy of Fallot may occur as an isolated condition, but is often part of a malformation syndrome, known as velocardiofacial or DiGeorge syndrome, which is associated with a deletion of chromosome 22q11.2.

[m]Intussusception is a condition in which a segment of the intestine invaginates into the adjoining intestinal lumen, causing bowel obstruction.

Infant Physical Exam

The examination of an infant is similar to that of the newborn. The differences and special features will be highlighted in this section. Infants 1 week to 6 months of age can be examined on the examination table with a caregiver standing nearby. It may be easier to perform part of the examination while the infant is in the caregiver's arms or lap. Infants 6 months to 1 year of age are best examined on the caregiver's lap. The examiner should also be seated at the infant's level.

Observation is a key element of the examination; the most meaningful assessments of the infant's respiratory state, or use of arms and legs, are often obtained when the infant is unaware of being observed. The more difficult and more invasive portions of the examination, such as the evaluation of the pharynx and the otoscopic examination, should be performed last, and therefore are described at the end of this section. To listen to the lungs and heart, take advantage of any time when the infant is quiet.

General Assessment

Start with observation as this step can reveal so much. Observe the infant's activity, alertness, and social responsiveness. Pay attention to the caregiver's interactions with the infant. Do they seem bonded or disconnected? Note the infant's coloring for worrisome signs of cyanosis and check for any signs of distress. These easily observable signs would necessitate immediate attention and management by the healthcare professional.

Skin

Inspect for dermatologic conditions. Note any rashes or lesions, whether new or preexisting. Rashes are very common in infancy and usually benign, but it is important to recognize when abnormal skin findings indicate a more serious condition.

Seborrheic dermatitis is the most common rash seen in the first two months of life; it begins at 2 to 4 weeks of age and subsides after 3 to 4 months of age. An initial manifestation is often a crusting of the scalp known as *cradle cap,* as shown in Fig. 24.19. The greasy, yellow or salmon-colored, nonpruritic, sharply delimited oval scales involve the scalp and face, especially the forehead, eyebrows, nasolabial folds, and retroauricular folds. When more widespread on the trunk, lesions may appear as erythematous macules, papules, and plaques. Fig. 24.20 shows seborrheic dermatitis in another patient. Notice the greasy papular eruption on the face of this 3-week-old infant. Seborrheic dermatitis may be differentiated from atopic dermatitis by its early onset, lack of pruritus, and scalp and diaper area involvement.

Atopic dermatitis, also known as *infantile eczema,* is very common in infants and begins at approximately 6 to 8 weeks of age. It is characterized by dryness of the skin, pruritus (though hard to tell in young infants), erythematous papules and vesicles, and, if infected, serous discharge, and crusting. The usual site in children 6 months of age is the face (Fig. 24.21), with the nose commonly spared (the *headlight sign*). The extensor surfaces of the arms and legs are the most common sites in 8- to 10-month-old infants, as seen in Fig. 24.22. Notice the exudative lesions on the lower extremity.

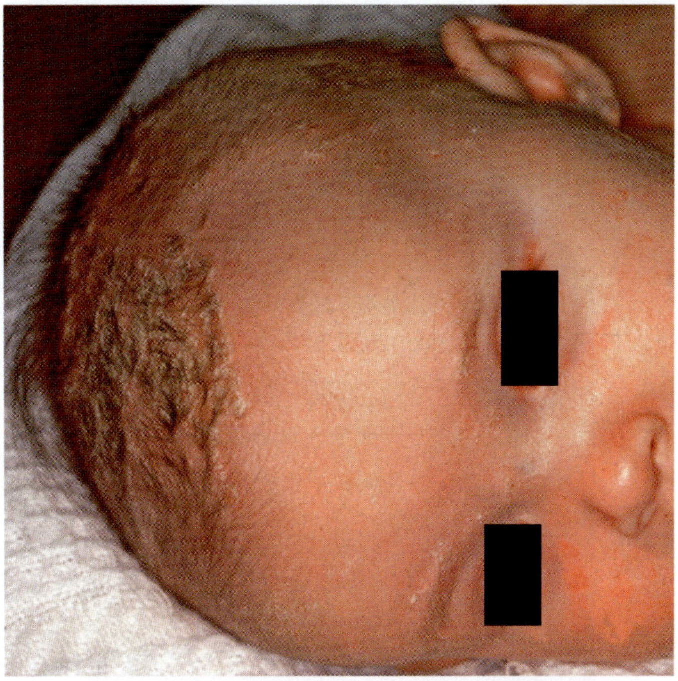

Fig. 24.19 Seborrheic Dermatitis of the Scalp, or Cradle Cap. (From Ferri FF: *Ferri's fast facts in dermatology*, 2019, Elsevier [chapter 3].)

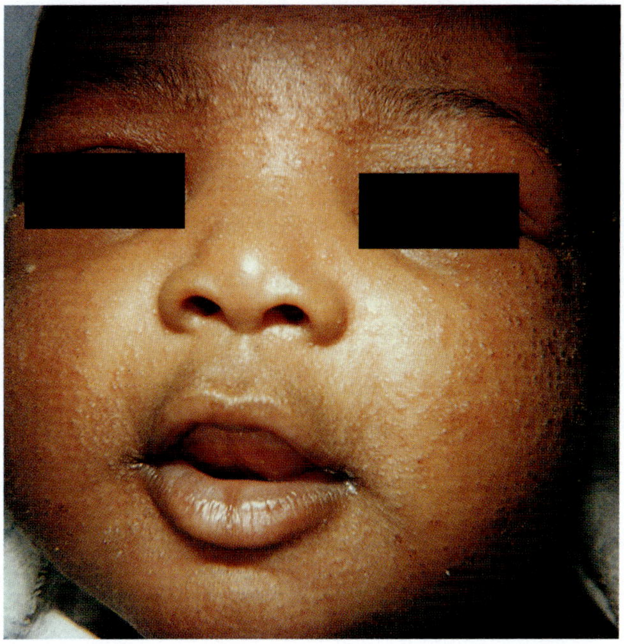

Fig. 24.20 Seborrheic Dermatitis on the Face of an Infant. (From Cohen BA: *Atlas of pediatric dermatology*, London, 1993, Wolfe Publishing.)

Palpate the skin and assess *skin elasticity*. Pull up 2.5 to 5 cm of skin over the abdomen and release it. It should quickly return to its former position. A decreased response is termed *tenting* and is suggestive of dehydration or malnutrition. Skin that seems excessively stretchy may be an indication of *Ehlers-Danlos syndrome,* a disorder of type I collagen that is a combination of hyperelasticity of skin with joint laxity and easy dislocation, with easy bruisability.

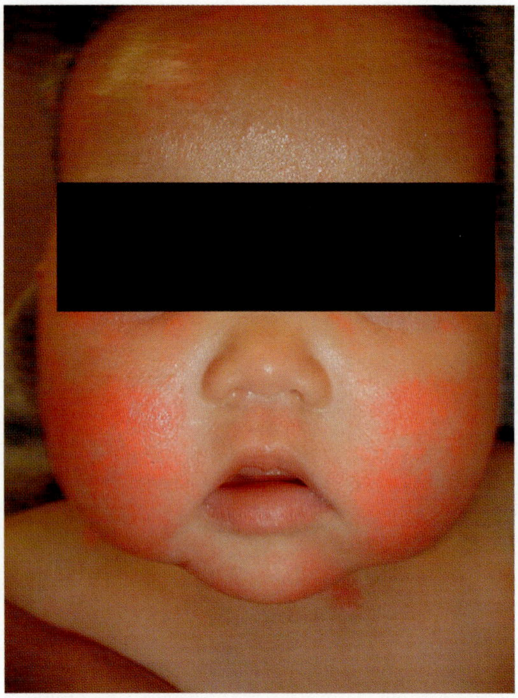

Fig. 24.21 Infantile Atopic Dermatitis on the Face. (From Kalavala M, Alfaham M, Shekariah T: *Paediatrics and child health*, vol. 21, 2010, Elsevier, pp. 112–118.)

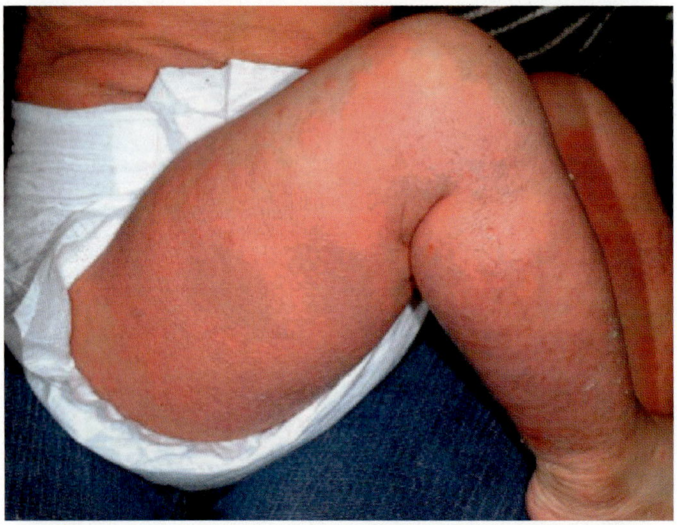

Fig. 24.22 Severe Infantile Atopic Dermatitis on the Extensor Surface of the Leg. (From Warner JO, Boner AL: *Allergy*, 2012, Elsevier, pp. 347–360 [chapter 18].)

Head

As previously described, plot the infant's head circumference on the standard growth charts. A head that is growing too rapidly should be evaluated for *hydrocephaly. Microcephaly* is a condition in which the head size is three standard deviations below the mean and is usually related to a defect in brain growth.

Observe the fontanelles. Are they still patent? As noted previously, the age at which closure of the fontanelles occurs is variable, with the posterior fontanelle closing earlier in life than the anterior. Premature closure of the anterior fontanelle, especially in a child with microcephaly, is another sign that brain growth might be impaired.

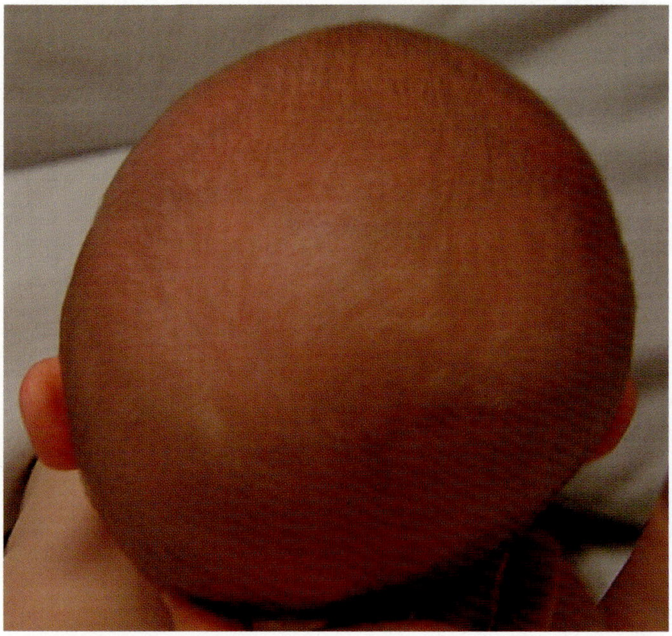

Fig. 24.23 Positional Plagiocephaly, Right Occiput. (From Lessard S, Gagnon I, Trottier N: Complementary therapies in clinical practice, 17(4):193–198, 2011. © 2011.)

Check for asymmetry. An unusual head shape may be due to *craniosynostosis,* premature closure of the sutures of the skull. As mentioned earlier in this chapter, craniosynostosis is a malformation caused by sutural closure at an unusually early age. Closure of the coronal sutures leads to *brachycephaly,* in which the head is short in the anteroposterior diameter and wider laterally. This is the opposite of the head shape that results from premature closure of the sagittal suture, a head that is long in the anteroposterior diameter and narrow laterally (a skull shape known as *dolichocephalic* or *scaphocephalic*). Premature closure of one lambdoid suture leads to posterior plagiocephaly that does not resolve on its own.

Another cause for asymmetry is a condition called *positional plagiocephaly,* which represents a deformational process caused by forces acting on the otherwise normal skull. It may become worse during the first few months of life because the infant will prefer to rest their head on one side as shown in Fig. 24.23. This position of comfort dictates which side of the occiput is more prominent. Since infants are put to sleep on their backs, positional plagiocephaly, with flattening of the occiput and friction alopecia in the area, has become more common. After 6 months, when the infant is able to turn over and sit unassisted, positional plagiocephaly gradually resolves.

Is the *face* symmetric? An easy way to detect facial paralysis is to observe the child when they cry. The weakened or paralyzed side appears expressionless in comparison with the normal side.

Eyes

In an infant older than 3 weeks of age, check the *pupillary responses.* Pupils should be equal, round, and equally reactive to light. A sluggishly reacting pupil is suggestive of congenital glaucoma.

The production of tears during crying begins at approximately 2 to 3 months of age, but the nasolacrimal duct is not fully patent until 5 to 7 months of age. If chronic tearing is present, the nasolacrimal duct may not be patent. In this case, massaging over the nasolacrimal sac may yield a purulent or mucoid discharge, which is suggestive of nasolacrimal duct obstruction.

Visual acuity is assessed by qualitative observations. By 4 weeks of age, the infant's eyes should be able to fixate on and follow a target through a brief arc. By 8 weeks of age, the child should be able to visually follow an object past the midline, coordinating eye movements with head turning. At 4 months of age, the normal infant can visually follow an object in all directions. Convergence is also present at this time. The presence of *optokinetic nystagmus* indicates a complete pathway from the retina to the occipital visual cortex. This response can best be elicited in children 3 months of age and older by using a long, striped cloth and passing it rapidly from one side to the other in the child's view. The development of nystagmus as the child attempts to maintain fixation on a stripe is the normal response, indicating normal visual pathways. At 5 to 6 months of age, the child should be able to focus on objects but is farsighted. The child should be able to reach out for an object and grasp it. Recognition of objects and faces by 4 to 6 months of age is suggestive of normal visual acuity.

Observe *ocular motility* in a child 3 months of age or older. Have the child visually follow an object into the various positions of gaze. Alignment of the eyes is best determined by the symmetry of the *corneal light reflex* and the *alternate cover test,* which are described below. The child is most susceptible to *amblyopia* within the first 2 years of life, although the risk is present until 6 to 7 years of age.

Strabismus is a condition where the eyes are misaligned where one or both eyes may turn inward, outward, up, or down, which are called eso-, exo-, hyper-, or hypotropia, respectively. Since extraocular muscles are still weak in newborns, misalignment of the eyes is common. By 4 months of age, they should have conjugate gaze and strabismus testing should start. It is crucial to detect strabismus early as if it goes undetected can lead to amblyopia, or vision loss, due to lack of visual input in the affected eye. This can first be determined by the corneal light reflex performed by shining a light on the infant's eyes and looking for a reflection from the cornea that is symmetrical in both eyes. If the light reflection is off center this can indicate the eye is deviated in the other direction as shown in Fig. 24.24. In addition, the cover test can be used to identify strabismus once the infant can fixate on an object. Have the infant fixate on an interesting object, such as a toy, and then alternately cover each eye. If the uncovered eye shifts as it fixates on the object, that is suggestive of possible strabismus. This is in contrast to *pseudostrabismus,* where the eyes appear to be crossed due to prominent epicanthal skin folds medially covering a part of the sclera. However, when the cover test is performed, there is no shift seen. An example of a cover test in a patient with true esotropia is found in Fig. 24.25.

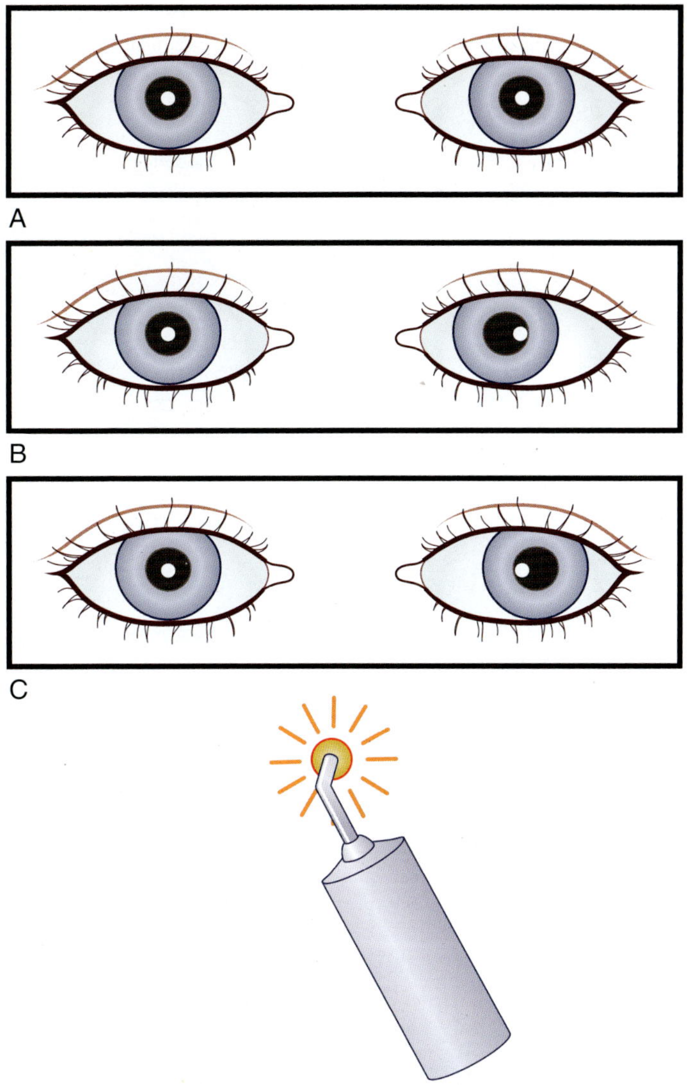

Fig. 24.24 The Corneal Light Reflex Demonstrating. (A) No deviation. (B) Left esotropia. (C) Left exotropia. (From Lavin PJM: *Bradley's neurology in clinical practice,* Published January 1, 2016, pp. 528–572.e2. © 2016.)

Another test to assess for strabismus is the *Bruckner test,* checking for red reflexes simultaneously in both eyes. The technique is the same as described in the newborn eye exam section to assess red reflex. In strabismus, the red reflex is asymmetrical and is brighter in the deviated eye.

It is critical to continue to assess the red reflex to screen for cataracts, glaucoma, and retinoblastoma even beyond infancy.

During the first 6 months, the connective tissue of the sclera becomes thicker, leading to the normal white color expected in an adult. Persistence of blue color of the sclera after 6 months of age is suggestive of the presence of a connective tissue disorder, such as *osteogenesis imperfecta* or *Ehlers-Danlos syndrome* (see Fig. 10.52).

Fundoscopy is not useful for detecting papilledema in an infant with an open fontanelle because an increase in intracranial pressure produces a bulging of the fontanelle, and even separation of the cranial sutures, *before* papilledema.

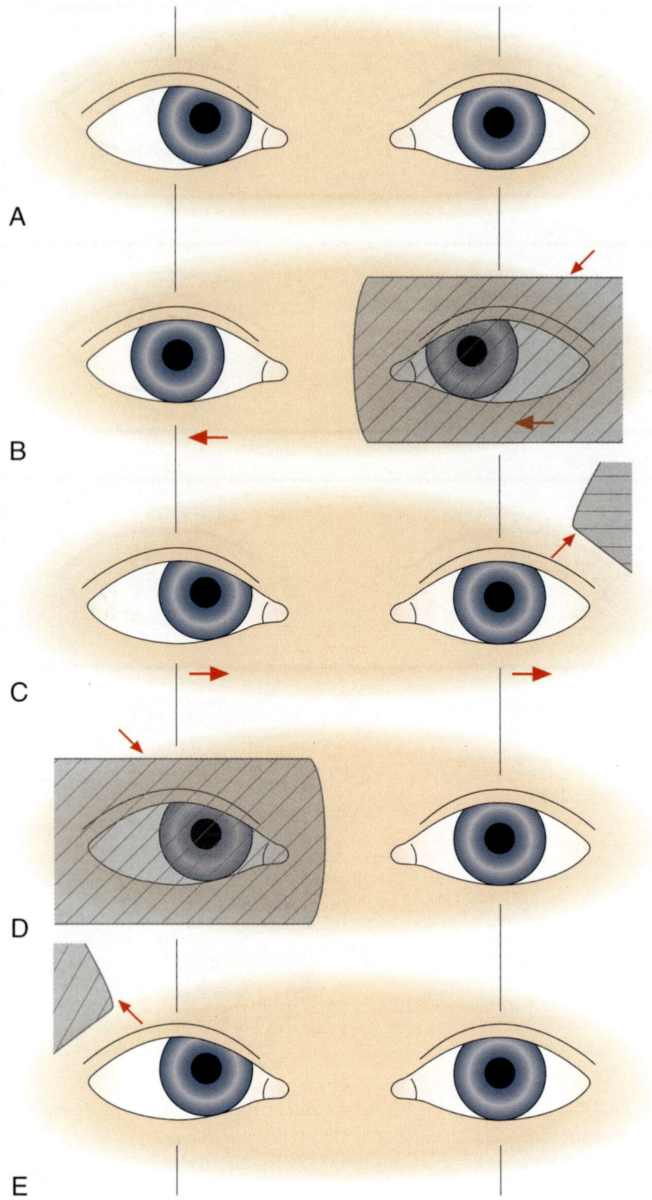

Fig. 24.25 **The Cover Test in a Patient With Right Esotropia.** (A) The right eye deviates inward slightly, but this may not be obvious. (B) As the left eye is covered, the right eye is seen to move out to take up fixation. Behind the cover, the left eye moves to the right. (C) As the left eye is uncovered, it moves out to take up fixation as it is the non-strabismic eye. (D) When the right eye is covered, the left eye does not move. (E) When the right eye is uncovered, neither eye moves. (From Barrett BT: *Clinical procedures in primary eye care*, Published January 1, 2014, pp. 147–208. © 2014.)

Nose

Elevate the tip of the nose to view the nasal septum, floor of the nose, and turbinates. Are any masses or *foreign bodies* present? A foreign body should be suspected in any child with a chronic unilateral nasal discharge, especially if it is foul-smelling.

Neck

Palpate for lymphadenopathy in the same areas as in the adult. It is common to feel small (<1 cm), firm, mobile lymph nodes in the anterior and posterior cervical chains in infants and young children due to frequent upper respiratory infections with reactive nodes. These types of nodes are commonly called "shotty" lymph nodes due to their features similar to buckshots.

Chest

The examination of the chest is best performed while the infant is either sleeping or being held by a caregiver.

Often the tracheal breath sounds, or even nasal and pharyngeal sounds, are transmitted down to the chest. This is confirmed by placing the stethoscope in front of the nose and hearing the same sounds. Do not misinterpret these sounds as crackles, and do not interpret the accompanying tactile sensation of "rattling" as abnormal fremitus.

Is the child in *respiratory distress*? The most important signs of distress are tachypnea, the use of accessory muscles, head bobbing, and flaring of the nasal alae. Intercostal retractions are also commonly present. Tachypnea may be a sign of congestive heart failure caused by an underlying congenital heart defect. Typically, the most common of these, a ventricular septal defect, may not cause any manifestations until the child is 6 weeks old or older (see the next section on the Heart).

Does the child have *stridor*, a high-pitched noise on inspiration? Stridor is indicative of tracheal narrowing, as in *croup*. See also Chapter 13, The Chest. Auscultate the lung fields. Is the child wheezing, which occurs on expiration? In children of this age, wheezing is often indicative of bronchiolitis, usually caused by a viral infection.

Heart

Inspect for *cyanosis*. If cyanosis develops within the first few days to weeks of life, there is probably a serious anatomic anomaly such as tetralogy of Fallot.

Inspect for evidence of *congestive heart failure*. The most important signs are persistent tachycardia, tachypnea, and an enlarged liver. A persistent tachycardia of more than 200 beats/min in newborns or more than 150 beats/min in children up to 1 year of age should alert the examiner. Feeding problems are often the first sign that an infant has heart failure. Such infants take a long time to feed, often more than an hour to take 2 or 3 ounces. The caregiver describes the child becoming "tired" or "out of breath" during feeding and having to stop to catch their breath after every two or three sucks. Persistent diaphoresis and failure to thrive are also important signs associated with congestive heart failure. Observing a feeding may be extremely useful if heart failure is suspected. If heart failure develops, a structural defect such as a ventricular septal defect, patent ductus arteriosus, or coarctation of the aorta should be suspected. A truncus arteriosus also produces heart failure during this period, often with minimal cyanosis.

Palpate for the point of maximum impulse.

Auscultate as in newborns. S_3 and S_4 may be normal in this age group. As previously noted, the clinical significance of a murmur, especially in the first few weeks of life, must be carefully assessed. See Tables 24.10 and 24.11 at the end of this chapter for a summary of innocent and pathologic murmurs heard in the pediatric age group.

Palpate for the femoral pulses as discussed previously.

Abdomen

Inspect, auscultate, percuss, and palpate the abdomen, using light and deep palpation, checking for any masses. In infants with idiopathic hypertrophic *pyloric stenosis,* infants present with projectile, nonbilious vomiting. Assess for large peristaltic waves moving from the left to the right in the upper abdomen. These are easier to note during or after a feeding. A mass, which consists of the enlarged pylorus, referred to as the "olive," is also sometimes observed or palpated. This may be easier to palpate with the infant suspended in the examiner's hands in the prone position.

Palpate for the *liver, spleen,* and *kidneys.* The estimated liver span of a 6-month-old infant varies from 7.1 to 7.5 cm, and the edge may be palpable up to 2 cm below the costal margin. At 1 year of age, the span is approximately 8 cm. It may be difficult to assess tenderness in this age group as palpation alone may elicit discomfort or crying.

Genitalia

Inspect the external genitalia as previously described in the newborn genitalia examination sections. Is diaper rash present? *Diaper dermatitis* is the most common rash in infants and typically results from irritation of the skin that is in direct contact with the urine and stool in the diaper. These areas include the buttocks, genitalia, lower abdomen, and upper thighs whereas the skin folds are unaffected. The skin findings can range from mild erythema of the skin or erythematous papules to painful erosions and nodules. Fig. 24.26 shows a child with irritant diaper dermatitis. With basic skin care and barrier creams, diaper dermatitis generally lasts for a few days.

However, if it persists longer than that, there may be secondary infection with *Candida albicans. Candidal diaper infections* cause bright or deep erythematous plaques in the diaper area along with satellite papular lesions and pustules along the periphery as shown in Fig. 24.27. In addition, candidal infections do not spare the skin folds. They require treatment with topical antifungal creams.

In male infants, the foreskin is not fully retractable until 3 years of age or later. Do not forcefully retract the foreskin. If you do manage to retract it, be sure you return it to its original location; otherwise, you may cause *paraphimosis,* a situation in which the retracted foreskin impedes venous drainage of the glans and results in progressive edema and pain. Diaper rash can cause *balanitis,* which is an acute inflammation of the glans penis. In boys who are uncircumcised, *phimosis,* the pathologic inability to retract the foreskin, may develop after balanitis.

Musculoskeletal Examination

Palpate the *clavicle.* At 1 month of age, the presence of a callus formation is suggestive of a healing clavicular fracture.

The *hips* must be reexamined for dislocation at every routine visit for the first year of life to look for DDH. The Ortolani and Barlow techniques have been described in the neonatal section. After 4 months of age, a dislocated hip can no longer move in and out of the socket, and so these tests are not useful. Instead, the examiner should try to fully abduct both hips. If DDH is present the hip does not fully abduct. Additionally, when there is unilateral DDH, there will be thigh-length discrepancy, making Galeazzi, described previously, and Klisic tests useful maneuvers to suggest DDH. To perform the *Klisic test,* the examiner places the finger on the anterior superior iliac spine and the middle finger on the greater trochanter and draws an imaginary line between these two points. If this line points toward or above the umbilicus, then the Klisic test is negative, and the infant does not have DDH. However, if the imaginary line goes below the umbilicus, that indicates that the hip is dislocated.

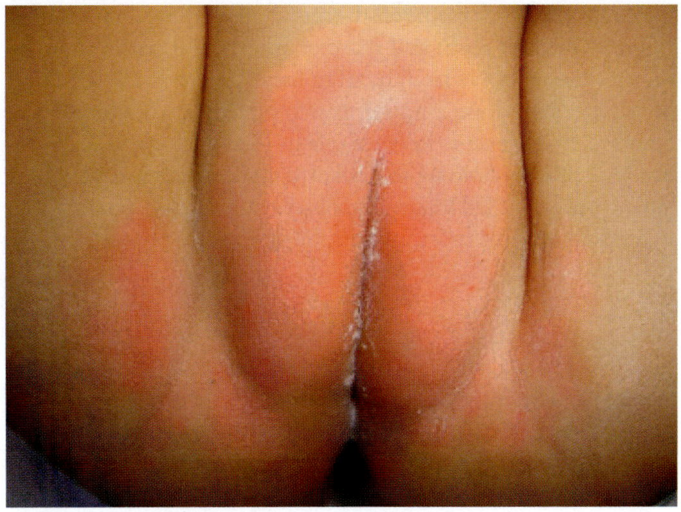

Fig. 24.26 Irritant Diaper Dermatitis. (From Matiz C, Eichenfield LF: *Treatment of skin disease: comprehensive therapeutic strategies*, Published January 1, 2018, pp. 203–205. © 2018.)

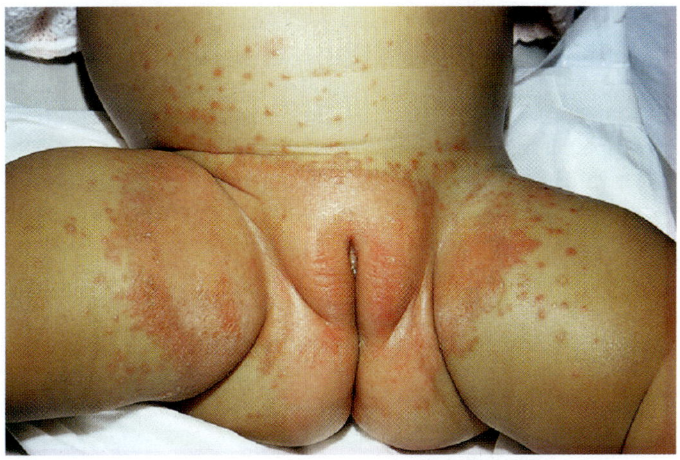

Fig. 24.27 Candidal Diaper Dermatitis. *(Reused with permission from Shah BR, Laude TA: Atlas of pediatric clinical diagnosis, 2000, Elsevier, Saunders.)*

Neurologic Examination

By the fourth month, when the supine infant is pulled into a sitting position, no head lag should be present. Many other infantile reflexes have disappeared by 4 months, most notably the Moro reflex. See prior discussion of infantile reflexes, including typical times they extinguish, in the newborn neurologic examination section. By the eighth month, the infant should be able to sit without support.

Coordination of the hands begins at approximately 5 months, when infants can reach and grasp objects. By 7 months, they can transfer these objects from hand to hand. At 8 to 9 months, they should be able to use a pincer grip to pick up small objects. The *parachute reflex* occurs in older infants (8 to 12 months). This reflex is elicited by holding the infant upright and then, simulating having the infant fall forward to observe the arms extending as if to break a fall. This reflex appears before the onset of walking.

Ears

Otoscopy is one of the most difficult skills to learn in infants and toddlers, and it is also one of the most important because these are the ages when otitis media is most prevalent. Many children do not like their ears to be examined, and this part of the exam often provokes resistance and crying. Therefore, it is best to save this part of the exam for the end so that other parts of the examination can be evaluated without the patient being upset.

The child can either be placed prone on the examination table or held by a caregiver. Fig. 24.28 demonstrates how to position the child in the caregiver's lap. To examine the ear, gently pull the pinna backward to move the acoustic meatus in line with the auditory canal. The pinna is pulled down until a child is approximately 4 to 6 months of age; afterward, pulling up, as in adults, usually provides the best visualization. Hold the otoscope near the eyepiece rather than the end and use the little finger to rest on the patient's cheek to prevent injury if the patient turns the head. While looking into the otoscope, carefully insert the otoscope with the correct sized ear speculum into the ear canal, angling it slightly toward the patient's nose to follow the canal. Carefully move the otoscope to different angles to view the canal walls and tympanic membrane. Pneumatic otoscopy (see Chapter 11, The Ear and Nose) is an important skill for detecting mobility of the ear drum. To check for mobility of the tympanic membrane, create an airtight seal with the speculum and squeeze the bulb of an insufflator to apply positive and negative pressures. Fig. 24.29 demonstrates the positioning of the examiner's hands. Notice how the hands are braced against the child's head, as well as the correct position for holding the pneumatic bulb. The *tympanic membrane* should be easily visualized unless cerumen is present. Any cerumen should be removed by someone experienced in doing so.

Upon examination of the ear, the examiner should look for landmarks like the manubrium and short process of the malleus, light reflex (cone of light), pars tensa, and pars flaccida. Note the tympanic membrane's contour (normal, retracted, full, or bulging), color (gray, yellow, pink, amber, white, or red), translucency, and mobility. A normal tympanic membrane is pink/gray in color, translucent, in a neutral position, and mobile with air inflation as illustrated in Fig. 24.30.

Evidence of a middle ear effusion (fluid in the middle ear) on examination include air-fluid levels, an opaque tympanic membrane, a full or bulging position, or decreased or absent mobility on pneumatic otoscopy. To diagnose an *acute otitis media (AOM)*, there should be a middle ear effusion and evidence of acute inflammation such as moderate to severe bulging of the tympanic membrane as seen in Fig. 24.31 or new onset of otorrhea not due to acute otitis externa. Another way to diagnose AOM is if there's mild bulging of the tympanic membrane AND recent (<48 hours) onset of ear pain (holding, tugging, rubbing of the ear in a nonverbal child) or intense erythema of the tympanic membrane. In many young children, the eardrum may be red from crying or fever without middle ear infection. Therefore,

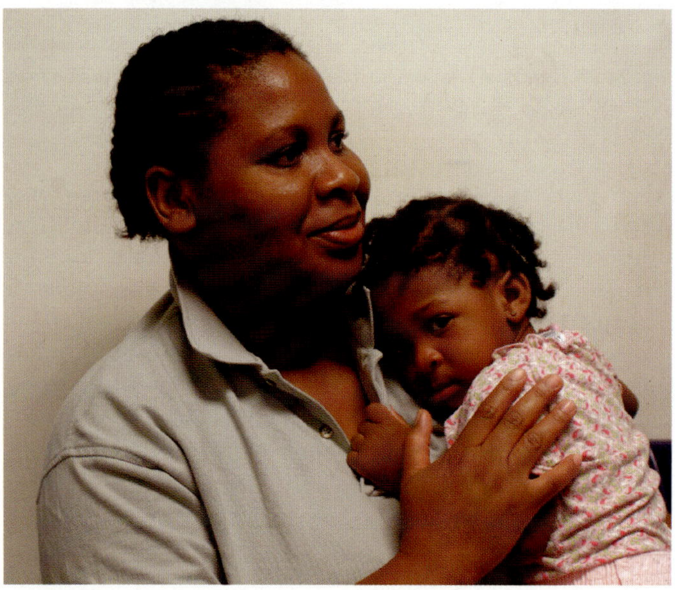

Fig. 24.28 Positioning of the Child for Otoscopic Examination. There are many ways to position the child in the caregiver's lap, which provides the child with some security. The child should be upright so that the examiner can brace the child's head against the caregiver's chest. The caregiver needs to hold the child's hands so that they do not grab the otoscope. If necessary, the child's legs can be scissored between the caregiver's legs.

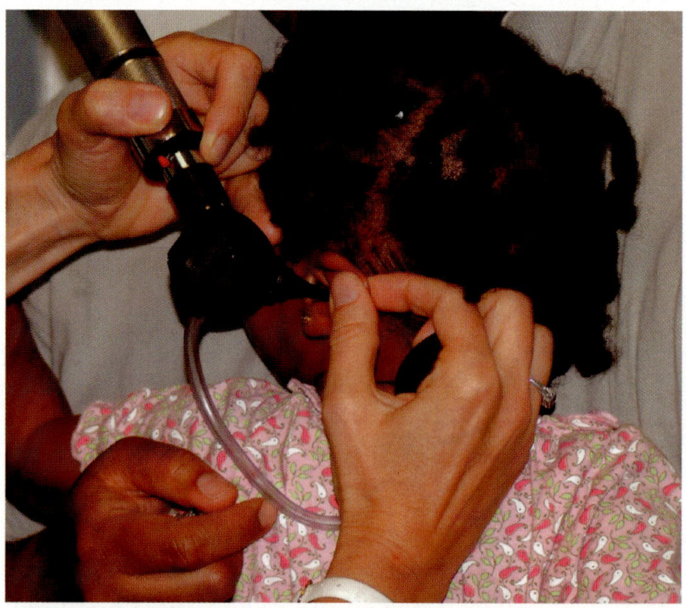

Fig. 24.29 Positioning of the Examiner's Hands for Otoscopic Examination. Note that the little finger of the hand holding the otoscope is braced against the child's head. (The examiner is left-handed.) The first two fingers of the other hand retract the pinna, while the remaining fingers are wrapped around the bulb of the insufflator, prepared to squeeze the bulb if the examination warrants.

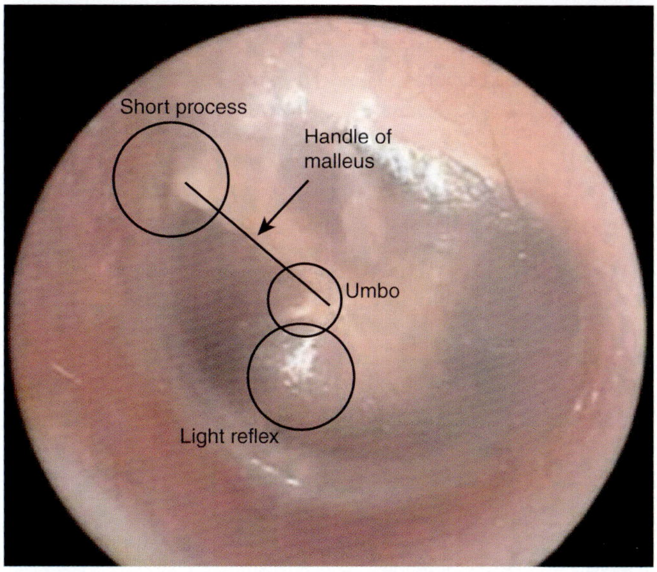

Fig. 24.30 Normal Tympanic Membrane With Labeled Landmarks. (From Casey JR, Bluestone CD: *Feigin and Cherry's textbook of pediatric infectious diseases*, 2018.])

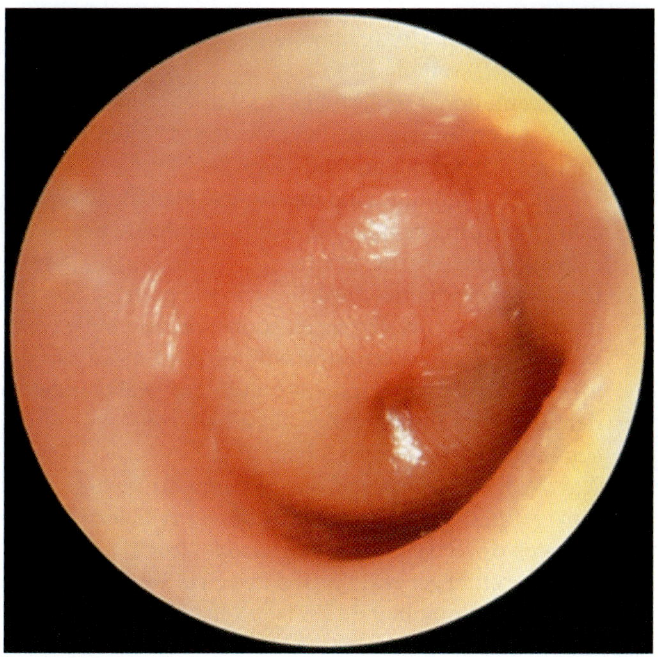

Fig. 24.31 Acute Otitis Media With Bulging, Opaque Tympanic Membrane.

healthcare professionals should *not* diagnose AOM in children who do not have a middle ear effusion based on exam, pneumatic otoscopy, and/or tympanometry. Otitis media with effusion (OME) is a condition where there is fluid in the middle ear without evidence of acute inflammation, as shown in Fig. 24.32.

Oropharynx

The examination of the mouth and pharynx is the last part of the examination in this age group. If the patient is crying from the ear examination, it will be possible to get a good look into the mouth and pharynx.

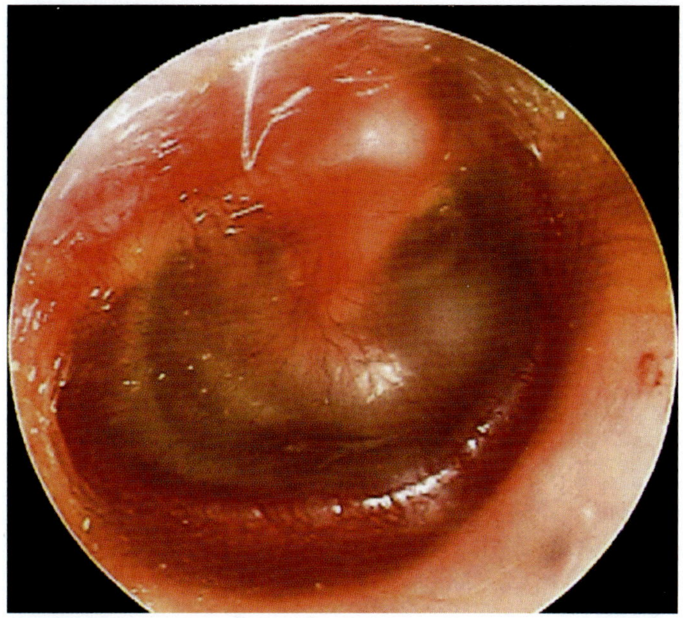

Fig. 24.32 Otitis Media With Effusion, Semiopaque Tympanic Membrane but Not Bulging. (From Kerschner J, Preciado D: *Otitis media.* In Kliegman R, editor: *Nelson textbook of pediatrics*, ed 20, Philadelphia, 2016, Elsevier, p. 3090.)

The child should be seated on the caregiver's lap, with the caregiver holding the child's head. It is usually possible to examine a crying infant without using the tongue depressor. A frightened child who is holding their mouth firmly closed can be examined if someone occludes the nares; this will make the child open the mouth. Enlist the caregiver as the nose-holder if this technique must be used. The tongue depressor can then be slipped into the side of the mouth and then rotated over the tongue.

Are any *teeth* present? The first teeth to erupt are the lower central incisors, at about 6 to 10 months. Fig. 24.33 illustrates the chronology of primary teeth eruption. Salivation is temporarily increased with the eruption of new teeth. Sometimes bruising of the gum is visible when a tooth is erupting.

EARLY CHILDHOOD: 1 YEAR TO 4 YEARS

Early Childhood History

In this next period, attention is placed on language development, social skills, and early school experience. The expected explosion of language in years 2 and 3 of life requires caregiver input and close monitoring. In infancy, children use sounds to mimic words, as well as using gestures to communicate, and by approximately 12 months of age, children usually speak their first word, usually "dada" or "mama." By 15 months of age, children are expected to say between 3 and 10 words, and by 2 years of age, their vocabulary may contain more than 200 words; it is at this age that we expect children to be able to put two or more words together in a phrase, such as "mama go" or "Up me!" By 3 years of age, children are able to put together sentences of five or six words from a 1500-word vocabulary and should be 75% intelligible to an adult who does not know the child; by 4 years, they should be fully intelligible.

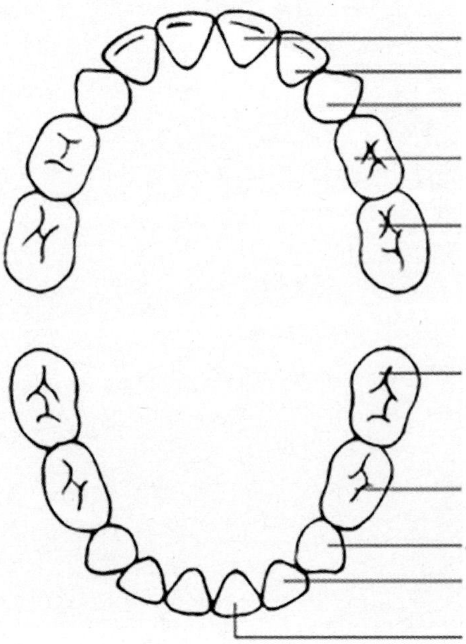

Upper Teeth	Erupt	Shed
Central incisor	8–12 months	6–7 years
Lateral incisor	9–13 months	7–8 years
Canine (cuspid)	16–22 months	10–12 years
First molar	13–19 months	9–11 years
Second molar	25–33 months	10–12 years

Lower Teeth	Erupt	Shed
Second molar	23–31 months	10–12 years
First molar	14–18 months	9–11 years
Canine (cuspid)	17–23 months	9–12 years
Lateral incisor	10–16 months	7–8 years
Central incisor	6–10 months	6–7 years

Fig. 24.33 Chronology of Primary Teeth Eruption. (From https://www.mouthhealthy.org/en/az-topics/e/eruption-charts. © 2023 American Dental Association. All rights reserved. Reprinted with permission.)

During this period of early childhood, isolated language delays as well as more global social concerns may become apparent. With the current prevalence of autism spectrum disorder (ASD) in the United States at 1 in 36 children, according to the CDC,[14] it is essential to act on concerning behaviors that have been reported or observed. These behaviors include, but are not limited to, a toddler not pointing to indicate wants; not turning to name being called; not making eye contact; not having joint attention (shared attention between two people and an object such as a child, parent, and book); and having a speech delay. A formal screening for ASD is recommended at 18 months, for example, with the use of the M-CHAT questionnaire.[15] Early identification of ASD or any developmental delays is essential as early intervention with multiple therapies can significantly improve the outcome of these children.

Finally, this is a period to also concentrate on healthy eating, encouraging physical activity and keeping the child safe as they explore their environment. As the toddler exerts their independence, using proper and productive discipline techniques must be stressed.

- Diet
  - What are the child's eating habits like?
  - Is the child drinking water (encourage) or juice (discourage)?
  - Is the child eating foods from all four food groups or have they gotten pickier?
  - Does the family eat meals together?
- Elimination
  - Any concerns about stool consistency or frequency?
  - Is the child toilet training or toilet trained?
- Sleep
  - Where does the child sleep? (e.g., crib, toddler bed, regular bed, co-sleeping?)
  - Is the child still napping?
- Development/behavior (examples with progression over this time period) (see Table 24.1)
  - Social/emotional milestones (points to show interest, notes when others are hurt or upset, follows simple routines when told, pretend play)
  - Language/communication milestones (Mama/dada specifically, increasing number of words, combines two words, asks questions, says sentences)
  - Cognitive milestones (Imitates chores, pretend play, follows one then two step instructions, copies circle, names some colors, draws a person with three or more parts
  - Motor/physical development milestones (walks independently, drinks from a cup, kicks a ball, runs, jumps, uses spoon then fork, catches a ball)
  - Any temper tantrums? (This is common in toddlers as they exert their independence but can't always express themselves verbally yet—"*the terrible twos*"!)
  - Does the child get any physical exercise? Watch screens or use phones/computers?
  - Is the child getting ready for school?
- Social
  - What are the childcare arrangements?
  - Are social support services needed?
  - Any changes in the living situation?
  - Are there any high-risk conditions in the home? (i.e., domestic violence, food insecurity, home dangers)
- Screenings: Development, autism, lead, anemia, tuberculosis, vision (starting at age 3), hearing (starting at age 4), oral health
- Anticipatory guidance (here are some examples)
  - Use appropriate-size rear-facing car seat until age 2 years and then forward-facing, in back seat
  - Avoid screens and other digital media; encourage physical activity, unstructured play time, human interactions;

after 2 years of age limit to 1 hour high-quality, shared media use

- Read nightly, stimulate language by talking to child throughout the day
- Put small objects, medications, cleaning fluids out of reach or locked up, know poison control number
- Remove firearms from home; if necessary, store unloaded and locked
- Provide a smoke-free environment
- Use gates to block stairs or rooms with danger
- Once teeth erupt, brush twice a day and find a dental home
- Use timeouts, not physical means, to discourage undesired behaviors
- Praise positive behaviors for reinforcement

Review of Systems

A child 1 to 4 years of age is becoming verbal and can contribute to the ROSs. They may start to report sore throat, ear pain, chest pain, leg pain, or headache. The Wong-Baker FACES Pain Rating Scale[n] is one of several tools to help the examiner rate pain in a young child as young as 3 years old who might not be able to articulate the severity of the pain. Other questions to add to the child's ROSs include questions about snoring and loss of bowel or bladder control in a child who has been toilet trained. Most children have achieved daytime control by 4 years of age, although only approximately half of children are dry at night by then. Restless sleep, including nightmares, night terrors, and sleepwalking are not uncommon at this age.

Early Childhood Physical Exam

See Video 24.2.

It is useful to spend time observing the child at play while interviewing a caregiver. It is also rewarding to allow a toddler to play with a stethoscope, tongue blade, or penlight to "make friends" with the equipment that will be used later in the physical examination.

For an adequate examination, the child needs to be relaxed. With children in this age group, it is important to speak softly and demonstrate the parts of the examination on dolls or toy animals, or on the caregiver. Allowing the child to hold the stethoscope or penlight often distracts them enough so that other parts of the examination can be performed. The child soon learns that the light and stethoscope need not be feared. Play with the child. Show interest in their toys. Have the child "blow out" the light. Let the child use the stethoscope as a telephone. Above all, *talk* to the child. It is amazing how easily an examination can be performed while telling a young child a simple fantasy about imaginary animals. Ask the child questions about these characters. A reassuring voice goes a long way in making the child comfortable. Throughout the examination, describe to the child what is being done, such as, "Now I'm going to listen to your heart beating." Children also seem to be reassured by conversations with their caregivers during the examination. Children younger than 3 years of age are best examined on the caregiver's lap; try to stay at the child's level.

The child should be completely undressed for the examination. If the child is modest, respect the child's privacy. Provide a gown or remove only the clothing that is necessary for each part of the examination. Recover that area before moving on. Modesty varies greatly among children in this age group. If the child is on an examination table, have the caregiver stand at the child's feet. Any child in respiratory distress is easiest to examine in the position of most comfort, usually sitting.

In a child who appears to be *apprehensive,* auscultation of the heart and lungs should be performed *first* because this requires the child's cooperation and should be performed early when the child may be more cooperative. Because the sight of medical instruments is likely to frighten a child, use them last.

General Assessment

Observe the child's behavior. This may be the most important source of information about their neurologic and musculoskeletal systems.

Skin

The examination of the skin is the same for children as for adults.

Careful descriptions of the numerous rashes seen in this age group are paramount for diagnosis. There are many exanthematous diseases of childhood. These rashes may consist of macules, papules, vesicles, pustules, or petechiae. See Table 24.9 at the end of this chapter for a summary of important viral and bacterial exanthems.

Impetigo is one of the most common skin conditions of children in this age group. It is a highly contagious, superficial skin infection caused by group A β-hemolytic streptococcus, *Staphylococcus aureus,* or both, and is more common in summer. The primary lesion is a vesicopustule; once it has ruptured, it produces a honey-colored crust surrounded by a rim of erythema. Bullous impetigo results in vesicles or larger bullae. The lesions may be seen on any part of the body, but the face is a common location. The child pictured in Fig. 24.34 has the classic weeping, encrusted lesions of impetigo.

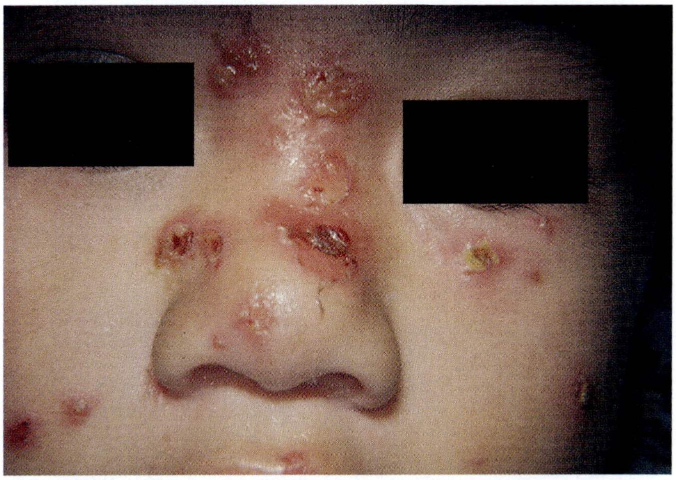

Fig. 24.34 Impetigo. (From Shah BR, Laude TA: *Atlas of pediatric clinical diagnosis*, Philadelphia, 2000, WB Saunders.)

---

[n]https://wongbakerfaces.org/

Head

Inspect the shape of the head. Look for signs of trauma.

Palpate over the *maxillary sinuses* in children older than 2 years. Tenderness may indicate sinusitis.

Inspect the area of the *parotid glands.* Localized swelling can best be detected by telling the child to look up to the ceiling while they are seated. Note any swelling below the angle of the jaw. Palpate the area. An enlarged parotid gland often pushes the lobe of the ear away from the side of the head; this can be seen when the child is observed from behind.

Neck

Inspect the size and shape of the neck. Palpate the *thyroid gland.* This is usually best done by using your thumb and index finger to feel for the gland while the child is in a supine position. Check for a *thyroglossal duct cyst.* The child in Fig. 24.35 has a midline thyroglossal duct cyst. See also Chapter 9, The Head and Neck.

Examine the *lymph nodes.* All the chains (as indicated in Chapter 9, The Head and Neck) must be examined. Small, <1 cm in diameter, movable, nontender, discrete nodes are commonly found. Warm, tender nodes are usually indicative of infection. Palpate the anterior and posterior triangles for lymphadenopathy as in adults. Anterior cervical adenopathy is associated with inflammation of the sinuses, ears, teeth, or pharynx.

Any child with an acute febrile illness with irritability should be examined for *nuchal rigidity,* resulting from meningeal irritation. The Brudzinski and Kernig tests are described in Chapter 21, The Nervous System, and become more reliable in this age group. Nuchal rigidity can sometimes be detected by encouraging the child to look at something below them; the natural tendency is to flex the neck, but such a movement is avoided with meningeal irritation.

Chest

Inspect the shape of the chest. Does the child have a *pectus excavatum* or *pectus carinatum*? The former, also known as "funnel chest," is the most common anomaly of the anterior chest wall and is caused by aberrant growth of the sternum and ribs, which leads to a sunken appearance; the latter, known as "pigeon chest," is caused by a protrusion of the sternum and ribs. Both of these conditions usually occur as an isolated defect; however, both can occur in connective tissue disorders, such as Marfan syndrome.

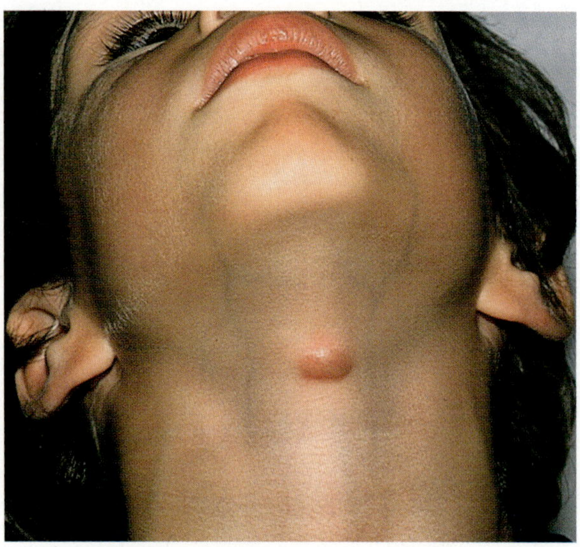

Fig. 24.35 Thyroglossal Duct Cyst.

Auscultation needs to be done systematically, but it can be difficult, and patience is required. If a child is asked to "take a deep breath," the child frequently holds the breath; instead, demonstrate taking deep breaths and tell the child to imitate. Alternatively, ask the child to "blow out the birthday candles." It may be helpful to examine the heart first before the child starts taking deep breaths as they may not understand when to stop. Are the breath sounds normal? Are there any adventitious sounds? Breath sounds in children sound louder than those in adults as a result of the chest configuration.

If indicated, percuss the chest, using the same technique as in adults. Because the chest wall is thinner in children than in adults, the percussion notes are more resonant in children. Percuss gently because overly vigorous percussion may produce vibrations over a large area and obscure an area of dullness.

Heart

In the cardiac examination of a young child, follow these procedures:

1. Inspect the precordium.
2. Palpate for any lifts, heaves, or thrills.
3. Auscultate in the same areas described in Chapter 14, The Heart. Describe any murmurs or abnormal sounds.
4. Palpate the femoral pulses.

Abdomen

The examination of the abdomen is often one of the earlier parts of the examination of a young child because this requires no instruments other than the stethoscope and is usually painless. An anxious child 2 or 3 years of age can be examined in the caregiver's lap: By leaning back in the chair, the caregiver acts as the examining table, with the supine child semi-reclined against the caregiver's chest and abdomen. An adequate abdominal examination on a child may require repeated "visits" to that part of the examination, until the child is relaxed with the process.

Inspect the abdomen. As children grow older, the protuberant abdomen becomes more scaphoid, except in children who are obese. Tell the child to cough. Are there any bulging masses at the umbilicus?

Auscultate for peristaltic sounds. Are any *bruits* present? The presence of an abdominal bruit may be suggestive of coarctation, especially in the presence of upper extremity hypertension and reduced or delayed femoral pulses. Use the stethoscope to listen over the kidneys posteriorly. The presence of a bruit in this location is suggestive of renal artery stenosis.

Percuss the abdomen for abnormal dullness.

Light palpation is performed as described in the adult examination. Is tenderness noted? Observe the patient's face while palpating. Facial expressions are more useful than asking the child, "Does this hurt?" Children are often very ticklish; if you sandwich the child's hand between your two hands as you examine, the child's tendency to giggle diminishes. Alternatively, light palpation can be done with the stethoscope after listening to the bowel sounds. Deep palpation is also performed as in adults.

Palpate the *liver* and *spleen* as described in Chapter 17, The Abdomen. The mean liver span of a 3- to 5-year-old is approximately 8.6 cm. Begin palpation for organomegaly well down in the lower abdomen and work your way up. Otherwise, you risk missing the edge of a markedly enlarged liver or spleen.

The *kidneys* may be palpable by ballottement in children up to 5 to 6 years of age. Place your left hand under the right costal margin at the costovertebral angle. Your right hand is placed over the midposition of the right abdomen. Tap firmly on the abdomen to try to feel the size of the kidney. The hands should be reversed to feel the left kidney.

Inspect the *anus.* Is diaper rash present in a child who is not yet toilet trained? Is there evidence of excoriations? Pinworm infestation commonly causes pruritus and excoriations.

Rectal examination is usually not part of the standard examination in this age group. Only children with abdominal pain or symptoms referable to the lower gastrointestinal tract require a rectal examination. Instruct the child to lie on their side, knees drawn up, facing the caregiver at the side of the table. Tell the child that the examination will be like "taking your temperature." You should use your fifth finger, gloved and well lubricated, for the examination. Tenderness and sphincter tone are determined, as well as the presence of a mass.

Genitalia

Inspect the external genitalia as previously described in prior genitalia examination sections.

Palpate the *testicles.* Are both present in the scrotum? In this age group, the testicles can often become retracted into the inguinal canal. Warm hands and a warm room often aid in this exam. If one or both testicles are not felt in the scrotum, try manipulating the testicle from the inguinal area into the scrotum. Having the patient stand up may facilitate the exam. If that maneuver fails, tell the child to sit on a chair with their feet on the seat. Instruct them to grab their knees. Repeat the palpation. This additional abdominal pressure may force a retracted or undescended testicle into the scrotum. Another useful maneuver to counteract an active cremasteric reflex is to have the child lie down supine and flex their leg at the knee, placing their foot on the opposite leg. This "tailor position" brings the tendon of the sartorius muscle over the inguinal canal and prevents an active reflex from retracting the testicle.

Palpation for an *inguinal hernia* can usually be performed in children 4 years of age and older. The procedure is the same as in adults and should be performed with the child standing.

If the child is female, inspect the *vaginal area.* Is a *rash* present? Rashes may be related to bubble baths. Is a *discharge* present? A discharge in girls aged 2 to 6 years may be related to a foreign body in the vagina or poor hygiene. A nasal speculum can be used by an experienced examiner to inspect the vagina for the cause of the discharge. Look for a smooth vaginal opening.

Musculoskeletal Examination

Observe the *gait* by telling the child to walk back and forth with shoes or socks on. Having the child walk on a cold floor without socks or shoes may distort the gait. "Intoeing" and "out-toeing" are common in children. Most such gaits are physiologic variants that arise from in utero positioning and resolve spontaneously during the active growing period. Intoeing in the toddler age group is most often due to *internal tibial torsion.* When observing the child's gait, the patellae will be facing forward, as the problem lies below the knee, but the toes will turn in.

Tell the child to stand in front of you and inspect the legs. Is bowing present? Commonly, a child may appear bowlegged *(genu varum)* for 1 to 2 years after starting to walk. Knock-knees *(genu valgum)* frequently follow bowing and are seen in children 2 to 4 years of age. The normal gait of a child 2 to 4 years of age is wide-based, with a prominent lumbar lordosis.

As limp is always a concerning symptom in young children, the entire lower extremity from the toes to the hip should be examined in a limping child. Look for evidence of trauma, localized bone tenderness, joint or leg swelling, or skin changes. Children with abnormalities of the hip frequently localize the area of discomfort to the knee. Any child concerned with knee pain must have their hips fully assessed. The presence of a limp and knee pain in a child 3 to 8 years of age, especially a boy, is suggestive of *Legg-Calvé-Perthes disease,* which is aseptic necrosis of the femoral head. Septic hip is another concerning cause of limp in this age group. Patients will be ill-appearing with high fever, have limited range of motion, and will keep the hip abducted and externally rotated in a position of comfort. This should be distinguished from *transient synovitis*, a benign, self-limited cause of limp in this age group. The classic presentation is milder symptoms and limited range of motion in a well appearing child with a preceding viral infection. This condition affects boys more commonly than girls.

Neurologic Examination

See Video 24.3.

The development of speech and the ability to manipulate small objects, throw a ball, feed and dress oneself, and understand simple directions are the best indicators of a normally developing nervous system. Deep tendon reflexes are usually not tested unless there is reason to suspect a developmental abnormality or an acute insult to the central nervous system (infection or trauma). If they are tested, use the same techniques as described in Chapter 21, The Nervous System.

Eyes

Visual acuity in children aged 1 to 3 years is assessed by their ability to identify brightly colored objects and to circumnavigate the exam room. Routine visual acuity testing should begin when the child is approximately 3 years of age, with an appropriate Snellen eye chart. Pediatric eye charts use pictures or the "tumbling E" as shown in Fig. 24.36. Average visual acuity for a 3-year-old child is 20/40; at age 4 to 5 years, it is 20/30. Instrument-based screening, like the photoscreener, while not testing visual acuity, can identify problems that can cause amblyopia

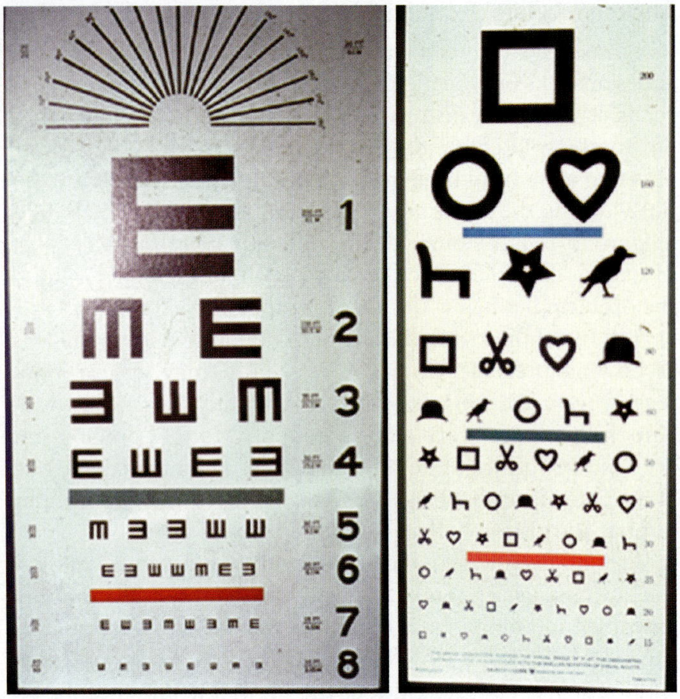

Fig. 24.36 **Pediatric Eye Charts.** (From Kaiser PK, Friedman NJ: *Massachusetts eye and ear infirmary illustrated manual of ophthalmology*, 2014, pp. 565–612.)

such as astigmatism or refractive errors in young or uncooperative children.

Darken the room and compare the red reflex in the two eyes simultaneously. Any asymmetry in the red reflex suggests a refractive error, tumor, or other "amblyogenic" problem that warrants a referral to an ophthalmologist.

Check *ocular movements.* Are the eyes straight? Be aware that a child with large epicanthal folds that partially cover the globe may be thought to have strabismus. The eyes should be parallel in all fields of gaze. Check the corneal light reflex and cover test as previously described.

Is the conjunctiva red? One of the most common eye problems in this age group is *red eye.* The causes are numerous and include conjunctivitis, obstruction of the nasolacrimal duct, chalazion, local trauma, allergy, and toxin exposure. Is there discharge from the eye?

Nose

Inspect the tip of the nose. Is there a permanent transverse crease near the lower part of the nose directing the tip upward? This is commonly seen in allergy sufferers. This unmistakable sign is caused by the *allergic salute:* using a palm or an extended forefinger to rub the nose upward and outward.

Elevate the tip of the nose and inspect the nasal mucosa. Are secretions present? Purulent secretions from above and below the middle turbinate may be suggestive of sinusitis. Watery discharge may be indicative of allergy or viral upper respiratory infection. Swollen, boggy turbinates are seen in response to seasonal or environmental allergies. Epistaxis is usually caused by local trauma and is quite common in preschool- and school-aged children. In children with head trauma, the presence of a clear discharge from the nose is suggestive of cerebrospinal fluid leakage. Check for *nasal polyps.* These may be associated with allergies or cystic fibrosis.

Ears

Is any *discharge* present? Purulent discharge may be due to a perforated tympanic membrane resulting from excess pressure buildup of fluid in AOM or exudate seen in otitis externa (or swimmer's ear). Eczema may cause flaking and cracking behind the ears. A bloody discharge may be caused by irritation, injury, a foreign body, or a basilar skull fracture.

Use the otoscope to inspect the *external canal* and *tympanic membrane.* A cooperative 2- to 3-year-old child may be either sitting or lying prone or supine on the examination table with the head turned to one side. An uncooperative child can be held upright or prone in a caregiver's arms. The otoscope should be held as indicated previously. Use the largest speculum possible.

Palpate the *mastoid process.* Is it tender? Tenderness is suggestive of mastoiditis, which may be associated with redness of the mastoid and forward displacement of the pinna, most obvious when the child is viewed from behind.

Are *posterior auricular lymph nodes* present? These nodes are classically found in children with rubella. They are also found in children with measles, roseola, chickenpox, or inflammation or infections of the scalp as in tinea capitis.

Check *hearing.* Formal, office-based hearing testing, or audiometry, begins at age 4.

Hearing is necessary for the normal development of language. If hearing loss is suspected, or the child has language delay, the child should be scheduled for full audiometric testing as soon as possible.

Oropharynx

As previously mentioned, the evaluation of the mouth and pharynx is usually the last part of the examination of the small child.

Inspect the *lips* for any lesions and color.

Tell the child, "Open your mouth. I am going to count your teeth." Inspect the *teeth* for number and caries. The first lower molars erupt at approximately 14 to 18 months of age. (See Fig. 24.33 for timing of eruption of full primary dentition.) By 3 years of age, children should have their full set of 20 primary teeth. Flattened edges are seen in children who grind their teeth.

Multiple caries, especially of the upper incisors, are often an indication of *milk caries,* also known as *nursing bottle caries.* They are caused by the child going to sleep with a bottle of milk or juice or breast in the mouth. The fermentable carbohydrates in these cariogenic fluids constantly bathe the teeth while the infant is asleep, interact with *Streptococcus mutans* and other microorganisms in the mouth, and result in acid demineralization of the susceptible tooth enamel. Untreated carious destruction progresses through the enamel, dentin, and pulp, producing *periapical abscesses.* The maxillary anterior teeth are the first to be affected. The mandibular teeth are the least affected. Fig. 24.37 shows severe milk caries that necessitated removal of all the child's primary dentition. Always look for a

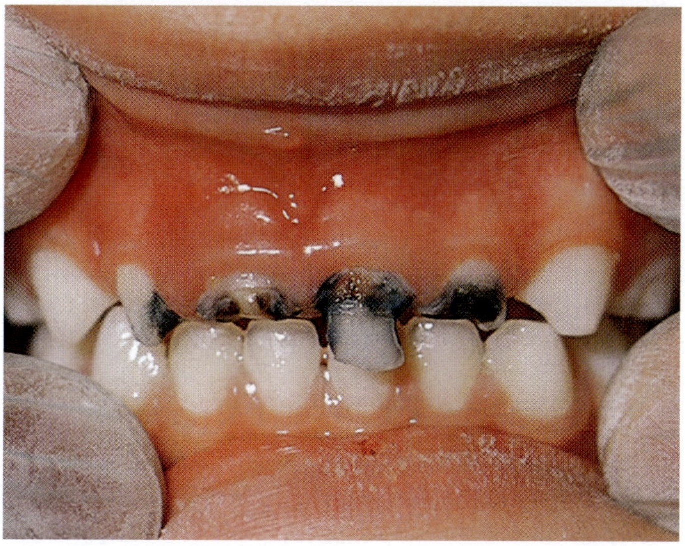

Fig. 24.37 Milk Caries. (From Eisen D, Lynch DP: *The mouth: diagnosis and treatment*, St. Louis, 1998, Mosby.)

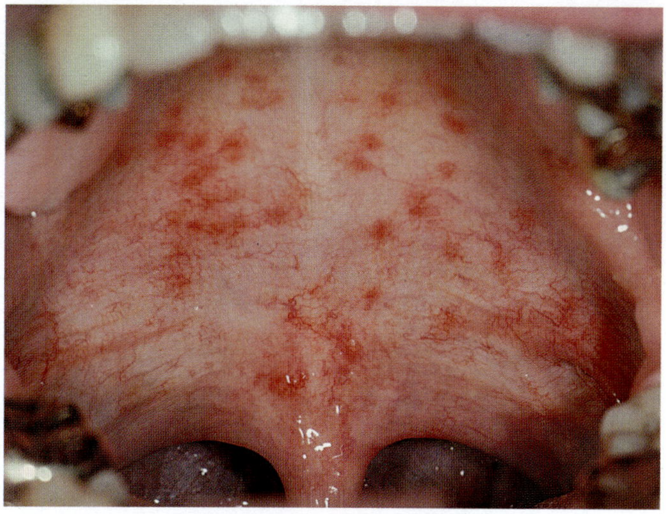

Fig. 24.38 Forchheimer Spots.

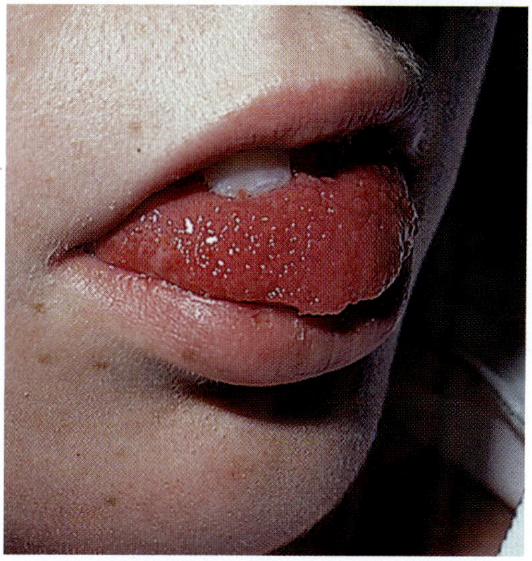

Fig. 24.39 Strawberry Tongue.

small pimple in the alveolar ridge above a damaged tooth; this is evidence of a *periapical abscess* and necessitates urgent referral for dental treatment.

Inspect the *bite*. Have the child bite down while you inspect the occlusion. Normally, the upper teeth override the lower teeth. Slight maxillary protrusion is termed *overbite* and is the normal position; mandibular protrusion is termed *underbite*. If the teeth don't meet, malocclusion is present which can result from frequent pacifier use.

Inspect the *gingivae* for any lesions. Inspect the *buccal mucosa*. In measles, on the second or third day of the disease, pinpoint white spots are often seen on the buccal mucosa opposite the lower molars. These spots are called *Koplik spots* and are pathognomonic for measles. Vesicles on an erythematous base are suggestive of *herpes simplex* infection. Similar vesicles on the soft palate and tonsillar pillars are suggestive of *herpangina* caused by coxsackievirus infections. Dusky red 1- to 3-mm spots on the buccal mucosa and palate are an early sign of rubella. These diffusely scattered oral lesions, known as *Forchheimer spots*, appear on the posterior hard and soft palates and develop at the end of the prodromal stage or at the beginning of the cutaneous eruption. Fig. 24.38 shows Forchheimer spots of rubella.

Inspect the *tongue*. *Geographic tongue*, also known as *benign migratory glossitis*, is a normal variation where the surface of the tongue has mildly depressed lesions with irregular borders (see Fig. 12.25A). Dryness is seen in dehydration and in chronic mouth breathers. Strawberry tongue, as shown in Fig. 24.39, is distinctive with increased redness of the tongue associated with prominent inflamed papillae and is indicative of several conditions such as scarlet fever and Kawasaki disease (KD).

The child should be seated during this part of the examination for best visualization of the posterior pharynx. Tell the patient that you are going to look in their throat and that they should open the mouth as widely as possible. If the child is extremely uncooperative, have the child lie on their back on the examination table. The caregiver should stand at the head of the table, raise the child's hands over the head, and squeeze the child's elbows against the head so that the head does not move. The examiner can then lean over the child, holding a tongue blade in one hand and a light in the other.

Inspect the *posterior pharynx*. Inspect the size of the *tonsils*. Tonsillar size is estimated on a scale from 1+ to 4+, whereby 4+ indicates that the tonsils meet in the midline. "Kissing" tonsils (see Fig. 12.41) may be indicative of obstructive apnea. Is a purulent exudate present? Are *petechiae* present? Streptococcal pharyngitis is often associated with petechiae on the palate. Fig. 24.40 shows the tonsillar exudate of streptococcal pharyngitis.

Inspect the *posterior pharyngeal wall*. A cobblestone appearance is suggestive of chronic postnasal drip.

MIDDLE CHILDHOOD: 5 YEARS TO 10 YEARS

Middle Childhood History

During this next period, as the child ventures out into the world and takes on more of a role in their own well-being, the

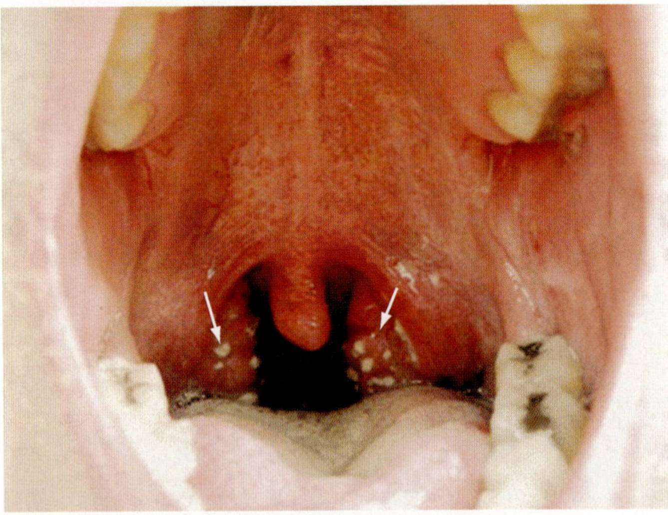

Fig. 24.40 Streptococcal Pharyngitis Showing Exudate on the Tonsils. (From Bryant AE, Stevens DL: *Mandell, Douglas, and Bennett's principles and practice of infectious diseases*, Published January 1, 2015, pp. 2285–2299.e4. © 2015.)

pediatric healthcare professional has the opportunity to help the child, along with the caregiver, make health-promoting decisions. Guidance about healthy diet and exercise, appropriate digital media exposure and use, and social interactions with friends, adults, and strangers can be directed to the caregiver(s) and child. For the school-aged patient, the child's social, motor, and language development, as well as emotional maturation, are reflected in current behavior, so it is important to get the caregiver's view of the child's demeanor, personality, and behavior. Also, school becomes a central focus of the child's life both academically and socially. Successes and challenges in school performance should be identified and addressed early. Student struggles could be due to anything from a learning disability to attention-deficit/hyperactivity disorder (ADHD),[o] anxiety, or depression, to troubles in the home. School-aged children should also start to develop their own interests and hobbies and take a role in chores around the house. Some older school-aged children may start to go through puberty and will need guidance on that.

- Diet
  - What types of food does the child eat? Drink?
  - What does the child eat at school? After school?
  - Any snacks or unhealthy or fast foods?
- Elimination
  - Any concerns about stool consistency or frequency?
  - Is the child having regular bowel movements? It is common to see constipation in school-age children who don't like to use the school bathroom.
- Sleep
  - Where does the child sleep?
  - Is the child getting enough sleep?
  - Any sleep problems? (e.g., may see nightmares, night terrors, sleepwalking)
- School/activities
  - Where does the child go to school? In what grade is the child (is it appropriate for age?)
  - Is the child in regular education class or is there an Individualized Education Program (IEP) in place to provide additional services or special education classes?
  - How is the child doing in school?
  - Any concerns (from caregivers or teachers) about academic performance? About behavior in the class?
  - Any bullying?
  - How much time does the child spend on screens daily?
  - Are there limits on media use, phones, video games? Are parental controls set up?
  - Ask the child about their friends, hobbies, activities
- Social
  - What are the after school childcare arrangements?
  - What type of relationship does the child have with other family members, friends?
  - Are social support services needed?
- Screenings: Tuberculosis, mental health, vision, hearing, oral health, substance use
- Anticipatory guidance (here are some examples)
  - Car safety
  - Street safety
  - Set limits on television and other digital media (avoid during mealtimes, within 1 hour of bedtime, unsupervised use); make a media use plan
  - Internet safety
  - Brush teeth twice a day
  - Remove firearms from home; if necessary, store unloaded and locked
  - Provide smoke-free environment
  - Sunscreen use outdoors
  - Stranger danger, inappropriate touching

Review of Systems

School-aged children are becoming more independent and able to describe their own symptoms. They may have chronic somatic concerns such as headaches, stomach pain, or leg pains that often have a partly psychosocial component. A relevant history of the circumstances in which these concerns occur can help tease out the triggers. Other items to add to the ROSs for children aged 5 to 10 years include persistent sneezing and nasal itching, itchy eyes, snoring, disturbed sleep, daytime somnolence, chest pain, exercise-induced cough or wheezing, nocturnal cough, palpitations, polyuria, polydipsia, syncope, persistent sadness or worry, sports injuries, and concussion.

Middle Childhood Physical Exam

It is usually easy to examine children between 5 to 10 years of age. They understand the purpose of the examination and rarely present any problems. It is often helpful to engage the child in conversation regarding school, friends, or hobbies. Conversation helps relax the child even if they do not appear apprehensive.

[o]ADHD is a chronic condition marked by persistent inattention, hyperactivity, and sometimes impulsivity. ADHD begins in childhood and often lasts into adulthood. As many as two out of every three children with ADHD continue to have symptoms as adults.

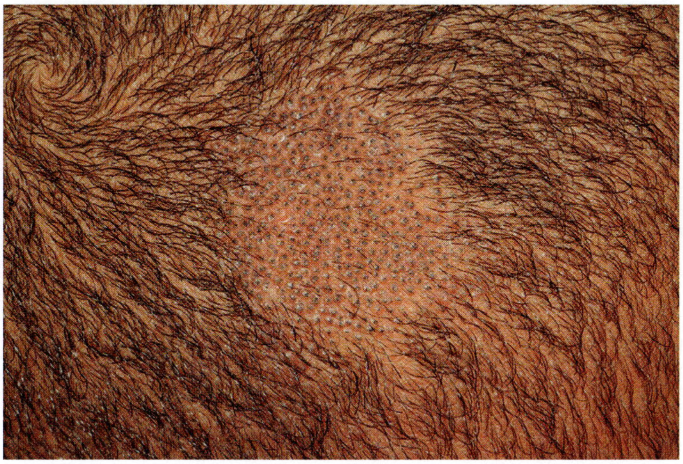

Fig. 24.41 Tinea Capitis. (From Gupta PS, Mbuyi N: *Ferri's clinical advisor 2019*, pp. 1369–1371.e1. © 2019.)

Allow the child to wear a gown or drape. The order of the examination is essentially the same as in adults. If the child is concerned with pain in a certain area, that area should be examined last. As with younger children, brief explanations about each part of the examination should be given to older children.

General Assessment

As with other age groups, note the general appearance of the school-aged child, including body habitus and general assessment of development and nourishment.

Skin

Are any *rashes* present? Persistent dandruff may be *tinea capitis.* Circular areas of alopecia on the scalp, especially with broken-off hairs, known as the black dot appearance are likely due to tinea capitis as shown in Fig. 24.41. Reactive occipital lymph nodes are often present. Eczema, or atopic dermatitis, is very common at this age and is most noticeable on flexor surfaces, such as the antecubital and popliteal fossae. It appears as pink, scaly plaques that are universally pruritic. Patients with atopic dermatitis tend to have an extra groove of the lower eyelid, called the *atopic pleat*. Atopic dermatitis is often found in children with other atopic diseases such as asthma, food allergies, or seasonal allergies. Fig. 24.42 shows a child with atopic dermatitis.

Check the back of the neck for *acanthosis nigricans,* a thickened, hyperpigmented plaque found in patients who may have insulin resistance.

Eyes

The examination of the eyes is essentially the same as in adults, with emphasis on *visual acuity.* A test with a standard Snellen eye chart is necessary. A two-line difference in acuity between the eyes warrants a referral to an ophthalmologist. Children in this age range may start becoming cooperative with a complete fundoscopic exam.

Confrontation visual field testing is performed only in children 5 years of age and older in whom there is a suspicion of decreased acuity or an intracranial mass. The test is conducted as in adults, except that a small toy is used instead of finger counting. The toy is brought in from the periphery of the child's vision, and the child is instructed to tell the examiner when they see it.

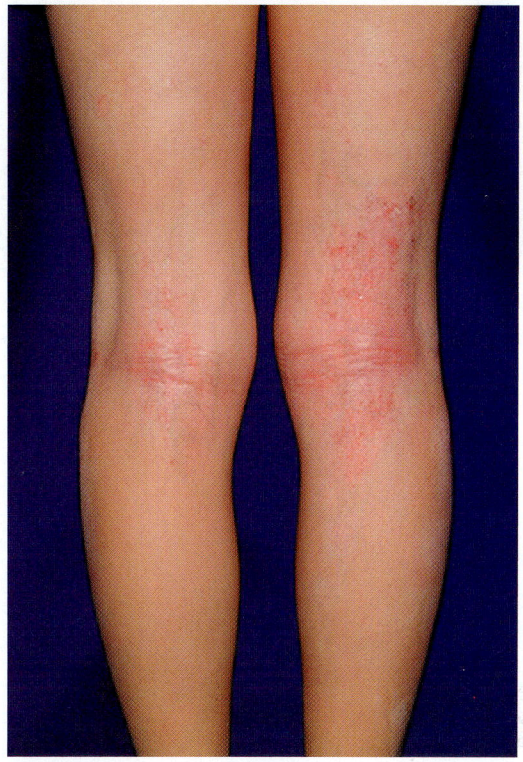

Fig. 24.42 Atopic Dermatitis in a Child. Note the characteristic involvement of the popliteal fossae. (From Paller AS, Mancini AJ: *Hurwitz clinical pediatric dermatology*, 2016, pp. 38–72.e7. © 2016.)

Ears

The examination of the ears is the same as in adults, with emphasis on *auditory acuity.* Audiometric testing should be performed on all school-aged children.

Nose

The examination of the nose is essentially the same as in adults.

Oropharynx

The *teeth* should be examined with regard to their condition and spacing. Have the child bite down and observe the *bite.* During this period children will start shedding primary teeth and permanent teeth will come in. See Fig. 24.33 for ages of primary teeth shedding. Fig. 24.43 illustrates the chronology of eruption of the permanent teeth.

The remainder of the exam is the same as in adults.

Neck

Palpate the *thyroid* for nodules. The thyroid is rarely palpable in children in this age group.

Palpate for *lymphadenopathy.* Anterior cervical nodes are seen in association with upper respiratory infections and dental infections. Posterior adenopathy is seen with infections of the

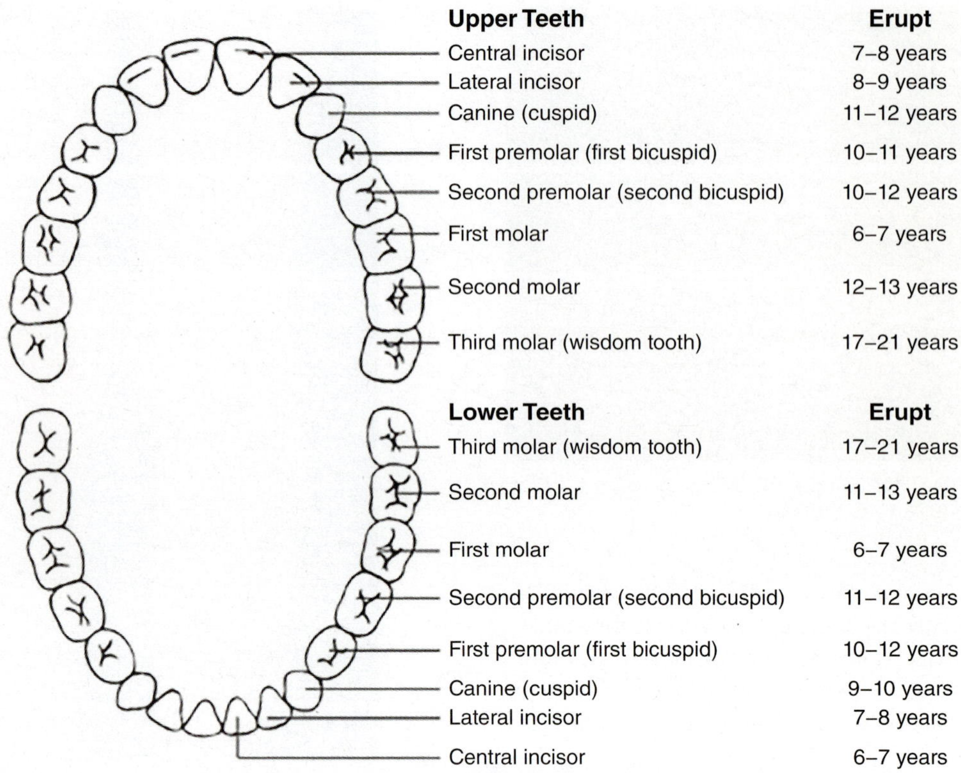

Fig. 24.43 Chronology of Eruption of the Permanent Teeth. (From https://www.mouthhealthy.org/en/az-topics/e/eruption-charts. © 2023 American Dental Association. All rights reserved. Reprinted with permission.)

middle ear and scalp. Generalized adenopathy is seen in viral diseases such as infectious mononucleosis, measles, and human immunodeficiency virus (HIV). Nodes that need further evaluation include those which are greater than 1 cm, tender, rubbery, fixed, or growing fast due to concerns for hematologic malignancies such as leukemia or lymphoma.

Chest

The examination of the chest is the same as in adults. See the discussion of Tanner staging of breast development in the genitalia section of the adolescent exam later in this chapter.

Heart

The examination of the heart is the same as in adults.

Abdomen

The order of the abdominal examination is the same as in adults. The average span of the liver at 7 to 9 years of age is 10.5 cm; at 12 years of age, the span is approximately 11.5 cm.

Genitalia

The age of development of secondary sexual characteristics varies greatly. As indicated in Chapter 16, The Breast, development of the breasts in females may begin as early as 8 years of age and continues for the next 5 years. The development of pubic hair in females occurs at around the same time. Testicular development in males begins somewhat later, at approximately 9 to 10 years of age. Pubic hair starts to develop in males at approximately 12 years of age and continues to develop in the ensuing years. The growth of the penis begins about a year after the beginning of testicular enlargement, at 10 to 11 years of age. Whereas the growth spurt in females occurs at approximately 12 years of age, early in their pubertal development, this spurt is not seen until approximately 14 years of age in males, when the genital changes are fairly well advanced.

The child should be given a gown to preserve modesty. Inspect the *external genitalia.* Is *pubic hair* present? What are the *sex maturity ratings? Are any lesions present? Is there evidence of sexual abuse*? For further information regarding sex maturity ratings in males and females, see genitalia section under the adolescent physical examination later in this chapter.

Palpate the testes. Is an *inguinal hernia* present?

Pelvic examinations are not routine in this age group unless clinically indicated and should be performed by an experienced examiner. Vaginal bleeding in females younger than 9 years of age is most often a result of infection from foreign objects or less commonly from trauma.

Musculoskeletal Examination

The musculoskeletal examination of children may detect *scoliosis.* Scoliosis is the most common spinal deformity, especially in pubertal girls. Have the patient stand with the back exposed to the waist. Inspect the back. Are the shoulders, or scapulae, at the same height? Is the occiput aligned over the intergluteal cleft? Ask the child to bend down and try to touch the toes, allowing the arms to hang freely. A unilateral elevation of the ribs is seen in patients with scoliosis. This is shown in Fig. 24.44. Scoliosis screening is recommended for females at age 10 and 12, and males once at age 13 or 14 years.[16]

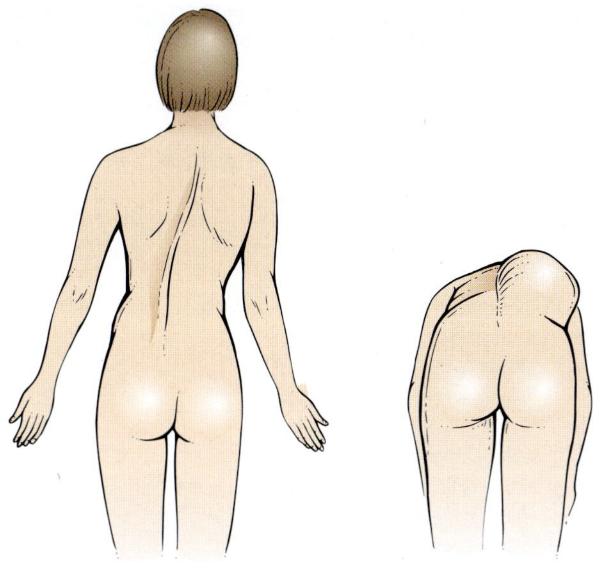

Fig. 24.44 Scoliosis. Note asymmetry of hips and shoulders when standing and asymmetry of ribs on forward bending.

Observe the child's gait. Intoeing in this age group is most often due to *femoral anteversion*. If present, both the knees and the feet are turned in since the legs are rotated inward at the level of the hip.

Neurologic Examination

The neurologic examination is essentially the same as outlined in Chapter 21, The Nervous System. However, in children in this age group, the complete neurologic examination is indicated only when there is evidence of developmental abnormalities, an acute insult to the central nervous system, or a concern such as headache.

ADOLESCENCE: 11 YEARS TO 21 YEARS

Adolescent History

Sexual maturation, or puberty, begins at approximately 10 to 11 years of age in most females and 11 to 12 years of age in most males. Adolescence is often considered the transitional stage from puberty to adulthood, although some consider adolescence the transition from childhood to adulthood. In fact, there is no one scientific definition of the period of adolescence. It is a stage of physical, cognitive, psychological, social, and emotional development and is roughly considered the period between 11 and 21 years of age.

During adolescence, individuals become increasingly conscious of their body image. They develop their sexual, gender, racial, and ethnic identities. They explore their own values, ethics, and spirituality. While adolescents are learning what makes them unique, they also have an increased need to "fit in." Therefore, identity formation can be especially challenging for individuals who feel different from others because of their cultural, ethnic, gender, or sexual identity. Peer relationships become increasingly important. School responsibilities increase. Many adolescents experiment with drugs and alcohol. The adolescent years also have unique stresses and pressures. Parents, guardians, and other caring adults play vital roles in providing support and helping adolescents achieve their best on their way to adulthood.

The American Academy of Child and Adolescent Psychiatry has described the developmental characteristics of adolescents in three substages specific to physical, cognitive, and social-emotional development as shown in Table 24.6.

Pre-teens and teenagers can usually provide their own history so questions should be directed toward them. Caregivers may supplement answers or voice their own concerns. Early in the visit, it is vital to establish the ground rules about confidentiality with both the caregiver and the teenager, as well as support the caregiver's role in their adolescent's healthcare. It should be explained that one-on-one time with the healthcare professional is routine for all children starting at age 11 to 12 and is not being done due to concerns about this patient. For instance, the healthcare professional may say something like, "*For someone your child's age, it's very important to have a private visit with the doctor, just as it would be for you with your doctor. I will keep what we talk about confidential unless something comes up that is acutely life-threatening. While it's crucial that I keep what I'm told confidential, I also encourage my teenaged patients to share with their parents what they have told me.*" After the interview with both the caregiver and teenager, the caregiver should be asked to leave the room, which provides an opportunity to discuss confidential matters with the adolescent privately. The presence of the caregiver during the physical exam should be a shared decision with the patient.

- Diet
  - What is your diet like?
  - What did you eat yesterday?
  - Do you drink soda? Water?
- Elimination
  - Any problems using the bathroom?
- Sleep
  - Are you getting enough sleep?
  - What time do you go to sleep? Wake up?
- School/Activities (will also be covered with teen in HEEADSSS exam)
  - What school do you attend? How was the transition to middle school or high school?
  - Any concerns (from caregivers or teachers) about academic performance? About behavior in the class?
  - Any bullying?
  - How much time is spent on screens daily?
  - Are there limits on media use, phones, video games? Are parental controls set up?
  - Any physical activity/exercise?
- Screenings: Tuberculosis, mental health, vision, hearing, oral health, sexually transmitted infections (STI) (once the adolescent is sexually active)
- Anticipatory guidance (here are some examples)
  - Healthy diet; drink water
  - Physical exercise 60 min/day
  - Internet safety; avoid cyberbullying, sexting, sharing personal information
  - Oral health

TABLE 24.6 Stages of Adolescence

Stages of Adolescence	Physical Development	Cognitive Development	Social-Emotional Development
Early adolescence Approximately 11–13 years of age	Puberty: grow body hair, increase perspiration and oil production in hair and skin Girls—breast and hip development, onset of menstruation Boys—growth in testicles and penis, wet dreams, deepening of voice Tremendous physical growth: gain height and weight	Growing capacity for abstract thought Mostly interested in present with limited thought to the future Intellectual interests expand and become more important Deeper moral thinking	Struggle with sense of identity Feel awkward about one's self and one's body; worry about being normal Realize that parents are not perfect; increased conflict with parents Increased influence of peer group Desire for independence Tendency to return to "childish" behavior, particularly when stressed Moodiness Rule- and limit-testing Greater interest in privacy Growing sexual interest
Middle adolescence Approximately 14–18 years of age	Puberty is completed Physical growth slows for girls, continues for boys	Continued growth of capacity for abstract thought Greater capacity for setting goals Interest in moral reasoning Thinking about the meaning of life	Intense self-involvement, changing between high expectations and poor self-concept Continued adjustment to changing body, worries about being normal Tendency to distance selves from parents, continued drive for independence Driven to make friends and greater reliance on them, popularity can be an important issue Feelings of love and passion Increased sexual interest
Late adolescence Approximately 19–24 years of age	Young females, typically, are physically fully developed Young males continue to gain height, weight, muscle mass, and body hair	Ability to think ideas through from beginning to end Ability to delay gratification Examination of inner experiences Increased concern for future Continued interest in moral reasoning	Firmer sense of identity, including sexual identity Increased emotional stability Increased concern for others Increased independence and self-reliance Peer relationships remain important Development of more serious relationships Social and cultural traditions regain some of their importance

Adapted from the American Academy of Child and Adolescent Psychiatry: Facts for Families.

- Remove firearms from home; if necessary, store unloaded and locked
- Provide smoke-free environment
- Sunscreen use outdoors; seat belts use in cars
- Privately
  - Risks of/avoid cigarettes, vaping, alcohol, drug use
  - Dangers of impaired driving
  - Pubertal changes
  - Reproductive health, safe sex, contraception, sexually-transmitted illness (STI) prevention, Ok to say no.

Chapter 33, Clinical Ethics and Professionalism, provides additional information on privacy, confidentiality, informed consent, and shared decision making with adolescents.

Social History

Once the examiner is alone with the adolescent patient, it is crucial to ensure confidentiality with the teenager, while also spelling out any limits to confidentiality. Each state in the United States has laws and regulations regarding consent and confidentiality for minors. In general, it is important to assure the teenager that any information that they share with the healthcare professional will remain confidential unless there is a threat to the patient's safety or the safety of others. Once this confidentiality agreement is established, it is easier to proceed with asking questions to explore the patient's adolescent social history. It is essential to remain nonjudgmental during this discussion so as to gain the patient's trust and openness.

This part of the interview is also an opportunity for patients to ask questions or raise concerns that are more private or personal in nature that they do not want to share with their caregivers. The conversation should start by asking patients if they have anything they want to discuss. Furthermore, this alone time will be an important chance to educate these patients about avoidance of high-risk behaviors and personal safety.

The ***HEEADSSS*** *mnemonic* is a useful tool for remembering the main topics for private adolescent interviews. It has been updated over the years to include advances in technology and media. Beginning with more neutral questions about home, education, eating, and activities can promote the teenager's comfort.

The letters in HEEADSSS stand for the **H**ome environment, **E**ducation and employment, **E**ating, peer-related **A**ctivities, **D**rugs, **S**exuality, **S**uicide/depression, and **S**afety from injury and violence. Sample questions for each item can be found in Table 24.7. An alternative version of the adolescent social history questions is SSHADESS,[17] a strength-based psychosocial assessment: **S**trengths, **S**chool, **H**ome, **A**ctivities, **D**rugs/substance use, **E**motions/eating/depression, **S**exuality, **S**afety.

TABLE 24.7 The HEEADSSS Psychosocial Interview for Adolescents

	Potential First Line Questions	Questions if Time Permits or if Situation Warrants Exploration
Home	Who lives with you? Where do you live? What are relationships like at home? Can you talk to anyone at home about stress? (Who?) Do you have a smartphone or computer at home? What do you use it for? (May ask this in the activities section.)	Have you moved recently? Have you ever had to live away from home? (Why?) Have you ever run away? (Why) Do you feel safe at home?
Education and employment	Tell me about school. Is your school a safe place? Have you been bullied at school? Do you feel connected to your school? Do you feel as if you belong? Are there adults at school you feel you could talk to about something important? (Who?) Do you have any failing grades? Any recent changes? What are your future education/employment plans/goals? Are you working? Where? How much?	How many days have you missed from school this month/quarter/semester? Have you changed schools in the past few years? Tell me about your friends at school. Have you ever had to repeat a class/grade? Have you ever been suspended? Expelled? Have you ever considered dropping out? How well do you get along with the people at school? Work? Have your responsibilities at work increased? What are your favorite subjects at school? Your least favorite subjects?
Eating	Does your weight or body shape cause you any stress? If so, tell me about it. Have there been any recent changes in your weight? Have you dieted in the last year? How? How often?	What do you like and not like about your body? Have you done anything else to try to manage your weight? Tell me about your exercise routine. What do you think would be a healthy diet? How does that compare to your current eating patterns? Does it ever seem as though your eating is out of control? Have you ever taken diet pills?
Activities	What do you do for fun? How do you spend time with friends? Family? (With whom, where, when?) Some teenagers tell me that they spend much of their free time online. What types of things do you use the Internet for? How many hours do you spend on any given day in front of a screen, such as a computer, TV, or phone?	Do you participate in any sports? Do you regularly attend religious or spiritual activities? Have you messaged photos or texts that you have later regretted? Can you think of a friend who was harmed by spending time online? How often do you view pornography (or nude images or videos) online? What types of books do you read for fun? How do you feel after playing video games? What music do you like to listen to?
Drugs	Do any of your friends or family members use tobacco? Alcohol? Other substances? Do you smoke or vape? Do you drink alcohol? Do you use marijuana in any form, take other substances, energy drinks, steroids, or medications not prescribed to you?	Is there any history of alcohol or misuse of substances in your family? Does anyone at home use tobacco? Do you ever drink or misuse substances when you're alone? (Assess frequency, intensity, patterns of misuse, and how patient obtains or pays for drugs, alcohol, or tobacco.)
Sexuality	What is your gender identity? Have you thought about your gender recently? What pronouns do you typically use? What pronouns would you like me to use today? Have you ever been in a romantic relationship? Are you attracted to anyone now? Tell me about the people that you've dated. To whom are you attracted? Have any of your relationships ever been sexual relationships (such as involving kissing, touching or more)? Tell me about your sexual practices. Have you had penile-vaginal, anal, or oral sex?	Are your sexual activities enjoyable? Have any of your relationships been abusive? What does the term "safer sex" mean to you? Have you ever sent unclothed pictures of yourself on e-mail or the Internet? Have you ever been forced or pressured into doing something sexual that you didn't want to do? Have you ever been touched sexually in a way that you didn't want? Have you ever been raped, on a date or any other time? How many sexual partners have you had altogether? (Females) Have you ever been pregnant or worried that you may be pregnant? (Males) Have you ever gotten someone pregnant or worried that might have happened? What are you using for birth control? Are you satisfied with your method? Do you use condoms every time you have intercourse? What gets in the way? Have you ever had a sexually transmitted infection or worried that you had an infection?

Continued

TABLE 24.7 **The HEEADSSS Psychosocial Interview for Adolescents—cont'd**

	Potential First Line Questions	Questions if Time Permits or if Situation Warrants Exploration
Suicide and depression	Do you feel "stressed" or anxious more than usual (or more than you prefer to feel)? Do you feel sad or down more than usual? Are you "bored" much of the time? Are you having trouble getting to sleep? Have you thought about hurting yourself or someone else? Tell me about a time when someone picked on you or made you feel uncomfortable in person or online.	Tell me about a time when you felt sad while using social media. Does it seem that you've lost interest in things that you used to really enjoy? Do you find yourself spending less time with friends? Would you rather just be by yourself most of the time? Have you ever tried to kill yourself? Have you ever hurt yourself (by cutting yourself, for example) to calm down or feel better? Have you started using alcohol or drugs to help you relax, calm down, or feel better?
Safety	Have you ever been seriously injured? (How?) How about anyone else you know? Do you always wear a seatbelt in the car? Have you ever met in person (or plan to meet) with anyone whom you first encountered online? Do you send text messages while driving? Have you ever ridden with a driver who was drunk or high. When? How often? Is there a lot of violence at your home or school? In your neighborhood? Among your friends?	Do you use safety equipment for sports and/or other physical activities (for example, helmets for biking or skateboarding)? Have you ever been in a car or motorcycle accident? (What happened?) Have you ever been picked on or bullied? Is that still a problem? Have you gotten into physical fights in school or your neighborhood? Are you still getting into fights? Have you ever felt that you had to carry a knife, gun, or other weapon to protect yourself? Do you still feel that way? Have you ever been incarcerated?

Adapted from https://www.contemporarypediatrics.com/view/heeadsss-30-psychosocial-interview-adolescents-updated-new-century-fueled-media. Accessed October 3, 2023.

The more sensitive subjects of drugs, sexuality, suicide/depression, and safety will be further elaborated on later.

Drugs

Asking about cigarettes, substance misuse, and alcohol use broaches a potentially sensitive subject, and there are many ways to introduce it. For younger adolescents, it may be better to ask if any of their friends drink alcohol or use drugs. They may be more likely to talk about their friends' behaviors and habits, and that may open an opportunity for the healthcare professional to inquire about the patient's experiences. For older teenagers, it may be possible to simply ask about substance misuse and alcohol use more directly with good results. However, it is important to be aware of what kind of substances youth are experimenting with and using and being aware of the nicknames used by teens. See e-Appendix B, Commonly Misused Substances.

If the teenager does report drinking or using drugs, then it is necessary to explore how much, how often, and whether there have been negative consequences (i.e., losing consciousness, a "driving while intoxicated" offense, or a suspension from school).

Remember that nicotine and other chemicals in tobacco are drugs. Ask about cigarette use, including age of initiation, frequency, and quantity of use. It is also important to inquire about vaping (using electronic cigarettes), as this has become an epidemic in the adolescent population with marketing and products directed at this age group.[18] Due to the addictive nicotine ingredients, youth who use e-cigarettes are more likely to use cigarettes or tobacco products in the future. In 2016, the U.S. Surgeon General issued a report[19] that stated that youth should not use e-cigarettes due to their dangerous health effects.

Many outpatient healthcare professionals use a brief, validated screening tool, **CRAFFT** (**C**ar, **R**elax, **A**lone, **F**orget, **F**riends, **T**rouble) to assess for risk of a serious misused substance.[20]

The goal of asking about drugs and alcohol in the adolescent social history is to identify those patients who may have a problem and encourage them to discuss this with their caregivers so that they have support and potentially access to treatment. The healthcare professional can serve as a facilitator in these conversations. However, this subject can remain confidential if there is no immediate danger to the patient or others.

Sexuality

Talking about sexuality may very well be the most sensitive part of the history. Younger adolescents may have many questions about puberty and the changes that they are experiencing in their bodies and socially. In addition, adolescence is a time when people are forming their gender identity and exploring sexual attraction. These topics can be delicate and require special attention to make sure the patient feels comfortable answering questions about them.

Avoid making assumptions based on general appearance. Explore gender identity with some of the suggested questions in Table 24.7. If the patient does not understand the questions, ask more specifically if they identify as cisgender, transgender, nonbinary, or something else or if they identify as a girl, a boy, neither, or something else. See Chapter 26, The Transgender Patient, for additional information.

There are many ways to introduce the topic of sexual activity. For instance, normalize the question: "I know that lots of people your age are thinking about having sex. How about you?" It may also be very helpful to explain why the healthcare professional "needs to know": "To understand what is causing your pain,

I need to know something about your sexual experiences." It is useful to be explicit: Something like "Have you ever had sex?" is more likely to reveal more relevant information than "Are you sexually active?" The teenager may answer no to the second question because they have not had sex in 2 weeks. It is also important to phrase questions without heterosexual bias. Try to use inclusive language in all of your history questions.

- "Are you dating anyone?" rather than "Do you have a boyfriend?"
- "To whom are you attracted?" rather than "Are you attracted to boys, girls, or both?
- "How would you label your sexual orientation?" rather than "Do you identify as gay or straight?"

Ask the teenager about their sexual practices, including penile-vaginal, anal, oral and nonpenetrative sex. It is also important to find out what the teenager knows about contraception and STIs. Many teenagers do not have an adult that they can get reliable information from about fertility and sexual health, and therefore they rely on their friends or the Internet where information can be erroneous. Ask about the teenager's personal history of contraceptive use and STIs. It is important to let teenagers know that healthcare professionals can be a confidential resource for reproductive health information and services. It is important to be familiar with state confidentiality laws.[21]

Suicide/Depression

Screening for depression merits special emphasis. Suicide is one of the top three causes of death among teenagers; therefore, it is imperative to screen for depression and suicidality at every visit with a teenager. Several screening tools are available. Box 24.7 provides the Patient Health Questionnaire 2 (PHQ-2), which is a brief and easily administered tool.

If the teenager admits to a depressed mood, then the next critical step is to probe further by asking directly if they have had thoughts of harming or killing themselves. Suicidal ideation on the part of a teenager is an indication to break confidentiality, so as to get the adolescent prompt mental healthcare. This is also the same if the teenager poses a threat to the safety of others.

Safety

It is important to realize that the major causes of morbidity and mortality in teenagers are unintentional injuries, suicides, and homicides. Safety refers not only to personal safety practices, such as using a seat belt or wearing a bike helmet, but also to the risk of violence in interpersonal relations: at home, with an intimate partner, at school, or in the community. It is also important to assess the teenager's access to weapons. Knowing what kinds of resources are available in the community is also helpful in counseling teens about safety.

BOX 24.7 Patient Health Questionnaire 2 (PHQ-2)

Over the last 2 weeks how often have you been bothered by any of the following problems?	Not at all	Several days	More than half the days	Nearly every day
Little interest or pleasure in doing things	0	1	2	3
Feeling down, depressed, or hopeless	0	1	2	3

A cut-off score ≥ 3 is positive

Review of Systems

The ROSs for the adolescent is almost the same as for the adult. Of note, questions about menstruation, including menstrual cramps or premenstrual symptoms; about sexual function and symptoms of STIs; about possible pregnancy; and about sports injuries, mood disorders, and thought disorders become relevant with the adolescent patient and should be discussed privately.

Adolescent Physical Exam

The physical examination of adolescents is essentially the same as that of adults. It is appropriate for the examiner to ask the caregiver to leave during the examination. However, some adolescents prefer to have their caregiver present for the examination; therefore, ask the patient their preference. As mentioned previously, for examination of breasts or genitals, it is recommended to have a chaperone.

Because the examination is so similar to that of adults, only the dissimilarities are described in this section.

General Assessment

As with other age groups, note the general appearance of the pre-adolescent or adolescent patient. A lot can be gleaned from observation, including affect and signs of physical and emotional distress.

Skin

Examination of the skin of adolescents usually reveals evidence of *pubertal changes*. These include acne, areolar pigmentation, functioning of the apocrine sweat glands, pigmentation of the external genitalia, and development of axillary and pubic hair.

Abdomen

The abdominal examination is the same as in adults. The liver span of 15- to 17-year-olds is about 12 cm.

Genitalia (Including Breasts)

Sex maturity ratings for males and females were established by J. M. Tanner in 1962. In males, the growth of pubic hair and the development of the penis, testes, and scrotum are used to assign a sex maturity rating from 1 to 5. The examiner should record two ratings: one for the pubic hair and one for the genitalia. If the development of the penis differs from that of the testes and scrotum, the two ratings should be averaged.

The Tanner sex maturity ratings for females are based on the growth of pubic hair and the development of the breasts. Five stages are observed for each. The examiner should record two ratings: one for the breasts and one for the pubic hair.

The Tanner sex maturity ratings for breast development in females are illustrated and summarized in Fig. 24.45A. The Tanner sex maturity ratings for pubic hair development in males and females are illustrated and summarized in Fig. 24.45B. The

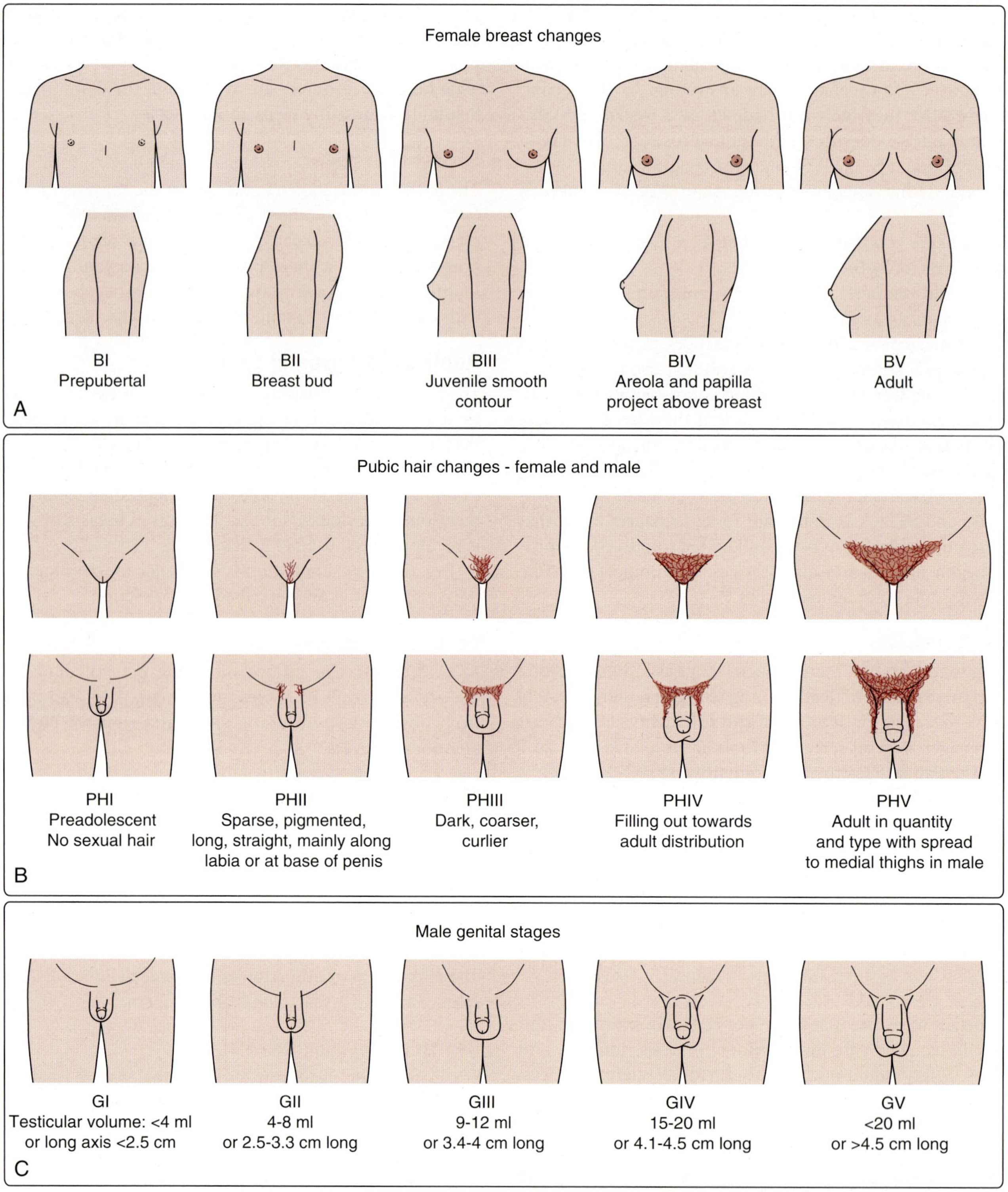

Fig. 24.45 **Tanner Stages of Development.** (A) Breast development in females. (B) Pubic hair development in males and females. (C) Male genital development. Tanner stages I (prepubertal) to V (adult); B (breast), PH (pubic hair), G (male genital). (Reused from Rodgers A, Salkind J: *Crash course: paediatrics*, ed 5, 2019, Elsevier.)

Tanner sex maturity ratings for genital development in males are illustrated and summarized in Fig. 24.45C.

The examiner should evaluate the patient and explain to them about the body changes that are related to normal puberty. For example, breast development occurs in both males and females. A male with unilateral gynecomastia who is at Tanner stage 3 or 4 can be reassured that this change is part of normal puberty and will be transient. Asymmetric breast development in females is common. Reassure the patient that puberty is progressing normally.

Routine pelvic examinations for initiation of contraception is unnecessary, and Pap smear screens do not start until age 21.

If an internal pelvic examination is necessary due to genital concerns for a female adolescent, an extremely gentle approach is required. Use of a small-sized speculum often renders the examination less uncomfortable.

Musculoskeletal Examination

Adolescents often have musculoskeletal complaints either due to periods of rapid growth or from injuries, especially due to sports involvement. Knee pain in an adolescent is usually the result of trauma. Partial avulsion of the tibial tubercle associated with a painful swelling in that area is called *Osgood-Schlatter disease.* This common condition is seen more frequently in athletic pubertal males and is usually self-limited. Hip pain or knee pain referred from the hip may result from a *slipped capital femoral epiphysis* (SCFE). Patients with SCFE have limited internal rotation of the involved hip, and compulsory movement of the hip into external rotation as the leg is passively flexed at knee and hip is very suggestive of SCFE. SCFE is more common during the pubertal growth spurt and in obese adolescents.

Scoliosis often progresses rapidly during the pubertal growth spurt.

If the adolescent is seeking medical clearance for competitive sports, it is necessary to perform a comprehensive preparticipation physical examination (PPE) to assess cardiac, neurologic, and musculoskeletal health. A comprehensive history and physical exam form for this purpose is available.[22,23]

CLINICOPATHOLOGIC CORRELATIONS

Child Maltreatment

Child maltreatment is pervasive around the world and is defined as the abuse and neglect of children. Abuse can take on several forms, including physical abuse, sexual abuse, emotional or psychological abuse, and neglect. Child maltreatment can have immediate effects such as injuries or death. In the U.S., over 1750 children die per year due to child abuse or neglect, and children younger than 3 years of age account for 66% of these deaths. But in addition to mortality, there are serious long-term consequences of abuse and adverse health outcomes, such as depression, substance abuse, obesity, high-risk sexual behaviors, and unplanned pregnancies. People who were abused as children are at risk for continuing the cycle of violence by being the perpetrator or ongoing victim of abuse. There are individual (both of the caretaker and of the child), community, and societal characteristics that increase the risk for child maltreatment (Table 24.8), and it is important for healthcare professionals to be aware of these when assessing the socioeconomic environment of each child.

Child maltreatment is a worldwide problem, but often hidden and unrecognized. Therefore, it is imperative to take notice of clues in both the history and physical examination that raise the suspicion for abuse, as all healthcare professionals are mandated by law to report these concerns to the authorities and/or child protective services. If a child comes to medical attention with a suspicious injury, the AAP recommends that the healthcare professional consider abuse if any of these red flags are present in the history[24]:

1. "There is either no explanation or a vague explanation given for a significant injury;
2. There is an explicit denial of trauma in a child with obvious injury;
3. An important detail of the explanation changes in a substantive way;
4. An explanation is provided that is inconsistent with the pattern, age, or severity of the injury or injuries;
5. An explanation is given that is inconsistent with the child's physical and/or developmental capabilities;
6. There is an unexplained or unexpected notable delay in seeking medical care; or
7. Different witnesses provide markedly different explanations for the injury or injuries."

TABLE 24.8 Key Risk and Protective Factors for Child Maltreatment at Each Level of the Socioecological Model

	Key Risk Factors	Key Protective Factors
Individual level[a]	• Child age • Special healthcare needs or disabilities	• Self-regulation skills • Social competence • Adaptive functioning • Self-esteem
Interpersonal level	• Family poverty and material hardships • Parental mental health disorders • Parental substance use disorders • Parental intimate partner violence	• Supportive, nurturing parental relationships • Parents having social and emotional support from family and friends
Community level	• Neighborhood crime and violence • Concentrated disadvantage	• Neighborhood social cohesion and control • Availability of health, social, and educational services
Societal level	• Economic policies and trends • Gender inequality	• Paid parental level • Earned Income Tax Credits • Increases in minimum wage • Fewer restrictions on welfare benefits

[a]Individual level protective factors are those that promote resilience among children who have experienced maltreatment.

Reused with permission from Austin AE, Lesak AM, Shanahan ME: Risk and protective factors for child maltreatment: a review, *Curr Epidemiol Rep* 7(4):334–342, 2020. doi:10.1007/s40471-020-00252-3.

Similarly, the AAP describes physical findings that are red flags for abuse[24]:

1. "ANY injury to a young, preambulatory infant, including bruises, mouth injuries, fractures, and intracranial or abdominal injury
2. Injuries to multiple organ systems
3. Multiple injuries in different stages of healing
4. Patterned injuries
5. Injuries to nonbony or other unusual locations, such as over the torso, ears, face, neck, or upper arms
6. Significant injuries that are unexplained
7. Additional evidence of child neglect"

We will focus on signs of abuse that can be detected on physical examination.

Bruises are the most common sign of physical abuse. Despite being generally easy to see, they are often missed as a sentinel injury in children who die or nearly die from abuse. Because bruising can be common in children, it is important to know which ages, locations, and patterns of bruising are suggestive of physical abuse. In children who can walk, the most common places to have bruising related to normal activity are the knees and shins or bony prominences like the forehead. A useful mnemonic to help healthcare professionals identify bruises that are suggestive of abuse is "TEN 4," which stands for:

T: torso;

E: ear;

N: neck; and

4: in children less than or equal to 4 years of age and ANY bruise in an infant under 4 months of age.

See Fig. 24.46 for examples of inflicted bruises in these areas.

It is important to note that some medical conditions do predispose a person to have easy bruising, such as coagulopathies and vasculitides, and a workup for these conditions may be warranted when evaluating a child for physical abuse.

Bite marks are also concerning for abuse. Human bite marks should be suspected when ecchymosis, lacerations, or abrasions are found in any oval shape. Tooth marks by the canine teeth are the most prominent part of a bite. It might be possible to identify the perpetrator with the help of dental professionals by assessing the size, dentition characteristics, arch form, and intercuspid distance.

Accidental burns in childhood can be common, therefore it is important to try to determine when a burn is a result of abuse. Inflicted tap water scalds, including immersions, are the most common type of nonaccidental burn injury. A large circular-type burn with sharp lines of demarcation on the genitalia, buttocks, and thighs may result from the infant's immersion in scalding water. A lower extremity burn is shown in Fig. 24.47. Burns by a hot object, such as irons, radiators, or cigarettes are well-circumscribed with the outline of the hot object. Fig. 24.48 shows the typical appearance of specific types of burns. Small, circular, punched-out lesions of uniform size may represent

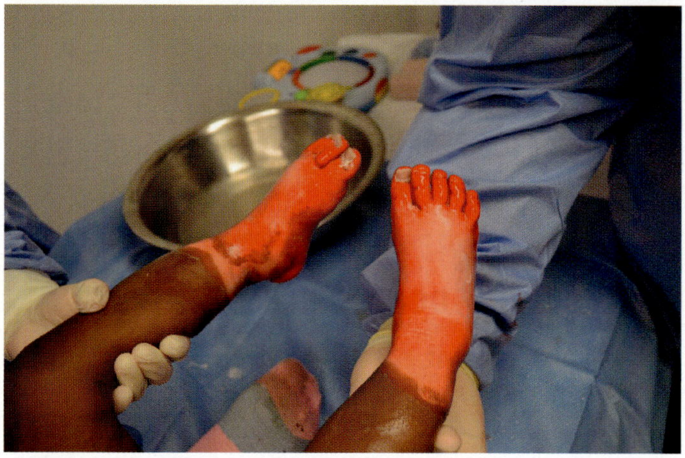

Fig. 24.47 Immersion Burn in a Stocking Distribution of the Lower Extremities. (From Letson MM, Tscholl JJ: *Clinical pediatric emergency medicine. Bruises, burns, and other blemishes: diagnostic considerations of physical abuse*, vol. 3(3), September 1, 2012.)

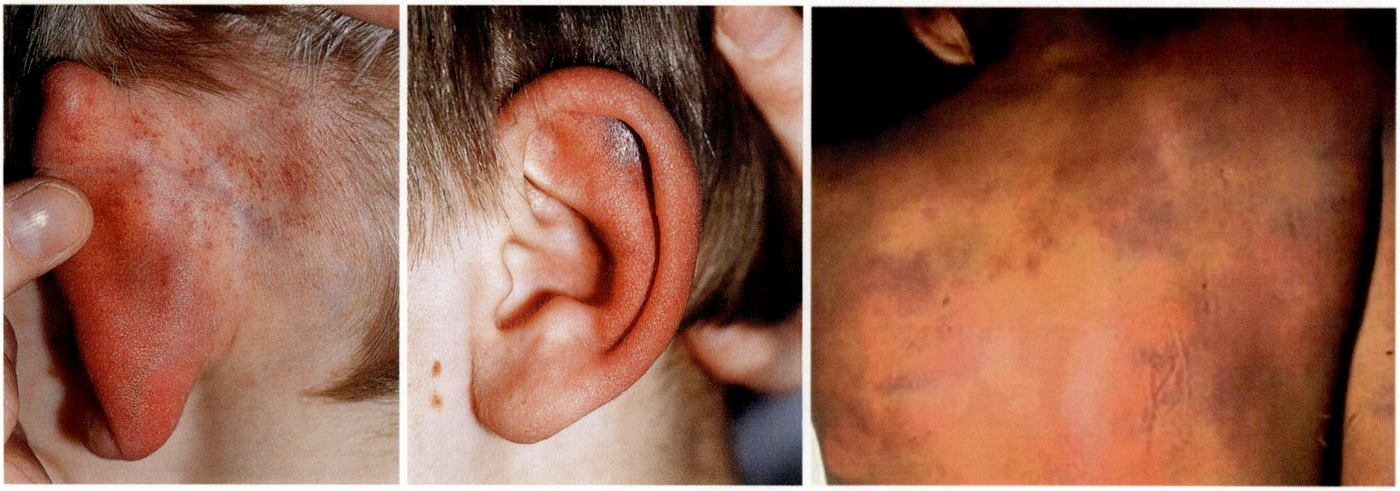

A B C

Fig. 24.46 (A and B) Bruising and petechiae of the pinna and post auricular area in a 6-year-old boy, consistent with a hand slap by an adult. (C) Bruising from a belt and belt buckle on the back of an 8-year-old boy. (A, B from Hobbs CJ, Wynne JM: *Physical signs of child abuse*, © 2001 WB Saunders. C, Courtesy Sharon Ann Raimer, MD.)

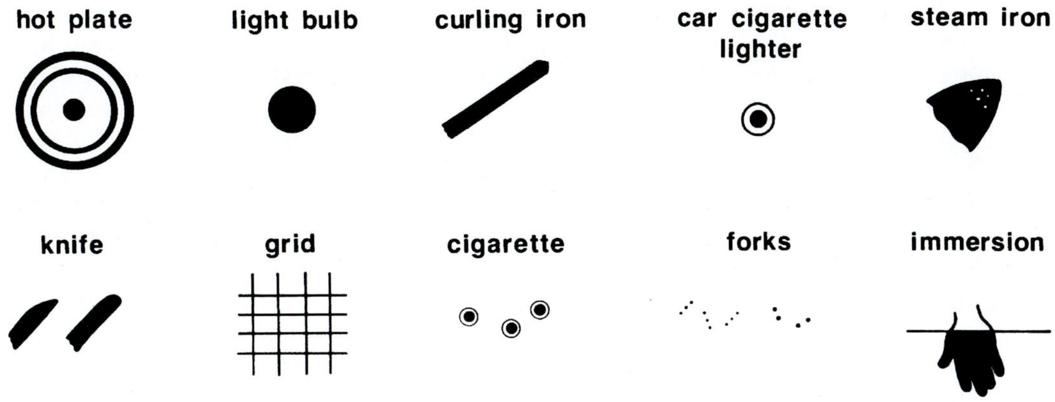

Fig. 24.48 Burn Patterns. (From Johnson CF: Inflicted injury versus accidental injury, *Pediatr Clin North Am* 37(4):807, 1990.)

cigarette burns. Due to delays in seeking medical care, inflicted burns can be more severe.

Acute fractures in childhood are most commonly a result of accidental trauma, but healthcare professionals must be vigilant so as not to miss the cases when physical abuse is the cause. In general, children who have suffered a recent fracture have pain, swelling, and may refuse to use the affected part of the body. It is important to inspect the skin surfaces looking for signs of "grab marks" that could suggest a mechanism where the child was pulled forcefully or twisted to fracture the bone. The absence of bruising, however, does not exclude a fracture or grabbing.

Abusive head trauma (AHT) is the most common reason for death from child physical abuse and occurs most frequently in infants. Some infants might present with swelling on the scalp due to some blunt injury, but often times infants found to have intracranial injuries due to AHT have no neurologic symptoms, making the diagnosis challenging. Signs of head trauma in infants can range from being absent, mild, or nonspecific to severe presentations of altered mental status or death. If abuse is suspected in an infant, neuroimaging is indicated. In addition, indirect ophthalmoscopy examination looking for retinal hemorrhages is required when there is concern for AHT. The severity, location, depth, and extent of the retinal hemorrhages (Fig. 24.49) may help differentiate between AHT and nonaccidental trauma. This examination is preferably done by an ophthalmologist with pediatric experience or retinal expertise.

Another form of child maltreatment is sexual abuse. Worldwide, 18% of females and 8% of males report they suffered child sexual abuse. The most important signs of abuse include difficulty walking, vaginal discharge, anal infections, genital irritation or swelling, torn or stained underclothes, vaginal or anal bleeding, and bruises. When sexual abuse is suspected, it is important to conduct a thorough examination of the child to assess for all types of injuries since children who are sexually abused are also at risk for physical abuse or neglect. If there are reported symptoms of genital or anal pain or bleeding, an anogenital examination should be performed to ensure the child does not require acute interventions.

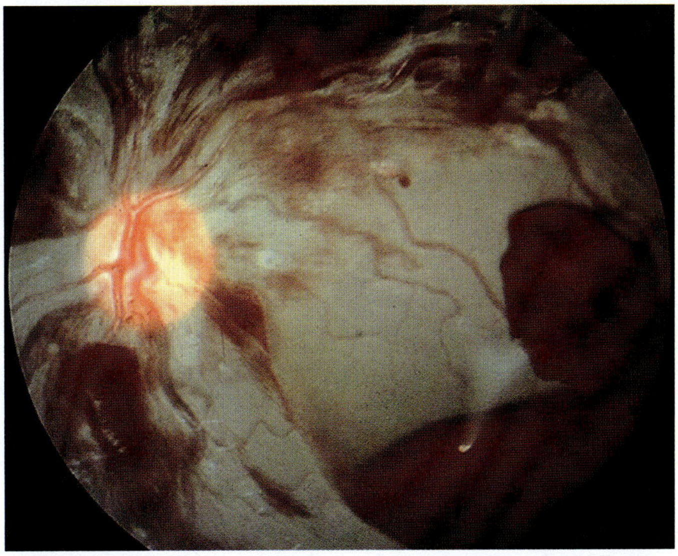

Fig. 24.49 Retinal Hemorrhages in an Infant Who Suffered From Abusive Head Trauma.

Most children who have been sexually abused exhibit no physical findings, even those who have been sexually penetrated. The tissue in the anogenital region tends to heal quickly and completely when injury occurs. Therefore, it must be noted that a normal physical examination of the genitals and anus does not rule out sexual abuse.

It is crucial that an experienced healthcare professional performs the anogenital examination if sexual abuse is suspected, and that the number of anogenital examinations is limited to what is necessary. If the abuse occurred a while ago and the child is currently asymptomatic, it might be appropriate to defer the examination and refer the child to a specialty center for medical evaluation of abuse.

A child who has been sexually or physically abused may exhibit behavior changes such as aggression, moodiness, irritability, withdrawal, regression, memory loss, insecurity, and clinginess. In addition, the child may experience nonspecific symptoms, such as loss of appetite, headache, or stomach problems. The child may want to bathe excessively or not at all and may become frightened of medical examinations. Some children may exhibit precocious sexual behaviors. An older child in school may exhibit a drop in academic performance, prevarication, stealing, or even running away from home.

Vascular Anomalies

Vascular anomalies range from simple skin changes to more serious and potentially life-threatening conditions. Historically, the nomenclature to name these entities was merely descriptive of appearance, which frequently led to incorrect diagnosing and subsequently to improper evaluation and mismanagement. Therefore, the International Society for the Study of Vascular Anomalies (ISSVA) devised a classification framework using consistent terminology that could be used and shared across disciplines that manage vascular anomalies, including general practitioners, surgeons, and pathologists. As previously mentioned in the chapter, the nomenclature is now based on clinical characteristics, such as cellular makeup and natural clinical progression. The broad categories are vascular tumors, simple malformations, combined vascular malformations, anomalies of major named vessels, and vascular malformations associated with other anomalies.

Vascular tumors are categorized as benign, locally aggressive or borderline, or overtly malignant. The most common vascular tumors, and tumors of infancy, are infantile hemangioma (IHs). They are made of proliferating endothelial cells and typically appear on the skin within the first few weeks after birth, slowly enlarge over several months, and then typically involute spontaneously. Depending on morphology and distribution of the IH, it can be further classified as focal, multifocal, segmental, or indeterminate. In addition, the IH can be described as superficial, deep, or mixed depending on the location in the skin or hypodermis. See Fig. 24.50 which shows an IH in proliferative phase and involution phase.

In contrast, congenital hemangiomas (CHs) are less common than IHs and are fully grown and present at the time of birth. Depending on their type, they can involute quickly, usually within a year, stay the same size, or partially regress.

Vascular malformations are relatively static anomalies and are subclassified as simple malformations, combined malformations, malformations of major named vessels, and malformations associated with other anomalies. Simple malformations include lesions composed of one type of vessel, such as veins, capillaries, or lymphatics. In addition, arteriovenous malformations (AVMs), composed of malformed arteries, veins, and capillaries, are also classified as simple malformations and can be aggressive. There is direct communication between the arteries and veins leading to shunting. See Figs. 24.51 and 24.52.

Combined vascular malformations contain two or more vascular malformations in one. Malformations of major named vessels impact large caliber arteries, veins, or lymphatics. The final classification is vascular malformations associated with other anomalies, including anomalies of the bone, soft tissue, or viscera.

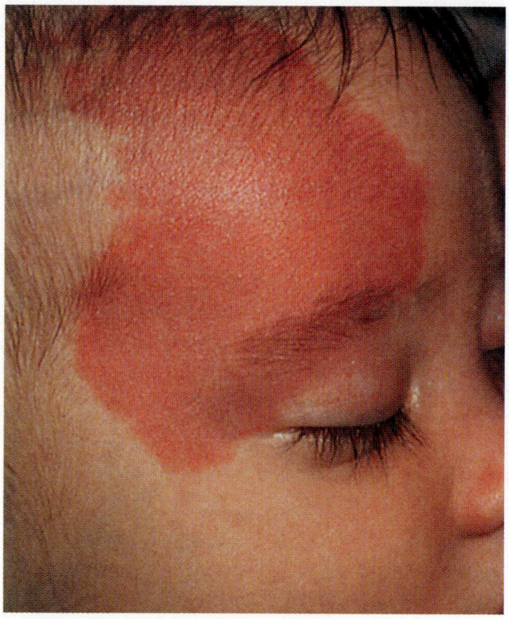

Fig. 24.51 Capillary Malformation. (From Cohen BA: *Atlas of pediatric dermatology*, London, 1993, Wolfe Publishing.)

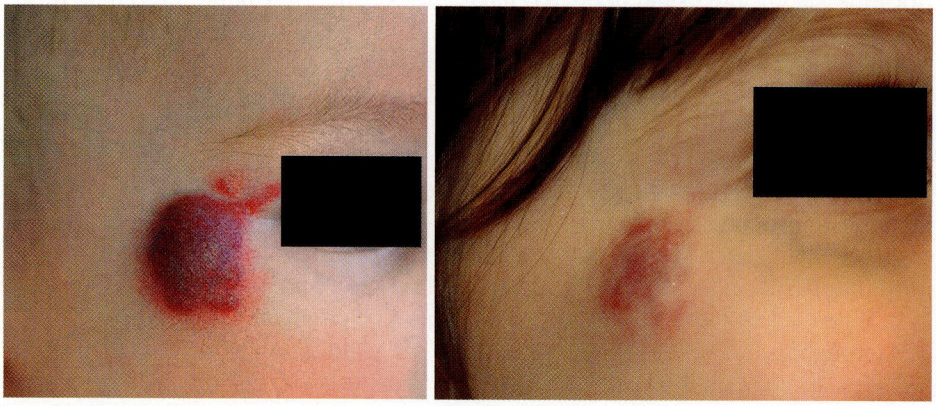

A B

Fig. 24.50 Infantile hemangioma in proliferative phase (A) and involution phase (B). (From *Pediatric Clinics of North America*. Holland, Kristen E, MD; Drolet, Beth A. Published October 1, 2010. Volume 57, Issue 5, Pages 1069–1083. © 2010.)

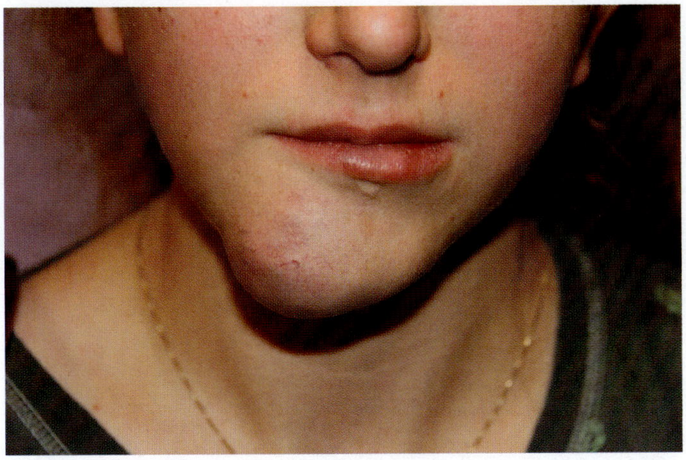

Fig. 24.52 Cutaneous Arteriovenous Malformation on this Child's Chin, Which is a Pulsatile Mass. (From McCormick AA, Grundwaldt LJ: Zitelli and Davis' *atlas of pediatric physical diagnosis*, 2018, pp. 378–393. © 2018.)

Kawasaki Disease

Kawasaki disease (KD), or mucocutaneous lymph node syndrome, is an acute febrile illness of young children. Almost all affected children are younger than 5 years, and most are younger than 3 years. The annual incidence in the United States is estimated to be about 9–20 per 100,000 children less than 5 years of age. The illness may occur more commonly during winter and spring. The cause is unknown, although the seasonal peaks suggest that infectious agents may trigger the inflammatory response in KD. Males are affected more than females, and the overall frequency is highest among Asians. KD is the most frequent cause of acquired heart disease in developed countries.

The histopathologic condition is a vasculitis of medium-sized, extraparenchymal arteries with a predilection to aneurysmal disease of the coronary arteries. Coronary artery lesions occur in <5% of cases of KD, and giant aneurysms in 1%. Although most individuals recover without sequelae, death occurs in <0.5% of patients as a result of coronary arteritis, most commonly in cases with giant aneurysms. Early intervention with intravenous gamma globulin and aspirin has been shown to significantly reduce coronary abnormalities.

The diagnostic criteria for KD are clinical and are as follows:

- Fever for at least 5 days
- Presence of four of the following:
  - Bilateral nonpurulent conjunctival injection (limbic-sparing 90%)
  - Changes in the lips and mucosa of the oropharynx (not discrete oral ulcers or tonsillar exudates)
  - Changes of the extremities (e.g., edema of hand and feet, erythema of palms and soles)
  - Polymorphous exanthem (not bullous or vesicular), desquamation usually starts in perineal region
  - Cervical lymphadenopathy, usually unilateral in the anterior cervical chain, must be nonfluctuant, nontender, and greater than 1.5 cm in size

The fever in KD is high, typically >102.2°F (>39°C) and is abrupt in onset and refractory to antipyretics. It is usually the first sign and lasts for at least 5 days. Within a few days, an irregular, morbilliform, macular eruption develops over the trunk and legs. Palm, sole, and fingertip desquamation occurs 10 to 18 days after the onset of fever; this is one of the most characteristic features of the disease. Desquamation also commonly occurs in the inguinal and perineal area and may precede extremity changes. The conjunctiva becomes injected, and punctate redness of the palate and strawberry tongue (see Fig. 24.39) develop. Peripheral edema and asymmetric cervical lymphadenopathy are seen early in the disease in 75% of patients. Arthritis is present in many cases. Fig. 24.53 shows the many physical exam findings in KD.

Healthcare professionals must also consider a condition referred to as incomplete (atypical) KD when a patient has some of the clinical features of KD but does not meet criteria for diagnosis. In these cases, laboratory tests contribute to the diagnosis of KD, whereas an echocardiogram showing coronary artery aneurysms is confirmatory. Incomplete KD is more common in infants and older children, and they are at greater risk for developing coronary artery lesions.

Conditions to consider in the differential diagnosis of KD include Multisystem Inflammatory Syndrome in Children (MIS-C) appearing after infection with COVID-19, infections caused by Epstein-Barr Virus, measles, adenovirus, enterovirus, Rocky Mountain Spotted Fever, or other conditions such as Stevens-Johnson syndrome.

Exanthematous Diseases

Exanthematous diseases of childhood are extremely common and are mostly caused by viruses. There are now immunizations for many of the classic childhood exanthems. In the early years of the 20th century, pediatricians frequently referred to many childhood diseases by number. *Scarlet fever* and *measles* were numbers one and two, respectively; rubella became known as the third disease; the fourth disease was probably a combination of scarlet fever and rubella and did not represent a distinct entity; the fifth disease was *erythema infectiosum,* and the sixth disease was *roseola.* Other common viral exanthems include *varicella, coxsackie,* and *herpes simplex.* Table 24.9 summarizes these exanthematous diseases of childhood.

Pediatric Murmurs

Heart murmurs are common in the pediatric age group. Some are serious, but many normal preschool children have a short, musical systolic murmur at the lower left sternal border. Tables 24.10 and 24.11 summarize the more common murmurs and associated findings.

Telephone Triage

See Video 24.4.

Healthcare professionals are often asked to provide medical assistance by speaking to patients and their families by means of a telephone conversation. The telephone interview video shows a pediatrician taking a call from a mother seeking guidance about her 3-year-old daughter, who has vomiting and diarrhea.

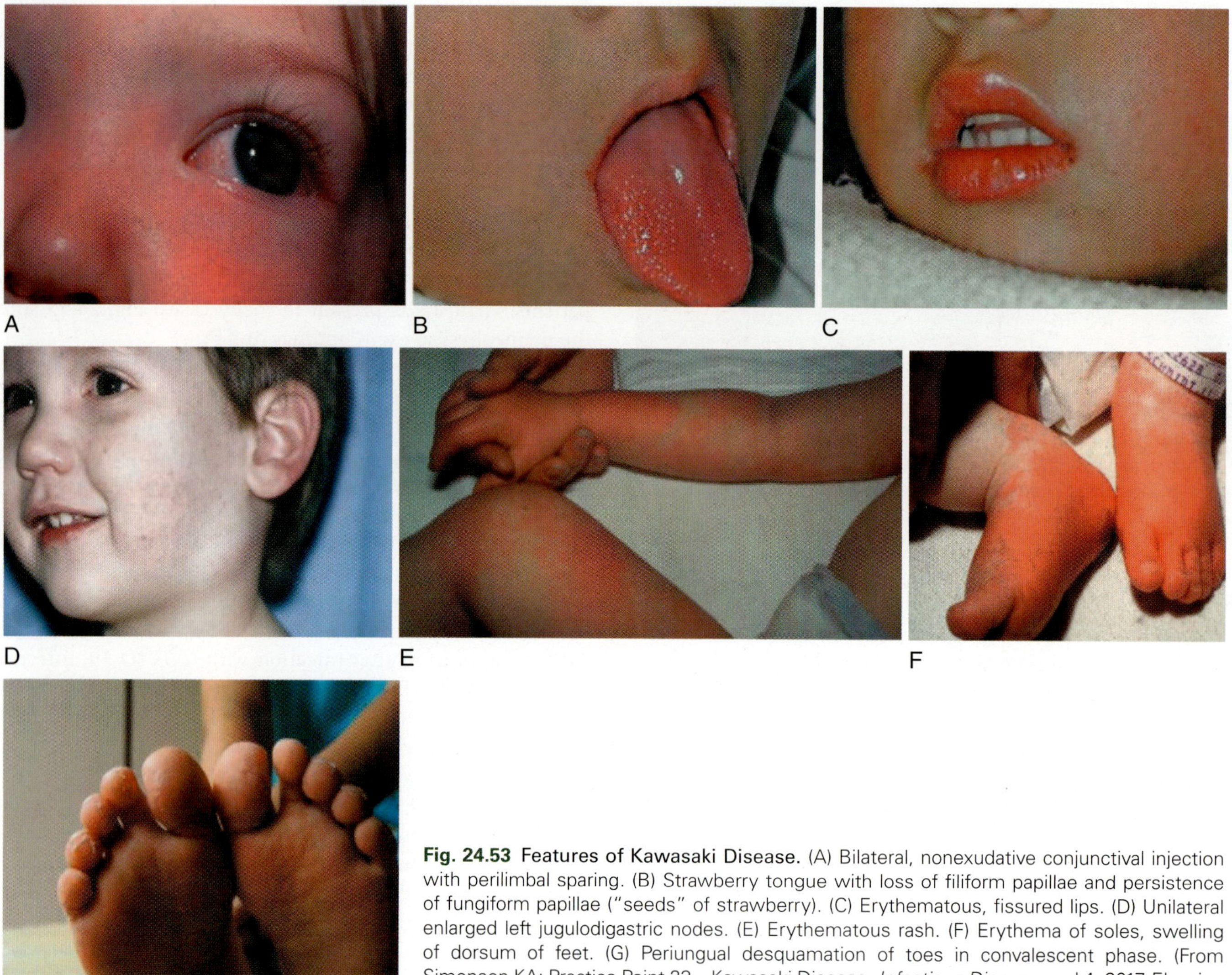

Fig. 24.53 **Features of Kawasaki Disease.** (A) Bilateral, nonexudative conjunctival injection with perilimbal sparing. (B) Strawberry tongue with loss of filiform papillae and persistence of fungiform papillae ("seeds" of strawberry). (C) Erythematous, fissured lips. (D) Unilateral enlarged left jugulodigastric nodes. (E) Erythematous rash. (F) Erythema of soles, swelling of dorsum of feet. (G) Periungual desquamation of toes in convalescent phase. (From Simonsen KA: Practice Point 23—Kawasaki Disease. *Infectious Diseases*, ed 4, 2017, Elsevier, pp. 640–642.e1.)

TABLE 24.9 Exanthematous Diseases of Childhood

Disease	History	Cutaneous Findings	Location and Progression	Other Findings	Comments
Scarlet fever Fig. 24.54	School-age children Acute onset of fever, sore throat Often associated with abdominal pain and/or vomiting, and headache Lack of rhinorrhea and cough Rash appears 12–48 h after onset of symptoms	Multiple, very fine pink or red papules Density of papules give sandpaper texture Known as scarlatiniform rash Blanches with pressure Prominent in skin folds	Starts in groin/axillae Progresses to cover the trunk May see on the face Extremities last, spares palms and soles	Circumoral pallor Strawberry tongue Late desquamation of fingers/toes Linear petechiae in antecubital fossae known as Pastia lines	Caused by exotoxins produced by Group A β-hemolytic strep Less virulent than in the past
Measles (Rubeola) Fig. 24.55	Contact with measles case including via travel, as it is one of the most contagious of all infectious diseases Unimmunized 3–4 days prodromal period with high fever, chills, malaise, headache Cough, coryza, and conjunctivitis develop before the rash in this period	Erythematous maculopapular rash Becomes dense with coalescing of lesions May appear purplish or hemorrhagic As rash fades becomes brown	Starts on the face, scalp, behind ears Spreads quickly from head caudally down body and to extremities	Ill-appearing child Enanthematous lesions called Koplik spots in prodromal period Appear as pinpoint white spots on the buccal mucosa opposite the lower molars	Caused by measles virus Vaccine preventable Main complications are pneumonia and encephalitis

TABLE 24.9 Exanthematous Diseases of Childhood—cont'd

Disease	History	Cutaneous Findings	Location and Progression	Other Findings	Comments
Rubella (German measles) Fig. 24.56	Mild constitutional symptoms with low-grade fever possible Rash may be first sign of disease Adolescents and adults, especially females, may have arthralgia and/or polyarthritis	Rose-/pink-colored maculopapular rash Does not coalesce	Starts on the face and spreads downward Becomes generalized over 24 h Rash lasts a median of 3 days	Lymphadenopathy may precede rash and last a week Posterior auricular and suboccipital nodes most often involved but can be generalized Intraoral Forchheimer spots may be found during prodromal period; appear as diffuse dusky red 1- to 3-mm spots on the buccal mucosa and palate (see Fig. 24.36)	Caused by rubella virus Vaccine preventable Main complication is congenital rubella syndrome
Fifth disease (Erythema infectiosum) Fig. 24.57	Seen in preschool and school-aged children Starts with asymptomatic "slapped cheek" appearance on the face Fever absent or low grade	Erythematous maculopapular, lacy, serpiginous, blanching rash on the trunk and extremities Usually asymptomatic, sometimes pruritic	Starts on trunk, spreads outward Lasts days to weeks or months Intensity waxes and wanes Becomes more prominent with heat exposure (bathing, sunlight)	Intense erythema of cheeks	Caused by parvovirus B19 Mild, self-limited illness in healthy children Can cause aplastic anemia in patients with sickle cell disease Harmful to the fetus in the first trimester of pregnancy
Roseola infantum (Exanthem Subitum) Fig. 24.58	3–5 days of high fevers with no other symptoms Fever breaks abruptly and rash develops Seen in infants and toddlers	Pink, red maculopapular rash	Starts on neck, scalp, and trunk Spreads to face and extremities Resolves quickly in 1–2 days	Erythematous tympanic membranes common Lymphadenopathy is a later finding	Most frequent cause is human herpesvirus 6 (HHV-6) Usually benign self-limited illness, though visits to emergency department common for fever
Chickenpox (Varicella) Fig. 24.59	Prodrome of fever, headache, malaise Highly pruritic rash starts within 24 h	Vesicles on an erythematous base ("dew-drop on a rose petal") Lesions of different stages at development are present at the same time	Crops of vesicles appear over a few days Start as macules, progress to papules, vesicles, and pustules then crusting Starts on trunk, face, centrifugal spread	Monitor for superinfected lesions caused by scratching	Caused by varicella zoster virus Vaccine preventable Teratogenic in 1st trimester Complications include cellulitis, pneumonia, and encephalitis
Hand-foot-mouth disease Fig. 24.60	Typically seen in summer and autumn in young children Starts with mouth or throat pain with refusal to eat Fever may be present Prodrome may include fussiness or gastrointestinal symptoms	Vesicular rash on hands, feet, and buttocks Nonpruritic, nontender lesions	Macular, papular, or vesicular lesions may be present Involves palms, soles Can spread up hands to arms and up foot to legs	Oral lesions start as red macules that progress to vesicles with surrounding erythema, then rupture into superficial ulcers Lesions on tongue, buccal mucosa, and palate	Caused by enteroviruses, most commonly coxsackie A16 and enterovirus A71 Can see oral lesions without skin lesions and vice versa
Herpes simplex gingivostomatitis Fig. 24.61	Prodrome of fever and irritability Acute phase of painful oral lesions lasts 4–9 days and is self-limited Seen in toddlers and school-aged children Occurs any time of the year	In primary infection, can have extensive perioral and intraoral vesicles, pustules, and erosions Gingivae become markedly edematous and erythematous and bleed easily	Oral, perioral, and gingivae Vesicles rupture and become encrusted Desquamation and healing are usually complete in 10–14 days	Cervical and submaxillary lymphadenopathy are common Signs of dehydration due to refusal to drink secondary to pain	Caused by herpes simplex virus type 1 (HSV1) Can recur throughout life as reactivation episodes that are less severe

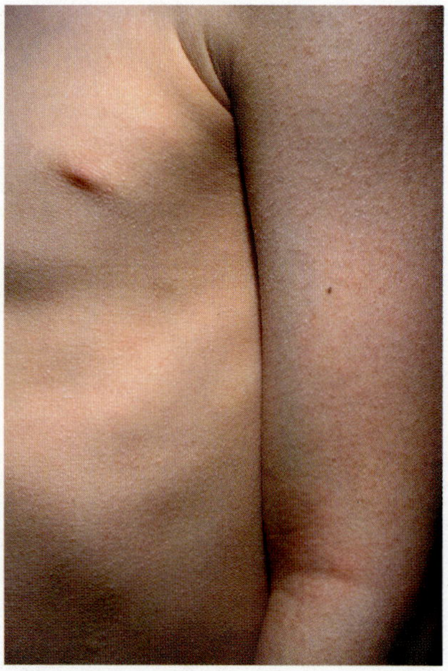

Fig. 24.54 Scarlet Fever. Note the numerous tiny papules giving a sandpaper-like texture to the skin. (From Habif TP: *Clinical dermatology*, 2016, pp. 534–576. © 2016.)

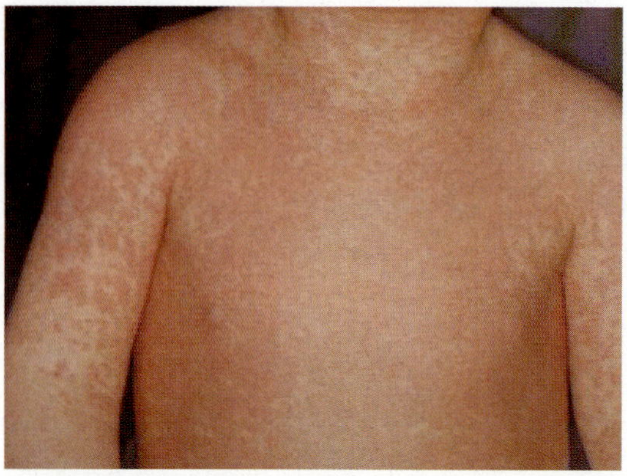

Fig. 24.55 Measles. Note the diffuse red maculopapular rash that coalesces. (From Bryant PA, Sharland M: *Medicine*, 37(12):686–690, 2009. © 2009.)

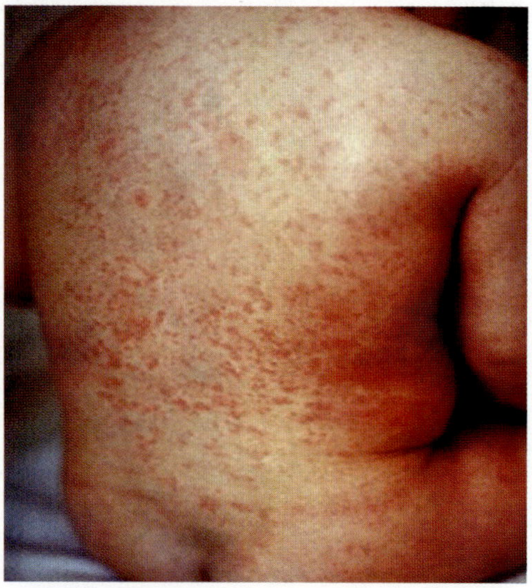

Fig. 24.56 Rubella. Fine pink-reddish maculopapular rash of rubella that does not coalesce. (From the Centers for Disease Control and Prevention Public Health Image Library, ID #: 712.)

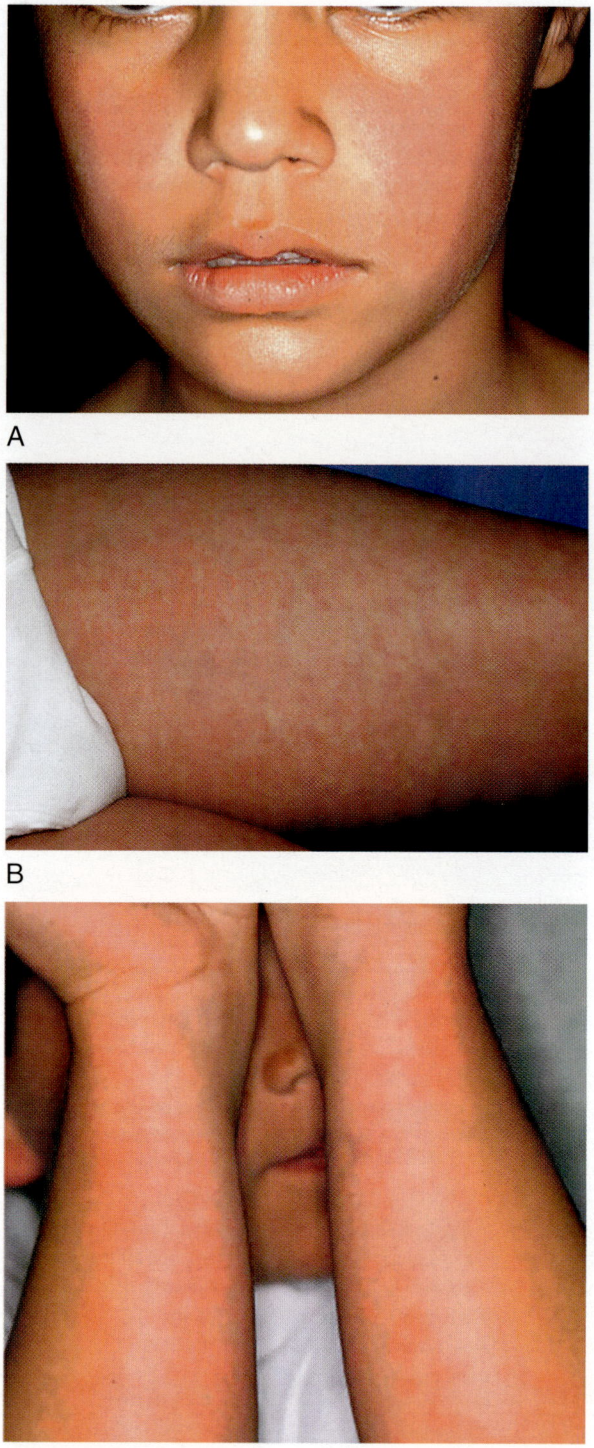

A

B

Fig. 24.57 Fifth Disease. (A) Bright red macular erythema on the cheeks. (B) Lacy, reticulated erythematous eruption on the thigh and (C) on the arms. (A, Courtesy Louis A. Fagola, Jr., MD; B, Courtesy Julie V. Schaffer, MD; C, Courtesy Kalman Watsky, MD. From *Dermatology*. Mancini AJ, Shani-Adir A, Sidbury R, editors: Published January 1, 2018, pp. 1425–1446. © 2018.)

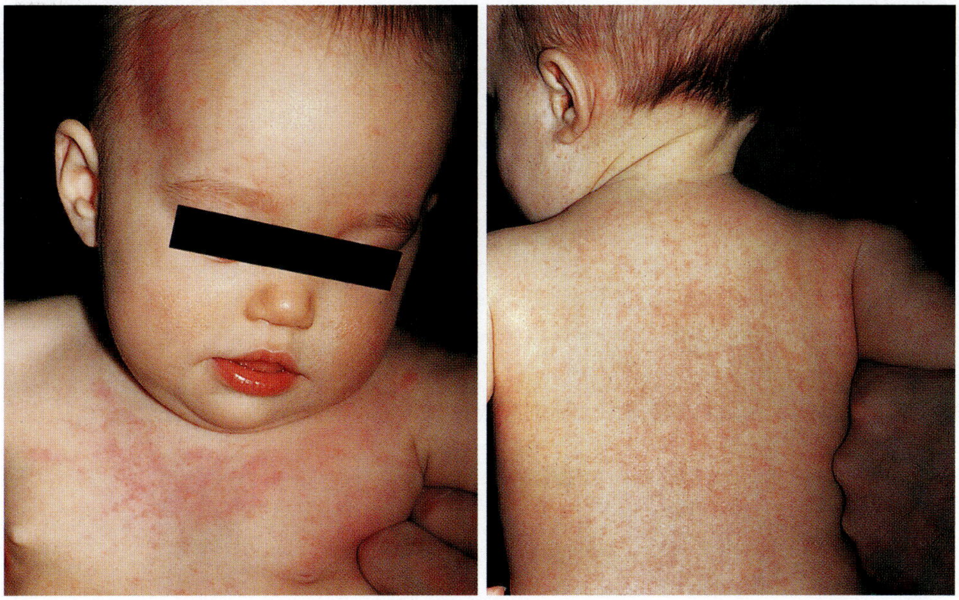

Fig. 24.58 Roseola. Discrete, rose-pink macules. It may be generalized at first or may start centrally and spread centrifugally. Scalp involvement is prominent. (From Michaels MG, Williams JV: *Zitelli and Davis' atlas of pediatric physical diagnosis*, 2018, pp. 455–509. © 2018.)

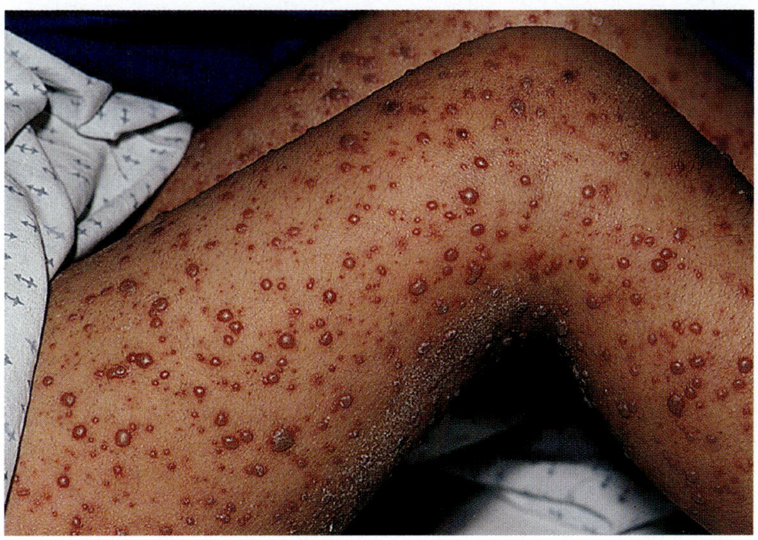

Fig. 24.59 Varicella. Note multiple vesicles and lesions at different stages.

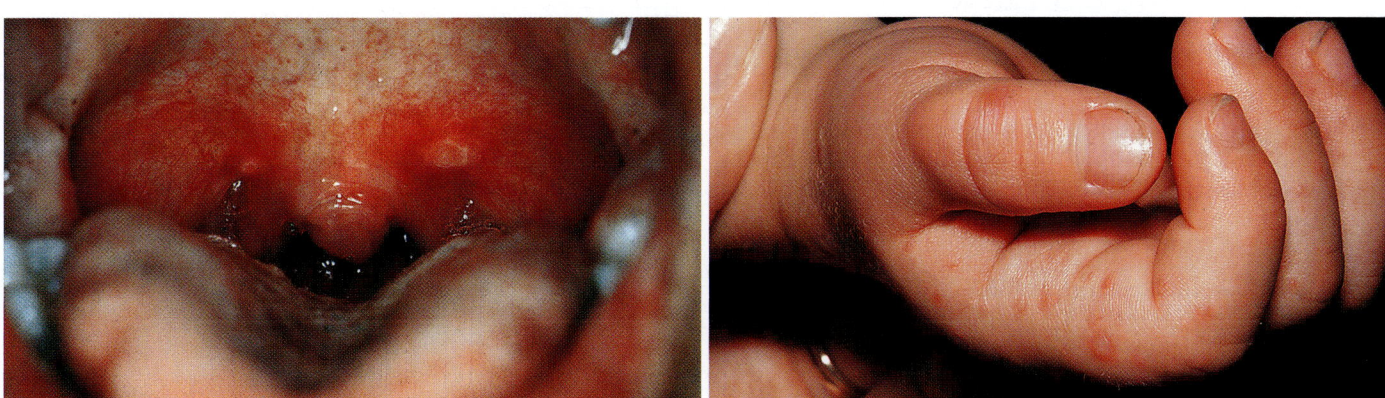

A B

Fig. 24.60 Coxsackie. (A) Shallow, yellow ulcers surrounded by red halos on the soft palate. Thick-walled, gray vesicles on an erythematous base on the palmar, plantar, and interdigital surfaces of the hands (B) and feet

Continued

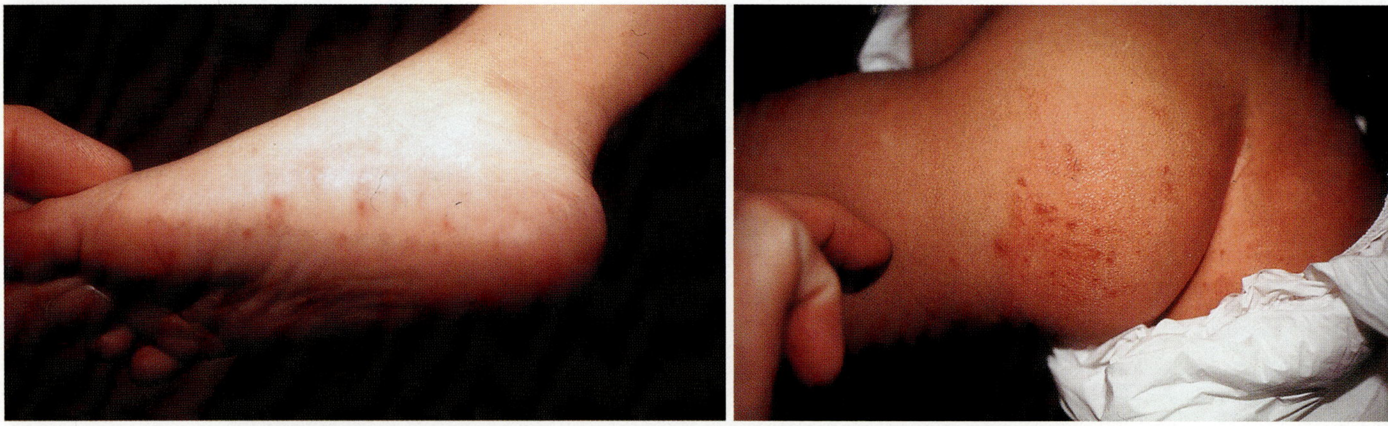

C D

Fig. 24.60, cont'd (C) and the buttocks (D). (From Michaels MG, Williams JV: Zitelli and Davis' *atlas of pediatric physical diagnosis*, 2018, pp. 455–509. © 2018.)

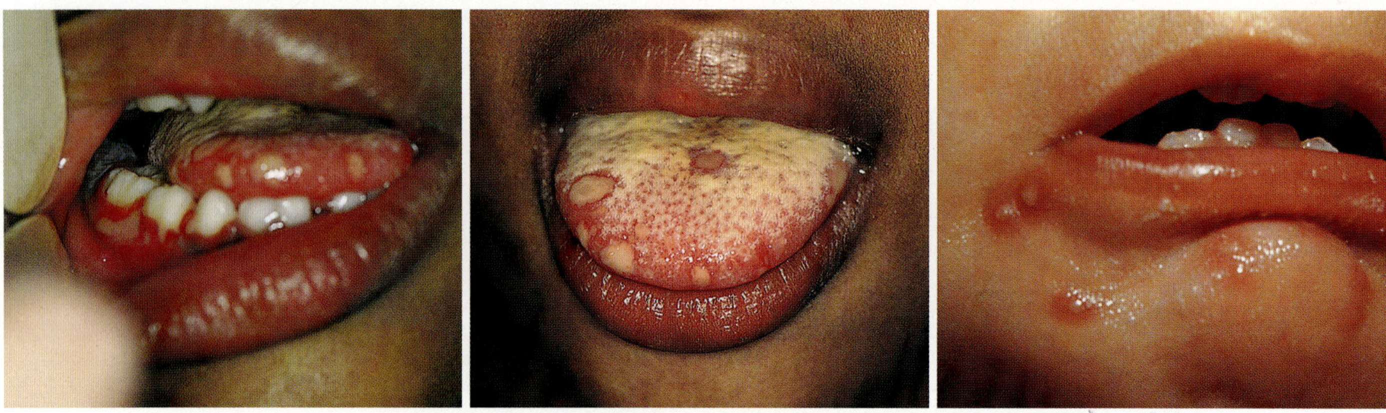

A B C

Fig. 24.61 Herpetic Gingivostomatitis. (A) Discrete mucosal ulcerations and diffuse gingival erythema, edema, and friability. (B) Numerous yellow ulcerations with thin red halos are seen on the patient's tongue as well. (C) Perioral thick-walled vesicles on an erythematous base. (From Michaels MG, Williams JV: Zitelli and Davis' *atlas of pediatric physical diagnosis*, 2018, pp. 455–509. © 2018.)

SAMPLE DOCUMENTATION OF A NEWBORN'S HISTORY AND PHYSICAL EXAM[p]

History

The patient is a 3610 g male infant born via uncomplicated NSVD on 1/1/01 at 1:00 a.m. at 38 weeks 6 days gestation to a 27-year-old G3 P1011 mother with a history of mild asthma. Her prenatal history is significant for gestational diabetes, controlled by diet. The mother is GBS+, had no intrapartum fever, and received penicillin ×3 doses prior to delivery. Her other prenatal lab results were normal, including HepBSAg-, HCV-, HIV-, Measles immune, Rubella immune, Varicella immune, GC and CT-, rapid plasma regain (RPR)-; HgbAA, Pb <1, blood type A+. She had normal ultrasounds. NIPS low risk. Rupture of membranes was 1 hour before delivery, and the fluid was clear. The baby's Apgar scores were 9 and 9.

The mother lives with her husband and 3-year-old son in an apartment in good condition and works as a teacher. She smoked cigarettes until her first pregnancy and denies any other substance use. The baby breastfed in the delivery room.

[p]CT, Chlamydia; GBS, group B strep; GC, gonorrhea; G3P1001, gravida3 para1001; HCV, hepatitis C virus; HepBSAg, hepatitis B surface antigen; HIV, human immunodeficiency virus; NIPS, noninvasive prenatal screening; NSVD, normal spontaneous vaginal delivery; Pb, lead; RPR, rapid plasma reagin.

Physical Exam

General: Well-appearing newborn male infant in no acute distress; no dysmorphic features

Weight 3610 gm (70th percentile)

Length 50 cm (52th percentile)
Head circumference 35 cm (66th percentile)

Vital signs: Temp 98.2°F Pulse: 140 Resp: 40 O_2Sat: 98%

HENT: Normocephalic, anterior fontanel open and flat, posterior fontanel open and flat. Auditory canals normal. Palate intact. Mucous membranes moist. Oropharynx free of lesions.

Eyes: No ptosis, conjunctiva clear, PERRL. Red reflexes present bilaterally.

Neck: Supple, FROM, no webbing or masses noted. No clavicular crepitus.

Cardiovascular: Regular rate and rhythm, normal S1 S2, no murmur. Femoral pulses are symmetrical and of normal intensity.

Pulmonary/Chest: Lungs clear to auscultation, no rhonchi, rales, wheezing.

Abdominal: Soft, +BS, Non-tender, non-distended without masses or hepatosplenomegaly. 3 vessel umbilical cord.

Genitourinary: Normal male genitalia, urethral meatus at tip of glans, testicles descended bilaterally, anus normally placed.

Musculoskeletal: No deformities noted. Full ROM in all major joints. Hips stable. Negative Ortolani and Barlow. Spine straight. No sacral dimples, tufts, or deformities.

Skin: Skin is intact without lesions or rashes. No jaundice.

Neurological: Alert, intact suck, grasp, and Moro reflexes, normal muscle tone throughout, face and movements of extremities are symmetrical.

TABLE 24.10 Characteristics of Innocent Heart Murmurs

Type	Description	Age at Detection	Can Sound Like
Aortic systolic murmur	Systolic ejection murmur best heard over the aortic valve	Older childhood into adulthood	—
Mammary artery souffle[a]	High-pitched systolic murmur that can extend into diastole; best heard along the anterior chest wall over the breast	Rare in adolescence	Arteriovenous anastomoses or patent ductus arteriosus
Peripheral pulmonary stenosis	Grade 1 or 2, low-pitched, early- to mid-systolic ejection murmur heard over axilla or back	<1 year	Pulmonary artery stenosis or normal breath sounds
Pulmonary flow murmur	Grade 2 or 3, crescendo-decrescendo, early- to mid-systolic murmur peaking in mid-systole; best heard at the left sternal border between the second and third intercostal spaces; characterized by a rough, dissonant quality; loudest when patient is supine and decreases when patient is upright and holding breath	All	Atrial septal defect or pulmonary valve stenosis
Still murmur	Grade 1 to 3, early systolic murmur; low to medium pitch with a vibratory or musical quality; best heard at lower left sternal border; loudest when patient is supine and decreases when patient stands	Infancy to adolescence, often 2 to 6 years	Ventricular septal defect or hypertrophic cardiomyopathy
Supraclavicular/ brachiocephalic systolic murmur	Brief, low-pitched, crescendo-decrescendo murmur heard in the first two-thirds of systole; best heard above clavicles; radiates to neck; diminishes when patient hyperextends shoulders	Childhood to young adulthood	Bicuspid/stenotic aortic valve, pulmonary valve stenosis, or coarctation of the aorta
Venous hum	Grade 1 to 6 continuous murmur; accentuated in diastole; has a whining, roaring, or whirring quality; best heard over low anterior neck, lateral to the sternocleidomastoid; louder on right; resolves or changes when patient is supine	3 to 8 years	Cervical arteriovenous fistulas or patent ductus arteriosus

[a]Mammary artery souffle murmur is caused by blood flow in the arteries and veins leading to and from the breasts.
Frank JE, Jacobe KM: Evaluation and management of heart murmurs in children, *Am Fam Physician* 84(7):793–800, 2011.

TABLE 24.11 Prevalence and Characteristics of Pathologic Heart Murmurs

Type of Structural Heart Lesion	Prevalence Among Children With Congenital Heart Disease (%)	Symptoms and Clinical Course	Characteristics
Ventricular septal defect	20 to 25	Small defects: usually asymptomatic Medium or large defects: CHF, symptoms of bronchial obstruction, frequent respiratory infections	Small defects: loud holosystolic murmur at LLSB (may not last throughout systole if defect is very small) Medium and large defects: increased right-to-left ventricular impulses; thrill at LLSB; split or loud single S_2; holosystolic murmur at LLSB without radiation; grade 2 to 5; may also hear a grade 1 or 2 mid-diastolic rumble

Continued

TABLE 24.11 **Prevalence and Characteristics of Pathologic Heart Murmurs—cont'd**

Type of Structural Heart Lesion	Prevalence Among Children With Congenital Heart Disease (%)	Symptoms and Clinical Course	Characteristics
Atrial septal defect	8 to 13	Usually asymptomatic and incidentally found on physical examination or echocardiography; large defects can be present in infants with CHF	Grade 2 or 3 systolic ejection murmur best heard at ULSB; wide split fixed S_2; absent thrill; may have a grade 1 or 2 diastolic flow rumble at LLSB
Patent ductus arteriosus	6 to 11	May be asymptomatic; can cause easy fatigue, CHF, and respiratory symptoms	Continuous murmur (grade 1 to 5) in ULSB (crescendo in systole and decrescendo into diastole); normal S_1; S_2 may be "buried" in the murmur; thrill or hyperdynamic left ventricular impulse may be present
Tetralogy of Fallot	10	Onset depends on severity of pulmonary stenosis; cyanosis may appear in infancy (2 to 6 months of age) or in childhood; other symptoms include hypercyanotic spells or decreased exercise tolerance	Central cyanosis; clubbing of nail beds; grade 3 or 4 long systolic ejection murmur heard at ULSB; may have holosystolic murmur at LLSB; systolic thrill at ULSB; normal to slightly increased S_1; single S_2
Pulmonary stenosis	7.5 to 9	Usually asymptomatic but may have symptoms secondary to pulmonary congestion	Systolic ejection murmur (grade 2 to 5); heard best at ULSB radiating to infraclavicular regions, axillae, and back; normal or loud S_1; variable S_2; systolic ejection click may be heard at left sternal border and may vary with respiration
Coarctation of the aorta	5.1 to 8.1	Newborns and infants may present with CHF; older children are usually asymptomatic or may have leg pain or weakness	Systolic ejection murmur best heard over interscapular region; normal S_1 and S_2; decreased or delayed femoral pulse; may have increased left ventricular impulse
Aortic stenosis	5 to 6	Usually asymptomatic; symptoms may include dyspnea, easy fatigue, chest pain, or syncope; newborns and infants may present with CHF	Systolic ejection murmur (grade 2 to 5) best heard at upper right sternal border with radiation to carotid arteries; left ventricular heave; thrill at ULSB or suprasternal notch
Transposition of the great arteries	5	Variable presentation depending on type; may include cyanosis or CHF in first week of life	Cyanosis; clubbing of nail beds; single S_2; murmur may be absent or grade 1 or 2 nonspecific systolic ejection murmur; may have a grade 3 or 4 holosystolic murmur at LLSB and mid-diastolic murmur at apex
Total anomalous pulmonary venous connection	2 to 3	Onset of CHF at 4 to 6 weeks of age	Grade 2 or 3 systolic ejection murmur at ULSB; grade 1 or 2 mid-diastolic flow rumble at LLSB; wide split fixed S_2
Tricuspid atresia	1.4	Early-onset cyanosis or CHF within the first month of life	Cyanosis; clubbing of nail beds; normal pulses; single S_2; holosystolic murmur at LLSB or midsternal border; murmur may be absent; mid- diastolic flow murmur at apex may be present
Hypoplastic left heart syndrome	Rare	May be asymptomatic at birth, with cyanosis and CHF developing with duct closure	Hyperdynamic precordium; single S_2; nonspecific grade 1 or 2 systolic ejection murmur along left sternal border
Truncus arteriosus	Rare	Onset of CHF in first few weeks of life; minimal cyanosis	Increased cardiac impulses; holosystolic murmur (ventricular septal defect); mid-diastolic rumble

CHF, Congestive heart failure; *LLSB*, lower left sternal border; *ULSB*, upper left sternal border.
Frank JE, Jacobe KM: Evaluation and management of heart murmurs in children, *Am Fam Physician* 84(7):793–800, 2011.

REVIEW QUESTIONS

1. What are unique considerations of the pediatric physical examination?

A. The power of observation cannot be overemphasized
B. The approach and sequence of the pediatric exam may need to be altered
C. Normal ranges for vital signs varies by age
D. Some physical exam maneuvers or findings are only found in children
E. All of the above

2. All of the below signs are included in the initial assessment of a newborn, EXCEPT:

A. Color
B. Muscle tone
C. Reflex irritability
D. Blood pressure
E. Respiratory effort

3. **Characteristics of *caput succedaneum* include all of the following, EXCEPT:**
   A. Swelling over the vertex of the skull
   B. Swelling due to subperiosteal hemorrhage limited to one cranial bone
   C. Swelling resolves in the first few days of life
   D. Swelling crosses the suture lines
   E. Swelling that is related to the birth process during a vertex delivery
4. **How do you elicit the Galant reflex in a neonate?**
   A. Place the examiner's thumb on the plantar surface of the foot directly under the toes
   B. Stroke the corner of the infant's mouth or cheek
   C. Stroke one side of the back along a paravertebral line 2 to 3 cm from the midline going from the shoulder to the buttocks
   D. Support the infant's body in the right hand and support the head with the left hand. The head is suddenly allowed to drop a few centimeters, with immediate resupport by the examiner's hand
   E. Allow the dorsum of one of the infant's feet to touch the undersurface of a tabletop lightly
5. **What physical exam maneuvers help to detect developmental dysplasia of the hips?**
   A. Ortolani
   B. Barlow
   C. Galeazzi
   D. Klisic
   E. All of the above
6. **Tanner sex maturity ratings are based on:**
   A. Growth of pubic hair
   B. Development of the penis, testes, and scrotum
   C. Development of breasts
   D. All of the above
   E. None of the above
7. **Which locations of bruises are suggestive of abuse in children less than or equal to 4 years of age?**
   A. Ear
   B. Neck
   C. Torso
   D. All of the above
   E. None of the above
8. **The following are diagnostic criteria for Kawasaki disease, EXCEPT:**
   A. Bilateral nonpurulent conjunctival injection
   B. Changes in the lips and mucosa of the oropharynx
   C. Edema of hand and feet, erythema of palms and soles
   D. Polymorphous exanthem
   E. Cervical lymphadenopathy smaller than 1.5 cm in size
9. **What are the cutaneous findings for scarlet fever?**
   A. Erythematous maculopapular rash. Becomes dense with coalescing lesions. May appear purplish or hemorrhagic. As rash fades, it becomes brown.
   B. Multiple, very fine pink or red papules. Density of papules gives sandpaper texture. Blanches with pressure. Prominent in skin folds.
   C. Rose-/pink-colored maculopapular rash. Does not coalesce.
   D. Erythematous maculopapular, lacy, serpiginous, blanching rash on the trunk and extremities. Usually asymptomatic, sometimes pruritic.
   E. Vesicular rash on hands, feet, and buttocks. Nonpruritic, nontender lesions.
10. **What are the characteristics of a murmur caused by a small ventricular septal defect?**
   A. Systolic ejection murmur heard best at left upper sternal border radiating to infraclavicular regions, axillae, and back
   B. Systolic ejection murmur best heard over interscapular region
   C. Systolic ejection murmur best heard at right upper sternal border with radiation to carotid arteries
   D. Loud holosystolic murmur at left lower sternal border
   E. Continuous murmur in left upper sternal border

REFERENCES

Available online.

BIBLIOGRAPHY

Available online.

25

The Geriatric Patient

Mark H. Swartz

To care for those who once cared for us is one of the highest honors.

Tia Walker (1970–current)

VIDEOS

Video 25.1 Interviewing a patient with a cognitive impairment
Video 25.2 Discussing advance directives
Also, see
Video 21.1 Assessing mental status

GENERAL CONSIDERATIONS

Every day, 10,000 people in the United States reach the age of 65. This means that seven people officially become geriatric patients every minute. As we move into the 2030s, the numbers are expected to continue rising due to the aging Baby Boomer generation. This phenomenon is known as "The Silver Tsunami," and it has a significant impact on the healthcare industry in the United States.[1] According to the Social Security Administration's Cohort Life Tables,[2] people who are 40 years old today will likely live to be 80 years old, and females are more likely than males to live to celebrate a 100th birthday. Geriatric patients in the United States use more than one-third of all healthcare services, and healthcare professionals spend over half of their time caring for them. The American Geriatrics Society estimates that approximately 30% of this population requires a geriatrician's care. However, there is a national shortage of healthcare professionals trained in this medical subspecialty. To care for the 12 million older adults in the country, about 17,000 geriatricians are needed. Presently, there are only around 7500 practicing board-certified geriatricians in the United States. The current life expectancy in the United States is 76.1 years for males and 79.5 years for females. When one combines this lack of access to healthcare professionals for our frailest patients with the need for healthcare access and understanding for the many older adults who are aging more successfully, it is imperative that all healthcare professionals understand the basic history and physical exam of the older adult patient and the important ways that this assessment differs from younger patients.

THE GERIATRIC ASSESSMENT

A comprehensive geriatric evaluation includes a geriatric assessment, which goes beyond the traditional history and physical examination. It involves evaluating a patient's functional ability, physical health, cognitive status, mental health, and socioeconomic circumstances, with the goal of improving the patient's overall quality of life and achieving patient-centered care. The evaluation is conducted using a multidisciplinary approach and can be performed in a healthcare professional's office. A *comprehensive geriatrics assessment* is usually done at the specialist level, either in the outpatient office of a geriatrics healthcare professional or in the inpatient hospital setting as a consultative service. Parts of the evaluation are sometimes administered by different members of the patient's healthcare team, including physical and occupational therapists, social workers, dieticians, pharmacists, and nurses. Assessments may involve a range of healthcare professionals, including audiologists, dentists, podiatrists, and opticians. Conducting a comprehensive geriatric assessment in a busy outpatient setting can be challenging, therefore some healthcare professionals opt for a "rolling" assessment. This approach involves dividing the assessment into different parts and conducting them over multiple visits.

The comprehensive geriatric assessment[3] is a multidisciplinary approach to identifying medical, functional, and psychosocial problems in seniors, and the results are used to develop an individual treatment plan to maximize function, health, and quality of life. Not all patients, however, will benefit from this tool, as some patients are too frail to benefit or, conversely, not frail enough.[4] There are no validated criteria to determine which patients will clearly benefit from the assessment, but most programs target the following criteria[5]:

- Age
- Medical comorbidities (e.g., cancer, chronic obstructive pulmonary disease [COPD], heart failure)
- Psychosocial disorders (e.g., depression, social isolation)
- Specific geriatric conditions or syndromes. Geriatric syndromes are multifactorial problems frequently seen in older adults. This category includes cognitive impairment from dementia or delirium, incontinence, malnutrition, falls, gait disorders, pressure ulcers, fatigue, dizziness, sleep problems, and sensory disorders.
- Previous or predicted high healthcare utilization (e.g., after multiple recent admissions to the hospital or before a planned hospitalization)

- Change in living situation. Many seniors face changes in their living situation as part of transitions in care. This may be when a patient leaves a hospital setting to pursue inpatient rehab or moves from living at home independently to an assisted living setting.

CORE COMPONENTS OF A COMPREHENSIVE GERIATRICS ASSESSMENT

The following list outlines some of the most commonly used parts of a geriatric patient assessment. However, it's worth noting that this list is not exhaustive. Depending on the multidisciplinary components of the healthcare site, other tests may be included in the assessment process. These might include visual and hearing testing, an evaluation of spiritual support, or even a driver safety assessment.

Functional Capacity Assessment

The measurement of functional status is crucial in geriatric medicine as it assesses an individual's ability to perform essential daily activities, commonly referred to as *activities of daily living* (ADL). These activities are divided into three groups:

- **Self-care ADLs** include dressing, bathing, transferring from bed to chair, toileting, grooming, and feeding oneself.
- **Instrumental ADLs** include meal preparation, managing finances, using the phone, taking medications, doing housework, shopping, and managing transportation.
- **Mobility ADLs** specifically look at walking from room to room, climbing stairs, and walking outdoors.

Assessing the functional capacity of a patient involves exploring whether they are able to perform certain activities independently or if there have been any recent changes in how these activities are carried out. A decline in ADL function in an older adult can indicate that a change in living situation may be necessary. This change may involve obtaining in-home help, pursuing rehabilitation efforts, or even moving to a facility that can provide the required care. Bathing is usually the ADL most associated with disability and is often the main reason why older adults are referred to home care services.

There is a physical testing component involved in examining the functional status of geriatric patients. It is important to evaluate the usage of any assistive devices, such as canes and walkers, and observe the patient while they walk and use these devices. This observation can provide valuable insights. For instance, some patients may use a walker that once belonged to their spouse because they require additional physical support, and the device was already available in their home. When medical equipment is not used properly, it may be because the patient is using the wrong device for their specific problem. The device may often not be adjusted to the appropriate height requirements. However, these concerns can be easily addressed and corrected during the patient encounter. To determine the correct height of a cane, ask the patient to stand with their arms relaxed at their side. The top of the cane should be at the crease of their wrist. Physical therapists are extremely helpful in advising on the right appliance and fit. For example, a patient who has issues with balance and needs more support with standing probably should not use a rollator.[a] This patient would likely benefit more from a standard walker.

An important performance-based test is the "*Timed Get Up and Go Test.*" To perform this test, the patient rises from a chair, walks 10 feet, turns back to the chair, turns again, and sits down. Completing this sequence in less than 10 seconds would translate to normal function. Patients who take longer than 20 seconds to complete this sequence require further evaluation and may be at risk for a decline in their overall ADLs. Performing this test in the office is easy, allowing healthcare professionals to watch their patients walk. This activity alone is very powerful. Very often, in a busy outpatient practice, patients are seated in an exam room waiting for their healthcare professional to arrive for their appointment, making it possible for a professional to never see how their patient ambulates. This would be a critical miss in geriatrics. Assessing gait leads to an important database of information ranging from fall risk to disease diagnosis. For example, Parkinson disease patients have a very typical gait. They walk with small shuffling steps, and there may be a generalized slowness. Many ambulate with short steps that eventually become faster. This is called a "*festinating gait.*"

Other easy-to-incorporate office-based assessments include simply asking your patient to rise from a seated position with their arms folded across their chest, thus not allowing the patient to use their arms for support in the process. This allows the healthcare professional evaluator to assess weakness at the hip and knee flexor joints and quadriceps strength. This is also highly predictive of future disability and offers a clear place to intervene with physical therapy for improvement in function. **The single strongest predictor of future disability and death, however, is gait speed.** It has even been proposed as a possible geriatric vital sign. A patient who can walk 50 feet in a hallway in less than 20 seconds would have no impairment.[6] It is crucial to inquire whether the patient has experienced any falls in the past year and gather detailed information about these incidents. It has been reported that almost one-third of older adults living in the community fall every year. To prevent future falls, it is important to identify the reasons behind the occurrences and take necessary measures to modify the surrounding circumstances. Exercise, physical therapy, and vitamin D supplementation have been linked to reducing the risk of falls in patients aged 65 and above.

Nutritional Assessment

It is recommended to measure the weight of the patient during every visit. If there is an unintentional loss of more than 5% of body weight within 6 months or if the BMI is less than 20, further investigation is necessary. Weight loss may be a sign of underlying malignancy in older patients, but there are also several other reasons for unintentional weight loss that can be

[a]A rollator is an ambulatory device that consists of a frame with three or four large wheels, handlebars, and a built-in seat, which allows the user to stop and rest when needed.

treated. The "*Meals on Wheels*" mnemonic is an easy way to remember these factors, which are often multifactorial[7,8]:

- **M:** Medication effects
- **E:** Emotional problems, especially depression
- **A:** Anorexia nervosa, alcoholism
- **L:** Late-life paranoia
- **S:** Swallowing disorders
- **O:** Oral factors (e.g., poor fitting dentures and caries)
- **N:** No money
- **W:** Wandering and other dementia-related behaviors
- **H:** Hyper- or hypothyroidism, hyperparathyroidism, and hypoadrenalism
- **E:** Enteric problems
- **E:** Eating problems (inability to feed oneself)
- **L:** Low salt/cholesterol diet restriction effect
- **S:** Social problems (isolation, unable to access preferred foods) and stones

Cognitive Assessment

Among Americans, 6.7 million are living with Alzheimer disease. This number is expected to grow to 13.8 million by 2060, barring the development of medical breakthroughs to prevent, slow, or cure Alzheimer disease. In fact, every 65 seconds, someone in the United States develops the disease. The number of people living with the disease doubles every 5 years beyond age 65. The vast majority of these patients are over the age of 65 years. Essentially, 1 in every 10 people over the age of 65 years in the United States has Alzheimer dementia. The prevalence increases with increasing age, affecting a third of the patients over the age of 85.[9] Alzheimer dementia is the most common type of dementia. When one considers the additive effects of other common dementias (e.g., vascular dementia, Parkinson disease—related dementia, and Lewy body dementia), along with some of the less common etiologies, the prevalence approaches 40% to 50% of the population at age 90. In 2020 and 2021, when COVID-19 entered the ranks of the top 10 causes of death, Alzheimer disease was the seventh-leading cause of death. Total payments in 2023 for healthcare, long-term care, and hospice services for people aged 65 and older with dementia were more than $345 billion in the United States.

Screening for cognitive compromise is essential. Patients with cognitive impairment are at increased risk for adverse outcomes, including delirium, accidents, medication nonadherence, and worsening disability. Early detection of dementia and mild cognitive impairment (MCI) is important because early treatment initiation is beneficial to patients. Additionally, there are many ways that healthcare professionals can intervene to improve the quality of life, safety, and support for these patients.

See Video 21.1.

There are quite a few validated tools available to make a quick office-based assessment:

The Mini-Cog Assessment Instrument for Dementia

There are two parts to this assessment: the *three-item word recall* and the *clock-drawing test*. The *three-item word recall test* is the best way to screen for cognitive impairment. The examiner will say three words to the patient and ask them to repeat them. The patient will then be asked to recall the three words after a minute has passed.

The *clock-drawing test* looks specifically at visual-spatial and executive function skills. The patient will be asked to draw a clock face, put all the numbers in the right place, and draw the hour and minute hands at either 2:50 or 11:10.

The Mini-Cog Assessment is easy to give, can be given by any healthcare team member, and is not dependent on the patient's level of education or native language. It only takes about 3 minutes to complete. Step-by-step instructions on administering and scoring this test are available at https://mini-cog.com.

Montreal Cognitive Assessment

The Montreal Cognitive Assessment (MoCA)[10] was developed as a screen to better detect MCI, which previously was harder to detect using available assessment tools. In fact, the MoCA is more sensitive for detecting MCI and Alzheimer disease than the Mini-Mental Status Examination (MMSE). It is a 12-item test with a maximum score of 30 and takes about 10 minutes to administer. Any member of the healthcare team can administer it. It tests recall, orientation, executive function, verbal fluency, orientation, attention, naming, repetition, abstraction, and visuospatial skills. The full version is available at www.mocatest.org.

Saint Louis University Mental Status Examination

The Saint Louis University Mental Status Examination (SLUMS)[11] is another test developed to screen for MCI and dementia. Its sensitivity and specificity are similar to the MMSE overall, but it appears that the SLUMS is better at picking up mild neurocognitive disease than the MMSE is. The SLUMS is an 11-item test with a 30-point score possibility. It looks at orientation, recall, naming, attention, calculation, and executive function. It takes 7 minutes to administer and can be administered by other healthcare team members. It has been translated into many languages and is available at https://www.slu.edu/medicine/internal-medicine/geriatric-medicine/aging-successfully/assessment-tools/mental-status-exam.php.

Folstein Mini-Mental Status Examination

This test was the first test of its kind for cognitive impairment. It is dependent on the level of education achieved, age, and race. It is a 19-item test with a score of up to 30 points. The test examines orientation, registration, naming, visuospatial skills, recall, attention, language, and the ability to carry out a three-step command. The MMSE takes about 10 minutes to administer and can be administered by other healthcare team members. It is available only by purchase at www.minimental.com.

Animal-Naming Test

This is a quick office-based screen to look at executive function, a skill that is often the first to be affected by cognitive change, and often in subtle below-the-radar ways. To perform the animal-naming test, the healthcare professional asks the patient to name as many four-legged animals as possible in 1 minute's time. A normal result is the ability to name more than 21 animals in 1 minute. Patients who name less than 15 are likely to be cognitively impaired and are 20 times more likely to have Alzheimer disease when compared to a patient who is able to name more than 20 animals in the same amount of time.[12]

See Videos 21.1.

Psychological Assessment

Depression is not a normal part of aging. However, it is estimated that 1 in 10 older adults seen in the primary care setting would meet the criteria for major depressive disorder. Many others would present with more subclinical findings: low energy, insomnia, or somatic concerns. The presence of even subclinical depression increases the risk of disability and declining function. Concurrent depression makes it harder for seniors to recover from acute illness over time. Untreated depression is also associated with leads to social, cognitive, and quality of life decline, as well as increased healthcare utilization and suicide.[13] Screening for depression should be part of any office-based geriatrics assessment. In a busy office setting, taking the time to ask only one screening question—"Do you often feel sad or depressed?"—can, at the very least, identify patients who would need further evaluation. The two most common office-based screening tools are the *Geriatric Depression Scale* (GDS) and the *Patient Health Questionnaire* (PHQ). The GDS exists in long (30-question) and short (15-question) forms. Both versions are assessment tools only and are not meant to substitute for a diagnostic interview and further evaluation. The GDS does not screen for suicidality. Both forms are available and translated into many languages at https://web.stanford.edu/~yesavage/GDS.html. The PHQ-2[14] is a two-question version of the PHQ. It asks about feelings of depression and hopelessness as well as the ability to gain pleasure from or be interested in doing things over this time period. It is scored on a 0- to 6-point scale. A score of 3 or higher should prompt further evaluation with the PHQ-9 scale. The PHQ-9 is a valid and reliable tool to measure the severity of depression, and it has the advantage of being able to be self-administered.[15]

Medication Reconciliation

Older adults in America use one-third of all of the drugs prescribed in the country. The average older adult takes at least five prescription medications.[16] Seniors are also high utilizers of supplements, complementary alternative medicine, and other over-the-counter preparations. Medication reconciliation should be performed at every visit with an older adult patient and at every transition point in care. It is not uncommon to uncover errors of duplication or omission as well as significant adverse medication interactions. The easiest way to do this is through a "brown bag" review: simply ask the patient to bring everything they are taking to the office in a brown bag. Patient- or family-prepared medication lists are also helpful, but you may need to ask specifically about supplements and over-the-counter preparations, as many patients will leave these off a "traditional" medication list.

See Video 25.1.

Social Assessment

Several elements to a social assessment are important to consider in an initial or follow-up encounter with an older adult. Here are some of those elements and some sample questions that prompt a deeper exploration:

- **Cultural background:** Are there cultural issues involved in the understanding or meaning of illness? Are there important cultural issues to understand about your own interactions with a particular patient and their family? What is the patient's preferred language? See also Chapter 5, Anti-Racist and Anti-Oppressive Clinical Skills.
- **Spiritual background:** How does religion and spirituality play into medical decision making for this patient? How does it affect the way in which they view their own illness?
- **Home safety:** What is the setup in the home? Is the patient's bedroom on the ground floor? How many stairs are involved in gaining entry to the home? Are there railings or grab bars? What kinds of equipment does the bathroom have? Have there been any accidents? Are there throw rugs that are not secured?
- **Finances:** How does the patient pay for your medications? How do they pay for food? Are they responsible for paying their own bills? Are there gaps in what they can afford that are concerning to them?
- **Screening for elder abuse:** Does the patient feel safe in the home? Is it difficult to explain physical findings or accidents? What is the interaction between family members or caregivers and the patient? Is the patient dressed appropriately for the weather? Do they have all the necessary food, medication, and services? Are there any signs of neglect? It's important to think not just about physical abuse but also emotional and financial abuse. Ask about internet usage. Older adults are often the target of online financial fraud or mail fraud.
- **Examining the structure of the patient's personal support system:** Do they need or have a caregiver? What is the level of caregiver burden/stress? Are there resources this patient may be eligible for to extend the reach of their caregiver?

GOALS OF CARE AND ADVANCE CARE PREFERENCES

Discussing the goals of care and advance care preferences with patients is an essential aspect of providing excellent primary care. It is recommended to have these conversations as part of routine outpatient visits. Ask if the patient has designated a healthcare proxy, who can make medical decisions on their behalf if they are unable to do so. Additionally, inquire if the patient has a living will or a *Provider Order for Life-Sustaining Treatment (POLST)*. These documents are crucial, so make sure to add them to the patient's medical record and review them periodically to ensure that preferences have not significantly changed. If the patient does not have these documents, take the time to explain their significance and direct them to resources that can help them complete their advance care plans. Refer to Chapter 33, Clinical Ethics and Professionalism, for more information.

See Video 25.2.

STRUCTURE AND PHYSIOLOGIC CHARACTERISTICS

This section covers some of the anatomic and physiologic changes attributed to aging, as well as some of the physical findings that result.

Skin

There is atrophy of the epidermis, hair follicles, and sweat glands, which results in thinning skin. The skin becomes fragile and discolored. Wrinkling and dryness result from reduced skin turgor. In addition, the nails become thin and brittle, with marked ridging. The dermis has decreased vascularity, which contributes to prolonged healing time. Common pigmentary changes include the development of *senile lentigines*, or "liver spots." These brown macules are commonly found on the backs of the hands, forearms, and face. They are caused by localized mild epidermal hyperplasia associated with increased numbers of melanocytes and increased melanin production. Fig. 25.1 shows senile lentigines on the hand of an 87-year-old female.

Another common skin change is *senile (solar) keratosis*, which is a well-defined, raised papule or plaque of epidermal hyperkeratosis. The surface scale varies in color from yellow to brown. These lesions are common on the face, neck, trunk, and hands. Fig. 25.2 shows several senile keratoses on an 82-year-old male.

There is commonly a degeneration of the elastic fibers and collagen of the skin, resulting in a loss of elasticity and the development of senile purpura. These purple macules, commonly seen on the backs of the hands or on the forearms, result from blood that has extravasated through capillaries that have lost their elastic support. Fig. 25.3 shows senile purpura on the forearm of a 90-year-old female.

Sebaceous gland hyperplasia, especially on the forehead and nose, is common. These yellowish glands range in size from 1 to 3 mm and have a central pore. It is important to differentiate these benign lesions from basal cell carcinomas.

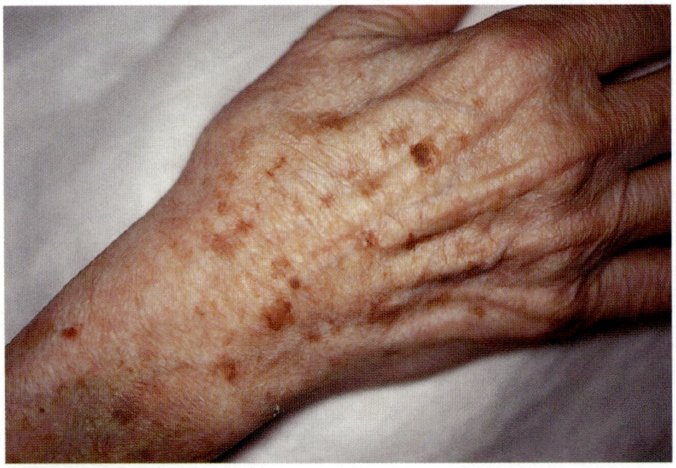

Fig. 25.1 Senile lentigines in an 87-year-old female. Notice the well-demarcated, brownish-black macules.

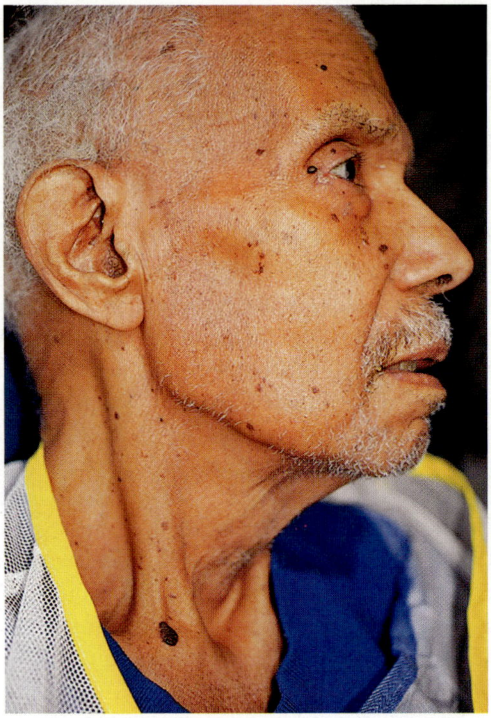

Fig. 25.2 Raised senile keratoses on the face and neck of an 82-year-old male.

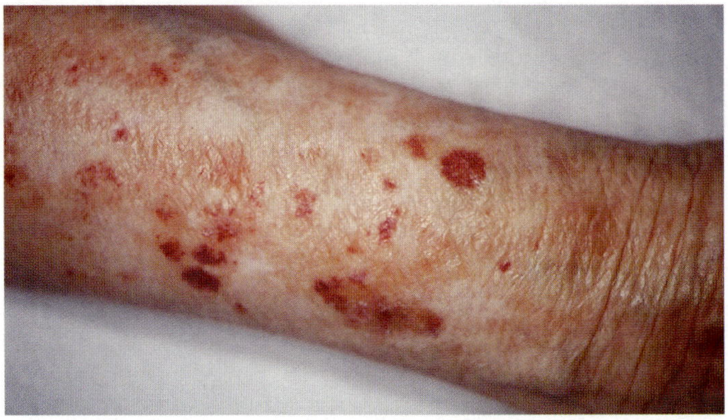

Fig. 25.3 Senile purpura on the forearm of a 90-year-old female. Note the red macules and the loss of turgidity of the skin.

Hair loses its pigment, commonly resulting in "graying" of the hair. With the reduction in hair follicles, hair loss is all over the body: head, axilla, pubic area, and extremities. With the reduction in estrogens, an increase in hair may actually develop in many older females, especially on the chin and upper lip. Chin hairs on a 79-year-old female are shown in Fig. 25.4.

As a result of the reduction in subcutaneous tissue, there is less insulation and less padding over bony surfaces. This predisposes older people to hypothermia and the development of pressure sores or pressure ulcers. Fig. 25.5 shows a pressure sore that developed on an 85-year-old male within 1 week. He had been seen 1 week earlier when a small, intact erythematous area was noticed over his sacral area. He was brought back to the emergency department 7 days later with the decubitus ulcer seen in the figure. The ulceration eroded through the skin and

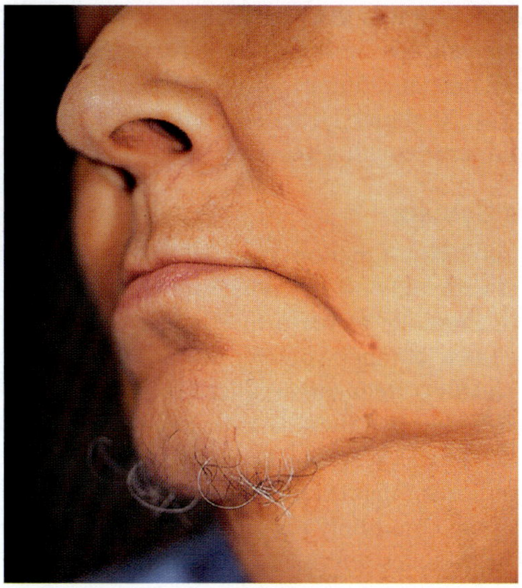

Fig. 25.4 Chin hairs on a 79-year-old female.

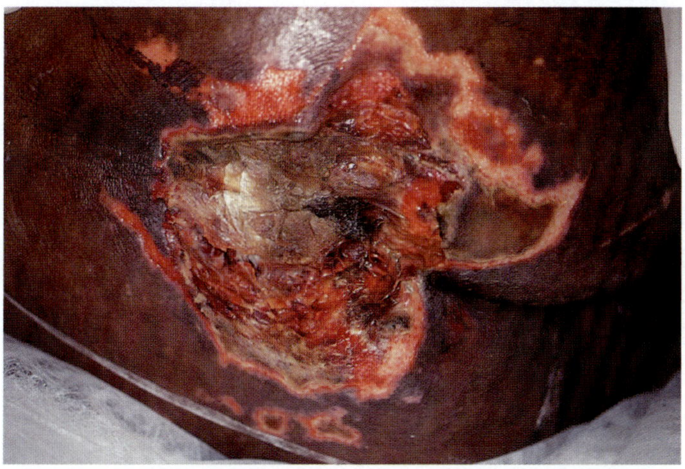

Fig. 25.5 A stage IV pressure sore in the sacral area of an 85-year-old male. Note the sacrum *(white area)* and necrotic surrounding muscles.

muscle, into the sacrum, and into the bowel, with the development of a rectovesicular fistula.

Eyes

As a result of a reduction of orbital fat, the eyes appear sunken. Laxity of the eyelids, or senile ptosis, often develops. Entropion (see Fig. 10.19) or ectropion (see Fig. 10.20) may develop, caused by the lower eyelids falling inward or falling away, respectively. There may also be a clogging of the lacrimal duct, resulting in epiphora or tearing. Fatty deposits in the cornea may produce an arcus senilis, as seen in Figs. 10.57 and 10.58. Inadequate production of mucous tears by the conjunctiva may predispose persons to corneal ulcers, exposure keratitis, or dry eye syndrome (see Chapter 10, The Eye).

An accumulation of yellow pigment in the lens alters color perception. A loss of elasticity in the lens results in presbyopia. Nuclear sclerosis of the lens develops into cataract formation. Patients experience decreased visual acuity and commonly are concerned with sensitivity to glare from interior lights, sunlight, or floor reflection.

Degenerative changes in the iris, vitreous humor, and retina may impair visual acuity, reduce the fields of vision, and lead to the development of floaters (muscae volitantes). Senile macular degeneration (see Figs. 10.125 to 10.127) and retinal hemorrhages are other medically significant causes of decreases in visual acuity.

Ears

Degeneration of the organ of Corti may result in presbycusis, an impaired sensitivity to high-frequency tones. Patients experience slow, progressive hearing loss with a consistent pattern of pure tone loss. Otosclerosis may produce conductive deafness, as does the excessive cerumen accumulation so commonly seen in older individuals. A degeneration of the hair cells in the semicircular canals may produce vertigo.

Nose and Throat

Atrophic changes occur in the mucosa of the nose and throat. Taste and especially smell may be altered, particularly in institutionalized individuals. A decrease in mucous production predisposes older patients to upper respiratory infections. A loss of elasticity in the laryngeal muscles may produce tremulousness and high voice pitch.

Mouth

Loss of teeth from dental caries or periodontal disease is common. Gingival recession may produce problems with dentures and a malalignment of the bite. Atrophic changes in the salivary glands cause mouth dryness, known as xerostomia, a common concern among older adults.

Lungs

A loss of elasticity in the pulmonary septa and atrophy of the alveoli cause coalescence of the alveoli, with a reduction in vital capacity and oxygen diffusion. There are decreases in forced vital capacity and expiratory flow rate. A degeneration of bronchial epithelium and mucous glands increases the susceptibility to infections. Skeletal changes also contribute to a decrease in vital capacity.

Cardiovascular System

A loss of elasticity of the aorta may cause aortic dilation. The semilunar and atrioventricular valves may degenerate and become regurgitant. Alternatively, these valves may become sclerotic, which causes stenosis of the valves. Degeneration or calcification of the conducting system may cause heart block or arrhythmias.

Noncompliance of the peripheral arteries may cause hypertension with a widened pulse pressure. Systolic blood pressure rises progressively with age, whereas diastolic pressure levels off in the sixth decade of life; these developments lead to an increased prevalence of isolated systolic hypertension. Coronary atherosclerosis may produce angina, myocardial infarction, or nonspecific symptoms such as confusion or tiredness.

There are also decreases in plasma volume, ventricular filling time, and baroreflex sensitivity.

Breasts

The amount of glandular tissue decreases, and fatty deposits replace the tissue. As a result of a loss of elastic tissue, the breasts become pendulous, and the ducts may be more palpable.

In males, gynecomastia may result from a change in the metabolism of sex hormones by the liver (see Fig. 16.21).

Gastrointestinal System

Atrophy of the gastrointestinal mucosa occurs with a reduction in the number of stomach and intestinal glands, causing alterations in secretion, motility, and absorption. Changes in elastic tissue and colonic pressures may result in diverticulosis, which can lead to diverticulitis. Pancreatic acinar atrophy is common, as are decreases in hepatic mass, hepatic blood flow, and microsomal enzyme activity. These decreases result in an increased half-life of lipid-soluble drugs.

Genitourinary System

There is a decrease in the number of glomeruli and a thickening of the basement membrane in Bowman capsule, resulting in a reduction in renal function. Degenerative changes occur in the renal tubules, which themselves are reduced in number. Renal blood flow is reduced to half by 75 years of age. Vascular changes may also contribute to a reduced glomerular filtration rate.

In males, prostatic atrophy or prostatic hypertrophy develops. Benign prostatic hypertrophy is present in 80% of all males older than 80 years. The penis decreases in size, and the testicles hang lower in the scrotum.

In postmenopausal females, the reduction in estrogen is associated with an increase in susceptibility to osteoporosis. The labia and clitoris are reduced in size, and the vaginal mucosa becomes thin and dry. The uterus and ovaries also decrease in size.

As discussed previously, pubic hair decreases in amount and becomes gray.

Endocrine System

There is a decreased metabolism of thyroxine and a decreased conversion of thyroxine to triiodothyronine. Because of a reduction in pancreatic β-cell secretion, hyperglycemia may result. The hypothalamus and the pituitary gland secrete reduced amounts of hormones. An increase in the secretion of antidiuretic hormone and atrial natriuretic hormone may alter fluid balance. There are also increased levels of norepinephrine.

Musculoskeletal System

There is general atrophy of muscles, causing a decline in strength. Muscle wasting is commonly seen in the distal extremities, especially in the dorsal interosseous muscles.

Osteoclastic activity is greater than osteoblastic activity. Enlarging the cancellous bone spaces and thinning of the trabeculae result in osteoporosis. Kyphosis and a loss of height are common (see Fig. 13.6). Degenerative changes and a loss of elastic tissue occur in joints, ligaments, and tendons. This frequently results in joint stiffness. Degenerative changes in bone may result in bone cysts and erosions, making these bones prone to fracture. Osteoarthritis is common. Thinning of cartilage and synovial thickening produce joint stiffness and pain. Range of motion is also reduced, perhaps because of pain. Fig. 20.70 shows Heberden and Bouchard nodes in an 86-year-old female with osteoarthritis.

Nervous System

Changes in brain function may adversely affect cognition. Significant variability exists among individuals, and many older individuals continue to perform at levels comparable with or exceeding those of much younger people.

Brain weight is frequently reduced by 5% to 7% due to atrophy of selected areas. There is a decrease in blood flow to the brain by 10% to 15%. Vascular changes of atherosclerosis can result in multiple infarcts or transient ischemic attacks.

Reflexes are commonly reduced; the gag reflex is frequently absent. The Achilles tendon reflex is often symmetrically reduced or absent. Primitive reflexes, such as snout or palmomental, may be present in normal older adults.

Hematopoietic System

There is an increase in the amount of marrow fat and a decrease in the amount of active bone marrow.

Immune System

There is a decreased number of newly formed T lymphocytes and a reduced capability of T lymphocytes to proliferate in response to mitogens or antigens. Humoral immunity is impaired, and suppressor T lymphocytes are decreased in number.

BASIC PRINCIPLES OF GERIATRIC MEDICINE

Many medical problems in geriatrics can be categorized as geriatric syndromes. These problems have more than one cause and may involve multiple parts of the body. The concept of geriatric syndromes means that although there may be one end presentation identifiable to the examiner, there are multifactorial reasons for its existence. There are also four common underlying features that many geriatric syndromes[17] share as likely risk factors for their development: older age, baseline cognitive impairment, functional impairment, and impaired mobility.

Common geriatric syndromes include:

- Urinary incontinence
- Falls
- Weight loss
- Delirium
- Dementia
- Syncope
- Dizziness
- Pressure ulcers
- Frailty

Medical problems in older adults, especially frail older adults, present differently than they do in younger patients. First, there is an *altered manifestation of disease*. The actual symptom may not be a symptom of the organ system involved with the disease. For example, if a person in their 50s were to have a heart attack, the individual, unless diabetic, would usually suffer from chest pain. This is not the case in the geriatric age group. It is well documented that 70% of nondiabetic individuals older than 70 years of age do not have chest pain with a myocardial infarction. Such patients may present instead with breathlessness, falling, confusion, or palpitations.

Another illustration of this alteration in symptoms is the geriatric patient with diabetes mellitus. Ordinarily, because of a lack of insulin, younger patients become acidotic and ketotic, with a smell of ketones on their breath. They may also exhibit shallow, rapid respirations. Older patients with uncontrolled diabetes mellitus may not become ketotic and acidotic. Instead, the syndrome of hyperosmolar, nonketotic coma may ensue. These patients, who do not have the smell of ketones on their breath and are not acidotic, are hyperosmolar and may have serum glucose levels in excess of 600 to 700 mg/dL. They may even present in a coma.

A geriatric patient with hyperthyroidism might not present with the tachycardia, sweats, or anxiety states that are seen in younger individuals with increased thyroid activity. The geriatric patient may instead appear depressed and apathetic. An older patient with acute appendicitis might not suffer from abdominal pain, and an older patient with pneumonia might not have shortness of breath; confusion may be the only symptom.

An older patient with pneumonia may not present with typical symptoms such as cough, fever, or chills, but instead show impaired cognitive function. Impaired cognitive function is also commonly found in geriatric patients with urinary tract infections.

A second principle in geriatric medicine is the *nonspecific manifestation of disease*. When an older person becomes ill, a family member may report as the main concern that the patient "just hasn't gotten out of bed" or "just aren't themself." The patient may spend more time in bed, appear exceptionally tired, or not eat and drink as usual. The presentation may consist of only nonspecific concerns.

A third principle is the *underreporting of illness*. When an interviewer asks a geriatric patient about various symptoms, the patient may fail to report blindness caused by a cataract, deafness caused by otosclerosis, pain in the legs at night, urinary incontinence, constipation, confusion, etc. The geriatric patient may believe these symptoms are normal for a 75- or 80-year-old. Abdominal pain and other gastrointestinal concerns, such as increased gas, are commonly mistaken by geriatric patients as a normal part of aging. Sometimes, a patient may say, "Nothing can be done about it, so I don't want to bother anyone by mentioning it."

A fourth principle is the recognition that *multiple pathologic conditions may be present* in a geriatric patient. This has clear implications when deciding on a treatment course, including possible planned procedures and prescribing medications. One medication may have deleterious effects on a particular patient, depending on the constellation of other medical problems. Of course, this can occur with any patient, but it is more likely in older patients with several pathologic conditions. Similarly, it is important to remember this principle when ordering tests. *Consider what you plan to do with the result before ordering a test. If the patient and family do not plan to act on a result, do not do the test.* Remember, not all medical tests are innocuous and noninvasive. For example, IV contrast dye, used to obtain a CT scan, can adversely affect the kidneys of an already compromised patient. Consider the patient and family goals of care before the evaluation of a particular symptom!

Finally, what is the patient's *chief concern*? This is sometimes called "*the myth of the chief concern*." Many geriatric patients do not have a single concern. There may be several problems related to their many conditions. In fact, as already discussed, if a chief concern is given, it may bear no relationship to the organ system involved. *Be careful in evaluating the chief concern when dealing with older patients.* Keep in mind the concept and complexity of geriatric syndrome.

THE GERIATRIC EXAMINATION

The physical examination of the geriatric patient is no different from that already described in this book. Special attention, however, should be given to the following areas.

It can be a bit uncomfortable for elderly patients to undress during a medical examination, especially if the examiner is much younger. Therefore, it is important to respect their modesty and only expose the area that needs to be examined. Additionally, it is recommended to ensure that the room is warm, as older individuals tend to get cold easily. Lastly, keep in mind that putting on a gown or robe may not be easy for an older patient who may have limited mobility due to conditions such as arthritis.

Assessment of Vital Signs

Perform a routine evaluation, including orthostatic changes in pulse and blood pressure. Be careful if the patient is concerned with dizziness or chest discomfort. If this occurs, have the patient lie down immediately. Obtain body temperature. If the patient is hypometabolic, as happens in hypothyroidism or in exposure hypothermia, the temperature may be less than 96.8°F (36°C). In the geriatric population, a normal temperature is commonly found in patients with severe infections. Accurate weights should be documented and observed over time.

Skin

Observe the skin for any malignant changes, pressure sores, evidence of pruritus, and ecchymoses suggestive of falls or abuse.

Head, Eyes, Ears, Nose, Throat, and Neck

Evaluate the patient for any evidence of skull trauma. Palpate the superficial temporal arteries, which are located anterosuperior to the tragus. In patients who have a concern of visual symptoms, headaches, or polymyalgic symptoms, polymyalgia rheumatica or temporal (giant cell) arteritis should be suspected (see "Clinicopathologic Correlations" at the end of this chapter).

Is entropion (see Fig. 10.19) or ectropion (see Fig. 10.20) present? Determine visual acuity if this was not already tested. Eye movement should be checked for gaze palsies. The ability to gaze upward declines with increasing age. Are cataracts present (see Figs. 10.72 and 10.73)? Examine the retina if a cataract does not exist. Is macular degeneration present (see Figs. 10.125 to 10.127)?

Is cerumen impacted in the external canal (see Fig. 11.4)? Evaluate auditory acuity if this was not already done.

Ask the patient to remove any dentures, if present. Examine the mouth for dryness, lesions (see Figs. 12.16, 12.17, and 12.20), condition of teeth, oral ulcers (see Fig. 12.45), and malignancies (see Figs. 12.50 and 12.52 to 12.54). Poor-fitting dentures may cause difficulty eating and chewing, which may lead to weight loss. Examine the tongue for malignancy (see Fig. 12.52).

Auscultate the neck. Are carotid bruits present? Make sure that you listen to the neck for carotid bruits before palpating the carotid! Palpate the thyroid. Are nodules present? Is the thyroid diffusely enlarged?

Breasts

Examine the breasts for dimpling, discharge, and masses. The incidence of breast cancer increases with advancing age. The incidence is the highest among females 85 years of age and older (see Fig. 16.6).

Chest

Inspect the shape of the chest. Is kyphoscoliosis present? Auscultate the chest. Are any adventitious sounds present?

Cardiovascular System

Evaluate the point of maximum impulse. Is it displaced laterally? Auscultate the heart in the four main positions. Are any murmurs, rubs, or gallops heard? Systolic murmurs are heard in 55% of all older adults.

Are the peripheral pulses present? Loss of peripheral pulses is common and may have little clinical significance, especially if the patient is not concerned with intermittent claudication. Is there evidence of peripheral vascular disease?

Abdomen

Perform routine palpation and percussion of the abdomen. Is the bladder enlarged? Is a pulsatile abdominal mass present? Palpate for inguinal and femoral hernias. Is there evidence of urine leakage on the undergarments? Perform a rectal examination. Examine the stool for blood. In a man, is the prostate enlarged?

Musculoskeletal Examination

Examine the joints. Ask the patient to stand up from a seated position and observe for any difficulties. Can the patient lift their hands over the head to brush their hair?

The extremities should be examined for arthritis, impaired range of motion, and deformities. The feet should be inspected for nail care, calluses, deformities (see Figs. 20.64 and 20.77), and ulceration (see Figs. 8.127 and 20.78). Evaluate the peripheral pulses.

Neurologic Examination

Evaluate mental status if this was not already done. Check vibration sense. Lack of vibration sense is the most common deficit in otherwise healthy older individuals. Test reflexes: asymmetry suggests stroke, myelopathy, or root compression. Evaluate for rigidity. Cogwheel rigidity is suggestive of Parkinson disease. Perform the Romberg test. Evaluate gait. Evaluate motor strength, tone, and rapid alternating movements.

CLINICOPATHOLOGIC CORRELATIONS

Among the elderly, various organ system issues are commonly encountered. This section provides a brief overview of several common disorders and functional states that are prevalent among older individuals.

Senile macular degeneration affects almost 10% of the elderly population, with more females being affected than males. It is the leading cause of legal blindness in the United States. The condition is characterized by a painless and gradual loss of central vision, which makes it difficult for patients to read. However, since only the macula is involved, peripheral vision remains unaffected, and complete blindness does not occur. You can refer to Figs. 10.125 to 10.127 for more information.

Temporal arteritis and *polymyalgia rheumatica* are medical conditions that are unique to the elderly population. These conditions are thought to be related to a disease called giant cell arteritis (GCA), which is an inflammatory disease that affects the blood vessels, a condition known as vasculitis. GCA mostly affects the large and medium arteries in the head, particularly the branches of the external carotid artery. The name GCA reflects the type of inflammatory cell involved as seen on a biopsy. It is more common in females than males by a ratio of 2:1 and more common in those of Northern European descent and those residing at higher latitudes. The mean age of onset is older than 55 years of age, and it is rare in those individuals less than 55 years of age. See Chapter 10, The Eye, for more information on these conditions.

The symptoms of temporal arteritis include headache, which is frequently associated with scalp tenderness; the temporal artery may also be tender. There are several generalized symptoms as well, such as fever, weight loss, anorexia, and fatigue. Visual disturbances (see Chapter 10, The Eye) include loss of vision (see Fig. 10.129), blurred vision, diplopia, and amaurosis fugax. Sometimes, patients may also have concerns of pain on chewing food. The diagnosis is made from temporal artery biopsy, which has a sensitivity of 90% and a specificity of 100%.

It is estimated that 40% to 50% of patients with temporal arteritis also suffer from *polymyalgia rheumatica*. This condition is more common in females than in males. People with polymyalgia rheumatica often experience symmetric pain and stiffness in the neck, shoulders, lower back, and pelvic girdle, especially in the morning. They may find it difficult to brush their hair. The upper extremities' proximal muscle groups and pelvic girdle are commonly affected.

Pressure sores, or pressure ulcers, are serious problems that can lead to pain, a longer hospital stay, and a slower recovery. They are caused by unrelieved pressure that results in damage to underlying tissue. They affect more than 2.5 million individuals yearly in the United States alone. The annual healthcare expenditures for these lesions are estimated to be between

$9.1 and $11.6 billion. Since 2008, the Centers for Medicare and Medicaid Services (CMS) have discontinued hospital payments for charges related to the development of hospital-acquired ulcers. This is significant when considering the cost of a hospital stay involving a pressure ulcer can reach $700,000. More than 17,000 legal cases are filed each year that are related to the development of pressure sores and related morbidity and mortality.[18] Bacteremia and deep-tissue injury are commonly associated problems, and osteomyelitis occurs in more than a quarter of all patients with nonhealing pressure ulcers. Studies have shown that there has been a decrease in the overall prevalence of pressure sores as well as hospital-acquired pressure sores in recent years. This is related to more aggressive and earlier therapy.[19]

Pressure ulcers result from prolonged pressure over bony prominences (see Fig. 25.5). A pressure ulcer starts as reddened skin but gets progressively worse, forming a blister, an open sore, and a crater. The most common places for pressure ulcers are over bony prominences (i.e., bones close to the skin) such as the elbows, heels, hips, ankles, shoulders, back, sacrum, and back of the head. The pressure causes a decrease in perfusion to the area, leading to the accumulation of toxic products, with subsequent necrosis of skin, muscle, subcutaneous tissue, and bone. Moisture caused by fecal or urinary incontinence or perspiration is also implicated because it leads to maceration of the epidermis and thus allows tissue necrosis. Shearing force is also a factor. Shear is generated when the head of a bed is elevated, causing the torso to slide down and transmit pressure to the sacrum. Poor nutritional status and delayed wound healing are other significant contributing factors.

Pressure ulcers are staged to classify the degree of damage observed. The four clinical stages of pressure ulcers are as follows:

- **Stage I:** Nonblanching erythema of intact skin; the heralding lesion of skin ulceration
- **Stage II:** Partial-thickness skin loss involving epidermis or dermis; ulcer extending up to subcutaneous fat
- **Stage III:** Full-thickness skin loss involving damage or necrosis of subcutaneous tissue without involving muscle or bone
- **Stage IV:** Full-thickness skin loss with extensive destruction, tissue necrosis, or damage to underlying muscle, bone, or supporting structures

Ulcers covered by superficial necrosis must undergo debridement before they can be staged. The patient in Fig. 25.5 presented with a stage I pressure sore, and 1 week later, when this photograph was taken, the sore had rapidly advanced to a stage IV lesion. The patient died of sepsis 4 days after the photograph was taken.

Prevention of pressure ulcers is extremely important in the care of bedridden or chair-bound patients. Repositioning or rotating the patient at least every 2 hours, minimizing moisture and shear forces, practicing basic skin care, and improving the nutritional state are important care measures to ensure. Skin should be cleansed at the time of soiling and at routine intervals. Care should be used to minimize the force and friction applied to the skin.

Urinary incontinence is an important problem in the geriatric age group. It occurs in 15% to 30% of community-dwelling individuals 65 years of age and older. Among institutionalized patients, the prevalence is 40% to 60%. Approximately 12 million adults in the United States have urinary incontinence. It is most common in females older than 50 years. There are many causes of urinary incontinence, including decreased bladder capacity, increased residual volume, medications, diabetes, and pelvic relaxation. In females, thinning and drying of the skin in the vagina or urethra may cause urinary incontinence; in males, an enlarged prostate gland or prostate surgery can cause urinary incontinence. The major transient causes of urinary incontinence can be remembered by the mnemonic "DIAPPERS":

- **D:** Delirium or dementia
- **I:** Infections (urinary)
- **A:** Atrophic vaginitis or urethritis; atonic bladder
- **P:** Psychologic causes such as depression, prostatitis
- **P:** Pharmacologic agents such as anticholinergics, psychotropics, alcohol, diuretics, opiates, and α-adrenergic agents
- **E:** Endocrine abnormalities such as diabetes and hypercalcemia
- **R:** Restricted mobility
- **S:** Stool impaction

There are four types of urinary incontinence: stress, urge, overflow, and functional. In *stress incontinence,* urine leaks because of sudden pressure on the lower abdominal muscles, as during coughing, laughing, or lifting a heavy object. It is very common in females. *Urge incontinence* occurs when the need to urinate comes on too fast before the patient can get to a toilet. Urge incontinence is most common in older persons and may indicate kidney or bladder infection. *Overflow incontinence* is a constant dripping of urine caused by an overfilled bladder. This type of urinary incontinence often occurs in males and can be caused by an enlarged prostate gland or tumor. Diabetes or certain medicines may also cause this problem. *Functional incontinence* occurs when the patient has normal urine control but has trouble getting to the bathroom in time because of arthritis or other conditions that make it hard to ambulate.

Dementia is characterized by an acquired and persistent impairment in short- and long-term memory and other disturbances, such as impairment in language (e.g., reading, writing, fluency, naming, repetition), concentration ability, visuospatial function (e.g., drawing, copying), emotions, and personality, despite a state of clear consciousness. A diagnosis of dementia requires evidence of decline from previous levels of functioning and impairment in multiple cognitive domains for at least 6 months to support the diagnosis. Despite its prevalence, dementia is often unrecognized in its early stages. As mentioned previously, dementia is not a single disease but a nonspecific syndrome with many etiologic factors. The onset and course of the symptoms often provide clues to the cause of dementia. A sudden onset is almost always related to a cerebrovascular accident. A subacute, insidious course may be related to a tumor, Creutzfeld-Jakob disease, or Alzheimer disease. Dementia with rigidity and bradykinesia is strongly suggestive of Parkinson disease. Dementia in association with urinary incontinence and a spastic, magnetic gait is seen in normal-pressure hydrocephalus. The development of cognitive compromise after a fall should raise suspicion of a subdural hematoma. Vivid visual hallucinations and behavioral disturbance are associated with Lewy body dementia.[b]

Finally, *falls* are the leading cause of fatal and nonfatal injuries for American older adults.[20] One in every four older adults will experience a fall each year. Every 11 seconds, a senior is treated in an emergency room for a fall. The total cost of fall-related injury care in the United States annually is approximately $50 billion. As the population ages with the "silver tsunami," this cost is expected to rise to more than $67 billion. Falls are associated with a recurrent fear of falling. This cycle leads to decreased activity and an eventual increased risk of falling for an individual. Patients with falls risk injury obviously, but also isolation, depression, functional decline, and feelings of helplessness. One fall per 10 results in a hip fracture. The most profound effect of falling is the loss of independent functioning. Of persons who fracture a hip, 25% require lifelong nursing care, and approximately 50% of older adults who sustain a fall-related injury are discharged to a nursing home instead of returning home.

Falls are clearly associated with the use of sedative-hypnotic agents and major tranquilizers. The Beer Criteria[21] is an updated guideline to assist clinicians in the use of potentially inappropriate medication use in older adults. Consulting the Beer Criteria and critically looking at the reasons older adults are taking specific medications is an important part of geriatric medicine. In fact, deprescribing[c] is common in geriatrics.

Several modifiable risk factors have been identified with falling. These include lower-body weakness and problems with walking and balance. The healthcare professional should try to encourage older patients to improve their lower body strength and balance through regular physical activity. Physical therapy interventions can be greatly beneficial. Tai chi is an exercise program that has also been shown to be very effective. All healthcare professionals must also carefully review all of a given patient's medications to reduce side effects and interactions. Finally, approximately half to two-thirds of all falls occur in and around the home. Therefore, it makes sense to reduce potential home hazards. Oftentimes, home-based physical therapy or nursing referrals can help identify potential fall hazards in the home and guide patients in ways to correct them. Possible home safety improvement suggestions would include removing tripping hazards such as throw rugs, using nonslip mats in the bathtub, installing grab bars next to the toilet and in the bathtub, installing handrails on both sides of stairways, and improving lighting throughout the home.

[b]Lewy body dementia is the second most common type of progressive dementia after Alzheimer disease. Protein deposits, called Lewy bodies, develop in nerve cells in the brain regions involved in thinking, memory, and motor control.

[c]Deprescribing is the process of intentionally stopping a medication or reducing its dose to improve the person's health or reduce the risk of adverse side effects.

CONCLUSION

In conclusion, the comprehensive assessment of geriatric patients is an indispensable tool in providing holistic and patient-centered care. The geriatric assessment, encompassing components such as cognitive function, functional status, medication review, and social support, serves as a valuable roadmap in tailoring interventions to the unique needs of older individuals. Understanding the physiological changes associated with aging, from alterations in organ function to shifts in metabolism, is essential for healthcare professionals navigating the intricacies of geriatric medicine. Discussing advance care preferences is essential to effective communication with geriatric patients. The basic principles of geriatric medicine have been discussed in detail, and it is important to understand them when practicing with our senior patients. The geriatric physical exam, with its focus on vital signs, mobility, sensory function, and nutritional status, unveils valuable insights into the overall health of older adults. As we delve into some of the clinicopathologic correlations, bridging the gap between clinical findings and underlying pathophysiology, a more nuanced understanding of geriatric syndromes emerges. In embracing the multidimensional nature of geriatric care, healthcare professionals are better equipped to optimize the well-being and quality of life for our aging population.

ACKNOWLEDGMENT

The author would like to acknowledge the contributions of previous edition co-author, Jessica L. Israel, MD.

REVIEW QUESTIONS

1. **Which of the following is part of the geriatric assessment?**
   - **A.** Patient's functional ability
   - **B.** Physical health
   - **C.** Cognitive status
   - **D.** Socioeconomic circumstances
   - **E.** All of the above
2. **Which of the following is NOT an activity of the self-care ADLs?**
   - **A.** Dressing
   - **B.** Meal preparation
   - **C.** Bathing
   - **D.** Transferring from bed to chair
   - **E.** Toileting
3. **Which of the following statements is NOT true?**
   - **A.** Patient weight should be measured at all visits.
   - **B.** Unintentional weight loss of more than 3% of body weight in 12 months should prompt further workup.
   - **C.** Underlying malignancy is a common reason for weight loss in the elderly.
   - **D.** The "*Meals on Wheels*" mnemonic is an easy way to remember the reasons for weight loss in the elderly.
   - **E.** The inability to feed oneself is a cause of weight loss.

4. **Which of the following is NOT a test for cognitive assessment?**
   A. Mini-Cog Assessment
   B. Montreal Cognitive Assessment
   C. Animal-naming test
   D. Folstein Mini-Mental Examination
   E. Vanderbilt Mental Status Examination
5. **Which of the following is NOT a common geriatric syndrome?**
   A. Urinary incontinence
   B. Frailty
   C. Pressure ulcers
   D. Diarrhea
   E. Syncope
6. **Which of the following symptoms is common in a geriatric patient with pneumonia?**
   A. Chest pain
   B. Confusion
   C. Cough
   D. Fever
   E. Rigors
7. **Which of the following is NOT a basic principle of geriatric medicine?**
   A. Altered presentation of disease
   B. Nonspecific manifestation of disease
   C. Underreporting of illness
   D. Multiple pathologic conditions
   E. Sundowning
8. **Stage IV of pressure ulcer development consists of:**
   A. Full-thickness skin loss
   B. Extensive destruction
   C. Tissue necrosis
   D. Damage to underlying muscle, bone, or supporting structures
   E. All of the above

REFERENCES

Available online.

BIBLIOGRAPHY

Available online.

26

The Transgender Patient

Sky Kihuwa-Mani and Joshua D. Safer

"Never take for granted things we're told to be the utmost truth, because I have found throughout the last few chapters of my existence, that society has it backward."

Te Manahou Mackay, Māori model and transgender female (1999–current)

GENERAL CONSIDERATIONS

Historically, the recognized biology connected to sexual reproduction was limited to external genitalia facilitating the mixing of gametes. Like with other biology, greater complexity has been appreciated over time, including the observation of chromosomes, genes, and other coding factors that may relate to visible anatomy, gender identity, and sexual orientation. Further, like with other biology, the independent components of sexual reproduction may not align in all individuals. Transgender individuals in particular have incongruity between their sex recorded at birth (a surrogate for the genitals observed at birth by physical exam) and their gender identity, which may be explained by genetic and environmental factors leading to a behavioral identity that does not match anatomy.

The History of Transgender Medicine

Awareness of gender identity has been apparent to different cultures worldwide in different iterations and at different time points in history. Classic examples include Hijra[a] in India, Māhū[b] in Hawaiian and Pacific Islander cultures, and Lhamana[c] among Zuni pueblo people of the Southwestern United States.

[a]The Islamic New Year, Al-Hijra, marks the journey of Muhammad from Mecca to Medina, where he fled persecution and established the first Islamic state. The term "Hijra" means migration. In colloquial Hindi, the term "hijra" is used to refer to intersex people. Hijras are typically born male but present themselves in traditionally feminine ways through their clothing and behavior. Some choose to undergo a castration ceremony as an offering to the Hindu goddess Bahuchara Mata, while others are born intersex.

[b]Historically the term *māhū,* meaning in Hawaiian *"in the middle,"* referred to people recorded male at birth, but in modern usage, *māhū* can refer to gender diversity. In Hawaiian culture, there are three genders: "kane" (male), "wahine" (female), and lastly, māhūs, who are known to be in the middle. Māhūs embrace both feminine and masculine traits. Māhūs hold a place of respect within Hawaiian culture and community.

[c]In Zuni culture, there is a group of individuals assigned male at birth known as *Lhamana* who take on the social and ceremonial roles that are traditionally performed by females. They wear a mix of male and female clothing and work in the areas that are typically occupied by Zuni females. Lhamana are highly respected for their artistic skills and often serve as mediators and teachers in their community.

The history of transgender medicine in modern medicine dates to at least the 19th and early 20th centuries. One of the first Americans widely known to have undergone a gender-affirming medical intervention of some form was Alan Hart, a physician himself, who was born in 1890 and who underwent a hysterectomy to align his body with his gender identity in 1917.

The Institut für Sexualwissenschaft was established in Berlin, Germany, in 1919 by Magnus Hirschfeld and became the mecca of transgender medicine. It was there that gender-affirming hormone therapy and so-called "sex change" surgeries were first pioneered. The father of modern plastic surgery, Sir Harold Gillies, is credited with developing the first penile inversion flap vaginoplasty technique in 1946 for transfeminine patients. This innovation laid the groundwork for the many hybrid graft-flap techniques that are considered the gold standard in transfeminine genital reconstruction today.

Today, transgender medicine can be an interdisciplinary care framework that sees patients for everything from mental health to primary care, spiritual health, surgical management, and more. This chapter is designed to introduce readers to the basics of transgender medicine, to dispel myths and misconceptions about this patient population, and to provide a roadmap to working with transgender patients.

Definitions

To ensure effective communication and respectful care, healthcare professionals should familiarize themselves with key terminology related to gender diversity. This section presents a comprehensive list of definitions that will aid in fostering a better understanding of transgender patients' experiences and healthcare needs (Table 26.1).

Pronouns and Proper Usage

Respecting a person's gender identity is at the core of providing appropriate and respectful healthcare. Healthcare professionals should always inquire about a person's pronouns during an initial interaction and allow patients to express their gender identity on their own terms. Assumptions should not be based on appearance, mannerisms, or legal documentation (see Box 26.1).

Many people are still unclear about the appropriateness of using they/them/their in the singular. We provide a few common

TABLE 26.1 Glossary of Terms Related to Transgender Medicine

Term	Definition
Gender/Sex	Both are broad terms to describe biological characteristics, self-identification, expression, and social roles that are male, female, or some variation or combination. In colloquial English, gender is often used as a synonym for sex. Some trans patients may make a distinction between gender—as their role in society, and sex—as their biological alignment with male or female. Healthcare professionals should use more specific language when referring to these characteristics and should clarify with patients what they mean when they use one or the other.
Gender Identity	Gender identity is an individual's internal sense of how they align with categories of male, female, neither, or both. It may be reflective of someone's internal sense of sex—male or femaleness, both, or neither.
Gender Expression	How a person conveys their gender identity through appearance, dress, name, pronouns, mannerisms, and speech.
Transgender, Transexual, Trans, TGD, Nonbinary, Genderqueer	Describes individuals whose internal sense of gender identity does not align with their sex recorded at birth (usually based on the appearance of physical characteristics). Conversely, transexual has been used by older generations of trans females and is increasingly used by younger binary trans people to make a distinction between those who undergo medical transition and those who do not. The latter two genderqueer and TGD are often used by individuals seeking to recognize a spectrum beyond male and female. Transgender and gender diverse (TGD) is an abbreviation that stands for trans and gender diverse and has been accepted in academic writing as an appropriate umbrella term to describe the many categories of people who are not cis.
Transfeminine, trans female	Describes a person with a female or feminine gender identity who was recorded male at birth.
Transmasculine, trans male	Describes a person with a male or masculine gender identity who was recorded female at birth.
Gender Dysphoria	Refers to the discomfort some may feel due to the disconnect between their gender identity and their sex recorded at birth. Not all trans persons necessarily experience gender dysphoria, though insurance often still requires a formal diagnosis of gender dysphoria to reimburse services related to transition. ICD-11 will have the term *gender incongruence* in a sexual health chapter that will work better than ICD-10 where *gender dysphoria* sits as a mental health code. Many endocrinologists code for what they're doing directly (e.g., androgen excess, hypogonadism) to have a medicine code to use for billing, etc.
Transition, Gender Affirmation, Gender Confirmation	Describes the steps taken to change an individual's gender expression and how their gender is perceived in alignment with their gender identity. May include changes to grooming, dress, name and pronouns, mannerisms, and speech. Medically can include gender affirming hormone therapy and surgery.
Cisgender, Nontransgender	Both terms to refer to individuals whose gender identity aligns with their sex recorded at birth. Cis is an appropriate abbreviated form of cisgender.
Bottom Surgery	Colloquial term used by trans people to refer to genital reconstruction related to gender affirming care, including vaginoplasty, metoidioplasty, phalloplasty, and sometimes hysterectomy and orchiectomy. Historically and inappropriately referred to as "the surgery." Healthcare professionals should avoid this kind of trivializing language.
Top Surgery	Colloquial term used by trans people to refer to chest reconstruction related to gender affirming care, including chest masculinizing mastectomy and breast augmentation with implantation.

BOX 26.1 Pronouns in Practice

Some non-transgender patients may respond with confusion or negativity when asked their pronouns. Healthcare professionals should be equipped to handle these situations sensitively and appropriately.

Consider,

"Hello, my name is [full name] and I am a [role] here at [healthcare center]. My pronouns are she, her, and hers. If you are comfortable sharing, may I ask what pronouns you use?"

If a patient becomes frustrated, you may respond,

"I apologize for upsetting you. My job is to treat all patients with respect and that means not making assumptions that could be hurtful."

BOX 26.2 Examples of the Singular "They"

"It looks like someone left their bag here. Do you know where they went?"

"Where did that customer go? I forgot to give them something."

"We are hiring a new manager. They will need to have experience to qualify for this role."

"A new teacher is coming to our school. They are here for an interview with the principal." [1]

examples of singular they/them/theirs from mainstream vernacular. These and sentences like these are enough evidence that they, them, and their are already used to refer to a single individual in our current mainstream vernacular (see Box 26.2). See also Chapter 1, The Interviewer's Questions, and Chapter 23, The Pregnant Patient.

GENERAL EVALUATION

A common theme throughout this chapter is an emphasis on the healthcare professional's sensitivity and flexibility. Indeed, when working with transgender populations like with all patients, professionals should navigate their interactions with humility and respect. It is good practice for healthcare professionals to be collaborators in all patient care, but this can be especially visible when working in developing fields like gender-affirming care. Many trans patients are very familiar with the latest literature and techniques and are ambitious in pursuing novel therapies. Professionals should be cautiously cooperative when navigating these discussions.

Healthcare professionals should be familiar with the vulnerability of transgender patients—for instance, the prevalence of sex work among transfeminine patients—and informed about best practices when working with patients who are sexually or socially vulnerable. Trauma-informed care should be employed as a best practice.

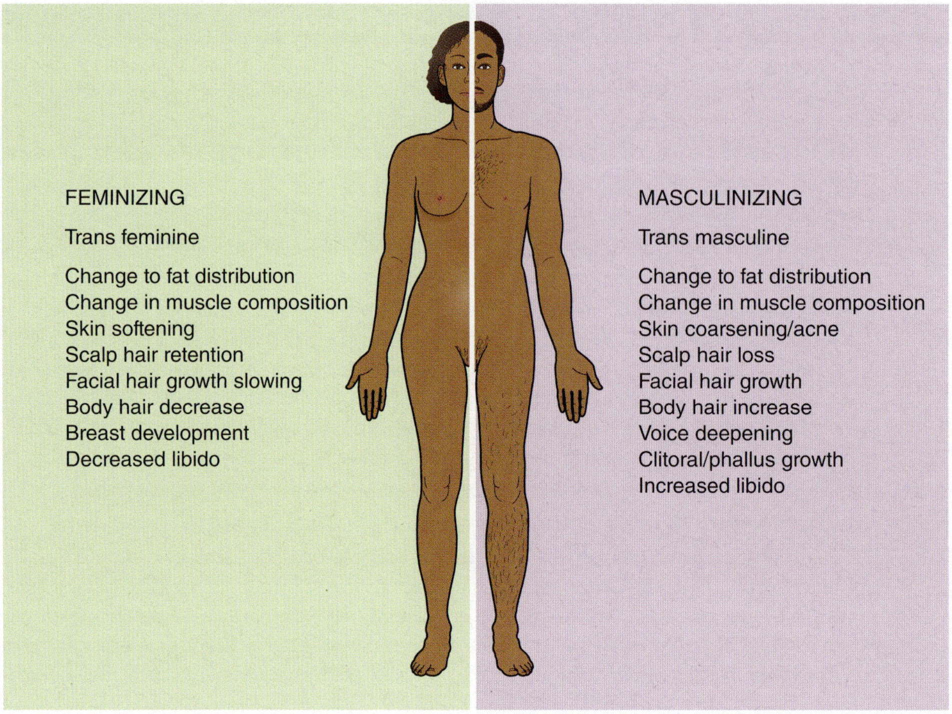

Fig. 26.1 Tissues Where Gender-Affirming Hormone Therapy (GAHT) Can Typically Have Impact.

Counseling should be approached with sensitivity and respect. For example, heterosexual trans females should be counseled about HIV PrEP[d] when their risk factors are determined to be sufficiently high, analogous to counseling for a heterosexual cisgender female typically based on social history.

A thorough sexual history will include questions about occupation, number and sex of sexual partners, specific activities and organs used, use of protective barriers or other health protective strategies, and history of sexually transmitted infections.

GENDER-AFFIRMING HORMONE THERAPY

Gender Affirming Hormone Therapy (GAHT) is sought by some trans individuals to better align other biology with gender identity. GAHT allows for exogenous control of sex steroids in a person's body. GAHT is a safe and effective treatment in the management of trans patient care.[2-6] Note also that *trans and gender diverse (TGD)* patients are a varied and heterogeneous group. Treatment is customized to the individual rather than limited to rigid protocols (see Fig. 26.1).

Additionally, healthcare professionals should be aware of the natural variations in secondary sex characteristics among diverse ethnic groups, to provide culturally sensitive care. For example, transmasculine patients with genetic ancestry among the original peoples of East Asia may have a lower likelihood of developing facial hair. Hence, healthcare professionals should consider counseling tailored to the patient's specific needs and expectations. Because gender-affirming care is a developing field, professionals should be flexible and may need to make extra effort to be current when treating TGD patients (see Box 26.3).[7]

BOX 26.3 Gender Identities Beyond Western Medicine

Healthcare professionals may encounter patients who can be described as transfeminine or transmasculine but who, for any combination of reasons, do not seek medical intervention. Sometimes these patients have sincerely held cultural or spiritual beliefs concerning their identity that transcends Western medicine.

For example, an Anishinaabe person recorded male at birth may identify as *ikwewaadizi* in their traditional worldview but use the term two-spirit or even transfeminine when articulating their gender identity to a non-Anishinaabe person. For others, it may be a personal choice, and they feel that accepting their femininity or masculinity and living with or without a different gender presentation is enough for them. Still, for others, it may be that they lack the education or access to medical intervention that they would otherwise accept or desire, due to a myriad of reasons that can range from social isolation and socioeconomic status to unmanaged mental health morbidities.

Healthcare professionals should seek to understand patients and their experiences. Professionals who are comfortable should be open to educating patients about the widespread availability and safety of GAHT but should never pressure patients to, nor dissuade patients from, pursuing medical intervention. Healthcare professionals should ensure that patients are counseled regarding their options.

"Two-spirit" refers to a person who identifies as having both a masculine and a feminine spirit, and is used by some Indigenous people to describe their sexual, gender and/or spiritual identity.

[d]PrEP (pre-exposure prophylaxis) can reduce a patient's chance of getting HIV from sex or injection drug use. When taken as prescribed, PrEP is highly effective for preventing HIV. There are two pills approved for use as PrEP: Truvada® and Descovy®. Truvada® is for people at risk through sex or injection drug use. Descovy® is for people at risk through sex. It is not for people recorded female at birth who are at risk for HIV through receptive vaginal sex. Apretude® is the only injection approved for use as PrEP. It is for people at risk through sex who weigh at least 77 pounds (35 kg).

BOX 26.4 Trans Broken Arm Syndrome

Another thing to be aware of in your general evaluation of trans patients is what has been termed Trans Broken Arm Syndrome. This refers to the scenario where trans patients seeking medical attention for a specific concern are dismissed, and their symptoms are attributed to their trans identity.[8]

For example, a transgender patient presents to the emergency department with a broken arm. During their workup, the healthcare professional learns they are receiving GAHT. The provider attributes their broken arm to presumed side effects of the GAHT, such as premature osteoporosis.

This unfortunate situation highlights the need for healthcare professionals to recognize and address the unique needs of transgender patients in a respectful and unbiased manner.

To mitigate the risk of Trans Broken Arm Syndrome, healthcare professionals should create a warm and inclusive environment where patients can express their concerns in their own words, free of assumptions and bias.

TRANS BROKEN ARM SYNDROME

TGD individuals face significant barriers to healthcare access. The *Trans Broken Arm Syndrome* refers to the medical discrimination faced by TGD patients. In this form of discrimination, healthcare professionals make incorrect assumptions about a patient's medical condition based on their gender identity or medical history. This often leads to invasive questioning and misattribution of medical issues, causing harm and distress to the patients. TGD individuals require equitable healthcare just like anyone else. All healthcare professionals need to be trained to treat and respect the whole person (see Box 26.4).

EVALUATION OF THE TRANSFEMININE PATIENT

Evaluation of the Transfeminine Patient on Gender-Affirming Hormone Therapy

For most transfeminine patients, GAHT will be an initial tool to help align other biology with gender identity. GAHT for transfeminine patients usually consists of an estrogen administered orally, transdermally, or by injection, alone or in combination with an adjunct anti-androgen like spironolactone, GnRH[e] agonist or progestin, or cyproterone acetate. Estrogens serve the dual purpose of potently suppressing testosterone via a central mechanism and of acting as the necessary circulating sex steroid for good bone health. Adjunct agents are used to decrease the required dose of estrogen therapy because exogenous estrogens have been associated with venous thromboembolic risk in a dose-dependent manner.[9]

Decreasing testosterone in the presence of sufficient estrogen can be expected to soften skin, decrease acne, induce fat redistribution to a more "female" pattern, stimulate breast development, and decrease the development of spermatozoa.[10-12]

[e]GnRH (gonadotropin hormone–releasing hormone) is the key regulator of the reproductive axis. This hormone ultimately regulates puberty onset, sexual development, and ovulatory cycles.

Feminizing hormones do not alter the voice, and they do not alter bone structure.[f]

At least one group has observed that initiating GAHT during the early stages of puberty results in hip bone geometry consistent with the gender identity, e.g., trans girls with hip geometry similar to cis girls.[13] One group investigating hip bone geometry in adult transgender people found no difference after GAHT, though this study did not measure cis controls.[14]

Healthcare professionals should counsel patients about what is known regarding the effects of feminizing GAHT and the limitations in current knowledge and monitor patients for novel changes to broaden and enrich the medical literature regarding gender-affirming care.

Evaluation of the Transfeminine Patient, Postoperative Care

Modern surgical intervention to reconfigure the penis into a vagina began in the early 1900s. Today, the *penile inversion flap vaginoplasty* is widely considered the standard in transfeminine genital reconstructive surgery (see Fig. 26.2).[15] While many surgeons have moved away from lining the vaginal canal with the pedicled penile skin flap, it is still the predominant method to utilize the foundational elements of penile flap to the posterior perineum as the basis for constructing a cosmetically acceptable vulva.[16]

Because of the homology of the penis and vulva, most gynecological considerations are relevant for the transfeminine patient who has undergone vaginoplasty. After vaginoplasty, transfeminine care can be within the scope of gynecology with appropriate training. Symptoms of sexually transmitted infections such as chlamydia and gonorrhea in patients with reconstructed vulvas mirror those seen in patients with natal vulvas.

One important difference between neovaginas and natal vaginas is the histological composition of the lining of the vaginal canal. There has been debate concerning the lining of the penile inversion flap vaginal canal and whether the keratinized epithelium undergoes metaplasia to a more mucosal composition. The limited available data suggest that metaplasia of the keratinized epithelial lining of the neovagina may not occur unless mucosal tissue is proximally available.[17] Thus, healthcare professionals examining post-vaginoplasty transfeminine patients should ascertain the exact surgical procedure performed and use this information accordingly. Discharge from a keratinized epithelium-lined vaginal canal may be cause for concern and should be investigated.

Post-vaginoplasty care management requires that patients regularly insert stents, often called dilators, into the neovagina, to maintain the neovaginal depth and width during healing. The most common complication following vaginoplasty of any canal construction is neovaginal stenosis.[18] This typically results from poor dilation or complete cessation of dilation. Healthcare professionals managing the care of transfeminine patients who have undergone vaginoplasty should be familiar

[f]For this reason, some transfeminine patients may opt for facial reconstructive surgery, known colloquially as facial feminization surgery or FFS. Although seemingly cosmetic, this is a medically necessary procedure.

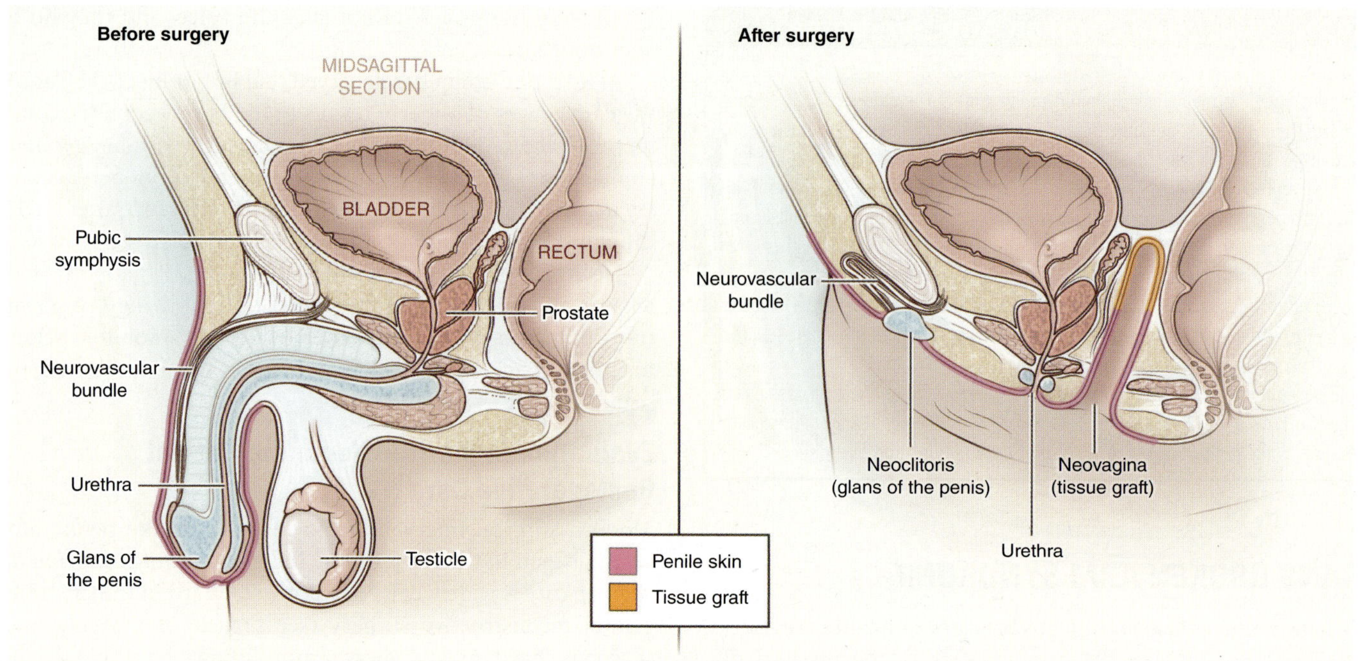

Fig. 26.2 Common Approach to Vaginoplasty. (Reused with permission from Safer JD, Tangpricha V: Care of transgender persons, *N Engl J Med* 381(25):2451–2460, 2019. doi:10.1056/NEJMcp1903650. PMID: 31851801.)

TABLE 26.2 Neovaginal Dilation Schedule

	1 Month Post-Op	2 Months Post-Op	3 Months Post-Op	6 Months Post-Op	Life
Frequency of Dilation	4×/day	3×/day	2×/day	1×/day	Weekly

with the necessity for lifelong dilation and the appropriate schedules for dilation (see Table 26.2).

Other common complications include the development of granulation tissue, hematoma, and/or wound dehiscence, particularly of the posterior introitus. More serious complications include rectovaginal fistula (typically associated with intraoperative damage to the rectum) and partial or complete graft loss of the neovaginal lining either due to poor anastomosis, poor oxygenation of the wound bed, or excessive graft tension.

Although data are few, it has been proposed that the type of vaginoplasty performed is associated with the type of microenvironment. Hence, peritoneal graft (i.e., tunica vaginalis) or flap (i.e., Davydov) vaginoplasty may be associated with a higher incidence of mucosal metaplasia and natal-like flora; penile inversion flap with or without scrotal grafting may be associated with a lower incidence of histological changes and penile prepuce-like flora; and colon flap vaginoplasty may be associated with gut-like flora of the neovagina.[19,20]

At least one paper has reported the possibility of neovaginal candidiasis in post-vaginoplasty patients.[21] Post-vaginoplasty transfeminine patients with symptoms of neovaginal candidiasis should be treated appropriately.

Current literature does not support Pap smears for transfeminine patients with neovaginas. Cancers of the neovagina are rare and typically HPV-related.[22] Speculum exams to visualize the vaginal canal and assess the lining for neoplasia may be appropriate.

One unique consideration of transfeminine gynecologic care is the clinical management of the prostate. In most surgeries, the prostate is relocated to the anterior wall of the vaginal canal when the pocket for the vaginal canal is dissected through the fascial layer between the rectum and prostate. Although rare, prostate cancer is reported in transfeminine people who have undergone vaginoplasty.[23] Digital examination of the prostate may be performed intravaginally when indicated.[24]

EVALUATION OF THE TRANSMASCULINE PATIENT

Evaluation of the Transmasculine Patient on Gender-Affirming Hormone Therapy

GAHT for transmasculine patients usually consists of testosterone (Table 26.3). Testosterone stops menstrual cycles and decreases the ovaries' ability to make estrogen. The goal of masculinizing hormone therapy is the development of male secondary sex characteristics and the suppression/minimization of female secondary sex characteristics.

Testosterone therapy can result in masculinization of the voice, increased body hair growth rate/amount, changes in body odor, increased sebaceous secretion with an associated increase in acne, onset of male-pattern facial hair growth, male pattern baldness for patients with genetic predisposition, and enlargement of the glans clitoris. Some patients also report mood changes and vaginal atrophy. At least one observational cohort study reports that prolonged androgen therapy may not appear to have a deleterious effect on gamete production.[26]

Evaluation of the Transmasculine Patient, Postoperative Care

For transmasculine patients, there are two types of genital reconstruction: metoidioplasty and phalloplasty.

TABLE 26.3 Gender-Affirming Hormone Therapy (GAHT) for Transmasculine Patients[25]

Agent	Route of Administration
Buccal testosterone (e.g., Striant®)	Buccal
Nasal testosterone (e.g., Natesto®)	Nasal
Pellet testosterone (e.g., Testopel®)	Subdermal
Testosterone gel (e.g., AndroGel®, Fortesta®, Testim®, Vogelxo®)	Topical
Testosterone solution (e.g., Axiron®)	Topical
Testosterone cypionate, testosterone enanthate, testosterone undecanoate	Intramuscular or subcutaneous injection

Metoidioplasty involves surgically freeing the clitoral tissue from the pubis, using the hood and proximal minora to construct a penile shaft. The urethra may be lengthened to meet the neopenis glans by mucosa grafting, typically with buccal or vaginal epithelium. A scrotum can be constructed by joining the majora together with sutures. Some patients may opt for testicular implants. Nearly all patients who could achieve orgasm through clitoral stimulation prior to surgery are also able to achieve orgasm through neopenis glans stimulation. Complications are generally less common than in phalloplasty, but key complications can include urinary incontinence, urinary retention, and urethral fistulas. Patients reporting symptoms of sexually transmitted illness (STI) should be evaluated appropriately.

Phalloplasty utilizes free flaps to construct a neophallus (see Fig. 26.3).

Historically, the flap has been harvested from the radial forearm because of its fat composition and neurovascular supply. Other sites are also used, including pedicled anterolateral thigh flaps or pudendal thigh flaps.[27,28] Because of the nature of this procedure, three surgeries may be required to achieve a functional and aesthetically acceptable phallus. These stages are, in general:

1. Creation of the neophallus and neourethra in phallus
2. Creation of the penis glans, scrotoplasty, and connection of the neourethra to the bladder

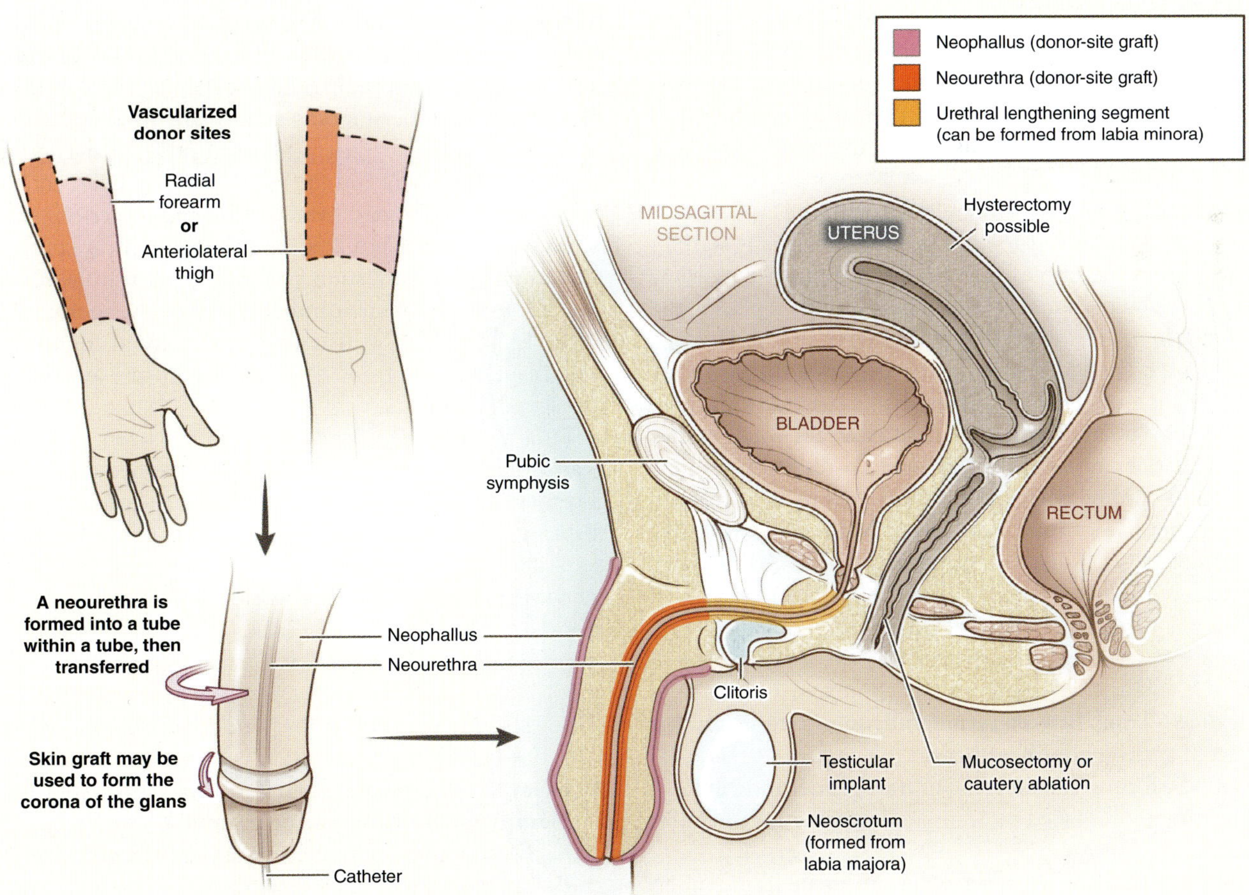

Fig. 26.3 Common Approach to Phalloplasty. (Reused with permission from Safer JD, Tangpricha V: Care of transgender persons, *N Engl J Med* 381(25):2451–2460, 2019. doi:10.1056/NEJMcp1903650. PMID: 31851801.)

3. Erectile and testicular prostheses
4. (If necessary) Further cosmetic refinement of the glans, scrotum, and pubis
5. (If necessary) Medical tattooing

Phalloplasty has the advantage of creating a phallus, which is of a typical adult male length compared to metoidioplasty. However, results are affected by body fat percentage and BMI of the patient undergoing the procedure. It is not uncommon for surgery to result in a neophallus that is much larger in circumference than what is typical for cis males. Complications are common, occurring in up to 51% of patients, including urethral strictures and fistulas. Devastating complications include complete loss of the phallus due to poor vascularization or other vascular insult, which is estimated to occur in 1.7% of patients according to one study.[29] Healthcare professionals evaluating patients who have undergone phalloplasty should ascertain the length of time since the procedure, with awareness of the risk of vascular insult in the early postoperative weeks. Professionals should be diligent in assessing patients for fistula and stricture. After undergoing all stages and after adequate healing, patients may experience other typical ailments of the penis. Patients in this late group who report symptoms of sexually transmitted infections should be evaluated appropriately.

EVALUATION OF THE PATIENT STOPPING CARE OR CHANGING GOALS

Several studies suggest that the vast majority (>98.3%; 98%[30]; 98.6%[31]) of patients starting GAHT continue it. Among those patients who choose to cease GAHT, the overwhelming majority (82.5%) report social discord as the reason for their decision.[32]

Regret following surgery is even lower, with the latest meta-analysis reporting a pooled regret rate of 1%.[33] This is significantly lower than the rate of regret for other major surgeries, including knee replacement (6%–30%),[34] hip replacement (4.8%),[35] and thoracic and abdominal surgery (37.6%).[36]

If a patient wishes to return to the presentation they had prior to entering care, they should not be dissuaded from their decision. It may be appropriate to first ascertain whether the patient is experiencing social issues, such as difficulty finding a job, difficulty finding romantic partners, loss of close friends or family due to rejection, lack of access to adequate care, and other social stressors. Continue to provide appropriate, supportive care that meets patient goals.

MENTAL HEALTH EVALUATION

In the context of transgender healthcare, mental health evaluation plays a crucial role in ensuring comprehensive and holistic care for transgender patients.

One important aspect addressed in mental health evaluation is the concept of minority stress. Transgender individuals often encounter discrimination, stigma, and social rejection due to their gender identity, which can contribute to higher rates of mental health issues.

The mental health evaluation process should be conducted by healthcare professionals who possess expertise in transgender healthcare and are sensitive to the unique experiences and challenges faced by transgender patients. Creating a therapeutic relationship built on trust and understanding is essential to ensure that transgender individuals receive appropriate support and care for their mental health needs.

CONCLUSION

In conclusion, healthcare for the transgender patient is multifaceted and deeply personal, marked by unique medical, psychological, and social considerations. Throughout this chapter, we have explored the challenges and complexities faced by transgender individuals as they navigate their healthcare experiences.

We began by acknowledging the importance of cultural sensitivity among healthcare professionals, recognizing that respectful and inclusive care is essential to fostering trust and improving health outcomes for transgender patients. We delved into the significance of understanding gender identity, gender incongruence due to a misalignment between one's gender identity and recorded sex at birth, and the role of medical interventions, such as hormone therapy and gender-affirming surgeries.

As we move forward, it is crucial for healthcare professionals to continue their education and training in transgender healthcare, to promote an environment of respect, dignity, and inclusivity. Empathy, active listening, and cultural humility should remain at the forefront of every healthcare encounter with transgender patients.

Finally, while significant progress has been made in recent years in recognizing and addressing the healthcare needs of transgender individuals, there is still much work to be done. By fostering a healthcare system that values diversity and ensures equitable access to quality care, we can contribute to a more inclusive and compassionate world for all patients.

REVIEW QUESTIONS

1. **What does "Trans Broken Arm Syndrome" refer to in the context of transgender healthcare?**
   A. A medical condition specific to transgender individuals
   B. Discrimination faced by transgender patients in healthcare
   C. A rare syndrome affecting bone health in transgender patients
   D. Misattribution of medical issues to a patient's gender-affirming treatment
   E. A term describing the emotional distress experienced by transgender patients
2. **What is the primary goal of masculinizing hormone therapy for transmasculine patients?**
   A. Development of female secondary sex characteristics
   B. Suppression of male secondary sex characteristics
   C. Development of male secondary sex characteristics
   D. Suppression of female secondary sex characteristics
   E. No effect on secondary sex characteristics

3. **What does "cisgender" mean in the context of gender identity?**
   A. Describes individuals whose gender identity aligns with their sex recorded at birth
   B. Describes individuals who do not identify strictly as male or female
   C. Describes individuals who have undergone gender-affirming surgeries
   D. Describes individuals who identify as both male and female
   E. A term used to describe transgender individuals
4. **What is the purpose of neovaginal dilation for transfeminine patients post-vaginoplasty?**
   A. To increase the sensitivity of the neovagina
   B. To maintain neovaginal depth and width during healing
   C. To reduce the risk of neovaginal stenosis
   D. To promote mucosal metaplasia in the neovagina
   E. To prevent the development of granulation tissue
5. **What is the goal of feminizing hormone therapy for transfeminine patients?**
   A. Development of male secondary sex characteristics
   B. Suppression of female secondary sex characteristics
   C. Development of female secondary sex characteristics
   D. Suppression of male secondary sex characteristics
   E. No effect on secondary sex characteristics
6. **What does the term "two-spirit" refer to in some Indigenous cultures?**
   A. A spiritual leader in the community
   B. A contemporary term used to describe gender-diverse individuals
   C. A warrior in the tribe
   D. A term used to describe cisgender individuals
   E. A term used to describe transgender individuals
7. **What is the primary objective of a mental health evaluation in transgender healthcare?**
   A. Prescribe hormone therapy
   B. Determine gender identity
   C. Address minority stress and mental health issues
   D. Evaluate physical health
   E. Provide counseling for family members
8. **What role does cultural humility play in transgender healthcare?**
   A. It ensures that healthcare professionals are well-versed in all cultural practices.
   B. It encourages healthcare professionals to recognize their own biases and engage with diverse cultural backgrounds respectfully.
   C. It promotes cultural assimilation among transgender patients.
   D. It involves enforcing cultural norms within healthcare settings.
   E. It discourages cultural diversity within healthcare practices.
9. **What is the purpose of a "metoidioplasty" in gender-affirming surgeries?**
   A. To construct a neophallus using a free flap
   B. To remove breast tissue
   C. To create a neophallus using clitoral tissue
   D. To increase testosterone levels
   E. To elongate vocal cords
10. **Which surgical procedure results in a neophallus of typical adult male length?**
    A. Chest reconstruction
    B. Metoidioplasty
    C. Phalloplasty
    D. Vaginoplasty
    E. Penile inversion flap

REFERENCES

Available online.

27

The Acutely Ill or Injured Patient

Mark H. Swartz and Paul E. Phrampus

There is no thing more precious here than tyme.

Saint Bernard (1090–1153)

The purpose of this chapter is to provide a practical approach to treating patients who are acutely ill or injured. The focus is on conducting a prioritized assessment and diagnostic considerations rather than providing therapy. This chapter is intended for healthcare professionals who work in traditional healthcare environments such as clinics, doctor's offices, and hospitals. We also emphasize the importance of those who may provide care for patients outside of medical settings or those who act as good samaritans and help someone in need while not at work.

When dealing with patients who are acutely ill or injured, time is often of the essence. It's important to have a well-organized and structured approach to quickly assess the patient's condition. This will enable you to administer the appropriate life-saving treatments, identify the necessary resources, and create an optimal environment for providing the best possible care.

When it comes to evaluating patients who are acutely ill, the process is different from evaluating stable patients. The focus is on identifying any potential issues with the patient's bodily functions that may require immediate intervention to prevent further harm or death. This is done while the final diagnosis is being investigated. Acute illnesses may present with similar symptoms, which makes it important to investigate and identify the root cause of the problem. However, in some cases, the treatment must begin immediately to prevent any complications.

When evaluating patients who are acutely ill, it is always important to **ensure your own safety first**. Then, think about what the most serious threat to the patient's life is, and do what you can to stabilize it. Make sure you have gathered all the necessary resources you may need to care for the patient. Finally, consider the most likely cause of the illness and make sure to rule out any potential causes.

When providing medical care in the field, it is crucial to assess the situation quickly to determine the exact resources necessary to take care of the patient(s) properly. Calling for extra resources promptly can often make a significant difference in saving a life. It is important to realize that there is always an inherent delay in the response time of additional care team members. Identifying the patient's situation at the scene may help determine the mechanisms of injury to assist in the diagnostic workup and treatment for the patient.

PERSONAL SAFETY

It is important to note that when discussing the care for acutely ill and injured patients, healthcare professionals should prioritize their own safety and well-being. Protecting oneself from pathogen exposure, as well as from trauma or additional injuries, is of utmost importance.

When caring for a patient who is acutely ill, there is a high risk of exposure to body fluids and communicable diseases. If the patient has an altered mental status, the initial responder should take precautions in case the patient becomes aggressive or violent. In the case of an injured patient, the initial healthcare professional should ensure that the scene is safe before beginning to care for the patient to prevent harm to themselves.

Standard precautions (see Chapter 6, The Physical Examination) should always be taken to minimize the possibility of contamination and exposure. The potential for concern should be evaluated to determine the appropriate precautions needed. Wearing protective gloves is certainly considered a minimum step. Still, as the potential for contamination escalates, consideration should be given to masks with eye shields, protective gowns, respiratory masks, and so on, which are appropriate for the situation.

The safety of the care environment should always be a primary consideration. Having adequate police, security, or additional personnel to ensure that the environment is safe for healthcare professionals is paramount. This is especially true in the prehospital care environment, particularly at the scene of an automobile accident, where the first instinct is to help the patient.

As you approach the apparent patient, always evaluate to determine whether you are in a safe environment; if not, protect yourself and your patient to limit exposure to possible injury before providing care. Assess environmental hazards, the potential of agitation from a delirious patient, acting aggressively, and other personnel hazards such as family members and bystanders. There are rising amounts of reports of violence against healthcare professionals, thus such an assessment is crucial to safety.

Although it is rare, there may be situations where a rescuer could be harmed or killed while providing care. In such cases, the rescuer should wait until the situation is safe before providing aid. For instance, if a patient is trapped in a car in a busy traffic lane after a car accident, the rescuer should not provide first aid until safety flares or cones are placed to prevent further accidents. Other hazards, such as downed power lines, must also be taken into account. In an active shooter situation, the care of the injured cannot begin until the scene has been secured properly by police personnel.

APPROACH TO THE UNCONSCIOUS PATIENT

The initial task for the healthcare professional in approaching most, if not all, patients in acute situations involving an unconscious patient is first to ensure that they are not in cardiopulmonary arrest. If so, the initial priorities are summoning help and performing cardiopulmonary resuscitation (CPR). If the patient does not need CPR, immediate identification of the causes of their non-responsiveness should be initiated through an organized two-step approach to the rapid patient assessment, including a primary and secondary survey.

When caring for the acutely ill outside the traditional care environment, particular attention should be paid to the primary survey. This organized approach helps identify the major threats to life first. The acceptable approach to these acute, undefined encounters is to consider the patient unstable until you can confirm, through a series of diagnostic steps, that the patient is well enough for you to take the time to perform a more rigorous and complete physical examination and document a complete history.

CURRENT CARDIOPULMONARY RESUSCITATION GUIDELINES

For the unconscious patient who is determined to be in cardiac arrest, the healthcare professional should initiate CPR according to the guidelines set by the American Heart Association (AHA). Cardiac arrest survival is directly related to how fast high-quality chest compressions (CPR) are started, along with defibrillation by an automatic external defibrillator (AED) as early as possible.

Chest compressions provide blood flow to the heart and brain during a cardiac arrest. Research has shown that delays or interruptions to compressions significantly reduce survival rates. Additional research demonstrates increased survival from cardiac arrest correlating with the onset of defibrillation, if appropriate. Starting CPR with chest compressions can effectively circulate blood to the victim's brain and heart sooner, with the principal goal of maintaining some amount of oxygenated blood circulating through the brain.

Initiating ventilation is less critical, as victims will have oxygen remaining in their lungs and bloodstream for the first few minutes after a cardiac arrest.

Fig. 27.1 shows the AHA CPR overview for adults. Fig. 27.2 shows the AHA CPR overview for children.

Current AHA guidelines make recommendations based on whether the lay rescuer is trained in CPR or not. According to the 2020 AHA Guidelines, the sole lay rescuer trained in CPR should do four basic things:

- Ensure scene safety
- Call for help/activate emergency response
- Start and continue compression-only CPR
- Send a second person to find an AED

On the other hand, when a patient is in cardiac arrest and there are two or more rescuers who are trained in CPR (and/or working in the healthcare environment), add rescue breathing and aggressive use of an AED via a second rescuer/team of rescuers in this sequence:

- Ensure scene safety
- Call for help/activate resuscitation team
- Apply AED as soon as available
- Start two-rescuer CPR using a ratio of 30 chest compressions to two rescue breaths

In the early days of CPR, an original A-B-C (airway, breathing, circulation) sequence was taught. However, it was later realized that survival rates improved with early chest compressions. Chest compressions were often delayed while the responder opened the airway to give mouth-to-mouth breaths or retrieved a barrier device or other ventilation equipment. Since 2010, the AHA Guidelines have recommended an overall change in the mnemonic to *C-A-B*. By changing the sequence to C-A-B, chest compressions can be initiated sooner, and ventilation is delayed only minimally until completion of the first cycle of chest compressions (30 compressions should be accomplished in approximately 18 seconds).

C-A-B

Compressions: Push hard and fast on the center of the victim's chest.

Airway: Tilt the victim's head back and lift the chin to open the airway.

Breathing: Give rescue breaths.

CARDIOPULMONARY RESUSCITATION SURVEY

Because of the time sensitivity associated with interrupted blood flow to the brain and vital organs, it is safest to suspect cardiac arrest in any patient who is not obviously interacting with their environment. Performing a quick rapid assessment can oftentimes easily rule out cardiac arrest.

As you approach the patient, observe the scene and surroundings for potential hazards. Then, observe the patient closely and look for spontaneous breathing or movements. If these are not discernible, stimulate the patient by gently shaking and talking loudly to them while asking, *"Are you okay?"*

If there is no response or evidence of spontaneous breathing, call for help in any way you can without leaving the patient; it is unlikely that you can manage the entire resuscitation by yourself. If another person is available, have them locate the nearest AED.

Determine whether there is spontaneous cardiac function by feeling for a carotid pulse for 10 seconds or, in an infant, by

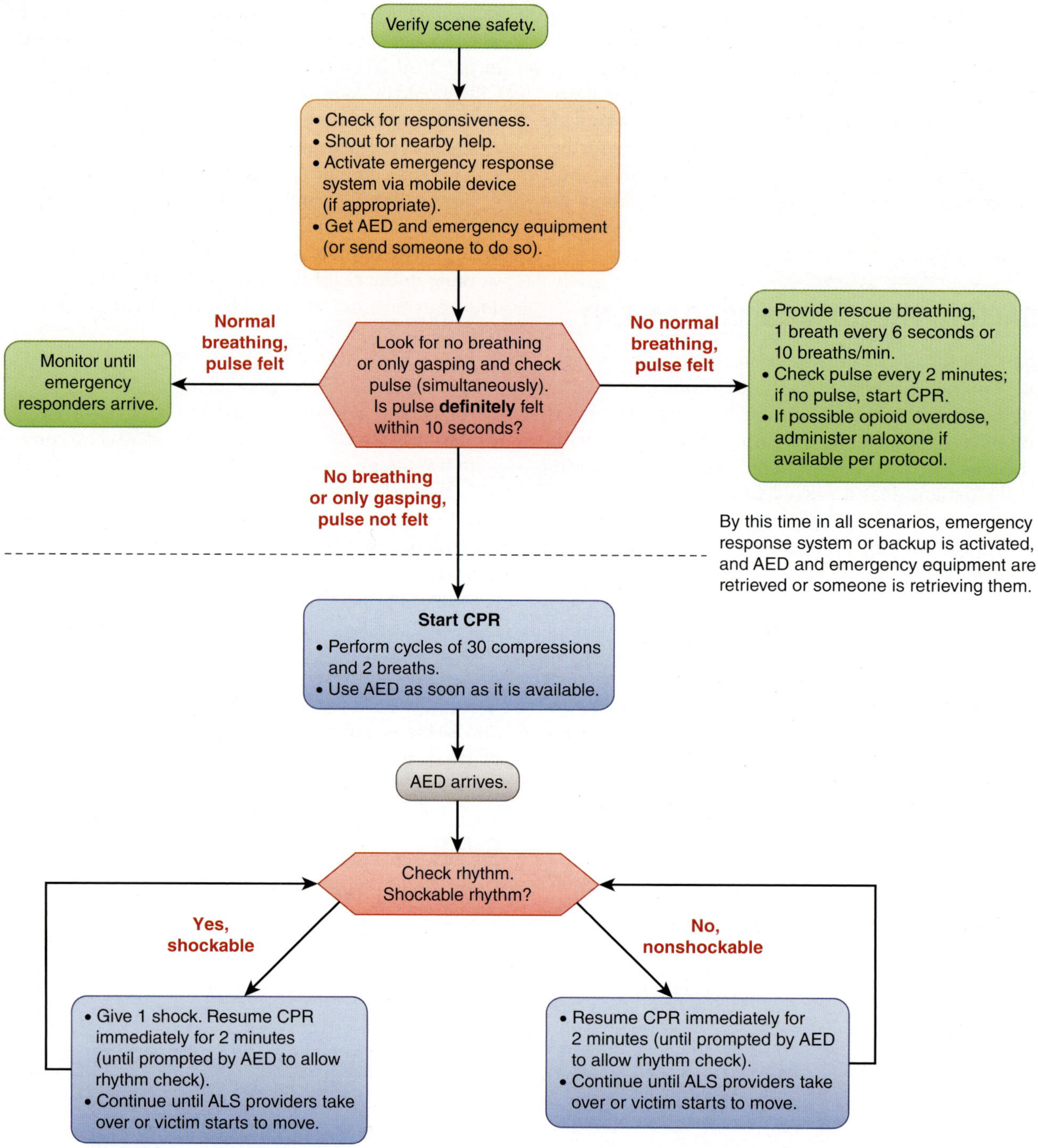

Fig. 27.1 **Adult Basic Life Support Algorithm for Healthcare Professionals.** AED indicates automated external defibrillator; ALS, advanced life support; and CPR, cardiopulmonary resuscitation. (Reprinted with permission Circulation. 2020;142:S366-S468. ©2020 American Heart Association, Inc.)

palpating the arm for a brachial artery impulse. If there is no pulse, begin external chest compressions, at least 100 per minute.

To open an unconscious victim's airway, hyperextend the head and lift the patient's chin; place one hand on the patient's forehead and the other behind the patient's occiput, and tilt their head backward. This maneuver moves the tongue away from the back of the throat, allowing air to pass around the tongue and into the trachea. Caution should be exercised with any patient who has a suspected neck injury, such as someone in a serious car crash. With such a patient, try to open the airway by lifting the chin and jaw without tilting the head backward; grasp the lower teeth and pull the mandible forward. If necessary, tilt the head back very slightly. If a patient wears dentures, remove them only if they occlude the airway.

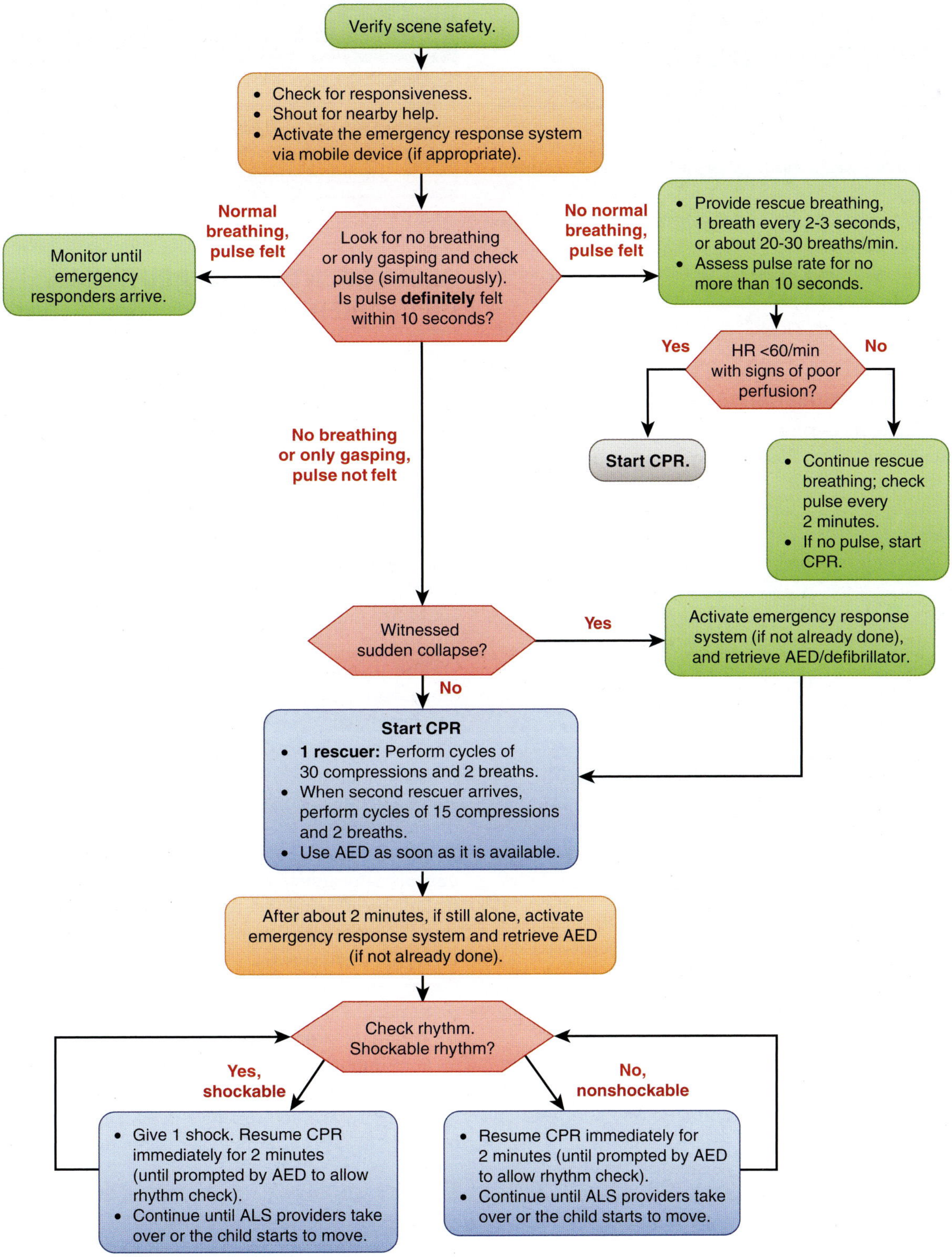

Fig. 27.2 Pediatric Basic Life Support Algorithm for Healthcare Professionals—Single Rescuer (American Health Association). AED indicates automated external defibrillator; ALS, advanced life support; CPR, cardiopulmonary resuscitation; and HR, heart rate. (Reprinted with permission Circulation. 2020;142:S469-S523. ©2020 American Heart Association, Inc.)

SUMMARY OF CARDIOPULMONARY RESUSCITATION GUIDELINES FOR ADULTS, CHILDREN, AND INFANTS

Check

- **If unresponsive:** No breathing or no normal breathing (only gasping)
  - Try to get the person to respond; if they don't, roll the person onto their back.
  - Call 911 or ask others to do so. Get the AED if available and return to the patient.
  - If a second rescuer is available, send them to get help and the AED.

Cardiopulmonary Resuscitation

- Attach and use AED as soon as available.
- Start chest compressions. Place the heel of your hand on the center of the patient's chest.
- Put your other hand on top of the first with your fingers interlaced.
- Push the chest at least 2 inches, 30 times in the center of the chest.
  - Push two-handed, with one hand on top of the other.
- Push at a rate of **at least 100** compressions per minute.
- Allow complete chest recoil after each push.
- Limit interruptions in chest compressions to less than 10 seconds.
- Open the patient's airway.
- Head Tilt–Chin Lift: Tilt the head back and lift the chin.
- Pinch closed the nose of the patient.
- Take a normal breath and cover the patient's mouth with your own to create an airtight seal, and then give two 1-second breaths.
- The patient's chest should rise with each breath.
- Use a barrier device if available.

Continue Sets of 30 Pushes and 2 Breaths

- Continue compressions and breaths—30 compressions, 2 breaths—until help arrives.
- CPR ratio for CPR is 30 compressions to 2 breaths.
- In two-person CPR, the rescuers should change positions every 2 minutes to avoid fatigue and a deterioration in the chest compression quality.
- Attach and use AED as soon as available.

A summary of key basic life support components for adults, children, and infants (excluding newborn infants) is available at https://heartcprtrainingcenter.com/pdf/2020BLSSummary.pdf (accessed July 24, 2024)

There is continued emphasis on providing high-quality chest compressions. Remember to:

- Get an AED
- Push hard
- Push fast

Box 27.1 summarizes the components of high-quality chest compressions.

BOX 27.1 Components of High-Quality Chest Compressions

Ensuring chest compressions of adequate rate
Ensuring chest compressions of adequate depth
Allowing full chest recoil between compressions
Minimizing interruptions in chest compressions
Avoiding excessive ventilation

ASSESSMENT OF THE ACUTELY ILL OR INJURED PATIENT

The assessment of the acutely ill patient involves moving through a series of simple evaluations, which are grouped into two categories termed the *primary* and *secondary surveys*. The primary survey is a check for conditions that are an immediate threat to the patient's life. This initial assessment should take no longer than 20 to 30 seconds. The initial part of the primary survey should rule out cardiac arrest and the need for immediate CPR. The remainder of the primary survey is to identify and begin emergency treatment of immediate threats to life if identified. The secondary survey is a check for conditions that could become life-threatening problems if not recognized and attended to.

The primary and secondary surveys are used for both adult and pediatric patients, as well as for medical and injury-related problems. During the primary survey, the treatment process may be integrated into the diagnostic process. For example, if the patient is not breathing, ventilation should begin immediately before you move on to the next diagnostic step.

The first task is to recognize when a patient is acutely ill. An unusual appearance or behavior may be the only sign. These include breathing difficulties, clutching the chest or throat, slurring of speech, confusion, unusual odor to the breath, sweating for no apparent reason, or uncharacteristic skin color (e.g., pale, flushed, or bluish). For example, in cases of traumatic injury, there may be obvious signs such as unresponsiveness, gasping for breath, or profound bleeding.

It is important to remember that an acutely ill patient is anxious and frightened; a calm and reassuring voice can go a long way toward comforting the patient. Caring for a relaxed patient is always easier than caring for an anxious one.

Primary Survey

Once it has been determined that the patient does not need CPR, attention should then turn to ascertain whether key life-sustaining functions are adequate and stable, or whether augmentation or other supportive measures are necessary.

The primary or initial survey developed by the American College of Surgeons (ACS) for the Advanced Trauma Life Support Guidelines is an excellent starting point for an organized rapid assessment to identify and begin treatment for potentially critically injured trauma patients, and it also works well for acute illness.

It uses a familiar mnemonic, ABCDE, for the initial or primary survey. During the evaluation of the primary survey, it is important to remember that if you find a significant problem, you should begin to initiate treatment before moving on, if possible.

A—Airway

Assessment of airway begins by assessing if the patient has a patent airway. This can be accomplished by observing if the patient has any obvious obstruction to the airway. In addition to observing, listening for sounds of obstruction can also be useful. Sounds such as gurgling or stridor can indicate partial upper airway obstruction.

Assessing the airway's overall patency can often be accomplished by asking the patient what their name is. If they can speak, the airway is open. When assessing the airway, one should be alert for signs of obstructions, potential obstructions, and associated signs and symptoms. It is important to remember that the **most common cause of airway obstruction in the unconscious patient is the patient's own tongue.** If the patient has no suspicion of neck injury, tilting the head backward to help move the tongue off the posterior pharynx can alleviate this situation.

Pay close attention to obstruction of the airway. Common findings in trauma are obstructions that may include vomit, teeth, or other foreign bodies, which should be removed immediately, when possible.

In trauma patients, it is important to try to maintain the alignment of the cervical spine during all aspects of the primary survey so the head tilt method is *not* used. In such cases, the jaw thrust is used to move the tongue. Immobilize the patient's head and neck by using boards, tape, bulky dressings, or towels or by assigning someone to hold the head immobile. Once a patient is immobilized, removal of these measures requires careful decision making.

If airway patency remains a problem, endotracheal intubation or the placement of a breathing tube by qualified professionals may need to be accomplished, depending on the clinical setting.

B—Breathing

Assessment of the adequacy of breathing and respirations is the second step to the primary survey. During this phase, evaluating for signs and symptoms of respiratory distress and identifying life-threatening injuries associated with the pulmonary system in trauma patients is undertaken.

Ensure the chest is rising and falling, note the approximate frequency, and determine whether the patient is breathing too fast, too slow, or just about normal. Observe for signs and symptoms of respiratory distress, such as accessory muscle use of the chest wall and or accessory muscle use in the neck area. Patients in respiratory distress will often have increased respiratory rate with an exaggeration of the use of the neck and chest wall muscles. A brief auscultation of the lung sounds to ensure air flows in both lungs is usually accomplished during this phase.

Noting the overall integrity of the chest wall and rib cage is important. Observing for paradoxical motion, meaning the unusual, asymmetric movement of the chest wall during respirations, can indicate a flail chest. In this case, there are many rib fractures that allow for a portion of the chest wall to be free-floating. This is an indication of significant trauma. Listening for gurgling or extraneous air movement can be clues to the serious underlying injury.

Pneumothorax is the collapse of a lung away from the chest wall. It can occur spontaneously or as the result of trauma. Pneumothorax can be classified as open, meaning an air leak communicating with the outside, or closed, which may occur because of a lung laceration from a rib fracture. They are often identified by findings of an absence or decreased volume of lung sounds on the side of the pneumothorax. The conscious patient with a pneumothorax may be concerned with sharp pain associated with inspiration. Palpation of the chest wall may reveal *subcutaneous emphysema*, which is air from the pleural space that has leaked into the subcutaneous skin surfaces. Subcutaneous emphysema is classically described as feeling like the crunch of Rice Krispies beneath your fingers.

An open pneumothorax, otherwise known as a *sucking chest wound*, allows air to enter the pleural space, leading to collapse of the underlying lung (producing a pneumothorax). It can be identified by a sucking sound or bubbling of blood in a chest wound associated with the patient's breathing. If identified, the wound should be covered with an occlusive dressing.

In trauma patients with severe respiratory distress, unconsciousness, or cardiac arrest, consideration must be given to the potential diagnosis of a *tension pneumothorax*. Tension pneumothorax occurs when an air leak in the lung causes a lung collapse and a pressure to build up on the injured side. As the pressure builds, the injured side encroaches on the uninjured side, leading to the lung's inability to expand. It also creates external pressure on the heart, which delays filling from the central venous system. This can evolve rapidly to severe shock and lead to death if untreated.

Tension pneumothorax should be suspected immediately by the absence or decrease of breath sounds on the side of the pneumothorax, profound distention of the jugular veins, and diminishing blood pressure. An extremely late finding of tracheal deviation away from the injured side can be found in advanced tension pneumothorax. If tension pneumothorax is suspected in a critically ill trauma patient, a needle decompression of the chest wall should occur immediately. Tension pneumothorax can rapidly cause severe shock and death if left untreated.

C—Circulation

In this step of the primary survey, the healthcare professional is trying to determine a rough estimate of the cardiopulmonary system with regard to circulation and blood pressure. Attempting to stabilize end-organ perfusion, such as the brain, heart, and lungs, is key to survival for the critically ill and injured.

Initially, attempting to palpate the radial pulse is a key physical exam component to completing this step. The radial pulse check can yield considerable amounts of information during the assessment of a critically ill patient. Noting the pulse rate (i.e., too fast, too slow, or approximately normal) and the quality of the pulse provides significant information. A rapid, thready pulse can indicate shock. Knowing that **if the radial pulse is palpable, the systolic blood pressure can be estimated to be at least 80 mm Hg.** If the radial pulse is not palpable, immediately assess the femoral pulse, which approximates the systolic pressure at 70 mm Hg if it is present.

It is important to remember that during the primary survey, we would not be taking a detailed measurement of the heart rate or ascertaining the blood pressure. We are using our clinical judgment to provide estimates to determine if there are any life-threatening conditions requiring immediate treatment.

While assessing the pulse checks, simultaneously note the skin color, moisture, and color. Pale, sweaty, cool skin findings are signs of shock and hypoperfusion that result from the activation of the sympathetic nervous system. If the patient's skin is warm, dry, and of normal color, it is likely that oxygenation and flow of blood to the periphery are adequate.

In shock, peripheral blood flow is shunted centrally; thus, skin changes are early indicators of hypovolemic or cardiogenic (i.e., low cardiac output) shock. Key diagnostic skin signs associated with these major acute cardiopulmonary derangements are gray, mottled, or cyanotic color; cold skin temperature; and markedly sweaty skin. The last sign, termed *diaphoresis*, is caused by activation of the sympathetic nervous system by any major threat to homeostasis.

In trauma patients, it is important to also assess for signs of life-threatening external bleeding, arterial or venous, which should be brought under control if identified. It is important to carefully inspect the seriously injured patient for external bleeding so that it does not go undiagnosed. Particular attention must be paid if the patient is wearing thick or multiple layers of clothing that can obscure bleeding.

Direct pressure over bleeding is the best first step to control it. If severe bleeding of an injured extremity persists, a tourniquet should be rapidly applied to bring major bleeding under control. Caution should be exercised when putting pressure on large bleeding areas of deformed extremities, as bone shards and fragments from open fractures can injure the rescuer.

D—Disability

Overall, mental status can be a key indicator of end-organ perfusion of the brain and serve as an important baseline test of trauma patients who are having an evolving mental status change secondary to brain injury. Central nervous system function is noted in this phase by the use of a simplified mental status evaluation process using the mnemonic known as ***AVPU***. The AVPU mnemonic for level of consciousness is as follows:

A: Patient is ***a***lert
V: Patient responds to a ***v***erbal stimulus
P: Patient responds to a ***p***ainful stimulus
U: Patient is ***u***nresponsive

E—Expose

More specific to trauma patients, depending on the clinical setting, it is necessary to expose the patient as much as possible to try and further identify any further threats to life. The clothes and other debris raise the possibility of concealing major bleeding, open chest wounds, and other physical examination signs, such as large areas of contusions, which can be clues to major internal injuries. After the assessment, it is important to cover the patient to minimize the loss of body heat.

Vital Signs

Assess and reassess vital signs. Once the steps of the initial survey are completed as described earlier, formal measurement of the vital signs should be performed. These include a detailed measuring of the patient's heart rate, respirations, blood pressure, and mental status. Depending on the clinical setting and the availability of equipment, vital signs should also include body temperature and pulse oximetry readings.

If a vital sign is abnormal, begin to treat the abnormality to bring it back to normal. For example, if the patient is breathing spontaneously at a rate of only 5 breaths/min, augment and assist the patient's breathing so that the depth and rate of breathing are normalized. Assisting ventilations can be accomplished by applying interspersed mouth-to-mouth ventilations if a barrier protective device is available. Employing a bag-valve-mask device or performing endotracheal intubation and placing the patient on a ventilator may also be indicated. The exact therapy will vary widely depending on the clinical setting and the experience of the healthcare professional, as well as the resources immediately available.

In a similar manner, the blood pressure can be supported by simply raising the legs, which returns the blood stored in the lower extremity venous system back into the central circulation. Establishing intravenous access should occur rapidly depending on the clinical setting.

In trauma patients, particular attention should be given to keeping external bleeding controlled, reevaluating for developing tension pneumothorax, and considering the need for immediate blood transfusions.

Once you believe that the patient is no longer in imminent risk of death or further instability, it is appropriate to move on to the secondary survey.

Secondary Survey

History

Documenting the history of an acutely ill or injured patient conforms closely to the documentation of the standard history, although it is usually abbreviated and focused on allowing rapid diagnostic and management decisions to be made.

In the secondary survey, obtain a history from the patient, the patient's relatives, emergency department personnel, or bystanders. The secondary survey is a systematic method for determining whether other conditions or injuries are present and necessitate urgent attention. This survey consists of a rapid interview, a vital signs check, and a focused physical examination. The mnemonic ***SAMPLE*** can be helpful in gathering pertinent information:

S: ***s***igns and symptoms associated with the illness
A: ***a***llergies
M: ***m***edications currently being taken; medication changes
P: ***p***ast medical history
L: ***l***ast meal
E: ***e***vents preceding the medical event

The utilization of the SAMPLE survey is important to try and uncover the details that will allow for identification or diagnosis of the underlying cause of the patient's acute illness or injury that will allow for appropriate further testing and or initiation of treatment. For example, the identifying in the history that a patient has had several days of fever, cough, and loss of appetite may indicate that the underlying illness may be pneumonia.

In dealing with a trauma patient, identifying the mechanism of injury is helpful. Did the patient sustain blunt trauma, such as an automobile accident, or was a weapon used that may have caused a penetrating injury? In the case of a vehicular accident, ascertain whether the patient was restrained with seatbelts, whether or not there was airbag deployment, the patient's position in the vehicle, and whether or not they were ejected from the vehicle. Attempt to identify if there was a loss of consciousness, which may indicate a head injury such as a concussion.

In trauma patients who are alert, asking them to identify the area associated with pain may help direct the physical examination further. In general, the secondary assessment of the patient involves examination of three main regions: the head and neck, the torso, and the extremities.

Secondary Survey Physical Examination

Head and neck. Look at the victim's face. In the acutely ill, a patient's sunken eyes and profoundly dry mucous membranes, along with cracked lips, can indicate severe dehydration. Are the mucous membranes pale? This could help identify critical anemia. Evaluate skin color and temperature.

In the trauma patient, is there evidence of *raccoon eyes* or *Battle sign?* A patient with raccoon eyes is shown in Fig. 10.32. Periorbital ecchymoses, or raccoon eyes, are seen 6 to 12 hours after a fracture of the base of the skull. Battle sign is ecchymosis behind the ear caused by basilar skull or temporal bone fractures; this sign may take 24 to 36 hours to develop.

The examination of the eyes for pupillary size and responsiveness to light is actually part of the neurological examination; it is usually performed when examining the face. Are the pupils equal? Are the pupils pinpoint? Is there a unilateral dilated pupil? Are the pupils fixed? Table 27.1 reviews the eye signs in a comatose patient.

With the emergence of the opioid epidemic, particular attention should be paid to identifying pinpoint pupils in a person who is unconscious with respiratory depression. If suspected, and the patient still has a pulse, rescue breathing with barrier protection should be started immediately. Summoning help is critical, and the administration of naloxone (Narcan®) may correct the problem. Patients who are at risk for opioid overdose may have been prescribed naloxone in an auto-injector that may be carried on the person or be available in their home. Fig. 27.3 shows the recommended AHA algorithm for an opioid-associated emergency for healthcare professionals.

Is there bleeding or discharge from the ears, nose, or mouth? If an otoscope is available, check to see if there is blood trapped behind the tympanic membrane, a finding known as *hemotympanum*. In trauma, this is another sign of a significant skull fracture.

TABLE 27.1 Eye Signs in a Comatose Patient

Eye Sign[a]	Possible Causes
Pupils reactive, eyes directed straight ahead, normal OCR[b]	Toxic or metabolic cause
Pinpoint pupils	Narcotic/opioid poisoning (OCR intact) Pontine or cerebellar hemorrhage (OCR absent) Thalamic hemorrhage Miotic eye drops
Disconjugate deviation of eyes	Structural brainstem lesion
Conjugate lateral deviation of eyes	Ipsilateral pontine infarction Contralateral frontal hemispheric infarction
Unilateral dilated, fixed pupil with no consensual responses	Supratentorial mass lesion Impending brain herniation Posterior communicating aneurysm
Bilateral midposition pupils, fixed pupils	Midbrain lesion Impending brain herniation
Raccoon eyes (periorbital ecchymoses), Battle sign	Fracture of the base of the skull or facial bones

[a]Eye signs are difficult to evaluate in patients with artificial lenses, prosthetic eyes, contact lenses, or cataracts or after cataract surgery.
[b]"Doll's eyes": Rotate the head quickly but gently from side to side. In an unconscious patient with an intact brain stem, the eyes move conjugately in a direction opposite the head turning. This is known as the oculocephalic reflex (OCR).

Palpate the head. Note for signs of crepitus, bleeding, or scalp hematoma.

Inspect the posterior neck for tenderness in the midline of the spine or any step-offs of the spinous processes of the posterior cervical spine. Inspect the anterior neck: note if the trachea is deviated to one side and the level of distention of the neck veins. If both findings are positive, suspect a chest injury, such as a tension pneumothorax. Palpate the neck for crepitus, which is indicative of air under the skin from a pneumothorax or leak of the lung.

If there is no tenderness of the neck, the patient has no other painful injuries, and they are not intoxicated, ask them to move their neck through a full range of motion slowly. Have the patient stop if pain is encountered.

Chest. Conducting a detailed examination of the chest is important in the critically ill or injured patient. Auscultation of the breath sounds in detail and noting the quality of the findings can provide vital clues. Rales, rhonchi, and wheezing can be signs of underlying pulmonary or cardiac conditions leading to the patient's illness.

In trauma patients, the presence or absence of breath sounds should be frequently evaluated, as should observation of the symmetrical rise and fall of the chest. As mentioned earlier, paradoxical or abnormal chest movement with respirations may indicate a flail chest, which should be stabilized. If the patient seems to be worsening with regard to respiratory status, re-check the breath sounds, the chest wall for subcutaneous emphysema, and oxygen saturation levels if the equipment is available.

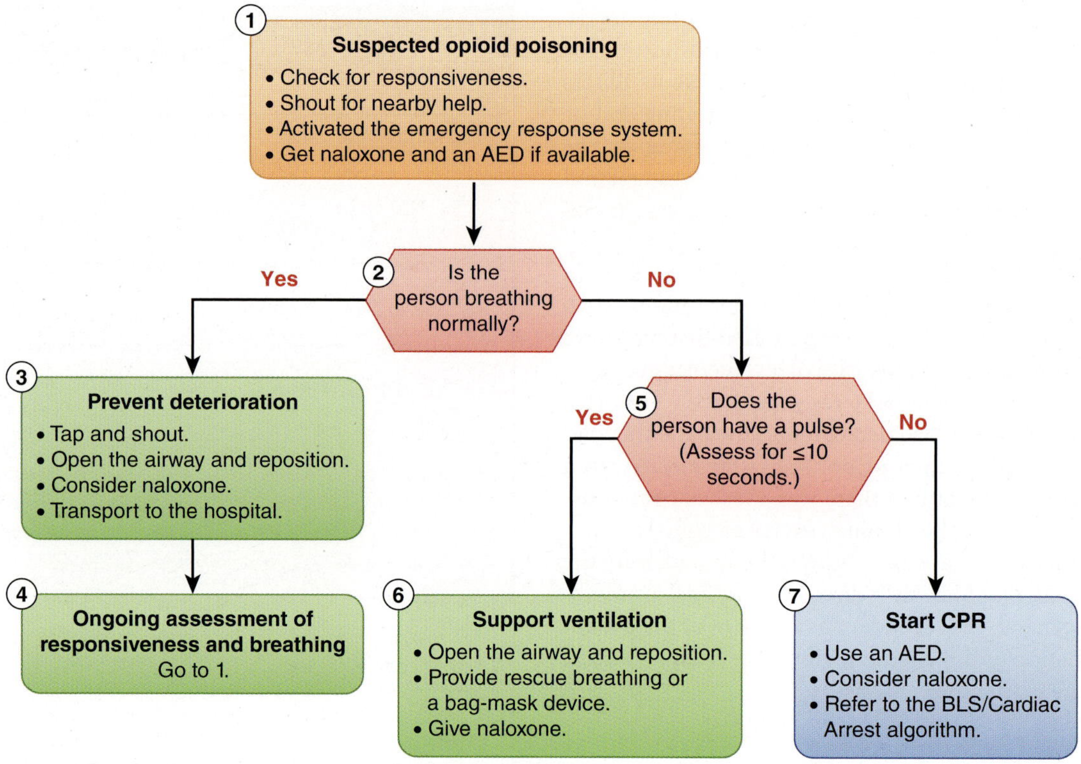

Fig. 27.3 Opioid-Associated Emergency for Healthcare Professionals Algorithm (American Heart Association). AED indicates automated external defibrillator; BLS, basic life support; and CPR, cardiopulmonary resuscitation. (Reprinted with permission Circulation. 2020;142:S469-S523. ©2020 American Heart Association, Inc.)

Heart sounds should be auscultated, with any major findings of tachycardia, murmurs, rubs, or gallops noted. Muffled heart sounds, particularly if combined with distended jugular veins, may be a sign of cardiac tamponade, another rapidly life-threatening condition that can be caused by significant trauma and insidiously in some medical conditions.

Abdomen. Inspect the abdomen. Is abdominal distention present? Are bowel sounds present? Gently palpate the abdomen, quadrant by quadrant, noting the presence of tenderness. **If the patient is a female of childbearing age, always consider the possibility that she may be pregnant.**

In trauma patients, be alert for evidence of blunt abdominal trauma, such as focal areas of tenderness, ecchymosis, abrasions, contusions, or the presence of an open abdominal wound. *Cullen sign* is a bluish discoloration around the umbilicus indicative of intra-abdominal bleeding or trauma, as shown in Fig. 27.4. A seatbelt sign—a horizontal line of ecchymosis, possibly accompanied by a diagonal line across the mid-chest—is a sign of injury from the seatbelt. This indicates considerable amounts of force were transferred to the patient's thorax and abdomen. *Grey Turner sign* is ecchymotic discoloration around the flanks, which is suggestive of retroperitoneal bleeding. Fig. 27.5 shows an example of the Grey Turner sign. Swelling or ecchymosis often occurs late; therefore, its presence is extremely important. Both Cullen and Grey Turner signs are late signs of injury. The absence of them should not delay diagnostic workup to continue if clinically indicated.

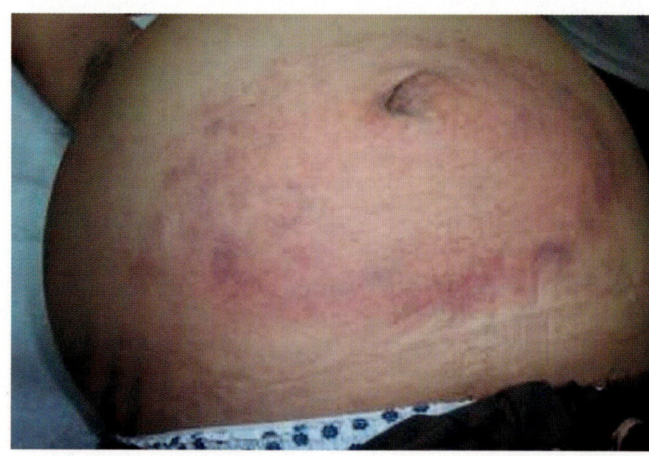

Fig. 27.4 Cullen Sign.

The most commonly injured abdominal organ in adult blunt trauma is the liver and should be considered when the patient has right upper quadrant pain. In contrast, left upper quadrant pain is suspicious for splenic injury and may have radiation to the left shoulder.

Inspect the anus and the perineum. Perform a rectal examination to assess anal sphincter tone, to determine whether blood is present, and to verify that the prostate is in its normal position.

Pelvis. Use the heels of your hands to apply gentle downward pressure on the anterior superior iliac spines and on the

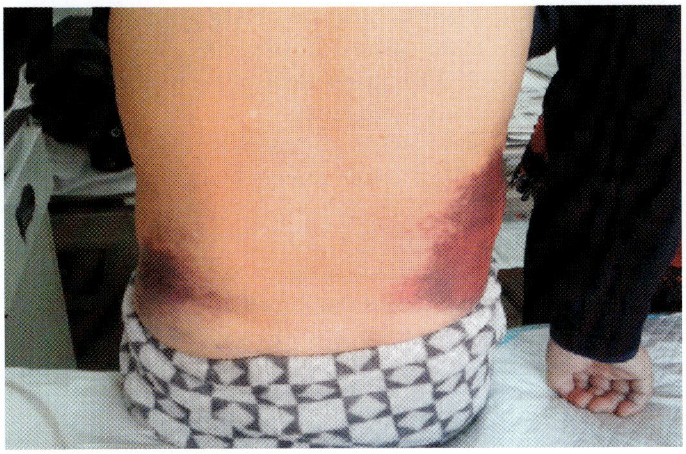

Fig. 27.5 Grey Turner Sign.

symphysis pubis. Is tenderness present? Is there any abnormal motion? If so, there may be a fracture of the pelvic ring. Inspect the urethral meatus for the presence of blood. If found, this can be a further indication of pelvic or bladder trauma.

Extremities. For acutely ill patients, inspecting the distal extremities should include observations associated with indicators of adequate circulation. The temperature, color, moisture, and finding of capillary refill should be evaluated. *Capillary refill* is an assessment of perfusion. It is the time required for a patient's skin color to return to normal after the nail bed has been pressed. The normal refill time is less than 2 seconds. Prolongation of the capillary refill indicates perfusion abnormalities.

If there is suspicion of underlying infection, checking the nail beds for splinter hemorrhages can be useful; if found, they may indicate endocarditis. Another finding of bacterial endocarditis is Janeway lesions, which are nontender hemorrhagic macules located on the palms and soles.

In patients with major trauma, there should be an examination of the major bones and joints to assess the stability of structure and assessment of function. Noting major deformities of long bones and joints is important. Splinting deformed long bones can assist in reducing blood loss associated with fractures and control pain. If significant deformity of a long bone is noted, one should assess pulses and neurological function distal to the injury.

Whether or not there is a deformity, a distal neurovascular examination of each extremity that notes the motor, sensory, and vascular function should be assessed and documented.

Back. Inspect the back, looking for obvious signs of injury. In trauma situations, this is best performed with a coordinated *log-roll* of the patient, with someone at the head to maintain the alignment of the cervical spine. To do this, you need at least four care team members: one to control the head and neck, two to roll the patient onto the side, and one to examine the back cautiously.

The entire spinal column of the back should be palpated. Note acute point tenderness, particularly in the mid-line, along with any spinal step-offs (bony prominences or depressions) that can indicate serious spinal fractures. Fig. 27.6 demonstrates the log-roll positions. Note the presence of any signs of injury, such as bleeding, contusions, abrasions, or focal areas of pain.

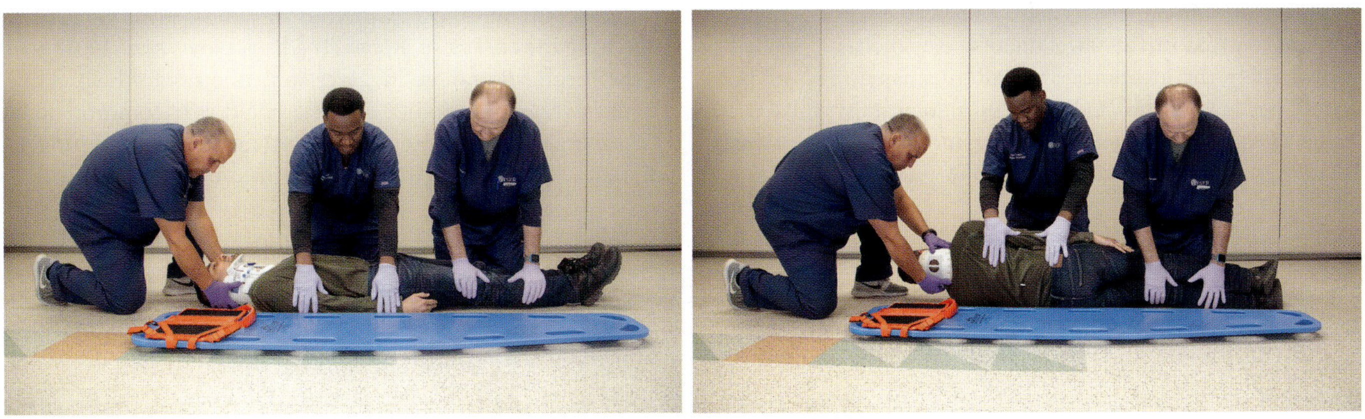

A B

Fig. 27.6 Log-Roll Procedure. (A) Positioning for log-rolling. (1) Apply a cervical spine immobilization device and place the patient's arms at the side. Note that one healthcare professional (HCP) maintains cervical immobilization manually throughout this procedure. (2) Three HCPs can be positioned at the side of the patient at the level of the chest, hips, and lower extremities while the long spine board is positioned on one side of the patient. (3) Check the patient's arm on the side of the HCPs for injury before log-rolling the patient, and then align the lower extremities. Note: The HCP at the lower extremities holds the patient's lower leg and thigh region, the HCP at the hips holds the patient's lower legs and places the other hand on top of the patient's buttocks, and the HCP at the chest holds the patient's arms against the body and at the level of the lower buttocks. (B) Log-rolling the patient. (4) On command from the HCP at the head, all HCPs rotate the patient toward themselves, keeping the body in alignment. (5) The HCPs then reach across with one hand and pull the board beneath the patient's arm. (6) On command from the HCP at the head, they gently roll the patient onto the board and then roll the board to the ground. (7) If the patient is expected to be transported further, strap the patient's torso and extremities securely to the board and immobilize the head until injury to the cervical spine has been safely ruled out.

THE PEDIATRIC EMERGENCY

Pediatric patients have less reserve capacity to compensate for dysfunction of the cardiopulmonary systems. When assessing an acutely ill child, a well-taken history from the parents can often narrow down the diagnosis. Overall, you should approach the pediatric emergency as you would an emergency in an adult from an organizational standpoint. In particular, the primary assessment of an acutely ill or injured child is the same as that of an adult.

The most dangerous, common, life-threatening pediatric emergencies result in *respiratory distress*. For this reason, it is recommended that *all acutely ill pediatric patients be placed on supplemental oxygen as soon as it is available*.

Respiratory distress in a pediatric patient may arise from various conditions resulting from upper or lower airway disease. Common pediatric respiratory problems of the upper airway include croup (i.e., laryngotracheobronchitis), epiglottitis, foreign bodies, and bacterial tracheitis. Lower airway obstruction may result from asthma, pneumonia, bronchiolitis, and foreign bodies.

The hallmarks of respiratory distress are tachypnea, nasal flaring, retractions, cyanosis, head bobbing, prolonged expiration, and grunting. Children with upper airway disease often exhibit stridor, a sound heard on inspiration associated with partial airway obstruction. See Chapter 13, The Chest. A child with severe distress may be in the tripod position, leaning forward onto an outstretched arm to improve respiration. If this position is noted and accompanied by drooling, it is a finding associated with epiglottitis, a condition that can rapidly progress to respiratory failure. In cases of suspected epiglottitis, it is crucial to keep the patient as calm as possible while initiating treatment to avoid further swelling of the epiglottis.

Fortunately, the incidence of epiglottitis has decreased, presumably because of the *Haemophilus influenzae* type B (HIB) vaccine. ***If epiglottitis is suspected, do not examine the airway without being prepared to provide airway stabilization on an emergency basis.*** Manipulating the child's airway or causing them to become more agitated can lead to complete airway obstruction. Table 27.2 compares some of the important differences between epiglottitis and croup.

Foreign body aspiration is common between the ages of 1 to 2 years. In a child, consider foreign body aspiration in the following situations:

- Choking is present
- Cough after playing with an object
- Sudden onset of stridorous (high-pitched inspiratory sound) breathing
- Unequal breath sounds
- The child becomes cyanotic

If the patient loses the ability to move air, indicated by lack of cough, inability to speak, or inability to remain conscious, emergency attempts at clearing the airway should be undertaken. Immediately place the child face down, with the head lower than the torso, over your arm, which is placed on your thigh. Support the child's head by holding their jaw. Deliver five forceful back blows with the heel of your other hand between the child's scapulae. Turn the child onto the back while holding the child's head. Place two fingertips on the middle portion of the sternum, one fingerbreadth below the nipples. Depress the sternum 1 inch. Repeat this maneuver up to five times. Attempt to remove any visible material from the pharynx. Repeat the back blows and chest thrusts until the object is dislodged.

If the child becomes unconscious, check the mouth for a foreign body and then perform mouth-to-mouth breathing. Gently tilt the child's head back while placing the other fingers under the jaw at the chin and lifting the chin upward. Seal the child's mouth and nose with your mouth. Deliver two breaths, watching the chest rise. Repeat the back blows and chest thrusts if the breaths do not go in. Have someone call for help.

Dehydration is another important and very common pediatric emergency. The most common causes are vomiting and diarrhea. In a child with mild dehydration (<5%), there may

TABLE 27.2 Differentiation Between Epiglottitis and Croup

Characteristics	Epiglottitis	Croup
Cause	*Haemophilus influenzae* type B	Viral, usually parainfluenza virus
Age of child	Any age (peak, 3–7 years)	3 months to 3 years
Clinical appearance	Extremely ill ("toxic")	Not extremely ill
Season	No seasonal predominance	Autumn and winter
Clinical onset	Rapid	Insidious
Upper respiratory tract infection	Rare	Common
Fever	>104°F (40°C)	<103°F (39.5°C)
Sore throat	Severe	Variable
Cough	Less severe symptoms throughout the day	"Barking"-type cough during the night
Drooling	Prominent	None
Stridor	On inspiration	On inspiration and expiration
Position	Sitting forward with neck extended and mouth open	Variable
Epiglottis	Bright red	Normal

be only a slight decrease in mucous membrane moisture. In severe dehydration (15%), the following are commonly found:

- Parched mucous membranes
- Crying with no tears
- Markedly decreased skin turgor
- Sunken fontanelles
- Sunken eyeballs
- Tachypnea
- Capillary refill longer than 2 seconds
- Cool and clammy skin
- Orthostatic hypotension: systolic pressure less than 80 mm Hg
- Tachycardia: heart rate faster than 130 beats/min
- Dry diaper due to decreased urination

Immediate intravenous infusion of isotonic fluids should be started in children with severe dehydration with initial doses aimed at 20 mL/kg of body weight followed by frequent reassessments.

The secondary assessment outlined earlier and the AVPU mental status documentation mnemonic are just as important for children as for adults and should be frequently reevaluated in critically ill children.

CONCLUSION

In conclusion, this chapter has provided an overview of the critical considerations and strategies essential for effectively managing patients facing sudden and severe medical conditions or injuries. By delving into the principles of rapid assessment, timely intervention, and multidisciplinary care coordination, healthcare professionals are better equipped to navigate the complexities of acutely ill or injured patients. Emphasizing the significance of clear communication, swift decision making, and a holistic approach to patient well-being, this chapter serves as a valuable resource for healthcare professionals seeking to enhance their skills in emergency care. As we navigate the dynamic landscape of healthcare, the insights gained from this chapter underscore the importance of continuous learning and adaptability in delivering optimal outcomes for acute, critically ill patients.

REVIEW QUESTIONS

1. **What is the first priority for a healthcare provider regarding scene safety when they find a patient in an emergency situation outside of their workplace?**
   - **A.** Assess the patient's injuries
   - **B.** Call for additional help
   - **C.** Ensure the safety of the scene for themselves and the patient
   - **D.** Move the patient to a safer location
   - **E.** Begin CPR immediately
2. **A healthcare provider finds a patient with no pulse. What is the recommended action regarding chest compressions?**
   - **A.** Begin chest compressions immediately at a rate of 100-120 per minute
   - **B.** Check for a pulse again after 30 seconds
   - **C.** Wait for emergency services to arrive
   - **D.** Administer two breaths before starting compressions
   - **E.** Perform abdominal thrusts
3. **What is the correct ratio of compressions to breaths in CPR for an adult?**
   - **A.** 15:1
   - **B.** 30:2
   - **C.** 20:2
   - **D.** 25:1
   - **E.** 30:1
4. **How should a healthcare provider assess the ABCs (Airway, Breathing, Circulation) in an unconscious patient?**
   - **A.** Check for breathing, then circulation, then airway
   - **B.** Open the airway, check for breathing, then assess circulation
   - **C.** Assess circulation first, then airway, then breathing
   - **D.** Check for responsiveness, then breathing, then circulation
   - **E.** Look for chest movements, then check pulse, then open the airway
5. **What does the SAMPLE acronym stand for when taking a patient's history?**
   - **A.** Signs, Allergies, Medications, Past medical history, Last oral intake, Events leading up to the incident
   - **B.** Symptoms, Allergies, Medications, Past injuries, Last oral intake, Events leading up to the incident
   - **C.** Signs, Allergies, Medications, Past medical history, Last oral intake, Examination findings
   - **D.** Symptoms, Allergies, Medications, Previous episodes, Last oral intake, Examination findings
   - **E.** Signs, Allergies, Medications, Past injuries, Last meal, Events leading up to the incident
6. **Which lung finding is most indicative of a tension pneumothorax?**
   - **A.** Crackles in the affected lung
   - **B.** Dullness to percussion over the affected lung
   - **C.** Absence of breath sounds on the affected side
   - **D.** Rhonchi on the affected side
   - **E.** Wheezing on the affected side
7. **What does the presence of abdominal bruising longitudinally across the lower abdomen potentially indicate after a car accident?**
   - **A.** Rib fractures
   - **B.** Bladder injury
   - **C.** Liver laceration
   - **D.** Potential internal abdominal injury from the seatbelt
   - **E.** Pelvic fracture
8. **In pediatric dehydration, what is the recommended initial fluid bolus?**
   - **A.** 10 ml/kg
   - **B.** 15 ml/kg
   - **C.** 20 ml/kg
   - **D.** 25 ml/kg
   - **E.** 30 ml/kg

9. Which of the following signs is not consistent with dehydration in the pediatric patient?

A. Decreased Skin Turgor
B. Bulging fontanelles (Correct)
C. Sunken Eyes
D. Tachypnea
E. Capillary refill longer than 2 seconds

10. Which of the following is an appropriate initial assessment for a lay rescuer at the scene of an emergency?

A. Call 911 immediately, then perform a full physical exam
B. Ensure their own safety, then check for responsiveness (Correct)
C. Begin chest compressions immediately
D. Administer rescue breaths first
E. Move the patient to a safer location

BIBLIOGRAPHY

Available online.

SECTION 5

Putting the Data to Work

28

Precision, Accuracy, and Critical Thinking in Clinical Assessment

Mark H. Swartz

Medicine is a science of uncertainty and an art of probability. One of the chief reasons for this uncertainty is the increasing variability in the manifestations of any one disease.

Sir William Osler (1849–1919)

ART, SCIENCE, AND OBSERVATION

This chapter is one of the most important chapters in the book as it covers the methods and concepts of evaluating signs and symptoms involved in diagnostic reasoning. The earlier chapters cover the scientific aspects of medicine, such as techniques for conducting interviews and physical examinations. Making the best decision in uncertain situations is the art of medicine, but there are rules and standards that guide this practice, which are the main focus of this chapter.

The primary steps in this process involve the following:

- Data collection
- Data processing
- Problem list development

Data collection is the product of the history and the physical examination. Additional test results, including blood chemistry profiles, complete blood cell counts, bacterial cultures, electrocardiograms, and chest radiographs, can supplement these findings. The history is the most important element of the database, making up around 70% to 75% of the problem list. Physical examination findings add an extra 20% to 25%. Laboratory and other test results account for less than 10% of the database.

Data processing is the clustering of data obtained from the history, physical examination, and laboratory and imaging studies. Patients often experience multiple symptoms and signs of a disease rather than just one. During a physical examination, the examiner may identify several related signs. The goal is to connect these clues into a meaningful pathophysiologic relationship, which is essentially data processing. It takes an astute observer to do this job effectively.

For example, suppose the interviewer obtains a history of dyspnea, cough, earache, and hemoptysis. Dyspnea, cough, and hemoptysis can be grouped together as symptoms suggestive of cardiopulmonary disease. Earache does not fit with the other three symptoms and may indicate another problem. For another patient who is concerned of epigastric burning relieved by eating and whose stool is found to contain blood, this symptom and this sign should be studied together. These data suggest an abnormality of the gastrointestinal tract, possibly peptic ulcer disease.

Although patients usually have multiple symptoms or signs from a pathologic condition, they may not always manifest all the symptoms or signs of the disease being considered. For instance, the presence of polyuria and polydipsia in a patient with a family history of diabetes is adequate to raise the suspicion that a lateral rectus muscle palsy may be related to diabetes, even if diabetes has not previously been diagnosed in this patient. In another patient, a 30-pound weight loss, anorexia, jaundice, and a left supraclavicular lymph node suggest gastric carcinoma with liver metastasis to the porta hepatis. This illustrates the concept of data processing multiple symptoms into a single diagnosis. The process has sometimes been likened to the rule of *Occam's razor*[a]: The simplest theory is preferable—in this case, all the symptoms can be explained by one diagnosis. Simply stated, the simplest explanation is preferable to one that is more complex. Healthcare professionals often use Occam's razor, which means they look for the simplest possible explanation for a patient's multiple symptoms and focus on the most probable causes. As another example, if a patient experiences loss of smell, headache, fever, and sneezing during the COVID-19 pandemic, the most likely explanation is that they have COVID-19 rather than a less common illness. This method avoids excessive treatment, panic, and risky interactions among various treatments. Although it is a useful rule to remember, it is not always applicable.

Problem list development summarizes a patient's physical, mental, social, and personal conditions that affect their health. It may include a diagnosis or a symptom or sign that cannot be grouped with other data. For each problem, the date of development is recorded. The list is arranged in order of importance, reflecting the healthcare professional's understanding of the patient's problems. An example of a problem list can be found in Table 28.1.

When a symptom or sign is related to a specific problem, it is called a *pertinent positive* finding. This means it is a sign or symptom that is expected based on the patient's chief concern. For example, if a male patient is concerned with excruciating back pain radiating to his testicle and has a history of gout and increased uric acid levels, he may suffer from renal colic due to a uric acid kidney stone. On the other hand, the absence of a

[a]The principle of Occam's razor, also known as the law of parsimony, originates from philosophy and is credited to William of Ockham, a 14th-century theologian, philosopher, and Franciscan friar.

TABLE 28.1 Example of a Problem List

Problem	Date	Resolved
1. Chest pain	12/25/2022	
2. Acute inferior myocardial infarction	1/30/2019	2/15/2019
3. Colon cancer	4/30/2017	6/3/2017
4. Diabetes mellitus	2010	
5. Hypertension	2004	
6. "Red urine"	6/10/2017	7/1/2017
7. Distress over son's substance use disorder	11/2021	

symptom or sign that would suggest a diagnosis is called a *pertinent negative* finding. This is just as important as a pertinent positive finding because it can help rule out certain diagnoses. For instance, a female with weight loss and a tremor who denies having a history of tachycardia or warm intolerance is less likely to have hyperthyroidism compared to a patient who has a history of tachycardia or warm intolerance.

In any database, it's crucial to have the patient's demographic information, including their sex, age, ethnicity, and area of residence. For instance, a male with a bleeding disorder since birth is likely to be diagnosed with hemophilia. Someone experiencing exertional chest pain at the age of 65 is statistically more likely to be suffering from coronary artery disease. Similarly, a 26-year-old African American patient with severe bone pain may be diagnosed with sickle cell anemia. And someone living in the San Joaquin Valley with pulmonary symptoms may have coccidioidomycosis. Although this information can help suggest a unifying diagnosis, it's essential to note that the absence of the "usual" finding should not entirely rule out a diagnosis. Additionally, it's crucial to be aware of bias, as discussed in Chapters 5 and 33, which address mitigating racism and bias in clinical medicine. Bias refers to the inclination or prejudice for or against a diagnosis, person, or group, which can be unfair.

A well-known phrase states that "common diseases are common." This highlights the importance of not jumping to rare diagnoses when a more common one may be the cause of a patient's symptoms. However, if common explanations cannot fully explain the situation, it may be necessary to consider less common diagnoses. Additionally, it is worth noting that unusual symptoms of common diseases are more frequently encountered than typical symptoms of rare diseases.

Although rare diseases may be uncommon, they can still greatly impact the individuals who have them. If a patient experiences symptoms and signs of an uncommon condition, they may be among the 1 in 10,000 who are affected by it. However, statistics based on population groups can still be helpful in making clinical decisions for individual patients.

DIAGNOSTIC REASONING FROM SIGNS AND SYMPTOMS

In the field of medicine, making decisions with complete certainty is rarely possible. The decision making process involves *weighing probabilities*, which is the likelihood that a particular proposition is true. Only when the symptoms, signs, and test results are crystal clear can a healthcare professional be entirely confident in a diagnosis, but this is a rare occurrence. Therefore, healthcare professionals must make the "best" decision based on current knowledge and research.

Both signs and symptoms, as well as laboratory test results, are held to the same rules and standards of evidence for diagnostic reasoning. However, it is important to note that signs and symptoms make up the majority (90%) of the developing problem list, compared to laboratory test results, which only account for less than 10%.

Sensitivity and Specificity

Throughout this text, signs and symptoms have been described often according to their *operating characteristics:* sensitivity and specificity. These operating characteristics, which apply also to laboratory tests, indicate the usefulness of the sign, symptom, or test to the healthcare professional in making a diagnosis. *Sensitivity* is sometimes called the true positive (TP) rate or the percentage of patients with the disease who test positive on the test. Sensitivity, therefore, is based solely on patients with the disease. *Specificity* is sometimes called the true negative (TN) rate or the percentage of patients who do not have the disease who test negative on the test. Specificity, therefore, is based only on individuals without the disease. A *false-positive (FP)* finding refers to a positive test result in an individual without the disease or condition. Thus, a sign, symptom, or test with 90% specificity can correctly identify 90 of 100 normal individuals; findings in the other 10 individuals are FP, and the FP rate is 10%. If a test result or observation is negative in a person with the disease, the result is termed *false negative (FN)*.

The *2 × 2 table* is useful for representing the relationship of a test, symptom, or sign to a disease.

D+ indicates the presence of the disease

D− indicates the absence of the disease

T+ is a positive test result or the presence of a symptom or sign

T− is the absence of a positive test result or the absence of a symptom or sign

Each of the cells of the table represents a set of patients. Consider the following 2 × 2 table:

	With disease D+	Without disease D–
Test positive T+	True positive (TP)	False positive (FP)
Test negative T–	False negative (FN)	True negative (TN)

Sensitivity is defined as the number of TP results divided by the number of patients with the disease (i.e., the total of the TP and the FN results):

$$\text{Sensitivity} = \text{TP/(number of patients with the disease)}$$
$$= \text{TP/(TP + FN)}$$

Specificity is defined as the number of TN results divided by the number of patients without the disease (i.e., the total of FP results and TNs):

$$\text{Specificity} = \text{TP/(number of patients without the disease)}$$
$$= \text{TP/(FP + TN)}$$

Substituting numbers:

	D+	D–
T+	65 (65%) (TP)	100 (10%) (FP)
T–	35 (35%) (FN)	900 (90%) (TN)
	100	1000

The *upper left cell* of the 2 × 2 table (TP) indicates that 65 of 100 patients with a certain disease (65%) had a certain positive test result or symptom or sign. Thus, the test has a TP rate of 0.65, or a sensitivity of 65%.

The *lower right cell* of the 2 × 2 table (TN) indicates that 900 of 1000 individuals without the disease (90%) did not have a positive test result or symptom or sign. Thus, the test has a TN rate of 0.90, or a specificity of 90%.

The FP rate is 0.10, meaning that 100 of 1000 in the normal population (10%) had the finding for some reason, without having the disease in question. This is shown in the *upper right cell.*

Finally, the *lower left cell* indicates that the test result, symptom, or sign is absent in 35 of 100 patients with the disease. Thus, the FN rate is 35%.

Note that the TP rate plus the FN rate equals 1; the FP rate plus the TN rate also equals 1. If the disease is aortic stenosis and the symptom (test condition) is syncope, then according to the preceding table, 65% of patients with aortic stenosis have syncope, and 35% do not; 90% of individuals without aortic stenosis do not have syncope, and 10% do.

Likelihood Ratios

Regarding diagnostic tests, we often use sensitivity, specificity, and positive and negative predictive values to describe their properties. However, these measurements only reflect the characteristics of a population and aren't easily applicable to individual patients. That's why *likelihood ratios (LR)* are a more practical approach to interpreting diagnostic test results and are immediately relevant in a clinical setting. In most cases, a useful test will have a high positive LR and a small negative LR.

When evaluating a symptom, sign, or test, it is important to consider both sensitivity and specificity. These values can be high or low, and they measure different properties. Therefore, a symptom, sign, or test can have high sensitivity and high specificity, low sensitivity and low specificity, high sensitivity and low specificity, or low sensitivity and high specificity.

Healthcare professionals commonly encounter the challenge of interpreting diagnostic test results in their clinical practice. It's important to note that these results are not always definitive. A negative test doesn't necessarily guarantee the absence of a disease, and some positive results may be inaccurate. Additionally, the implications of a test result may vary depending on the prevalence of the disease. For instance, chest pain is more likely to indicate coronary artery disease in an older male than in a young female.

Sensitivity and specificity are often combined to form the LR,[1] which provides a unitary measure of the operating characteristics of a sign, symptom, or test. LRs are independent of disease prevalence.

Imagine a patient takes a diagnostic test and the results are positive. If the test were perfect, it would mean that the patient definitely has the disease (TP). However, sometimes patients without the disease also test positive (FP), which prevents the healthcare professional from making a definite conclusion. To address this, we must adjust the TP rate by the FP rate. This is done mathematically by dividing one rate by the other (the LR).

The LR is the likelihood that a given test result would be expected in a patient with the disease compared to the likelihood that that same result would be expected in a patient without the disease. How likely is it that a patient has a disease or condition? It is a ratio of the probability that a test result is correct to the probability that the test result is incorrect. Mathematically, the positive LR is defined as the ratio of the TP rate to the FP rate as indicated here:

$$\textbf{Positive likelihood ratio} = \frac{\text{probability of positive test in those with disease}}{\text{probability of positive test in those without disease}}$$

$$= \text{TP rate / FP rate}$$

$$= \text{sensitivity / (1– specificity)}$$

The LR is used to assess how good a diagnostic test is and to help select an appropriate diagnostic test(s) or sequence of tests.

As indicated, a *positive predictive LR* is the proportion of patients *with* the disease with a finding divided by the proportion of patients *without* the disease who also have the finding.

A *negative predictive LR* is the proportion of patients *with* the disease who do *not* have a finding divided by the proportion of patients *without* the disease who also do *not* have the finding. Therefore,

$$\textbf{Negative likelihood ratio} = \frac{\text{probability of negative test in those with disease}}{\text{probability of negative test in those without disease}}$$

$$= \text{FN rate / TN rate}$$

$$= \text{(1− sensitivity) / specificity}$$

In the preceding example of syncope and aortic stenosis, where sensitivity = TP rate = 0.65, and 1 − specificity = FP rate = 0.10, the positive LR would be equal to 0.65/0.10, or 6.5. In other words, a positive sign, symptom, or test result is 6.5 times more likely in patients with disease than in individuals without disease. In the example, the occurrence of syncope would be 6.5 times greater in patients with aortic stenosis than in individuals without it.

Tests or signs with LRs greater than 1.0 are generally highly useful because they provide considerable confidence in diagnostic reasoning. The greater the LR, the more likely is the argument *for* the disease. The closer the LR is to 0.0, the more likely is the argument *against* the disease.

Ruling In and Ruling Out Disease

Sensitivity and specificity (and the LR) refer to properties of the symptom, sign, or test result that are invariant across different populations. This is true even though particular populations may differ regarding the prevalence of the disease or condition in question. Sensitivity is based solely on patients with disease, and specificity is based solely on individuals without disease. Thus, the relative sizes of the two groups—with disease and without disease—in the population of concern, which is the basis for the computation of prevalence, play no role in the computation of sensitivity and specificity. Sensitivity and specificity are simply the operating characteristics of the test and as such provide general information about the usefulness of the test for diagnostic reasoning *with any population of patients.* In actual clinical practice, however, the healthcare professional is concerned with the individual patient and whether that patient's test results are predictive of disease. How certain can the healthcare professional be that a patient has a disease if the test result is positive or if a symptom or sign is present? How certain can a healthcare professional be that a person is healthy if a negative test result or a symptom or sign is absent? Typically, these questions are answered by computing the positive and negative predictive values, which are based on sensitivity and specificity, but also consider the prevalence of disease in the population of which the patient is a member.

First, however, consider two cases of diagnostic reasoning in which clinical decisions can be based on only the knowledge of sensitivity and specificity. If the sensitivity of a given symptom, sign, or test is quite high, 90% or greater, and the patient has a negative result, the healthcare professional can somewhat confidently rule out disease because so few patients with disease have a negative test result (<10%). Sackett[2] devised the following acronym for this special case: **Sen**sitive signs when **N**egative help rule **out** the disease **(SnNout)**. In the absence of a highly sensitive sign, a person is most likely not to have the disease. The second case occurs if the specificity of a given test, symptom, or sign is quite high, 90% or greater, and the patient has a positive result. The healthcare professional can then somewhat confidently rule in disease because so few individuals without disease have a positive test result (<10%). Sackett's acronym for this case is **Sp**ecific signs when **P**ositive help rule **in** the disease **(SpPin)**. In the presence of a highly specific sign, a person is most likely to have the disease.

Predictive Values

SnNout and SpPin are quite useful in the previous two cases, but usually, the healthcare professional wants to predict the actual probability of disease for a patient with a positive result or the probability of no disease for an individual with a negative result. The former is estimated by the *positive predictive value (PV+),* which is the probability that subjects with a positive screening test will truly have the disease. It is equal to the number of TP findings divided by the total number of positive result findings in the population of which the patient is a member (the TP findings plus the FP findings):

$$\textbf{PV+} = \text{TP/all positive findings} = \text{TP/(TP + FP)}$$

The positive predictive value is the *frequency of disease* among patients with positive test results. For the patient, how worried should the patient be?

The *negative predictive value (PV−),* which is the probability that subjects with a negative screening test do not have the disease, is equal to the number of TN results divided by the total number of negative results in the patient's population (the TN findings plus the FN findings):

$$\textbf{PV−} = \text{TN/all negative findings} = \text{TN/(TN + FN)}$$

The negative predictive value is the *frequency of nondisease* in individuals with negative test results. Stated another way, it is the probability of not having the disease if the test result is negative or if the symptom or sign is absent. For the patient, how reassured should the patient be?

For example, assume that the 2 × 2 table discussed earlier represents the entire population of interest to the healthcare professional. The PV+ is calculated as:

$$\text{PV+} = 65/(65+100) = 0.39$$

and the PV− is calculated as:

$$\text{PV−} = 900/(35+900) = 0.96$$

Thus, the predicted probability that a person with a positive result in fact has the disease is 39%. The predicted probability that a person with a negative result does not have the disease is 96%. In this example, the probability that a patient with syncope actually has aortic stenosis is only 39%, whereas the probability that a person without syncope does not have aortic stenosis is 96%. The high PV− of 96% is consistent with the high test specificity of 90%.

Pretest probability is the probability of a patient having a disease before a diagnostic test result is known. It represents the probability that a specific patient with a specific history has a specific diagnosis. It can be calculated as the total TP + FN divided by the total sample (TP + FP + FN + TN). For example, a 59-year-old male with chest pain has a higher pretest probability for coronary artery disease than a 21-year-old female. The pretest probability of pneumonia is higher in a person with cough and fever who is immunosuppressed than in a 20-year-old previously healthy college student with cough and fever.

Prevalence

Clearly, the sensitivity and specificity of a sign, symptom, or test are important factors in predicting the probability of disease, given the test results. So too is the prevalence of the disease in the population of which the patient is a member. The *prevalence of disease* refers to the proportion with disease in the population of interest. In a 2 × 2 table that represents the entire population (or a representative sample), prevalence is equal to the number with disease (TP + FN) divided by the total number in the population (TP + FP + FN + TN). Again, assuming that the preceding 2 × 2 table represents the entire population of concern, prevalence is calculated as follows:

$$\text{Prevalence} = (65 + 35)/(65 + 100 + 35 + 900)$$
$$= 100/1100 = 0.09$$

Among this population, 9% have the disease in question.

Two intuitive examples illustrate the role of prevalence in predicting the probability of disease. Consider the value of the symptom of chest pain for predicting the probability of coronary artery disease. The first patient is a 65-year-old male with chest pain. The prevalence of coronary artery disease in 65-year-old males is high. Therefore, the presence of chest pain has a high positive predictive value for this patient, and it is probable that coronary artery disease exists in this patient. However, the absence of chest pain has a low negative predictive value, indicating that, because the prevalence is high, coronary artery disease may exist even in the absence of symptoms.

In contrast, consider the positive predictive value of chest pain in a 20-year-old female. Among females in this age group, the prevalence of coronary artery disease is low, so the probability that this patient's chest pain represents coronary artery disease is low. The presence of chest pain in a 20-year-old female has a low positive predictive value. However, the absence of chest pain has a high negative predictive value, indicating that coronary artery disease is unlikely to be present.

Fig. 28.1 illustrates how changes in disease prevalence affect predictive values. The most significant increase in the positive predictive value of a sign, symptom, or test occurs when the disease is less common. At this end of the curve, small changes in prevalence produce great changes in the positive predictive value. Conversely, the most significant increase in the negative predictive value occurs when the disease is most prevalent. Slight decreases in the prevalence of common diseases produce significant increases in the negative predictive value. The higher the prevalence is, the higher the positive predictive value is and the lower the negative predictive value is.

Differences in prevalence rates may be related either to the clinical setting in which the patient is seen or to the specific demographic characteristics of the patient. For example, a healthcare professional performing routine examinations in an outpatient clinic will find a prevalence of disease different from that found by a healthcare professional working only with inpatients in a hospital specializing in that disease. The *demographic characteristics* of the patient refer to age, gender, and race, and these characteristics play a major role in the prevalence of many diseases. Both the clinical setting and the characteristics of the patient help determine the usefulness of the sign, symptom, or laboratory test because they affect both the positive and the negative predictive values of the finding.

Bayes Theorem

Bayes theorem is a way of finding a probability when we know certain other probabilities. It is an evidence-based theorem.

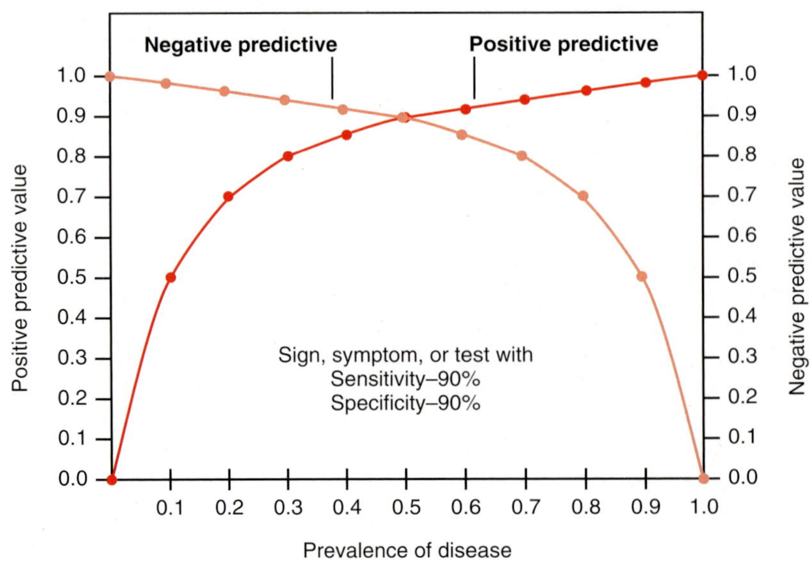

Fig. 28.1 Effect of Changing Disease Prevalence on Predictive Values.

How much can one trust the evidence available? Bayes theorem,[b] or Bayes law, is a mathematical formula for calculating conditional probabilities. A *conditional probability* is the probability of an event occurring, given that another event has occurred. The vertical line in a mathematical expression ("|") tells the reader that one is speaking about a conditional probability. A *prior probability* is an initial probability value originally obtained before any additional evidence is obtained. A *posterior probability* is a probability value that has been revised by using additional evidence that is later obtained. The Bayes theorem computes how to adjust the prior probability into the posterior probability; what should one believe after one has the evidence?

The probability of a hypothesis "B," conditional on some new piece of evidence "A," is written:

$$P(B \mid A)$$

Here is an example of the Bayes theorem:

If we have two events A and B, and we are given the conditional probability of A given B, denoted P(A|B), we can use Bayes theorem to find P(B|A), the conditional probability of B given A.

$$\text{Bayes Theorem: } P(B \mid A) = \frac{P(A \mid B)P(B)}{P(A \mid B)P(B) + P(A \mid B')P(B')}$$

Where P(B′) is the probability of B not occurring.

In other words, the formula states using exercise stress testing ("A") and coronary artery disease ("B") as examples:

What is the probability of having disease (B, coronary artery disease) *given a positive test* (A, exercise stress test)*?* This is what we want to determine. How likely is it that a patient has coronary artery disease with a positive exercise stress test? P(B|A)

What is the probability of having a positive test (A, exercise stress test) *given that the patient has disease* (B, coronary artery disease)*?*

(true positive) P(A|B)

What is the probability of having the disease (B, coronary artery disease)*?* P(B)

What is the probability of <u>*not*</u> *having a disease* (B′, no coronary artery disease)*?* P(B′)

What is the probability of a positive test (A, *exercise stress test*) *given that the patient does* <u>*not*</u> *have disease* (B′, no coronary artery disease)*?*

(false positive) P(A|B′)

Nomogram

The Bayes theorem formula may be inconvenient and cumbersome for readers and users of epidemiologic information. A nomogram is a graphical calculator that is a useful and convenient way to perform common calculations without remembering formulae. The use of Bayes nomogram has simplified diagnostic test information and is now frequently used by healthcare professionals who may be unaware of the formula involved in the conversion.

To simplify matters, a Bayes nomogram[c] is given in Fig. 28.2, which can be copied and used in the clinic or office. The nomogram provides the predictive values (post-test probability) without requiring the calculations of the Bayes theorem. To use the nomogram, first locate on the relevant axes the points that correspond to (1) the prevalence of disease for the patient's population (pre-test probability) and (2) the LR for the sign, symptom, or test. Recall that the LR is the ratio of the TP rate (sensitivity) to the FP rate (1 − specificity). Next, place a straight edge on the nomogram to connect the points. The PV+ (post-test probability) is given by the point at which the straight edge intersects the predictive value axis. For example, if the **prevalence = 0.80** and **LR = 0.65/0.10 = 6.50**, the **PV+ = 0.96**. To determine the PV−, use 1 − prevalence and TN rate divided by FN rate instead of prevalence and the LR.

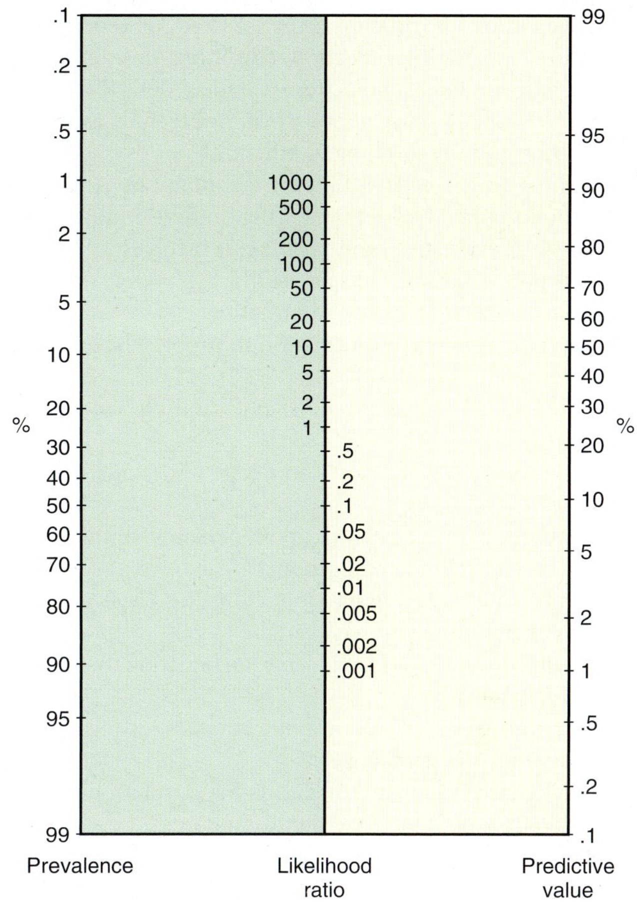

Fig. 28.2 Nomogram for Applying Likelihood Ratios. (Adapted from Haynes RB, Sackett DL, Guyatt GH, et al: *Clinical epidemiology: how to do clinical practice research*, ed 3, Philadelphia, 2005, Lippincott Williams & Wilkins.)

CRITICAL THINKING

What is *critical thinking*? Basically, it's ensuring we have good reasons for our beliefs. Scriven and Paul[d] described critical thinking as "the intellectually disciplined process of actively and skillfully conceptualizing, applying, analyzing, synthesizing,

[b]Named after 18th-century British mathematician Thomas Bayes.

[c]This nomogram illustrates how a LR (either positive [LR+] or negative [LR-]) associated with a diagnostic test is used to transform a pre-test probability (prevalence) into a post-test probability (predictive value).

[d]A statement by Michael Scriven and Richard Paul, presented at the 8th Annual International Conference on Critical Thinking and Education Reform, Summer 1987.

and/or evaluating information gathered from, or generated by, observation, experience, reflection, reasoning, or communication, as a guide to belief and action." Chaffee[3] described critical thinking as "making sense of our world by carefully examining our thinking, and the thinking of others…"

According to the revised Bloom's taxonomy by Anderson,[4] critical thinking involves remembering, understanding, applying, analyzing, evaluating, and creating. It involves:

- Knowledge of specific facts and skills
- Comprehension of existing information
- Application of known information to problem solve in new situations
- Analysis of new information and finding evidence to support it
- Creative synthesis of prior knowledge and skills into new knowledge and skills
- Evaluation of results based upon personal opinions and values resulting in the end product

Paul and Elder[5] described eloquently the "well-cultivated critical thinker as a person who can:

1. Raise vital questions and problems, formulating them clearly and precisely
2. Gather and assesses relevant information, using abstract ideas to interpret it effectively
3. Come to well-reasoned conclusions and solutions, testing them against relevant criteria and standards
4. Think open-mindedly within alternative systems of thought, recognizing and assessing, as needs be, their assumptions, implications, and practical consequences
5. Communicate effectively with others in figuring out solutions to complex problems

Critical thinking is, in short, self-directed, self-disciplined, self-monitored, and self-corrective thinking. It requires rigorous standards of excellence and mindful command of their use. It entails effective communication and problem-solving abilities and a commitment to overcome our native egocentrism and sociocentrism.

People who are critical thinkers do not simply accept ideas and assumptions without question. Instead, they carefully examine them to determine if they are accurate and complete. They are open to the possibility that the ideas, arguments, and findings may not be correct. Critical thinkers approach problems in a systematic way and use analysis to find solutions rather than relying on intuition or instinct.

Critical thinking revolves around *creative thinking*. A notable instance of creative thinking occurred on January 15, 2009, in New York City. US Airways Flight 1549 departed from LaGuardia Airport en route to Charlotte, North Carolina. Shortly after takeoff, the Airbus A320, powered by two turbofan engines, struck a flock of Canada geese at an altitude of 2818 ft (859 m), losing all engine power. Unable to reach any airport, Captain Chesley (Sully) Sullenberger had only 208 seconds to devise a plan and solve the problem. Despite never having attempted a water landing before, he successfully executed an emergency landing on the Hudson River near midtown Manhattan, and all 150 passengers, three flight attendants, pilot, and first officer survived (Fig. 28.3) and were rescued by nearby

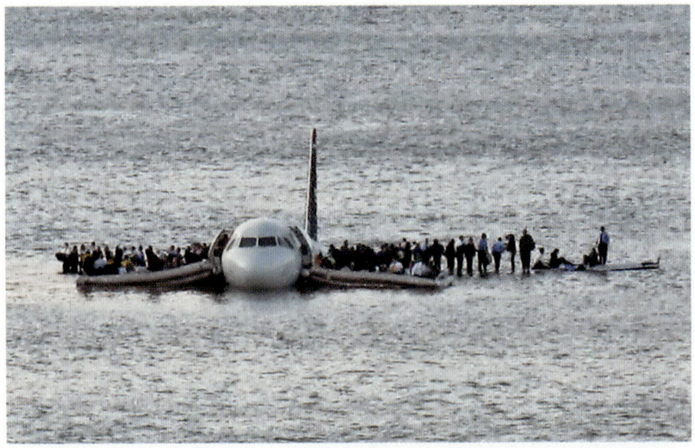

Fig. 28.3 US Airways Flight 1549 after emergency water landing in the Hudson River. (Reused with permission from AP Photo/Steven Day.)

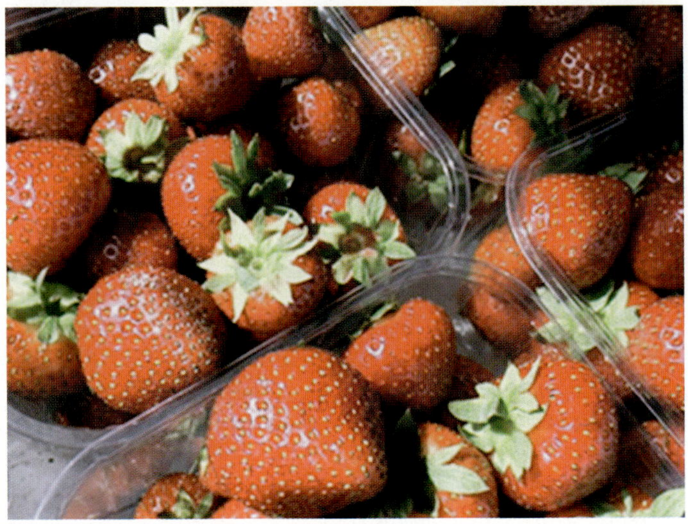

Fig. 28.4 What Are These?

boats. There were only a few minor injuries! It was the first officer's first A320 assignment as a pilot flying! This incredible event, which became known as "the miracle on the Hudson", highlights the importance of critical thinking, which involves not only acquiring knowledge but also knowing how to apply it effectively.

In the field of medicine, intuition is frequently utilized. Intuition is an unconscious and swift way of knowing something without the need to perceive or discover it through conscious reasoning. Essentially, it is the ability to immediately comprehend something, as if the brain is on autopilot. Look at Fig. 28.4. It's easy to recognize what it depicts without thinking about it. Now, observe Fig. 28.5. What are these objects, and how are they used? Although you may not have seen them previously, your prior experience with similar items will supply the answers. This same principle applies when examining patients. Consider the signs shown in Figs. 28.6 and 28.7. You can quickly discern that the skin lesion indicates Lyme disease, while the eye finding is an arcus senilis. Your familiarity with these clinical findings allows you to make an accurate diagnosis without additional

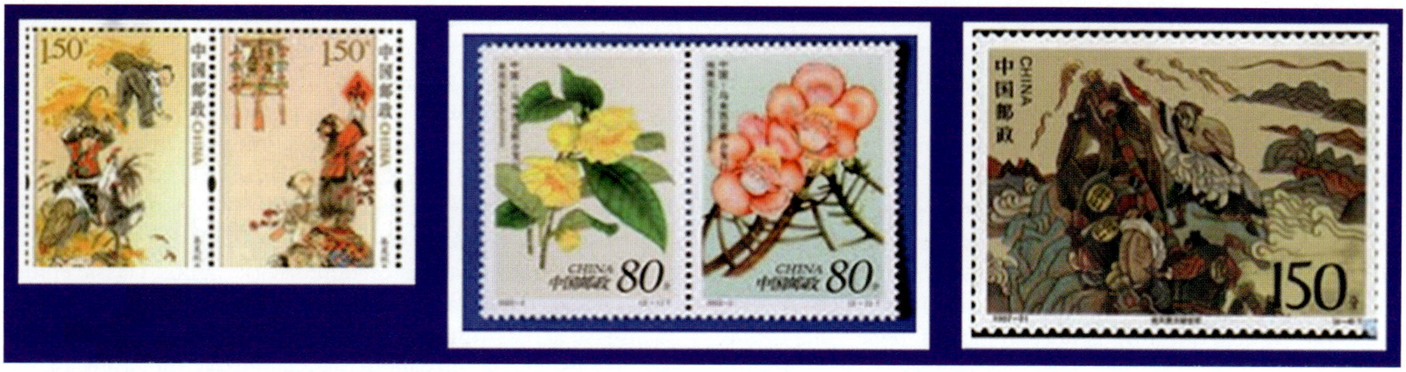

Fig. 28.5 What Are These and What Do You Do With Them?

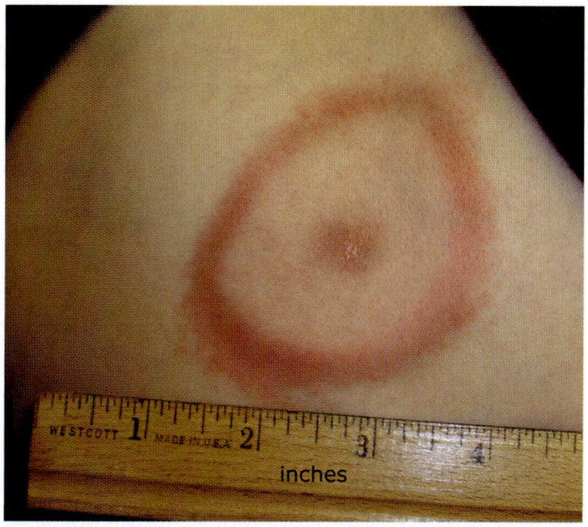

Fig. 28.6 Erythema Migrans of Lyme Disease: Site of the Tick Bite.

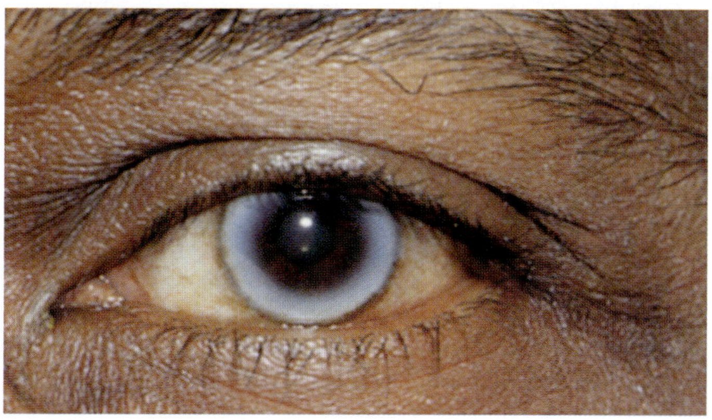

Fig. 28.7 Arcus Senilis. (From Kanski JJ, Nischal KK: *Ophthalmology: clinical signs and differential diagnosis*, St. Louis, 2000, Mosby.)

information. This is an example of pattern recognition, a skill we all employ in clinical decision making.

In the field of clinical medicine, arriving at a diagnosis is not always so straightforward. It requires careful questioning and gathering relevant information. This involves using *metacognition*, which is the act of critically thinking about one's own thinking. Metacognition involves planning, monitoring, and assessing one's own understanding and performance. By reflecting on our own thoughts, we gain insight into our needs, feelings, and behaviors. It's like having a running conversation we have in our mind sounding out ideas, weighing the pros and cons, and making informed decisions and plans.

The six objectives for critical thinking involve:

1. Identifying the main question or problem
2. Gathering relevant data to the main question or problem
3. Interpreting the data effectively
4. Recognizing assumptions, alternate points of view, and biases
5. Developing conclusions
6. Describing implications

Always ask yourself the following questions that are the universal intellectual standards of critical thinking:

1. Clarity—*Can one elaborate further on the point?*
2. Accuracy—*Can one check that information?*
3. Precision—*Can one provide more details to support the information?*
4. Relevance—*How is the answer connected to the problem?*
5. Depth—*How does the answer address the complexities of the problem?*
6. Breadth—*Does one need to consider another point of view?*
7. Logic—*Does this really make sense?*
8. Fairness—*Is this answer free of biases and preconceptions?*

Several pitfalls can hinder critical thinking. One of the most significant is the failure to use logic. Another pitfall is the reliance on tradition as an argument, which can lead to the flawed reasoning of "We've always done it that way!" Additionally, making hasty generalizations without considering all the evidence can undermine critical thinking. To avoid these pitfalls, a critical thinker should avoid jumping to conclusions and carefully consider all available evidence.

Martin Luther King, Jr. said, "Education must enable one to sift and weigh evidence, to discern the true from the false, the real from the unreal and the facts from the fiction. The function of education, therefore, is to teach one to think intensively and to think critically."

THE RATIONAL CLINICAL EXAMINATION

In 1992, the *Journal of the American Medical Association*[6] initiated a series of groundbreaking articles entitled *The Rational*

Clinical Examination.[7] This scholarly, evidence-based series of articles underscore the points made in this chapter: namely, that signs and symptoms provide critical information in diagnostic reasoning and that the operating characteristics (sensitivity and specificity) of the signs and symptoms must be considered in the reasoning process, as must the prevalence of the disease in question. In other words, the clinical examination can and should be more rational, based on empirical evidence of the predictive value of signs and symptoms used in diagnostic reasoning. In each issue of the series, a specific clinical question is posed (such as "*Does This Child With High Blood Pressure Have Secondary Hypertension?* March 28, 2023)[8] and the current evidence that is needed to answer the question is presented. A reference listing of the *JAMA Rational Clinical Examination Series* can be found in Appendix F.[8]

The rational clinical examination is part of a broader movement called *evidence-based medicine,* which "de-emphasizes intuition, unsystematic clinical experience, and pathophysiologic rationale as sufficient grounds for clinical decision making and stresses the examination of evidence from clinical research." The evidence-based approach to the practice of clinical medicine has its origins in clinical research generated within the relatively new field of *clinical epidemiology.* In the past, epidemiology was concerned with the causes of diseases, and hence the interest was in establishing that exposure to certain risk factors caused certain diseases. Thus, classic epidemiology has been characterized as the study of the distribution of disease across time, place, and people. Clinical epidemiology has expanded this focus to encompass the study of the entire clinical process, including diagnosis, treatment, prognosis, prevention, evaluation of healthcare services, and risk-benefit analysis. Evidence from clinical research in these areas will be used to provide an empirical base for rational clinical practice, including diagnostic reasoning, as the "art" of clinical decision making becomes more of a science.

REVIEW QUESTIONS

1. **A problem list contains a summary of which of the following?**
   A. Physical examination
   B. Mental status
   C. Social history
   D. Personal conditions
   E. All the above
2. **Which of the following statement is true?**
   A. Decisions in medicine can rarely be made with 100% certainty.
   B. Probability is defined as the likelihood that a proposition is false.
   C. Signs and symptoms account for about 65% of the developing problem list.
   D. Sensitivity is sometimes called the true negative rate.
   E. Specificity is sometimes called the true positive rate.
3. **Which statement about likelihood ratios is *false?***
   A. A positive predictive likelihood ratio is the proportion of patients with the disease with a finding divided by the proportion of patients without the disease who also have the finding.
   B. A negative predictive likelihood ratio is the proportion of patients with the disease who do not have a finding divided by the proportion of patients without the disease who also do not have the finding.
   C. Tests or signs greater than 0.5 are useful because they provide considerable confidence in diagnostic reasoning.
   D. The likelihood ratio is the likelihood that a given test result would be expected in a patient with the disease compared to the likelihood that the same result would be expected in a patient without the disease.
   E. The likelihood ratio is the true positive rate to the false positive rate.
4. **Which of the following statements about predictive values is *false?***
   A. The positive predictive value is the probability that subjects with a positive screening test will truly have the disease.
   B. The negative predictive value is the probability that subjects with a negative screening test will not have the disease.
   C. The negative predictive value is the frequency of no disease in individuals with negative test results.
   D. Pretest probability is defined as the probability of a patient not having the disease before a test result is known.
   E. A healthcare professional wants to predict the actual probability of disease with a positive test result.
5. **Which of the following statements about Bayes theorem is *false?***
   A. Bayes theorem is a way of finding a probability when we do not know other probabilities.
   B. A conditional probability is the probability of an event occurring given that another event has occurred.
   C. A prior probability is an initial probability value originally obtained before any additional evidence is obtained.
   D. A posterior probability is a probability value that has been revised by using additional evidence that is obtained later.
   E. Bayes theorem computes how to adjust the prior probability into the posterior probability.
6. **Which of the following statements about critical thinking is *false?***
   A. Critical thinking is basically making sure that we have good reasons for our beliefs.
   B. It includes knowledge of specific facts and skills.
   C. It includes gathering and assessing relevant information using abstract ideas to interpret it effectively.
   D. It is self-directed, self-disciplined, self-monitored, and self-corrective thinking.
   E. Intuition is rarely used in clinical medicine.
7. **Which of these statements about critical thinking is correct?**
   A. Identifying the main question of the problem
   B. Gathering relevant data to the main problem or question

C. Developing conclusions
D. Describing implications
E. All of the above

8. **Which of the following types of statements is the universal intellectual standard of critical thinking?**
A. Clarity
B. Precision
C. Relevance
D. Logic
E. All of the above

9. **Which of the following statements about metacognition is *false?***
A. Metacognition is critically thinking about thinking.
B. It refers to the processes used to plan, monitor, and assess one's own understanding and performance.
C. It reflects on our own thoughts to gain insight into our own needs.
D. Recognizing immediately yellow sclera as jaundice is an example of metacognition.
E. Healthcare professionals always need to use metacognition in evaluating patients.

REFERENCES

Available online.

BIBLIOGRAPHY

Available online.

29

The Clinical Record

Mark H. Swartz

May I never forget that the patient is a fellow human creature in pain. May I never consider the patient merely a vessel of disease.

From Oath of Maimonides (1135–1204)

PUTTING THE HISTORY AND PHYSICAL EXAMINATION TOGETHER

This book covers both history-taking and physical examination techniques. Chapters 1–5 delve into history-taking techniques, while Chapters 6–21 focus on various components of history and physical examination. Chapter 22 outlines a comprehensive approach to conducting a physical examination and documenting it. Chapters 23–27 discuss the evaluation of specific patients, and Chapter 28 covers data gathering, analysis, and critical thinking. This chapter provides guidance on integrating the patient's history and physical examination into one comprehensive statement.

In writing up the history and the physical examination, the examiner should follow several rules:

- Record all pertinent data.
- Avoid extraneous data.
- Use common terms.
- Avoid nonstandard abbreviations.
- Be objective.
- Use diagrams when indicated.

When documenting a patient's medical record, it is important to refrain from including comments on their behavior or attitudes unless they are medically or scientifically relevant. It is important to accurately describe all parts of the examination that were performed and note any that were deferred. It is more precise to state specific findings rather than make general statements. Additionally, it is not necessary to list all possible abnormalities if they are not present. By stating that a particular area is normal, it is implied that the examiner inspected it and did not find any concerning issues. **Remember that the patient's medical record is a legal document that should be accurate and objective.**

Let's revisit the case of Mr. John Doe, whose interview was previously recorded in Chapter 4, Putting the History Together. In the next section, we will provide a detailed account of his medical history and physical examination.

Patient: John Doe[a]

Date of Visit: July 19, 2024

History

Source

Self, reliable.

Chief Concern

"Chest pain for the past 6 months."

History of Present Illness

This is the first St. Mary's Hospital admission for this 45-year-old lawyer with atherosclerotic coronary artery disease. The patient's history of chest pain began 4 years before admission. He described the pain as a "dull ache" in the retrosternal area, with radiation to his left arm. The pain was provoked by exertion and emotions. On July 15, 2022, Mr. Doe suffered his first heart attack while playing tennis. He had an uneventful hospitalization in Kings Hospital in New York City. After 6 days in the hospital and 4 weeks at home, he returned to work. The patient suffered a second heart attack 6 months later (January 9, 2023), again while playing tennis. The patient was hospitalized in Kings Hospital, during which time he was told of an "irregularity" in his heart rate. Since then, the patient has not experienced any palpitations, nor has he been told of any further irregularities.

Over the past 6 months, Mr. Doe has noted an increase in the frequency of his chest pain. The pain now occurs 4 to 5 times a day and is relieved within 5 minutes with 1 or 2 nitroglycerin tablets under his tongue. The pain is produced by exercise, emotions, and sexual intercourse. The patient also describes 1-block dyspnea on exertion. The patient relates that 6 months ago, he could walk 2 or 3 blocks before becoming short of breath.

[a]This name is fictitious. Any similarity to any person living or dead with this name is purely coincidental.

Although the patient shows significant denial of his illness, he is anxious and depressed.

The patient has currently been admitted for elective cardiac catheterization.

Past Medical History

General: Good.

Past illnesses: History of untreated hypertension for years (blood pressure not known); no history of measles, chickenpox, mumps, diphtheria, or whooping cough.

Injuries: None.

Hospitalizations: Appendectomy, age 15 years, Booth Memorial Hospital in Rochester, New York (Dr. Ralph Meyers, surgeon).

Surgery: See Hospitalizations.

Allergies: None.

Immunizations: Salk vaccine for polio, tetanus vaccine, both as a child; no adverse reactions remembered.

Substance abuse: A 40-pack-year (2 packs a day for 20 years) history of smoking; stopped smoking after first heart attack; marijuana on rare occasions in past; drinks alcohol "socially" but also admits to feeling the need for a drink as the day goes on (CAGE score, 1); denies use of recreational drugs.

Diet: Mostly red meat, with little fish in diet; 3 cups of coffee a day; recent decrease in appetite, with a 10-pound weight loss in past 3 months.

Sleep patterns: Recently, falls asleep normally but awakens around 3 AM and cannot go back to sleep.

Current medications:

- Metoprolol, 50 mg once daily
- Amlodipine 2.5 mg once daily
- Nitroglycerin, 1/150 grains prn chest pain
- Chlor-Trimeton, for colds
- Aspirin, for headaches
- Multivitamins with iron, daily

Family History (Fig. 29.1)

Father, 75, diabetes, broken hip
Mother died, 64, stomach cancer
Brother, 45, heart attack at age 40
Sister, 37, alive and well
Son, 15, alive and well
Wife, 41, alive and well

There is no family history of congenital disease. No other history of diabetes or cardiac disease. No history of renal, hepatic, or neurologic disease. No history of mental illness.

Psychosocial History

"Type A" personality; born and raised in Middletown, New York; family moved to Rochester, New York, when Mr. Doe was 13 years of age; patient moved to New York City after high school; college and law school in New York City; he is now a senior partner of a law firm for which he has worked for the past 17 years; married to Emily for the past 13 years; was an active tennis player before second heart attack; before 6 months ago, enjoyed the theater and reading.

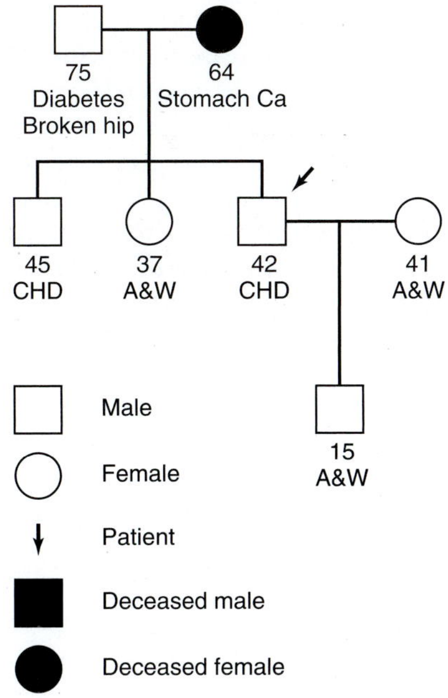

Fig. 29.1 Family Tree of Patient John Doe. *A&W,* Alive and well; *Ca,* cancer; *CHD,* coronary heart disease.

Sexual, Reproductive, and Gynecologic History

Patient was born male; thinks of himself as male. Is exclusively heterosexual, with one partner, his wife. He has one son, age 15 years. Recently, because of angina, the patient has stopped having sexual relations. He has noted that for the past 2 years, his erections have been "less hard."

Review of Systems

General: Depressed for the past 6 months as a result of his ill health.

Skin: No rashes or other changes.

Head: No history of head injury.

Eyes: Wears glasses for reading; no changes in vision recently; saw ophthalmologist 1 year ago for routine examination; no history of eye pain, tearing, discharge, or seeing halos around lights.

Ears: Patient not aware of any problem hearing; no dizziness, discharge, or pain present.

Nose: Occasional upper respiratory infection, two or three times a year, lasting 3 to 5 days; no hay fever, sinus symptoms.

Mouth and throat: Occasional sore throats and canker sores associated with colds; no difficulty in chewing or eating; brushes and flosses twice a day; sees dentist twice a year; no gingival bleeding.

Neck: No masses or tenderness.

Chest: History of occasional blood-tinged sputum and cough in the morning when patient was smoking, but not recently; last chest x-ray film 1 year ago, was told it was normal; 1-block dyspnea on exertion (as noted in History of Present Illness); no history of wheezing, asthma, bronchitis, or tuberculosis.

Breasts: No masses or nipple discharge noted.

Cardiac: As noted in History of Present Illness.

Vascular: No history of cerebrovascular accidents or claudication.

Gastrointestinal: Recent decrease in appetite with 10-pound weight loss in past few months; uses no laxatives; no history of diarrhea, constipation, nausea, or vomiting; no bleeding noted.

Genitourinary: Urinates four to five times a day; urine is light yellow in color, never red; nocturia ×1; no change in stream; no history of urinary infections; no sexual intercourse in past 6 months, owing to angina during sex; no history of venereal disease.

Musculoskeletal: No joint or bone symptoms; no weakness; no history of back problems or gout.

Neurologic: No history of seizures or difficulties in walking or balance; no history of motor or sensory symptoms.

Endocrine: No known thyroid nodules; no history of temperature intolerance; no hair changes; no history of polydipsia or polyuria.

Psychiatric: Depressed and very anxious about his ill health; also anxious about the results of the upcoming cardiac catheterization; asked, "What's going to happen to me?"

Physical Examination

General appearance: The patient is a 42-year-old, slightly obese white male who is lying in bed. He appears slightly older than his stated age. He is in no acute distress but is very nervous. He is well groomed, cooperative, and alert.

Vital signs: Blood pressure (BP), 175/95/80 right arm (supine), 175/90/85 left arm (supine), 170/90/80 left arm (sitting), 185/95/85 right leg (prone); heart rate, 100 and regular; respirations, 14.

Skin: Pink; no cyanosis present; 5 to 7 nevi (each 0.5 to 1.5 cm in diameter) on back, most with hair; normal male escutcheon.

Head: Normocephalic, without signs of trauma.

Eyes: Visual acuity with reading glasses using near card: right eye (OD) 20/40, left eye (OS) 20/30; confrontation visual fields full bilaterally; extraocular movements (EOMs) intact; pupils are equal, round, and reactive to light (PERRL); eyebrows normal; conjunctivae pink; discs sharp; marked arteriovenous (AV) nicking present bilaterally; copper wiring present bilaterally; a cotton-wool spot is present at 1 o'clock position (superior nasal) in the right eye and at 5 o'clock position (inferior temporal) in the left eye; no hemorrhages are present.

Ears: Normal position; no tenderness present; external canals normal; Rinne test, air conduction (AC) greater than bone conduction (BC) bilaterally; Weber test, no lateralization; both tympanic membranes appear normal, with normal landmarks clearly seen.

Nose: Straight, without masses; patent bilaterally; mucosa pink, without discharge; inferior turbinates appear normal.

Sinuses: No tenderness present over frontal or maxillary sinuses.

Mouth and throat: Lips pink; buccal mucosa pink; all teeth in good condition, without obvious caries; gingivae normal, without bleeding; tongue midline and without masses; uvula elevates in midline; gag reflex intact; posterior pharynx normal.

Neck: Supple, with full range of motion; trachea midline and freely mobile; no adenopathy present; thyroid not felt; prominent "a" wave seen in neck veins while lying at 45 degrees; neck veins flat while sitting upright.

Chest: Normal anteroposterior (AP) diameter; symmetric excursion bilaterally; normal tactile fremitus bilaterally; chest resonant bilaterally; clear on percussion and auscultation.

Breasts: Normal male, without masses, gynecomastia, or discharge.

Heart: Point of maximum impulse (PMI), fifth intercostal space, midclavicular line (5ICS-MCL); S_1 and S_2 normal; normal physiologic splitting present; a loud S_4 is present at the cardiac apex; no murmurs or rubs are heard (Fig. 29.2).

Vascular: Pulses are present and symmetric down to the dorsalis pedis bilaterally; no bruits are present over the carotid or femoral arteries; no abdominal bruits are present; no edema is present.

Abdomen: A well-healed appendectomy scar is present in the right lower quadrant (RLQ); the abdomen is slightly obese; no masses are present; no tenderness, guarding, rigidity, or rebound is present.

Rectal: Anal sphincter normal; no hemorrhoids present; prostate slightly enlarged and soft; no prostatic masses felt; no stool in ampulla.

Genitalia: Circumcised male with normal genitalia; penis normal without induration; testicles, 4 × 3 × 2 cm (right) and 3 × 6 × 4 cm (left) with normal consistency.

Lymphatic: No adenopathy noted.

Musculoskeletal: There are several stony-hard, slightly yellowish, nontender masses over the extensor tendons on the patient's hands; normal range of motion of neck, spine, and major joints of upper and lower extremities.

Neurologic: Oriented to person, place, and time; cranial nerves II to XII intact (cranial nerve I not tested); gross sensory and motor function normal; cerebellar function normal; plantar reflexes down; gait normal; deep tendon reflexes as in Table 29.1.

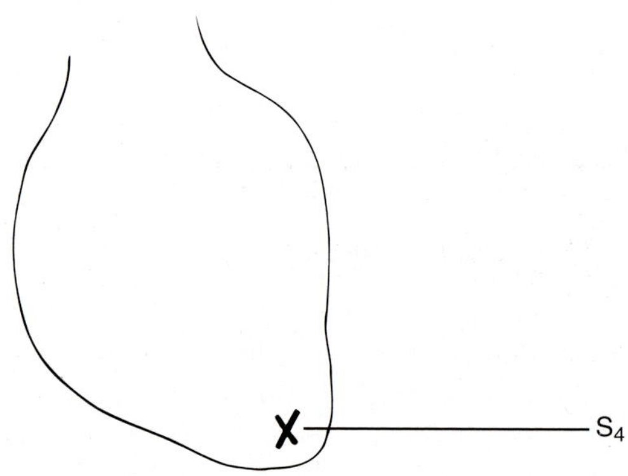

Fig. 29.2 Diagram Showing Location of Abnormal Cardiac Findings in Patient John Doe.

TABLE 29.1 Deep Tendon Reflexes of Patient John Doe

Side	Biceps	Triceps	Knee	Achilles
Right	2+	2+	2+	1+
Left	2+	2+	1+	1+

Reflex scoring: 2+, normal; 1+, diminished.

Summary

Mr. Doe is a "type A" 42-year-old male with a history of coronary artery disease, status post (S/P)[b] two myocardial infarctions in July 2022 and January 2023, with current admission for elective cardiac catheterization. His risk factors for coronary artery disease are untreated hypertension and a long history of cigarette smoking. The patient has a brother who suffered a myocardial infarction at the age of 40 years. His cardiac medications are metoprolol 50 mg daily, amlodipine 2.5 mg daily, and nitroglycerin as needed.

Physical examination reveals a slightly obese male with hypertension and its associated early to intermediate funduscopic changes. Cardiac examination reveals a loud fourth heart sound, suggesting a noncompliant (stiff) ventricle. This may be a manifestation of ischemic heart disease or ventricular hypertrophy secondary to hypertension. Although the patient is not aware of any lipid abnormalities, numerous tendinous xanthomata on the hands are present, which are strongly suggestive of hypercholesterolemia, an additional risk factor for premature coronary artery disease.

Problem List

When Mr. Doe visits a healthcare professional, they refer to a list of his health problems called a "problem list" (Table 29.2). The list includes the dates when each problem was identified and resolved, and it's regularly updated. The healthcare professional creates a plan to resolve each issue, and there are four components to this plan.

- **S**ubjective data
- **O**bjective data
- **A**ssessment
- **P**lan

This is the **SOAP format**,[c] which is a method used to update subjective and objective data, assess a problem, and plan for its resolution. When writing a progress note, it's important to include the date, time, writer's name, and service used by the patient. It's also helpful to list antibiotics and their course dates, as well as other medications and their doses. For patients who have undergone surgery, it's important to indicate the postoperative time on the top of the note (e.g., "Postop Day 3").

When gathering information from patients, it's important to ask about their ***subjective*** **experiences**. This includes how they're feeling, what symptoms they're experiencing, and what they've been eating. It's also crucial to note if they're not allowed to eat due to being NPO.[d]

[b]*S/P* is an abbreviation for "status post," referring to a state that follows a medical intervention or a medical condition.

[c]The creation of the SOAP (Subjective, Objective, Assessment, and Plan) note and the problem-oriented medical record was a significant turning point in the healthcare industry. Dr. Lawrence Weed, who developed the SOAP note, questioned traditional medical documentation and pushed for a scientific framework to support clinical reasoning in the 1950s. His paper, "*Medical Records That Guide and Teach*" (NEJM, 1968), is widely cited in the field of informatics, having been referenced thousands of times.

[d]NPO is an acceptable Latin abbreviation for "(take) nothing by mouth."

TABLE 29.2 Problem List for Patient John Doe

Problem	Date	Resolved
1. Chest pain	2018	
2. Myocardial infarction	July 15, 2022	3 weeks later
3. Myocardial infarction	January 9, 2023	3 weeks later
4. Hypertension	Years	
5. Smoking	1999	July 15, 2022
6. Dyspnea on exertion	6 months ago	
7. Depression	3 months ago	
8. Weight loss	3 months ago	
9. Sleeping abnormality	3 months ago	
10. Diet modification	3 months ago	
11. Appendectomy	1993	
12. Headaches	About 1996	
13. Tendinous xanthomata	?	
14. S4 gallop	?	

Additionally, ask about their sleeping patterns, ability to walk, and any issues with urination or bowel movements.

When a patient says they are "not doing well," avoid including that statement in your notes. This could be misinterpreted as your own assessment. Instead, ask the patient to describe why they feel that way.

When gathering information about a patient, it is important to focus on **objective data**. This includes information from physical exams, lab tests, and radiographic studies. To ensure accuracy, vital signs and fluid intake and output should be recorded, especially if the patient is on a diuretic regimen or not allowed to eat. It is also important to note any changes in the patient's condition and record daily weights, if applicable. When documenting physical examination findings, include only relevant positive and negative information.

As a summary of the patient's progress or problem, the **assessment** reflects your impression of how they are doing and any changes since the previous day.

Your **plan** outlines the actions you will take to address each problem. This could involve continuing, starting, or stopping medication; ordering laboratory tests; obtaining test results; consulting with others; and providing education to the patient or their family.

When writing a SOAP note, it's not necessary to provide as much detail as you would in an admitting note. Abbreviations[1] can be used, but, as mentioned previously, it's important to keep in mind that different medical specialties may use different abbreviations. For example, PND is commonly used as an abbreviation for paroxysmal nocturnal dyspnea in most medical services, but in an ear, nose, and throat service, it refers to postnasal drip (or discharge). Similarly, the abbreviation MS can stand for multiple sclerosis, mitral stenosis for a cardiologist, morphine sulfate for a pharmacist or anesthesiologist, or musculoskeletal for an orthopedist or rheumatologist.

The length of notes varies depending on the specialty. Medical notes tend to be longer while surgical notes are shorter, but you can ask the house staff team for guidance. Generally, professional students' notes are more detailed than those of the house staff.

ELECTRONIC MEDICAL RECORD AND ELECTRONIC HEALTH RECORD

Electronic medical record (EMR) systems are "electronic records of health-related information on an individual that can be created, gathered, managed, and consulted by authorized clinicians and staff within one healthcare organization."[2] These systems can facilitate workflow and improve the quality of patient care and patient safety. The records contain information about the patient's demographics, medical history, and billing details. As of 2023, 88.2% of office-based physicians and 96% of hospitals[3] in the United States were using an EMR provider system[e] according to the National Electronic Health Records Survey.[4]

EMRs offer several **advantages,** including the ability to maintain detailed patient records, facilitate the sharing of patient data, enhance the quality of care, and increase convenience and efficiency. There are several **risks** associated with using EMR. These risks can be categorized into user-related issues, financial issues, and design flaws that hinder their effectiveness in providing healthcare services. EMR systems are often targeted in healthcare breaches. Other risks include privacy concerns, susceptibility to hacking, loss or destruction of data, and inaccuracies during the transition from paper records to electronic records.

Some people use the terms "electronic medical record" (EMR) and "electronic health record" (EHR) interchangeably, but they are different. **Electronic health records (EHRs)** are essentially upgraded versions of EMRs, as they provide all the same functions plus additional features. They serve as a digital representation of a patient's medical history and chart. EHRs are a way to share a patient's records with authorized healthcare professionals. They provide a comprehensive view of a patient's health, beyond just the clinical data collected in the provider's office. EHRs[f] are designed to be shared with other healthcare professionals, like laboratories and specialists, so they contain information from all healthcare professionals involved in the patient's care. This information can travel with the patient to any location in the United States. EHR adoption in United States hospitals has increased from 72% to 96% in the past 10 years.

It is important to remember that the chart is a legal document. While presenting, it is recommended to be confident but also conservative in the chart, ensuring that the facts are clearly stated. Avoid mentioning other healthcare professionals' opinions in your notes. **Allow the facts in the chart to speak for themselves.**

PROTECTING PATIENT'S RIGHT TO PRIVACY

HIPAA is the **H**ealth **I**nsurance **P**ortability and **A**ccountability **A**ct of 1996, also known as Public Law 104-191.[5] HIPAA legislation is a law in the United States that aims to protect the privacy and security of medical information. It sets national standards for safeguarding patients' personal or protected health information, including their name, address, birth date, social security number, physical and mental health conditions, care provided, and payment information. Providers who violate HIPAA may face substantial fines.

As a healthcare professional, it is crucial to respect your patients' privacy rights and always maintain patient confidentiality. This means refraining from discussing any patient-related information in public areas such as the hallway, waiting room, or elevator. Whether intentional or not, any unauthorized disclosure of patient information is a violation of HIPAA regulations. When disposing of paper-based protected information, make sure to use electronic shredding machines instead of simply throwing it in the trash. For more information on patient privacy and confidentiality, please refer to the section entitled "Privacy and Confidentiality" in Chapter 33, Clinical Ethics and Professionalism.

REFERENCES

Available online.

BIBLIOGRAPHY

Available online.

[e]Some EMR provider systems are EpicCare, Cerner Ambulatory, DrChrono, and eClinicalWorks,

[f]Some EHR provider systems are Epic, athenahealth, Allscripts, Kareo, Cerner, and eClinicalWorks.

30

The Focused History and Physical Examination

Mark H. Swartz

All we know is still infinitely less than all that still remains unknown.

William Harvey (1578–1657)

VIDEOS

Video 30.1 A focused history and physical exam

GENERAL CONSIDERATIONS

Mastering the art of conducting a thorough patient history and physical examination is crucial for healthcare professionals. It allows them to quickly understand a patient's needs and educate them properly. However, it takes time and practice to become proficient in this skill. Once a healthcare professional is confident with the complete history and physical examination, they can then focus on extracting the most relevant components for a more targeted and efficient examination.

Although it would be great if healthcare professionals could dedicate 45 to 60 minutes to new patients, they usually only have about 10 to 15 minutes per encounter due to time constraints. Therefore, acquiring the skills to conduct a thorough and focused medical history and physical examination is crucial. Even though most professional schools do not teach these skills, it is essential to learn how to document medical histories and conduct physical exams in a focused and efficient manner.

When conducting a medical interview, it's important to *begin with open-ended questions* and find out the reason the patient is seeking medical attention. Later, it can be helpful to ask the patient, "What do you think is happening?" This can reveal any underlying conflict or anxiety and help the patient share their actual problem. It's best to let the patient speak without interruption and avoid using leading or biased questions.

The process of conducting a thorough patient history and physical exam requires a variety of skills but can be challenging to teach. It involves combining scientific knowledge with effective communication and logical reasoning to ask relevant questions about the patient's health.

In Chapter 28, Precision, Accuracy, and Critical Thinking in Clinical Assessment, it was explained that diagnoses are often not straightforward. The symptoms and medical history of patients can vary greatly and may not fit the typical pattern expected for a certain condition. For example, a 64-year-old male with a history of hypertension and hypercholesterolemia may not always present with crushing chest pain secondary to an acute myocardial infarction; a 41-year-old overweight female with severe right upper quadrant pain may not always experience accompanying nausea or radiating pain to her right shoulder secondary to an acute cholecystitis! Healthcare professionals commonly face uncertainty when diagnosing patients and must evaluate the likelihood of a particular medical condition. This uncertainty is present in most cases they will encounter.

Even with advanced technology, healthcare professionals still rely on their judgment when making clinical decisions. Deciding when to use further testing and when to be cost-conscious can be challenging. Creating a standard approach for dealing with medical problems and uncertainty is difficult. Good medicine involves using available data to make informed decisions. The first step is to gather important details about the patient's medical problem or reason for seeking medical attention.

When conducting a focused history and physical examination, it's crucial to explore the patient's main concern, medical history, allergies, family and social history, occupation, and sexual history. **It is important to note that a focused examination doesn't stop at one diagnosis, and a differential diagnosis must be considered**. During the physical examination, it's necessary to examine the body part(s) or system(s) directly involved in the medical issue. However, it's also important to evaluate other organ systems. For example, a patient with chest pain requires a full cardiac examination, as well as an examination of the legs for peripheral pulses and edema, auscultation of the lungs, auscultation and palpation of the carotid artery, evaluation of liver size, and ophthalmoscopic examination for related vascular changes.

Once you have completed a clinical evaluation, you should only order tests to confirm your clinical impression or if it will impact your decision-making. Remember that *common symptoms are more likely to indicate a common condition*,[a] whereas uncommon symptoms are more likely to be an uncommon manifestation of a common condition rather than an entirely rare condition.

[a]There is a famous quote by J.C. Peters that says, "*When you hear hoofbeats in Central Park, think horses, not zebras!*" **Common things are common!** Central Park is in the center of Manhattan in New York City.

ILLUSTRATIVE CASE

The History of Mr. Roger Stern[b]

Let's take the case of Mr. Roger Stern as an example. He's a 29-year-old male who has come to the emergency room with chief concern of "diarrhea and abdominal pain." What could be causing these symptoms? There are many possibilities to consider, such as genetic disorders, infectious diseases, immune system disorders, tumors, environmental factors, nutritional issues, vascular problems, or traumatic injuries. These could be acute or chronic conditions (Video 30.1).

Now try to narrow down the possible diagnoses by starting the **interview:**

Where is the pain in your abdomen?

Right here (pointing to his lower abdomen).

How long have you been having the abdominal pain?

I have been having diarrhea and abdominal pain for the past 3 months.

What was the reason you came in today?

I saw some blood mixed in the stools, and I got very scared.

I can understand your concern. It's good that you came in today. We will do everything possible to help you. Can you describe the pain?

It's crampy and comes in waves. I also have this bloating sensation in my abdomen all the time. It's as if gas is always there.

What makes the pain better?

It's hard to say… Not much.

What makes it worse?

I don't really know… Perhaps anxiety?

Has there been a change in your life that has created more anxiety?

I guess my job has been rather stressful. I don't get along well with my bosses.

What type of work do you do?

I am a legal assistant.

On a scale of 1 to 10, with 10 being the worst, how would you describe the pain?

I guess the pain is about 5 to 7.

How does the pain affect your lifestyle?

I do go to work, but it's tough getting up all the time to go to the bathroom and making excuses.

When you have the pain in your abdomen, do you have pain in any other area of your body at the same time?

No, I don't think so.

Have you noticed that the pain is worse when you're hungry or after meals?

No, it just comes and goes and is not related to eating.

Now let's talk about the diarrhea. Can you describe it for me?

The stool is very loose and sometimes watery. And today there was *blood* in it.

Was there blood in the toilet bowl?

No. It was kind of wrapped with the stool.

How many times did you see blood with your stool?

Three times!

[b]This name is fictitious. Any similarity to any person living or dead with this name is purely coincidental.

Is there mucus in the stool?

Yes, often. It's kind of stringy.

Is the stool formed?

Not really.

About how many bowel movements do you have a day?

About 8 to 10 for the past week.

Does the stool float?

No.

Does it smell strange?

No. *[pause]* Doc, do you think I have cancer?

Mr. Stern, it's too early to say. I need to ask you some more questions, perform a physical examination, and do other tests. When we have all the tests back, I will be in a better position to advise you. At this time, however, there are many things that it could be. Let me ask you a few more questions. Have you had a fever?

No. I don't think so.

Have you noticed that milk or milk products make the diarrhea worse?

No.

Have you noticed that wheat, oat, barley, or rye products make the diarrhea worse?

No. I love bread and wheat products. They don't seem to make things worse.

Do you drink alcohol?

Not really. Maybe one beer over the weekend at most.

Have you had abdominal pain in the past?

I first noticed abdominal pain with watery diarrhea about 15 months ago.

What happened then?

I was traveling with a friend to Central America.

Did you see a doctor?

No.

Did you take any medications?

My friend gave me some Pepto-Bismol® and Imodium® for the pain and diarrhea.

Did it help you?

The pain persisted on and off for about 3 weeks and then disappeared.

Do you take other medications?

No. I have been in good health otherwise. I have no other problems.

Have you had other episodes of abdominal pain?

The pain and diarrhea returned about 3 months ago, but the diarrhea was no longer watery. The stool was just very loose.

Have you seen any doctor about this problem?

Yes, I saw a local doc about 3 weeks ago who gave me some antibiotic for it.

Do you remember the name of the antibiotic?

It was Flagyl.

Did it help you?

No. In fact, it seemed to make it worse, so I stopped taking it after 5 or 6 days.

Do you have nausea?

Not really.

Any vomiting?

No.

How's your diet?

I think okay, but recently I'm not too hungry because of the abdominal pain and diarrhea.

Has there been any change in your weight?

I've lost maybe about 5 pounds in the past month.

Does anyone else in your family have a similar problem?

No.

Have you ever had surgery?

No.

Tell me about your parents' health.

My mom is 54, and she's fine. My dad died about 15 months ago from a sudden heart attack. He was 56. I miss him a lot.

I am sorry to hear about your father.

Thanks.

Do you have any siblings?

Yeah, I have an older brother who's fine. He's 31.

Do you use any recreational drugs?

Marijuana about once or twice a month.

Anything else?

No.

Do you have any allergies?

No.

Are you sexually active?

Yeah.

Are your partners male, female, or both?

Only women. I've got a great relationship going on now. I've been living with my girlfriend for the past 8 months. I sure hope it continues.

Do you use protection?

Condoms all the time!

Mr. Stern, I just have a few more general questions before I begin the physical examination. Have you ever had a problem with your eyes?

Eyes… yeah. When I was 19 years old in college, I had iritis in my right eye.

Tell me more about that.

I had real bad pain in my right eye, and it got real red. I saw the eye doc, who gave me steroids to take for about 4 weeks. I also remember that I had to wear sunglasses most of the time because the light really bothered me. I got better in about 3 weeks. I took all the meds because I didn't want that to come back again! Thank God it never came back!

Any history of back problems?

Yeah, I've had low back pain for several years since, I guess, I was 21. I think it's from too much bowling.

Did you ever see a doctor about it?

No. I just take some aspirin or Tylenol, which helps it.

Have you had any oral ulcers or mouth sores?

Not really.

Any urinary problems?

Nope.

Any rashes?

No.

Any chest pain?

No.

Any shortness of breath?

No.

In summary, Mr. Stern, a 29-year-old male, is seeking medical evaluation for a history of abdominal pain and diarrhea. The patient experienced his first episode of pain about 15 months ago while on a trip to Central America. Although the pain disappeared, it returned about 3 months ago. Today, the patient noticed red blood mixed with his stool and sought medical attention. The patient describes the pain as crampy, mostly felt in his lower abdomen. The pain is relieved with defecation, and the patient describes it as about a 5 to 7 on a scale of 10. The patient has also been experiencing bloating in his abdomen. He has not experienced any nausea or vomiting and denies being febrile. Over the past month, he has experienced a 5-pound weight loss. About 3 weeks ago, Mr. Stern saw a local physician who prescribed an antibiotic, which seemed to make things worse. Consequently, he stopped taking the medication after 5 or 6 days. The symptoms have persisted, with the patient experiencing about 8 to 10 bowel movements each day for the past week. He has also noticed some stringy mucus mixed in with the stool. The stools do not float, and he does not have any sensitivity to lactose or gluten (wheat, oat, barley, or rye products).

He is not taking any medications. He does not have any known allergies.

He lives with his girlfriend of 8 months and always uses condoms for sexual protection. He enjoys smoking marijuana about once or twice a month. He denies using any other misused substances. He works now as a legal clerk.

His mother is 54 years old and is in good health. His father died at age 56 from a sudden heart attack about 15 months ago. He has an older brother, age 31, who is healthy.

It is important to note that he experienced iritis in his right eye at the age of 19, which was treated with steroids and sunglasses for a period of 4 weeks. The condition improved after about 3 weeks. He also has a history of occasional low back pain that he believes is due to bowling and started when he was around 21 years old.

DIAGNOSTIC EVALUATION

After speaking with Mr. Stern, there are several possible diagnoses to consider. These include inflammatory bowel disease (IBD), irritable bowel syndrome, traveler's diarrhea, pseudomembranous colitis, celiac disease, and giardiasis. Based on his history of iritis and low back pain, IBD is a likely possibility. IBD includes Crohn disease and ulcerative colitis, which are quite common with an annual incidence of 3 to 10 new cases per 100,000 people in the U.S. Patients with IBD often experience extraintestinal inflammatory complications, including ocular manifestations in 5% of cases and ankylosing spondylitis in 5% to 10%. Mr. Stern did indicate a history of iritis at age 19. A non-deforming, large-joint, asymmetric arthritis is the most common complication, occurring in 20% of cases. However, Mr. Stern does not have a history of this type of arthritis. Genetic disorders are not likely as his symptoms started at age 27 or 28. It is unlikely that the problem is caused by viral or bacterial gastroenteritis because it has persisted for a long time, despite having traveled to Central America 15 months ago. Infections such as *Salmonella*, *Shigella*, and *Campylobacter* enterocolitis typically cause fever and last for a short duration of 3 to 6 days, although *Campylobacter* infection may cause a more protracted diarrheal illness. It is unlikely that the patient is suffering from antibiotic-associated colitis (pseudomembranous colitis) since most of the symptoms appeared before the recent prescription of antibiotics. The patient's age and medical history make it unlikely that he has colorectal carcinoma, although this still remains to be a possibility. While giardiasis is still a possibility, it is lower on the list of potential diagnoses. This is because most patients with giardiasis experience malabsorptive diarrhea, which is not a symptom displayed by this patient. Additionally, lactase deficiency is common in patients with giardiasis, but the patient denies having any intolerance to milk. Using condoms regularly during sexual activity with only females can reduce the risk of contracting acquired immunodeficiency syndrome (AIDS)-related diarrheal illness in males. AIDS patients have a high likelihood of experiencing malabsorptive syndromes and diarrheal illnesses, which can affect up to 50% of patients. Malabsorptive syndromes are characterized by the inability to absorb nutrients such as fats, vitamins, and minerals. Symptoms can include chronic diarrhea and flatulence, but the primary indicator is excessive fecal fat content or steatorrhea. The patient, Mr. Stern, denies experiencing steatorrhea symptoms such as floating stools. Although celiac disease is a chronic condition, the patient's insensitivity to gluten makes it an unlikely diagnosis. The patient's age and lack of other medical conditions make vascular disorders improbable.

The Physical Examination of Mr. Roger Stern

Based on the history, the focused physical examination of Mr. Stern should include the following (see Video 30.1):

- General appearance for signs of wasting, jaundice
- Inspection of skin for rashes
- Inspection of the mouth for oral ulcers
- Inspection of the abdomen
- Light palpation of the abdomen in all four quadrants after auscultation
- Deep palpation of all four quadrants
- Percussion of the abdomen
- Evaluation of liver size
- Rectal examination and evaluation for fecal occult blood
- Evaluation of sacroiliac joints for tenderness

After performing these physical examination maneuvers, you should be able to narrow down or confirm the most likely diagnosis. Always obtain as much information as possible. You can always narrow down your differential diagnosis.

It is a difficult task to obtain a good, focused history and perform a good, focused physical examination. It requires an excellent knowledge of physical diagnosis, pathophysiologic processes, and epidemiologic data to home in on the important aspects of the patient's medical problem.

BIBLIOGRAPHY

Available online.

31

Artificial Intelligence in Clinical Encounters: Opportunities and Challenges

Joy J. Jiang, Lili Chan, and Girish N. Nadkarni

AI is not meant to replace caregivers, but those who use AI will probably replace those who don't.[1]

Bertalan Meskó (1984–current)

In previous chapters, you learned about the healthcare professional and patient interaction for obtaining a detailed medical history and performing a physical examination. **Artificial intelligence (AI)** will likely significantly impact these interactions in the future. In the following sections, we review AI concepts and discuss how AI impacts healthcare professional–patient interactions now and in the future.

GENERAL CONSIDERATIONS

AI refers broadly to the development of computer systems that can perform tasks that typically require human intelligence (Fig. 31.1). In the context of medicine, AI involves the application of models, also known as algorithms, to analyze data and make informed decisions or predictions. These algorithms can process vast amounts of information coming from different sources, such as medical images, patient records, and research data. AI in medicine aims to enhance clinical practice, improve patient outcomes, and optimize healthcare processes by assisting in disease detection, personalizing treatment recommendations, and enabling more efficient healthcare delivery. From 2018 to 2023, there were 84 randomized control trials involving AI algorithms across the world.[2]

Machine learning (ML) refers to the subset of AI techniques that allow machines to learn from medical data and make predictions or assist in clinical tasks based on that learning. There are two major types of ML: supervised and unsupervised learning. In **supervised learning,** algorithms are trained on datasets that are labeled to create models that relate input to the outcome and then used to predict or classify outcomes in new unlabeled data. In **unsupervised learning,** algorithms are used to identify structures, such as clusters of similar data points, in unlabeled data.

Deep learning (DL) is a subset of ML that utilizes neural networks to detect patterns in massive datasets. Just as the human brain is composed of interconnected neurons that work together to process and transmit information, a **neural network** consists of artificial **neurons**, also known as nodes or units, that are interconnected in layers. The artificial neuron receives input, transforms information, and outputs results. These neurons communicate with each other by sending signals through the connections, known as weights. These neurons are arranged into layers, and the combination of these layers is called "deep," giving rise to the term DL.

Natural language processing (NLP) is a branch of AI that gives a computer the ability to understand text and spoken words. **Large language models (LLMs)** are DL models trained to produce text. LLMs are "foundation models" that are large pretrained AI systems, meaning that they have been trained on enormous bodies of text to learn semantic relationships. They can be repurposed with minimal effort across numerous domains and diverse tasks. In recent years, LLMs have exploded onto the market, and multiple ways of using LLMs in medicine have been proposed.

Reinforcement learning (RL) is a type of ML in which an agent learns how to make decisions through interaction with an environment. The agent takes actions within the environment and receives feedback in the form of rewards or penalties based on the outcomes of those actions. The goal of the agent is to develop a policy that maximizes the cumulative rewards it receives over time by exploring the environment, trying different actions, and learning from the consequences of those actions. Through this trial-and-error process, the agent gradually develops a sense of which actions are more likely to lead to favorable outcomes. While its use has yet to emerge in clinically deployed algorithms, RL remains an area of active investigation.

Key Terms and Concepts

To understand this chapter, there are various important terms and concepts listed in Table 31.1. These terms and concepts will provide the fundamental basis for the applications that will be discussed.

Evaluation of ML Algorithm Performance

When evaluating ML models, it is essential to consider various performance metrics. Common metrics are outlined later and should be used under specific circumstances (Fig. 31.2). No single metric is necessarily better, and often an evaluation using multiple metrics is used to provide a comprehensive understanding of model performance.

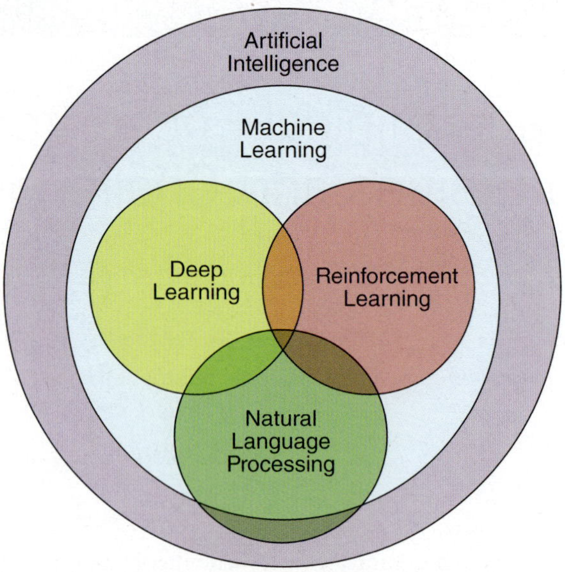

Fig. 31.1 Overall Taxonomy of AI Categories.

Accuracy measures overall correctness, calculating correctly classified instances to the total number of instances. It can be misleading when dealing with imbalanced datasets in which there is an unequal representation of different classes. When there is a disproportionate representation of one class in comparison to others, a model may demonstrate high accuracy even if it were to predict incorrectly on the minority classes. For example, if a model were to predict whether a person from the general population will experience acute myocardial infarction in a 1-year time

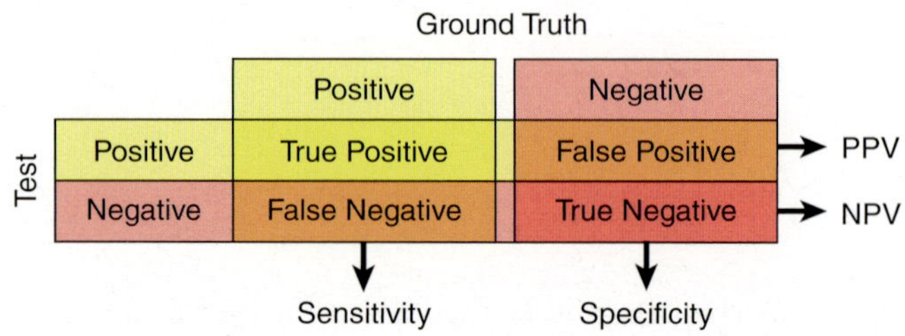

Fig. 31.2 Calculation of Select Performance Metrics.

TABLE 31.1 Key Terms and Concepts

Term	Definition
Artificial intelligence (AI)	Field of computer science that develops systems and algorithms capable of performing tasks that typically require human intelligence, such as learning, problem solving, and decision making
Bias	Decision making that can result in unfair or inaccurate outcomes for certain sociodemographic groups
Deep learning (DL)	Subfield of machine learning that involves training and deploying artificial neural networks with multiple layers to automatically learn and extract complex patterns and representations from data
Explainability	Ability to understand decisions made by AI
F1 score	Metric that combines precision and recall into a single value, providing a balanced measure of a classification model's accuracy by considering both the false positives and false negatives
Machine learning (ML)	Subfield of artificial intelligence that focuses on developing algorithms and models that enable computer systems to learn from and make predictions or decisions based on data, without explicit programming
Natural language processing (NLP)	Field of artificial intelligence that deals with the interaction between computers and human language, enabling machines to understand, interpret, and generate human language in a meaningful way
Negative predictive value (NPV)	Metric that measures the proportion of instances correctly predicted as negative out of all instances predicted as negative, indicating its ability to avoid false negatives
Neural network	Computational model inspired by the human brain consisting of interconnected nodes or neurons that process and transmit information to perform tasks such as pattern recognition and data analysis
Precision (also positive predictive value [PPV])	Metric that measures the proportion of true positives among the predicted positive cases by a diagnostic model, indicating its ability to accurately identify cases without many false positives
Recall	Metric that measures the proportion of true positives identified by a diagnostic test or model, indicating its ability to capture and detect the relevant cases without many false negatives
Receiver Operating Characteristic Curve (ROC)	Graphical representation that illustrates the performance of a binary classification model by plotting the true positive rate against the false positive rate at various classification thresholds
Reinforcement learning (RL)	Subfield of machine learning where an agent learns to make decisions by interacting with an environment and receiving rewards or penalties for its actions
Sensitivity	Metric that measures the proportion of true positives correctly identified by a diagnostic test or model, indicating its ability to accurately classify individuals with the condition or trait of interest
Specificity	Metric that measures the proportion of true negatives correctly identified by a diagnostic test or model, indicating its ability to accurately classify non-affected individuals
Supervised learning	Machine learning approach in which a model is trained using labeled data, where input-output pairs are provided, to enable it to make accurate predictions or classifications on unseen data
Unsupervised learning	Machine learning approach in which a model analyzes unlabeled data to discover hidden patterns, relationships, and structures without predefined output labels

frame, it could have an artificially high accuracy by predicting that all patients will not experience myocardial infarction.

Precision, or **positive predictive value (PPV)**, measures the proportion of positive predictions made by the model that are correct, representing the ratio of true positives to total predicted positives (also see Chapter 28, Precision, Accuracy, and Critical Thinking in Clinical Assessment). Precision is advantageous when false positives have notable consequences. However, it does not remark on false negatives.

Meanwhile, **negative predictive value (NPV)** is used to measure the proportion of negative predictions made by the model that are correct. NPV is particularly important in situations in which false negatives may have serious consequences. For example, if a model is intended to predict disease presence, false negatives can result in missed illnesses.

Recall is also known as **sensitivity** or **true positive rate,** representing discrimination of all positive cases by determining the ratio of true positives to all to actual positives. Recall does not consider false positives. High recall may indicate many false positives and lead to low precision.

Specificity, or **true negative rate**, measures the correct identification of negative cases, calculating the ratio of true negatives to all actual negatives. However, specificity does not consider the number of false negatives. A model that has a high specificity value but misses a significant number of positive cases will lead to a low recall rate.

These metrics can be combined to produce measures that balance trade-offs. The **F1 score** is a combination of precision and recall, calculating the harmonic mean of precision and recall by way of assessing both false positives and false negatives simultaneously. F1 score considers precision and recall equally. Depending on the application, precision or recall might be more important, such that F1 score might not capture the desired balance. When F1 score is high, both precision and recall are high, but when F1 score is low, it is unclear which measure is low.

Area Under the Receiver Operating Characteristic Curve (AUROC) evaluates model discrimination between true positive rate and false positive rate across various classification thresholds. It provides an aggregate measure of the model's performance but does not automatically account for the specific classification threshold that should be chosen in practice and is sensitive to class imbalance.

Area Under the Precision-Recall Curve (AUPRC) evaluates performance based on precision and recall across different classification thresholds, particularly in cases of imbalanced datasets. AUPRC is particularly useful in scenarios where positive cases are rare or when the focus is on minimizing false positives.

When evaluating ML models, considering these performance metrics collectively enables a comprehensive understanding of model strengths and weaknesses, which can assist in selecting the most appropriate model for specific clinical applications.

HISTORY TAKING

Obtaining an accurate history is a crucial initial step in determining the patient's problems. Traditionally, the history is obtained directly from the patient during the encounter. However, the rise of AI in medicine has enabled information sharing to occur before and after the encounter. New tools have been developed to assist healthcare professionals in obtaining histories, reducing administrative workload, and diagnosing diseases. In the following section, we provide a brief overview of how AI can be integrated into healthcare professional–patient interactions. Fig. 31.3 summarizes the applications of ML to history taking.

Before the Encounter

Chatbots

Chatbots are computer programs that use AI, specifically LLMs, to simulate human conversations. They are often delivered via text or email. You have likely encountered chatbots on many Internet websites where they are used to answer frequently asked questions. In 2023, ChatGPT® become a popular, publicly available chatbot designed to provide insightful and context-aware responses to a wide range of queries for assisting with complex tasks across various domains.[3] In the healthcare field, several companies have developed healthcare chatbots to aid patients.

No-shows are frequent and negatively impact resource allocation and delays in patient diagnosis or treatment.[4] Forgetting appointments and patient scheduling conflicts are contributors to no-shows.[5,6] Prior research has demonstrated that reminder phone calls can significantly reduce no-shows.[7] Northwell Health has deployed chatbots to aid in reducing no-shows for colonoscopies. Florence® is another healthcare chatbot that can remind patients of appointments and medication consumption.

More advanced chatbots are assisting in providing patient education. For example, the World Health Organization acquired Florence® to provide medical advice on stress management, diet, and tobacco cessation. Others have developed AI-powered symptom checkers to help patients diagnose their disease and connect with healthcare professionals. While some are text-based only, more advanced ones, such as those developed by Sensely/ADA, can take speech, images, and videos as input.

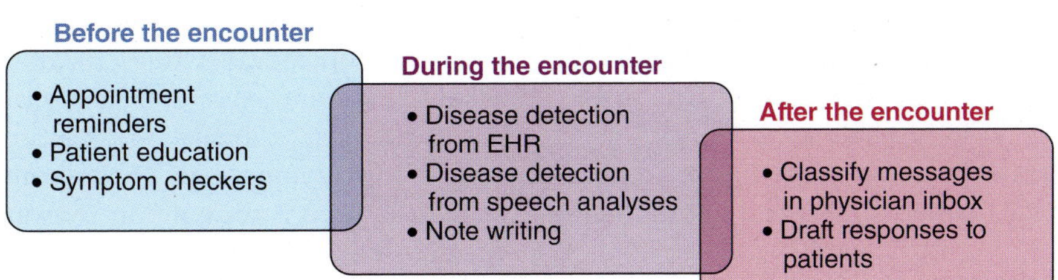

Fig. 31.3 Examples of ML Applications to History Taking.

Given the availability of these AI-powered resources, the history portion of the visit is partially acquired even before the visit begins. A subgroup of patients will also have conducted their own research and bring in their findings for discussion with their healthcare professionals. In one Pew Research Study, 35% of U.S. adults used Google to identify a medical condition.[8] Other research found moderate acceptability of medical chatbots, particularly for minor health concerns that would not require a physical examination.[9] A study that compared the healthcare professional to AI-generated responses to patient questions from an online forum found that evaluators preferred the chatbot response to healthcare professional responses 79% of the time.[10] The chatbot response was rated to have higher quality and more empathy than healthcare professionals. However, chatbots are not foolproof. ChatGPT® is known to produce ***hallucinations***,[a] responses that sound factual despite being false. In this situation, healthcare professionals must dispel misinformation while not dismissing the patient, which can lead to patients becoming defensive and fracture the patient–doctor relationship.

During the Encounter

Automated Disease Detection

An electronic health record (EHR) is multimodal and includes structured data (e.g., vital signs and laboratory data), unstructured data (e.g., progress notes), waveform data, and medical imaging. ML can leverage EHR information to provide various benefits for patients. By analyzing large volumes of patient data, ML algorithms can identify patterns and correlations that may not be easily discernible to healthcare professionals. This can enable early detection and prediction of diseases, personalized treatment recommendations, and improved clinical decision making. ML models can also assist in risk stratification, identifying patients who are at higher risk for certain conditions or adverse events, and allowing for targeted interventions and preventive measures.

The results of ML models are generally delivered to healthcare professionals as clinical decision support systems (CDSS). CDSS are intended to aid in medical decision making with targeted clinical knowledge, patient information, and other health information.[11] Given the near-universal use of EHR in the U.S., CDSS are available in most clinics and healthcare systems.[11,12]

CDSS are classified into two types: knowledge-based and non-knowledge-based. A knowledge-based system uses a rules-based algorithm whereby the system will evaluate if the rule is met and then enact an action or output. A common example of knowledge-based CDSS is one developed to check for drug-drug interactions.[11,13] These types of CDSS incorporate drug safety software that provides checking for dosing, duplication of therapies, and interaction checking. They can be deployed as active alerts to healthcare professionals. Another CDSS includes the detection of diseases, such as in-hospital acute kidney injury (AKI). Implementation of CDSS into practice has had mixed results.[14,15] A non-knowledge-based CDSS still requires access to patient data but relies on AI or statistical algorithms to make determinations instead of following an expert-derived rule. The machine can learn via both supervised and unsupervised learning. Some popularly cited examples of non-knowledge-based CDSS include the detection of hospital-acquired pressure ulcers and the creation of adaptive order menus.[16,17]

[a]A hallucination refers to when an AI model makes up false information or facts that aren't based on real data or events.

Few non-knowledge-based CDSS have been implemented into clinical practice because the decisions made by these models lack human interpretability. One that has been successfully deployed at Duke University was Sepsis Watch®.[18] Sepsis Watch® was developed to improve the detection and management of sepsis, a life-threatening medical emergency caused by the body's extreme response to an infection, in patients admitted to the emergency department (ED). The model is a DL model that combines multitask Gaussian processes and recurrent neural networks. Patient demographics, comorbidities, and laboratory results were used as features for the model. Development and implementation at their single center took over 2 years of time and an estimated 8000 hours of personnel time.

Companies have also developed similar risk prediction tools using AI to provide better risk assessment for disease progression. Renalytix is one company that focuses on improving the prediction of the progression of diabetic kidney disease.[19] The product KidneyIntelX® inputs patient characteristics and laboratory information into a random forest ML model to predict the progression of diabetic kidney disease. The model has superior performance compared to clinical models, AUC of 0.77 for the random forest model compared to 0.661 for the clinical model in the validation cohort. Their model was tested at the Mount Sinai Health System and demonstrated that the return of model results along with clinical guidelines and education support resulted in changes in the clinical management of patients with early diabetic kidney disease.[20]

Note Writing

Healthcare professionals document their findings in progress notes and these notes serve as communication to other healthcare professionals and for billing purposes. One study found that healthcare professionals spend nearly two hours on EHR and other desk work per one hour of patient direct care.[21] Several companies have AI-based speech-to-text software to aid with healthcare professional documentation.[22-24] The use of voice-to-text software will theoretically allow the healthcare professional to spend more time with the patient and reduce time with documentation. The potential of speech recognition software was demonstrated in an observational study of simulated patient-healthcare professional interactions where healthcare professionals were asked to compare note writing by typing vs. speech recognition.[25] The researchers found that despite similar documentation times, dictated notes were longer, had fewer errors, and were of better quality. In an assessment of healthcare professionals' preference for speech recognition compared to typing, half of the healthcare professionals preferred the speech recognition software.[26] However, there was no change in data entry times, quality of care or documentation, or impact on workflows.

While the prior studies evaluated speech recognition in a simulation environment, one study conducted a randomized controlled trial on the effect of a voice-generated electronic note system compared to usual documentation practices on generating inpatient progress notes.[27] They did not find any difference in their outcomes of time between when patients were seen on rounds and when progress notes were viewable by others, healthcare professional satisfaction, or note quality. In their qualitative analysis of healthcare professional satisfaction with the note-writing process, healthcare professionals cited interruptions in workflow and poor performance of the voice recognition software as reasons for overall poor satisfaction. Currently, in a controlled setting speech recognition for healthcare professional documentation demonstrates promise. However, multiple logistical barriers including improved performance of voice recognition models and better accessibility of software must be addressed before more widespread clinical implementation. New to the market are ambient clinical intelligence solutions such as Nuance Dragon Ambient eXperience (DAX)®.[28] DAX® captures dialogues between the patient and healthcare professional during the encounter and then uses AI to convert this to a clinical note. This has resulted in patients finding their healthcare professionals to be more engaged, allowed healthcare professionals to see more patients, and decreased wait times to see healthcare professionals.[29]

Healthcare professionals spend significant amounts of time reviewing the EHR to update themselves on the patient's other healthcare encounters. LLMs can be used to provide a summary of the patient's medical records.[30] LLMs such as ChatGPT® can also be asked specific questions, such as if the patient was admitted to the hospital since the last encounter. This can provide a more comprehensive overview of the patient's health status and save healthcare professionals' time.

Automated Disease Detection From Spoken Language

The breakdown of linguistic skills is characteristic of several neurologic and psychiatric conditions. AI can be used to identify abnormalities in structured or spontaneous speech during the patient-healthcare professional encounter.

One area of focus has been the identification of dementia, particularly dementia of Alzheimer type (DAT). DAT is characterized by breakdowns in semantic processing, shallow vocabularies, and word-finding difficulties. Early in the disease course, deficits may be noticed by family members but not by healthcare professionals. Current methods to identify DAT involve structured interviews; however, they may fail to identify patients with early disease. Therefore, there is growing interest in developing AI algorithms for the automated detection of DAT. Several studies have developed ML algorithms to identify patients with DAT using transcriptions of voice recordings.[31-33] In other studies, researchers used features extracted from audio recordings and features from transcriptions to develop classifiers for identifying various dementia types.[34-36]

Another area of focus has been on psychiatric illnesses. Despite mental health disorders affecting 25% of adults in the United States, diagnosis is challenging as they rely on reports from affected individuals or their caregivers, which is prone to recall bias, cognitive limitations, and social stigma. Many studies have examined acoustic features and speech analysis in psychiatric conditions, with depression, schizophrenia, and bipolar disorder being the most frequently researched.[37] Data generated from international workshops and competitions such as the Audio/Visual Emotion Challenge and Workshop along with open access recordings such as the Distress Analysis Interview Corpus have enabled the training of different AI algorithms for disease mental health illness detection and monitoring.[36,38,39]

Ultimately, the goal is for these algorithms to be deployed in the clinical setting during the healthcare professional-patient encounter for automatic detection of diseases. Unfortunately, in our review of the literature, the algorithms that currently exist are trained on audio recordings from answers to prompted research questions or formal neuropsychological testing.[40] Most are internally validated but lack external validation. Therefore, it is unclear how these models would perform in a patient encounter.

After the Encounter

The healthcare professional receives messages from patients via electronic inbox. Family healthcare professionals spend 1 to 1.5 hours daily on their inboxes and receive an average of 100 messages daily during working hours.[41,42] The COVID-19 pandemic required healthcare professionals and patients to rapidly switch to online care, which has led to a drastically increased number of messages that are routed to healthcare professionals to address.[43] Research suggests that healthcare professionals who spend the most time on EHR work after hours have higher odds of exhaustion and burnout.[44] Novel methods to address this increased workload are needed.

One proposal is to have non-healthcare professional team members manage messages that require low medical decision making. AI can be trained to classify patient messages. Sulieman et al. used multinomial naïve Bayes and random forest to classify 500 surgical patient messages into four groups based on the complexity of decision making.[45] The ML approaches outperformed the models without ML, with precision ranging from 0.5 to 0.67 and recall ranging from 0.5 to 0.88. Another approach developed by Cronin et al. was to develop ML algorithms to automatically classify patient messages by types of consumer health information needs: clinical information, medical, logistical, and social needs.[46] Their models had good performance with the highest AUC of 0.914 achieved using a random forest model for identifying posts for logistical needs. Automatic classification can serve two purposes: (1) workload reduction and (2) faster response times to patients.

In addition to automatic classification, LLMs can be used to respond to patient messages. LLMs such as ChatGPT® are not authorized to provide medical advice. However, with the use of carefully crafted prompts, ChatGPT® can be used to draft messages to patients.[47] Examples of appropriate use may be providing patient education regarding their new diagnoses tailored to the patient's reading level. Additionally, they can be used to generate patient instructions in a reassuring and empathetic tone. In addition to patient-facing tasks, LLMs can be used to handle administrative tasks such as helping draft emails for prior authorizations or suggestions for the use of specific billing codes. However, text produced by LLMs will require the oversight and review of healthcare professionals to ensure results are factual and free of hallucinations.

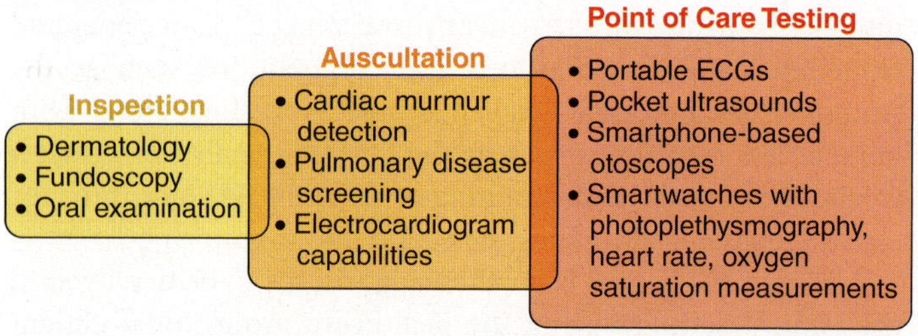

Fig. 31.4 Examples of ML Applications to the Physical Examination.

Physical Examination

The physical exam is a pillar of the diagnostic evaluation. Physical examination maneuvers requiring pattern recognition and abnormality detection can be improved by AI algorithms. Such algorithms can be trained on and applied to enhance select procedures, such as inspection and auscultation. Furthermore, DL can potentially enable these components of the physical exam to take place outside of the healthcare professional's office, especially in settings with limited infrastructure. Fig. 31.4 summarizes the applications of ML to enhancing and extending the physical examination.

Before and After the Encounter

Augmentation of wireless diagnostic tools with AI models to provide rapid point-of-care assessment has become an area of active research, making it possible for data collection for healthcare monitoring to occur during daily life. AI algorithms can analyze and interpret test results obtained from such devices in real time, detecting anomalies or deviations from expected patterns. When predetermined thresholds are exceeded, AI algorithms can provide alerts to healthcare professionals. Further, AI algorithms can optimize the workflow and efficiency of point-of-care testing by analyzing patterns and historical data by predicting the time needed for specific tests or suggesting optimized testing sequences.

In the future, patients may present to their appointments with questions or concerns raised by their wearable device. Moreover, such information could be leveraged to augment the physical exam outside of the scheduled encounter. Therefore, it is critical for healthcare professionals to be able to respond to queries, evaluate the nature of data captured by the wearable, and integrate relevant information into their patient assessment.

Certain technologies have already reached commercial distribution. Wireless diagnostic tools such as the AliveCor® (Mountain View, CA) enabled electrocardiogram (ECG), pocket ultrasounds (Butterfly Network, Guilford, CT), and smartphone-based otoscopes (Cellscope®, San Francisco, CA) increase the opportunity for data interpretation that could impact clinical decision making, with information gathered beyond in-person physical examination.[48] In particular, AI algorithms have now been increasingly applied to wearable technologies.[49]

Smartwatches are a mainstay of research in the wearables space. ECG-enabled devices are becoming more effective in the detection of arrhythmias, ischemia, QT-interval prolongation, electrical abnormalities associated with sudden cardiac death, and LVEF.[50-52] This technology became particularly useful during the COVID-19 pandemic. The FDA issued Emergency Use Authorizations for using mobile devices to monitor QT intervals in patients taking certain medications and for detecting low LVEF as a potential complication of COVID-19.[49,53] International efforts are also underway to utilize ECGs for diagnosing COVID-19 and assessing cardiac involvement.[49]

AI approaches can also analyze signals other than the ECG, such as photoplethysmography (PPG) signals from smartwatches to detect conditions like atrial fibrillation (AF). The 2019 WATCH AF trial aimed to compare the diagnostic accuracy of a smartwatch-based algorithm using photoplethysmographic signals with cardiologists' diagnosis by electrocardiography (ECG) for detecting AF.[54] The study involved 672 hospitalized subjects and utilized a commercially available smartwatch to record PPG pulse waves along with an Internet-enabled mobile ECG. Out of the 650 subjects with cardiologists' diagnoses, 508 subjects were suitable for analysis. The PPG algorithm demonstrated a sensitivity of 93.7%, a specificity of 98.2%, and an accuracy of 96.1% in detecting AF.

Heart rate variability (HRV) is another metric obtained from smartwatches, and its analysis is the centerpiece of studies conducted under the Warrior Watch project at the Icahn School of Medicine at Mount Sinai. One such study aimed to evaluate the use of HRV collected by the Apple Watch to identify and predict COVID-19 and its associated symptoms among healthcare workers.[55] HRV measurements were taken throughout the study, and daily surveys assessing infection and symptom-related questions were obtained. The analysis revealed that the mean amplitude of the circadian pattern of the standard deviation of the interbeat interval of normal sinus beats differed between individuals with and without COVID-19. Furthermore, significant changes in the mean and amplitude of this circadian pattern were observed before and after a COVID-19 diagnosis, as well as on the first day of reporting COVID-19-related symptoms compared to symptom-free days.

Multiple sources of information from the smartwatch can be integrated. For example, one study aimed to evaluate the feasibility of using the Huawei smartwatch for remote monitoring of patients who underwent transcatheter aortic valve replacement (TAVR).[56] A total of 100 patients with severe aortic stenosis who received TAVR were enrolled in the study. Vital signs such as heart rate, rhythm, oxygen saturation, and activity were continuously recorded using the smartwatch. Single-lead ECGs were also recorded multiple times per day in the week following TAVR discharge and at least twice a week for the next month. A designated healthcare team member remotely monitored the data from the smartwatch and provided healthcare when necessary. Out of the 34 patients who experienced cardiac events after discharge, the smartwatch detected and confirmed 76.0% of these events. Six patients were readmitted to the hospital for arrhythmia events detected by the smartwatch, and four of them received pacemaker implantation. The remaining 28 patients received telemedicine monitoring instead of in-person visits. The study also observed new-onset left branch bundle block in 48 patients, which recovered spontaneously in 30 patients and detected new-onset atrial fibrillation in 4 patients.

These developments illustrate the potential of digitally delivered AI technologies for timely deployment and large-scale implementation at the point of care. As these devices become more common, equitable access must be a forefront consideration for all patients, regardless of socioeconomic status. AI algorithms can integrate point-of-care results with other patient data, such as EHR, imaging results, or laboratory data, for comprehensive analysis. By combining multiple sources of information, AI can generate insights, support data-driven decision making, and identify patterns or trends that may not be apparent from individual tests alone.

During the Encounter

Inspection

In the context of inspection, AI algorithms can help to identify lesions, provide quantitative metrics, and aid in accurate diagnosis. While DL has particularly revolutionized areas such as radiology and intravascular imaging, AI algorithms can be trained to classify lesions into different categories for the primary care space. A DL model can be trained on a dataset of labeled images to identify whether an image contains a certain abnormality or condition, learning to recognize patterns and features within the images that are indicative of specific classes.

Dermatologic examinations have benefited from AI in the identification of melanocytic lesions. One study investigated the benefits of dermatologists collaborating with a market-approved convolutional neural network (CNN) in classifying melanocytic lesions.[57] The CNN achieved comparable sensitivity, higher specificity, and higher diagnostic accuracy compared to dermatologists working alone. Moreover, when dermatologists collaborated with the CNN, their diagnostic performance significantly improved, and the higher specificity of the CNN helped guide dermatologists to excise fewer benign nevi. Dermatologists with less experience in dermoscopy showed the most significant improvement when working with the CNN.

AI algorithms are also under active investigation for use in fundoscopic examinations for automated analysis of retinal diseases, such as retinopathies and macular degeneration. For example, one study compared standard widefield fundus imaging with low field-of-view, inexpensive, smartphone-based fundus imaging (SBFI) systems used by an operational technician-led telemedicine program in India in the ability to screen for retinopathy of prematurity (ROP).[58] The results showed that humans paired with autonomous AI-based systems were able to accurately identify cases requiring treatment for ROP using only SBFI photos with a sensitivity of 100% and specificity of 83.5%.

Finally, oral and oropharyngeal squamous cell carcinoma (OPSCC) screening can be facilitated by AI. For example, a multistage, multicenter study investigated the use of an inexpensive smartphone-based oral cancer probe, furnished with a proprietary DL algorithm designed for screening in high-risk populations in areas with limited resources.[59] Probe input combined with information about OPSCC risk factor tabulations are analyzed to provide triage guidance, with PPVs, NPVs, sensitivities, and specificities in the range of 81% to 95%.

Classification algorithms are most encountered in trials for clinical implementation. AI algorithms are also under development to reconstruct or enhance medical images to improve their quality, as well as detect and localize specific objects or regions of interest. These models are under active investigation for real-life deployment, but they serve as examples of types of technology that could be incorporated into physical exam procedures of the future.

Auscultation

Auscultation is one of the key components of the physical exam. However, auscultation is a highly subjective process and can be highly dependent on the healthcare professional's training and experience. AI algorithms can address this gap. They can be trained to analyze recorded body sounds, such as heart or lung sounds, to classify them into different categories or identify specific abnormalities. This can aid in the detection of conditions such as heart murmurs and arrhythmias or abnormal lung sounds associated with respiratory disorders. These models can be integrated into digital stethoscopes that have built-in sensors to capture body sounds and can transmit the recorded sounds to an AI algorithm for real-time feedback and interpretation. AI-enabled auscultation can be particularly valuable in telemedicine settings, where sounds can still be transmitted to healthcare professionals for remote analysis.

In one clinical trial, the performance of a DL algorithm was assessed to detect murmurs and clinically significant valvular heart disease using recordings from a commercial digital stethoscope platform. The algorithm was trained using over 34 hours of previously recorded heart sound data and tested on 962 patients in a clinical study. The algorithm demonstrated a sensitivity of 76.3% and a specificity of 91.4% for detecting murmurs. When excluding softer murmurs, sensitivity increased to 90.0%. The algorithm also showed high sensitivity and specificity for detecting moderate-to-severe aortic stenosis and mitral regurgitation. The study suggests that DL algorithms can serve as valuable clinical support tools for screening cardiac murmurs caused by valvular heart disease.[60]

Digital stethoscopes are not just limited to the analysis of sounds, as they can now be equipped with ECG capability. In another prospective multicenter clinical trial, researchers assessed an algorithm called AI-ECG, which analyzed single-lead ECG recordings, to screen for reduced left ventricular ejection fraction (LVEF) of ≤40% in patients with heart failure using single-lead ECG inputs obtained through an ECG-enabled stethoscope examination.[61] The study included a racially diverse population and found that AI-ECG accurately detected reduced LVEF using single-lead inputs, with the highest accuracy observed at the pulmonary valve position. Combining inputs from multiple positions further improved accuracy. These findings suggest that AI-ECG can be a valuable tool for point-of-care screening of reduced LVEF using single-lead ECGs, potentially enabling earlier detection and treatment in primary care settings.

CHALLENGES

The hope promised by AI in improving healthcare must be separated from the hype. While AI has shown immense potential in revolutionizing the healthcare industry by streamlining history-taking and physical exam procedures, it is essential to approach these advancements with a critical lens. The hype surrounding AI in healthcare often obscures the complexities and challenges of bias, implementation, data privacy concerns, and ***explainability.***[b]

Additionally, AI must be trained and deployed deliberately and thoughtfully, benefiting the outcomes of all patients without bias or discrimination. Starting in 2022, section 1557 of the Affordable Care Act (ACA) has prohibited discrimination in covered health programs and activities based on various factors such as race, sex, color, national origin, age, or disability.[62] This ruling has prompted reevaluating how ML models are developed and implemented in clinical settings.

While it can be difficult to identify sources of bias and discriminatory outputs in AI algorithms, healthcare organizations are required to take responsibility for ensuring that these algorithms are carefully evaluated within the context of their practice. This involves healthcare professionals assessing available algorithms, establishing protocols for detecting and addressing potential bias, and implementing effective oversight mechanisms to ensure fair and meaningful outcomes.

For ML algorithms to perform optimally, they must be developed using large and diverse groups of people. However, sharing data across different institutions can be challenging for several reasons, such as the maintenance of patient privacy. As a result, some healthcare systems have de-identified their data and made them publicly available or created programs that collect data nationally. Federated learning is another approach that enables the creation of prediction models without moving data out of their respective institutions.[63,64]

Despite the existence of many published models, only a few are used in clinical practice. One of the reasons for this may be the lack of understanding of the models and what drives them, or otherwise termed as explainability. Healthcare professionals are unlikely to trust models that do not provide information about which features contribute to their predictions. Lack of explainability by models can lead to ambiguous culpability when incorrect decisions are made.

Finally, it is important to note that while AI algorithms can support medical decision making, they should be seen as tools to assist healthcare professionals rather than supplant them. Disruptions to patient-healthcare professional relationships can occur with increased automation, which can lead to weaker rapport as well as mistrust of the healthcare system depending on the accuracy of the AI. The final interpretation and decision making should involve the patient insight and priorities, clinician considerations of exam findings, and AI-generated insights. Therefore, as its applications to medicine currently stand, AI should be used to make clinical decisions only with the input of healthcare professionals.

ETHICAL CONSIDERATIONS

As the use of ML in medicine increases, concerns about the privacy and confidentiality of patient data have also risen. Patients may not be aware of the secondary use of their EHR data and may be unable to opt out. Moreover, **bias** in ML models occurs when the model produces results that are systematically prejudiced due to flawed assumptions.[65] Models that are trained on one population may perform well in that population but poorly in others. Additionally, during data collection or cleaning, feature selection may introduce unintended bias. This can lead to missing data in EHR that is not missing at random and can introduce bias in the models. To mitigate bias, researchers should develop models in representative populations, carefully select data features, and use tools like the Prediction Model Risk of Bias Assessment Tool (PROBAST) to help identify bias in models.[66]

Moreover, hallucinations can have ethical implications. They can contribute to lead to incorrect decisions as well as potentially reinforce bias and amplify discrimination. These hallucinations occur due to a multitude of reasons, including limitations in data quality, model complexity, generalization capabilities, insufficient testing, and malicious actors launching adversarial attacks. It is especially critical for healthcare professionals to learn about the algorithm that they employ and engage in their clinical training to ward off the occurrence of hallucinations and ensure the responsible and safe use of AI.

CONCLUSIONS

The implementation of AI into the history and physical exam is heralding a new era of personalized medicine. AI is revolutionizing healthcare by offering advanced capabilities in data analysis, pattern recognition, and decision support. This data-driven approach integral to AI models allows for a more comprehensive and nuanced understanding of individual patients, promising workflow improvements and better support for resource-limited settings. Additionally, automation permitted by AI liberates time once devoted to routine or repetitive tasks and offers the opportunity for healthcare professionals to focus on the actual art and science of medicine. Finally, leveraging AI algorithms enables healthcare professionals with powerful tools to provide a better standard of care for our patients, assisting and not overthrowing human oversight.

As healthcare professionals, we must embrace these technological advancements and educate ourselves about the potential of AI in transforming our practice. While AI in the history and physical exam holds tremendous promise, it is essential to approach its implementation with caution and ethical considerations. By staying informed and continuously educating ourselves, we can effectively utilize AI tools and integrate them into our workflow. It is equally important to educate our patients about the role of AI in their care, emphasizing its potential benefits and addressing any concerns they may have.

DISCLAIMER

The authors do not have any financial interests or investments in the aforementioned products and provide them as examples that may be encountered in the clinical space.

[b]Explainability, also known as "interpretability," is the concept that a machine learning model and its output can be explained in a way that "makes sense" to a human being at an acceptable level.

REVIEW QUESTIONS

1. **What does machine learning (ML) refer to in the context of artificial intelligence (AI)?**
   - **A.** The process of teaching machines how to replace human decision making
   - **B.** The development of machines that can independently learn from data and improve their performance
   - **C.** The creation of machines with human-like emotions
   - **D.** The study of how machines can mimic physical movement
   - **E.** The design of computer programs that learn exactly like humans
2. **What is the difference between supervised and unsupervised learning?**
   - **A.** Supervised learning necessitates hands-on manipulation during training, while unsupervised learning does not.
   - **B.** Supervised learning requires labeled data, while unsupervised learning does not.
   - **C.** Supervised learning is used for classification tasks, while unsupervised learning is used for regression tasks.
   - **D.** Supervised learning uses neural networks, while unsupervised learning uses decision trees.
   - **E.** Supervised learning is faster and more accurate than unsupervised learning.
3. **Which of the following is an example of a healthcare application that would benefit from supervised learning?**
   - **A.** Identifying patterns in unstructured medical text data
   - **B.** Discovering clusters of similar patient populations
   - **C.** Reducing high-dimensional images into simpler representations
   - **D.** Segmenting medical images to identify abnormalities
   - **E.** Predicting the risk of readmission for heart failure patients
4. **Which of the following performance metrics is most suitable for evaluating machine learning models when dealing with imbalanced datasets?**
   - **A.** Accuracy
   - **B.** F1 score
   - **C.** AUROC (Area Under the Receiver Operating Characteristic Curve)
   - **D.** AUPRC (Area Under the Precision-Recall Curve)
   - **E.** NPV (Negative Predictive Value)
5. **Clinical Decision Support Systems (CDSS) rely on which type of machine learning?**
   - **A.** Supervised
   - **B.** Unsupervised
   - **C.** Either supervised or unsupervised learning
   - **D.** Reinforcement learning
   - **E.** None of the above
6. **Which of the following is an example of supervised learning applied to auscultation methods?**
   - **A.** Classifying heart sounds as normal or abnormal based on labeled audio recordings
   - **B.** Analyzing lung sound data to identify patterns and clusters of similar sounds
   - **C.** Applying machine learning to optimize the positioning of a stethoscope for sound capture
   - **D.** Predicting the patient's numerical age based on auscultation findings
   - **E.** Clustering sounds extracted from lung auscultation
7. **Outside of a patient encounter, according to the text, which of the following ML methods is most appropriate to manage messages?**
   - **A.** Provide automated answers by feeding the question into ChatGPT and returning that response
   - **B.** Train the algorithm from a corpus of 1000 patient response emails that have been previously written by healthcare professionals
   - **C.** Create an algorithm to stratify severity of response and discard low acuity responses
   - **D.** Implement a model to detect the patients' primary concern and automatically return the top five Google search results
   - **E.** Classify patient messages by types of consumer health information needs: clinical information, medical, logistical, and social needs
8. **Which of the following scenarios could introduce bias into a ML model in a medical context?**
   - **A.** Analyzing model performance by sociodemographic subgroups of patients
   - **B.** Using a dataset with a balanced representation of different medical conditions
   - **C.** Training the model on data from a diverse range of patients
   - **D.** Incorporating input from multiple medical professionals to validate the model's predictions
   - **E.** Collecting data only from a single demographic group, such as young adults
9. **What is explainability in the context of ML?**
   - **A.** The ability of an ML model to predict outcomes accurately
   - **B.** The process of simplifying complex ML algorithms to make them easier to implement
   - **C.** The practice of disclosing proprietary algorithms to the public
   - **D.** The ability to interpret and understand the decisions and reasoning of ML models
   - **E.** The clarity with which an ML algorithm can describe its reason for a prediction
10. **Which of the following is not an ethical consideration in ML?**
    - **A.** Patient data privacy and confidentiality
    - **B.** Bias in machine learning models
    - **C.** Representativeness of data population
    - **D.** Use of secondary data for research without consent
    - **E.** None of the above

REFERENCES

Available online.

32

Telehealth: Adapting Clinical Assessment

Lisa Zickuhr, Jason R. Kolfenbach, and Marcy B. Bolster

Tell me and I forget, teach me and I may remember, involve me and I learn.

Benjamin Franklin (1706–1790)

INTRODUCTION

The development of videoconferencing technology and growing access to broadband (high-speed) Internet service now permit clinical assessment of patients outside the traditional office or hospital-based settings. Telehealth involves using digital technologies and communication to support remote evaluation and management of health-related conditions, as well as foster the patient–healthcare professional relationship. Telehealth services include both synchronous and asynchronous modalities, such as real-time video visits, audio-only encounters, secure messaging platforms, and more. The utilization of telehealth to conduct real-time video visits has the potential to improve access to subspecialty care for patients living in rural and/or underserved areas, as well as those with reduced healthcare access due to mobility or transportation concerns. Additionally, face-to-face encounters in the office (including travel time to and from the clinic, parking, check-in, vital sign measurement, clinical encounter, and check-out) represent a significant time investment that may pose a risk to their employment. In addition, some clinical encounters may focus solely on patient counseling regarding diagnosis, prognosis, or treatment and may be appropriate (and more efficiently conducted) via telehealth.

Telehealth introduces new opportunities for patients and healthcare team members. Still, it also presents differences compared to the office-based environment that requires clinicians to familiarize themselves with the platform and adapt their clinical assessment. Remote clinical assessment may have legal implications in some states for new patient encounters or when the originating site (location of patient) in a telehealth visit is in a different state from the healthcare professional. The telehealth environment also requires adaptation of the history and physical exam, allows for the integration of longitudinal data in the form of remote patient monitoring (RPM), and has implications on post-visit care coordination and vulnerable patient populations. In this chapter, we will discuss the impact of telehealth on each of these domains of clinical assessment and describe how healthcare professionals may integrate this technology to enhance patient care.

GETTING STARTED

The first basic requirement for conducting a virtual visit is the telehealth platform. In many instances, the platform is embedded within the electronic health record (EHR). Alternatively, separate software may be required to provide Health Insurance Portability and Accountability Act (HIPAA)-compliant videoconference capabilities. Patient consent to conduct the visit in the telehealth setting is also required and often obtained by the clinic staff prior to the visit. State and federal laws regulating telehealth delivery impact several important scenarios, such as new patient encounters, mental health visits, and visits conducted when the patient is located in the home, a non-clinic location, and/or in a different state from the healthcare professional. State laws specify that a healthcare professional must have a separate license to practice medicine in the state where the originating telehealth site is located (location of patient), even if the healthcare professional is conducting the visit from their home state. The laws impacting telehealth have evolved since the onset of the COVID-19 pandemic and differ amongst states within the United States as well.[1] Given this changing landscape, it is requisite that healthcare professionals and healthcare systems stay abreast of the laws surrounding telehealth to ensure compliance with federal and state regulations.

Before initiating the telehealth visit, healthcare professionals should organize their workstations to ensure optimal video quality (e.g., lighting, camera positioning), privacy, and reduced opportunities for distraction or interruption. Similarly, it can be helpful for patients to become familiar with the videoconferencing platform and organize their workstations with attention to these aspects as well. The clinic staff may reach out to patients in advance of their appointment to provide information or a checklist to prepare for the telehealth visit. Several nonprofit organizations have developed materials to guide patients through the process of preparation.[2] Similar to in-person visits, patients should be encouraged to bring a list of questions they would like to discuss with their healthcare professionals, medication lists and/or bottles, and any logs of data (such as RPMs, see page 707) to be discussed during the visit. Once the telehealth visit has begun, the healthcare professional should ensure patient comfort with the platform, review expectations for the visit, and outline a backup plan should the video conference call be interrupted.

TAKING THE PATIENT'S HISTORY

The patient's history is an essential part of every patient care visit, whether conducted in person or via telehealth. History-gathering primarily aims to describe the symptoms and concerns prompting the patient to seek medical evaluation. It also includes delineating the distinguishing elements of the patient's presentation. The patient's history may become even more important for medical decision making during telehealth encounters because of the limitations of the virtual physical examination.

Healthcare professionals employ similar techniques when gathering patient histories across clinical settings while applying nuanced skills to optimize history-taking during telehealth. For example, the patient's history will flow most naturally after the healthcare professional ensures the patient's comfort with the telehealth platform and establishes rapport using "webside" rather than bedside manner. The healthcare professional can then most effectively elicit the patient's concerns and symptoms for the telehealth care encounter. Professionals first should identify the patient's primary reason for the visit, recognizing that more than one symptom may have prompted the patient's presentation. Next, patients and professionals engage in dialogue to delineate the patient's symptoms, including distinguishing characteristics such as when the symptoms started and how often they occur, as well as their severity, precipitating and alleviating factors, and any associated symptoms. The mechanics of listing the patient's symptoms and describing them are essentially the same when conducted during in-person and telehealth encounters. However, one of the greater challenges in history-taking during a telehealth encounter is the healthcare professional's ability to convey empathy when not in the same room with the patient. This challenge permeates the entire telehealth visit and emphasizes the importance of adapting interpersonal and communication skills to this setting.

WEBSIDE MANNER

Webside manner is the telehealth equivalent of bedside manner, whereby patients and healthcare professionals establish rapport and therapeutic relationships during telehealth encounters. Telehealth reduces communication through nonverbal methods, especially body language because patients and healthcare professionals are situated in different locations. For example, the key elements of bedside manner and establishing rapport with a patient seem more natural when sitting in an exam room with a patient where a professional can make eye contact, can reach out to touch the hand of a person struggling with personal or family problems, adopt open positioning of the body to provide body language of understanding, willingness to listen, time, and demonstrate empathy. Webside manner, instead, relies more heavily on the nonverbal cues of facial expressions, head positioning within the camera screen, making eye contact via the camera with the patient, and other subtle elements of body language conveyed via telehealth. Healthcare professionals must transform their skills to optimize communication in the telehealth setting, elevate the sense that the patient is being heard, advance a shared approach to decision making, and enhance the rapport established between patient and healthcare professional.

Empathy, the emotional mechanism that bridges the distance between patients and professionals, is a central component of professionalism.[3] The development of empathetic communication skills for healthcare professionals focuses on four main pillars, including (a) being present, (b) taking the patient's perspective, (c) demonstrating empathetic listening, and (d) acknowledging the patient's feelings (Fig. 32.1).[4]

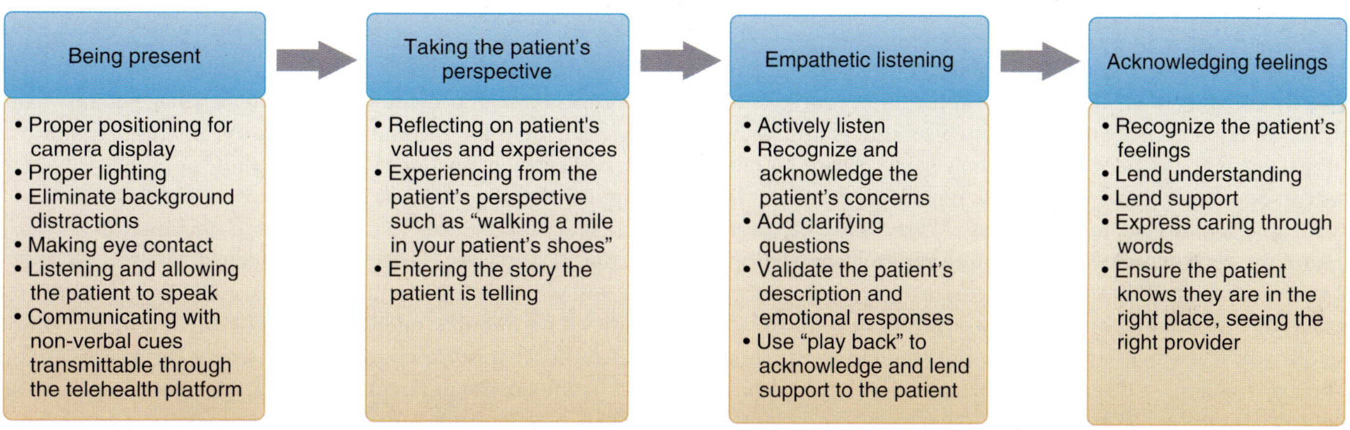

Fig. 32.1 Core pillars for developing and expressing empathy in telehealth encounters. There are four main areas of focus for developing empathy for an in-person or telehealth visit. These include (1) being present; (2) taking the patient's perspective; (3) demonstrating empathetic listening; and (4) acknowledging the patient's feelings. Suggestions for development of each of these pillars are included. (Adapted from Bolster MB, et al. Crossing the virtual chasm: practical considerations for rethinking curriculum, competency, and culture in the virtual care era, *Acad Med* 97(6):839–846, 2022. doi:10.1097/ACM.0000000000004660.)

BEING PRESENT

Many features relate to being present (Fig. 32.1), including listening to the patient and allowing the patient to speak freely. There are unique aspects of being present that are characteristic of the telehealth visit. First, it is essential that the patient feels comfortable conversing with their healthcare professional. During a telehealth visit, proper camera positioning should be ensured on the computer or phone, so the professional can look directly at the camera and make eye contact with the patient. Healthcare professionals also should avoid malpositioning the camera in ways that would produce too much "headspace" with the healthcare professional's face being outside of the center of the patient's screen. Of equal importance is the lighting to optimize the healthcare professional's face; front-lighting, with a lamp located behind the screen, will optimally illuminate the healthcare professional's face. Eliminating background distractions may entail using a virtual background, as warranted, and minimizing ambient noise. Making each of these steps requisite and streamlined for each visit enables the healthcare professional to be present and focus on the patient during the telehealth visit. Furthermore, strong telehealth interpersonal communication skills enable the healthcare professional to demonstrate empathy with body language that is available to the screen interactions, such as an appropriate smile or downward casting of the eyes for a sad moment.

TAKING THE PATIENT'S PERSPECTIVE

This feature of the telehealth visit has similarities to the interactions characteristic of in-person visits, such as reflecting on the patient's values and experiences and acknowledging the patient's unique experience (Fig. 32.1) with the axiom of "walking a mile in your patient's shoes." This element is essential to bring the healthcare professional into the story of the patient and fosters establishing rapport between professional and patient[3,5]; it is imperative that it is included in the telehealth encounter.

EMPATHETIC LISTENING

Empathetic listening (Fig. 32.1) entails the demonstration of active listening and ensuring, with appropriate questioning, that the patient feels not only heard but also understood. When appropriate, as the patient conveys their story, clarifying questions can be posed to query a patient's emotional reaction. This may include something along the lines of "I see how you carried tremendous responsibility as the caregiver to your [parent]; perhaps you can share with me how you felt with their peaceful passing" or "After being separated from your [sister] for so long, how did you feel when you learned that she had a recurrence of breast cancer?" Of great importance is the healthcare professional's ability to summarize, "playback," and demonstrate acknowledgment and support for the patient.

ACKNOWLEDGING FEELINGS

Acknowledgment of the patient's feelings (Fig. 32.1) heightens the patient's sense of connection and rapport with the healthcare professional. With this element, the professional offers not only recognition of feelings but also understanding and support. The professional may label a patient's feelings as "You seem saddened by this event" and can comment further to add support with something like, "And that is very appropriate for what you have been through." Similarly, the healthcare professional can express caring words and ensure that the patient knows they are in the right place to get help. It can be validating and helpful for patients, particularly when there is uncertainty about a diagnosis, prognosis, or management plan, to hear, "You are in the right place. We are on the same team, and together, we will work through this."

While these features of empathy are accomplished as part of competent healthcare professional practice, their essential role within a telehealth visit enriches the encounter. It uses the telehealth visit to enhance the care provided.

PHYSICAL EXAM

Despite potential limitations, the telehealth environment can provide opportunities to derive meaningful insight from the physical exam. Some elements of the exam (inspection, palpation, auscultation, percussion) are more amenable than others to telehealth, but adaptations to each of these techniques can be effective. Visual inspection is perhaps the most translatable exam technique that can be performed via telehealth utilizing video technology. Many dermatologic conditions can be effectively diagnosed via visual inspection alone, and experience in teledermatology with both synchronous video conferencing and asynchronous "store-and-forward" visits dates back prior to the year 2000.[6,7] Studies have shown favorable results, with good agreement between telehealth and in-office diagnoses in most studies.[8] Visual inspection using video-conferencing technology can be effective for evaluation of the head/ears/eyes/nose/throat region as well. However, significant limitations may be encountered in the setting of poor lighting (for example, in the mouth) or inability to focus on very close images. In addition, visual inspection of the blood vessels in the neck (assessing for jugular venous distension and variation in the waveforms of the neck veins), chest/thorax, abdomen (distension, periumbilical varices), and limbs (redness, swelling, and deformity of the joints) can all provide significant data. Image quality can be degraded by poor Internet connectivity; in these scenarios, it can be helpful for patients to upload photos of the involved site, if appropriate, to the EHR portal.

Inspection can also be used to obtain information on muscle strength, joint range of motion, and gait analysis as part of a detailed neurologic and musculoskeletal exam. Numerous studies have demonstrated the utility of the neurologic exam in telehealth settings for cognitive assessment (primarily utilizing data from questionnaires), identification of movement disorders such as Parkinson disease, and evaluation of patients with multiple sclerosis.[8,9] In some situations, a healthcare professional may work with another trained healthcare professional at the originating site with the patient, serving as a *telepresenter* and performing a *facilitated exam*. Telestroke, also called stroke telemedicine, clinics provide access to experts in neurology for patients living in rural and underserved areas, with studies suggesting good agreement with face-to-face encounters in evaluating the National Institutes of Health (NIH) stroke scale. Similarly, good agreement between exam findings elicited in telehealth and office-based encounters has been shown to assess low back pain, knee, ankle, and shoulder pain (weaker agreement for shoulder assessment), and post-knee arthroplasty rehabilitation assessments, among others. Palpation of the joint area to assess for swelling, tenderness, and crepitus is not possible in the telehealth space without the utilization of an on-site examiner. However, self-palpation by the patient can be used to identify focal sites of muscle or joint tenderness. In addition, other members of the healthcare team (registered nurses, for example) at the originating site can function as telepresenters and receive advanced training on ways to elicit data from the musculoskeletal exam and relay that information to specialty healthcare professionals at the distant telehealth site. Self-palpation can also be used to assess for abdominal tenderness or rebound, pitting edema, or unequal arterial pulses; self-percussion can help elicit tympany over the abdomen.

Auscultation is an important component of the cardiopulmonary exam and may be obtained in telehealth through a facilitated exam using advanced technology such as a digital stethoscope. In this scenario, a telepresenter would place the digital stethoscope over the chosen area to auscultate bruits and murmurs or help identify arrhythmias. Studies have demonstrated the high accuracy of the telehealth exam in comparing these findings to the office-based exam.[8,9] Vital signs, including heart rate and blood pressure, can also be obtained by the telepresenter and used to inform subsequent evaluation and management plans. Finally, data from wearable devices or home measurement logs (see next section on Remote Patient Monitoring) can be incorporated by the healthcare professional to aid in the overall assessment of the patient. Table 32.1 outlines an organ-system based physical exam that may be adapted for telehealth.

REMOTE PATIENT MONITORING

RPM, or telemonitoring, involves digital transmission of health-related data from external devices (smartphone applications, wearable biosensors, continuous blood glucose monitoring, pulse oximetry, etc.) to healthcare professionals to aid in the assessment of patients (Table 32.2).[10,11] This area of medicine has grown substantially over the past 15 years, most prominently in the fields of cardiology, endocrinology (diabetes and obesity), and pulmonology. The most common platforms for data transmission include wireless devices and smartphone applications. The information from RPM may improve the quality of assessment data (via collection of a larger amount of longitudinal data across time points) and allow for earlier disease intervention by alerting clinicians to worrisome changes that may occur between clinic appointments. The utilization of RPM has been perhaps most impactful in the management of chronic disease (congestive heart failure, coronary artery disease, diabetes, obesity, COPD), where frequent reassessment and adjustment of management plans are critical.

TABLE 32.1 Physical Exam Elements and Adaptations for Telehealth Visits

Organ System	Adaptation to Telehealth	Potential Limitations
Head, eyes, ears, nose, and throat	Visual inspection Visual acuity at 12 inches Telepresenter otoscope evaluation	Poor lighting intra-oral exam Magnification of image with video may be difficult
Skin	Similar to in-person evaluation	Poor Internet connectivity; consider patient uploading of photos
Cardiovascular	Visual inspection of neck veins Patient self-palpation of pulses, assessment for leg edema Telepresenter with digital stethoscope, vital sign assessment	Neck vein evaluation not optimal in upright position May be no option for telepresenter
Pulmonary	Visual inspection for work of breathing, accessory muscle use Telepresenter with digital stethoscope, vital sign assessment	May be no option for telepresenter
Abdominal	Visual inspection, patient self-palpation	Sensitive elements such as rectal exam not amenable
Genitourinary	———	Sensitive elements not easily amenable
Neurologic	Visual inspection for movement disorders Visual inspection and motor evaluation for stroke evaluation Patient report of changes in sensation on exam	Stroke evaluation typically done in conjunction with telepresenter
Psychiatric	Questionnaires for cognitive status	If baseline cognitive issues may have significant challenges with telehealth platform
Musculoskeletal	Visual inspection of joint Assessment of range of motion Patient self-directed provocative maneuvers (e.g., impingement testing such as Hawkin's maneuver) Self-palpation to identify site of maximal discomfort	Maneuvers that require passive range of motion not possible if no telepresenter or other person to assist Some areas (feet, knees, hips) more challenging to visualize during telehealth, some maneuvers (straight leg raise) challenging to perform
Extremities	Visual inspection for swelling, discoloration Patient self-palpation for pitting edema, assessment of pulses	Lower extremity visualization challenging (remove shoes, socks, clothing, change camera or body position to visualize)

TABLE 32.2 Different Modalities of Remote Patient Monitoring (RPM)

Data Measured	Device Recorder	Example Disease Application
Patient reported outcomes: subjective assessment of patient experience	Smartphone applications, personal digital assistants (PDAs)	Mental health conditions Fatigue, pain, or QOL measurement in RA
Body weight	Smartphone applications	Obesity, CHF
Activity levels	Smartphone applications, wearable biosensors	Obesity, cardiovascular conditions
Heart rate, BP	Wearable biosensors	Cardiovascular conditions, diabetes, CKD
Blood sugar	Continuous blood glucose monitoring	Diabetes
Oximetry, heart rate, BP	Wearable biosensors	COPD
CPAP monitoring	Wearable biosensors	OSA
Cardiac rhythm event recorder	Loop memory recorder, event recorder	Cardiac arrythmias

BP, blood pressure; CHF, congestive heart failure; CKD, chronic kidney disease; COPD, chronic obstructive pulmonary disease; CPAP, continuous positive airway pressure; OSA, obstructive sleep apnea; QOL, quality of life; RA, rheumatoid arthritis.

PRECEPTING THE VISIT

The approach to precepting telehealth visits shares similarities with in-person care. With any patient care visit, it is essential that the precepting faculty member have an opportunity to speak to and ask questions of the patient as well as examine the patient. The format in which learners present patients may vary between in-person and telehealth care encounters, and a well-planned workflow can optimize the experience for the patient, learner, and preceptor.

The precepting experience begins prior to the arrival of the patient. The trainee should "huddle" with the preceptor in advance of the patient care visit to share any background information the faculty preceptor may already have, and this may include information from prior visits, interactions with the faculty member, or outside records. The expected workflow for the telehealth visit can also be described to the learner, identifying the experience as (1) a shadowing opportunity, (2) precepting "outside the room," or (3) webside precepting. Proactively determining this pathway will ensure that all participants, including the learner, the preceptor, and the patient, are well informed.

Within a telehealth encounter, a shadowing experience would involve the student joining the video conference platform once the faculty preceptor has obtained permission from the patient for the student to participate. The student and faculty member could participate on the same screen, side by side, with the student being invited to physically sit in the room or office with the preceptor once the patient's permission has been granted. The student would observe the interactions between the patient and preceptor, and the student should be offered the chance to ask their own questions of the patient and similarly offer any thoughts about the patient's evaluation and management.

The "outside the room" precepting model[12] is comparable to the same format with an in-person encounter. The student independently conducts the history and physical examination within the video conference platform. The student then places the patient in the virtual waiting room, or the student physically leaves the room to meet with the faculty preceptor "outside the room" to review the patient's history and exam findings. Often, with this model, the faculty member asks questions of the student and offers teaching points before "entering the room," at which time the faculty member will elicit their own history and exam findings. The faculty preceptor and student then enter the telehealth encounter together, providing time for the faculty member to elicit history and exam findings, followed by the faculty preceptor and student discussing the patient's evaluation, including testing and disease management with the patient. The assessment of the patient could be provided by the student to the patient, using direct observation by the preceptor, or the preceptor could lead it.

The webside precepting model takes a patient-centered approach and interweaves patient care with precepting. In this model, the student first independently evaluates the patient on the video conference platform and then invites the faculty preceptor to join. The faculty member can join virtually, revealing three windows on the video conference platform, or the preceptor can join the student in the same room, sitting side by side for the telehealth visit. The student then presents the patient's history and exam findings to the preceptor while the patient listens, offering the patient the opportunity to both hear their own story (which patients seem to enjoy) as well as the chance for the patient to provide additional information. The preceptor can then ask clarifying questions; there is no need to repeat the questioning for the entire patient history because, together, the patient and faculty member have witnessed the story as told by the student. With the webside presentation, the preceptor and student may then discuss the patient's assessment, management plans, and next steps in front of (on the screen with) the patient, as with a "thinking out loud" approach. Alternatively, they may place the patient in the virtual waiting room to discuss the patient and then bring the patient back to the video conference space to review the evaluation and management plans. The faculty preceptor or the student may then explain the evaluation and next steps, offering an opportunity for direct observation by the preceptor of the student performing this important communication step.

Webside precepting fosters opportunities for the direct observation[13] of trainees' behaviors, skills, and communication. The telehealth visit offers a unique opportunity for a faculty preceptor to observe a trainee, with video and microphone off, as "a fly on the wall," offering an enriched opportunity for timely and actionable feedback. Due to logistical challenges and time constraints, this form of evaluation and subsequent feedback is often underutilized.

SHARED DECISION MAKING DURING TELEHEALTH

Shared decision making is the process through which patients and healthcare professionals work together to create plans that best align with patients' preferences.[14] Shared decision making benefits patient care in several ways, including upholding patient autonomy and improving medical adherence, patient satisfaction, healthcare utilization, and health equity.[15] Almost all patient encounters incorporate shared decision making, and telehealth skills are required to implement the process in the virtual setting.

The steps patients and professionals follow when sharing decisions are generally the same when conducted in person or virtually.[15] First, patients and healthcare professionals agree that a decision needs to be made. This may be in reference to diagnostic evaluation, treatment strategies, or even whether to conduct the next encounter in person or virtually. Next, professionals list options while patients relay their preferences, an exchange conducted through shared conversation with both parties contributing ideas. Finally, patients and healthcare professionals select a decision and create a plan. Patients and their healthcare professionals may finalize some choices in one visit, while other decisions may extend over multiple encounters. When conducted virtually, these steps draw upon the telehealth skills discussed throughout this chapter, including establishing webside manner and rapport, communicating virtually, accessing and using high-quality telehealth technology, and implementing health systems that support telehealth.

Telehealth is a tool that can optimize shared decision making in certain scenarios but may weaken efficacy in others, as outlined in Table 32.3.[15] Healthcare professionals must

TABLE 32.3 Optimization and Potential Challenges of Shared Decision Making During Telehealth

Factor	Description
Factors Where Telehealth Optimizes Shared Decision Making	
Patient–Professional Relationship	Established patients with whom healthcare professionals are confident in their diagnoses, physical examination findings, and understanding of patients' personal tendencies enrich shared decision making during telehealth.
Communication	Verbal communication is accentuated during telehealth, necessitating strong verbal communication skills on behalf of patients and healthcare professionals.
Patient Education	Telehealth platform tools, such as screen sharing, chat function, virtual decision aids, and after visit summaries, facilitate virtual patient education.
Time	Telehealth workflows minimize registration and rooming procedures, thereby maximizing time patients spend with healthcare professionals sharing decision making. Secure messaging and follow-up telehealth encounters expand the time during which patients can make decisions.
Technology	High quality telehealth devices dependably transmit audio and visual signals through which shared decision making occurs. Familiarity using telehealth technology facilitates shared decision making.
Healthcare System	Patient-specific factors: Telehealth helps patients overcome determinants of health, such as travel limitations, childcare needs, and work requirements, so that they may engage in shared decision making. Clinic workflows: Patient guidance, technology support during telehealth encounters, and contingency planning for technology failures each support access to telehealth care and shared decision making. Insurance policies: Policies that provide coverage for telehealth encounters enable virtual shared decision making.
Factors Where Telehealth Challenges Shared Decision Making	
Patient–Professional Relationship	New or established patients with whom healthcare professionals are uncertain of the diagnosis, baseline physical examination, or personal tendencies will reduce patients' and healthcare professionals' confidence in their shared decision making. Emotionally charged decisions are difficult to make during telehealth.
Communication	Non-verbal communication focuses on facial expressions during videoconference encounters, limiting the use and interpretation of non-verbal cues outside of the camera's window. Barriers to verbal communication, such as patient–healthcare professional language discordance, hinder shared decision making. Patient environmental distractions, such as work or childcare responsibilities, setting, and location, may interfere with shared decision making during telehealth.
Virtual Physical Examination	The virtual physical examination relies upon inspection or another person's (e.g., patient, care partner, telepresenter) interpretation of tactile findings as well as optimal camera angles and lighting during the telehealth encounter. Shared decision making is impaired if the healthcare professional must complete a hands-on examination or cannot inspect the examined area virtually, thereby reducing the exam's contribution to shared decision making.
Technology	Limited access to, familiarity with, and quality of telehealth technology will impair shared decision making.
Healthcare System	Patient-specific factors: Determinants of health, such as poor health literacy, or increased acuity of the patient's condition, may require in-person shared decision making. Medical policies: Licensing laws limit healthcare professionals' practice to specified regions, preventing shared decision making during telehealth when patients are not within those boundaries.

competently identify decisions that can be made successfully during telehealth versus requiring an in-person encounter, weighing the facilitating and prohibiting factors. For example, compare patients A and B. Both patients live 4 hours from the clinic and have poorly controlled diabetes that requires shared decision making to modify treatment plans. Patient A was diagnosed with diabetes 6 months ago, is comfortable uploading continuous glucose monitoring data into the EHR, is in the process of adapting their lifestyle to diabetes (making dietary changes and learning how medications influence their blood sugars), and has never before participated in a videoconference encounter. On the other hand, patient B was diagnosed with diabetes 10 years ago, intermittently records their blood sugars on a written log, successfully completed a videoconference encounter last month, and has been hospitalized four times in the past year, most recently 4 weeks ago, for episodes of hyperglycemia.

Both patient scenarios depict factors facilitating shared decision making during a telehealth encounter, such as patient A's ability to provide glucose readings electronically and their general level of health literacy, and patient B's long-standing diagnosis, as well as previous experience with telehealth. Similarly, both patient scenarios contain factors that may prevent shared decision making during telehealth. Namely, patient A's recent diagnosis of diabetes, ongoing education towards self-management, and unfamiliarity with telehealth, and patient B's heightened acuity of diabetes with recent hospitalization concerning health literacy and reduced engagement in their care. Technology support embedded within telehealth workflows and virtual patient education tools can be used to help overcome patient A's barriers to shared decision making. In contrast, for patient B, the reliance on verbal communication in telehealth (with diminished non-verbal cues) may limit the ability of the healthcare professional to convey the severity of the disease, engage the patient in discussion regarding management options and preferences, verify shared understanding, and successfully finalize decisions. Therefore, at this time, patient A appears to be better suited for shared decision making in the context of a telehealth visit.

VISIT COORDINATION

Telehealth introduces new components throughout the clinical workflow.[16] At the beginning of a telehealth encounter, patients must provide consent prior to receiving telehealth care and, if they are new to telehealth, be oriented to the platform. The patient's location must also be verified as private and safe before proceeding with telehealth care delivery. Telehealth workflows that integrate these tasks during virtual registration streamline the process and increase clinical efficiency. During the visit, healthcare professionals confirm that the patient's symptoms and condition are suitable for telehealth, perhaps redirecting the patient to an in-person clinic appointment or, more acutely, receiving evaluation and treatment in an urgent care or emergency setting. Professionals and patients also create care plans that mitigate potential social and structural barriers to care, ensuring the patient has access to the needed diagnostic and therapeutic measures and planning the next follow-up appointment in person or virtually to meet patient- and disease-specific needs. For example, a patient due for diagnostic testing at the time of their next appointment may be better suited for an in-person encounter, while a patient who plans to provide an update on medication tolerance can be scheduled for telehealth follow-up. After the encounter, healthcare professionals who need to inform other members of the healthcare team may do so differently than they would during in-person visits. Secure messaging among healthcare staff, inviting other members of the team into the telehealth encounter, or handing off the virtual visit to another team member can enhance communication, inclusion, and teamwork among collaborating healthcare professionals.

HEALTH EQUITY AND TELEHEALTH

Telehealth can enhance or hinder health equity depending on patient context and telehealth utilization processes.[17] Significantly, telehealth expands access to care, especially among patients with work responsibilities, childcare needs, or travel barriers. Telehealth transmits care to patients in resource-poor locations where healthcare professionals may be scarce. For some patient populations, telehealth increases privacy around their health concerns, protecting people from having to notify employers, friends, or family that they seek health services.

On the other hand, telehealth may impede health equity, resulting in worse outcomes for some patients. Patients lacking access to high-quality bandwidth and other requisite technology for telehealth may be limited to audio-only encounters, which reduces the utility of virtual physical examination maneuvers and visual aids for patient education. People with disabilities may require adaptive equipment to successfully engage in the telehealth platform, while older adults may need additional support using requisite technology. Those with language barriers may experience a disadvantage because of telehealth's strong reliance on verbal communication. Patients without a private space in which to conduct telehealth encounters may withhold their full participation or be at risk of suffering a breach of confidentiality.

The U.S. Department of Health and Human Services lists several recommendations for augmenting health equity during telehealth care, including training professionals and staff in cultural humility and structural competence, asking patients about their access to technology and safe, private spaces, providing interpreters and other supportive services for people with language barriers, using images and words in virtual communications, and providing technology assistance for those who need it.[17]

CONCLUSION

Telehealth is a useful tool that can enhance access to healthcare and reduce health disparities when utilized correctly. Healthcare professionals must acquire unique abilities specifically tailored for telehealth to communicate effectively with patients, conduct appropriate clinical assessments, and develop care plans that align with patients' preferences and conditions. By doing so, healthcare professionals can provide secure, efficient, and patient-centered telehealth services that optimize outcomes.

REVIEW QUESTIONS

1. **Verification of which of the following factors at the beginning of a patient encounter is unique to telehealth and not required for in-person visits?**
   A. Obtaining consent for treatment
   B. Ensuring the patient is in a safe and private location
   C. Reconciling medications
   D. Reviewing allergies
2. **Which statement best describes the utilization of telehealth for shared decision making?**
   A. The steps of shared decision making are different during telehealth compared to in person.
   B. Telehealth enhances shared decision making for all patients.
   C. Patient context must be considered to optimize the utilization of telehealth when making decisions regarding patients' care.
   D. Telehealth streamlines decision making into a single encounter.
3. **You are evaluating a patient with hypertension and congenital deafness who communicates through American Sign Language and lip reading in clinic. The blood pressure is 156/73 mm Hg, and you decide to increase the patient's amlodipine from 5 mg daily to 10 mg daily. The patient has a blood pressure cuff at home. Which plan would be best for the patient's next follow-up encounter?**
   A. A videoconference telehealth encounter with a family member interpreting American Sign Language
   B. An audio-only telehealth encounter using a teletypewriter
   C. An in-person encounter with an American Sign Language interpreter present during the encounter
   D. An in-person encounter with an American Sign Language interpreter present remotely through tablet videoconferencing
4. **Which of the following determinants of health has research shown to reduce patients' access to telehealth care?**
   A. Access to broadband Internet
   B. Childcare responsibilities
   C. Lack of transportation
   D. Food insecurity
5. **Which of the following factors is *not* a potential limitation to participation in telehealth care?**
   A. Patient location is in a different state from healthcare professional conducting visit
   B. Patient is scheduled for a new patient visit with a specialist
   C. Patient location poses challenging transportation obstacles to office location
   D. Patient has new onset lightheadedness in setting of known cardiac arrythmia
6. **Which of the following options best describes the function of a *telepresenter?***
   A. An on-site healthcare professional present with a patient during a telehealth visit who can obtain vital signs, perform a facilitated exam, and help coordinate visit activities
   B. A healthcare professional who summarizes a patient case and poses a clinical question to a specialty provider in hopes of obtaining recommendations for patient care
   C. A healthcare professional who sets up the video telecommunications platform for a patient to conduct the telehealth visit
   D. A patient who relays their medical history and history of present illness within the telehealth environment
7. **Which of the following terms best describes the form of patient assessment involving digital transmission of health-related data from external devices to healthcare professionals?**
   A. Telepresenter
   B. Facilitated physical exam
   C. Shared decision making
   D. Remote patient monitoring
8. **Which of the following represents a difference between reliably obtaining a detailed patient history during an in-person visit compared to during a telehealth visit?**
   A. Patient's presenting symptom(s)
   B. Duration of current symptom(s)
   C. Severity
   D. No difference
9. **Which of the following enhances the healthcare professional's ability to express empathy within a telehealth videoconference visit?**
   A. Using a virtual background with a setting of a hospital clinic room scene
   B. Using dim lighting instead of a well-lit videoconference setting
   C. Ensuring proper positioning of the camera to permit ease for eye contact
   D. Allowing the patient to speak for 12 seconds, before asking the first question, as they report their current symptoms
10. **An in-person bedside presentation is most similar to a telehealth videoconference visit that is characterized by which one of the following?**
   A. Inviting the preceptor into the videoconference platform to present the patient's history and physical examination findings with the patient having video and microphone on
   B. Shadowing a faculty preceptor
   C. Presenting the patient's history and physical examination using the videoconference platform with the patient waiting in the waiting room
   D. A "huddle" that occurs prior to the patient's scheduled visit

REFERENCES

Available online.

SECTION 6

Analyzing Ethical Issues in Clinical Medicine

33

Clinical Ethics and Professionalism

Patrick D. Herron

I will use treatment to help the sick according to my ability and judgment, but never with a view to injury and wrongdoing. And whatsoever I shall see or hear in the course of my profession in my discourse with others ... I will never divulge, holding such things to be holy secrets.

From The Physician's Oath, Hippocrates (460–377 BCE)

INTRODUCTION

Bioethics is the study of ethical issues emerging from advances in science and medicine. This includes moral deliberation on the intersection of societal views of healthcare, law, and moral philosophy. The field of bioethics is quite expansive as it applies to all aspects of human development, our interaction with our environment, and the use of technology. The term "medical ethics" or "clinical ethics" more specifically examines issues related to patient–healthcare professional encounters. All health professions cite the importance of ethical behavior as an attribute of professionalism, but how such behavior ought to be demonstrated is often not included in guidelines for its professionals. Legislative regulations and court rulings also provide guidance to healthcare professionals, but laws vary in regard to jurisdiction from state to state and may change over time to reflect shifting societal perspectives. Sometimes these legal differences result in healthcare professionals and trainees experiencing moral distress if they believe their ethical duty conflicts with legal obligations.

Medical professionalism and ethics are often conflated as they are each used as defining attributes of one another. Professionalism encapsulates those virtues that foster a healthcare professional's ability to recognize, understand, and apply the skills necessary to honor their ethical obligations. Patients and society hold healthcare professionals to a high standard of ethical behavior, an attribute that is expected of their chosen profession. Healthcare professionals face challenging issues every day in the scope of their work with patients. The concerns of patients frequently extend beyond their physical symptoms to include psychosocial needs, socioeconomic challenges, and social justice concerns to name only a few of the compounding issues that are commonly seen as ethical issues requiring attention. Some of these issues appear to have easy answers as to what should be done, but the lack of easily or equitably accessible solutions can be difficult to overcome. There are other issues that remain controversial because there is no clear discernment as to what is the ethically appropriate course of action. When faced with a moral dilemma regarding the care of a patient, the study of bioethics, and more specifically the use of ethics analysis, can help healthcare professionals determine if a proposed course of action is ethically obligatory, ethically permissible, or ethically impermissible. Clinical ethics training offers healthcare professionals the skills to recognize, understand, and consider appropriate solutions to address and resolve ethical dilemmas when they arise in patient care or amongst professionals when in conflict with one another.

This chapter will highlight some moral frameworks and bioethics concepts that may be used when faced with professional and ethical conflicts related to patient care. An advanced study of bioethics is recommended for all healthcare professionals in training and as part of their continuing professional development requirements.

PRINCIPLISM

Principlism is a decision-making approach based on the four principles of **autonomy**, **beneficence**, **non-maleficence**, and **justice**. It offers a method of analysis by utilizing widely accepted norms of moral agency (the ability of an individual to make judgments of right and wrong) to identify ethical concerns and determine acceptable resolutions for clinical dilemmas.

Autonomy refers to respecting the decisional capacity of an adult person's ability to make reasoned informed choices and to take actions based on their personal values and beliefs. This principle is the basis for the doctrine of informed consent in medical care and human subjects research. In westernized cultures, autonomy is often focused on a person's individualism. In other cultures, autonomy can be inclusive of a person's family, shared group identity, and/or community. The principle recognizes that all adult persons have autonomy, and it is our ethical duty as healthcare professionals to honor and promote it. As a principle, autonomy does not apply to infants and children as they have not reached the age of majority, or age of legal adulthood (often 18 years) as it is recognized or declared in law.

While laws may arbitrarily determine the age of adulthood to be equivalent to a specific biological age, it is ethically permissible to consider an adolescent's intellectual ability and maturity to participate in their health decisions on the basis of the adolescent's emerging or developing autonomy. Some states legally permit adolescents to make some of their own healthcare decisions independently of their parents or guardians. A more detailed discussion on pediatric ethics is included later in this chapter.

Beneficence refers to the balancing of the potential benefits of treatment against the potential risks and burdens experienced by the patient. Healthcare professionals should act in a way that benefits the patient as well as take the necessary steps to prevent or mitigate harm. This principle applies not only to the healthcare needs of individuals but is applicable to communities and society at large.

Non-maleficence means preventing or mitigating the causation of harm or injury either through action or inaction. It is presented sometimes in contrast to the principle of Beneficence, but they are intended to be complementary to one another. Many medically indicated and beneficial treatments may result in some harm, even if minimal, but the harm should not be disproportionate to the benefits of treatment. This principle is frequently invoked as "*Do No Harm*" in regard to medical errors committed by healthcare professionals.

Justice honors the position that patients in similar circumstances should be treated in a similar manner. It requires that we advocate for a fair or equitable distribution of benefits, risks, healthcare costs, and resources. Justice applies not only to medical care provided at the bedside but more broadly across our healthcare system, laws, and policies that govern access to healthcare.

Principlism Case Example

Mei is a 39-year-old female with a mild intellectual disability. She is admitted to the hospital with an ovarian cyst. The cyst is blocking Mei's ureter and if left untreated will result in renal failure. Mei will need an operation to remove the cyst. She is very uncomfortable in a hospital setting and has always had a heightened fear of needles. Mei indicated clearly that she does not want a needle inserted for the anesthetic required before attempting to surgically remove the cyst. The attending physician is concerned that if the cyst is not removed soon, Mei will develop renal failure and require dialysis, which would involve the regular use of needles and be very difficult to carry out given her known fear of needles and overall discomfort with hospitals. The anesthesiologist is concerned that if Mei does not cooperate with the procedure, she will need to be physically restrained to prevent injury. Mei has lived independently her entire adult life but has an adult sister who visits once a week to help with managing Mei's finances. The sister is adamant that Mei should receive treatment. Should the surgeon perform the operation despite Mei's objections?

Respect for **Autonomy** entails taking into account and giving consideration to the patient's views on their treatment. Autonomy is not an all-or-nothing concept. Mei may not be fully capacitated (capable of a particular action or legally competent to act in a particular way) in regard to this specific decision, but this does not mean that her views should not be respected. Mei has expressed her wishes clearly; she does not want a needle inserted for the anesthetic. An autonomous decision does not have to be the "correct" decision from an objective viewpoint, otherwise individual needs and values would not be respected. However, an autonomous decision is an *informed* decision. Has Mei been given enough information in a manner that she comprehends the situation and consequences of her decisions?

Healthcare professionals should act in a manner that benefits the patient. This principle of **Beneficence** may clash with the principle of Autonomy if the patient makes a decision that a healthcare professional does not think is in the best interests of the patient. Here, we should consider both the long-term and short-term effects of overriding Mei's views. In the short term, Mei will be frightened to have a needle inserted in her arm and to be in the hospital. This may lead Mei to distrust healthcare professionals and be reluctant to seek medical help or cooperate in the future. In the long term, there will be a benefit to Mei having her autonomy overridden. Without treatment, Mei will suffer serious and long-term health problems that will likely require greater medical intervention (ongoing dialysis) than the treatment required now (operation). The benefits of acting would need to be weighed against the consequences of failing to respect Mei's autonomy. The question of Mei's capacity to make her own decisions is central to the ethical dilemma as the law protects the rights of capacitated patients from being overridden even if it is seen by healthcare professionals as being in the patient's best interests.

The ethical principle of **Non-Maleficence** focuses on possible harm to the patient. We can foresee that Mei would be harmed by forcibly restraining her to insert the needle for anesthesia. On the other hand, if she is not treated now, Mei's condition will worsen, and she would require ongoing dialysis a number of times per week. If Mei does not cooperate with dialysis treatment, it would be difficult to administer treatment safely, and she may need to be restrained. Ethics analysis requires us to reflect on which course of action would result in the *greatest* harm. That process relies on assumptions such as how successful is the operation likely to be and how likely is it that Mei will comply with dialysis?

We know very little about the extent of Mei's intellectual disability in regard to her decision-making capacity. The principle of **Justice** requires us to be mindful that patients with disabilities are among those viewed as being from vulnerable populations. Such individuals often have health conditions that are exacerbated by unnecessarily inadequate healthcare or whom are not treated equitably due to their underlying medical conditions. This principle is also drawn upon when questions of cost effectiveness of the treatment options are raised by healthcare professionals and/or the impact of the decision about their treatment has on the availability of treatment for others (e.g., awaiting dialysis). While associated healthcare costs are sometimes relevant, consideration of this specific issue may not have as significant a role in the deliberation of what ought to be done in regard to Mei's situation. It is also important to reflect on whether the same consideration would be raised if Mei was not a person with a disability.

Ethics Analysis

Principlism can provide a sound and useful way of analyzing ethical dilemmas, but it does not provide a unique answer to an ethical dilemma. The four principles are sometimes referred to as the *prima facie* principles, meaning that a principle is binding unless it conflicts with another moral principle, as depicted in the ethics analysis regarding Mei. In such situations, healthcare professionals deliberate on possible interventions using ethics analysis as a guide toward treatment approaches. It is a common misconception that the principle of Autonomy should take priority over the others. This is a westernized perspective to be mindful of when working with patients and colleagues with non-westernized views of healthcare. The four principles are not intended to be hierarchical but should be given equal consideration when faced with ethical uncertainty. Ethics analysis can help healthcare professionals formulate questions that will aid them in determining if an action is *ethically obligatory*, *ethically permissible*, or *impermissible*. It is possible to have more than one ethically permissible decision or course of action among all available options.

- **Ethically Obligatory:** means that a healthcare professional has an ethical obligation to perform an action. It is not only right to do it, but it would be wrong not to do it. For example, we might say it is ethically obligatory for parents to care for their children, not only because it is right for them to do it but also because it is wrong for them not to do it. The children would suffer and die if their parents did not care for them. We, as a society, hold the consensus view that parents are ethically obligated to care for their children.
- **Ethically Permissible:** actions are neither right nor wrong to do them or to not do them. Sometimes described as ethically "neutral," because it is. We might say that having plastic surgery is ethically permissible because it is not wrong to have the surgery (it is not impermissible) but neither is it ethically necessary (obligatory) to have the surgery.
- **Ethically Impermissible:** refers to those actions that are wrong to do and situations in which it would be right not to perform an action. For example, we would say that murder is ethically impermissible.

Principlism is only one of several ethics analysis frameworks used in the study and practice of clinical ethics. Many bioethicists incorporate multiple concepts and approaches of ethical inquiry when considering ethical and moral conflicts. The following sections are summarizations of various ethical theories, frameworks, and analytic tools available for exploration and addressing ethical dilemmas in medicine.

MORAL PHILOSOPHY: DEONTOLOGY VS. UTILITARIANISM

Moral philosophy is a discipline that examines the nature of morality and the theories that are used to arrive at decisions about what a person ought to do and why. Clinical ethics incorporates frameworks from these philosophical theories, including deontology and utilitarianism. Developed by the moral philosopher Immanuel Kant, ***deontology*** is sometimes referred to as Kantian or duty-based ethics. He defined that the morality of an act is based solely on the nature of the action regardless of the consequences or any other factors. As it applies to healthcare, decisions ought to be made on what is in the best interest of the patient. Deontology views actions as either right or wrong without any regard to contextual features. An example sometimes used is that of the Ten Commandments (e.g., "Honor your father and mother"; "Do not kill"; "Do not steal"). We can easily point to deontology's influence in healthcare in regard to promoting "truth telling" with patients. What should a healthcare professional do though if the truth might cause harm to the patient or others? A commonly cited criticism in relation to the moral imperative of truth telling (i.e., do not lie) is the hypothetical scenario in which you are hiding someone from a murderer. The murderer comes to your home and asks if a person, their intended victim, is there. Kantian ethics would consider the moral thing to do would be telling the truth, regardless of the consequences.

Utilitarianism is a consequentialist moral theory that emphasizes efforts to maximize the overall good. Consequentialism, as an ethical theory, is concerned only with the consequences of an action. Applying a utilitarian framework for decision making entails an analysis with the goal of achieving the greatest benefit for the greatest number of persons. It is the consequence, or outcome of the decision, that determines the morality of the action. Examples of utilitarian approaches include institutional requirements for vaccinations and reporting communicable disease infections to public health authorities. While some believe such mandates limit expression of personal choice and may pose harm, the benefits resulting from those requirements are seen as promoting the greater good and thus morally (ethically) permissible. A counterpoint critique of a utilitarian approach that has been depicted in popular culture is how healthcare professionals may act in the aftermath of public health disasters by triaging patients based on the amount of limited resources required to ensure likelihood of survival. Such practices may violate one or more of the four principles that guide our conception of a medical standard of care while creating significant moral distress for the healthcare professionals involved.

CASUISTRY

A case-based approach to addressing ethical conflicts, *casuistry* utilizes an inductive method of reasoning and decision making. It offers an alternative to principlism, deontological ethics, and utilitarianism. This method shares many contextual features with medical and legal decision making. Appropriate actions depend on the specific features of a case. Popularized as a tool specifically for clinical ethics by Jonsen, Siegler, and Winslade, it asks healthcare professionals to examine ethical dilemmas within the framework of four categories intrinsic to every clinical encounter (see Table 33.1).

Utilizing a casuist approach to ethics analysis:

1. Evaluate the facts under each topic and identify the salient features of the case.
2. Identify relevant paradigm cases; cases with similar features that have been debated and decided by the general public and medical and legal communities at a national level.

TABLE 33.1 **Casuistry's Four-Box Approach**

Medical Considerations	**Patient Preferences**
1. What is the medical problem? Is the problem Acute? Chronic? Critical? Reversible? Urgent? Terminal? 2. What are the goals of treatment? Goals of care? 3. In what circumstances are further medical treatments not indicated? 4. What are the probabilities of success for various treatment options? 5. How can this patient benefit from medical and nursing care? How can harm be avoided?	1. Has patient been informed of risks and benefits of treatment? Does patient understand the information and give consent? 2. Does patient have decisional capacity? Is the patient legally competent? ***(FYI: there is a difference between these two terms)*** 3. What treatment preferences has the patient stated? 4. If incapacitated, has the patient expressed prior preferences? 5. Who is the appropriate surrogate decision maker if the patient lacks capacity? What standards should govern their decisions? 6. Is the patient unwilling or unable to comply with standard medical treatment? If so, why?
Quality of Life	**Contextual Features**
1. What are prospects, with or without treatment, for a return to normal life? What physical, cognitive, and socioeconomic effects might the patient experience even if treatment succeeds? 2. Could anticipated quality of life be undesirable for a patient who cannot make or express their own judgement? 3. What biases might prejudice the medical team's judgement of a patient's future quality of life? 4. What ethical issues arise concerning improving or enhancing a patient's quality of life? 5. Do quality-of-life assessments raise any questions that might contribute to a change of treatment plan, such as forgoing life-sustaining treatment? 6. Are there plans to provide pain relief and provide comfort if a decision is made to forgo life-sustaining interventions? 7. Is medically assisted death ethically or legally permissible? 8. What is the legal and ethical status of suicide?	1. Are there professional, interprofessional, or business interests that might create conflicts of interest in the clinical treatment of patients? 2. Are there stakeholders other than the healthcare professional and patient, such as family members, who have a legitimate interest in the clinical decision? 3. What are the limits imposed on patient confidentiality by the legitimate interests of third parties? 4. Are there financial factors that create conflicts of interest in clinical decisions? 5. Are there problems of allocation of resources that affect clinical decisions? 6. Are there cultural or spiritual factors that might influence clinical decisions? 7. What are the legal issues that might affect clinical decisions? 8. Are there considerations of clinical research and medical education that affect clinical decisions? 9. Are there considerations of public health and safety that influence clinical decisions? 10. Does institutional affiliation create conflicts of interest that might influence clinical decisions?

3. Develop a justified plan of action, drawing on the expert opinion from paradigm cases adapted for the specific features (the context) of that particular case.

One of the limitations of casuistry is that it may yield different conclusions depending on which paradigms or features individuals prioritize in their analysis. This makes it difficult to achieve consensus on complex or controversial issues.

PRIVACY AND CONFIDENTIALITY

One of our most valued human rights is the right to privacy. Whatever information about ourselves that we willingly choose to share with others is a selective process integral to our personal integrity. Violations of a person's privacy deprive them of one of our most fundamental freedoms. Privacy rights can be either positive or negative. Positive rights of privacy concern an individual's choice to determine who has access to and may share information about themselves with others. Negative rights of privacy encapsulate the right to be left alone or our right to noninterference from others. Privacy applies not only to knowledge of information, but visual images, auditory recordings, written documentation, and access to one's person (e.g., blood, DNA swabs, urine sample).

An individual's right to privacy is recognized and protected by confidentiality. Respecting one's privacy through confidentiality is based on the fiduciary relationship (in which one person places special trust, confidence, and reliance in and is influenced by the other who has a duty to act for their benefit) between healthcare professionals and patients. This applies to many different types of relationships beyond the scope of healthcare, including the law, pastoral care, and financial relationships with whom individuals establish bonds of trust. The duty to respect the privacy of patients is among the earliest professional obligations of physicians as reflected in the Hippocratic Oath. In modern times, expectations for privacy and confidentiality are set forth through laws and codes of professional ethics. This applies to not only physicians but also any individual with access to patient health information. Confidentiality is not limited to the provision of healthcare services. Human subjects research also requires adherence to privacy laws and regulatory oversight of how information about persons must be protected. Given the complexity of our healthcare system and the number of individuals interacting with patients and their information, the concept of privacy and confidentiality has dramatically changed in the era of electronic medical records. Rather than contribute to a false sense of secrecy, healthcare professionals should be transparent with patients regarding privacy policies. Patients should be informed that the provision of their care requires numerous individuals to have access to their health information. Regardless of the number of persons having access to medical information, healthcare professionals and trainees have a shared ethical obligation to maintain confidentiality by adherence to institutional safeguards and standards of professionalism.

Disclosure and Duty to Warn

Patients need to be able to trust that healthcare professionals will not reveal health information, especially sensitive and personal information, that has been shared in confidence. Healthcare professionals have a duty to protect the privacy and confidentiality of patient disclosures. Patients retain the right to decide whether and how that information may be shared. In the United States, such actions are regulated through the Health Insurance Portability and Accountability Act of 1996 (HIPAA). This federal law applies to all forms of communication, including data privacy and security provisions for safeguarding medical information that is stored online or in printed form.

There are circumstances in which a healthcare professional is permitted to share relevant or pertinent health information without the specific consent of the patient. The most common reason being consultation with other healthcare professionals for the purpose of providing care or for healthcare operations regarding the patient. Other examples include requests from appropriate authorities (e.g., law enforcement agencies) when disclosure may be required to mitigate or prevent a potential threat when in the healthcare professional's judgment there is a reasonable probability that:

- The patient may seriously harm themselves.
- The patient may inflict serious physical harm on an identifiable individual or individuals.

INFORMED CONSENT

The *doctrine of informed consent* is based upon the right of every individual to determine what shall be done to their body in connection with medical treatment and/or medical research. Informed consent is not a document but a *process* of informing, verifying understanding, and obtaining permission from an individual. In the clinical setting, this involves healthcare professionals seeking permission to treat patients who, by consenting, agree to accept known risks in anticipation of potential benefit to themselves through treatment. It is rooted in both a legal and ethical right the patient has to direct what happens to their body and from the ethical duty of the physician to honor and promote the autonomy of a patient by involving them in their healthcare.

> *Every human being of adult years and sound mind has a right to determine what shall be done with his own body; and a surgeon who performs an operation without his patient's consent commits an assault, for which he is liable in damages.*
>
> ***Justice Benjamin Cardozo, 1914***

The process and elements for informed consent to participate in human subjects research are defined and guided by governmental regulation and institutional policies, which include collaboration with Institutional Review Boards (IRBs) who must review and approve research protocols. The specifics of legal requirements and the IRB process will not be discussed in this chapter. Instead, we will examine informed consent as it relates to patient care. The doctrine of informed consent has evolved over the past century to incorporate legal requirements established by courts. In addition to several prominent court rulings that established precedent, there were other influential societal changes, including the civil rights and civil liberties movements, increased interest in advocating for patient rights, and greater access to medical information by patients.

Elements of Informed Consent

The goal of the consent process is for the patient to have an opportunity to be a well-informed participant in their healthcare. A valid informed consent process must include several elements (see Box 33.1), and the patient must be able to demonstrate that they have the requisite **decisional capacity** (see Table 33.2) to actively participate in an informed consent process.

Types of Consent

Healthcare professionals and patients use the term "consent" so frequently that there is sometimes confusion as to its usage in regard to clinical care. Many of the routine tasks performed in the course of medical care do not require the same level of attention as the informed consent process described earlier. We sometimes refer to this as **implied consent** or the granting of permission for medical care without a formal process (i.e., you make a primary care appointment to get a checkup during which the physician performs a physical examination and draws blood for lab tests, but the healthcare professional doesn't ask you for consent for each component of the office visit). The patient permits or **assents** to these tasks to be done without having participated in a formal informed consent process. One way to think about the distinction is that these are tasks with a very low level of risk and generally considered to be the only or best approach available. In an emergency situation, when a patient is unconscious or conscious but incapacitated, and there is no family member (surrogate decision maker) present or available for permission, the patient's consent for treatment is **presumed** rather than obtained if the available emergency treatment will prevent death, disability, or severe harm. How

BOX 33.1 Elements of Informed Consent Process

- Disclosure of relevant information including:
  - Nature of the treatment (therapy) or test being considered
  - Benefits, risks, and consequences of the intervention being considered
  - The alternatives and their benefits, risks, and consequences
- An assessment of the patient's understanding of relevant information
- The patient is able to make a decision that is voluntary and without coercion

TABLE 33.2 Criteria for Decisional Capacity Assessment

Clinical Standards for Decisional Capacity	How To Facilitate Assessment of Decisional Capacity
The patient makes and communicates a choice • Factors that can affect ability to choose: neurological impairment, denial, anxiety • Factors that affect communication: sedation, need for ventilator support	• Utilize various forms of communication that will maximize patient's ability to express choice (verbal, written, use of interpreter) • Enlist family with patient's permission • Healthcare professionals can present choice and ask patient if they agree or disagree • Patients may reconsider choice as new information is learned; this is not the same as being indecisive
The patient understands the following information • The medical situation and prognosis • Recommended course of treatment • Alternatives to treatment • Risks, benefits, and consequences of each alternative	• Healthcare professionals should provide clear explanations in appropriate language (non-technical terms, "bleeding" vs. "hemorrhage") • Asking the patient to share their understanding of their current health with you
The patient is able to appreciate consequences • The patient can describe how the outcomes of a decision would affect their life: "If I have the amputation, I may not be able to walk, but I won't be in pain anymore" • Also known as "insight" • Examples of patients without this: paranoid patient, 'you are plotting against me!', patient who denies illness	Ask questions that assist patients in clarifying their appreciation: • What do you believe will happen if you are not treated? • How do you think surgery will help (or harm) you? • Why do you think your doctor has recommended this treatment?
The patient's reasoning to make a choice • Focus is not on the outcome but on the process by which patient reached it • Should reflect patient's values/goals • It is consistent with patient's values/goals • May be difficult to articulate, often based on intuition or emotional response • Decision is not the result of a delusion • spiritual faith/belief vs. delusion	Utilize attentive empathy and nonjudgmental inquiry with patients • Tell me how you reached your decision? • What is it that makes this option a better choice than the other option? • Enlist support and input from those who know the patient well

does a healthcare professional know when they have provided sufficient information about a proposed clinical treatment or intervention? While there are variations in definition, the law in most states and medical literature agree on the following approaches:

- ***Professional Standard:*** Also referred to as the "*reasonable physician standard*." Healthcare professionals must disclose all information that similarly situated professional colleagues would disclose about a proposed procedure. This standard is often viewed as inadequate since research has shown that many healthcare professionals tell the patient minimal information. This standard may be insufficient for informed consent if the focus is on the healthcare professional's perspective rather than on what the patient needs to know.
- ***Reasonable Person Standard:*** Healthcare professionals must disclose all information that a reasonable person would find meaningful in making a decision whether to consent to a proposed procedure. In other words, what would the average patient need to know to be an informed participant in the decision? This is the most often relied-upon approach.
- ***Subjective Standard:*** Healthcare professionals must disclose information that an individual patient would desire to know whether to consent to a proposed procedure. This standard is the most challenging to incorporate into practice since it requires tailoring information to each individual patient's preferences or needs.

Power Dynamic Between Healthcare Professionals and Patients

While engaging in an informed consent process, healthcare professionals have the ability to exert undue influence while providing information to patients. Healthcare professionals should be mindful of this inequality that exists and be cautious not to permit any of the following from impeding a patient's autonomy. Healthcare professionals should never use **coercion,** or the use of a credible and severe threat of harm or force, to control a patient. Any use of **manipulation,** in which a healthcare professional gives information to the patient either selectively or through emphasizing or deemphasizing some information, violates the patient–healthcare professional relationship. Examples of such tactics may include lying, omitting vital information, or deliberately deceiving. This is always ethically suspect, even if the healthcare professional believes such behavior will benefit the patient by misleading them into accepting their medical recommendation.

Healthcare professionals may utilize **persuasion** (i.e., attempt to encourage a person to accept or reconsider a decision to decline) if they believe a specific recommendation is in the patient's best interest. Patients recognize that healthcare professionals have relevant expertise and advice about their care, and expect their healthcare professionals to be forthright with recommendations. While very rare, healthcare professionals may withhold information if they believe disclosure of specific information would severely harm the patient or undermine an informed decision-making process. This is referred to as **therapeutic privilege,** and while under rare circumstances it might be considered permissible, it is not typically endorsed given the concerns for possible misuse by healthcare professionals as a form of medical paternalism (i.e., attitude in which healthcare professionals disregard preferences of patients and instead substitute their own judgment in lieu of the patient).

How Does Informed Consent Apply to Children?

Previously, we discussed the principle of Autonomy and its limitation with infants, children, and adolescents. In most states, 18 years is the age of majority, and thus, consent must be obtained from the patient's parent or legal guardian prior to that age. Either parent or legal guardian (if more than one) may provide consent for treatment. The exception to this practice is if the parents are not married. There may be circumstances in which one parent of a minor patient has temporary or permanent limited parental authority due to custodial decrees. Healthcare professionals may request documentation of custodial agreements to ensure treatment decisions are made appropriately. This helps to facilitate the patient–healthcare professional–parental relationship and ensure the bests interests of the child (patient) are being promoted.

Many children, due to their lack of maturity, do not have the required decisional capacity to provide informed consent. Since consent, by definition, is given for an intervention for oneself, parents are not providing informed consent but informed permission for treatment. For some older children and adolescents, participation in their healthcare decisions can be highly beneficial for their maturation and development. While this is not the same as legally providing consent, obtaining assent from a minor patient should always be sought in addition to the authorization of legal surrogates. While a specific age provides clear guidance as to when a patient may be treated as an adult, there are many minors who are capable of doing so before the age of 18. In recognition of this, the mature minor doctrine qualifies a minor to make decisions about their own health and welfare if they can show that they are mature enough to make a decision independently. Not all states recognize the mature minor doctrine. In the states where it is legally permitted, the mature minor doctrine takes into consideration the age and situation of the minor to determine maturity, in addition to behavior and conduct that may demonstrate their maturity. Adolescents and mature minors are permitted to provide informed consent if they have been legally emancipated through the court system. In many states, they may provide consent for matters regarding sexual and reproductive health, substance use disorders, and mental health (see Table 33.3). Healthcare professionals have an obligation to be familiar with legal requirements and exemptions for treatment decisions. Consulting with your institution's office of legal affairs or risk management is recommended if you are uncertain what the law allows for patients under the age of majority.

Shared Decision Making With Children and/or Adolescent Patients

Children and adolescents with the developmental ability to understand their medical condition and prognosis should be permitted to engage with their parents and healthcare professionals regarding healthcare decisions. In addition to the

TABLE 33.3 Mature Minor Doctrine: Examples of Medical Treatments That May Be Applicable

Reproductive Healthcare	• Contraceptive care and counseling, including emergency contraception • Pregnancy tests and options counseling • Abortion services
Prenatal Healthcare	• Medical, dental, health and hospital services relating to prenatal care • Labor and delivery services • All medical care for themselves and their child, once the child is born

STI Screening and Treatment	• HIV testing and treatment
	  • For emergency care; or
	  • If parental involvement is impossible or could cause harm; and
	  • Minor is sufficiently mature to follow the treatment regimen
	• Regardless of age or mature minor exemption, guidelines for reporting of communicable diseases to public health department still required

Treatment Following Sexual Assault	• May include consent or refusal of all post-sexual assault care
	  • Medical services, even if minor generally could not consent on their own (e.g., treatment of injuries)
	  • Forensic evidence collection
	  • Rape crisis counseling

Drug and Alcohol Treatment	• May include confidential alcohol and substance use disorder counseling • May include consent to medical treatment for substance use disorder
Mental Health	• May include consent to mental health counseling • May include consent to inpatient mental health treatment
Emergency Medical Treatment	Regardless of whether your state has in place mature minor laws, parental consent is not required in cases of medical emergency. Records of emergency treatment are generally disclosed to a parent unless the healthcare professional is concerned that disclosure may harm the minor patient.

examples of when minor patients might be legally permitted to make their own health decisions, it is ethically permissible, and many would concur advisable, to allow minors to participate in healthcare discussions and treatment decisions even if not allowed by law.

DECISIONAL CAPACITY

In the United States and many other countries, legal standards presume that adult persons, and *sometimes* children under the age of majority, are capable of making their own healthcare decisions. Questions regarding a patient's ability to make decisions often raise ethical concerns for healthcare professionals. For a patient to consent to treatment, they must demonstrate decisional capacity. Complicating matters is the conflation of medical and legal concepts regarding decision making. Terminology such as **capacity** or incapacity is often used interchangeably with **competence** or incompetence. Understanding the meaning and appropriate usage is important when applying them to the assessment of a patient. Competency refers to a legal context. An individual may be determined to be incompetent by a judge in a court of law if the individual is unable to take care of themselves and/or manage their finances, assets, and/or property. Such decisions are typically made in consultation with healthcare professionals having requisite training. A legal declaration of incompetency revokes an individual's rights. This may include the right to vote, have a driver's license, or control property transfer rights. In such cases, courts will appoint a legal guardian to oversee and supervise care and decision making for such individuals.

Capacity may sometimes be used in a legal context to describe the cognitive or physical limitations of an individual's functionality. While this is one of the ways in which the term is used across both fields, it is more commonly associated with medical assessments by healthcare professionals to determine a patient's ability to participate in medical decision making (see Table 33.2). The reason for such assessments may be due to either permanent or temporary deficits in psychophysiological processes. Healthcare at every level is about decisions, informed consent is a constant requirement, and capacity is the cornerstone of informed consent. Capacity may be diminished at times due to a multitude of factors (see Box 33.2).

BOX 33.2 Factors Affecting Decisional Capacity

- Any medical condition that inhibits cognitive activity and/or psychological state can lead to diminished capacity
  - Fever
  - Hypoxia (oxygen deficiency)
  - Delirium
  - Sedation
  - Fear, anxiety, denial
  - Inadequate pain management
- Other than patients with advanced, severe dementia, there is generally no clinical correlation between a specific diagnosis and a loss of decisional capacity

It is important to recognize this, to find ways to enhance capacity if medically symptomatic, and to remember that capacity is decision specific and not generalizable. Patients may have the ability to make some treatment decisions (i.e., low risk of potential harm with expectation of benefit) but have difficulty making other decisions (i.e., high risk of potential harm with uncertainty of benefit). A patient's capacity may also fluctuate at times so it is important to continuously re-assess.

Capacitated patients may either accept or refuse medical treatment regardless of the benefit it may offer to the patient. Healthcare professionals frequently assume patients to have capacity, even when they may not or it may be impaired due to their illness. Special attention must be provided to ensure that healthcare professionals do not assume that passive compliance with treatment means that the patient has provided informed consent. It is often not until there is disagreement with a treatment recommendation that a patient's ability to make their own health decisions is questioned by healthcare professionals. This sometimes reflects the inequality in the relationship between patients and healthcare professionals, and the patient's vulnerability due to this power imbalance.

ADVANCE DIRECTIVES

Whenever a patient does not have the decisional capacity to make either a specific healthcare decision or multiple decisions, there are several options available to consider. If a patient has completed an advance directive (sometimes referred to as either a healthcare proxy document or power of attorney [POA] document) naming a healthcare agent to serve as their surrogate decision maker, the healthcare professional can work together with the agent to ensure that the patient's values and preferences are being respected (Fig. 33.1). The healthcare agent (i.e., surrogate decision maker) is whom the patient has voluntarily designated to make decisions on their behalf. In some states, the terms "healthcare proxy" and "POA" refer to both the document and the person named in the document. Relevant medical information that would have been shared with the patient may also be shared with the healthcare agent making decisions. Patients may also have completed an advance directive referred to as a living will that may elaborate or clarify in more detail the specific types of medical treatment or interventions they would accept if unable to make their own decisions. A living will may be very helpful if the details outlined in the document are relevant and applicable to the patient's current medical status and prognosis. If it is not, the document may still offer some insight into the patient's values and preferences, but that could be left to interpretation and not as useful as intended. A very common problem is that many patients do not have such documentation and/or have not discussed with family members or friends what they would like to happen if they were unable to speak for themselves or make their own decisions. These types of situations may apply to elderly patients or those who have experienced chronic illness, but there are many previously healthy younger adults who may have unexpected medical illnesses or who have had an accident that has rendered them

Health Care Proxy Form

YOUR BIRTH DATE
_____/_____/_____

(1) I, ____, residing at ____________________
(PRINT your name)

____
(Street) (City or Town) (State)

appoint ____
(Name of person you choose as Agent/Proxy)

of ____
(Street) (City/town) (State) (Phone)

as my health care agent to make any and all health care decisions for me, except to the extent that I state otherwise. This proxy shall take effect only when and if I become unable to make my own health care decisions.

(2) Optional: Alternate Agent/Proxy

If my Agent is unwilling or unable to serve, then I appoint as my Alternate Agent:

____, of
(Name of person you choose as Alternate Agent)

____.
(Street) (City/town) (State) (Phone)

as my health care agent to make any and all health care decisions for me, except to the extent that I state otherwise.

(3)

Unless I revoke it or state an expiration date or circumstances under which it will expire, this proxy shall remain in effect indefinitely. (*Optional: If you want this proxy to expire, state the date or conditions here.*) This proxy shall expire (*specify date or conditions*):

____

____

____

(4) Optional:

I direct my health care agent to make health care decisions according to my wishes and limitations, as he or she knows or as stated below. (*If you want to limit your agent's authority to make health care decisions for you or to give specific instructions, you may state your wishes or limitations here.*) I direct my health care agent to make health care decisions in accordance with the following limitations and/or instructions (*attach additional pages as necessary*):

____

____

In order for your agent to make health care decisions for you about artificial nutrition and hydration (*nourishment and water provided by feeding tube and intravenous line*), your agent must reasonably know your wishes. You can either tell your agent what your wishes are or include them in this section.

(5) Your Identification (please print)

Your Name ____

Your Signature________________________________ Date____________________

Your Address____

(6) Optional: Organ and/or Tissue Donation

I hereby make an anatomical gift, to be effective upon my death, of: (*check any that apply*)

☐ Any needed organs and/or tissues
☐ The following organs and/or tissues________________________________

____

☐ Limitations____

If you do not state your wishes or instructions about organ and/or tissue donation on this form, it will not be taken to mean that you do not wish to make a donation or prevent a person, who is otherwise authorized by law, to consent to a donation on your behalf.

Your signature ________________________________ Date ________________

(7) Statement by Witnesses

(*Witnesses must be 18 years of age or older and cannot be the health care agent or alternate.*)
I declare that the person who signed this document is personally known to me and appears to be of sound mind and acting of his or her own free will. He or she signed (or asked another to sign for him or her) this document in my presence.

Date ________________________
Name of Witness 1 (*print*)

____
Signature

____

Address_______________________

Date ________________________
Name of Witness 2 (*print*)

____
Signature

____

Address_______________________

Fig. 33.1 Healthcare Proxy Form.

incapacitated. Healthcare professionals should consider initiating conversations with patients about the values and preferences and goals of care (see Video 25.2). These conversations can sometimes be difficult for patients and healthcare professionals, but they are necessary and beneficial to the patient.

SURROGATE DECISION MAKING

When a patient without capacity does not have a designated healthcare agent or any type of advance directive, steps must be taken to ensure that the patient is able to access and benefit from medical care. At times, the most appropriate intervention required may be to help facilitate the restoration of the patient's capacity (i.e., the patient with fever is delirious; treatment of fever will resolve delirium and the patient will regain capacity). This is not always possible and, in such situations, it is necessary to rely on a surrogate decision maker.

Traditionally, we have looked to "next of kin" or family members of patients to make surrogate treatment decisions. This ambiguous designation has allowed healthcare professionals some latitude in choosing between a spouse, adult children, siblings, companions, etc. In recent years, many states have enacted surrogate decision-making laws to help formalize the process for healthcare professionals to determine who should be the designated person to act as a surrogate if a patient has not named a surrogate or provided instructions for medical treatment. This can be beneficial when there is disagreement amongst family members, partners, friends, etc. However, it may not always be helpful for some patients because the most appropriate surrogate may not be someone with a biological or legal relationship to the patient, but a trusted friend. Before identifying who the most appropriate surrogate would be, a healthcare professional should ascertain who knows the patient's values and preferences best.

Substituted Judgment

Oftentimes, there is no written documentation providing clear instructions regarding healthcare decisions. Persons serving in the role of surrogate decision maker are obligated to use *substituted judgment* to make decisions that the patient, being represented, would have made if they were capable of doing so. Surrogate decision makers may require assistance from healthcare professionals in fulfilling this role by asking them to reflect on the patient's prior experiences and whether any previous statements or perspectives expressed by the patient might provide insight regarding the circumstances at hand. This can sometimes be challenging for the surrogate given the need for interpretation and uncertainty to know what the right thing to do would be for the patient.

Best Interest Standard

If it is not possible to effectively apply a *substituted judgment* approach, it is ethically permissible to utilize a *best interest* standard. Deliberating on what is in another person's best interest can be difficult to do in practice if the patient's values and preferences are unknown and cannot be inferred. Clinical ethics consultation can help address these issues and can offer ethically appropriate recommendations to guide the decision-making process with surrogates. A best interest standard examines the following aspects of the patient's situation:

- The patient's prognosis with and without intervention
- The potential benefit of available treatments and degree of benefit in regard to prognosis
- The patient's pain and suffering
- Whether the interventions will mitigate or exacerbate the patient's pain and suffering
- Quality of life as experienced by the patient

Parental Decision Making

Parents have the legal right to consent to medical treatment on behalf of their children. That includes the right to accept treatment that is offered; decline treatment (withhold); or discontinue treatment (withdraw), even if such treatment may be life-sustaining. This is ***not*** an absolute right though, as there are exceptions if such decisions are not in the child's best interest. Healthcare professionals have an ethical and legal duty to advocate for the best interests of the child whenever parental decisions are considered imprudent, neglectful, abusive, or potentially dangerous to the child's health and well-being. Healthcare professionals may override parental decisions if such decisions place the child at significant risk of serious harm. If the decision to override a parental decision cannot be mediated among the parents and medical staff, legal recourse may be required through court order decisions and/or invoking the need to report to state child protective services.

ETHICAL ISSUES AT THE END OF LIFE

While ethical dilemmas may arise with any patient across their lifespan from infancy through adulthood, ethical conflicts concerning medical decisions for patients at the end of life are the most common in clinical ethics. Conflicts may arise when there is disagreement or uncertainty as to what the best course of treatment is for the patient. The principles of beneficence and non-maleficence require that healthcare professionals recommend only those treatments and interventions that will benefit the patient and refrain from those that will not improve outcomes, especially if it may cause suffering. If a patient or their family member asks that "everything be done," healthcare professionals should seek to understand what that means to the patient or their family member. Another way of processing such requests is to reframe it as everything that is medically appropriate be done. Inquiring about a patient's values and preferences will facilitate communication as it will help to elicit the needs of the patient and will provide an opportunity to clarify any medical facts regarding the effectiveness of treatment options and the associated risks involved. Some patients' values are closely aligned with religious and/or cultural beliefs. Healthcare professionals should never assume to understand an individual's belief system as many people incorporate multiple perspectives and may not hold the same view as other members of their community or agree with all aspects of their religion's doctrine. Inquiring about the patient's beliefs in a respectful and non-judgmental manner will enhance the patient's relationship.

If a patient or their family request to continue with medical treatment that is not recommended, the healthcare professional has an ethical duty to understand the perspective of the patient or surrogate decision makers. This may require reviewing their understanding of the patient's medical status and considering whether the request being made is aligned with the patient's values and preferences. It may be the recommendation of the medical staff to withhold non-beneficial treatment or to withdraw treatment if it has not proven to be or no longer continues to be an effective intervention. In such situations, many bioethicists hold the view that withholding of treatment and the withdrawal of treatment to be ethically equivalent actions. There are often different types of moral distress associated with these different actions, however, and such conversations should be conducted with sensitivity and compassion. Collaborating with colleagues who have specialized training in clinical ethics can help elucidate the ethical and moral concerns associated with such clinical care situations and offer ethically permissible recommendations to the healthcare professionals responsible for the care and treatment of the patient.

ETHICS COMMITTEES AND CLINICAL ETHICS CONSULTATION

Given the ethical complexity that can arise in clinical practice, healthcare professionals and patients may require assistance with resolving these issues. In the United States, The Joint Commission, a nonprofit organization responsible for the accreditation of more than 20,000 healthcare organizations and programs, requires healthcare institutions to provide a mechanism for addressing ethical issues. The process by which this is done is left to the discretion of the institution. Some utilize ethics committees, while others have clinical ethics consultants to aid employees, patients, and families as needed. The purpose of an ethics consultation or an ethics committee is to analyze and present recommendations to resolve ethical dilemmas. Ethics consultants are trained to gather information and seek clarification of the medical facts of the case as a first step. Identifying relevant stakeholders is a key function of the ethics analysis process. Consultants or committee members are expected to remain objective or neutral in their role so as to not impose their own personal views. Ethical conflict is sometimes the result of ineffective communication and/or interpersonal dynamics, which may require mediation skills. Individuals serving in the role of clinical ethics consultants or committee members include physicians, nurses, social workers, chaplains, and any number of healthcare professionals. Bioethics is an interprofessional field that includes philosophers, community members, advocates, and members of the legal profession. While The Joint Commission does not set forth specific criteria, clinical ethics consultation requires a combination of clinical expertise and/or formal bioethics education and training.

SUMMARY

In conclusion, the study of clinical ethics and professionalism is essential for healthcare professionals as it forms the cornerstone of patient-centered care and trust in the healthcare system. This chapter has delved into the fundamental principles that guide ethical decision making in clinical practice, emphasizing the importance of autonomy, beneficence, non-maleficence, and justice. Moreover, it has underscored the significance of professionalism in maintaining the integrity and reputation of healthcare professionals, emphasizing the values of honesty, accountability, and compassion. By understanding and adhering to these ethical and professional standards, healthcare professionals can ensure the highest quality of care, promote patient well-being, and foster a healthcare environment built on trust and respect. As we move forward in the ever-evolving landscape of healthcare, the principles discussed in this chapter will continue to serve as the ethical and professional compass guiding clinicians in their daily practice, ultimately benefiting both patients and healthcare professionals alike.

REVIEW QUESTIONS

1. **Michael Brown is a 27-year-old male with a known psychiatric history of schizophrenia and depression. He has an appointment at the hospital's outpatient primary care clinic for renewal of his prescription for asthma medication, which Michael reports has been worse due to his downstairs neighbors smoking on their balcony. Michael appears very angry and voices frustration about the smoking and how it is "slowly killing me!" You ask if Michael has tried talking with them to explain the situation and he replies, "if they don't stop, they won't need to worry about cigarettes killing them, I'll do it myself!" What is the most appropriate course of action for the patient's primary care physician?**
   A. Inform law enforcement of the threats made by the patient and provide the patient's home address.
   B. Maintain patient confidentiality but encourage the patient to make an appointment with their psychiatrist.
   C. Maintain patient confidentiality but admit the patient to the hospital for homicidal ideation.
   D. Notify the patient's next of kin to warn them of the threats Michael is making against his neighbors.
   E. Visit Michael's neighbors in person and warn them to stop smoking.

2. **A 23-year-old male was brought into the emergency room after being found unconscious by his roommate with deep cuts to both wrists. His roommate and the first responders were able to control the bleeding, but the lacerations are large and the physicians in the ER want to suture them. The patient, who is once again conscious, angrily refuses. The doctors explain that, without the sutures, there will be significant scarring. The patient nods and says he understands, but he doesn't need their help and doesn't want to be in the hospital.**

What is the most appropriate course of action at this time?

A. Given the fact the patient tried to commit suicide, he no longer has the capacity to refuse medical treatment.
B. Admit the patient for a 72-hour psychiatric observation.
C. Ask the roommate for contact information for a family member who can authorize consent for treatment.
D. Explain to the patient that the sutures will help prevent infection and promote faster healing, but if he still refuses, then do not suture the wounds.
E. Sedate the patient and call legal counsel to request a court order for medical treatment.

3. **Adam Sanchez, a 61-year-old male, was admitted to the intensive care unit after sustaining multiple injuries including severe head trauma after falling down a flight of stairs. He has been unconscious for the past 3 days with a significant subdural hematoma and increasing difficulty with breathing. The medical team recommends intubating the patient and putting him on a ventilator. The patient's long-term partner has been at the hospital every day since he was admitted. The partner agrees with the medical team's recommendation. Before the medical staff attempted the procedure, the patient's brother, who lives out of state, arrived. The brother has brought with him a copy of the patient's advance directive, which lists the brother as the patient's healthcare proxy. The brother tells the medical team they shouldn't put the patient on a ventilator because he "hated the idea of ever being hooked up to a machine." The patient's advance directive includes instructions that he would never want to be on a ventilator. The patient's partner asks if the team can at least try using the ventilator to see if he gets better one day. What is the most appropriate course of action at this time?**
   A. Honor the partner's request to intubate the patient and place him on the ventilator.
   B. Ask if there are any other family members who can corroborate the brother's statements.
   C. Continue to provide medical treatment, but follow the patient's instructions and do not intubate him.
   D. Petition for a court-appointed guardian to help resolve the conflict between the patient's brother and partner.
   E. Inform the brother that if he won't accept the medical team's recommendations, he should request a transfer to another hospital.

4. **Myles Bartram, age 54, was admitted to the hospital for gangrene on his right foot. This is Myles' fourth admission for the same medical problem, and he has left the hospital against medical advice each time to return to living in a shelter or in a local park. The vascular surgery team recommends a below-knee amputation, but Myles consistently refuses to consent to the procedure. The attending vascular surgeon states that the situation has become serious, and the surgeon is concerned that the patient will risk losing even more of his leg, or even death, without surgical treatment. The nursing team states that Myles is argumentative and often refuses to take medications or allow them to perform routine nursing care. Myles' doctor meets with him at bedside to ask some questions about why he is refusing. Myles can clearly explain his medical condition and he seems to understand the seriousness. When asked about treatment options, Myles states that surgery is one option and that the proposed amputation is expected to keep him from becoming more ill. When asked what that would mean in the long term, the patient tells the doctor that he does not want the amputation because he would not be able to walk through the park. Myles states that he will be better off with a "bum leg" if his pain can be controlled. What was the doctor attempting to assess in this encounter?**
   A. Myles' ability to appreciate quality of life considerations
   B. Myles' capacity to make informed medical decisions
   C. Myles' competence to make financial decisions
   D. Myles' intelligence to understand medical information
   E. Myles' attitude toward the nursing staff

5. **A 47-year-old is brought into the emergency department by two co-workers with complaints of headache, neck pain, fever, and a reported change in mental status and disorientation. After reviewing the results of a normal head CT scan, the medical team has determined that the patient requires an emergency lumbar puncture and intravenous antibiotics. The patient is very agitated and appears scared. They are physically pushing away any staff who attempt to get near them and preventing the physician from safely performing the lumbar puncture. Which of the following is an appropriate course of action?**
   A. Sedate the patient and perform the lumbar puncture.
   B. Wait for the patient's spouse to arrive to obtain consent for the procedure.
   C. Respect the patient's decision to refuse treatment.
   D. Ask one of the co-workers to sign for consent for the procedure.
   E. Wait until the patient is asleep before attempting to perform the lumbar puncture.

6. **Bernard Lee, an 88-year-old male with a medical history of diabetes, high cholesterol, and high blood pressure, is admitted to the hospital with pneumonia. He has a fever, and the doctors are worried that Bernard isn't getting enough oxygen. He appears uncomfortable but can talk, briefly stating, "I'm hanging in there, doc. Just a little under the weather, that's all." The doctors are worried that Bernard may need intubation and mechanical ventilation if he doesn't improve soon. The doctors will need Bernard's consent to be intubated or for other treatment, but they need to know if Bernard has the capacity to make medical decisions. Which of the following is most likely to impair Bernard's decision-making capacity at this time?**
   A. Hearing impairment
   B. Poor health literacy
   C. Age
   D. Lack of family
   E. Low blood oxygen levels

7. **A 9-year-old falls off their skateboard while attempting to jump the curb. They have a deep 2-inch cut on their right leg. A couple passing by helps them into a nearby urgent care clinic. One of the physicians evaluates the child and determines that the cut requires stitches. Which of the following is the most accurate statement?**
   A. Consent for treatment can be given by the couple since they assumed responsibility to bring them into the clinic.
   B. Consent for treatment is not required in an urgent care clinic.
   C. Consent for treatment must be obtained from both parents.
   D. Consent for treatment must be obtained from at least one of the parents.
   E. Consent for treatment can be given by the patient if they act mature enough.

8. **Which of the following would not be considered an element of decisional capacity?**
   A. Patient's willingness to express their values
   B. Patient's reasoning for a stated choice
   C. Patient's ability to communicate a choice
   D. Patient's demonstration of understanding of facts
   E. Patient's appreciation of the consequence of choice

BIBLIOGRAPHY

Available online.

A Journey Through Physical Diagnosis

Mark H. Swartz

Where the art of medicine is loved, there is also love for humanity.

Hippocrates (c. 460 BCE–c. 375 BCE)

As we conclude our journey through the pages of the *Textbook of Physical Diagnosis: History and Examination*, we reflect upon the timeless art and science of medicine that has been the cornerstone of healing for centuries. This textbook has served as your faithful guide, unveiling the secrets of the human body through the lens of history-taking and physical examination. It has equipped you with the skills and knowledge to decipher the intricate language of signs and symptoms, allowing you to paint a vivid picture of a patient's health.

In the ever-evolving landscape of medicine, the art of physical diagnosis remains as relevant as ever. Despite the remarkable advancements in technology and diagnostic tests, the power of a skilled healthcare professional's clinical skills cannot be overstated. It is a testament to the enduring value of communication skills, history-taking, and physical examination, practices that will continue to define the essence of healthcare for generations to come.

As you close this textbook, we hope you carry with you a deep appreciation for the history and traditions that have shaped modern medicine. Remember that every patient encounter is an opportunity to not only diagnose but also to connect on a human level, offering empathy and understanding in times of vulnerability.

The journey does not end here, for medicine is an ever-evolving field. New discoveries will reshape our understanding of disease, and emerging technologies will enhance our diagnostic capabilities. However, the core principles of physical diagnosis—listening, observing, and touching—will always remain at the heart of compassionate care.

May you continue to refine your skills, cultivate your knowledge, and approach each patient with the same dedication and reverence for the art of healing you have gained from this textbook. Your journey as a healthcare professional is a lifelong commitment to learning, growing, and, above all, making a positive impact on the lives of those entrusted to your care.

In closing, let the spirit of this textbook serve as a perpetual guide, reminding you that behind every symptom, every sign, and every examination, there is a unique story waiting to be heard, a life seeking relief and healing, and a professional with the power to make a difference.

Thank you for embarking on this journey of discovery, empathy, and healing. Your dedication to the art of physical diagnosis is a gift to your patients and the world of medicine.

I wish you great success in your chosen field!

Mark H. Swartz, MD

A APPENDIX

Answers to Review Questions

CHAPTER 1, THE INTERVIEWER'S QUESTIONS

1. B
2. D
3. D
4. E
5. E
6. C
7. D
8. E
9. C
10. D

CHAPTER 2, THE PATIENT'S RESPONSES

1. E
2. E
3. A
4. E
5. A
6. D
7. C
8. C

CHAPTER 3, UNDERSTANDING COMPLEMENTARY AND ALTERNATIVE MEDICINE

1. B
2. D
3. E
4. C
5. E
6. E
7. A
8. A
9. D
10. A

CHAPTER 5, ANTI-RACIST AND ANTI-OPPRESSIVE CLINICAL SKILLS

1. B
2. E
3. E
4. D
5. E
6. C
7. D
8. C
9. B
10. C

CHAPTER 6, THE PHYSICAL EXAMINATION

1. E
2. D
3. A
4. E
5. E
6. E
7. E
8. B
9. A
10. D
11. E
12. B
13. D
14. A
15. A

CHAPTER 7, ASSESSMENT OF NUTRITIONAL STATUS

1. D
2. D
3. C
4. A
5. E
6. C
7. E
8. B
9. D
10. D

CHAPTER 8, THE SKIN

1. D
2. B
3. C
4. A

5. C
6. B
7. D
8. C
9. C
10. A

CHAPTER 9, THE HEAD AND NECK

1. E
2. C
3. C
4. E
5. C
6. E
7. B
8. C
9. B
10. E

CHAPTER 10, THE EYE

1. D
2. C
3. B
4. A
5. B
6. E
7. A
8. D
9. B
10. C

CHAPTER 11, THE EAR AND NOSE

1. A
2. B
3. E
4. C
5. C
6. C
7. C
8. C
9. E
10. E

CHAPTER 12, THE ORAL CAVITY AND PHARYNX

1. C
2. C
3. B
4. A
5. E
6. A
7. E
8. D
9. E
10. E

CHAPTER 13, THE CHEST

1. C
2. D
3. A
4. D
5. C
6. C
7. D
8. A
9. A
10. E

CHAPTER 14, THE HEART

1. E
2. B
3. D
4. C
5. E
6. C
7. A
8. E
9. D
10. E
11. B

CHAPTER 15, THE PERIPHERAL VASCULAR SYSTEM

1. D
2. B
3. C
4. D
5. E
6. C
7. E
8. B
9. E
10. C

CHAPTER 16, THE BREAST

1. A
2. E
3. A
4. E
5. C
6. E
7. C
8. B
9. C
10. C

CHAPTER 17, THE ABDOMEN

1. C
2. B
3. A
4. C
5. E
6. C
7. A
8. E
9. B
10. E

CHAPTER 18, MALE GENITALIA AND HERNIAS

1. B
2. C
3. A
4. C
5. E
6. D
7. C
8. A
9. B
10. D

CHAPTER 19, FEMALE GENITALIA

1. B
2. B
3. C
4. C
5. B
6. B
7. C
8. E
9. D
10. C

CHAPTER 20, THE MUSCULOSKELETAL SYSTEM

1. E
2. C
3. B
4. A
5. C
6. E
7. C
8. D
9. B
10. E

CHAPTER 21, THE NERVOUS SYSTEM

1. A
2. E
3. E
4. C
5. E
6. A
7. A
8. B
9. E
10. D

CHAPTER 23, THE PREGNANT PATIENT

1. D
2. B
3. C
4. B
5. D
6. B
7. C
8. E
9. C
10. D

CHAPTER 24, THE PEDIATRIC PATIENT

1. E
2. D
3. B
4. C
5. E
6. D
7. D
8. E
9. B
10. D

CHAPTER 25, THE GERIATRIC PATIENT

1. E
2. B
3. B
4. E
5. D
6. B
7. E
8. E

CHAPTER 26, THE TRANSGENDER PATIENT

1. D
2. C
3. A
4. B
5. C
6. B
7. C
8. B
9. C
10. C

CHAPTER 27, THE ACUTELY ILL OR INJURED PATIENT

1. C
2. A
3. B
4. B
5. A
6. C
7. D
8. C
9. B
10. B

CHAPTER 28, PRECISION, ACCURACY, AND CRITICAL THINKING IN CLINICAL ASSESSMENT

1. E
2. A
3. C
4. D
5. A
6. E
7. E
8. E
9. D

CHAPTER 31, ARTIFICIAL INTELLIGENCE IN CLINICAL ENCOUNTERS: OPPORTUNITIES AND CHALLENGES

1. B
2. B
3. E
4. D
5. C
6. A
7. E
8. E
9. D
10. B

CHAPTER 32, TELEHEALTH: ADAPTING CLINICAL ASSESSMENT

1. B
2. C
3. C
4. A
5. C
6. A
7. D
8. D
9. C
10. A

CHAPTER 33, CLINICAL ETHICS AND PROFESSIONALISM

1. C
2. A
3. D
4. C
5. B
6. A
7. E
8. D
9. A

INDEX

Note: Page numbers followed by "f" indicate figures, "t" indicate tables, and "b" indicate boxes.

B

D

O

Q

T

U

V